The
Activator
Method

Second Edition

Arlan W. Fuhr, DC

President, National Institute of Chiropractic Research;
Senior Member, International Society for the Study of the Lumbar Spine;
Co-Founder and CEO, Activator Methods, Inc.
Phoenix, Arizona

Associate Editor

Rebecca S. Fischer, DC, FIACA

Secretary, Clinical Advisory Board
Senior Clinical Instructor, Activator Methods, International;
Private Practice, Doctor's Chiropractic Center, Inc.
Colorado Springs, Colorado

With 530 illustrations
Table in photographs courtesy of Lloyd Table Company

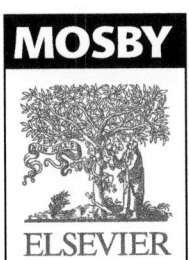

MOSBY

ELSEVIER

The Activator Method

Second Edition

The
Activator
Method

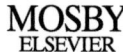

11830 Westline Industrial Drive
St. Louis, Missouri 63146

THE ACTIVATOR METHOD, EDITION 2   ISBN: 978-0-323-04852-1
Copyright © 2009, 1997 by Mosby, Inc., an affiliate of Elsevier Inc.

Notice

Neither the Publisher nor the Authors assume any responsibility for any loss or injury and/or damage to persons or property arising out of or related to any use of the material contained in this book. It is the responsibility of the treating practitioner, relying on independent expertise and knowledge of the patient, to determine the best treatment and method of application for the patient.

The Publisher

Library of Congress Control Number: 2007933194

Vice President and Publisher: Linda Duncan
Senior Editor: Kellie White
Senior Developmental Editor: Jennifer Watrous
Editorial Assistant: April Falast
Publishing Services Manager: Patricia Tannian
Senior Project Manager: Kristine Feeherty
Cover Designer: Paula Catalano
Text Designer: Paula Catalano

Working together to grow
libraries in developing countries

www.elsevier.com | www.bookaid.org | www.sabre.org

ELSEVIER   BOOK AID International   Sabre Foundation

To my wife, Judi, without whose help the
Activator Method would not have
survived in the world of chiropractic
as it is today. Her unconditional love carried me through
the most difficult times I have faced, both
personally and professionally.

Arlan W. Fuhr, DC

CONTRAINDICATIONS

See *Guidelines for chiropractic quality assurance and practice parameters: Proceedings of the Mercy Center Consensus Conference*, Gaithersburg, MD, 1993, Aspen.

It is recommended that the Activator Adjusting Instrument be used in adjusting procedures only by those who have received proper instruction from a chiropractic college that teaches the Activator Method or who have attended an Activator Methods Technique Seminar.

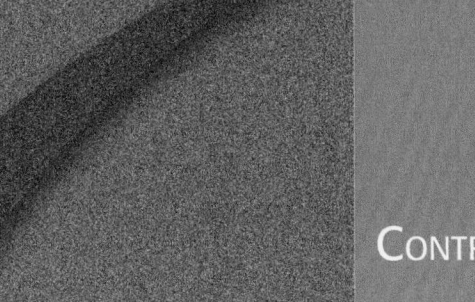

CONTRIBUTORS

James DeVocht, DC, PhD
Assistant/Associate Professor
Palmer Center for Chiropractic at Palmer
   College of Chiropractic
Davenport, Iowa

Rebecca S. Fischer, DC, FIACA
Secretary
Clinical Advisory Board
Senior Clinical Instructor
Activator Methods, International;
Private Practice
Doctors Chiropractic Center, Inc.
Colorado Springs, Colorado

Gregory N. Kawchuk, BSC, DC, MSc, PhD
Assistant Professor
Faculty of Rehabilitation Medicine
University of Alberta, Edmonton
Alberta, Canada

†Joseph C. Keating, Jr., PhD, LittD(hon), FICC(h)
Professor and NCMIC Historian of the
   Profession
Cleveland Chiropractic College;
Member, Board of Directors
Association for the History of Chiropractic
Kansas City, Missouri

Tianye Li
Undergraduate Student
University of Alberta, Edmonton
Alberta, Canada

Randall C. McLeod, DC, FCCRS(c), DACRB
Private Practice
Immanuel Healing Centre
Stony Plain, Alberta, Canada

Joel G. Pickar, DC, PhD
Professor
Palmer Center for Chiropractic Research
Davenport, Iowa

N.G. Narasimha Prasad
Associate Professor
Department of Mathematical & Statistical
   Sciences
University of Alberta, Edmonton
Alberta, Canada

Wally Schaeffer, DC
Private Practice
Schaeffer Chiropractic
Coralville, Iowa

Xue-Jun Song, MD, PhD
Department of Neurobiology
Parker College Research Institute
Dallas, Texas;
Jiangsu Province Key Laboratory of
   Anesthesiology
Xuzhou Medical College
Xuzhou, Jiangsu, China

Tasha Stanton
Graduate Student
University of Alberta, Edmonton
Alberta, Canada

Charlotte J. Watts, BS, DC, FICPA
Senior Clinical Instructor
Activator Methods, International;
Professor
Parker College of Chiropractic
Dallas, Texas;
Private Practice
Grand Prairie, Texas

Qiaohao Zhu
Statistician
Integrated Centre for Care
   Advancement through Research (iCare)
Capital Health
Edmonton, Alberta, Canada

---

†Deceased.

EDITORIAL COMMITTEE

Rebecca S. Fischer, DC, FIACA
Secretary
Clinical Advisory Board
Senior Clinical Instructor
Activator Methods, International;
Private Practice
Doctors Chiropractic Center, Inc.
Colorado Springs, Colorado

Peter Arizzi, DC, FIAMA
Senior Clinical Instructor
Activator Methods, International;
Arizzi Chiropractic Health & Wellness Center
Middleton, Massachusetts

Wayne A. Comeau, DC, DACBOH, FACC
Senior Clinical Instructor
Activator Methods, International;
Comeau Health Care Associates
Danvers, Massachusetts

Thomas R. De Vita, DC, FACC
Vice Chairperson
Clinical Advisory Board
Senior Clinical Instructor
Activator Methods, International;
Director
De Vita Chiropractic Office PC
Acton, Massachusetts

Richard Dussault, DC
Clinical Instructor
Activator Methods, International;
Private Practice
Centre Chiropratique Dussault
Longueuil, Quebec, Canada

Joseph B. Steinhouser, DC
Clinical Advisory Board
Senior Clinical Instructor
Activator Methods, International;
Private Practice
Lake Elsinore, California;
Instructor
Activator Methods, Inc.
Phoenix, Arizona

Lois E. Ward, DC
Clinical Advisory Board
Senior Clinical Instructor
Activator Methods, International;
Private Practice
Farmington, Missouri

Charlotte J. Watts, BS, DC, FICPA
Senior Clinical Instructor
Activator Methods, International;
Professor
Parker College of Chiropractic
Dallas, Texas;
Private Practice
Grand Prairie, Texas

Ronald (Chip) R. Weisel II, DC
Senior Clinical Instructor
Activator Methods, International;
Private Practice
Hartville, Ohio

Developmental Acknowledgments

A special thanks to the following individuals who contributed to the development of the Activator Method.

Frank Antonino, DC, Naperville, Illinois
Peter Arizzi, DC, Middleton, Massachusetts
Birger Baastrup, DC, Juneau, Alaska
Anthony J. Barone, DC, Lakewood, New Jersey
Scott D. Bautch, DC, Wausau, Wisconsin
Richard Boatright, DC, Pinetop, Arizona
Stephen Bradford, DC, West Sussex, United Kingdom
Richard R. Bray, DC, Windsor, Ontario, Canada
Paul C. Brooks, DC, Norway, Maine
Steven R. Conway, DC, Janesville, Wisconsin
William J. Coykendall, DC, Punta Gorda, Florida
Donald H. Dearth, DC, Tempe, Arizona
John DeLuca, DC, Belmar, New Jersey
David A. Dengler, DC, Albuquerque, New Mexico
Kurt J. Deutscher, DC, Athabasca, Alberta, Canada
Lisa M. Devlin, DC, Mountain View, California
Randy R. Dierenfield, DC, Ankeny, Iowa
D. Michael Dinkin, DC, West Hills, California
Richard P. Dussault, DC, Longueuil, Quebec, Canada
Aron W. Enns, DC, Abbotsford, British Columbia, Canada
John H.C. Ewart, DC, Pembroke, Ontario, Canada
Rebecca S. Fischer, DC, FIACA, Colorado Springs, Colorado
Dean A. Flora, DC, Saginaw, Michigan
Rex W. Fowler, DC, Jackson, Tennessee
Albert Gadomski, DC, Oldsmar, Florida
Edward J. Galvin, DC, Oswego, New York
Gary R. Gaulin, DC, Palm Desert, California
Jonathan Golub, DC, Seaford, New York
Lawrence L. Gray, DC, Scarborough, Maine
R. Dean Harman, DC, San Mateo, California
Dwight A. Hayden, DC, Findhorn, Moray, Scotland, United Kingdom

Gerald F. Hendrickson, DC, Oshkosh, Wisconsin
Michael P. Hergenroether, DC, Santa Barbara, California
Teresa C. Hill, DC, Sterling, Colorado
David R. Hughes, DC, Paulding, Ohio
Casey J. Iverson, DC, Grand Island, Nebraska
Irv Jacobs, DC, Van Nuys, California
Harlen H. Johnson, DC, Big Fork, Montana
Paul M. Kell, DC, San Diego, California
Ed Kinum III, DC, Scotia, New York
Ed Kinum, Sr., DC, Scotia, New York
Edward J. Klein, DC, Tujunga, California
Bradley P. Kristiansen, DC, Cedar Rapids, Iowa
Rick Ksenda, DC, Orange, California
Ward C. Lamb, DC, San Jose, California
Warren H. Landesberg, DC, Briarcliff Manor, New York
Donald C. Leary, DC, Salem, Oregon
Howard F. Lewis, DC, Fallston, Maryland
Richard E. Lind, DC, Orange, California
Jack Lube, DC, Tallahassee, Florida
T.J. McKay, DC, Calgary, Alberta, Canada
Roderic McLean, DC, Waratah, New South Wales, Australia
Sidney L. Mouk, DC, Baton Rouge, Louisiana
Gary Nadler, DC, Cottonwood, Arizona
Stephen A. Nedd, DC, Fort Myers, Florida
Linda J. Patterson, DC, Mesa, Arizona
Donald D. Pattison, DC, Albuquerque, New Mexico
Steven J. Pavia, DC, Monroe, New York
James J. Peck, DC, Andover, Massachusetts
Jane E. Perry, DC, Allen, Texas
Eric Petermann, DC, Phoenix, Arizona
Howard A. Pettersson, DC, Davenport, Iowa
Bradley S. Polkinghorn, DC, Santa Monica, California
Vernon S. Redd, DC, Albuquerque, New Mexico
David R. Reich, DC, Richmond Hill, New York

Richard A. Richett, DC, North Hampton, New Hampshire

Robert D. Ross, DC, Ephrata, Washington

Vernon M. Rowe, DC, Little Rock, Arkansas

Richard Roy, DC, Lasalle, Quebec, Canada

F. Rocco Ruggiero, DC, Napa, California

Dan J. Rutz, DC, Las Vegas, Nevada

Thomas H. Sawyer, DC, La Canada, California

Sid W. Schultz, DC, St. Cloud, Minnesota

Wayne P. Seddon, DC, Glen Roy, Victoria, Australia

Gordon L. Shepro, DC, Juneau, Alaska

Donald A. Sickmeyer, DC, Chester, Illinois

Ron Singleton, DC, Wenatchee, Washington

Malik Slosberg, DC, Pleasanton, California

Bart Smith, DC, Honolulu, Hawaii

Norman R. Smith, DC, Rockland, Maine

Joseph B. Steinhouser, DC, Lake Elsinore, California

Judith L. Steinhouser, DC, Laguna Hills, California

Leo B. Stouder, DC, Hollywood, Florida

Robin T. Swaim, DC, Oregon, Ohio

Myron W. Thatcher, DC, Ann Arbor, Michigan

John P. Thompson, DC, Apple Valley, Minnesota

Grant Thomson, DC, Banora Point, New South Wales, Australia

Charlotte J. Watts, DC, FICPA, Grand Prairie, Texas

Karl W. Weber, DC, Cooma, New South Wales, Australia

Ronald R. Weisel II, DC, Hartville, Ohio

Chris L. Wertin, DC, Lawrence, Kansas

John M. Wertin, DC, Manhattan, Kansas

Randall S. Widmaier, DC, Phoenix, Arizona

Michael W. Youngquist, DC, Willmar, Minnesota

Ann Zajac, DC, Tinley Park, Illinois

FOREWORD

At first I was surprised to receive an invitation from Arlan Fuhr, DC, to consider writing the foreword to the newest edition of his text, *The Activator Method*. However, knowing Arlan, it eventually made sense. Recognizing that I would not write about something I had not seen, Dr. Fuhr sent me all 17 chapters so that my commentary could be based on an actual review of the text. He wasn't seeking mere perfunctory comments—he wanted a real review. Still, given my strong advocacy for manual manipulation, I found it particularly strange that Dr. Fuhr would ask me to review his text. However, he is a risk taker and was convinced that the evidence would support a fair review. His thought was to ask someone who has a contrarian view and perhaps he would get a foreword that just might be objective.

Dr. Fuhr has an insatiable thirst for the truth, and in his search he was brave enough to go where the research took him regardless of whether or not it might prove counter to his beliefs. Anyone who has been around the profession for any length of time knows of the inextricable tie between Arlan and the Activator—a link that now spans 40 years. Despite the tie, Dr. Fuhr has provided funding for research and maintained a high level of integrity in the research he has conducted on and with the Activator instrument.

Despite my bias concerning manipulation by hand, I have been extremely impressed with two individuals whose names are affiliated with techniques or equipment in this profession, and I have so stated publicly many times. These two individuals are Arlan Fuhr, DC; and James Cox, DC. Both of these gentlemen have been strongly committed to the advancement of the profession, and both use mechanically assisted devices to help their patients. Perhaps the most impressive thing about these two individuals is the fact that they have spent their lives conducting research to investigate what they claim. They "put their money where their mouths are," and the profession has been the beneficiary of their efforts. As I look down the list of chapter authors, I cannot help but be impressed. From the "universal skeptic," Joseph Keating, PhD; to Joel Pickar, DC, PhD; Greg Kawchuk, DC, PhD; Xue-Jun Song, MD, PhD; Rebecca Fischer, DC; Wally Schaeffer, DC; and James DeVocht, DC, PhD, the choice of chapter authors predicts the quality that follows.

The previous text on Activator Methods was published a decade ago, and it was noteworthy then for its empirical orientation. This new edition does not disappoint, and it is impressive for its inclusion of a decade of new research that addresses the neurological mechanism of the adjustment. The reader can feel confident about the authors' commitment to the evidence.

As an older practitioner, now in my forty-fifth year, I am delighted that again the commentary in this new text does not skirt a major issue of concern to me and to a host of other practitioners. In his chapter, "Chiropractic Science: Toward Understanding Spinal Manipulation," Dr. Pickar clearly poses the question that I have asked many times: "Is the clinical encounter between the patient and the doctor affected by the method of delivery of the manipulative intervention?" In other words, is the adjustment alone the most important item in the patient encounter? The answer to this question requires further investigation.

Readers will find an interesting and informative history of the development of Activator Methods by Dr. Joe Keating. We tend to forget the turmoil, trials, and tribulations that each new idea, invention, or innovation can elicit, and the evolution of the Activator Method is no exception. In light of this rich history, I think I'll never look at an Activator Adjusting Instrument quite the same way again.

All the authors place a great deal of focus on the very essence of that complex being, which Dr. Joseph Janse referred to as "man the biped."

From the chapter on the temporomandibular joint by Wally Schaeffer, DC, on how this complex joint can and does have an impact on the global structure to the clear and informative aspects of spinal stabilization, this text has many wonderful "clinical pearls" for the practitioner to use in his or her practice. Throughout the text, the authors weave a recognition and appreciation of the complexity of the neurological chain of events requiring conscious and unconscious coordination through the neurological system. The text has a tremendous focus on the very complex biomechanical conditions that doctors of chiropractic encounter each day in their practices. The emphasis on mobility and the complex mechanisms of neural coordination was indeed enlightening. Stability and mobility of the locomotor system are clearly of primary concern, and the text illuminates how dysfunction and abnormal neuro-biomechanics can create the myriad dysfunctional disorders and their ramifications that are seen by doctors of chiropractic every day.

The chapters dealing with the tests, evaluations, and adjustments for the analysis of the human spine and extremities are very well written and easily understood. Whether the clinician is an experienced practitioner or a new graduate, the illustrations and commentary concerning the evaluation and treatment are equally relevant.

I have had the privilege to attend two Activator instructor conferences. Although I have been to many seminars in my lifetime, I wasn't sure what to expect at first. However, I was indeed surprised and pleased to see that the programs started on time, that the quality of the speakers was as good as any research symposium, and that the professionalism of the attendees spoke volumes about the intent to learn rather than the desire for continuing education credits. The professionalism in evidence at Activator seminars is reflected also in Dr. Fuhr's new text.

After reading this book I am certain you will come away with a better understanding of the entire Activator Method Analysis, but more important, you will have read a text that is backed more by sound research data than the charisma of the developer. It is time in our profession that we begin to ask the tough questions when we encounter unsubstantiated claims by individuals or groups offering "the answer." This book offers some of those answers, at least about Activator.

The Activator Method is a worthwhile read and provides some provocative thoughts concerning the things we do and see every day in our office. Dr. Fuhr has a lot of courage because if I were he, I do not know if I would have asked someone like me, who is partial to a nonmechanical method, to write the foreword. But then again, that is what makes Activator Arlan—and Arlan Activator.

Louis Sportelli, DC
Palmerton, Pennsylvania

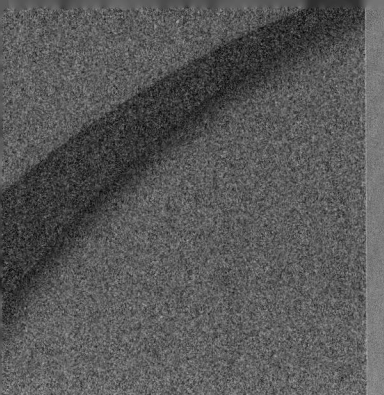

PREFACE

Ten years have passed since the first edition of the *Activator Methods Chiropractic Technique* was published. We never expected it to be the all-time best-selling technique book ever in chiropractic, but it has been. I think it was so successful because it was full of practical information for the student and the veteran practitioner.

I still believe the quote I made in the first paragraph of the first book: "If it isn't written down, it didn't happen" is as true today as it was 10 years ago. This really came through to me only this year, when I heard my minister explain the difference between the world's religions and cults. He explained that the world's greatest and lasting religions prevailed because of their written word. Likewise, the most studied chiropractic techniques will have a better chance of remaining so by virtue of their texts. It is for the future of the technique and future generations of doctors that we have taken so much time to write down all of our observations.

The one thing that really impressed me about this revision is the fact that we have come such a long way documenting our findings in 10 years with such limited resources. In the first book there were chapters, especially in the technique sections, that had very few references. In this revision we have succeeded in showing scientific progress in many areas.

The contributing authors in this edition are published scientists of the highest caliber, well known for their expertise throughout the scientific community. Most of them have a Doctor of Chiropractic degree, or a degree in medicine as well as a PhD in advanced study in their field. We believe this level of competency will give readers the best value for their time and money.

We have reorganized the book based on more than 40 years of teaching experience and what we've gleaned from past readers. The new book makes it easier for students to follow and apply the Activator Method clinically.

In the first edition I made the statement, "I find scientific investigation a bit like taking your clothes off in public." I still feel that way. For every question you answer, four more new questions appear. One of the definitions of being a profession is obtained when the profession and the people laboring in it contribute something new to the body of knowledge. In this textbook I truly believe we have accomplished that goal.

Arlan W. Fuhr

ACKNOWLEDGMENTS

This project required a group effort from many different people. First of all, I want to thank all of the contributing chapter authors who gave of their time and expertise to make this book a reality. All of the authors involved are very busy people who already had their schedules full when I prevailed upon them to contribute to this project. However, I strongly believe that we have recruited the best people in their respective fields to make this a first-rate textbook.

Next I want to thank the Associate Editor and Chairperson of the Editorial Committee, Rebecca Fischer. The number of hours she put in could never be calculated because it went beyond a time clock. We started by using GoToMeeting.com, which saved the day because she lives in Colorado and I live in Phoenix. We spent numerous hours staring at our computers and listening to each other on our speaker phones. Rebecca possesses not only a keen mind but also the ability to be extremely detailed. She persevered until the final edits were done and all the references and pictures were checked and rechecked, and she never once complained about the tedious nature of the work. This book would not have become what it is without her talent and dedication.

Next I would like to thank the editorial committee, which consists of field practitioners who have the greatest amount of clinical experience of any group in the actual application of the Activator Method. They not only use the Activator Method in their daily practices but are instructors as well. Because of this expertise, their input was invaluable. For them this was not a job but a labor of love, and no type of compensation would have been adequate.

I would also like to thank the many field doctors who contributed their findings over the years and have spent the time writing down their clinical observations.

A book is always easier when you have good editors. I was thrilled when Elsevier assigned Kellie White to this project. I worked with her on the first edition, and she is a real professional with a great deal of talent. Jennifer Watrous has been with this project from the beginning, and one could not find a harder working or more fun person. Kristine Feeherty was our final proof editor, and she was a taskmaster who set timelines and made us stick to them. To all of the Elsevier staff: You were great to work with.

Finally I would like to thank my wife, Judi, who heard more about this book than she ever wanted to but good naturedly kept encouraging me when I had a hundred other things on my plate. For that I thank her wholeheartedly.

Arlan W. Fuhr

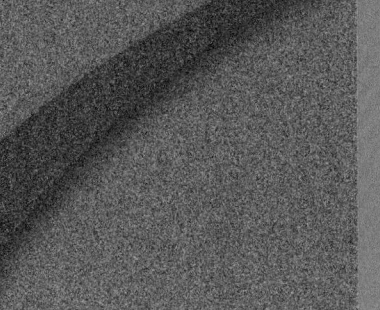

CONTENTS

The
Activator Method

SECTION I

INTRODUCTION TO THE ACTIVATOR METHOD

HISTORY OF A TECHNIQUE SYSTEM

Joseph C. Keating, Jr., and Arlan W. Fuhr

The saga of the Activator Method is multi-faceted. This account encompasses some of the several instruments used to treat the musculoskeletal system in various cultures and the careers of the founders of the Activator Method. The story includes the theoretical pathways that led to the development of many features of the Activator Method and the generations of Activator Adjusting Instruments that have emerged. The tale must also take into account the dissemination of the Activator Method within the chiropractic culture and the many people who have contributed to this effort; only a few of these folks can be mentioned here. Surely, a single chapter can do no more than focus on the highlights and leave the details to future raconteurs.

The Activator Method is referred to as a "technique." This term (sometimes written "technic") has multiple meanings and uses among doctors of chiropractic (DCs). *Technique* can refer to relatively circumscribed assessment procedures (as in passive motion palpation of joints) or to elaborate theories and methods for evaluating patients (as in applied kinesiology or the Meric system). Many if not most chiropractic techniques involve both assessment and treatment components, and the Activator Method is among this latter group. Accordingly, to address the history of the Activator Method, we must distinguish between its analysis and intervention aspects.

The Activator Method of joint analysis and diagnosis represents a unique contribution to the health care field, but many of its component procedures and its theoretical rationales can be found in prior literature and methods within the profession. Similarly, the Activator is not the first instrumental means of producing the segment-specific thrusting that DCs have traditionally prized so highly, but its ease of application and presumed safety have made it the most popular of mechanically assisted manual methods among healers. Its evolution is inextricably entwined with the careers of its inventors, Drs. Warren Lee and Arlan Fuhr. And because

a product, no matter how good, must find a market in order to be successful in the business sense, the story of the Activator Method is also a tale of the marketing and dissemination of the instrument and analysis strategies used within the chiropractic profession, as well as the reactions it has yielded.

BEFORE THE ACTIVATOR

Although adjusting instruments find their widest application among DCs, the use of objects and devices in the service of manual therapies is not unique to chiropractic. Hinojosa,[1] for instance, documents the application of sacred objects, *hueso* or *baq*, among the Maya bonesetters of Guatemala. A paper in the March 1935 issue of the National Chiropractic Association's *Journal* reported the purchase of a tool supposedly used by Montana's Crow Indian healers to relieve "stomach trouble and bowel trouble" by means of thrusts and massage of the spine.[2] These simple, hand-held percussive devices are a far cry from the Activator Adjusting Instrument (AAI), but they merit recognition as pre-chiropractic examples of manipulative tools.

The earliest known chiropractic version of instrument adjusting is credited to Duluth, Minnesota, resident Thomas H. Storey, DC, a former "vitapathic physician" (magnetic healer) turned chiropractor under the tutelage of D.D. Palmer.[3] Dr. Storey, a 1901 graduate of the Palmer School, introduced "some strange adjusting paraphernalia: a wooden mallet and stick."[4] Before relocating to Southern California in 1902, Storey introduced the new method to a number of Minnesota DCs, who "thus got to using the mallet and chisel to set the spine of the whole vertebral column ..."[4] (Figure 1-1).

Although the father of chiropractic did not initially approve of this innovation, on the grounds that it violated his meaning of chiropractic—done by hand—his curiosity was obviously stimulated. He authored a whimsical

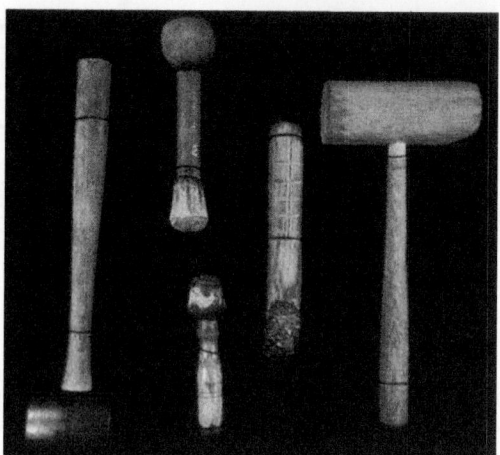

Figure 1-1   Early wooden chisels and mallets used by chiropractors for adjusting. *(Courtesy Palmer College of Chiropractic Archives.)*

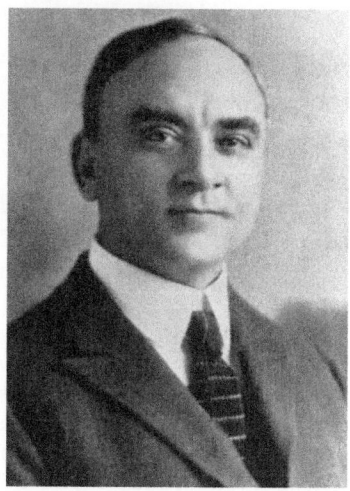

Figure 1-3   Charles A. Cale, DC, ND, circa 1928.

allegory of "A Spine Set Personified"[5] and included a photograph of Storey's simple tools in his classic 1910 tome.[6] According to an account passed along by T.F. Ratledge, DC, founder of the school that is today Cleveland Chiropractic College of Los Angeles, Old Dad Chiro made use of a "rubber hammer (pleximeter) with which he experimented adjusting vertebrae. This was used for the sole purpose of freeing the nerves from obstructive pressure" (Ratledge)[7] (Figures 1-2 to 1-4).

Dr. Storey employed his instrumental method of adjusting on his patient, Charles A. Cale, who would later (1911) establish the Los Angeles College of Chiropractic (LACC)[8] (Figures 1-5 and 1-6). Many years later, Cale's wife, Linnie, a chiropractor and osteopathic physician, recalled the primitive method:

> In 1895 she married Charles A. Cale. In 1900 they moved to California for their health. In 1904 they heard of a Dr. Storey who was practicing chiropractic in Los Angeles and who was a graduate of Dr. D.D. Palmer. They both took treatments of Dr. Storey and regained their health. Mr. Cale had stomach trouble. Quite sometime later his stomach trouble returned. He got down on his stomach on the floor and asked Dr. Linnie Cale to get one of the children's blocks and a hammer. He had her place the block in the region of the 5th and 6th vertebrae and hit it with the hammer. Doing this a few times relieved him of his stomach trouble. That was her first chiropractic adjustment, 55 years ago.[9]

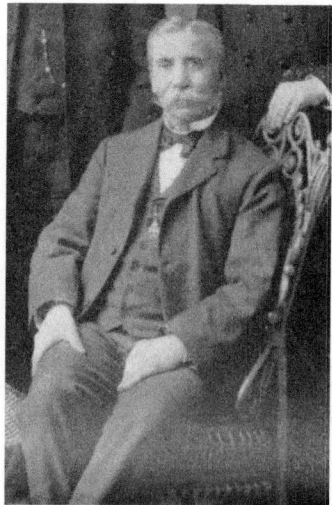

Figure 1-2   Thomas H. Storey, DO, DC, 1905.

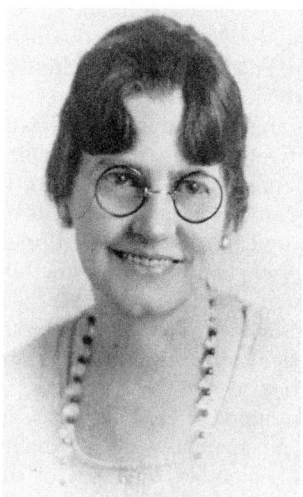

Figure 1-4   Linnie A. Cale, DC, DO, circa 1924.

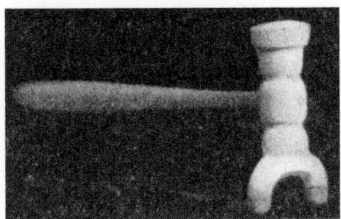

Figure 1-5 This simple concussor was offered by Dr. J.S. Riley (circa 1921) for tapping spinal joints.

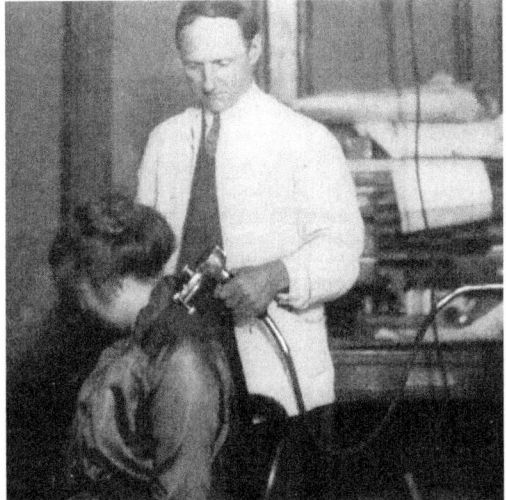

Figure 1-6 Dr. J.S. Riley employs a pneumatic concussor to treat a patient.

Instrument adjusting also found favor at the Palmer-Gregory College of Chiropractic in Oklahoma City. The school, founded circa 1907 by D.D. Palmer and Carver Chiropractic College alumnus Alva Gregory, MD, DC, gave impetus to a variety of "mixer" methods, among them concussion devices.[10] Spinal concussors were also propagated by the institution's vice president, Joe Shelby Riley, DO, DC, who marketed and taught the use of various thrusting machines. Riley's instruction in instrument adjusting extended beyond Oklahoma, for he established schools in Massachusetts[11] and the District of Columbia[12] in later years, and authored books that described his methods.

Dr. Gregory's influence also extended to Albert W. Richardson, DC,[13] purchaser of the LACC in 1913 and founder of various branches of the California Chiropractic College. B.J. Palmer, DC, reported that Richardson and his faculty at the San Francisco branch ran afoul of the law when a patient who had been treated with a "plesameter" and "mallet" filed charges

for assault.[14] The "developer of chiropractic" was pleased to report to his readers that the Palmer graduates of San Francisco had publicly declared that "No mallet or other instrument of any kind or character is ever used as a part of CHIROPRACTIC technique. Only the hands are used in giving a CHIROPRACTIC adjustment and they are not employed to strike, massage, stretch, twist or otherwise injure the patient."[14] The rationale for this dictum was not offered.

Albert Abrams, MD, former administrator of the Cooper Medical College (today, the Medical School of Stanford University), is perhaps best remembered for his creation of radionics. However, he came to D.D. Palmer's attention[6] because of his interest in "spondylotherapy,"[15,16] a form of manipulation involving stimulation of nerves for the treatment of disease (Figure 1-7, A):

> This hammer for evoking the vertebral reflexes (page 7), is called after the French neurologist, plexor of Dejerine. Although employed chiefly for diagnostic purposes, it may substitute a concussion-apparatus in spondylotherapy. Indeed, many physicians have used the plexor exclusively to attain their therapeutic results. The rubber affixed to the plexor is designed to give resiliency to the blow, an important desideratum in the elicitation of the reflexes.
>
> This pleximeter of metal, covered at one end with rubber, is employed concurrently with the plexor . . .[16]

Abrams promoted a variety of instruments, including pneumatic and electrical devices, and distinguished between the usefulness of vibratory vs. concussive stimulation (Figures 1-7, B, 1-8, and 1-9):

> Pneumatic hammer with concussors. This operates with a pressure of 40 pounds and yields a blow equivalent to 12 pounds.
>
> This hammer is very efficient but because it is noisy and compressed air is not always available, the electro-concussor of the author is preferable. . . .
>
> The author's electro-concussor. This apparatus was constructed for the purpose of securing percussion-effects and the latter only. Practically all the instruments designed for sismotherapy are mere vibrators and are *absolutely useless* for executing the methods of spondylotherapy. This electro-concussor is portable, and its flexible shaft is readily attached to an "AC" or "DC" motor. At a slight expense,

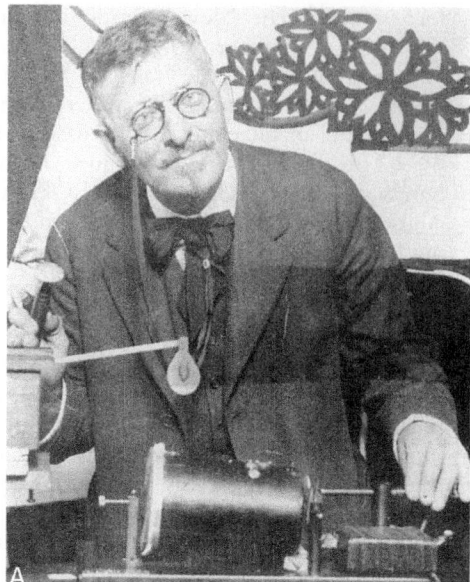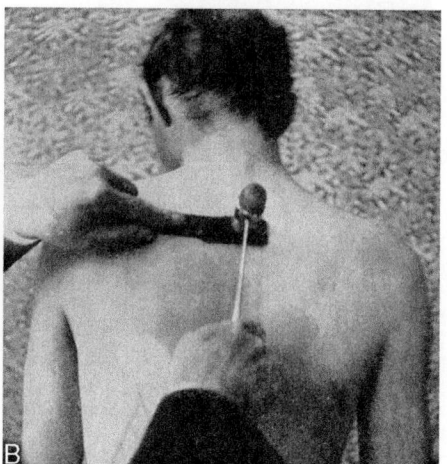

Figure 1-7 **A,** Dr. Albert Abrams with one of his many contraptions. **B,** Dr. Albert Abrams' use of "plexor and pleximeter." *(**B,** From Abrams A. Spondylotherapy: spinal concussion and the application of other methods to the spine in the treatment of disease. San Francisco: Philopolis Press; 1910.)*

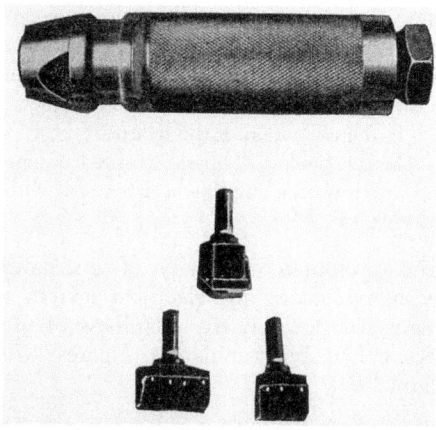

Figure 1-8 Dr. Albert Abrams' pneumatic hammer with concussors. *(From Abrams A. Spondylotherapy: spinal concussion and the application of other methods to the spine in the treatment of disease. San Francisco: Philopolis Press; 1910.)*

an extra motor may be purchased and as both motors are interchangeable, the apparatus may be used on either current. It is provided with two concussors which deliver blows to both sides of a spinous process.[16]

The use of manipulative devices was also popular among other drugless healers. The Zoe Johnson Company of St. Joseph, Michigan, marketed concussion and vibration devices and books on their application for many years.[17,18] Benedict Lust,

MD, ND, DC, the father of naturopathy in America, was happy to include advertisements for "Benko Hand Concussion Sets," which he marketed during the 1920s through 1940s in his widely distributed periodical, *Naturopath & Herald of Health* (Figure 1-10):

> SPINAL CONCUSSION
>
> Correct in Principle and Design
>
> Spondylotherapy, or the science of concussion of the spinal nerve centres, was originated and developed by Dr. Abrams, who has written a scientific treatise of considerable length on the subject. Of late, Dr. Alva Gregory and Dr. J.S. Riley have written much of value and interest concerning this new method . . . every practitioner of experience will confirm the statement that spinal concussion is one of the most powerful adjuncts to drugless therapy . . .[19]

Interest in mechanical forms of manipulation even captured the imagination of a few allopathic physicians (Figures 1-11 to 1-13):

> CLINICAL MEDICINE AND SURGERY
> Volume 43, Number 1
> Notes from International Medical Assembly
> Reported by George B. Lake, MD, Waukegan, Ill.
>
> . . . A more elaborate apparatus is the *Articulator* (shown in Fig. 3), which is intended to do, in an accurately regulated and scientific

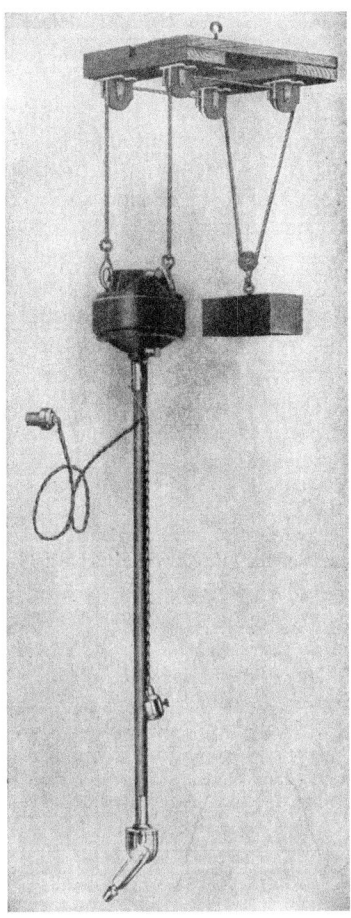

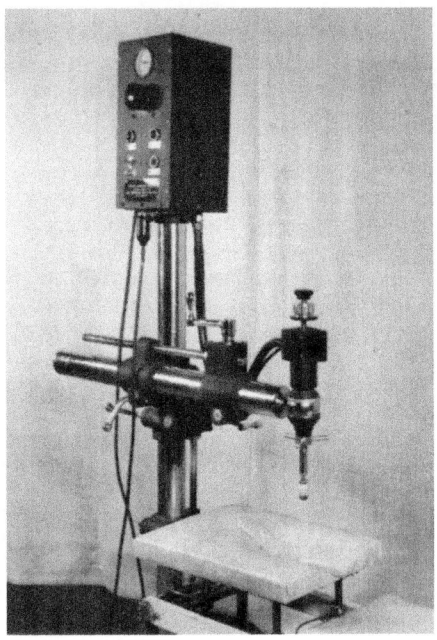

Figure 1-11 Spinal Adjusting Machine of Arden Zimmerman, DC, circa 1965.

Figure 1-9 Dr. Albert Abrams' electric concussor hammer. *(From Abrams A. Spondylotherapy: spinal concussion and the application of other methods to the spine in the treatment of disease. San Francisco: Philopolis Press; 1910.)*

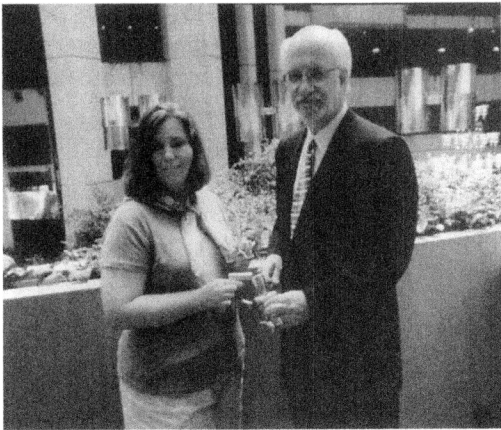

Figure 1-10 Palmer student Andrea Benko, granddaughter of Andrew Benko, an original founder of the Benko Hand Concussion Instrument, with Activator cofounder, Dr. Arlan Fuhr, who is holding one of the original instruments. *(Courtesy Arlan Fuhr.)*

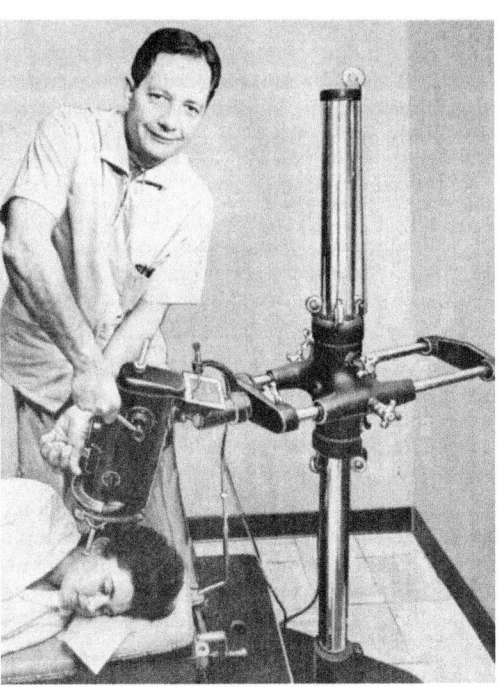

Figure 1-12 Futuramic Cervical Specific Instrument. *(From Advertisement for Futuramic Cervical Specific Instrument. Dig Chiropr Econ. 1968;10[4]:36.)*

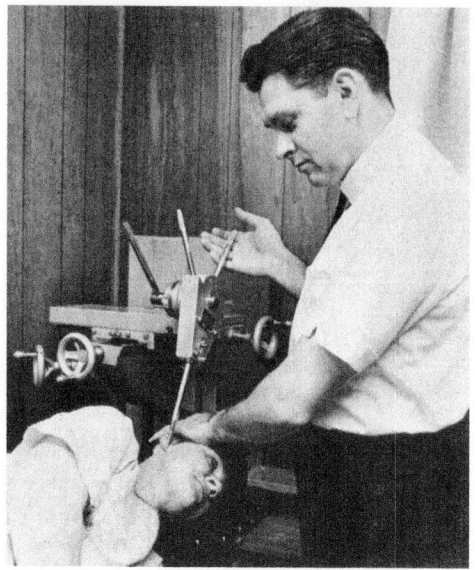

Figure 1-13 Image of an adjusting machine from an ad for the Pettibon Method. *(From Advertisement for the Pettibon Method. Dig Chiropr Econ. 1968;11[3]:52.)*

manner, everything that a chiropractor can do with his hands, and a good deal more. It is used in the treatment of fractures, sprains, dislocations, stiff joints (including those of the spine) and all other conditions where gentle, exact and rhythmic pulling and stretching of any part of the body is indicated.

Editorial Note—The Medical Profession once contended that the vertibrae [sic] could not be moved nor interfere with the transmission of nerve energy. Now they are recognizing this basic principle.[20]

Osterbauer and coauthors[21] suggested that development of "Hole-in-One" (HIO), an upper cervical adjusting strategy that involves a "toggle recoil" thrust, by B.J. Palmer, DC, gave impetus (unintentionally, no doubt) to the development of manipulative devices. The difficulties experienced by chiropractors as they attempted to skillfully perform this technique encouraged the development of mechanical devices that might serve the same purpose.[22,23] Some of this equipment resembled a punch-press that delivered a thrust very similar to "the force displacement pattern of the toggle mechanism."[23] Grostic reviewed the mechanical characteristics of several of these machines, including a "cam-stylus" adjusting instrument that can be motorized or computer operated, resulting in varying cam rotation speeds.[23] Exemplary of these are the Life College Adjusting Instrument and the Pettibon Adjusting Instrument.

Osterbauer and co-workers[21] also describe the Thrust Air Model 2001, a hand-held, "gun-styled" compressed air unit powered by a separate air compressor. Other hand-held mechanical adjusting instruments use two basic systems: solenoid-activated and spring-activated devices. "While both the solenoid and spring-activated units have similar kinetic energy–induced force displacement curves characteristic of such percussion devices, the solenoid type units are limited by the strength of the coil and whether or not the stylus is attached to the iron core or is free to move independently of it."[21] Examples of solenoid-activated devices are the Humber-King KH-4 Electronic Pulse and the Kinetic Precision Spinal Adjuster (Figures 1-14 to 1-16).

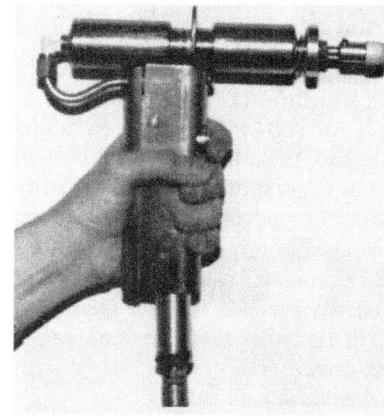

Figure 1-14 The Thruster, a pneumatic device, from an ad. *(From Advertisement for the Thruster Adjusting Instrument. Dig Chiropr Econ. 1985;28[1]:9.)*

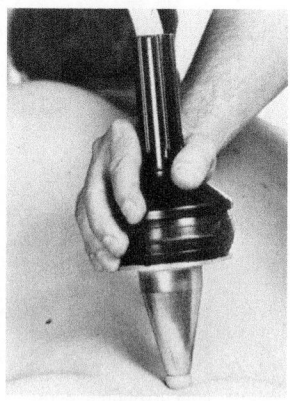

Figure 1-15 G-5 instrument from Standard Distributors delivers "nearly 4,000 oscillations per minute." *(From Advertisement: Controlling kinetic energy. J Fla Chiropr Assoc. 1970; Winter:25.)*

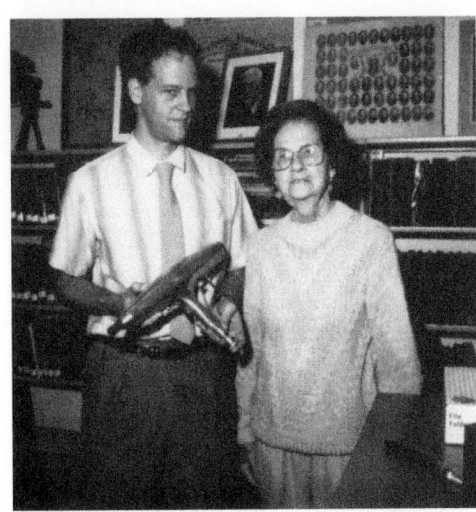

Figure 1-16 Student Charles Cushing and Dr. Vi Nickson display a pneumatic adjusting device. *(From Logan student honored by Alumni Association and Red Cross. Tower [Logan College] 1993;Summer:10.)*

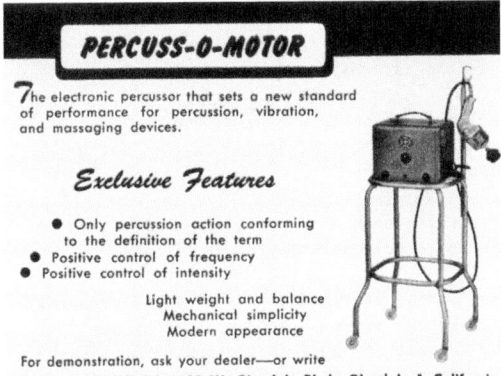

Figure 1-17 Advertisement for Percuss-O-Motor; from *Chirogram* for April 1951. *(Courtesy Southern California University of Health Sciences.)*

It is against this background of innovation and invention that the AAI made its debut in the late 1960s (Figure 1-17).

FOUNDERS OF ACTIVATOR

Born December 8, 1914, in rural Villard, Minnesota, Warren Clemens Lee enrolled at the Northwestern College of Chiropractic (NWCC) in Minneapolis and graduated on March 1, 1942.[24] Founded in 1941, the NWCC accepted a number of transfer students from the nearby Minnesota Chiropractic College (MCC)[25]; Warren Lee may have been one of these. Hugh B. Logan, DC, founder of the Logan Basic College of Chiropractic (LBCC) in St. Louis, had visited the MCC in 1941 and contemplated a contract to permit instruction in his proprietary method, Basic Technique (BT), within the MCC curriculum.[26] Dr. Lee had also received "advanced placement from Logan Basic College of Chiropractic (attended 01/42 to 08/42)"[24] (Figure 1-18).

After completing his studies in BT, Lee practiced as an associate of a St. Paul, Minnesota, chiropractor before establishing himself in his own practice in the southwestern Minnesota farm town of Redwood Falls in 1946. He supplemented his training in BT with the work of I.N. Toftness, DC, and radionics. Among his new patients in 1953 was a 13-year-old farm boy named Arlan William Fuhr (Figures 1-19 to 1-21).

Born September 2, 1939, in Sheridan Township, Minnesota, Arlan Fuhr was also the product of a rural background. The youngster suffered from chronic sore throats, and at age 13 was taken by his mother, a patient of Lee, to see the family chiropractor. Fuhr has a clear recollection of seeing his x-rays showing a "leaning tower spine" during his first visit to Dr. Lee's clinic. He received a dozen Toftness adjustments from an associate at Lee's facility, Dr. Wilson, and his throat difficulty resolved without recurrence. This happy outcome set the young man on an early career path: He resolved to become a chiropractor. He was strongly supported in this choice by his mother, despite discouragements received from some family members and grade school teachers.

Arlan enrolled at the University of Minnesota to take the pre-chiropractic, basic science course work required of licensed practitioners in Minnesota. He matriculated at LBCC the following year and believed he had found a new home. A special bond developed with the College's president, Vinton F. Logan, DC, and the future Dr. Fuhr fondly recalls his mentor's call for development of a "push-button Basic" to accelerate delivery of BT. Arlan would meet that challenge with the development of the Activator Method. He graduated from LBCC in 1961 (Figure 1-22).

Following a stint in the U.S. Navy, during which time he served on a wooden-bottomed minesweeper off the Cuban coast during the missile crisis of 1962, Arlan returned to Minnesota to practice. He accepted Dr. Lee's offer of an associateship in Redwood Falls. The duo found a common bond in Logan's teachings about the structural unity of the skeletal system and the effects of gravity on the spinal column. BT focused attention on the relationship of the sacrum to the pelvis and compensatory

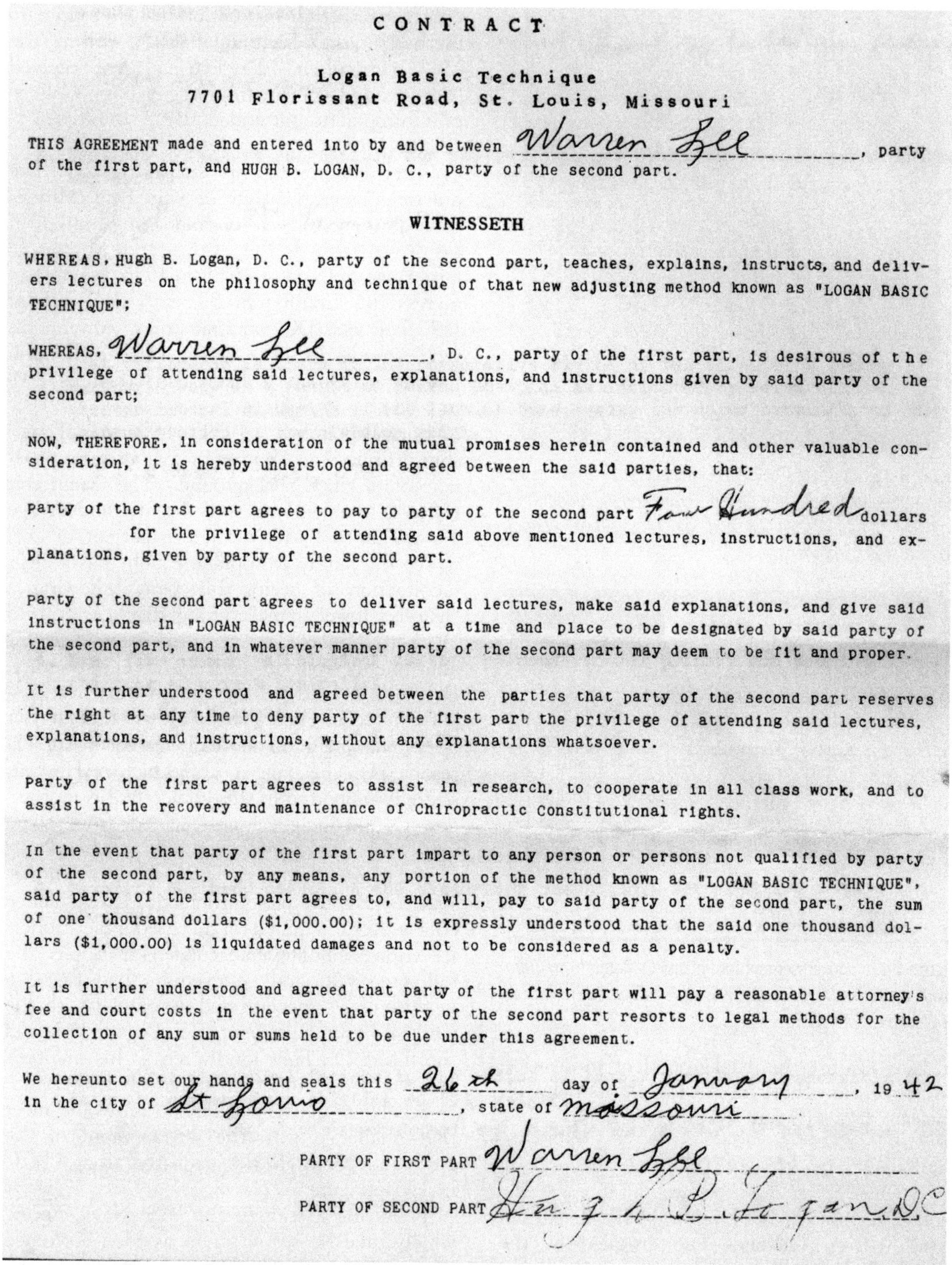

CONTRACT

Logan Basic Technique
7701 Florissant Road, St. Louis, Missouri

THIS AGREEMENT made and entered into by and between *Warren Lee*, party of the first part, and HUGH B. LOGAN, D. C., party of the second part.

WITNESSETH

WHEREAS, Hugh B. Logan, D. C., party of the second part, teaches, explains, instructs, and delivers lectures on the philosophy and technique of that new adjusting method known as "LOGAN BASIC TECHNIQUE";

WHEREAS, *Warren Lee*, D. C., party of the first part, is desirous of the privilege of attending said lectures, explanations, and instructions given by said party of the second part;

NOW, THEREFORE, in consideration of the mutual promises herein contained and other valuable consideration, it is hereby understood and agreed between the said parties, that:

Party of the first part agrees to pay to party of the second part *Four Hundred* dollars for the privilege of attending said above mentioned lectures, instructions, and explanations, given by party of the second part.

Party of the second part agrees to deliver said lectures, make said explanations, and give said instructions in "LOGAN BASIC TECHNIQUE" at a time and place to be designated by said party of the second part, and in whatever manner party of the second part may deem to be fit and proper.

It is further understood and agreed between the parties that party of the second part reserves the right at any time to deny party of the first part the privilege of attending said lectures, explanations, and instructions, without any explanations whatsoever.

Party of the first part agrees to assist in research, to cooperate in all class work, and to assist in the recovery and maintenance of Chiropractic Constitutional rights.

In the event that party of the first part impart to any person or persons not qualified by party of the second part, by any means, any portion of the method known as "LOGAN BASIC TECHNIQUE", said party of the first part agrees to, and will, pay to said party of the second part, the sum of one thousand dollars ($1,000.00); it is expressly understood that the said one thousand dollars ($1,000.00) is liquidated damages and not to be considered as a penalty.

It is further understood and agreed that party of the first part will pay a reasonable attorney's fee and court costs in the event that party of the second part resorts to legal methods for the collection of any sum or sums held to be due under this agreement.

We hereunto set our hands and seals this *26th* day of *January*, 19 *42* in the city of *St Louis*, state of *Missouri*.

PARTY OF FIRST PART *Warren Lee*

PARTY OF SECOND PART *Hugh B. Logan DC*

Figure 1-18   Contract to study Logan's Basic Technique, signed by Warren C. Lee and Hugh B. Logan on January 26, 1942. *(Courtesy Activator Methods International.)*

distortions. In these respects, BT followed the theoretical lead of Willard Carver, LLB, DC, whose "structural approach" to spinal analysis and adjusting stood in contrast to the segmentalism of traditional Palmer theory.[27,28]

Lee and Fuhr practiced their own integration of BT and Toftness methods, and they searched for practical methods by which to better determine patients' preadjustive and postadjustive spinal status. By 1965 Fuhr had grown interested

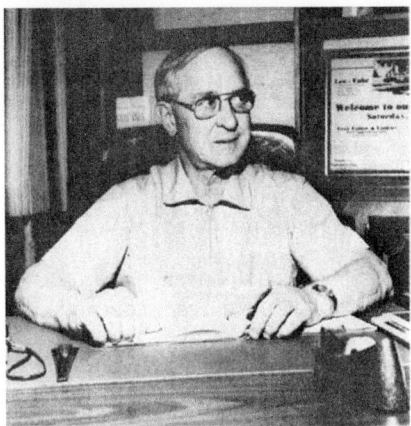

Figure 1-19 Dr. Warren C. Lee, circa 1977. *(Courtesy Activator Methods International.)*

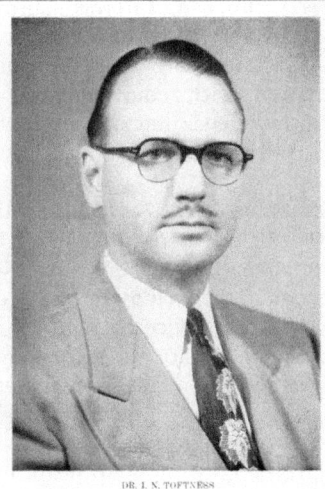

Figure 1-20 Dr. I.N. Toftness, from the cover of a Logan College periodical, 1951.

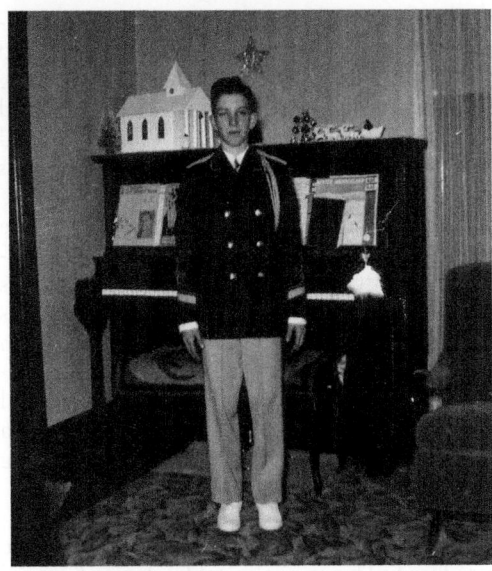

Figure 1-21 Arlan Fuhr, age 16, member of his high school band. *(Courtesy Arlan Fuhr.)*

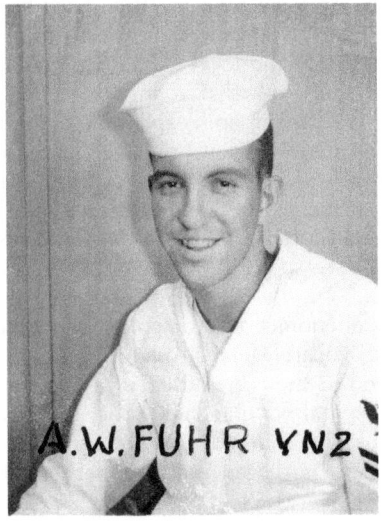

Figure 1-22 Dr. Arlan Fuhr in the Navy, 1961. *(Courtesy Arlan Fuhr.)*

in the leg length measurements and double thumb lock toggle adjusting procedures taught by Richard Van Rumpt, DC, in his Directional Nonforce Technique (DNFT) seminars. However, he was not comfortable with some of Van Rumpt's more esoteric procedures, particularly "dropping the bomb," in which the clinician observed relative leg lengths while silently asking Innate Intelligence to communicate the locations and listings of subluxations. This was beyond the pale of reason for Fuhr, who ceased attending the DNFT seminars in 1967.

In the late 1960s, while staffing a Minnesota Chiropractic Association blood pressure testing booth at the state fair in Minneapolis, Fuhr took

an additional step along the path toward what has become the Activator Method assessment method. An elderly woman came up to the booth and asked to have her blood pressure checked and began talking to Fuhr about chiropractic. She introduced herself as Mabel Derefield. Well known within the Palmer branch of the profession, the Derefield name meant nothing to the young Logan graduate, who was only half listening. However, when Dr. Derefield began to outline on a napkin a system of pelvic analysis while using a relative leg length measurement, Fuhr was intrigued. He later realized that the woman was a chiropractor and had given him a lesson in the Derefield Leg Check procedures, which she had developed with her husband. Lee and Fuhr incorporated these procedures into their patient examinations (Figure 1-23).

Lee and Fuhr were also influenced by the Truscott System of Angular Analysis and Controlled Adjusting.[29] Developed by Leon Lewis Truscott, DC, PhC, of San Jose, California, this method of spinal analysis involved leg length measurement at the adductor *tubercles*. According to Truscott, "Subluxations of the cervical vertebrae manifest themselves by producing a functional shortening of one leg, thus creating bodily imbalance."[29]

As Lee and Fuhr's leg length method of subluxation analysis evolved, new features were introduced. The specialty tables (manufactured by Tri W-G) that they had devised involved a manually operated foot piece, which required pulling it up with the left hand into the locked position. At some time in 1976, Fuhr began to notice a fairly constant, dull aching pain in his left rib cage at the level of the twelfth thoracic vertebra. Fuhr asked a young associate doctor for an adjustment and explained to him that when he raised his left arm over his head, the pain increased. The associate noticed that this maneuver seemed to dramatically shorten Fuhr's functional short leg. Thus was born the first Isolation Test, specific to the twelfth thoracic vertebra.

This phenomenon prompted development of other provocative maneuvers up and down the spine and in the extremities to test for subluxations of spinal vertebrae and other articulations. Subsequently, chiropractors who attended Activator seminars began sending in their clinical observations, which were tested by Lee and

Fuhr and eventually by a review panel made up of Activator Method instructors. The reviewers used these tests on their own patients and noted the results. Those that seemed "valid" were incorporated into the main body of the technique.

ACTIVATOR ADJUSTING INSTRUMENT

The assessment components of the Activator Method, derived from the concepts of Van Rumpt, the Derefields, and Truscott, evolved before the invention of the AAI. This instrument, which would become standard equipment for most members of the profession, had its origins in the physical stress that Lee and Fuhr experienced with repeated use of the thumb toggle adjustment. Although these maneuvers produced a fair degree of articular specificity, they also generated extreme fatigue, muscle strain, and frequent elbow injury caused by the elbows striking each other during rapid movement when thrusting into patients' spines. They sought an alternative means of producing a manipulation with equivalent or superior control of the speed, force, and direction of thrust, but without the wear and tear on the doctor.

In 1966 Steve Inglis, a local dentist, suggested that a dental impactor might provide a solution. This small instrument was designed to force amalgam into cavities in the teeth. Lee and Fuhr used the device to render thrusts to the joints of a few patients but believed that the impactor did not generate sufficient force to make a difference in their patients' conditions. Several other devices were tried but were consigned to the growing scrap heap, including a center punch (which required too much preload before firing), an instrument made by a patient, and another instrument developed by Frederick G. Proehl, BS, DC, a former basic science instructor at Logan College. None of these seemed to serve the purpose (Figure 1-24).

Another dentist-patient in the Lee-Fuhr Clinic, Dr. Stava of Marshall, Minnesota, offered a somewhat more promising contraption. He provided a surgical impact mallet that was used to split impacted wisdom teeth. The scalpel tip was replaced with a brake shoe rivet, and a small rubber doorstop was fastened to the end. This device tested successfully on patients, and the first functional ancestor of the modern AAI was born. Lee and Fuhr further modified this instrument and arranged for its manufacture by the Union Broach Company in New Jersey until 1976 (Figures 1-25 to 1-27).

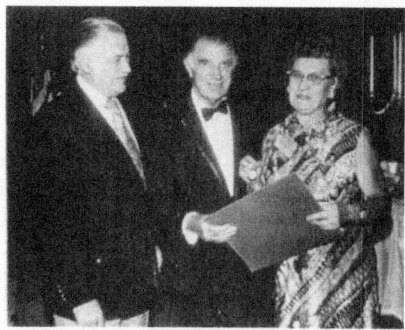

Figure 1-23   The Drs. Derefield with Palmer College president David Palmer, DC, 1971.

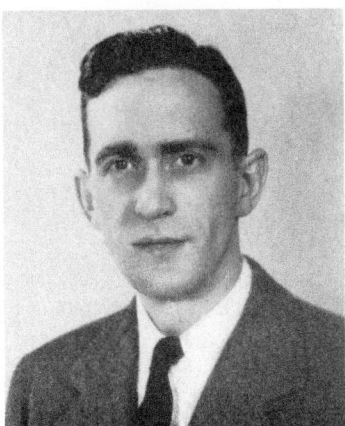

Figure 1-24 Dr. Freddy Proehl, from the 1950 issue of the Logan College yearbook, *Keystone*.

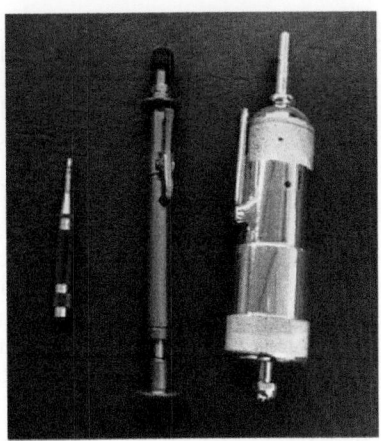

Figure 1-26 Early devices that preceded the Activator instrument. *(Courtesy Activator Methods International.)*

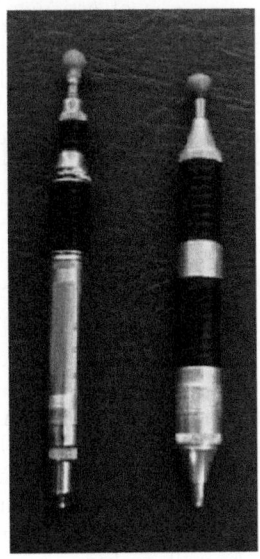

Figure 1-25 Dental amalgam snappers were precursors of the Activator Adjusting Instrument but were painful for patients. *(Courtesy Activator Methods International.)*

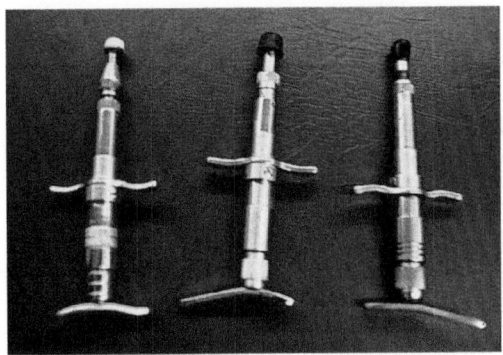

Figure 1-27 Early generations of the Activator Adjusting Instrument, derived from a surgical impact mallet, circa 1967. *(Courtesy Activator Methods International.)*

This early Activator Instrument tended to break under heavy usage. To the rescue came Freddy Hunziker, then a student at Cleveland Chiropractic College in Los Angeles. Hunziker worked nights in the Western Airlines machine shop, where he made use of the facilities to design and build a more reliable internal mechanism for the instrument. His version involved a hammer-anvil effect that produced a dependable and controlled force to osseous spinal structures.[30] Hunziker sold the patent rights for this design to Activator Methods, Inc., in 1976 and introduced Fuhr to a Swiss-American firm that was able to manufacture the AAI to a high standard of quality (Figure 1-28).

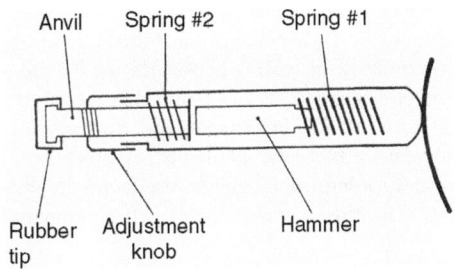

Figure 1-28 Schematic of mechanism of the Activator instrument. *(From Duell ML. The force of the Activator adjusting instrument. Dig Chiropr Econ. 1984;27[3]:17-9.)*

Production of this newly designed instrument began in 1976, but another dependability problem soon surfaced. The small springs inside the AAI lasted only 3 months under heavy usage. Credit for resolving this difficulty goes to Clark Bumgarner, DC, of Coffeyville, Kansas, who informed Fuhr in 1978 that the spring in a 29-cent Parker ballpoint pen worked well and lasted much longer.[30] The springs of all AAIs in stock were replaced by the Parker ballpoint springs until stronger springs could be inserted during the manufacturing process.

Activator Methods, Inc., was granted a patent for its AAI on September 26, 1978. The patent acknowledged that the purpose of the device was "to provide a manually manipulatable instrument capable of providing a dynamic thrust which includes a controlled force of adjustment applied at a precise and specific line of drive at a high speed" (U.S. Patent 4,116,235). The AAI was subsequently registered with the U.S. Food and Drug Administration pursuant to the Medical Practices Devices Act. This early generation of AAI remained the standard for the next 16 years (Figure 1-29).

By 1994, studies conducted by Tony Keller, PhD, at the University of Vermont had prompted further refinement in the AAI. Dr. Keller's investigations[31-34] suggested that an instrument re-equipped with a particular type of impedance head would significantly improve the frequency content of the force delivered to the spine.[33-35] Activator Methods, Inc., reported the following in the November/December 1994 issue of its periodical, the *Update* (Figure 1-30):

> Activator Methods commissioned the Vermont Orthopaedic and Biomechanic Consultants to test the original Activator instrument for the purpose of perfecting the design. One of the resulting improvements was a permanent cervical attachment which solved the common problem of the cervical tip loosening and losing line of drive when adjusting difficult contact points on the body. In addition, during the process of evaluation . . . we found that the white tip between the instrument and the cervical attachment had a dampening effect which lowered the energy delivered to the spine. In the case of the human spine, the resonant

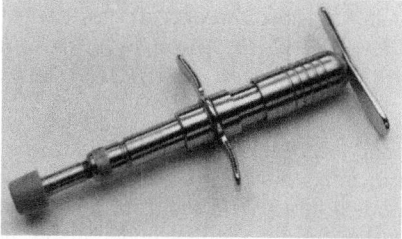

Figure 1-29 First mass-produced Activator Adjusting Instrument (AAI-1). *(Courtesy Activator Methods International.)*

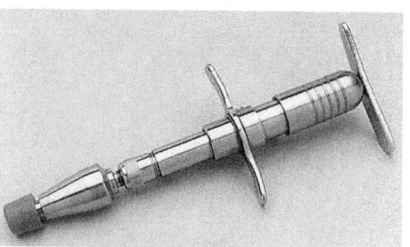

Figure 1-30 Next-generation Activator Adjusting Instrument (Activator II), circa 1994. *(Courtesy Activator Methods International.)*

frequency occurs at dynamic frequencies between 40-50 Hertz. At these frequencies, the posterior-anterior motion in response to the adjustment is at a maximum. The presence of the white tip caused the frequency content of the input energy to be reduced by approximately one-half.

To address this issue, we examined dynamic load input/acceleration response or impedance head interface (rigid vs. flexible) and impulse delivery technique (continuous vs. temporary contact). Our research revealed that a rigid interface, combined with a temporary contact impulse delivery procedure, resulted in significant improvement in the input frequency content. The new ACTIVATOR II encompasses these improvements.

Development of a third-generation AAI sought to overcome human error in the use of the adjusting device. In using the AAI-I and the AAI-II, the clinician compressed the internal springs of the instrument when they put too much pressure on the patient before delivery of the thrust. As well, each doctor created a different, often excessive preload pressure. This idiosyncratic compression of the internal springs caused the instrument to lose force and to reduce the speed of the thrust. Discussion of this preload problem with a consulting engineer prompted the idea of constructing an instrument with a rack built around it that would prevent the clinician from compressing the internal springs, thereby preserving force and speed. After several months of conversation and collaboration with the manufacturer, the AAI-III emerged as a "clinician-proof" adjusting tool with a rack and automatic preload (Figure 1-31, A and B).

The AAI-IV would further the refinements previously introduced. This fourth-generation Activator included a higher speed setting and lightened the preload for the very sensitive patient. This latest model was field-tested to

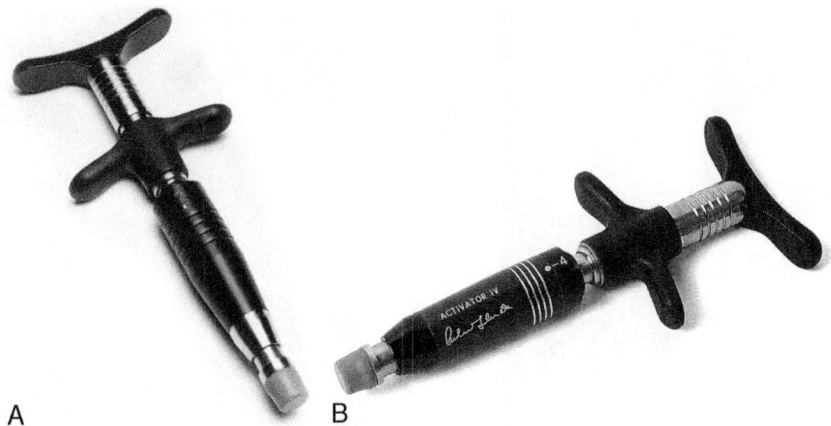

Figure 1-31 **A,** Third-generation Activator Adjusting Instrument. **B,** Fourth-generation Activator Adjusting Instrument. *(Courtesy Activator Methods International.)*

determine what would work best. As well, this latest model overcame a problem that had plagued the AAI for years. Most clinicians held the instrument between their trigger finger and their middle finger. However, some held it between their middle finger and their ring finger. If the latter method was used, it caused wear on the instrument. The solution was to allow the triggering handle to spin, in which case it made absolutely no difference how the Activator was held (Figure 1-32).

By late 1967, Lee and Fuhr had developed a method of biomechanical analysis and an adjusting instrument, but this technique package was as yet unnamed. Inspiration for the "Activator" brand came in part from the name of the company, Active-Aid, with whom they had contracted to produce a unique adjusting table. Lee and Fuhr had resisted any temptation to name their method after themselves, reasoning that the longevity of the technique then might be no greater than their life spans. At Logan, they had learned to adjust the vertebrae passively by using the apex Basic contact. Lee and Fuhr now believed that they were actively moving bones by using the low-force, high-

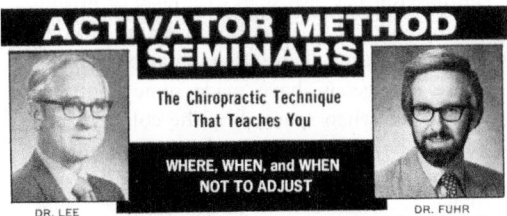

Figure 1-32 Advertisement for Activator Methods appearing in the September-October 1976 issue of *Digest of Chiropractic Economics.*

speed, mechanical adjusting instrument that they had developed; they were in effect "activating" the vertebrae. The "push-button Basic" that Vinton Logan had challenged students to develop would emerge as Activator Methods. Early promotions for the new method suggested that Activator practitioners would know "where, when, and when not to adjust."

ACTIVATOR METHODS ADJUSTING TABLE DEVELOPMENT

Similar to the AAI, development of the special tables employed in the Activator Method was prompted by need. Patients required a step stool to climb onto a 29-inch-high wooden bench–like table for leg check analysis and then were moved to the lower Zenith Hi-Lo tables for double thumb toggle adjustments. As well, Lee and Fuhr were fatigued by bending over adjusting tables. They realized that a less stressful method was needed for patients and for themselves.

In 1969 a motorized adjusting table was designed that took the patient from the standing to the prone position (and vice versa) and also raised the prone patient higher from the floor. Assessment and treatment now required the patient to mount just one table, and adjustments were administered with the clinician in a much more comfortable posture. A local manufacturer of physical therapy equipment, Active-Aid, began to produce the new adjusting table (Figure 1-33).

Difficulties with the motors that drove the Active-Aid tables prompted Lee and Fuhr to look for another manufacturer. While visiting the Active-Aid factory to discuss the problem, they picked up an advertising pamphlet for

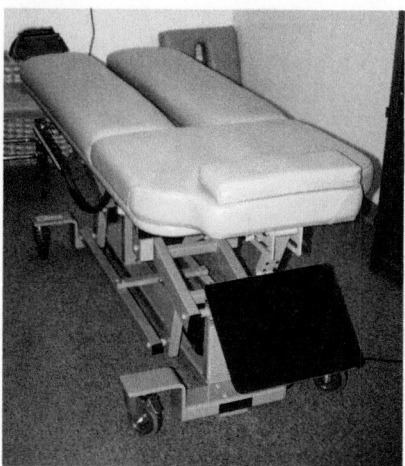

Figure 1-33 Eighth-generation Tri W-G table employed for Activator Methods Chiropractic Technique. *(Courtesy Activator Methods International.)*

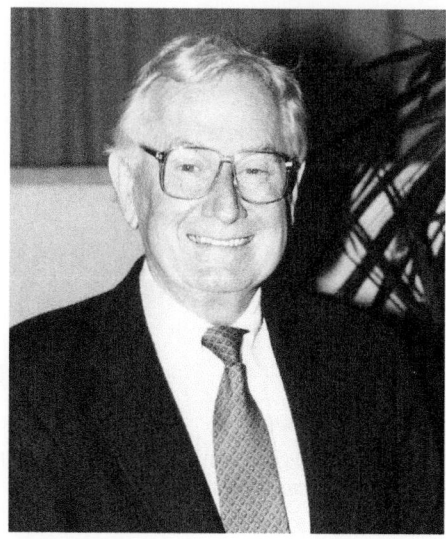

Figure 1-34 Bernard A. Coyle, PhD, circa 1995. *(Courtesy Bernard A. Coyle.)*

Tri W-G, Inc., a Valley City, North Dakota, manufacturer of physical therapy equipment. John Weber, president of Tri W-G, was contacted in 1971, and a visit to the plant was arranged. The relationship between the equipment manufacturer and the technique company was cemented when Fuhr's treatment of Weber's wife, whose recent back surgery had not resolved her pain, enabled her to walk for the first time in 6 weeks. Tri W-G developed a new, chiropractic division. When Activator Methods became an international company, Lloyd Table Company took over as the Activator table developer and distributor because of its capability for worldwide distribution.

ACTIVATOR METHOD INSTRUCTION

Weekend seminars have served as the primary mode of delivering instruction in the Activator Method. In the tradition of postgraduate education that has persisted throughout chiropractic history, Drs. Lee and Fuhr commenced to teach their new method to any interested chiropractor. This training began rather informally with a fellow Minnesota DC, who responded to rumors about the new technique and inquired of the Redwood Falls practitioners. By 1970 the pair had decided to offer the Activator Method on a regular basis to chiropractors near and far. The first of these seminars, which drew 10 curious doctors, was organized by two of Fuhr's former Logan classmates, Irvin Chessin DC, and Eric Perlman DC, and was held in Garden Grove, California, at the clinical offices

of Carl Remlin, DC. Instructional content included procedures for detecting subluxations by monitoring Leg Length Inequality and for making instrument-assisted adjustments of the pelvis and lower lumbar and upper cervical vertebrae. It was a humble beginning.

Weekend seminars in chiropractic have elicited criticism over the years, largely on the grounds that they are unregulated and offer instruction of unequal quality and sometimes dubious content. Nonetheless, many of the "brand named" techniques employed by DCs, some of which are taught in the accredited colleges, have their roots in private seminars. Nowadays, many of these seminars offer license renewal credit through co-sponsorship with a chiropractic school. Although chiropractic college faculty have sometimes questioned the appropriateness of technique entrepreneurs, sentiment toward technique seminars is not universally negative. Drs. Barney Coyle and Robert Tolar, former senior administrators at two chiropractic institutions, have opined the following (Figure 1-34):

> Enthusiasm has also sparked a bevy of private entrepreneurial educators, many of whom, despite making claims that have often been quite outrageous, have made some contribution, even when spurned by the colleges. Too seldom has there been an honest attempt to synthesize what is offered from diverse activity. It has been too easy to ignore them and shut the doors, thereby allowing some wisdom together with a liberal quantity of incoherent or forgettable material to fall outside.... A far

better approach for a college that values academic integrity is to allow persons prominent in the profession to make formal presentation on campus and to indulge in honest academic argument.[36]

Joseph Donahue, DC, suggests that private technique instructors have served a valuable role in professional development:

> I believe clinical entrepreneurs have historically filled a void. Considering the poor state of our colleges over most of the profession's history, chiropractic would not have survived without technique systems . . . Without a technique system to guide him/her the chiropractor was very likely to fail in practice. In many ways, chiropractic technique systems are necessary heuristic devices.[37]

Such issues were surely not a concern when Lee and Fuhr commenced seminar offerings in Minneapolis in 1971. Their intent was to disseminate what they believed was a worthy contribution to the clinical armamentarium of chiropractors. The following year saw their largest attendance to date—56 doctors—at an Activator Method offering in Columbia, South Carolina. And a window was about to open that would bring the new technique to the attention of a much wider segment of the profession.

In 1973 Fuhr presented the Activator Method at a seminar at the Baker Hotel in Dallas, Texas. Although only eight doctors were in attendance, one of them was Karl Parker, DC, a recent graduate of the Texas Chiropractic College and son of James W. Parker, DC, well known for his practice-building seminars. Very impressed with the Activator Method, the younger Dr. Parker visited the Lee-Fuhr Clinic in Redwood Falls in 1975 to observe the high-volume operation. Pleased with the encounter and what he had learned, Dr. Parker suggested that Lee and Fuhr might wish to attend one of his father's Parker seminars and consider joining the teaching staff of the Parker School for Professional Success (Figure 1-35).

Some time elapsed before Dr. Fuhr took up the offer. In the meanwhile, Dr. Lee offered Activator Method training in weekend seminars on the campus of Palmer College of Chiropractic and at hotels in Davenport, Iowa, and St. Louis; the latter presentations were well attended by Logan College students. The first international seminar in the Activator Method was presented by Dr. Lee at Bournemouth, England (home of the Anglo-European College

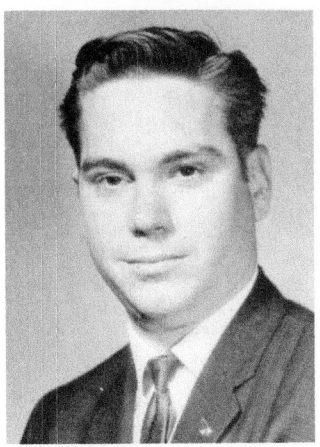

Figure 1-35 Texas Chiropractic College freshman, Karl Parker, from the 1966 edition of the College's yearbook. *(Courtesy Texas Chiropractic College.)*

of Chiropractic) in 1972; in 1974 Dr. Fuhr ventured to Sydney, Australia, where two weekend training sessions were provided.

In September 1976, Fuhr attended his first "Parker extravaganza" and, 2 months later, commenced instruction in the Activator Method as part of the Parker program. In the coming years, Activator Method instruction would become a regular feature of the Parker offerings. Fuhr was named a Parker Associate Lecturer (PAL) and, in this capacity, taught the Activator Method and practice management procedures. Although the Activator Method would continue to be taught in other venues, it was the Parker seminars that provided the "kick start" that brought the new method to the national attention of chiropractors and boosted attendance at Activator seminars.[30] Currently, Activator Method seminars are held in major cities across the United States, Canada, and Australia, and occasionally, in Europe, Japan, and Taiwan. In most instances, Activator Method training qualifies the participating chiropractor for license renewal credits (Figures 1-36 and 1-37).

Activator Methods' weekend seminars have evolved over the years and now comprise three sections (tracks). Track I introduces the basics of prone leg length measurements, Isolation Testing (from the pelvis to the occiput), and instrument-adjustment procedures for the same. Track II, which builds on the first module, reviews prone leg measurements and introduces Isolation Tests and adjusting procedures of a more advanced nature. The third module reviews the Track II material, introduces more specific isolation adjusting procedures, case management methods, treatment algorithms, outcome assessments, and credentialing for managed care requirements.

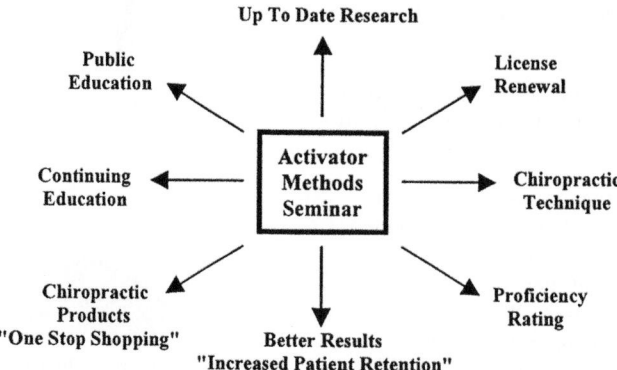

Figure 1-36   Services offered by Activator Methods, Inc., 1998. *(Courtesy Activator Methods International.)*

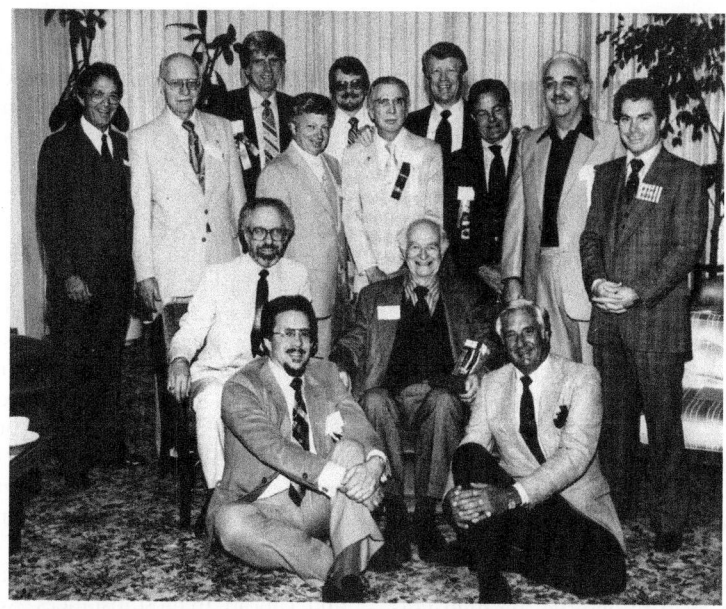

Figure 1-37   Instructors gather with Nobel laureate Linus Pauling, PhD, during a Parker seminar. *Standing left to right:* Bill Brown of the Parker School of Professional Success; Major Bertrand DeJarnette, DO, DC; John F. Thie, DC; Monte Greenawalt, DC; David Walther, DC; J. Clay Thompson, DC; Lamar Rosquist, DC; George J. Goodheart, DC; Glenn Stillwagon, DC; and Karl Parker, DC. *Seated on chairs, left to right:* Arlan W. Fuhr, DC, and Dr. Pauling. *Seated on floor, left to right:* David Denton, DC, and Russ Erhardt, DC, DACBR. *(Courtesy Activator Methods International.)*

The "proficiency rating" for Activator Method seminar attendees was introduced in the early 1980s, just as Dr. Lee chose to retire. Fuhr described the process in a 1985 newsletter:

> The Proficiency Ratings will continue to be given at all Activator sponsored seminars. About one quarter of the doctors attending have been taking the practical and oral test. . . . The doctors who pass are placed on our Preferred Referral Directory and those names are

the first to be given out in response to requests for referrals. All that is needed to keep current is to attend one seminar a year to be informed of new developments.[38]

This certification process was augmented by a subsequent category, "advanced proficiency rating," in the late 1980s. Activator Methods, Inc., established a referral network for patients and referred patients to proficiency-rated Activator practitioners in America, Europe, and

Australia during 1988-1994.[39] Today, because of the widespread use of the Internet, www.activator.com receives more than 1 million hits per month. There are now more than 2000 Activator proficiency rated doctors throughout the world who receive the benefit from this referral list. It was Dr. Fuhr's dream to use the Internet as a resource for patients to find qualified chiropractors who use a standardized procedure (Figure 1-38).

To facilitate the dissemination of the Activator Method, the company assembled a team of Activator instructors to provide didactic and experiential training in seminars around the world. An annual re-credentialing requirement for instructors was instituted in 1986, so as to enhance consistency in training content and methods wherever the Activator Method is taught. This recertification for instructors includes at least one annual meeting wherein standard methods are reviewed, new procedures are introduced, and published research findings related to the Activator Method are reviewed. Several of these instructors also constitute a clinical advisory board, which offers its perspectives to the company (Figure 1-39).

In 1999 Dr. Fuhr was married to Judith J. Hamilton, President of Hamilton Consulting, one of the top ten governmental relations firms in Phoenix, Arizona. Judi brought her organizational ability to Activator Methods International. It was from this expertise that a clinical advisory board was established, and the company was organized into regions throughout the world. Judi also formed a Business Advisory Board, which helps oversee the business aspects of the company. This turned Activator Methods International into a fully functional worldwide corporation (Figure 1-40).

The success of Activator Method instruction in terms of number of seminars and quality of instruction is attested to by the reception it has enjoyed within the chiropractic profession. An estimated 45,000 doctors worldwide make use of some or all of the Activator Method procedures,[40] although regional variation seems likely. Pedersen[41] estimated that European chiropractors employ the Activator Method in 14% of their cases. Surveys by the National Board of Chiropractic Examiners,[42,43] on the other hand, suggest that approximately half of all chiropractors make some use of Activator Method procedures in approximately 20% of their cases, making it one of the most popular of chiropractic techniques. These surveys have not differentiated between use of Activator analysis vs. use of the AAI. However, since 1967 an estimated 75,000 AAIs have been sold.[40]

Instruction in the Activator Method was accelerated by its introduction to the course offerings at various schools, beginning in 1980, when Logan College of Chiropractic offered the Activator Method as an elective. The Parker College of Chiropractic was the first institution to require instruction in the Activator Method of all doctoral students. Today, required or elective course work in the Activator Method is provided at many chiropractic schools (Table 1-1) and in postgraduate settings. On many college campuses, both those that include the Activator Method in their curricula and those that do not, Activator clubs are thriving. These clubs are generally headed by enthusiastic students and are guided by a faculty advisor who is proficient in the Activator Method (Figure 1-41).

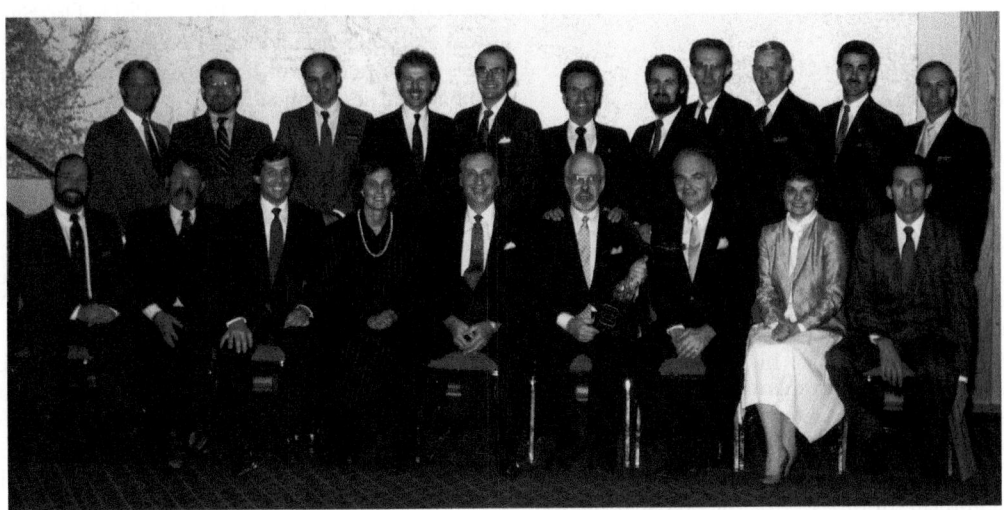

Figure 1-38   Activator instructors, 1986. *(Courtesy Activator Methods International.)*

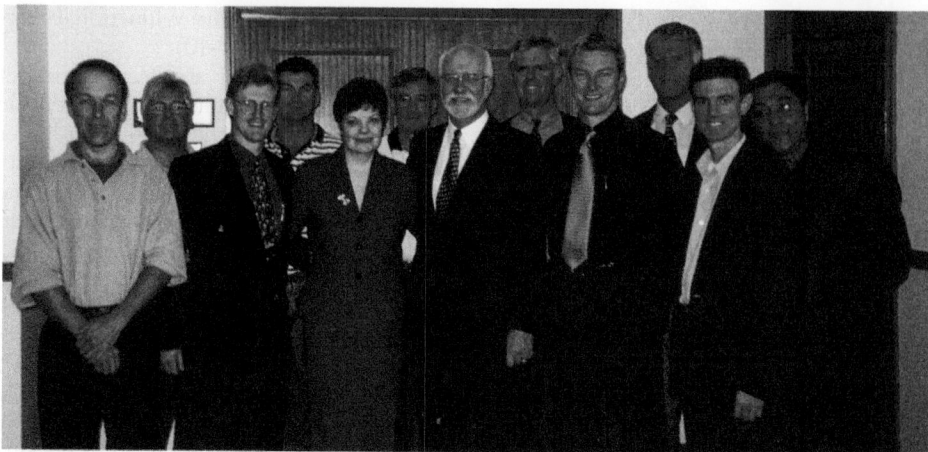

Figure 1-39   Drs. Lois Ward and Arlan Fuhr *(center)* meet with Australian Activator instructors, 2002. *(Courtesy Activator Methods International.)*

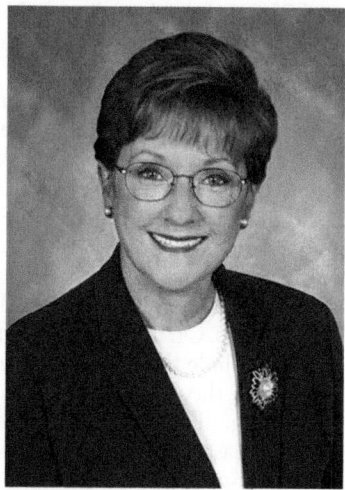

Figure 1-40   Judi Fuhr. *(Courtesy Activator Methods International.)*

ACTIVATOR METHODS, RESEARCH, AND CREDIBILITY

Since antiquity, spinal and articular manipulation has been practiced based on anecdote and private clinical experience. The earliest known systematic clinical trials of such methods did not appear until the latter half of the twentieth century.[44-51] The first randomized, controlled clinical trial of adjusting reported by chiropractors made its appearance in 1986.[52] The earliest known controlled study of instrument adjusting employed as active (as opposed to placebo) intervention was contributed by Yates and co-workers.[53]

The founders of the Activator Method took their clinical training during the preexperimental era in chiropractic. However, by the early 1980s

Fuhr had become concerned that anecdotes and informal clinical observations provided an insufficient basis for claims of efficacy and effectiveness for the Activator Method or any other form of manipulation. As well, the introduction of AAI had generated considerable controversy within the profession; some chiropractors voiced opinions that the device was hazardous to patients, and others considered an instrumental thrust a poor substitute for adjusting by hand. Although quite unprepared by his formal training, Fuhr chose to enter the research arena (Figures 1-42 and 1-43).

It was something of an ordeal for this research novice, who accepted a challenge from the president of TRI W-G, L. John Weber, to seek a federal grant to underwrite Activator research. Fuhr solicited the aid of immunologist Dennis Smith, PhD, and Logan College research administrator Barry P. Davis, PhD. Dr. Smith was self-taught in bioengineering but nonetheless led a successful grant-writing team, which submitted its application to the Small Business Innovative Research Grants Program of the National Institutes of Health (NIH). Their proposal sought funding to investigate the safety of the AAI with the use of a dog as the research subject. The project, conducted at Logan College and at the School of Comparative Medicine at St. Louis University, garnered $50,000 from the federal government. This was a miniscule amount by national standards but probably represented the first federal dollars received by any chiropractor-investigator. The study revealed "relative bone movement" as a result of thrusts with the AAI, thereby disconfirming critics' suggestion that the Activator Method did not "move a bone." This initial

Table 1-1   Instruction in the Activator Method at Various Chiropractic Colleges

College	Required in Doctoral Program	Elective in Doctoral Program	Postdoctoral (Relicensure) Offering	Activator Club*
Canadian Memorial Chiropractic College				X
Cleveland Chiropractic College of Kansas City		X	X	X
Cleveland Chiropractic College of Los Angeles		X	X	
Life University, Georgia		X	X	X
Life Chiropractic College West, California	X		X	
Logan College of Chiropractic, Missouri		X	X	X
New York Chiropractic College		X		X
Palmer College of Chiropractic, Iowa		X	X	
Palmer College of Chiropractic West		X		X
Parker College of Chiropractic, Texas		X		
Sherman College of Straight Chiropractic				X
Northwestern University of Health Sciences		X		
Texas College of Chiropractic	X			
Université du-Québec à Trois-Rivières, Canada		X		
Anglo European College of Chiropractic, England		X		
Macquarie University, Sidney, Australia		X		
Universidad Estatal del Valle de Ecatepec, Mexico City	X			

Compiled from Fuhr AW, Menke JM. Status of Activator Methods chiropractic technique, theory and practice. J Manipulative Physiol Ther. 2005;28(2):135.

*Activator clubs active as of Spring 2002 term.

research was published in the profession's preeminent scholarly periodical, the *Journal of Manipulative & Physiological Therapeutics*.[54,55] Whether relative bone movement is a necessary condition for therapeutic benefit remains undetermined.

Unsuccessful in his second grant application to the NIH, and now realizing the magnitude of the financial resources needed in the chiropractic research community, in 1987 Fuhr solicited the aid of his Activator instructors to establish a nonprofit research foundation, the

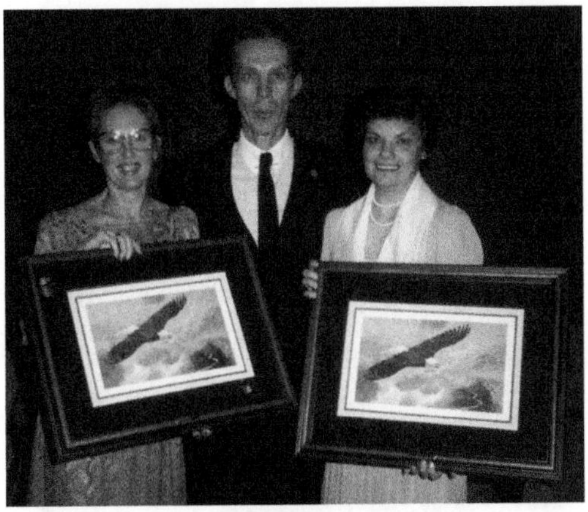

Figure 1-41   Michelle Petermann *(left)*, a longtime seminar staff member, is seen here with Drs. Gary and Lois Ward, Activator instructors, in 1985. *(Courtesy Activator Methods International.)*

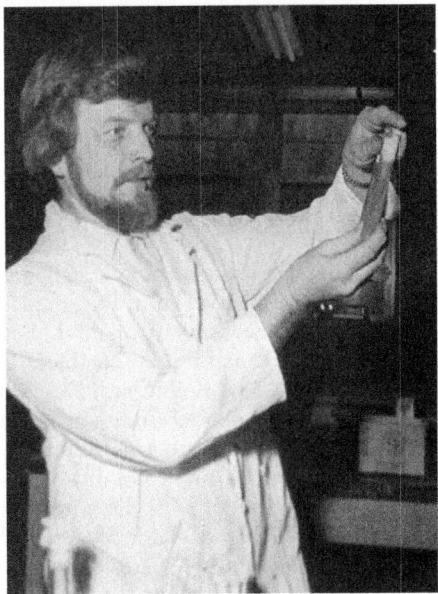

Figure 1-42   Dr. Barry Davis, from the 1975 edition of the Logan College yearbook, *Keystone.*

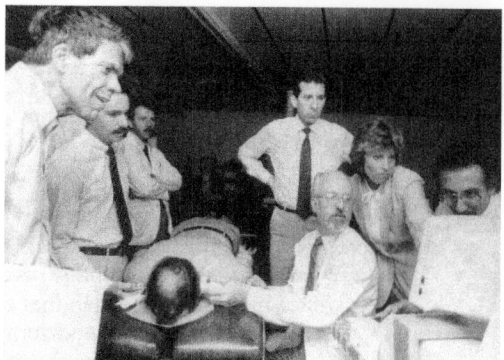

Figure 1-43 Dr. Dennis Smith is seen at far left during 1986 diagnostic studies with ultrasound equipment. *(Courtesy Activator Methods International.)*

National Institute of Chiropractic Research (NICR). The purposes of the NICR evolved somewhat over the years but were clearly stated in 1992:

> ... raise funds for fundamental scientific, clinical and historical research and scholarship in chiropractic. The NICR conducts research, and through a modest extramural grant-making program, has funded a number of research projects by other investigators. To date, funds have been awarded to investigators at Life Chiropractic College-West, Logan College of Chiropractic, Northwestern College of Chiropractic, the (Pacific) Consortium for Chiropractic Research, Palmer College of Chiropractic, Palmer College of Chiropractic/West, the University of the Pacific, and Arizona State University, among others. Awards have also been made to the Association for the History of Chiropractic and Palmer College of Chiropractic/West in support of projects in chiropractic history. The NICR is a member of the Association for the History of Chiropractic and the (Pacific) Consortium for Chiropractic Research. (Statement of Purpose, Activities & Affiliations, October 28, 1992)

The founding members of the NICR board of directors included Arlan W. Fuhr, DC, *President*, Tony Trimble, JD, *Secretary*, Donald J. Petermann, *Treasurer*, Donald G. Kimble, DC, Anthony Pavia, DC, and Lois Ward, DC. Since 1987 a number of talented individuals have contributed their expertise to this initiative as members of this board, most notably Bernard A. Coyle, PhD, Kenneth F. DeBoer, PhD, Robert A. Leach, DC, and Malik Slosberg, DC. The board was assisted at various times by employees Roy W. Hildebrandt, DC (founding editor of the *Journal of Manipulative & Physiological Therapeutics*), and Paul J. Osterbauer, DC,

MPH, a graduate of NWCC who served as research administrator for NICR in the late 1980s and early 1990s (Figures 1-44 to 1-46).

In its two decades of operation, the NICR has distributed slightly more than $690,000 in external grants and has supported a total of 262 scholarly presentations, books and chapters, and papers in scholarly and scientific periodicals (Box 1-1). The scope of the foundation's work has extended well beyond the questions posed by the Activator Method, and the NICR has been the most frequent source of funding for historical investigations in the profession.

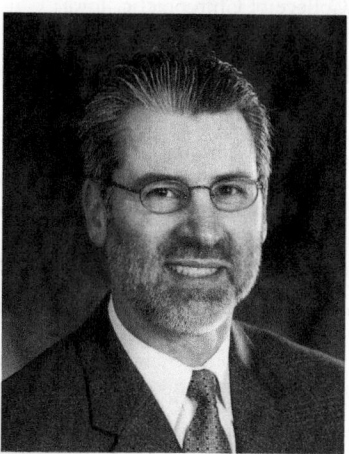

Figure 1-44 Thomas DeVita, DC, Activator instructor and vice president of the National Institute of Chiropractic Research, 2002. *(Courtesy Activator Methods International.)*

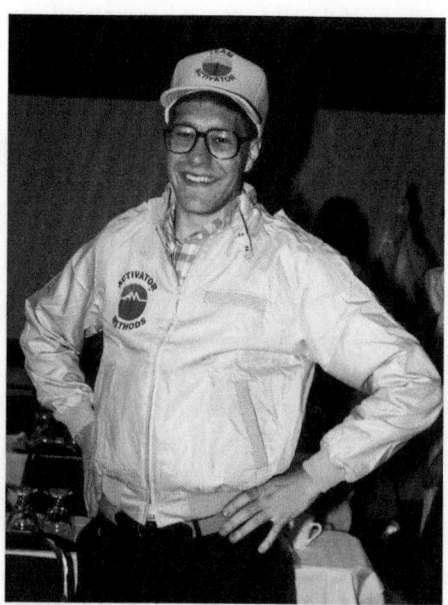

Figure 1-45 Dr. Paul Osterbauer, circa 1987. *(Courtesy Activator Methods International.)*

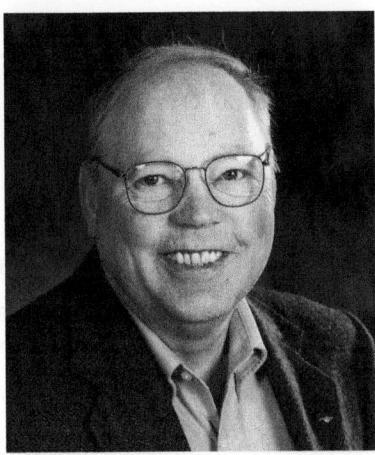

Figure 1-46 Dr. Ken DeBoer, member of the National Institute of Chiropractic Research board of directors, 2002. *(Courtesy Activator Methods International.)*

Box 1-1 **Periodicals in Which NICR-Supported Papers Have Been Published**
• *American Journal of Chiropractic Medicine* • *Chiropractic* • *Chiropractic History* • *Chiropractic Journal of Australia* • *Chiropractic Sports Medicine* • *Chiropractic Technique* • *D.C. Tracts* • *European Journal of Chiropractic* • *Journal of Biomechanics* • *Journal of Chiropractic Humanities* • *Journal of Manipulative & Physiological Therapeutics* • *Journal of Spinal Disorders* • *Journal of the American Geriatric Society* • *Journal of the Canadian Chiropractic Association* • *Philosophical Constructs for the Chiropractic Profession* (renamed *Journal of Chiropractic Humanities*) • *Psychophysiology* • *Skeptical Inquirer* • *Spine* • *Topics in Clinical Chiropractic*

NICR, National Institute of Chiropractic Research.

The Activator Method has become one of the most extensively studied technique systems in chiropractic, and the Activator company has been an active participant in the profession's emerging research community. Osterbauer et al. observed that since 1987,

AMI has participated in the research meetings of the California Chiropractic Foundation (Conference on Research and Education), the Consortium for Chiropractic Research, the Foundation for Chiropractic Education and Research (International Conference on Spinal Manipulation), and the several Consensus Conferences on Chiropractic Methods sponsored by the ACA Council on Technic. Concurrently, AMI has conducted a variety of clinical investigations. These studies have yielded numerous papers in the referred scientific literature and conference presentations and have inspired others to study the value of AMCT [Activator Methods chiropractic technique]. Interest in studying AMCT has resulted in interdisciplinary collaboration with the Departments of Bio-Engineering and Exercise Science and Sport of Arizona State University, the Harrington Arthritis Research Center, and the Department of Mechanical Engineering at the University of Vermont and the Vermont Space Grant Consortium in conjunction with the National Aeronautics and Space Administration.[35]

The company has made repeated efforts to ensure accessibility to practitioners of the knowledge base relevant to the Activator Method.[21,39,40] This literature garnered a "promising to established" rating for this form of instrument adjusting during the 1992 Mercy Center clinical guidelines consensus conference[56] and a similar rating from a consensus panel commissioned by the Canadian Chiropractic Association.[57]

Technique research in chiropractic is still very much "in its infancy."[58] The company has repeatedly acknowledged that, similar to most forms of manual healing, the Activator Method requires a greater number of well-controlled outcome studies.[40] That said, the Activator Method is one of the better studied methods of chiropractic care.[58] Nonetheless, controversy over instrument adjusting has persisted within the profession. In Saskatchewan, mechanical adjusting devices were banned by the licensing authority for a time, prompting a critical review of the evidence, which was conducted by a committee appointed by the provincial society.[59,60] The majority opinion was that mechanical adjusting procedures, in particular, the Activator, "were as effective as manual (HVLA [high-velocity, low amplitude]) procedures in producing clinical benefit and biological change."[59] However, a minority report reasserted that "there was not enough evidence to support or refute the efficacy" of instrument adjusting. And although most committee members argued that the AAI has "no more relative risk" than manual adjusting, a minority of the group believed that the evidence was too thin to justify a conclusion.[60] Because of this debate documented in the literature and its favorable outcome, Activator is approved for use in Saskatchewan today.

CONCLUSION

The Activator Method is part of the tradition of instrument adjusting in chiropractic dating to the first decade of the profession, and even farther back into antiquity. Credit for the origin of the AAI rests with two rural Minnesota practitioners; Activator Method assessment procedures have multiple conceptual roots, all of which are anchored in various subluxation theories. The growth of the Activator Method has been based primarily on patient and clinician satisfaction, but the Activator company has sought to hold its methods up to the critical scrutiny of scientific inquiry. Bioengineering research has suggested a number of mechanical improvements in the AAI over the years, and this work continues. A still meager clinical outcomes evidence base combined with clinician judgment has prompted generally favorable reviews of the Activator Method. This form of instrument adjusting has become usual and customary within the profession and is widely taught in chiropractic colleges and in postgraduate relicensure seminars. Much work remains to be done.

REFERENCES

1. Hinojosa SZ. The hands, the sacred, and the context of change in Maya bonesetting. In: Oths KS, Hinojosa SZ, editors. Healing by hand: manual medicine and bonesetting in global perspective. Walnut Creek (CA): AltaMira Press; 2004.
2. Dorn WH. Indian lore: crude use of chiropractic fundamentals centuries ago. Chiropr J (NCA). 1935;4(3):17-8.
3. Smith BA. Thomas Henry Storey, DO, DC, 1943 to 1923. Chiropr Hist. 1999;19(2):63-84.
4. Zarbuck MV, Hayes MB. Following D.D. Palmer to the west coast: the Pasadena connection, 1902. Chiropr Hist. 1990;10(2):17-22.
5. Palmer DD. A spine set personified. Chiropractor. 1905;1(11):30.
6. Palmer DD. The chiropractor's adjustor: the science, art and philosophy of chiropractic. Portland (OR): Portland Printing House; 1910. p. 20, 478.
7. Smallie P. Introduction to Ratledge files and Ratledge manuscript. Stockton (CA): World-Wide Books; 1990.
8. Keating JC, Phillips RB, editors. A history of Los Angeles College of Chiropractic. Whittier (CA): Southern California University of Health Sciences; 2001.
9. Dr. Linnie Cale honored. J Calif Chiropr Assoc. 1959;15(7):32.
10. Advertisement for Alva Gregory's Three Stroke Vibrator. American Drugless Healer. 1913;3(4):66.
11. Wardwell RB, Walter I. Chiropractic: history and evolution of a new profession. St. Louis: Mosby; 1992. p. 122-4.
12. Alloway WJ, Ronkin ME. The social anthropology of chiropractic in Washington, DC: project DC/DC. Chiropr Hist. 1982;2:6-11.
13. Ratledge TF. Letter to R.E. Mathis, DC, 14 September 1915. Ratledge papers, Cleveland Chiropractic College of Kansas City.
14. Palmer BJ. A bad penny always returns. Fountain Head News. 1918[A.C. 24](Oct 26); 8(7):5-6.
15. Abrams A. Spondylotherapy: spinal concussion and the application of other methods to the spine in the treatment of disease. San Francisco: Philopolis Press; 1910.
16. Abrams A. Spondylotherapy: physio- and pharmaco-therapy and diagnostic methods based on a study of clinical physiology. 5th ed. San Francisco: Philopolis Press; 1914.
17. Advertisement: Spring tonics for your practice. J Int Chiropr Congr. 1932;1(5):23.
18. Advertisement: Vita Motor. Chiropr J (NCA). 1935;4(3):39.
19. Advertisement for Benko Hand Concussion Sets. Naturopath. 1924;October:970.
20. Medical profession develops mechanical chiropractic adjusting machine. Sci Chiropractor. 1936;1(7):9.
21. Osterbauer PJ, Fuhr AW, Hildebrandt RW. Mechanical force, manually assisted short lever chiropractic adjustment. J Manipulative Physiol Ther. 1992;15(5):309-17.
22. Fuhr AW, Fuhr D. History. In: Fuhr AW, Colloca CJ, Green JR, Keller TS, editors. Activator methods chiropractic technique. St. Louis: Mosby; 1997.
23. Grostic JD. The adjusting instrument as a research tool. Chiropr Res J. 1989;1(2):47-55.
24. Healy J. Personal communication (E-mail to J.C. Keating). May 25, 2004.
25. Hinz D. Diversified chiropractic: Northwestern College and John B. Wolfe, 1941-1984. Chiropr Hist. 1987;7(1):34-41.
26. Regular meeting of the Board of Trustees of Logan Basic College of Chiropractic. January 2, 1941. Logan Archives.
27. Keating JC. Several pathways in the evolution of chiropractic manipulation. J Manipulative Physiol Ther. 2003;26(5):300-21.
28. Montgomery DP, Nelson JM. Evolution of chiropractic theories of practice and spinal adjustment. Chiropr Hist. 1985;5:70-6.
29. Truscott LL. Truscott compatibility tests. San Jose (CA): Self-published; 1956.
30. Richards DR. The activator story: development of a new concept in chiropractic. Chiropr J Aust. 1994;24(1):28-32.

31. Keller T, Nathan M, Kaigle A. Measurement and analysis of interspinous kinematics. Proceedings of the International Conference on Spinal Manipulation, Foundation for Chiropractic Education and Research; April 30–May 1, 1993; Montreal, Canada. p. 51-5.

32. Keller TS, Lehneman JB. Dependence of the delivered force on the force setting on the activator adjusting instrument: technical report. Phoenix (AZ): Activator Methods, Inc.; 1994.

33. Nathan M, Keller TS. Measurement and analysis of the in vivo posteroanterior impulse response of the human thoracolumbar spine: a feasibility study. J Manipulative Physiol Ther. 1994;17(7): 431-44.

34. Nathan M, Lehneman JB, Keller TS. The dynamic response of the human spine to low amplitude, high velocity posteroanterior thrusts. Proceedings of the International Conference on Spinal Manipulation; June 10-11, 1994; Palm Springs, CA. p. 87.

35. Osterbauer P, Fuhr AW, Keller TS. Description and analysis of Activator Methods chiropractic technique. In: Lawrence DJ, Cassidy JD, McGregor M, Meeker WC, Vernon HT, editors. Advances in chiropractic. Vol. 2. St. Louis: Mosby; 1995. p. 471-511.

36. Coyle BA, Tolar RL. Chiropractic education: fearless youth, yet new horizons and distant scenes. Top Clin Chiropr. 1995;2(2):31-40.

37. Donahue J. Reply to Dr. Bryner. J Can Chiropr Assoc. 1991;35(2):98-100.

38. Fuhr AW. Activator Update. 1985;12(4):13.

39. Fuhr AW, Colloca CJ, Green JR, Keller TS. Activator Methods chiropractic technique. St. Louis: Mosby; 1997.

40. Fuhr AW, Menke JM. Status of Activator Methods chiropractic technique, theory and practice. J Manipulative Physiol Ther. 2005;28(2):135.

41. Pedersen P. A survey of chiropractic practice in Europe. Eur J Chiropr. 1994;42(1):3-28.

42. Christensen MG, Morgan DR, Sieve YD, Townsend PD. Job analysis of chiropractic in Canada. Greeley (CO): National Board of Chiropractic Examiners; 1993. p. 84.

43. Christensen MG, Kerkhoff D, Kollasch MW, Cohn L. Job analysis of chiropractic. Greeley (CO): National Board of Chiropractic Examiners; 2000. p. 129.

44. Coyer AB, Curwin IHM. Low back pain treated by manipulation: a controlled series. Br Med J. 1955;1:705-7.

45. Fisk JW. A controlled trial of manipulation in a selected group of patients with low back pain favoring one side. N Z Med J. 1979;90:288-91.

46. Glover JR, Morris JG, Khosla T. Back pain: a randomized clinical trial of rotation manipulation of the trunk. Br J Industr Med. 1974;31:59-64.

47. Maitland GD. Low back pain and allied symptoms and treatment results. Med J Aust. 1957;2(24):851-4.

48. Parker B, Tupling H, Pryor D. A controlled trial of manipulation for migraine. Aust N Z J Med. 1978;8:589-93.

49. Rasmussen GG. Manipulation in treatment of low back pain (a randomized clinical trial). Manuelle Medizin. 1979;1:8-10.

50. Sims-Williams H, Jayson MI, Young SM, Baddeley H, Collins E. Controlled trial of mobilization and manipulation for patients with low back pain in general practice. Br Med J. 1978;2:1338-40.

51. Sims-Williams H, Jayson MI, Young SM, Baddeley H, Collins E. Controlled trial of mobilization and manipulation for low back pain: hospital patients. Br Med J. 1979;24:1318-20.

52. Waagen GN, Haldeman S, Cook G, Lopez D, DeBoer KF. Short-term trial of chiropractic adjustments for the relief of chronic low back pain. Manual Med. 1986;2(3):63-7.

53. Yates RG, Lamping NL, Abram NL, Wright C. Effects of chiropractic treatment on blood pressure and anxiety: a randomized, controlled trial. J Manipulative Physiol Ther. 1988;11(6): 484-8.

54. Fuhr AW, Smith DB. Accuracy of piezoelectric accelerometers measuring displacement of a spinal adjusting instrument. J Manipulative Physiol Ther. 1986;9:15-21.

55. Smith DB, Fuhr AW, Davis BP. Skin accelerometer displacement and relative bone movement of adjacent vertebrae in response to chiropractic percussion thrusts. J Manipulative Physiol Ther. 1989;12(1):26-37.

56. Haldeman S, Chapman-Smith D, Petersen DM, editors. Guidelines for chiropractic quality assurance and practice parameters. Proceedings of the Mercy Center Consensus Conference; Gaithersburg, MD. Aspen; p. 108-109.

57. Henderson D, Chapman-Smith D, Mior S, Vernon H, editors. Clinical practice guidelines for chiropractic practice in Canada Proceedings of a consensus conference commissioned by the Canadian Chiropractic Association; April 3-7, 1993; Glenerin Inn, Mississauga, Ontario, Canada; Toronto: Canadian Chiropractic Association; 1994. p. 110.

58. Gleberzon BJ. Chiropractic "name techniques": a review of the literature. J Can Chiropr Assoc. 2001;45(2):86-99.

59. Taylor SH, Arnold ND, Biggs L, Colloca CJ, Mierau DR, Symons BP et al. A review of the literature pertaining to the efficacy, safety, educational requirements, uses and usage of mechanical adjusting devices: Part 1 of 2. J Can Chiropr Assoc. 2004;48(1):74-88.

60. Taylor SH, Arnold ND, Biggs L, Colloca CJ, Mierau DR, Symons BP et al. A review of the literature pertaining to the efficacy, safety, educational requirements, uses and usage of mechanical adjusting devices: part 2 of 2. J Can Chiropr Assoc. 2004;48(2):152-79.

2 CHIROPRACTIC SCIENCE: TOWARD UNDERSTANDING SPINAL MANIPULATION

Joel G. Pickar

This chapter discusses the development of chiropractic science. It begins by posing a question. Indeed, the impulse for the scientific process is the desire to know; thus the question posed in the next sentence bears the effort of evoking and focusing a framework for understanding the mechanisms underlying the effects of chiropractic care. "How could a mechanical intervention, applied to the spine and which typically lasts but a fraction of a second (chiropractic spinal manipulation or adjustment), produce long-lasting clinical effects?" With this question as the backdrop for developing testable research hypotheses, our experimental work can bring us closer to an evidence-based, biological understanding of spinal manipulation. This is not knowledge for knowledge's sake but knowledge for the long-term goal of learning how best to apply our skills to improve the health of the public. This chapter addresses three areas of chiropractic research that may contribute data that will help us to answer this question.

As chiropractic science seeks to answer this fundamental question, we should be mindful that spinal manipulation is always delivered within the wider context of the patient's clinical encounter with his/her doctor. It is not yet clear whether or how these interactions and the physical procedures preparatory to chiropractic adjustment contribute to the effectiveness of the mechanical intervention itself. As research findings from both clinical and basic science laboratories are integrated into our understanding, we must remember that these laboratory-based mechanisms are layered onto potential effects that may stem from subjective and nonverbal communications involved in the clinical encounter itself.

PRINCIPLES

Painted upon a hallway wall that I often pass on my way to meetings, an epigram attributed to Dr. Clarence S. Gonstead reads, "Remember that chiropractic always works. When it does not seem to, examine your application but do not question the principle." Upon first reading this epigram, I shook my head with concern and discomfort. Its conclusion that chiropractic "always" works smacked of thinking that was both dogmatic and self-serving. It seemed rather nonspecific. In chiropractic, did Dr. Gonstead include adjustments provided to the spine and to the extremities, or did Dr. Gonstead refer to an application that included more than adjustments? By principle, was he referring to a metaphysical construct like the presence of an Innate Intelligence, or to a more biological construct that states that nerve interference has the capacity to affect homeostatic mechanisms? When I considered members of the profession, including doctors of chiropractic, teaching faculty, and chiropractic students, having fully internalized this idea, I envisioned its potential to curtail dialogue, discourage critical and analytical thinking, and sustain clinical decisions that might not reflect the patient's best interest. And yet, because of the epigram's location on the wall of the institution and the professional stature of its author, I felt compelled to consider how wisdom might be contained in the words. Did my original concern about the quote miss something important?

I undertook a thought experiment by asking myself at what conclusion I might have arrived had I read a similar epigram displayed on the walls of a Medical College: "Remember that medicine always works. When it does not seem to, examine your application but do not question the principle." Similar to my previous issue, this statement would raise the question of what is meant by "medicine"? Would this term refer to the use of drugs, the use of surgery, an allopathic philosophy, or something else? So, I began by equating medicine with the use of pharmaceuticals because this constitutes a substantial proportion of medical interventions. Thus the question then became, "Upon what principle is the use of drugs based?" The obvious answer was, "a chemical or biochemical principle." The use of drugs (or any chemical substances, for that matter, even botanicals) is predicated upon their ability to affect living systems through direct interaction with chemical processes and biochemical pathways.[1]

It would likely come as no surprise to you, the reader familiar with biology, that biochemistry constitutes one dimension of animate existence, and that the controlled and integrated activity of biochemical interactions underlies many aspects of physiological function. We know this because it has been demonstrated and confirmed time and time again through scientific investigation. As examples, catabolic pathways break down large organic molecules comprising food into smaller molecules, some of which are used to provide energy for physical activity such as muscle contraction. Anabolic pathways use the smaller molecules for building processes to achieve growth and repair. DNA is translated and transcribed into proteins through biochemical machinery that retrieves and bonds together amino acids. Endocrine and paracrine signaling molecules bind with cell-surface or intracellular receptors and change the activity of their target cells within an organ. Neurotransmitter molecules released from presynaptic neurons cross the synaptic cleft and bind to postsynaptic receptors, thus altering the neuronal activity of postsynaptic neurons.

Drugs affect physiological processes at the biochemical level. These are compounds whose shape and constituent molecules interact with biomolecules. They often bind to regulatory molecules, consequently activating or inhibiting normal body processes. For example, nonsteroidal antiinflammatory drugs such as aspirin, ibuprofen, and naproxen block the action of the enzyme cyclooxygenase. This enzyme catalyzes the conversion of arachidonic acid (a fatty acid cleaved from phospholipids of the cell membrane through the action of phospholipase A_2) into the paracrine signaling molecules prostaglandin and thromboxane A_2. These eicosanoids bind to cell-surface receptors whose activation contributes to hemostasis, the elaboration of pain, fever, and inflammation achieved through cell signaling pathways.[2] Should a drug not seem to work, the "biochemical principle" underlying its use would likely not be called into question. Consideration for its lack of effectiveness would be ascribed to alternate possibilities such as use of the wrong drug, use of the wrong dosage, the presence of competing biochemical interactions that negated the drug's influence, lack of specificity for the target ligand, the presence of a non–biochemically based problem (e.g., a broken bone), or the conclusion that we do not know enough about physiology to know which drug or drug combination to use.

Thus my thought experiment led to a fresh perspective on the petition to "remember that chiropractic always works. When it does not seem to, examine your application, but do not question the principle." The epigram was not necessarily a call for stagnation. It no doubt was based on experience that suggests that chiropractic care has contributed to the quality of people's lives. It was a statement that there is a principle upon which it must be based. It represented a challenge to us to fully explore, discover, and understand how it works. I then found it amusing that around the corner, in the same hallway that depicted the Gonstead epigram, an epigram from B.J. Palmer read, "When facts are known, knowledge exists. When we possess knowledge, a reliance on faith and beliefs can disappear, for one (facts) is the skeletal frame for the substance of the other (knowledge)." [Parentheses inserted by this chapter's author.] Together, these epigrams place value on the pursuit of knowledge, and this from individuals and an institution that historically laid great emphasis on the philosophy of chiropractic. Through scientific inquiry, we can identify the actual biological principle(s) that underlie the clinical successes of chiropractic, thereby improving its delivery in the service of public health. It is to this biological perspective that the remainder of this chapter now turns. We discuss here three principles that might contribute answers to the question, "How can a mechanical intervention applied to the spine that typically lasts but a fraction of a second (chiropractic spinal manipulation or adjustment) produce long-lasting clinical effects?"

Neuromechanical Principle

To the extent that the effects of chiropractic are based on a neuromechanical principle, the mechanical stimulus inherent to spinal manipulation would directly affect the nervous system in ways that mechanical inputs with slower time courses do not. Mechanical input would first affect the discharge of primary afferent neurons; this, in turn, would affect the discharge properties of second and higher order neurons of the central nervous system.[3-5] Because chiropractic spinal manipulation is inherently a mechanical intervention, the primary afferents most likely to respond are those neurons that are inherently sensitive to mechanical stimuli. This would include all group I (Aα) and II (Aβ) afferent fibers, as well as subpopulations from group III (Aδ) and IV (C) fibers.[6] In addition, subpopulations of group III and IV afferents not inherently sensitive to mechanical stimuli may become sensitized as the result of chemical changes in their local environment.[7]

Spinal manipulation may alter the discharge of all or some of these neuronal groups. However, our knowledge is sufficiently lacking in this area that we do not know whether spinal manipulation actually removes a source of mechanosensory input, such as a noxious, painful input, or adds a novel source of mechanosensory input.[8-10] From a research perspective, establishing this mechanism as contributing to a neuromechanical principle for chiropractic would involve determining how spinal manipulation directly affects the discharge of sensory nerves and central neurons.

If the therapeutic effects of spinal manipulation are mediated, even in part, by a neuromechanical principle, it seems reasonable to expect that primary afferent neurons that are stimulated by manipulation and sending of sensory information from paraspinal tissues would respond in some unique fashion to the time course of spinal manipulation. This consideration led to a series of experiments that examined the neural activity of a group of proprioceptors that innervate the paraspinal muscles, namely, muscle spindles and Golgi tendon organs. Both are activated by spinal manipulation.[11] Muscle spindles in lumbar paraspinal muscles respond in a nonlinear fashion, producing a high-frequency discharge when the speed of the manipulation approaches that provided clinically.[12,13] At comparable velocities, muscle spindles were more sensitive to lower amplitude spinal manipulations.[13] It was suggested that spinal manipulation may take advantage of an inherent property of muscle spindles wherein they exhibit nonlinear properties and show greater sensitivity to length changes that are small in magnitude and of increasing velocity.[13,14] Spinal manipulation may provide a unique neuromechanical signal in that it loads spinal segments at a critical velocity and with displacements that are small in amplitude, with which they do not get loaded through activities experienced with daily living. Despite these provocative findings and interpretations, it should be recognized that at this point in our knowledge, we do not know whether the discharge of muscle spindles is necessary or sufficient to elicit the beneficial effects of spinal manipulation.

If a neuromechanical principle is involved in the effects of chiropractic adjustment, then how can a brief, high-frequency neural discharge in primary afferent neurons have long-lasting effects on the nervous system? The answer may lie in the fact that synaptic function can be both use dependent and frequency dependent. Nearly two decades ago, several laboratories[15-17] showed that synaptic efficacy (the probability that a neuron will fire in response to a previous input) is affected by the history of high-frequency bursting from group Ia and group II muscle afferents whose effect lasts beyond the duration of the burst itself. For example, α-motoneurons that receive bursts of action potentials with short interspike intervals affect the magnitude of their postsynaptic potentials differently from bursts with longer interspike intervals. α-Motoneurons are bistable and can sustain plateau potentials, that is, they have depolarized membrane potentials above threshold. Brief periods of stimulation depolarize them to below threshold and switch them into a period of self-sustained firing.[18] Experiments in human muscle suggest that this phenomenon can have consequences for the normal production of muscle force.[19] Similarly, high-frequency stimulation of smaller diameter Aδ and C fibers also affects spinal synaptic transmission. Both long-term potentiation and depression may be produced.[20] (See Boal and Gillette[21] for an excellent review.) Effects can last up to 1 hour after the initial sensory barrage.[20,22] Although nothing is known about the discharge characteristics of Aδ and C fibers during impulse loading such as spinal manipulation, Aδ and C fibers are known to be responsive to slow, passive mechanical loads in the physiological range.[23,24]

In the central nervous system, Gillette et al.[25] demonstrated that non-noxious mechanical inputs to paraspinal tissues can turn off wide dynamic range and nociceptive-specific dorsal horn neurons that receive widely convergent input. This inhibition lasted only as long as neural input lasted, although it lasted longer in response to noxious mechanical input. In general, noxious mechanical input may turn off for longer periods of time dorsal horn neurons that are receiving sensory complex receptive fields.[26] Spinal manipulation has been shown to increase pain tolerance and pain threshold in humans and animals,[27-29] and the recent finding that monoamine receptors of neurons in the spinal cord contribute to the antihyperalgestic effects of joint mobilization in inflamed joints may be important in this regard.[30] In the human cortex, spinal manipulation of dysfunctional cervical joints produced changes in cortical responsiveness that outlasted the manipulation (by up to 20 minutes).[31] The attenuation of cortical somatosensory–evoked potentials may represent a sustained alteration in cortical somatosensory processing and sensorimotor integration. These considerations highlight the need for further investigation to explore the discharge characteristics of primary sensory afferents and the time course of responses from central neurons and circuits in response to high-velocity, low-amplitude spinal loading.

Biomechanical Principle

If a biomechanical principle contributes to the relationship between the short-lasting time course of a chiropractic spinal manipulation and its long-lasting clinical effects, then research efforts should seek to provide evidence that manipulation produces sustained biomechanical alterations in paraspinal tissues. It would seem reasonable to anticipate that biomechanical changes would be those expected from the high-velocity loading characteristic of the manipulation. Such primary, sustained biomechanical changes would likely have secondary and important effects on other systems as well, such as the nervous, circulatory, and immune systems.

Structural features of the spinal column are consistent with this principle and have led to several mechanistic theories.[32-37] Mechanical release of trapped meniscoids, discal material, or segmental adhesions from a rapidly applied load could evoke long-lasting changes in the distribution of stress and strain in paraspinal tissues, thereby altering segmental or regional spinal movement. This redistribution and altered movement could secondarily alter mechanosensory input from paraspinal tissues. Meniscoids do indeed exist within the lateral recesses of the facet joint. In addition, adhesions occur with both immobilization and inflammation.[38,39] Adhesions, fixations, or discal herniation may produce ectopic sources of neural activity. For example, dorsal roots and dorsal root ganglia (DRG) are more susceptible to the effects of mechanical compression than are axons of peripheral nerves because their function is impaired or altered at substantially lower pressures compared with peripheral nerves.[40,41] Applying as little as 10 mm Hg of pressure to the dorsal root reduces by 20% to 30% nutritional transport to peripheral axons.[42] Bove et al.[43] inflamed peripheral axons, which increased the spontaneous activity of group III and IV axons innervating deeper structures. Adhesions that form with inflammation could be a mechanical source of irritation. High-velocity spinal manipulation may release some mechanical connections. It has yet to be directly shown that a high-velocity manipulation changes any of these biomechanical-neural relationships.

Tissues are often characterized by their viscoelastic properties. In particular, viscoelastic stiffness is characterized by the relationship between load and displacement, and the effects of time on this relationship. As tissue becomes stiffer, the load developed for a small displacement becomes greater. When a viscoelastic tissue is displaced more quickly, the load developed is greater and the tissue becomes even stiffer. Structural features at both macroscopic and microscopic levels contribute to tissue stiffness, and several biomechanical tools have been used to measure the stiffness of spinal tissue.[44-48] Changes in spinal stiffness may be useful for diagnosing degenerative disc disease.[49] The reliability and sensitivity of these tools in assessing changes in stiffness subsequent to spinal manipulation are not yet clear.[50] If sustained changes in stiffness could be measured, this would provide direct support for a biomechanical principle. Demonstrating physiological responses to this biomechanical change would be an important next step.

Despite the short duration of a spinal manipulation, evidence suggests that mechanical changes in the facet joint capsule may outlast the duration of the manipulation. Using magnetic resonance imaging (MRI) scans in human subjects, Cramer et al.[51,52] showed that side-posture spinal manipulation accompanied by cavitation gaps in the facet joints increases the joint space to a greater extent than does side-posture positioning alone. Although the length of time between manipulation and the MRI scan was not reported, MRI scans were performed within 20 minutes after the manipulation was performed (personal communication). The synovial space of the lumbar facet joints increased in width by an average of 2.2 mm in subjects who were positioned in side posture and had received a side-posture spinal adjustment. By comparison, the joint space widened by only 1.5 mm (i.e., 0.7 mm less) in subjects who were positioned in side posture but did not receive a manipulation. This raises the possibility that muscles and connective tissues attached to the vertebra could be stretched for periods longer than the duration of the manipulation itself. Although not studied directly, according to biomechanical strain data from Khalsa's laboratory,[53] joint separations of these magnitudes appear sufficient to at least load facet joint tissues. The increased joint space would strain the facet capsule, inducing a biomechanical change that would outlast the manipulation itself. This mechanical change, in turn, could stimulate mechanically sensitive primary afferents with receptive endings in the facet capsule. It is interesting to note that distraction of the facet joint produced by intracapsular injection of a large volume of saline reduced reflex paraspinal muscle responses that accompanied stimulation of the intervertebral disc.[54]

Mechanochemical Principle

Over the past 20 years, interest in mechanochemistry has been growing. This field may offer some understanding of whether the short duration of a spinal manipulation could evoke long-lasting physiological changes. Mechanochemistry is the study of the effect that mechanical forces have on those biochemical processes that are not directly responsible for the regenerative signaling of the nervous system.[55] It involves the balance of tensile loading between outwardly directed forces from extracellular connections and intracellular osmotic pressure and inwardly directed forces from a cell's cytoskeleton, and the ability of these mechanical changes to directly activate biochemical processes. The neuromechanical principle discussed here states that many receptive endings of primary afferent neuronal cells are specialized to respond to mechanical changes in their environment. Such mechanical changes are transduced into action potentials. Frequency coding of these action potentials contains the information necessary to communicate those changes to the central nervous system. The behavior of many cells without these specializations can also be modified in response to mechanical stimuli. This mechanical change is transduced into biochemical activity. Some cellular activities reportedly affected by mechanical changes at the cell membrane include growth, differentiation, apoptosis, motility, transmembrane transport, signal transduction pathways, and nuclear activity, including gene expression.[56] Moreover, the extracellular matrix within which cells are embedded may contain binding sites and may act as a storage depot for immunomodulatory signaling molecules. Conformational changes in this matrix may lead to release of its stores or further access to binding sites.[57] Although a mechanochemical principle is ultimately expressed through biochemical processes, the mechanical change is the proximate cause for changes in cell activity.

If some effects of spinal manipulation are based on a mechanochemical principle, how does such a macroscopic event at the whole body level ultimately influence the microscopic level? Cells, tissues, and, ultimately, organs are constructed as structural hierarchies that are linked through connective tissue networks. Fascia is continuous throughout the organism, becoming confluent with the extracellular matrix at the cellular level and providing a structural framework. Adhesion molecules, in particular those from the integrin family, form an important mechanical link at the cell membrane between the extracellular matrix and intracellular structural elements, as well as between neighboring cells.[56] Some of these connections may provide specific pathways by which extracellular

mechanical loads are transferred to and influence intracellular structures. Thus macroscale loads likely influence the extracellular matrix through which the mechanical load may be transferred to and may influence cellular activity. Because tissues are viscoelastic, they become stiffer in response to a high-velocity load. Even relatively small macroscopic displacements could produce large mechanical loads at the cell membrane.

It has recently been suggested that a variety of body-based therapies may "work" via a mechanochemical principle.[55] Recent histological studies of acupuncture, which is not classically considered a body-based therapy, suggest that it could also have a mechanical component.[58] The sensation of *de Qi* by an individual who is receiving needle acupuncture is thought to indicate the success of the needle's application. On the part of the acupuncturist, this sensation is experienced as an increase in resistance as the clinician twists the needle. Twisting acupuncture needles appears to successively wind connective tissue in whirls, increasing the force necessary to remove the needles.[59,60] This mechanical phenomenon may underlie the sensation of *de Qi*. As needles penetrate the dermis, the windings of subdermal collagen may transmit a mechanical signal through deformation of the extracellular matrix. At present, this mechanism remains speculative. It is also worth considering that mechanically induced changes in the distribution of charged moieties of the extracellular matrix, such as the heparin sulfates, may affect cell behavior via conformational changes in voltage-sensitive proteins of the cell membrane.

CONCLUSION

The signature intervention offered with chiropractic care is spinal adjustment or manipulation. Most technique systems share this mechanical denominator, whereby loads are rapidly applied to paraspinal and spinal tissues. With nearly 100 technique systems in chiropractic recently identified,[61] is it reasonable to think that a common biological principle underlies their effectiveness? More than 90% of chiropractic patients receive a short-lever, high-velocity, low-amplitude thrust as part of their care.[62] Maneuvers of this sort may share common biological principles. This chapter discusses three biological principles that represent likely areas of exploration toward understanding how the mechanical characteristics of chiropractic spinal manipulation could produce longer lasting effects on physiological systems.

REFERENCES

1. Katzung BG. Basic principles: introduction. In: Katzung BG, editor. Basic and clinical pharmacology. Stamford (CT): Appleton & Lange; 1998. p. 1-8.

2. Foegh ML, Hecker M, Ramwell PW. The eicosanoids: prostaglandins, thromboxanes, leukotrienes, and related compounds. In: Katzung BG, editor. Basic and clinical pharmacology. Stamford (CT): Appleton & Lange; 1998. p. 304-18.

3. Korr IM. Proprioceptors and somatic dysfunction. J Am Osteopath Assoc. 1975;74(7):638-50.

4. Leach RA. The chiropractic theories. 4th ed. Philadelphia: Lippincott Williams & Wilkins; 2004.

5. Pickar JG. Neurophysiological effects of spinal manipulation. Spine J. 2002;2(5):357-71.

6. Lewin GR, Moshourab R. Mechanosensation and pain. J Neurobiol. 2004;61(1):30-44.

7. Kaufman MP, Rybicki KJ, Waldrop TG, Ordway GA. Effect of ischemia on responses of group III and IV afferents to contraction. J Appl Physiol. 1984;57(3):644-50.

8. Eldred E, Hutton RS, Smith JL. Nature of the persisting changes in afferent discharge from muscle following its contraction. In: Homma S, editor. Understanding the stretch reflex. New York: Elsevier; 1976. p. 157-83.

9. Buerger AA. Experimental neuromuscular models of spinal manual techniques. Manual Med. 1983;1:10-7.

10. Gillette RG. A speculative argument for the coactivation of diverse somatic receptor populations by forceful chiropractic adjustments. Manual Med. 1987;3:1-14.

11. Pickar JG, Wheeler JD. Response of muscle proprioceptors to spinal manipulative-like loads in the anesthetized cat. J Manipulative Physiol Ther. 2001;24(1):2-11.

12. Pickar JG, Kang YM. Paraspinal muscle spindle responses to the duration of a spinal manipulation under force control. J Manipulative Physiol Ther. 2006;29(1):22-31.

13. Pickar JG, Sung PS, Kang YM, Ge W. Thrust duration and amplitude affect the response of lumbar paraspinal muscle spindles to spinal manipulation under displacement control. Spine J. In press 2007.

14. Matthews PBC. Mammalian muscle receptors and their central actions. Baltimore: Williams & Wilkins; 1972.

15. Davis BM, Collins WF, Mendell LM. Potentiation of transmission at Ia-motoneuron connections induced by repeated short bursts of afferent activity. J Neurophysiol. 1985;54(6):1541-52.

16. Luscher HR, Ruenzel PW, Henneman E. Effects of impulse frequency, PTP, and temperature on responses elicited in large populations of motoneurons by impulses in single Ia-fibers. J Neurophysiol. 1983;50(5):1045-58.

17. Collins WF III, Honig MG, Mendell LM. Heterogeneity of group Ia synapses on homonymous alpha-motoneurons as revealed by high-frequency stimulation of Ia afferent fibers. J Neurophysiol. 1984;52(5):980-93.

18. Hounsgaard J, Hultborn H, Kiehn O. Transmitter-controlled properties of alpha-motoneurones causing long-lasting motor discharge to brief excitatory inputs. Prog Brain Res. 1986;64:39-49.

19. Collins DF, Burke D, Gandevia SC. Sustained contractions produced by plateau-like behaviour in human motoneurones. J Physiol. 2002;538 (Pt 1):289-301.

20. Randic M, Jiang MC, Cerne R. Long-term potentiation and long-term depression of primary afferent neurotransmission in the rat spinal cord. J Neurosci. 1993;13(12):5228-41.

21. Boal RW, Gillette RG. Central neuronal plasticity, low back pain and spinal manipulative therapy. J Manipulative Physiol Ther. 2004; 27(5):314-26.

22. Ikeda H, Asai T, Murase K. Robust changes of afferent-induced excitation in the rat spinal dorsal horn after conditioning high-frequency stimulation. J Neurophysiol. 2000;83:2412-20.

23. Wilson LB, Wall PT, Pawelczyk JA, Matsukawa K. Cardiorespiratory and phrenic nerve responses to graded muscle stretch in anesthetized cats. Respir Physiol. 1994;98(3):251-66.

24. Leshnower BG, Potts JT, Garry MG, Mitchell JH. Reflex cardiovascular responses evoked by selective activation of skeletal muscle ergoreceptors. J Appl Physiol. 2001;90(1):308-16.

25. Gillette RG, Kramis RC, Roberts WJ. Suppression of activity in spinal nocireceptive "low back" neurons by paravertebral somatic stimuli in the cat. Neurosci Lett. 1998;241(1):45-8.

26. Cadden SW. The ability of inhibitory controls to "switch-off" activity in dorsal horn convergent neurones in the rat. Brain Res. 1993;628 (1-2):65-71.

27. Terrett ACJ, Vernon HT. Manipulation and pain tolerance: a controlled study of the effect of spinal manipulation on paraspinal cutaneous pain tolerance levels. Am J Phys Med. 1984;63 (5):217-25.

28. Vernon HT. Pressure pain threshold evaluation of the effect of spinal manipulation on chronic neck pain: a single case study. J Can Chiro Assoc. 1988;32(4):191-4.

29. Song XJ, Gan Q, Cao JL, Wang ZB, Rupert RL. Spinal manipulation reduces pain and hyperalgesia after lumbar intervertebral foramen inflammation in the rat. J Manipulative Physiol Ther. 2006;29(1):5-13.

30. Skyba DA, Radhakrishnan R, Rohlwing JJ, Wright A, Sluka KA. Joint manipulation reduces hyperalgesia by activation of monoamine receptors but not opioid or GABA receptors in the spinal cord. Pain. 2003;106(1-2):159-68.

31. Haavik-Taylor H, Murphy B. Cervical spine manipulation alters sensorimotor integration: a somatosensory evoked potential study. Clin Neurophysiol. 2007;118(2):391-402.

32. Farfan HF. The scientific basis of manipulation procedures. In: Buchanan WW, Kahn MF, Laine V, Rodnan GP, Scott JT, Zvaifler NJ et al, editors. Clinics in rheumatic diseases. London: Saunders; 1980. p. 159-77.

33. Giles LGF. Anatomical basis of low back pain. Baltimore: Williams & Wilkins; 1989.

34. Lewit K. Manipulative therapy in rehabilitation of the locomotor system. Oxford: Butterworth-Heinemann; 1991.

35. Haldeman S. The clinical basis for discussion of mechanisms of manipulative therapy. In: Korr IM, editor. The neurobiologic mechanisms in manipulative therapy. New York: Plenum; 1978. p. 53-75.

36. Vernon H. Biological rationale for possible benefits of spinal manipulation. Rockville (MD): Agency for Health Care Policy and Research; 1997. Publication No. 98-N002105-115.

37. Rahlmann JF. Mechanisms of intervertebral joint fixation: a literature review. J Manipulative Physiol Ther. 1987;10(4):177-87.

38. Woo SL-Y, Matthews JV, Akeson WH, Amiel D, Covery FR. Connective tissue response to immobility: correlative study of biomechanical and biochemical measurements of normal and immobilized rabbit knees. Arthritis Rheum. 1975;18(3):257-64.

39. Videman T. Connective tissue and immobilization: key factors in musculoskeletal degeneration? Clin Orthop. 1987(221):26-32.

40. Rydevik BL. The effects of compression on the physiology of nerve roots. J Manipulative Physiol Ther. 1992;15(1):62-6.

41. Howe JF, Loeser JD, Calvin WH. Mechanosensitivity of dorsal root ganglia and chronically injured axons: a physiological basis for the radicular pain of nerve root compression. Pain. 1977;3(1):27-41.

42. Olmarker K, Rydevik B, Hansson T, Holm S. Compression-induced changes of the nutritional supply to the porcine cauda equina. J Spinal Disord. 1990;3(1):25-9.

43. Bove GM, Ransil BJ, Lin H-C, Leem J-G. Inflammation induces ectopic mechanical sensitivity in axons of nociceptors innervating deep tissues. J Neurophysiol. 2003;90(3):1949-55.

44. Owens EF, Jr, DeVocht JW, Wilder DG, Gudavalli MR, Meeker WC. The reliability of posterior-to-anterior stiffness measures in a population of patients with low back pain. J Manipulative Physiol Ther. 2007;30(2):116-23.

45. Kawchuk GN, Fauvel OR. Sources of variation in spinal indentation testing: indentation site relocation, intraabdominal pressure, subject movement, muscular response, and stiffness estimation. J Manipulative Physiol Ther. 2001;24(2):84-91.

46. Kawchuk GN, Fauvel OR, Dmowski J. Ultrasonic indentation: a procedure for the non-invasive quantification of force-displacement properties of the lumbar spine. J Manipulative Physiol Ther. 2001;24(3):149-56.

47. Keller TS, Colloca CJ, Fuhr AW. In vivo transient vibration assessment of the normal human thoracolumbar spine. J Manipulative Physiol Ther. 2000;23(8):521-30.

48. Latimer J, Lee M, Goodsell M, Maher C, Wilkinson B, Adams R. Instrumented measurement of spinal stiffness. Man Ther. 1996;1(4):204-9.

49. Kawchuk GN, Kaigle AM, Holm SH, Rod FO, Ekstrom L, Hansson T. The diagnostic performance of vertebral displacement measurements derived from ultrasonic indentation in an in vivo model of degenerative disc disease. Spine. 2001;26(12):1348-55.

50. Latimer J, Lee M, Adams RD. The effects of high and low loading forces on measured values of lumbar stiffness. J Manipulative Physiol Ther. 1998;21(3):157-63.

51. Cramer GD, Tuck NR, Jr, Knudsen JT, Fonda SD, Schliesser JS, Fournier JT et al. Effects of side-posture positioning and side-posture adjusting on the lumbar zygapophyseal joints as evaluated by magnetic resonance imaging: a before and after study with randomization. J Manipulative Physiol Ther. 2000;23(6):380-94.

52. Cramer GD, Gregerson DM, Knudsen JT, Hubbard BB, Ustas LM, Cantu JA. The effects of side-posture positioning and spinal adjusting on the lumbar Z joints: a randomized controlled trial with sixty-four subjects. Spine. 2002;27(22):2459-66.

53. Ianuzzi A, Little JS, Chiu JB, Baitner A, Kawchuk G, Khalsa PS. Human lumbar facet joint capsule strains: I. During physiological motions. Spine J. 2004;4(2):141-52.

54. Indahl A, Kaigle AM, Reikeras O, Holm SH. Interaction between the porcine lumbar intervertebral disc, zygapophysial joints, and paraspinal muscles. Spine. 1997;22(24):2834-40.

55. Ingber DE. The mechanochemical basis of cell and tissue regulation. Mech Chem Biosyst. 2004;1(1):53-68.

56. Ingber DE. Cellular mechanotransduction: putting all the pieces together again. FASEB J. 2006;20(7):811-27.

57. Gilat D, Cahalon L, Hershkoviz R, Lider O. Interplay of T cells and cytokines in the context of enzymatically modified extracellular matrix. Immunol Today. 1996;17(1):16-20.

58. Langevin HM, Yandow JA. Relationship of acupuncture points and meridians to connective tissue planes. Anat Rec. 2002;269(6):257-65.

59. Langevin HM, Churchill DL, Fox JR, Badger GJ, Garra BS, Krag MH. Biomechanical response to acupuncture needling in humans. J Appl Physiol. 2001;91(6):2471-8.

60. Langevin HM, Churchill DL, Cipolla MJ. Mechanical signaling through connective tissue: a mechanism for the therapeutic effect of acupuncture. FASEB J. 2001;15(12):2275-82.

61. Bergmann TF. Various forms of chiropractic technique. Chiropr Tech. 1993;5(2):53-5.

62. Christensen MG, Kerkhoff D, Kollasch MW, Cohn L. Job analysis of chiropractic 2005. Greeley (CO): National Board of Chiropractic Examiners; 2005.

3

VARIABILITY OF FORCE MAGNITUDE AND FORCE DURATION IN MANUAL AND INSTRUMENT-BASED MANIPULATION TECHNIQUES*

Gregory N. Kawchuk, N.G. Narasimha Prasad, Randall C. McLeod, Tasha Stanton, Tianye Li, and Qiaohao Zhu

Manipulation is a common therapeutic intervention that is used by different professions to treat patients with musculoskeletal conditions such as low back pain. Although attempts have been made to standardize the application of manipulation through clinical guidelines,[1-3] clinical responses to manipulation are known to vary.[4-8] The primary source of this variation is thought to be patient heterogeneity[9,10]; however, variation in the application of manipulation itself may be an additional factor. Indeed, prior investigations have reported that manipulation can vary significantly in terms of force magnitude,[11,12] force duration,[13] and the location of force application.[14] Although the clinical significance of these sources of variation is not yet understood, their reduction is presumed to be beneficial, as is the case with other physical interventions.[15-20]

One approach to reducing variability in manipulation would be to standardize its application through instrumentation—an approach taken with other therapeutic tasks for which human variability may be detrimental.[21-24] To this end, appropriate instrumentation now exists and represents the second most common approach for applying manipulative forces.[25] Unfortunately, little evidence suggests that these instruments reduce application variability compared with manual methods. Given this background, the goal of this study was to describe the variation in forces delivered through mechanical and manual methods of manipulation.

METHODS

Overview

Four operators used four different mechanical instruments to apply force to a uniaxial load cell. A different group of four operators used a

traditional manual technique to apply force to a sensor mat. Outcome variables obtained from each sensor included peak-to-peak force magnitude and peak-to-peak force duration.

Instruments

Clinicians who wish to apply forces by instrument have numerous choices of devices with which to do so. In addition, these instruments use different technologies (i.e., spring, compressed gas, and electromechanical) to generate force through a blunt stylus that contacts the skin. Given this selection, we adopted a pragmatic approach and tested a selection of instruments that represented each of these technologies. Although several spring-based instruments exist, the Activator IV (Activator Methods International, Phoenix, Ariz.) is arguably the most popular of these instruments. This instrument has four discrete force settings that act by limiting spring displacement. Only one compressed gas instrument was identified (Air Activator, Activator Methods International), which uses a valve to allow continuous adjustment of force magnitude between its minimal and maximal settings. Although many electromechanical instruments are available, we were able to identify only one that is capable of delivering single, noncyclic applications of force (Impulse, Neuromechanical Innovations, Phoenix, Ariz.). This instrument uses an electric switch to select between three discrete force settings that act to control a solenoid, an electromagnetic device (Table 3-1). Mean values and standard deviations (SDs) were attained for forces generated by four operators (two experts and two novices) with the use of four instruments (maximal force settings). Also shown are force data generated by four different operators who used a manual technique. To compare performance between two of the same type of instrument, a second spring-based device was selected, the Activator Signature, which differs from the Activator IV only in its outward appearance.

*Paper reproduced from J Manipulative Physiol Ther. 2006;29:611-8.

Table 3-1	**Mean Force and Duration**			

FORCE (N)

	Expert 1	Expert 2	Novice 1	Novice 2
Activator IV*	169.771 ± 8.589	177.585 ± 4.933	177.315 ± 4.604	174.334 ± 4.831
Air Activator*	207.331 ± 9.239	188.361 ± 12.045	210.593 ± 12.017	193.724 ± 13.357
Impulse*	174.554 ± 6.851	181.037 ± 6.053	163.058 ± 9.081	182.998 ± 4.978
Signature*	133.111 ± 3.941	133.131 ± 3.404	136.974 ± 3.579	136.934 ± 5.847

	Expert A	Expert B	Novice A	Novice B
Manual	253.654 ± 37.738	157.408 ± 24.624	256.773 ± 49.836	387.432 ± 61.526

DURATION (ms)

	Expert 1	Expert 2	Novice 1	Novice 2
Activator IV	1.098 ± 0.08	1.146 ± 0.03	1.266 ± 0.075	1.324 ± 0.086
Air Activator	0.856 ± 0.032	0.776 ± 0.018	0.86 ± 0.016	0.902 ± 0.011
Impulse	0.76 ± 0.086	0.656 ± 0.026	0.756 ± 0.016	0.77 ± 0.051
Signature	0.882 ± 0.049	0.966 ± 0.04	1.112 ± 0.06	1.246 ± 0.037

	Expert A	Expert B	Novice A	Novice B
Manual	66.924 ± 5.152	99.882 ± 13.897	164.228 ± 55.745	250.889 ± 87.429

*p ≤ .05 (significant difference).

Operators

Four individuals operated the four selected instruments. Two of the operators were considered to be "experts" because they use instrument-based force application in their practices on a daily basis and are certified by the manufacturer in the use of Activator instruments. The remaining two operators were considered to be "novices" because they do not use any of the instruments clinically, nor are they certified to do so. Four different individuals (called "operators" for convenience) were selected to apply forces manually. Two operators were considered to be "experts" because they use manual force application techniques in clinical practice and are licensed by their local jurisdiction to do so. The remaining two manual manipulators were considered to be "novices" because they do not possess training, experience, or licensure to perform manual applications of force.

Data Collection and Sensors

For the mechanical instruments, a single operator applied each instrument at its maximal force setting to a load cell (1 kN capacity;

Measurement Specialties, Hampton, Va.) fixed to a rigid surface. Each operator was allowed to practice using the instrument on the sensor before data were collected. Specifically, a single operator used a single instrument at its maximal force setting to perform 10 applications of force at 5-second intervals. The remaining operators then used the same instrument in the same manner before the next instrument was tested. Because forces applied by instruments typically occur over short durations[26] and are not associated with concurrent increases in contact area,[27] a single sensor system (i.e., a load cell) was used to achieve an adequately high sampling rate. After calibration, force versus time data were collected by a 16-bit analog-to-digital data collection system (National Instruments, Austin, Tex.) at 50 kHz.

For manual force applications, each operator performed 10 force applications at 5-second intervals on a 10 × 10 sensor mat (each sensor 1 cm²; Sensor Products Inc., Hanover, N.J.) mounted on a rigid surface. All operators contacted the mat using a reinforced single hypothenar hand orientation. For sufficient force magnitude to reach the sensor, without magnitude great enough to cause discomfort to the operator (given the rigid mounting of the sensor mat), operators were instructed to produce a "moderate" amount of force and were allowed to practice on the system before data collection was begun. Because the force durations of manually applied forces[28] can be almost two orders of magnitude larger than those applied by instrument,[26] force-recording equipment with high sampling rates is not required. This permits use of multiplexed sensor matrices, which can characterize changes in contact area known to occur with manual force applications.[14] The multiple-sensor mat used in this experiment was calibrated for a maximal pressure of 120 psi, and data were collected by the manufacturer's proprietary system at a maximal rate of 1000 Hz (Sensor Products Inc.).

Variables

From the load cell and sensor mat data, two primary variables were collected: peak-to-peak force magnitude (N) and force duration (millisecond). Force magnitude was calculated after any preapplication force was subtracted, with the difference of force occurring over the ascending limb of the force-time plot. Force duration was computed by counting the number of data samples occurring in the ascending limb, then dividing this figure by the collection rate.

Variation Analysis. For each primary variable (force and force duration), mean value and SD were calculated for all 10 trials generated from each unique combination of instrument and operator (16 instrument combinations and 4 manual combinations). As a general measure of variability in primary variables and to place data on a common reference scale, the SD of each instrument/operator combination was expressed as a percentage of its associated mean value. In addition, Levene's test was used as a measure of intraoperator variability wherein a p value greater than .05 described insignificant between-operator differences in within-operator variation for a given instrument.

Absolute Value Comparison. To determine whether different instrument operators generated different magnitudes of absolute force and force duration, we performed multiple comparisons on the primary variables for each operator pairing (six possible) for each instrument and for the manual technique. If Levene's test was insignificant (homogeneous within operator variation), the Tukey post hoc analysis was performed; if Levene's test was significant, the Tamhane post hoc analysis was performed.

RESULTS

General Results

Manual applications of force were generally greater in force magnitude and force duration than were those delivered by instrument (see Table 3-1 and Figure 3-1, A and B). The mean force for all manual applications was 264 N, and mean force duration was 145 milliseconds. For all instrument applications, the average force was 171 N, and average force duration was 0.963 milliseconds.

Variation Analysis

Although greater in magnitude, manual forces also displayed greater deviation from the mean value. On average, the SD for all manual applications represented 16% of the mean applied force and 23% of the mean force duration (see Table 3-1, Figure 3-1, Table 3-2, and Figure 3-2, A and B). For all instrument applications, the SD represented 4% of the mean applied force and 5% of the mean force duration (see Tables 3-1 and 3-2; see Figures 3-1 and 3-2). Results for Levene's test pertaining to intraoperator variability are described in Table 3-3. For the force variable, intraoperator variation for all instruments and for the manual technique was found not to differ between operators.

For force duration, the Impulse instrument and the manual technique were shown to have intraoperator variations that differed significantly between operators (p = .01 and p = .004, respectively).

Absolute Value Comparison

Multiple comparisons between any of six instrument operator pairings showed significant differences in the absolute force magnitudes and force durations produced (Table 3-4). For force magnitude, 9 of 24 instrument operator comparisons (38%) were found to differ significantly (p ≤ .05) in terms of absolute force produced. On further analysis, these differences were not found to be the result of any specific pairing of operators; significant differences in forces generated between expert operators with the same instrument were just as common as those between novice operators. With only one instrument, Activator IV, were all operators able to generate equal forces. Similar results for instrument operators were observed for force duration (Table 3-5); 18 of 24 between-operator comparisons (75%) were significantly different (p ≤ .05). For force

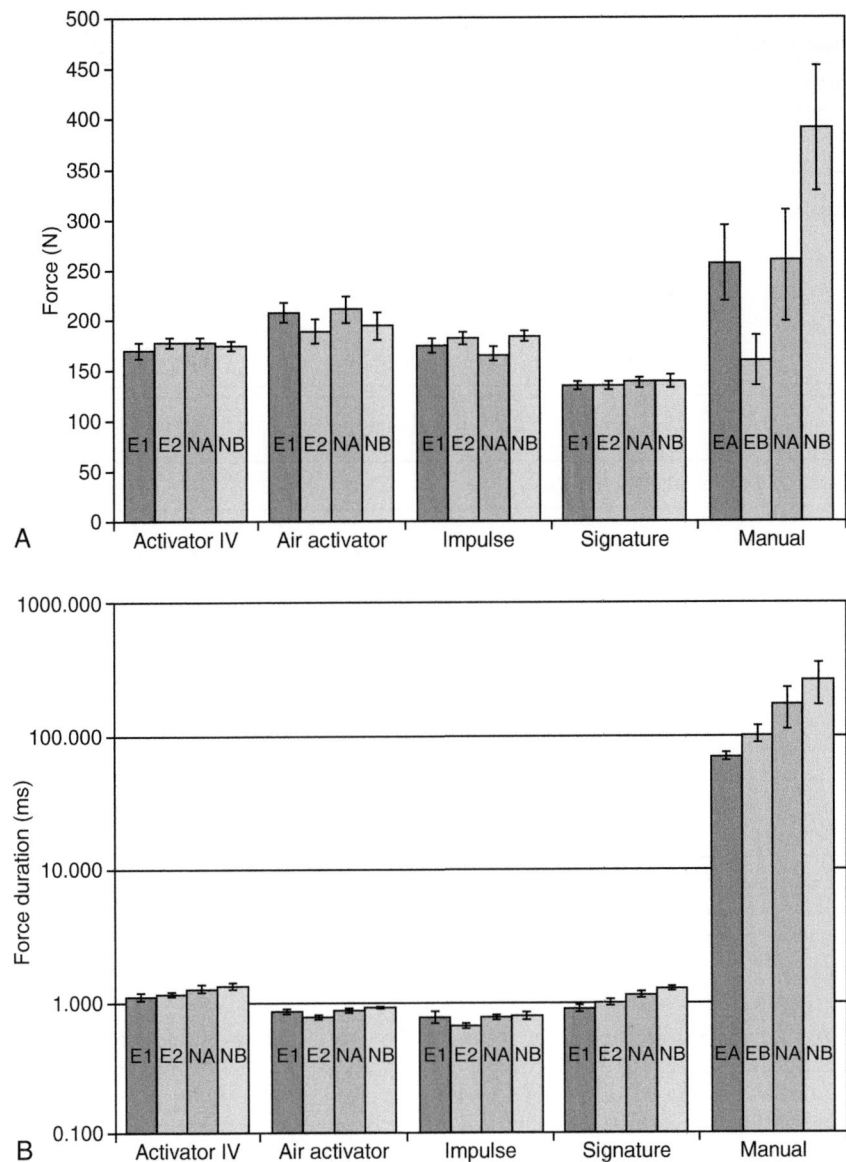

Figure 3-1 A, Mean forces and standard deviation (SD) bars of forces generated by four operators (two experts and two novices) who were using four instruments (maximal force settings), and four different operators (two experts and two novices) who were using a manual technique. **B,** Log plot of mean force durations and SD bars of force durations generated by four operators (two experts and two novices) who were using four instruments (maximal force settings) and a manual technique. *E1,* Expert 1; *E2,* expert 2; *N1,* novice 1; *N2,* novice 2 (for instrument operators). *EA,* Expert A; *EB,* expert B; *NA,* novice A; *NB,* novice B (for manual operators).

duration data, more significant differences were reported between expert operators than between novices.

DISCUSSION

As was the case in other investigations that studied manual force application,[11,29-33] we observed large variations in force magnitude and force duration. In general, the manual technique generated much greater between-operator differences in mean absolute force and in force duration compared with instruments. This was expected in that no objective target magnitude reference is available for manual operators other than instruction to provide some subjective level of force. This was also the case for SDs; the absolute SD for forces and force durations was

Table 3-2 Percent Deviations of Mean Force and Mean Duration

% DEVIATION OF MEAN FORCE (N)

	Expert 1	Expert 2	Novice 1	Novice 2
Air Activator IV	5.059	2.778	2.596	2.771
Air Activator	4.456	6.395	5.706	6.895
Impulse	3.925	3.343	5.554	2.720
Signature	2.961	2.557	2.613	4.270

	Expert A	Expert B	Novice A	Novice B
Manual	14.878	15.644	19.409	15.880

% DEVIATION OF MEAN DURATION (ms)

	Expert 1	Expert 2	Novice A	Novice B
Air Activator IV*	7.309	2.608	5.960	6.519
Air Activator*	3.783	2.368	1.899	1.259
Impulse*	11.302	4.014	2.087	6.685
Signature*	5.600	3.994	5.376	2.935

	Expert A	Expert B	Novice A	Novice B
Manual	7.699	13.913	33.944	34.949

Standard deviations, expressed as a percentage of the mean value, of force durations generated by four operators (two experts and two novices) who were using four instruments (maximal force settings) and a manual technique. Also shown are force data generated by four different operators who were using a manual technique.
*$p \leq 0.05$ (significant difference).

generally greater for the manual technique than for all instruments. It must be noted that comparison of absolute force between instrument and manual methods is difficult because contact areas may differ between the two approaches.[27]

Given these results, we would expect that the use of an instrument would reduce human inconsistency and would result in reduced variation among the primary variables. Specifically, we would expect that because the instrument has predefined force settings, the mean force generated between operators by any instrument should be much more similar than the mean force generated between manual operators who lack a common magnitude reference. Second, the use of a tool over a manual method should decrease output variability. To a large extent, these two expectations were met, but other considerations are relevant.

First, although the use of an instrument reduced variation in mean force and in force duration, variability was not completely eliminated.

The fact that two almost identical instruments (Activator IV and Activator Signature) produced different results underscores this point. As can be seen in the multiple comparison analysis, absolute force generated by any two operators for a given instrument resulted in significant differences in 9 (38%) of 24 possible pairings. For force duration, this difference reached 75%.

These between-operator differences in absolute force parameters are most likely explained by variations in application of the instrument, not by differences in the mechanism of the instrument. Although our data provide no direct proof that significant variation between instrument operators is the result of any specific factor, or that these factors occur globally with other instruments and operators, we observed that the angle of instrument inclination can change significantly between trials. Instrument angulation would act to decrease output in the load cell used in this experiment because any component of force that is not perpendicular

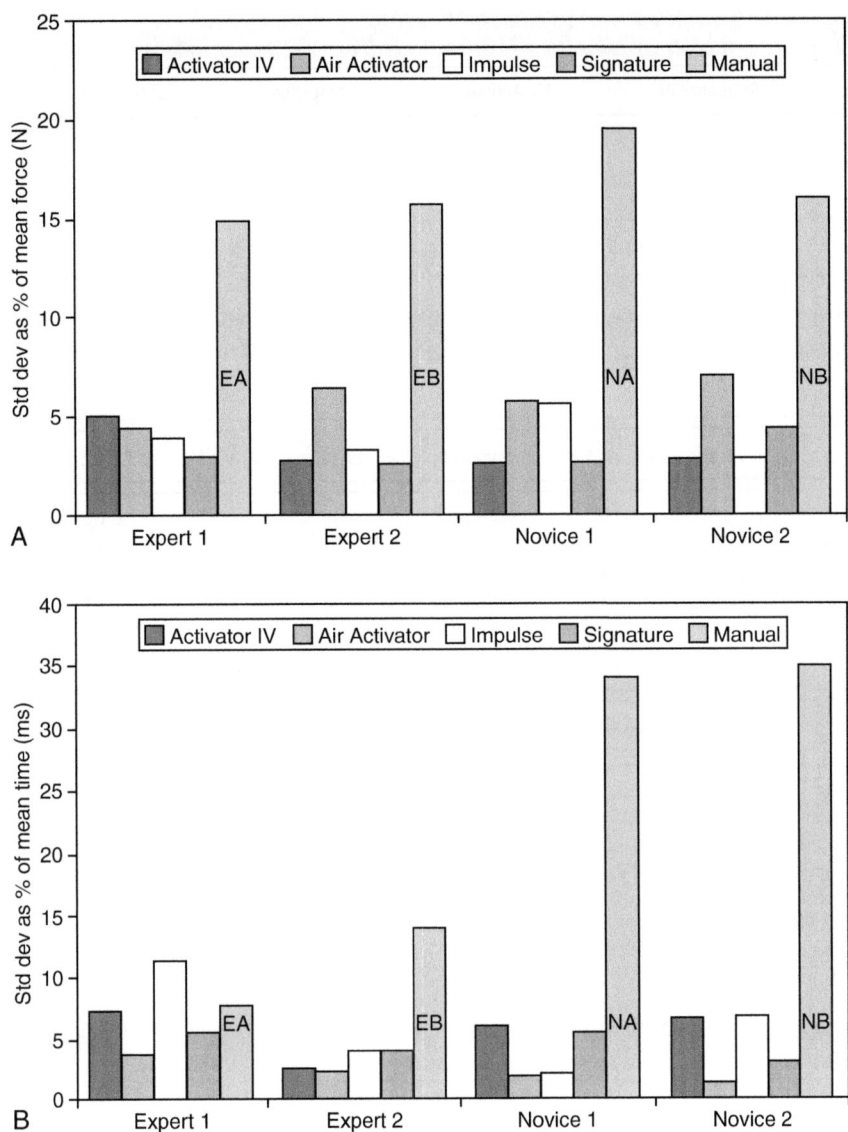

Figure 3-2 **A,** Standard deviations of forces generated by four operators (two experts and two novices) who were using four instruments (maximal force settings), and four different operators (two experts and two novices) who were using a manual technique, expressed as percentage of the mean force for each operator/instrument combination. **B,** Standard deviations of force durations generated by four operators (two experts and two novices) who were using four instruments (maximal force settings) and a manual technique (two experts and two novices), expressed as percentage of the mean force duration for each operator/instrument combination. *EA,* Expert A; *EB,* expert B; *NA,* novice A; *NB,* novice B.

to the surface of the load cell is lost in the output of the load cell. It was also apparent from our observations, and in speaking with the operators, that it was possible to hold the instrument in ways that alter the operator's opposition to instrument recoil—a phenomenon that we reproduced after data had been collected. Given these observations, we propose that these two factors—instrument angulation and opposition to instrument recoil—potentially influence the

variability of force-producing instruments and may be the underlying reason for our observation that different operators can produce different results with the same instrument.

Second, intraoperator variability for force magnitude, as measured by Levene's test, was found to be equal for any application method; operators of the manual technique were just as variable in producing force as were instrument operators. What is not described by Levene's test

Table 3-3 Intraoperator Variability

	Activator IV	Air Activator	Impulse	Signature	Manual
Force	0.654	0.513	0.331	0.189	0.09
Duration	0.185	0.103	0.004	0.531	0.01

Shown are the p values of Levene's test for homogeneity of variation in force and duration data among all operators for four instruments (maximal force settings). Also shown are data for four different operators who were using a manual technique.

Table 3-4 Comparison of Operator Parings (Force)

FORCE (N)

	Overall	E1 vs. E2	E1 vs. N1	E1 vs. N2	E2 vs. N1	E2 vs. N2	N1 vs. N2
Activator IV*	0.024*	0.034*	0.044*	0.364	1.000	0.624	0.692
Air Activator*	0.000*	0.005*	0.923	0.062	0.001*	0.747	0.014*
Impulse*	0.000*	0.180	0.006*	0.048*	0.000*	0.919	0.000*
Signature	0.075	1.000	0.253	0.253	0.213	0.213	1.000
	Overall	E1 vs. E2	E1 vs. N1	E1 vs. N2	E2 vs. N1	E2 vs. N2	N1 vs. N2
Manual	0.000*	0.000*	0.999	0.000*	0.000*	0.000*	0.000*

One-way analysis of variance of force magnitudes generated by four operators (two experts and two novices) who were using four instruments and four different operators who were using a manual technique.
For instruments for which intraoperator variation was homogeneous (Levene's test, Table 3-3), Tukey post hoc multiple comparison was performed (Activator IV, Air Activator, Signature); otherwise, Tamhane post hoc multiple comparison was performed (Impulse, Manual).
E1, Expert 1; E2, expert 2; N1, novice 1; N2, novice 2 (for instrument operators). EA, Expert A; EB, expert B; NA, novice A; NB, novice B (for manual operators).
*p ≤ .05 (significant difference).

Table 3-5 Comparison of Operator Parings (Duration)

TIME (ms)

	Overall	E1 vs. E2	E1 vs. N1	E1 vs. N2	E2 vs. N1	E2 vs. N2	N1 vs. N2
Activator IV	0.000*	0.448	0.000*	0.000*	0.003*	0.000*	0.284
Air Activator	0.000*	0.000*	0.974	0.000*	0.000*	0.000*	0.000*
Impulse	0.000*	0.000*	0.998	0.975	0.001*	0.000*	0.935
Signature	0.000*	0.000*	0.000*	0.000*	0.000*	0.000*	0.000*
	Overall	E1 vs. E2	E1 vs. N1	E1 vs. N2	E2 vs. N1	E2 vs. N2	N1 vs. N2
Manual	0.000*	0.503	0.001*	0.000*	0.044*	0.000*	0.000*

One-way analysis of variance of force durations generated by four operators (two experts and two novices) who were using four instruments and four different operators who were using a manual technique.
For instruments for which intraoperator variation was homogeneous (Levene's test, Table 3-3), Tukey post hoc multiple comparison was performed (Activator IV, Air Activator, Signature); otherwise, Tamhane post hoc multiple comparison was performed (Impulse, Manual).
E1, Expert 1; E2, expert 2; N1, novice 1; N2, novice 2 (for instrument operators). EA, Expert A; EB, expert B; NA, novice A; NB, novice B (for manual operators).
*p ≤ .05 (significant difference).

is the magnitude of that variability. Therefore intraoperator variation cannot be considered independently of the absolute magnitudes of variation. This is especially true in cases in which an absolute reduction in variation is needed to consistently achieve some clinically significant value.

Furthermore, given that it is generally accepted that manual techniques require training for specific performance levels to be attained,[29,30,34] we unexpectedly observed equality in intraoperator variability for force (including in comparisons of novice to expert). In only two cases was intraoperator variability found to differ significantly between operators for the force duration generated by the Impulse instrument and by the manual technique. At present, a satisfactory explanation for these observations is not available on the basis of our data.

Results from this work indicate that (1) force-producing instruments may produce different results in the hands of different operators, and (2) results imply that previous attempts to evaluate the performance of different instruments may be confounded by unreported variability within or between operators. It should be pointed out that differences in methods make it impossible to apply the results found in this study in reexamining the conclusions of prior studies. Therefore statements that appear in academic journals[35,36] or in manufacturer advertisements[37-39] that do not account for operator variability and that claim that specific instruments are superior because they generate greater force (or less) or reduce force duration (or increased) should be interpreted with caution.

CONCLUSION

Force-producing instruments reduce absolute variation in force magnitude and duration. This reduction is not so great as to eliminate significant differences in absolute force parameters observed to occur between some operators who use the same instrument. The clinical significance of these results has yet to be determined. Given these observations, prior (and future) claims of instrument superiority, which do not account for interoperator variability, should be considered with caution.

ACKNOWLEDGMENTS

This work was supported in part by the Canada Research Chairs Program (Ottawa, Ontario, Canada), the Whitaker Foundation (Arlington, Va.), and the Natural Sciences and Engineering Research Council of Canada (Ottawa, Ontario, Canada). The authors would like to acknowledge Activator Methods for supplying instruments for use in this study. The load cell described in this article was purchased by Activator Methods and was used on loan by the authors.

REFERENCES

1. International Chiropractic Association. Recommended clinical protocols and guidelines for the practice of chiropractic. Arlington (VA): International Chiropractic Association; 1992.
2. Haldeman S, Chapman-Smith D, Peterson DM. Guidelines for chiropractic quality assurance and practice parameters: proceedings of the Mercy Center Consensus Conference. Gaithersburg (MD): Aspen Publishers; 1992.
3. Henderson D, Chapman-Smith D, Mior S, Vernon H, editors. Clinical guidelines for chiropractic practice in Canada. Toronto, Ontario: Canadian Chiropractic Association; 1992.
4. Assendelft WJ, Morton SC, Yu EI, Suttorp MJ, Shekelle PG. Spinal manipulative therapy for low back pain. Cochrane Database Syst Rev. 2004;CD000447.
5. Astin JA, Ernst E. The effectiveness of spinal manipulation for the treatment of headache disorders: a systematic review of randomized clinical trials. Cephalalgia. 2002;22(8):617-23.
6. Bronfort G, Haas M, Evans RL, Bouter LM. Efficacy of spinal manipulation and mobilization for low back pain and neck pain: a systematic review and best evidence synthesis. Spine J. 2004;4(3):335-56.
7. Bronfort G, Nilsson N, Haas M, Evans R, Goldsmith CH, Assendelft WJ, et al. Non-invasive physical treatments for chronic/recurrent headache. Cochrane Database Syst Rev. 2004;CD001878.
8. Gross AR, Hoving JL, Haines TA, Goldsmith CH, Kay T, Aker P, et al. Cervical overview group: manipulation and mobilisation for mechanical neck disorders. Cochrane Database Syst Rev. 2004;CD004249.
9. Brennan GP, Fritz JM, Hunter SJ, Thackeray A, Delitto A, Erhard RE. Identifying subgroups of patients with acute/subacute "nonspecific" low back pain: results of a randomized clinical trial. Spine. 2006;31(6):623-31.
10. Childs JD, Fritz JM, Flynn TW, Irrgang JJ, Johnson KK, Majkowski GR, et al. A clinical prediction rule to identify patients with low back pain most likely to benefit from spinal manipulation: a validation study. Ann Intern Med. 2004;141(12):920-8.
11. Harms MC, Bader DL. Variability of forces applied by experienced therapists during spinal mobilization. Clin Biomech (Bristol, Avon). 1997;12(6):393-9.
12. Rogers CM, Triano JJ. Biomechanical measure validation for spinal manipulation in clinical settings. J Manipulative Physiol Ther. 2003;26(9):539-48.

13. Kawchuk GN, Herzog W, Hasler EM. Forces generated during spinal manipulative therapy of the cervical spine: a pilot study. J Manipulative Physiol Ther. 1992;15(5):275-8.

14. Perle SM, Kawchuk GN. Pressures generated during spinal manipulation and their association with hand anatomy. J Manipulative Physiol Ther. 2005;28(4):e1-7.

15. Bisbinas I, Belthur M, Said HG, Green M, Learmonth DJ. Accuracy of needle placement in ACJ injections. Knee Surg Sports Traumatol Arthrosc. 2006;14(8):762-5.

16. Boon JM, Abrahams PH, Meiring JH, Welch T. Lumbar puncture: anatomical review of a clinical skill. Clin Anat. 2004;17(7):544-53.

17. Chen L, Tang J, White PF, Sloninsky A, Wender RH, Naruse R, et al. The effect of location of transcutaneous electrical nerve stimulation on postoperative opioid analgesic requirement: acupoint versus nonacupoint stimulation. Anesth Analg. 1998;87(5):1129-34.

18. Edwards P. Promoting correct site surgery: a national approach. J Perioper Pract. 2006;16(2):80-6.

19. Franco CD. Posterior approach to the sciatic nerve in adults: is Euclidean geometry still necessary? Anesthesiology. 2003;98(3):723-8.

20. Wiklund CU, Romand JA, Suter PM, Bendjelid K. Misplacement of central vein catheters in patients with hemothorax: a new approach to resolve the problem. J Trauma. 2005;59(4):1029-31.

21. Lee S, Yang DS, Choi MS, Kim CY. Development of respiratory motion reduction device system (RMRDs) for radiotherapy in moving tumors. Jpn J Clin Oncol. 2004;34(11):686-91.

22. Jekelis AW. Increased instrument intelligence—can it reduce laboratory error? Biomed Instrum Technol. 2005;39(3):232-6.

23. Guchelaar HJ, Kalmeijer MD. The potential role of computerisation and information technology in improving prescribing in hospitals. Pharm World Sci. 2003;25(3):83-7.

24. Croswell RJ, Dilley DC, Lucas WJ, Vann WF. A comparison of conventional versus electronic monitoring of sedated pediatric dental patients. Pediatr Dent. 1995;17(5):332-9.

25. Christensen MG, Kerkhoff D, Kollasch MW. Job analysis of chiropractic. Greeley (CO): National Board of Chiropractic Examiners; 2000.

26. Fuhr AW, Smith DB. Accuracy of piezoelectric accelerometers measuring displacement of a spinal adjusting instrument. J Manipulative Physiol Ther. 1986;9(1):15-21.

27. Herzog W, Kats M, Symons B. The effective forces transmitted by high-speed, low-amplitude thoracic manipulation. Spine. 2001;26(19):2105-10.

28. Wood J, Adams A. Forces used in selected chiropractic adjustments of the low back: a preliminary study. Res Forum. 1984;1:16-23.

29. Descarreaux M, Dugas C, Lalanne K, Vincelette M, Normand MC. Learning spinal manipulation: the importance of augmented feedback relating to various kinetic parameters. Spine J. 2006;6(2):138-45.

30. Enebo B, Sherwood D. Experience and practice organization in learning a simulated high-velocity low-amplitude task. J Manipulative Physiol Ther. 2005;28(1):33-43.

31. Forand D, Drover J, Suleman Z, Symons B, Herzog W. The forces applied by female and male chiropractors during thoracic spinal manipulation. J Manipulative Physiol Ther. 2004;27(1):49-56.

32. Chiradejnant A, Latimer J, Maher CG. Forces applied during manual therapy to patients with low back pain. J Manipulative Physiol Ther. 2002;25(6):362-9.

33. Kawchuk GN, Herzog W. Biomechanical characterization (fingerprinting) of five novel methods of cervical spine manipulation. J Manipulative Physiol Ther. 1993;16(9):573-7.

34. Cohen E, Triano JJ, McGregor M, Papakyriakou M. Biomechanical performance of spinal manipulation therapy by newly trained vs. practicing providers: does experience transfer to unfamiliar procedures? J Manipulative Physiol Ther. 1995;18(6):347-52.

35. Colloca CJ, Keller TS, Black P, Normand MC, Harrison DE, Harrison DD. Comparison of mechanical force of manually assisted chiropractic adjusting instruments. J Manipulative Physiol Ther. 2005;28(6):414-22.

36. Fuhr AW, Menke JM. Status of Activator Methods chiropractic technique, theory, and practice. J Manipulative Physiol Ther. 2005;28(2):e1-e20.

37. Neuromechanical innovations, Impulse [homepage on the Internet]. Phoenix: Neuro-Mechanical Innovations; 2006 [cited 2006 April 18]. Available from: http://www.neuromechanical.com/index.php?option=com_content&task=view&id=32&Itemid=50.

38. Chiropractic Biophysics Online [homepage on the Internet]. JMPT publications: impulse fair best. Phoenix: Clinical Biomechanics of Posture; 2004-2006 [updated 2006 March 21; cited 2006 April 18]. Available from: http://www. idealspine. com/pages/ajcc_october_2005_impulse_ fairs_best_among_adjusting_instruments.htm.

39. The Integrator [homepage on the Internet]. The torque release technique. Miami Beach (FL): Holder Research Institute; 2001-2006 [cited 2006 April 18]. Available from: http://www.torque release.com/overview.htm.

Xue-Jun Song

PERIPHERAL AND SPINAL PAIN RECEPTORS

The spinal receptors, the dorsal root ganglion (DRG) neurons, and the dorsal horn neurons of the spinal cord convey peripheral information to the brain. DRG neurons conduct impulses from peripheral terminals to the spinal cord and then directly project to the higher levels of the central nervous system or are relayed by spinal dorsal horn neurons. Spinal dorsal horn neurons receive input from the central branch of axons of the DRG neurons and transfer this information to the brain or to other higher regions of the nervous system through their axons. The distinct cytoarchitecture and function of these spinal receptors are discussed in detail in this chapter.

Primary Sensory Neuron

Characteristics of the Primary Sensory Neuron. The primary sensory neurons—in this case, the DRG neurons—are pseudo-unipolar primary sensory neurons that convey somatosensory information from the body to the central nervous system. The morphology of the DRG neuron is well suited to its principal functions: stimulus transduction and transmission of encoded stimulus information to the central nervous system. DRG neurons differ in a variety of ways that reflect their distinct roles in sensation. Each cell can be distinguished by (1) the morphology of its peripheral terminal, (2) its sensitivity to stimulus energy, (3) the presence (or absence) of a myelin sheath, and (4) the diameters of its axon and cell body.

Cells can be divided into three groups according to the size of the cell body (diameter, μm): large cells, ≥50; medium-sized, 30 to 50; and small, 10 to 30. The peripheral branch and the central branch (dorsal roots) of the axon of the DRG cell compose the primary afferent fiber and transmit encoded stimulus information to the central nervous system. The terminal of the peripheral branch is the only portion of the DRG cell that is sensitive to stimulus energy. The peripheral terminal is a bare nerve ending or an end organ that consists of a non-neural capsule surrounding the axon terminal. The dorsal roots enter and terminate in the spinal cord or brainstem (Figure 4-1).

The axons of the DRG cells conduct action potentials to the central nervous system. The speed at which an afferent fiber conducts action potentials is related to the diameter of the fiber. The bigger the diameter, the faster the speed, and the sooner the central nervous system can act on the information. The conduction velocity (m/s) is approximately six times the axon diameter (μm) for large fibers and five times the diameter for thinly myelinated fibers. The factor for converting axon 125 diameter to conduction velocity is smaller (1.5 to 2.5) for unmyelinated fibers.[1,2]

Two distinct classification systems exist for afferent fiber innervation of skin versus muscle. The alphabetical scheme is used for cutaneous nerves, and the numerical classification typically is used for muscle afferents. Both nomenclatures are based on conduction velocity (or axonal diameter). The muscle afferent fibers include four types of axons: large myelinated (I), medium myelinated (II), small myelinated (III), and unmyelinated (IV) fiber. Aα, Aβ, Aδ, and C are also used. The cutaneous nerves have three groups: Aβ, Aδ, and C fibers.[1] In general, Aα and Aβ fibers are the axons of the large cells, the Aδ fibers are the axons of the medium-sized cells, and the C fibers are the axons of the small cells.[3-5] DRG cells, fiber diameters, and conduction velocities for the four types of axons are listed in Table 4-1.

According to responses to the variety of stimuli, DRG neurons can be divided into different types of nociceptive and non-nociceptive receptors.

Nociceptors. Nociceptors are the receptors that respond selectively to stimuli that can damage tissue. They respond directly to some noxious stimuli and indirectly to others by means of one or more chemical intermediaries released

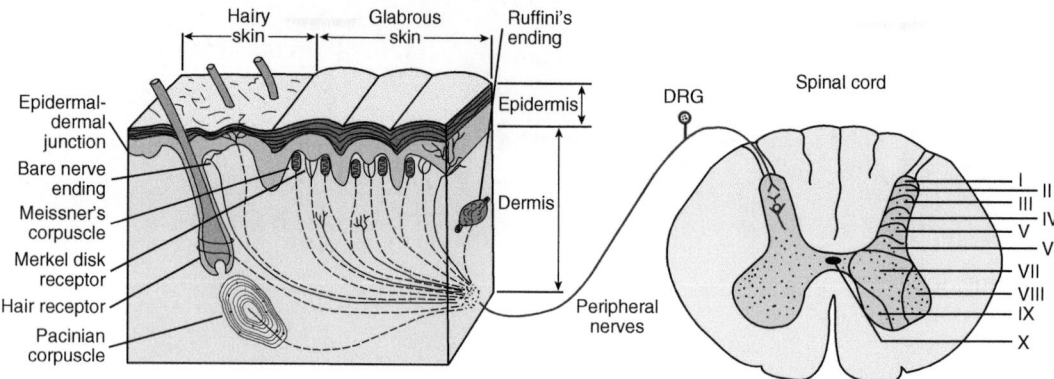

Figure 4-1 A model for accounting for the primary afferent pathways from the peripheral terminals to the spinal dorsal horn. *Left,* The location of various receptors in hairy and hairless (glabrous) skin of primates. Receptors are located in the superficial skin, at the junction of the dermis and the epidermis, and more deeply in the dermis and in subcutaneous tissue. Receptors of the glabrous skin include Meissner's corpuscles, located in the dermal papillae; Merkel's receptors, also located in the dermal papillae; and bare nerve endings. Receptors of the hairy skin include hair receptors, Merkel's receptors (having a slightly different organization than their counterparts in the glabrous skin), and bare nerve endings. Subcutaneous receptors, beneath both glabrous and hairy skin, include Pacinian and Ruffini's corpuscles. *Middle,* Dorsal root ganglia cells. The cell body lies in a ganglion on the dorsal root of a spinal nerve. The axon has two branches: The peripheral branch projects to the peripheral receptive fields, where its specialized terminal is sensitive to a particular form of stimulus energy; the other branch projects to the spinal cord or to higher levels of the central nervous system. *Right,* Columnar organization of the white matter and the butterfly-shaped gray matter of the spinal cord. The white matter is organized into three columns—dorsal, lateral, and ventral—that run parallel to the long axis of the spinal cord. The central gray matter is divided into ten layers (I to X) of functionally distinct nuclei. Laminae I to VI and lamina VII make up the dorsal horn and the intermediate zone, respectively. Laminae VIII and IX are equivalent to the ventral horn. Lamina X consists of the central canal. *(Modified from Haldeman S, editor. Principles and practice of chiropractic. 3rd ed. New York: McGraw-Hill; 2005.)*

Table 4-1	**Characteristics of Dorsal Root Ganglion Neurons and Their Axons**					
	Diameter of Cell Body (μm)	Cutaneous Nerve	Muscle Nerve	Axon Diameter (μm)	Myelinated (M) or Unmyelinated (UM) Axon	Peripheral Axon Conduction Velocity (m/s)
Large cell	≥50	Aα, Aβ	I, II	6-20	M	≥16
Medium cell	30-50	Aδ	III	1-6	M	2-15
Small cell	≤30 (usually 10-30)	C	IV	0.2-1.5	UM	0.4-2

from cells in the traumatized tissue. Four types of nociceptors are distinguished on the basis of properties of the stimuli [6-12]:

1. Mechanical nociceptors: activated only by strong mechanical stimulation, most effectively by sharp objects
2. Heat nociceptors: respond selectively to heat or cold. Heat nociceptors in humans respond when the temperature of their receptive field exceeds 45° C, the heat pain threshold. Both mechanical and thermal nociceptors have small-diameter, thinly myelinated Aδ or III fibers. Activation of these nociceptors is associated with sensations of sharp, pricking pain.

3. Cold nociceptors: respond to noxious cold stimuli (<5° C) and have small-diameter, unmyelinated C fibers
4. Polymodal nociceptors: respond to several different types of noxious stimuli, such as high-intensity mechanical, hot, cold, and chemical stimuli. Some naturally occurring agents such as the chemical mediators released from cells in damaged tissues—potassium, serotonin, bradykinin, histamine, prostaglandins, leukotrienes, and substance P—can activate or sensitize these nociceptors.[6,12,13] Polymodal nociceptors have small-diameter, unmyelinated C fibers.

Activation of these nociceptors results in slow-onset burning pain.

Both Aδ and C fibers are widely distributed in the skin, as well as in deep tissues. The viscera are innervated by DRG neurons with free nerve endings and have mechanosensory and chemosensory receptors.[6,14,15] Mechanosensory visceral afferents are similar to those in the skin and can be activated by distention and stretching of visceral muscle, which may evoke sensations of pain.[14-16] Chemosensory nerve endings are very important for monitoring visceral function and providing the afferent limb with many autonomic reflexes.[17]

Non-nociceptors. Non-nociceptors are those that respond to non-noxious stimuli, such as touch, warmth, cold, and limb proprioception. These receptors can be divided into cutaneous and subcutaneous mechanoreceptors, muscle and skeletal mechanoreceptors, and thermal and cool receptors. Virtually, all these sensations are mediated by the fast, myelinated Aα or Aβ fibers.

Cutaneous and Subcutaneous Mechanoreceptors. Three types of mechanoreceptors are located cutaneously or subcutaneously[18-20]:

1. Hair follicle receptors are the principal mechanoreceptors of the hairy skin, which covers most of the body. Three separate classes of receptors innervate different types of hair follicles: hair-guard, hair-tylotrich, and hair-down receptors.
2. Meissner's corpuscle and Merkel's receptor are the two principal types of mechanoreceptors in the superficial glabrous (hairless) skin. Meissner's corpuscle is a rapidly adapting receptor that responds at the onset, and often also at the termination, but not through the duration of the stimulus. Merkel's receptor is a slowly adapting mechanoreceptor that responds continuously to a persistent stimulus. Both receptors have specialized accessory structures that are thought to be mechanical filters that confer dynamic or static response specificity. Glabrous skin is a remarkably discriminating organ, and this sensitivity is most highly developed at the tips of the fingers.
3. Pacinian corpuscle and Ruffini's corpuscle: The former is a rapidly adapting receptor, and the latter is a slowly adapting receptor. Both receptors are located in subcutaneous tissue beneath hairy and glabrous skin. The receptive fields of Pacinian and Ruffini's corpuscles are larger than those of Meissner's corpuscles and Merkel's receptors in superficial skin (see Figure 4-1).

These mechanoreceptors can be activated when a long-lasting stimulus, such as a steady skin indentation, is presented. This stimulus first evokes the sensation of tapping or light contact, which may be mediated by rapidly and slowly adapting receptors. Rapidly adapting receptors stop firing after several hundred milliseconds. Meanwhile, slowly adapting receptors remain active, and a steady skin indentation is felt. The pure sensory experiences of steady skin indentation, flutter, and vibration are extremely different from the complex tactile sensations evoked by natural stimuli that humans usually encounter. Natural stimuli usually activate different combinations of mechanoreceptors rather than a single type of receptor.[10,21,22]

Muscle and Skeletal Mechanoreceptors. Four main types of peripheral receptors signal limb proprioception:

1. Mechanoreceptors—located in joint capsules
2. Muscle spindle receptors—mechanoreceptors in muscle that are specialized to signal the length, speed, and stretch of the muscle
3. Stretch-sensitive receptors—help to control the excess stretch or force
4. Golgi tendon organ—involved in muscle contraction

These receptors are important in limb proprioception and are essential for maintaining balance, controlling limb movement, and evaluating the shape of a grasped object.[21,23]

Warmth and Cool Receptors. Thermal sensations consist of separate senses of warmth and coolness. Warmth is mediated by thermal receptors that are selectively activated by temperatures ranging between approximately 32° C and 45° C. With progressively warmer stimuli, warmth receptors discharge at a greater rate. Discharge rate and perceived magnitude of warmth increase correspondingly.[18,21] At temperatures greater than approximately 45° C, warmth is not perceived, but instead pain. In this range of painful thermal stimuli—the range over which thermal nociceptors are active—the discharge of warmth receptors is actually reduced. Warmth is mediated by warm receptors, which have unmyelinated C fibers.[7,11] However, heat pain is mediated by nociceptors, as was described previously. Cool receptors discharge intensely when a cool stimulus (around 20° C to 25° C) is delivered to the receptive field, and the frequency of firing is proportionate to the rate and degree at which temperature is lowered. Cool is mediated by cool receptors, which consist of Aδ or II fibers.[21,24]

Dorsal Horn Neurons of the Spinal Cord

Anatomy of the Spinal Cord. The spinal cord is the first relay point for somatic sensory information that is being conveyed to the brain.

The spinal cord consists of a butterfly-shaped central gray area and a surrounding region of white matter. The central gray area contains the cell bodies of spinal neurons, and the white matter contains axons that ascend to or descend from the brain. Rexed[25] proposed that the gray matter of spinal cord consists of ten layers (laminae) that are based on neural cytoarchitecture. Later, the neurons were found to be functionally distinct and to exhibit different patterns of projections.[6,25] Laminae I through VI are equivalent to the dorsal horn, which contains interneurons and ascending projection neurons that relay peripheral sensory information to higher levels of the central nervous system. Lamina VII corresponds to the intermediate zone, which contains the autonomic preganglionic neurons and mediates a variety of visceral control functions; it also is made up of neurons that transmit afferent information to the cerebellum. Laminae VIII and IX are equivalent to the ventral horn, which contains interneurons and motor neurons that control muscles of the trunk and limbs. Lamina X consists of gray matter that surrounds the central canal[26] (see Figure 4-1).

We now look at the detailed functions of all laminae and the corresponding nuclei.[25,27] Lamina I, the marginal zone, is located in the most superficial region of the dorsal horn. Many Aδ fibers and the C fibers from muscles[27,28] terminate in this area and synapse with cells, which are nociceptive specific. This area is an important sensory relay for pain and temperature. Lamina II is also called the substantia gelatinosa (SG). The unmyelinated cutaneous C fibers terminate in this area,[27-29] which is isolated from the others because all SG cells are interneurons, and no axons project to other areas.[6,7,30] The axons of the cells in lamina I and the dendrites of the cells in the deeper laminae project to the SG area and synapse with SG neurons. SG is the most important area for integrating nociceptive information, as is described in the gate control theory of pain.[31] Laminae III, IV, V, and VI contain the nucleus proprius, which integrates sensory input with information that descends from the brain and the region of the base of the dorsal horn, where many of the neurons that project to the brainstem are located. Most Aβ, Aδ, and C fibers terminate in this area.[27-29] Wide dynamic range (WDR) neurons that receive and transmit both nociceptive and non-nociceptive information are located mainly in laminae I, IV, V, and VI.[27-29,31] Lamina VII contains Clarke's nucleus or cell column, which is present only in the thoracic and upper lumbar segments and relays information about limb position and

movement to the cerebellum. The intermediolateral nucleus or cell column, which is also located in the thoracic and upper lumbar segments, contains autonomic preganglionic neurons. Lamina VIII contains interneurons that are important in regulating skeletal muscle contraction. Lamina IX, the motor nucleus of the ventral horn, contains motor neurons that innervate skeletal muscles. Lamina X surrounds the central canal and receives afferent input similar to that of laminae I and II. Nociceptive neurons that receive nociceptive input from the joint are located primarily in this area.[6,31]

Spinal Dorsal Horn Neurons Relay Primary Afferent Fibers. Primary afferent fibers have their cell bodies in the DRG. Central axons enter the spinal cord through dorsal roots. Spinal dorsal horn neurons relay primary afferent fibers to the brain or to higher levels of the central nervous system. The different classes of primary afferent fibers that convey somatosensory modalities take specific routes and end in different regions of the spinal cord.[27-29] Collaterals of large-diameter Aβ fibers, which mediate tactile sense and limb proprioception, enter the lateral aspect of the dorsal columns, where they ascend to the medulla. Large-diameter fibers also give off collaterals that enter the dorsal horn from its medial aspect and terminate in the deeper laminae (III to VI) of the gray matter. Both Aδ and C nociceptive fibers, which mediate pain and temperature sense, ascend or descend for a few segments as part of the tract of Lissauer; axon collaterals synapse with neurons in the dorsal horn. Nociceptive fibers terminate primarily in the superficial dorsal horn at laminae I and II. Some Aδ nociceptive fibers also project more deeply and terminate in lamina V (see Figure 4-1). Nociceptive afferents form direct or indirect connections with three major classes of neurons in the spinal dorsal horn: (1) projection neurons that relay incoming sensory information to higher centers in the brain, (2) local excitatory interneurons that relay sensory input to projection neurons, and (3) inhibitory interneurons that regulate the flow of nociceptive information to higher centers.[6,31] As was described earlier, projection neurons that process nociceptive information are located mainly in laminae I and IV through VI; these convey primary input to the higher levels of the brain (details in the next paragraph).

Organization of afferent input to dorsal horn neurons is essential for interpreting some clinical pain syndromes. For example, referred pain, which arises from nociceptors in deep visceral structures but is felt at sites on the body surface, can be explained by the organization of cut-aneous and visceral somatic sensory systems (Figure 4-2).[9] Displacement of pain to certain areas of the body is stereotypical. For example, patients with myocardial infarction frequently report pain not only from the chest but also from the left arm.[9,32]

CENTRAL PROJECTIONS OF THE SPINAL RECEPTORS

The spinal sensory receptors convey impulses from peripheral terminals to the spinal cord, and then by means of dorsal horn neurons, project to higher levels of the central nervous system, either directly or by relay. Following is a discussion of the ascending pathways that convey somatosensory information to the cerebral cortex or to other higher centers in the brain. The ascending pathways that convey pain, thermal sense, touch, and proprioception also are discussed.

Ascending Systems That Convey Sensory Information to the Cerebral Cortex

In the dorsal column, the medial lemniscal and anterolateral systems (Figure 4-3) are the two major ascending systems that convey somatosensory information to the cerebral cortex.[9,21,26,33] These systems play an important role in the perception of various types of somatic sensations.

Dorsal Column–Medial Lemniscal System. This is a new system for the somatosensory modalities of discriminative touch and joint position and for the artificial sense of vibration. The system starts with the dorsal column, which originates from the ascending axons of large-diameter primary afferent fibers, the central branches of DRG cells, and the axons of neurons in laminae III and IV of the dorsal horn. Initially, this pathway runs ipsilaterally within the spinal cord. At upper spinal levels, the dorsal column separates into the gracile fascicle and the cuneate fascicle. The gracile fascicle ascends medially and contains fibers from the ipsilateral sacral, lumbar, and lower thoracic segments; the cuneate fascicle ascends laterally and includes fibers from the upper thoracic and cervical segments. The two bundles terminate in the lower medulla in the gracile nucleus and cuneate nucleus, respectively. The cuneate and gracile nuclei are located at about the same level in the caudal medulla. These two nuclei together are referred to as the dorsal column nuclei. Fibers from the dorsal column nuclei arch across the midline to form the

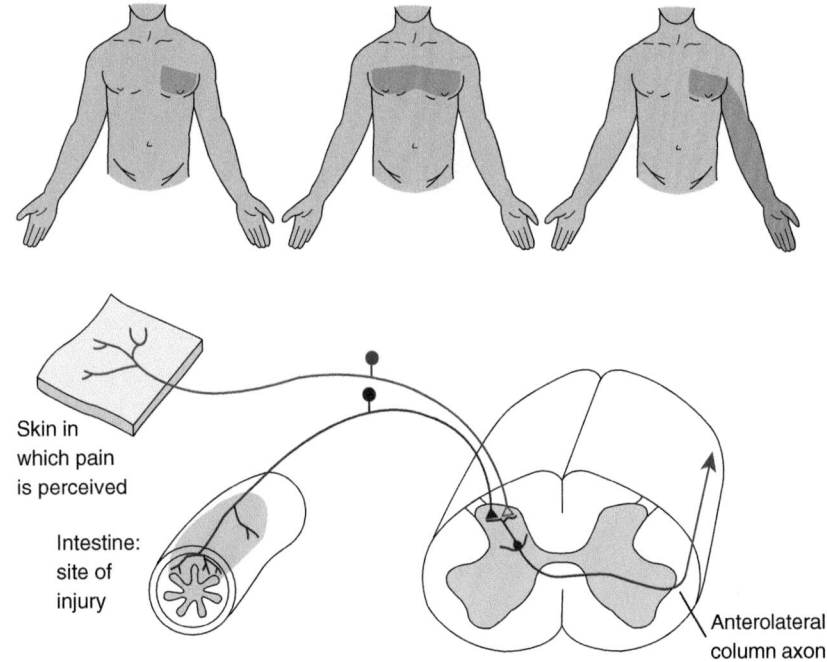

Figure 4-2 A model for accounting for referred pain: convergence of visceral and somatic afferents on the projection neurons in the dorsal horn of the spinal cord. Both visceral and somatic afferent fibers synapse with the same projection neurons, which convey the information to higher levels of the brain. Signals from nociceptors in the viscera can be felt as pain elsewhere in the body. The source of the pain can be readily predicted from the site of referred pain. *(Modified from Kandel ER, Schwartz JH, Jessell TM, editors. Principles of neural science. 4th ed. New York: McGraw-Hill; 2000.)*

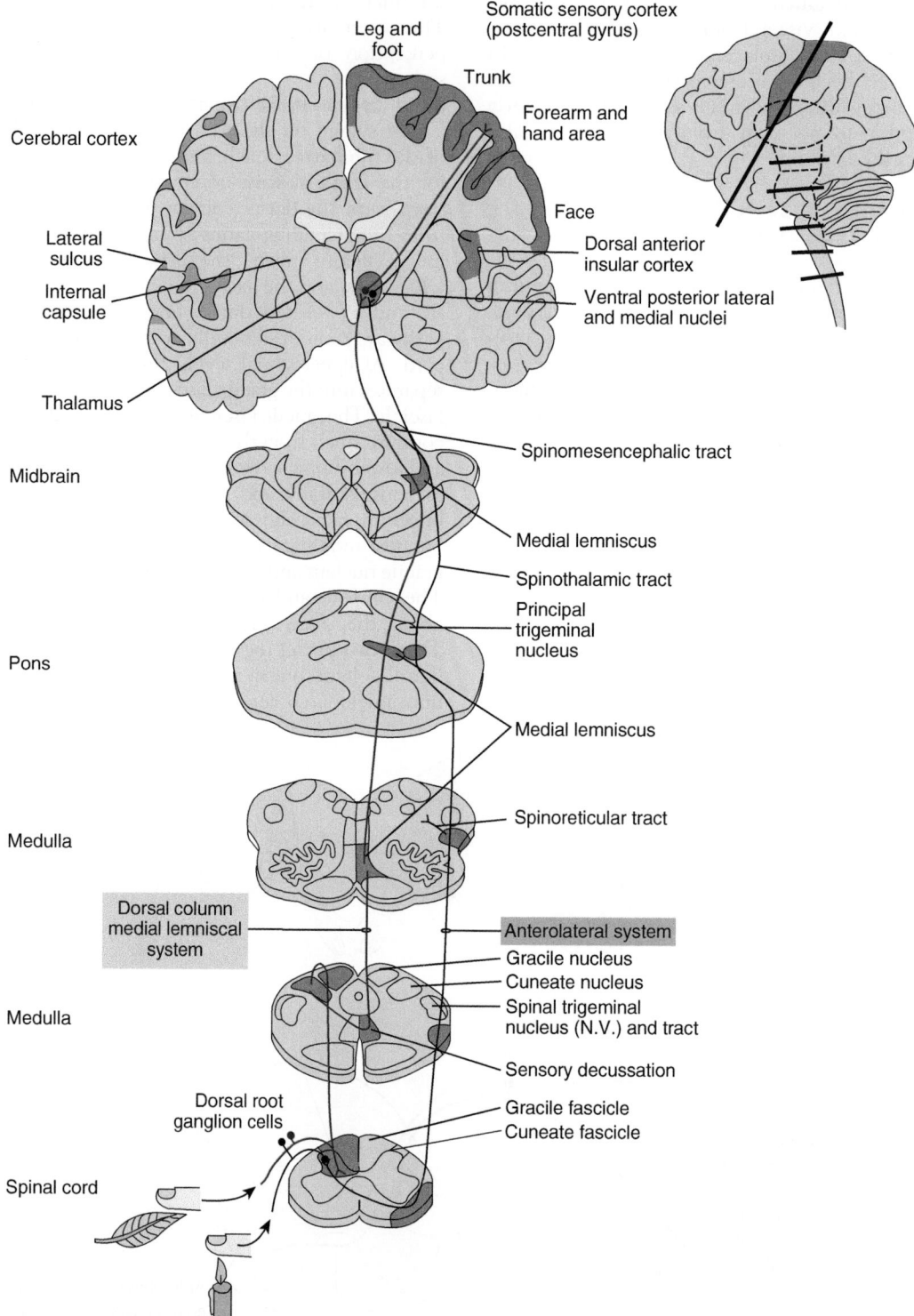

Figure 4-3   The dorsal column–medial lemniscal and anterolateral systems convey somatosensory information from the spinal cord to the thalamus and cerebral cortex. The dorsal column–medial lemniscal system *(orange)* conveys the tactile sensation and limb proprioception, and the anterolateral system transmits painful and thermal sensations to the thalamus. The anatomy of the pathways is shown on a series of brain slices. The top slice is a schematic oblique section through the postcentral gyrus, which is the location of the primary somatosensory cortex. The bottom five slices are schematic transverse sections through the brainstem and spinal cord at levels marked on the neuraxis. *(Modified from Haldeman S, editor. Principles and practice of chiropractic. 3rd ed. New York: McGraw-Hill; 2005.)*

medial lemniscus and ascend to the thalamus, where they synapse on neurons in the thalamus.

The pathways for proprioceptive information from the arms and legs to the medulla are somewhat different. The pathway for proprioception from the arm consists of axons in the cuneate fascicle synapse on neurons in a portion of the cuneate nucleus; axons project in the contralateral medial lemniscus. Proprioceptive information from the leg is transmitted by the neurons in Clarke's nucleus. Axons of these neurons synapse on neurons that are located in the contralateral medial lemniscus within the caudal medulla.

The thalamus transforms all sensory pathways with the exception of the olfactory system to the cerebral cortex. Somatic sensation is mediated by the ventral posterior nucleus. Axons of the neurons in the ventral posterior nucleus project to the primary somatosensory cortex through the posterior limb of the internal capsule. Axons from the thalamus terminate on pyramidal cells and also on interneurons in the primary somatosensory cortex. Primary and secondary somatosensory cortices and the posterior parietal cortex are the main regions of the cortex for the termination of fibers from the dorsal column–medial lemniscal system. Cortical neurons with axons or dendrites are oriented in columns. This columnar organization is an important feature of the cortical neurons that helps to limit the horizontal spread of afferent input to the cortex.

Anterolateral System. This is an older system that carries pain and temperature and some less discriminative forms of touch sensation. The system originates predominantly from neurons in lamina I and in deep laminae of the dorsal horn. The axons of these neurons cross the midline to the contralateral side of the spinal cord, usually within two to three segments above the level of entry of its peripheral fibers. This crossing occurs in the white matter at the front of the central canal and in commissural neurons and then ascends into the anterolateral portion of the lateral column. The reticular formation of the pons and medulla, the midbrain, and the thalamus are the brain regions in which most of the axons of the anterolateral system terminate.

The anterolateral system is composed of three ascending pathways: the spinothalamic, spinoreticular, and spinomesencephalic tracts. The spinothalamic and spinoreticular tracts mediate noxious and thermal sensations that are relayed from the periphery to the spinal cord by Aδ and C fibers. Axons in the spinoreticular tract end on neurons in the reticular formation of

the medulla and pons, which relay information to the thalamus and to other structures in the diencephalon. The spinomesencephalic (or spinotectal) tract terminates primarily in the tectum of the midbrain. The spinomesencephalic tract also projects to the mesencephalic periaqueductal gray matter, the region surrounding the cerebral aqueduct. In the medulla, the axons of the anterolateral system are located on the lateral margin and are separated from the medial lemniscus. In the pons, the anterolateral system and the medial lemniscus move closer together, and in the midbrain, the two systems are opposed in a more lateral position. Fibers of the anterolateral system synapse on neurons in three thalamic regions: the ventral posterior lateral nucleus, the intralaminar nuclei, and the posterior nuclei. Neurons of the ventral posterior lateral nucleus project only to the somatosensory cortical areas. The intralaminar nuclei project more widely to areas of the cortex and to the basal ganglia. The posterior nuclei project to regions of the parietal lobe outside the primary somatosensory area.

Essential differences between the dorsal column–medial lemniscal and anterolateral systems are compared and summarized in Table 4-2.

Ascending Pathways That Convey Nociceptive Information

Nociceptive information is carried from the spinal cord to higher centers in the brain through five major ascending pathways that originate in various laminae of the dorsal horn, as described by Willis (Figure 4-4) and others.[32,34] The ascending pathways that transmit pain are located primarily in the anterolateral system.

Spinothalamic Tract. The spinothalamic tract is the most prominent ascending nociceptive pathway in the spinal cord. It originates from nociceptive-specific and WDR neurons in laminae I[35] and V to VI of the dorsal horn. Axons of the dorsal horn neurons cross the midline, ascend in the anterolateral white matter on the contralateral side, and terminate in the thalamus. Experimental and clinical evidence has clearly shown that electrical stimulation of the spinothalamic tract results in pain, and lesions of this tract result in marked deficits in pain sensation.

Spinoreticular Tract. The spinoreticular tract originates from the axons of nociceptive neurons in laminae VII and VIII. This tract ascends in the anterolateral quadrant of the spinal cord and terminates in both the reticular formation and the thalamus. Most spinoreticular fibers project ipsilaterally; this is different from the

Origination	Dorsal Column–Medial Lemniscal	Anterolateral
Table 4-2 Comparison of the Dorsal Column–Medial Lemniscal and Anterolateral Systems		
Level of decussation	Large-diameter primary afferent fibers (central branches of dorsal root ganglion neurons) Neurons in laminae III and IV of the spinal dorsal horn Caudal medulla	Neurons in laminae I and IV-VI of the spinal dorsal horn Spinal cord (within 2-3 segments)
Termination in brainstem	Thalamus	Thalamus Hypothalamus Reticular formation of the pons and medulla
Terminations in cortex	Primary and secondary somatosensory cortices and posterior parietal cortex	Primary and secondary somatosensory cortices and posterior parietal cortex
Modalities	Tactile (discriminative touch, the artificial sense of vibration), proprioception (arm and joint position)	Pain Temperature sense Crude touch
Effects of hemisection of spinal cord	Loss of tactile sense and limb proprioception in ipsilateral arm and leg	Loss of pain and temperature sense in a few segments below the lesion in the contralateral arm and leg

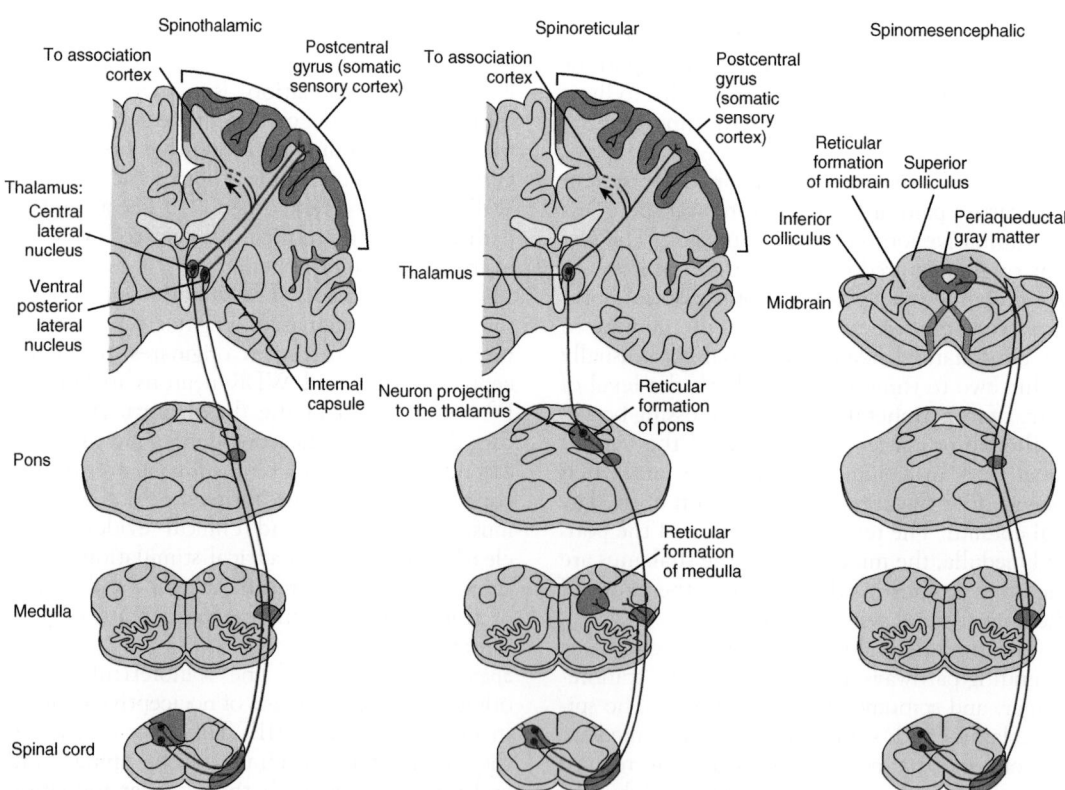

Figure 4-4 Three of the major ascending pathways that transmit nociceptive information from the spinal cord to the higher centers. *(Modified from Haldeman S, editor. Principles and practice of chiropractic. 3rd ed. New York: McGraw-Hill; 2005.)*

spinothalamic tract, in which almost all fibers cross the midline.

Spinomesencephalic Tract. The spinomesencephalic tract originates from nociceptive neurons in laminae I and V. It projects to the mesencephalic reticular formation, the lateral part of the periaqueductal gray region, and the parabrachial nuclei via the spinoparabrachial tract. Neurons of the parabrachial nuclei project to the amygdala, a major component of the limbic system that is involved in emotion. Therefore this pathway is thought to be involved in the affective component of pain. It is important to note that many of the axons of this pathway project in the dorsal part of the lateral funiculus, but not in the anterolateral quadrant.

Cervicothalamic Tract. This tract begins with the neurons in the lateral cervical nucleus, which is located in the lateral white matter of the upper two cervical segments of the spinal cord. Most neurons in lamina III or IV of the dorsal horn respond to tactile stimuli, but some also respond to noxious stimuli. These neurons project through the spinocervical tract, which runs in the dorsolateral spinal cord to the lateral cervical nucleus. The cervicothalamic tract crosses the midline and ascends in the medial lemniscus in the brainstem to midbrain nuclei and to the ventroposterior lateral and posterior medial nuclei of the thalamus.

Spinohypothalamic Tract. This pathway originates from axons of the neurons in laminae I, V, and VIII of the dorsal horn and projects directly to supraspinal autonomic control centers. The spinohypothalamic tract has been thought to be involved in the complex neuroendocrine and cardiovascular responses that follow noxious stimulation.

Nociceptive information is conveyed by the ascending pathways from the spinal cord to the thalamus. Of all the nuclei in the thalamus that process nociceptive information, the lateral and medial nuclear groups are the most important. The nuclei of the lateral nuclear group receive input via the spinothalamic tract, primarily from nociceptive-specific and WDR neurons located in laminae I and V of the dorsal horn. However, the nuclei of the medial nuclear group receive input primarily from neurons in laminae VII and VIII. The lateral thalamus is thought to mediate information about the location of an injury because these neurons have small receptive fields, as do the dorsal horn neurons that project to them. This information is then conveyed to consciousness as acute pain. Neurons in the medial nuclear group respond optimally to noxious stimuli and have widespread projections to the basal ganglia and many different cortical areas. Therefore the medial nuclear group may be involved in processing nociceptive information and in activating a nonspecific arousal system.

The thalamic nuclei then send nociceptive information to various regions of the somatosensory cortex. It is still unknown where and how nociceptive information is processed in the cortex. Using the imaging techniques of positron emission tomography (PET), Craig et al.[36-38] found that the cingulate gyrus and the insular cortex are involved in the response to nociception. The cingulate gyrus is a part of the limbic system that may be involved in processing the emotional component of pain. The insular cortex receives direct projections from the medial thalamic nuclei and from the ventral and posterior medial thalamic nucleus, and may contribute to the autonomic component of the overall pain response. In addition, some neurons in the somatosensory cortex have small receptive fields and respond selectively to nociceptive input, but they may not contribute to most clinical pain.[32]

Similar to nociceptive pain information, temperature sense is conveyed to the cortex in the anterolateral system.

CENTRAL RESPONSES TO NOCICEPTIVE INFORMATION

Complex connections exist among the primary afferent fibers, the second order neurons, various levels of the brainstem, and the somatosensory cortex. Varieties of somatosensory input are conveyed from the periphery to the brain along the different ascending pathways and systems to the brain. The primary somatosensory cortex (S-I), the secondary somatosensory cortex (S-II), and the posterior parietal lobe are the most important areas for receiving, processing, and integrating different somatosensory afferent information necessary for perception. The basic function of these pathways is to carry sensory discriminative and motivation-affective components of pain sensation. In addition, impulses in these pathways trigger both reflex motor and autonomic responses through their connections with specific nuclei. Furthermore, impulses in these pathways appear capable of activating the descending pain control or analgesic system. Central responses to pain stimulation are present, as are neurophysiological and neurochemical mechanisms for pain control. Touch is a complex topic that has been discussed in detail by Gardner and Kandel.[39]

The response of the brain to painful stimulation is extremely complex. Very few higher functions are not influenced to a greater or lesser extent by this super-powerful sensory stimulation. Some of the major areas of the brain that are affected by nociceptive input include reticular formation, thalamus, hypothalamus, limbic system, general cortex, parietal and temporal lobes, and primary somatosensory cortex. These affected areas in turn influence the response to pain stimulation.

General Arousal and Sensory Focusing

Being awake and alert is necessary for the cerebral cortex to analyze sensory stimulus and bring the sensation into consciousness. The brainstem reticular formation plays a very important role in maintaining the state of general wakefulness to focus attention on a particularly painful stimulus.

The reticular formation is a group of neurons found throughout the brainstem. From a ventral view of the brainstem, the reticular formation can be seen to occupy the central portion or core area of the brainstem from the midbrain to the medulla.[26] Fibers from the reticular formation ascend to the thalamus and project to various nonspecific thalamic nuclei. From these nuclei, fibers are distributed to the cerebral cortex, which is concerned with consciousness and has been called the ascending reticular activating system. Activation of this system causes generalized cerebral arousal. The reticular formation may also, at least in part, be responsible for the focusing of attention on specific sensations.[31,40,41] This arousal response can be obtained by stimulating the peripheral sensory receptors that connect directly with neurons in the reticular formation. The arousal response forms the basis for additional responses of the individual to nociceptive or non-nociceptive stimulation.

Emotional Response

The hallmark of pain is the distinctly unpleasant emotional experience. *Emotion* is defined as a strong feeling, an aroused mental state, or an intense state of drive or unrest directed toward a definite object and evidenced in both behavior and psychological changes (*Stedman's Medical Dictionary*). The limbic system has been thought to be responsible for this emotional sensation. The limbic system is the phylogenetically older part of the brain that includes cortical and noncortical (subcortical, diencephalic, and brainstem) structures. The paleospinothalamic tract,

the spinoreticular tract, and the multisynaptic ascending and descending propriospinal systems are the three pathways of the nonspecific motivational-affective system that pass information to the hypothalamus and the limbic system. This contributes to onset of emotional responses to noxious stimuli. Destruction of pathways or nuclei within the limbic circuit results in loss of the affective component to pain. When these connections have been surgically destroyed in humans through procedures such as orbitofrontal leukotomy or stereotactic surgery in attempts to reduce pain, patients have noted that they remain aware of the fact that something is wrong with the body, and they can localize the sensation (through an intact somatosensory cortex). These patients, however, no longer complain of discomfort or pain.[40-42]

Establishment of Memory Engram

The storage and retrieval of memory is of major importance in the interpretation of sensory input and allows an individual to correlate the nature, intensity, and associated sensations of the immediate stimulus with previous sensory experiences. This in turn leads to an appropriate response to the sensation. The major storage site for memory engram appears to be the temporal lobes, which receive thalamocortical projections from the medial thalamic nuclei.[40,41] Although the exact mechanism remains unclear, the establishment of memory engram for painful experiences has been noted to be a function of the intensity of the stimulus, the length of time the stimulus lasts, and the frequency with which it is repeated.[43]

Visceral-Hormonal Response

The visceral-hormonal responses to pain include cardiovascular, gastrointestinal, and hormonal changes that are manifested by increases in respiratory and heart rates, blood pressure, and gastrointestinal movement. Many of the cardiovascular and gastrointestinal responses are mediated by spinal or lower brainstem reflexes and are modified and coordinated, in turn, by the higher center in the cortex and the hypothalamus. The hypothalamus is one of the major centers involved in controlling sympathetic and parasympathetic activity, as well as hormonal function. The three motivational-affective pain pathways—paleospinothalamic tract, spinoreticular tract, and multisynaptic ascending and descending propriospinal systems—are also involved in regulating the visceral-hormonal response.[14,17]

Motor Response: Flexor Reflex and Crossed Extensor Reflex

In addition to the responses described earlier that are activated by noxious stimulation, motor responses are important in allowing the individual to escape from injury. Several spinal reflexes are directly involved in the responses of escaping from pain stimulation; these include the cutaneous reflexes, the flexor reflex, and the crossed-extensor reflex.[44,45] For example, when the skin of one foot of an individual is stimulated by a mechanical or a thermal noxious stimulus, the lower extremity undergoes a coordinated withdrawal. The flexor muscles contract and the extensor muscles relax, facilitating flexion of the joints, so as to allow escape from an injury. This coordinated reflex is called the flexor reflex. Meanwhile, extension of the contralateral leg is called the crossed-extensor reflex. This reflex causes the contralateral leg to bear the body's weight while the ipsilateral flexor reflex occurs. Both reflexes are mediated by polysynaptic pathways, and the integrative centers are found in the local spinal cord. These spinally mediated withdrawal reflexes can be reduced or blocked by the descending systems from the higher levels of the brain, such as that from the periaqueductal gray region, as discussed later in this chapter. In addition, the voluntary motor cortex may be involved in regulating spinal reflexes. The corticospinal neurons terminate on spinal motor neurons and interneurons in the spinal cord. These connections can gate reflex circuits, allowing voluntary movements to take advantage of spinal circuits because these circuits can link local sensory input to output.[46]

Hyperalgesia

Hyperalgesia is an extremely increased response to a stimulus that is normally painful. It has both peripheral and central origins. Changes in nociceptor sensitivity underlie primary hyperalgesia, and the hyperexcitability of spinal dorsal horn neurons underlies centrally mediated hyperalgesia.[47] Hyperalgesia is one of the major responses of the nervous system to repetitive noxious stimulation.

Upon repeated application of noxious stimuli, nearby nociceptors that were previously unresponsive to stimuli now become responsive. This phenomenon is called sensitization. The sensitization of nociceptors after injury or inflammation results from the release of a variety of chemicals by damaged cells and tissues in the vicinity of the injury. These substances include bradykinin, histamine, serotonin, prostaglandins, substance P, leukotrienes, and acetylcholine.[9,47]

Under conditions of severe and persistent injury, nociceptive C fibers fire repetitively, and the response of spinal dorsal horn neurons increases progressively. This phenomenon is called wind-up.[48,49] Wind-up is dependent on the release of glutamate from C terminals and the consequent opening of postsynaptic ion channels gated by N-methyl-D-aspartate (NMDA)-type glutamate receptors.[40] Therefore noxious stimuli can induce long-term changes and can produce hyperexcitability in the dorsal horn neurons. Profound alterations in biochemical properties and the excitability of dorsal horn neurons and of DRG neurons can lead to spontaneous pain and decrease the threshold for the production of pain.[4,5,50-52]

CENTRAL MECHANISMS FOR PAIN CONTROL

One of the remarkable discoveries in pain research is that pain can be controlled by central mechanisms. Nociceptive information is modulated by special circuits, nuclei, or pathways at different levels of the brain whose main function is to regulate the perception of pain.

Gate Control in the Spinal Cord

Nociceptive inputs from peripheral nociceptors to dorsal horn neurons of the spinal cord are regulated by the activity in other myelinated afferents that are not directly concerned with the transmission of nociceptive information. This idea that pain results from the balance of activity in nociceptive and non-nociceptive afferents was proposed by Melzack and Wall in 1965[31] and was called the gate control theory of pain. This hypothesis focuses on the interaction of four classes of neurons within the spinal dorsal horn: (1) nonmyelinated nociceptive afferents—C fibers; (2) myelinated non-nociceptive afferents—Aβ fibers; (3) projection neurons whose activity results in the sensation of pain—these neurons are located mainly in laminae V and I; and (4) inhibitory interneurons—in lamina II. The projection neuron is excited by both nociceptive and non-nociceptive neurons, and the balance of these inputs determines the intensity of pain. The inhibitory interneuron is spontaneously active and normally inhibits the projection neuron, thus reducing the intensity of pain. This inhibitory interneuron is excited by the non-nociceptive afferent but is inhibited by the nociceptive afferent. Therefore nociceptive afferents turn *on* and non-nociceptive afferents turn *off* a gate to the central transmission of noxious input. This circuit is potentially modulated by several central descending pathways.

This gate control theory provides a neurophysiological basis for the observations that a vibratory stimulus that selectively activates large-diameter non-nociceptive afferents can reduce pain, as can the use of transcutaneous electrical nerve stimulation (TENS), dorsal column stimulation, and techniques of acupuncture.[47,53,54]

Descending Nociceptive Control Pathways to the Spinal Cord

The gate control theory proposes that pain perception is sensitive to levels of activity in both nociceptive and non-nociceptive afferent fibers. It is also important to understand that nociceptive signals can be modulated at successive synaptic relays along the central pathway.

In experimental animals, stimulation of the periaqueductal gray region that surrounds the third ventricle and the cerebral aqueduct produced a profound and selective analgesia.[34,53] In human patients, stimulation of the periventricular gray region, the ventrobasal complex of the thalamus, or the internal capsule reduces the severity of pain.[9,55] This stimulation produces a profound suppression of activity in nociceptive pathways but does not change tactile sensations. The neural pathways that mediate this stimulation-produced analgesia have been defined as follows (Figure 4-5): Neurons in the periaqueductal gray matter, which usually do not directly project to the dorsal horn neurons of the spinal cord, make excitatory connections with neurons of the rostroventral medulla, in particular, with serotonergic neurons in the midline of the nucleus raphe magnus. Neurons of this nucleus project to the spinal cord via the dorsal part of the lateral funiculus and make inhibitory connections with the neurons in laminae I, II, and V of the dorsal horn. Stimulation of the rostroventral medulla inhibits dorsal horn neurons, including neurons of the spinothalamic tract that respond to nociceptive inputs. The other descending inhibitory systems originating in the noradrenergic locus ceruleus (LC) and other nuclei of the medulla and pons are also involved in suppressing the activity of nociceptive neurons in the dorsal horn.[47,56]

Contributions of Opioid Peptides to Endogenous Pain Control

It has been known that opiates such as morphine and codeine are effective analgesic agents. Microinjection of morphine, codeine, or other opiates directly into specific regions of the rat brain produces a powerful analgesia by inhibiting the firing of nociceptive neurons within the dorsal horn.[47,57-60] The periaqueductal gray region is among the most sensitive sites for eliciting such analgesia. This opiate-induced analgesia is involved in the same descending pathways, which originate from the periventricular gray region and from the noradrenergic LC and other nuclei of the medulla and pons, as described earlier. The brain contains specific receptors for opiates. Three major classes of opioid receptors have been identified: μ, δ, and κ.[61] The μ receptors are the most important in mediating analgesia and are highly concentrated in periaqueductal gray matter, the ventral medulla, and the superficial dorsal horn of the spinal cord; all are very important in regulating pain.[62,63] Naloxone, an antagonist of the opiate receptors, can bind the μ receptors and block the analgesia induced by morphine, an agonist of opiate receptors.[55,57] Three major classes of endogenous ligands for these receptors have been identified: enkephalins, β-endorphins, and dynorphins. Enkephalins are active at both μ and δ receptors, and dynorphin is a relatively selective agonist of the κ receptor.* Acupuncture or TENS can activate this endogenous opiate system to reduce the intensity of pain.

Several other important neurochemical agents, such as serotonin and norepinephrine, serve as primary neurotransmitters in both ascending and descending spinal pathways involved in the modulation of pain sensation.[61,65]

PROGRESS IN RESEARCH AND MANAGEMENT OF NEUROPATHIC PAIN

Acute physiological pain is "good" pain that can be well controlled with medicine or other countermeasures when necessary. However, so-called bad pain or chronic pain—particularly neuropathic pain—continues to pose major clinical challenges. It was estimated recently that chronic pain affects some 1.72 billion people a year worldwide, and it directly or indirectly causes losses of hundreds of billions of dollars annually. Many who suffer from chronic pain are told to learn to "live with it." Over the past two decades, many efforts have been put forth to understand mechanisms of chronic pain and to explore effective countermeasures.

Neurobiology of Neuropathic Pain
Conditions in Which Neuropathic Pain May Occur.
Painful neuropathic conditions may accompany a lesion of the peripheral and/or central

---

*References 47, 55, 57, 58, 60, 64.

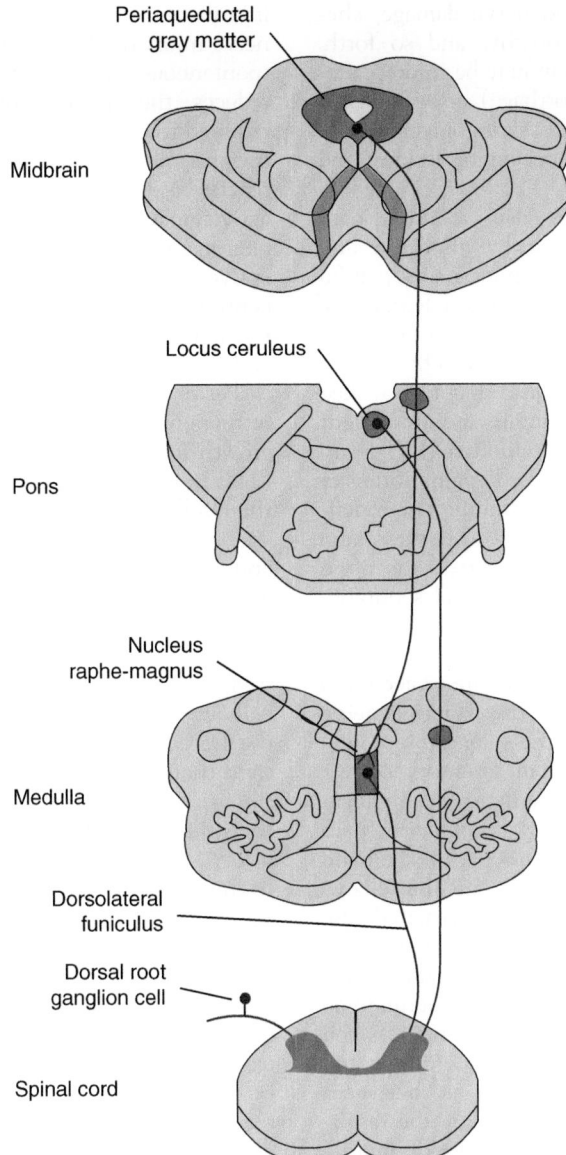

Figure 4-5 Two descending pathways regulate nociceptive neurons in the spinal cord. The pathways of the serotonergic periaqueductal gray region–nucleus raphe magnus–spinal dorsal horn and the noradrenergic locus ceruleus–spinal dorsal horn are involved in suppressing the activity of nociceptive neurons in the dorsal horn of the spinal cord. The former pathway arises in the midbrain periaqueductal gray region and projects to the nucleus raphe magnus and other serotonergic nuclei (not shown), then via the dorsolateral funiculus to the dorsal horn of the spinal cord. The second pathway arises from the noradrenergic cell groups in the pons and medulla and from the nucleus paragigantocellularis, which also receives input from the peripheral aqueductal gray region. In the spinal cord, these descending pathways inhibit nociceptive projection neurons through direct connections, as well as through interneurons in the superficial layers of the dorsal horn. *(Modified from Haldeman S, editor. Principles and practice of chiropractic. 3rd ed. New York: McGraw-Hill; 2005.)*

nervous system. The peripheral nerve may be damaged by the following traumatic conditions: iatrogenic nerve injury, ischemic neuropathy, nerve and/or root compression or entrapment, polyneuropathy (including hereditary, metabolic, toxic, inflammatory, infectious, paraneoplastic, and nutritional conditions in amyloidosis and vasculitis), plexus injury, stump and phantom pain after amputation, herpes zoster/postherpetic neuralgia, trigeminal and glossopharyngeal neuralgia, and cancer-related neuropathy due to neural invasion of the tumor, surgical nerve damage, radiation-induced nerve damage, chemotherapy-induced neuropathy, and so forth. The central nervous system may be injured after a stroke (infarct or hemorrhage) or by multiple sclerosis, spinal cord injury, syringomyelia/syringobulbia, epilepsy, space-occupying lesions, and so forth.

Characteristics of Neuropathic Pain. Painful neuropathies are characterized by allodynia and hyperalgesia, in addition to spontaneous painful syndromes. These are the common features of peripheral neuropathy in humans after nerve injury has occurred. *Allodynia* is defined as a pain or a nociceptive response that is provoked by normally innocuous stimuli, usually a light mechanical stimulus (tactile allodynia). *Hyperalgesia* is defined as increased pain intensity evoked by normally painful stimuli. These definitions were first given by Merskey and Bogduk.[66] Neuropathic pain states are often associated with nonpainful abnormal spontaneous and evoked sensory phenomena such as paresthesia and dysesthesia.

All types of neuropathic pain are projected to the innervation territory of the damaged nerve or pathway, according to the somatotopic organization of the primary somatosensory cortex. Examples of projected pain include pain localized to the amputated area in phantom pain and pain perceived in the ulnar part of the hand with ulnar nerve entrapment in the elbow. Nerve root compression from a herniated disc usually involves a combination of nociceptive pain in the area of the ruptured disc and neuropathic pain projected within the dermatome corresponding to the affected root(s). When nociceptors innervating the perineurium (the endings of the nervi nervorum) are activated during inflammation or compression, the resulting pain is nociceptive and is localized primarily to the site of the disturbance.[8,67]

Primary Sensory Neuron Mechanisms of Neuropathic Pain. Animal models of painful sequelae in humans after nerve injury have provided behavioral evidence for ongoing pain and cutaneous hyperalgesia. Animals that receive injury to primary sensory neurons—DRG neurons—exhibit behavioral symptoms of neuropathic pain manifested as mechanical and thermal hyperalgesia, or as allodynia. Injury to primary afferents distal to the DRG (i.e., the spinal[68] or sciatic nerve[69]) or to somata within the DRG[4,70,71] or dorsal rootlets[71] produces hyperalgesia accompanied with allodynia. Cellularly, increased excitability and other intrinsic alterations in membrane properties of DRG cells have been demonstrated after peripheral nerve injury or DRG compression. For example, nerve injury or DRG compression evokes ectopic spontaneous activity of the sensory neurons, reduces the amount of depolarizing current required to evoke an action potential, and lowers the action potential threshold and increases repetitive discharges.[3,5,71-73,75,76] Such abnormal activity and alteration of the excitability of sensory neurons, if they occur in the appropriate nociceptive afferent neurons, may maintain a state of central sensitization of nociceptive neurons in the dorsal horn; chronic pain and hyperalgesia and allodynia may result.

Peripheral axons of primary sensory neurons retrogradely transport cytokines, such as nerve growth factor (NGF) and tumor necrosis factor (TNF), from their peripheral targets back to their cell bodies (somata) in the DRG. Immune and Schwann cells, activated by axonal injury and inflammation, also release cytokines that may activate receptors or be taken up by injured and intact axons. This is likely to lead to the transport of signals to the somata, which may trigger additional cellular reactions such as glial cell activation and immune cell infiltration into the DRG.[77-81] Walters and Ambron[82] hypothesized that axon injury unmasks nuclear localization signals in certain axonplasmic proteins at the injured site. This causes proteins ("positive injury signals") to be transported retrogradely to the somata of sensory neurons and to activate transcription factors. These factors then induce the expression of early and late genes, which finally induce functional alterations.[83-85] These positive signals are coupled with negative signals that are produced by interrupted transport of trophic signals from peripheral targets to trigger alterations in expression of neuropeptides, receptors, and ion channels in neuronal somata.[86-88] For example, 2 weeks after transection of the sciatic nerve, DRG somata exhibit novel expression of a tetrodotoxin-sensitive (TTX-S) type III Na^+ current, a decrease in tetrodotoxin-resistant (TTX-R) Na^+ current,[87,89] a reduction in K^+ current,[90] and a reduction in an N-type component of high voltage–activated Ca^{2+} currents.[74,91] In addition, inhibitors of axonal transport can block axonal injury–induced hyperexcitability of sensory neurons.[85]

On the basis of these studies, we suggest that peripheral nerve injury or DRG somata compression activates positive injury signals that are transported retrogradely to the DRG soma to induce hyperexcitability. It is interesting to note that injury to the central branches of axons of DRG neurons may activate injury signals in the dorsal root that are transported primarily to central terminals in the spinal cord, rather than to DRG cells and their nuclei.[71] Studies have further shown that alterations in gene expression; alterations in expression of ion channels, receptors, and many peptides and other cytokines; inflammatory mediators; and nerve growth factors may contribute to the generation and development of allodynia and neuropathic pain.[86] These findings propose that increased excitability of DRG cells is associated with the generation and maintenance of neuropathic pain and plays an important role in allodynia and/or hyperalgesia.

Recent studies have suggested that altered gene expression occurs in sensory neurons,[92] especially large-diameter (Aβ) non-nociceptive sensory neurons in peripheral neuropathy.[93,94] Selective activation of these neurons causes mechanical allodynia and the release of neuropeptides such as substance P (SP) within the spinal cord.[95] Preprotachykinin, calcitonin gene-related peptide (CGRP), and SP mRNA are markedly upregulated in Aβ neurons[96-98] after peripheral nerve injury occurs. Innocuous stimulation-induced nociceptive neural response and allodynia and/or spontaneous pain can be attenuated by neurokinin-1 (NK-1) receptor antagonists.[99-101] These studies suggest that Aβ fibers, similar to C fibers, express SP via activation of the NK-1 receptor in the spinal dorsal horn neurons, and they appear to contribute to tactile allodynia. Our recent study provides direct evidence showing the functional roles of NK-1 receptors in the synaptic transmission of spinal dorsal horn neurons mediated by non-nociceptive input after peripheral nerve injury.[102] These studies have provided strong evidence to show that the intracellular signaling pathways (cyclic adenosine monophosphate/protein kinase A [cAMP/PKA] and cyclic guanosine monophosphate/protein kinase G [cGMP/PKG]) may greatly contribute to sensory neuron hyperexcitability and behavioral hyperalgesia after nerve injury or DRG compression.[103,104]

Spinal Mechanisms of Neuropathic Pain. Several hypotheses have been proposed concerning the way peripheral and central processing is altered following peripheral nerve injury, and how this may contribute to neuropathic pain. These possibilities primarily include descending facilitation from supraspinal levels,[105] altered signal transduction mechanisms,[106] long-term potentiation of neural synapse plasticity,[107] central sensitization,[108] decreased inhibitory mechanisms in the spinal dorsal horn,[109] and alterations in the primary sensory neurons such as ectopic spontaneous activity and neural hyperexcitability, as were discussed earlier.

In the spinal dorsal horn, three general mechanisms could potentially result in Aβ fiber–mediated neuropathic pain: central sensitization, disinhibition, and altered central circuitry. Central sensitization is a use-dependent form of plasticity.[110] Acute tissue-damaging stimuli activate nociceptors, which triggers a prolonged increase in the excitability of dorsal horn neurons. Nociceptors such as C fibers, by virtue of the slow synaptic currents they generate (which summate at low stimuli repetition rates to produce a marked buildup in the depolarization of spinal neurons), have the capacity to markedly elevate intracellular calcium levels through activation of ligand-gated ion channels that allow Ca^{2+} entry into the cells, particularly through the NMDA receptor, but also via voltage-dependent Ca^{2+} channels. Activation of metabotropic glutamate receptors (mGluR) and NK-1 metabotropic receptors by glutamate and substance P, respectively, will, via G protein–coupled signal transduction mechanisms, release Ca^{2+} from intracellular stores and also will elevate intracellular Ca^{2+} levels.[111] The elevated Ca^{2+} will in turn activate several calcium-dependent enzymes, including protein kinase C (PKC). PKC can phosphorylate the NMDA receptor. Phosphorylation of the NMDA receptor changes its properties such that the blockade of its ion channel by Mg^{2+}, which is normally present at resting membrane potentials, is reduced or eliminated.

This proposal has been evidenced by several lines of study and has been widely recognized. However, few electrophysiological studies have investigated spinal neurons in nerve injury models. It is unclear how changed neuronal responses and synaptic plasticity contribute to pain hypersensitivity. It is likely that central sensitization of spinal nociceptive neurons induced by the initial injury or by ongoing and/or ectopic activity in injured fibers is an important aspect of nerve injury pain.[112] Some studies have shown that the same conditioning stimulation fails to induce long-term potentiation (LTP) in the nerve-injured spinal cord,[113] although this LTP is evoked in the wider dynamic neurons of the spinal dorsal horn of normal animals. The threshold and peripheral receptive fields of C fibers and myelinated fibers become lower and bigger, and the baseline of the synaptic response tends to be higher, in rats with peripheral nerve injury.[99] These findings support the idea of pre-existing central sensitization of neurons. This sensitization is most likely to be triggered at the early period of nerve injury, such that additional increases in LTP are not attainable. Our recent unpublished studies have shown that this sensitization would happen within 2 hours after the initial injury. Additional studies have focused on this topic, and interesting new findings will be published shortly.

Changes in inhibitory activities in the spinal cord are of interest in the development of neuropathic pain. The inhibitory systems, including neurotransmitters and their receptors and interneurons, are found to be dysfunctional and to undergo degeneration and/or downregulation after nerve injury or damage. Decreases in tonic or phasic inhibition might contribute to pain hypersensitivity. Some studies have provided evidence that suggests this possibility.[86] Phasic and tonic types of inhibition are two major inhibitory controls that modulate the transmission of sensory information in the spinal dorsal horn. These inhibitory mechanisms operate via local interneurons and descending pathways from the brainstem via the classic inhibitory transmitters gamma-aminobutyric acid (GABA) and glycine, as well as through adrenergic, serotonergic, and enkephalinergic mechanisms. Both postsynaptic and presynaptic mechanisms are involved in the processing. Reconstruction of the patterns of primary afferents and of neurons within the dorsal horn following peripheral nerve injury is another possible mechanism underlying allodynia. Aβ fibers sprouting into the superficial laminae of the dorsal horn provide the basis for allodynia. This is an interesting idea that is supported[114-118] and is also challenged.[119] We have recently found that (1) peripheral nerve injury produces profound alterations in synaptic input to dorsal horn neurons mediated by non-nociceptive sensory neurons, and (2) activation of the NK-1 receptor may be involved in the enhanced synaptic response, thus contributing to tactile allodynia.[102] These findings support the general concept of phenotypical alterations in the dorsal horn of the spinal cord after peripheral nerve injury.

Recent studies have demonstrated that the Eph receptor tyrosine kinases and their ephrin ligands, which are involved in crucial aspects of nervous system circuit assembly during development, may regulate inflammatory pain processing.[120] We have recently provided strong evidence showing that ephrinB/EphB receptor signaling is involved in modulation of neuropathic pain after peripheral nerve injury.[121] Our new findings may reveal a novel mechanism underlying neuropathic pain in view of the development of the nervous systems and their damage,

and they strongly suggest that with ephrinB/EphB receptor signaling, probably other signals that are important to development[122] may be a new target of treatment for neuropathic pain. Another interesting finding is that activation of the spinal P2X4 receptor in hyperactive microglia is necessary for tactile allodynia and long-term plasticity in the dorsal horn of the spinal cord.[123,124]

Management of Neuropathic Pain

Neuropathic pain continues to pose clinical challenges. In the vast majority of cases, chronic neuropathic pain cannot be successfully treated with conventional analgesics and is resistant to oral opioids. Opioid sensitivity in neuropathic pain is a controversial issue within the scientific community. The array of therapeutic agents is multifaceted, but they are efficacious, to some extent, in only about half of patients. Effective new treatment strategies are desperately needed. Combinations of the treatments listed in the following paragraphs would benefit patients with neuropathic pain.[125]

Pharmacological Therapies. Choices may include opioids, antipyretic analgesics (nonsteroidals, acetaminophen, and phenazone derivatives), antidepressants (amitriptyline, maprotiline, selective serotonin reuptake inhibitors), anticonvulsants, local anesthetics, and mexiletine, baclofen, clonidine, ketamine, dextrorphan, and tramadol.

Psychological Treatments and Psychiatric Evaluation and Treatment. Be aware that neuropathic pain and other chronic pain are associated with a large number of psychiatric and psychological comorbidities, including depression, anxiety, drug dependence, somatoform disorders, and bipolar disorder.

Stimulation-Produced Analgesia. Several peripheral stimulation techniques that have been used to produce analgesia include TENS, acupuncture-like TENS, acupuncture, dry needle or electroacupuncture, vibration, and acupressure.

Surgical Pain Management. Surgical interventions include decompression, neuroma removal, neurotomy, glycerol injection, radiofrequency nerve/root lesion, dorsal root entry zone lesion, cordotomy, and stereotactic radiosurgery.

Traditional Chinese Medicine. See Complementary and Alternative Therapies.

Chiropractic and Spinal Manipulative Therapy. Recommended reading: Principles and practice of chiropractic. 3rd ed. New York: McGraw-Hill; 2005.

Activator-Assisted Spinal Manipulative Therapy. In addition to traditional manual spinal manipulative therapy (SMT), instruments such as the

Activator Adjusting Instrument have been used to produce spinal mobilization.[126] Activator was developed to precisely control the speed, force, and direction of adjustive thrusts, so a safe, reliable, and controlled force may be produced to adjust osseous spinal structures.[127,128] Activator evolved in response to current knowledge about biomechanical and neurophysiological categories of investigation. Under the biomechanical model, issues such as tissue compliance (stiffness), response to input force (impedance), and natural frequency resonance of the spine were explored. In neurophysiological investigations, threshold frequencies and minimal forces required for stimulation of joint mechanoreceptors were investigated.[126,129,130] We have recently documented potential mediating effects of SMT as performed with the Activator for pain and hyperalgesia produced by lumbar intervertebral foramen (IVF) inflammation in a small animal model; outcomes were assessed through behavioral, electrophysiological, and pathological approaches.[103]

Activator-assisted SMT applied on the L5, L6, or L5 and L6 spinous processes (Figure 4-6) can significantly reduce the severity and duration of thermal and mechanical hyperalgesia, as produced by IVF inflammation at L5. This effect may result from Activator-assisted SMT-induced faster elimination of inflammation and the recovery of excitability of inflamed DRG neurons attained by improving blood and nutrition supplements to the DRG within the affected IVF. This study suggests that manipulation of a specific spinal segment may play an important role in optimizing recovery from lesions involving IVF inflammation.

Complementary and Alternative Therapies. Complementary and alternative therapies (CATs) may be regarded as those that are used alongside conventional medicine, and alternative therapies as those used instead of conventional medicine. Be aware that the distinction is unclear between therapies considered to be CATs as opposed to mainstream medicine. Therefore some therapies described previously may be classified into conventional medicine and CATs. The National Center for Complementary and Alternative Medicine (NCCAM; part of the National Institutes of Health) classifies CATs into five categories:

1. Alternative medical systems are built on complete systems of theory and practice. Some are much older than conventional medicine (e.g., traditional Chinese medicine), and others have developed within Western culture (e.g., homeopathic medicine).

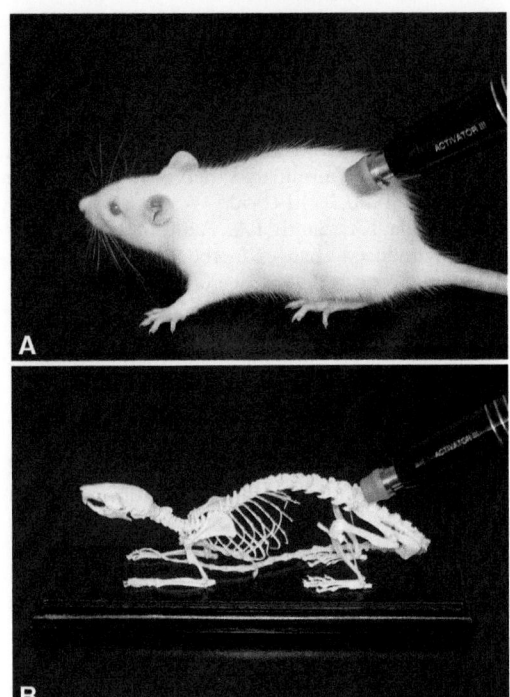

Figure 4-6 Methods of Activator-assisted spinal manipulative therapy applied to the lumbar spinous process in the rat. The location and direction of the Activator applied to the lumbar spinous process are shown in a real experimental rat **(A)** and in an artificial rat skeleton **(B)**. *(From Song XJ, Gan Q, Cao JL, Wang ZB, Rupert RL. Spinal manipulation reduces pain and hyperalgesia after lumbar intervertebral foramen inflammation in the rat. J Manipulative Physiol Ther. 2006;29[1]:5-13.)*

2. Mind-body interventions use techniques designed to enhance the mind's capacity to affect bodily function and symptoms. Some (e.g., cognitive-behavioral therapy) are mainstream; others are considered complementary and alternative medicine (e.g., mental healing).

3. Biologically based therapies use substances found in nature, such as herbs, foods, and vitamins. Some supplements are used in conventional medicine.

4. Manipulative and body-based methods are based on manipulation and/or movement of one or more parts of the body (e.g., chiropractic, osteopathy).

5. Energy therapies involve the use of energy fields. Biofield therapies affect energy fields that purportedly surround and penetrate the human body (e.g., Reiki, therapeutic touch). Bioelectromagnetics-based therapies involve the unconventional use of electromagnetic fields (e.g., magnetic fields).

REFERENCES

1. Kandel ER, Schwartz JH, Jessell TM. Principles of neural science. 3rd ed. Norwalk (CT): Appleton & Lange; 1992. p. 341-99.
2. Waxman SG. Determinants of conduction velocity in myelinated nerve fibers. Muscle Nerve. 1980;3(2):141-50.
3. Abdulla FA, Smith PA. Axotomy- and autotomy-induced changes in the excitability of rat dorsal root ganglion neurons. J Neurophysiol. 2001;85(2):630-43.
4. Song XJ, Hu SJ, Greenquist KW, Zhang JM, LaMotte RH. Mechanical and thermal hyperalgesia and ectopic neuronal discharge after chronic compression of dorsal root ganglia. J Neurophysiol. 1999;82(6):3347-58.
5. Zhang JM, Song XJ, LaMotte RH. Enhanced excitability of sensory neurons in rats with cutaneous hyperalgesia produced by chronic compression of the dorsal root ganglion. J Neurophysiol. 1999;82(6):3359-66.
6. Besson JM, Chaouch A. Peripheral and spinal mechanisms of nociception. Physiol Rev. 1987;67(1):67-186.
7. Campbell JN, Raja SN, Cohen RH, Manning DC, Khan AA, Meyer RA. Peripheral neural mechanisms of nociception. In: Wall PD, Melzack R, editors. Textbook of pain. 2nd ed. Edinburgh: Churchill Livingstone; 1989. p. 22-45.
8. Dubner R, Gebhart GF, Bond MR. Pain research and clinical management. Amsterdam: Elsevier; 1988.
9. Fields HL. Pain. New York: McGraw-Hill; 1987.
10. LaMotte RH. Can the sensitization of nociceptors account for hyperalgesia after skin injury? Human Neurobiol. 1984;3(1):47-52.
11. Light AR, Perl ER. Peripheral sensory systems. In: Dyck PJ, Thomas PK, Lambert EH, Bunge R, editors. Peripheral neuropathy. 2nd ed. Philadelphia: Saunders; 1984. p. 210-30.
12. Myers RR. The neuropathology of nerve injury and pain. In: Weinstein JN, Gordon SL, editors. Low back pain: a scientific and clinical overview Rosemont (IL): American Academy of Orthopaedic Surgeons; 1996. p. 247-64.
13. Junger H, Sorkin LS. Nociceptive and inflammatory effects of subcutaneous TNFalpha. Pain. 2000;85(1-2):145-51.
14. Joshi SK, Gebhart GF. Visceral pain. Curr Rev Pain. 2000;4(6):499-506.
15. Westlund KN. Visceral nociception. Curr Rev Pain. 2000;4(6):478-87.
16. Song XJ, Zhao ZQ. Involvement of NMDA and non-NMDA receptors in transmission of spinal visceral nociception in cat. Acta Pharmacol Sin. 1999;20(4):308-12.
17. Iversen S, Iversen L, Saper CB. The autonomic nervous system and the hypothalamus. In: Kandel ER, Schwartz JH, Jessell TM, editors. Principles of neural science. 4th ed. New York: McGraw-Hill; 2000. p. 965-69.
18. Iggo A, Andres KH. Morphology of cutaneous receptors. Annu Rev Neurosci. 1982;5:1-31.
19. Iggo A. Cutaneous and subcutaneous sense organs. Br Med Bull. 1977;33(2):97-102.
20. Johnson KO, Hsiao SS. Neural mechanisms of tactile form and texture perception. Annu Rev Neurosci. 1992;15:227-50.
21. Gardner EP, Martin JH, Jessell TM. The bodily senses. In: Kandel ER, Schwartz JH, Jessell TM, editors. Principles of neural science. 4th ed. New York: McGraw-Hill; 2000. p. 430-2.
22. Sur M, Wall JT, Kaas JH. Modular distribution of neurons with slowly adapting and rapidly adapting responses in area 3b of somatosensory cortex in monkeys. J Neurophysiol. 1984;51(4):724-44.
23. Solomonow M, Krogsgaard M. Sensorimotor control of knee stability: a review. Scand J Med Sci Sports. 2001;11(2):64-80.
24. Darian-Smith I, Goodwin A, Sugitani M, Heywood J. The tangible features of textured surfaces: their representation in the monkey's somatosensory cortex. In: Edelman G, Gall WE, Cowan WM, editors. Dynamic aspects of neocortical functions. New York: Wiley; 1984. p. 475-500.
25. Rexed B. The cytoarchitectonic organization of the spinal cord in the cat. J Comp Neurol. 1952;96(3):414-95.
26. Hendelman WJ. Atlas of functional neuroanatomy. Boca Raton (FL): CRC Press; 2001. p. 8-10, 96.
27. Light AR, Perl ER. Differential termination of large- and small-diameter primary afferent fibers in the spinal dorsal gray matter as indicated by labeling with horseradish peroxidase. Neurosci Lett. 1977;6:59-63.
28. Culberson JL, Brown PB. Projection of hindlimb dorsal roots to lumbosacral spinal cord of cat. J Neurophysiol. 1984;51(3):516-28.
29. Light AR, Perl ER. Spinal termination of functionally identified primary afferent neurons with slowly conducting myelinated fibers. J Comp Neurol. 1979;186(2):133-50.
30. Abrahams VC, Richmonds FJ, Keane J. Projection from C2 and C3 nerves supplying muscles and skin of the cat neck: a study using transganglionic transport of horseradish peroxidase. J Comp Neurol. 1984;230(1):142-54.
31. Melzack R, Wall PD. Pain mechanisms: a new theory. Science. 1965;150(699):971-9.
32. Jessell TM, Kelly DD. Pain and analgesia. In: Kandel ER, Schwartz JH, Jessell TM, editors. Principles of neural science. 4th ed. New York: McGraw-Hill; 2000. p. 385-99.
33. Martin JH, Jessell TM. Anatomy of the somatic sensory system. In: Kandel ER, Schwartz JH, Jessell TM, editors. Principles of neural science. 4th ed. New York: McGraw-Hill; 2000. p. 353-65.
34. Willis WD. Nociceptive pathways: anatomy and physiology of nociceptive ascending pathways. Philos Trans R Soc Lond B Biol Sci. 1985;308(1136):253-7.

35. Willis WD Jr, Zhang X, Honda CN, Giesler GJ, Jr. Projections from the marginal zone and deep dorsal horn to the ventrobasal nuclei of the primate thalamus. Pain. 2001;92(1-2):267-76.

36. Craig AD, Bushnell MC. The thermal grill illusion: unmasking the burn of cold pain. Science. 1994;26(5169):252-5.

37. Craig AD, Bushnell MC, Zhang ET, Blomqvist A. A thalamic nucleus specific for pain and temperature sensation. Nature. 1994;372(6508): 770-3.

38. Craig AD, Reiman EM, Evans A, Bushnell MC. Functional imaging of an illusion of pain. Nature. 1996;384(6606):258-60.

39. Gardner EP, Kandel ER. Touch. In: Kandel ER, Schwartz JH, Jessell TM, editors. Principles of neural science. 4th ed. New York: McGraw-Hill; 2000. p. 451-70.

40. Haldeman S. The neurophysiology of spinal pain. In: Haldeman S, editor. The principles and practice of chiropractic. 2nd ed. Norwalk (CT): Appleton & Lange; 1992. p. 165-83.

41. Saper CB. Brain stem modulation of sensation, movement, and consciousness. In: Kandel ER, Schwartz JH, Jessell TM, editors. Principles of neural science. 4th ed. New York: McGraw-Hill; 2000. p. 889-900.

42. Iversen S, Kupfermann I, Kandel ER. Emotional states and feelings. In: Kandel ER, Schwartz JH, Jessell TM, editors. Principles of neural science. 4th ed. New York: McGraw-Hill; 2000. p. 982-95.

43. Wyke B. Neurological aspects of low back pain. In: Jayson M, editor. The lumbar spine and back pain. New York: Grune & Stratton; 1976.

44. Pearson K, Gordon J. Spinal reflexes. In: Kandel ER, Schwartz JH, Jessell TM, editors. Principles of neural science. 4th ed. New York: McGraw-Hill; 2000. p. 713-35.

45. Sato A. Spinal reflex physiology. In: Haldeman S, editor. The principle and practice of chiropractic. 2nd ed. Norwalk (CT): Appleton & Lange; 1992. p. 91-2.

46. Krakauer J, Ghez C. Voluntary movement. In: Kandel ER, Schwartz JH, Jessell TM, editors. Principles of neural science. 4th ed. New York: McGraw-Hill; 2000. p. 756-79.

47. Basbaum A, Jessell TM. The perception of pain. In: Kandel ER, Schwartz JH, Jessell TM, editors. Principles of neural science. 4th ed. New York: McGraw-Hill; 2000. p. 477-9.

48. Dickenson AH. A cure for wind up: NMDA receptor antagonists as potential analgesics. Trends Pharmacol Sci. 1990;11(8):307-9.

49. Mendell LM. Physiological properties of unmyelinated fiber projections to the spinal cord. Exp Neurol. 1966;16:316-32.

50. Neumann S, Doubell TP, Leslie T, Woolf CJ. Inflammatory pain hypersensitivity mediated by phenotypic switch in myelinated primary sensory neurons. Nature. 1996;384(6607):360-4.

51. Woolf CJ. An overview of the mechanisms of hyperalgesia. Pulm Pharmacol. 1995;8(4-5): 161-7.

52. Woolf CJ. Pain. Neurobiol Dis. 2000;7(5):504-10.

53. Chang HT, Ji ZP, Huang JS. The study of acupuncture. Beijing: Science Press; 1986.

54. Zhang XT, Ji ZP, Huang JS. Acupuncture research. Beijing: Science Press; 1986.

55. Jessell TM, Kelly DD. Pain and analgesia. In: Kandel DD, Schwartz ER, Jessell JH, editors. Principles of neural science. 3rd ed. Norwalk (CT): Appleton & Lange; 1992. p. 392-5.

56. Kalra A, Urban MO, Sluka KA. Blockade of opioid receptors in rostral ventral medulla prevents antihyperalgesia produced by transcutaneous electrical nerve stimulation (TENS). J Pharmacol Exp Ther. 2001;298(1):257-63.

57. Akil H, Mayer DJ, Liebeskind JC. Antagonism of stimulation-induced analgesia by naloxone, a narcotic antagonist. Science. 1976;191:961-2.

58. Mansour A, Watson SJ, Akil H. Opioid receptors: past, present and future. Trends Neurosci. 1995;18(2):69-70.

59. Sohn JH, Lee BH, Park SH, Ryu JW, Kim BO, Park YG. Microinjection of opiates into the periaqueductal gray matter attenuates neuropathic pain symptoms in rats. Neuroreport. 2000;11(7):1413-6.

60. Unterwald EM. Regulation of opioid receptors by cocaine. Ann N Y Acad Sci. 2001;937:74-92.

61. Dubner R, Hargreaves KM. The neurobiology of pain and its modulation. Clin J Pain. 1989; 5(Suppl 2):S1-6.

62. Fields LH, Anderson SD. Evidence that raphe spinal neurons mediate opiate and midbrain stimulation-produced analgesia. Pain. 1978;5(4): 333-49.

63. Kuhar MJ, Pert CB, Snyder SM. Regional distribution of opiate receptor binding in monkey and human brain. Nature. 1973;245(5426): 447-50.

64. van Haaren F, Scott S, Tucker LB. Kappa-opioid receptor–mediated analgesia: hotplate temperature and sex differences. Eur J Pharmacol. 2000;408(2):153-9.

65. Messing RB, Lytle LD. Serotonin-containing neurons: their possible role in pain and analgesia. Pain. 1977;4(1):1-21.

66. Merskey H, Bogduk N. Classification of chronic pain: descriptions of chronic pain syndromes and definitions of pain terms. 2nd ed. Seattle: International Association for the Study of Pain Press; 1994. p. 222.

67. Hanson PT, Lacerenza M, Marchettini P. Aspects of clinical and experimental neuropathic pain: the clinical perspective. In: Hanson PT, Fields HL, Hill RG, Marchettini P, editors. Neuropathic pain: pathophysiology and treatment, progress in pain research and management. Vol. 21. Seattle: International Association for the Study of Pain Press; 2001. p. 1-18.

68. Kim SH, Chung JM. An experimental model for peripheral neuropathy produced by segmental spinal nerve ligation in the rat. Pain. 1992;50(3): 355-63.

69. Bennett GJ, Xie YK. A peripheral mononeuropathy in rat that produces disorders of pain sensation like those seen in man. Pain. 1988;33(1): 87-107.

70. Hu SJ, Xing J. An experimental model for chronic compression of dorsal root ganglion produced by intervertebral foramen stenosis in the rat. Pain. 1998;77(1):15-23.

71. Song XJ, Vizcarra C, Xu DS, Rupert RL, Wong ZN. Hyperalgesia and neural excitability following injuries to central and peripheral branches of axons and somata of dorsal root ganglion neurons. J Neurophysiol. 2003;89 (4):2185-93.

72. Devor M. The pathophysiology of damaged peripheral nerves. In: Wall PD, Melzack R, editors. Textbook of pain. 3rd ed. London: Churchill Livingstone; 1994. p. 79-100.

73. Stebbing MJ, Eschenfelder S, Habler HJ, Acosta MC, Janig W, McLachlan EM. Changes in the action potential in sensory neurones after peripheral axotomy in vivo. Neuroreport. 1999;10(2): 201-6.

74. Abdulla FA, Smith PA. Axotomy- and autotomy-induced changes in Ca^{2+} and K^+ channel currents of rat dorsal root ganglion neurons. J Neurophysiol. 2001;85(2):644-58.

75. Amir R, Michaelis M, Devor M. Burst discharge in primary sensory neurons: triggered by subthreshold oscillations, maintained by depolarizing afterpotentials. J Neurosci. 2002;22(3): 1187-98.

76. Amir R, Kocsis JD, Devor M. Multiple interacting sites of ectopic spike electrogenesis in primary sensory neurons. J Neurosci. 2005;25(10): 2576-85.

77. Wagner R, Myers RR. Schwann cells produce tumor necrosis factor alpha: expression in injured and non-injured nerves. Neuroscience. 1996;73(3):625-9.

78. Tonra JR, Curtis R, Wong V, Cliffer KD, Park JS, Timmes A, et al. Axotomy upregulates the anterograde transport and expression of brain-derived neurotrophic factor by sensory neurons. J Neurosci. 1998;18(11):4374-83.

79. George A, Schmidt C, Weishaupt A, Toyka KV, Sommer C. Serial determination of tumor necrosis factor-alpha content in rat sciatic nerve after chronic constriction injury. Exp Neurol. 1999;160(1):124-32.

80. Hu P, McLachlan EM. Macrophage and lymphocyte invasion of dorsal root ganglia after peripheral nerve lesions in the rat. Neuroscience. 2002;112(1):23-38.

81. Schäfers M, Geis C, Brors D, Yaksh TL, Sommer C. Anterograde transport of tumor necrosis factor-alpha in the intact and injured rat sciatic nerve. J Neurosci. 2002;22(2):536-45.

82. Walters ET, Ambron RT. Long-term alterations induced by injury and by 5-HT in Aplysia sensory neurons: convergent pathways and common signals? Trends Neurosci. 1995;18(3): 137-42.

83. Ambron R, Walters ET. Priming events and retrograde injury signals: a new perspective on the cellular and molecular biology of nerve regeneration. Mol Neurobiol. 1996;13(1):61-79.

84. Ambron RT, Zhang XP, Gunstream JD, Povelones M, Walters ET. Intrinsic injury signals enhance growth, survival, and excitability of Aplysia neurons. J Neurosci. 1996;16(23):7469-77.

85. Gunstream JD, Castro GA, Walters ET. Retrograde transport of plasticity signals in Aplysia sensory neurons following axonal injury. J Neurosci. 1995;15(1 Pt 1):439-48.

86. Hökfelt T, Zhang X, Xu ZQ, Ji RR, Shi T, Cirness J, et al. Phenotype regulation in dorsal root ganglion neurons after nerve injury: focus on peptides and their receptors. In: Borsook D, editor. Molecular neurobiology of pain, progress in pain research and management. Vol. 9. Seattle: International Association for the Study of Pain; 1997.

87. Waxman SG. The molecular pathophysiology of pain: abnormal expression of sodium channel genes and its contributions to hyperexcitability of primary sensory neurons. Pain. 1999;(Suppl 6): S133-40.

88. Waxman SG, Cummins TR, Dib-Hajj SD, Black JA. Voltage-gated sodium channels and the molecular pathogenesis of pain: a review. J Rehabil Res Dev. 2000;37(5):517-28.

89. Rizzo MA, Kocsis JD, Waxman SG. Selective loss of slow and enhancement of fast Na^+ currents in cutaneous afferent dorsal root ganglion neurones following axotomy. Neurobiol Dis. 1995;2(2):3-12.

90. Everill B, Kocsis JD. Reduction in potassium current in identified cutaneous afferent dorsal root ganglion neurons after axotomy. J Neurophysiol. 1999;82(2):700-8.

91. Baccei ML, Kocsis JD. Voltage-gated calcium currents in axotomized adult rat cutaneous afferent neurons. J Neurophysiol. 2000;83(4): 2227-38.

92. Xiao HS, Huang QH, Zhang FX, Bao L, Lu YJ, Guo C, et al. Identification of gene expression profile of dorsal root ganglion in the rat peripheral axotomy model of neuropathic pain. Proc Natl Acad Sci U S A. 2002;99(12):8360-5.

93. Moore KA, Kohno T, Karchewski LA, Scholz J, Baba H, Woolf CJ. Partial peripheral nerve injury promotes a selective loss of GABAergic inhibition in the superficial dorsal horn of the spinal cord. J Neurosci. 2002;22(15):6724-31.

94. Liu CN, Wall PD, Ben-Dor E, Michaelis M, Amir R, Devor M. Tactile allodynia in the absence of C-fiber activation: altered firing properties of DRG neurons following spinal nerve injury. Pain. 2000;85(3):503-21.

95. Obata K, Yamanaka H, Fukuoka T, Yi D, Tokunaga A, Hashimoto N, et al. Contribution of injured and uninjured dorsal root ganglion neurons to pain behavior and the changes in gene expression following chronic constriction injury of the sciatic nerve in rats. Pain. 2003;101(1-2):65-77.

96. Malcangio M, Ramer MS, Jones MG, McMahon SB. Abnormal substance P release from the spinal cord following injury to primary sensory neurons. Eur J Neurosci. 2000;12(1):397-9.

97. Marchand JE, Wurm WH, Kato T, Kream RM. Altered tachykinin expression by dorsal root ganglion neurons in a rat model of neuropathic pain. Pain. 1994;58(2):219-31.

98. Ma WY, Bisby MA. Increase of preprotachykinin mRNA and substance P immunoreactivity in spared dorsal root ganglion neurons following partial sciatic nerve injury. Eur J Neurosci. 1998;10(7):2388-99.

99. Pitcher GM, Henry JL. Nociceptive response to innocuous mechanical stimulation is mediated via myelinated afferents and NK-1 receptor activation in a rat model of neuropathic pain. Exp Neurol. 2004;186(2):173-97.

100. Cahill CM, Coderre TJ. Attenuation of hyperalgesia in a rat model of neuropathic pain after intrathecal pre- or post-treatment with a neurokinin-1 antagonist. Pain. 2002;95(3):277-85.

101. Meert TF, Vissers K, Greenen F, Kontinen VK. Functional role of exogenous administration of substance P in chronic constriction injury model of neuropathic pain in gerbils. Pharmacol Biochem Behav. 2003;76(1):17-25.

102. Zheng JH, Song XJ. αβ-Afferents activate neurokinin-1 receptor in dorsal horn neurons after nerve injury. Neuroreport. 2005;16(7): 715-9.

103. Song XJ, Wang ZB, Gan Q, Walters ET. cAMP and cGMP contribute to sensory neuron hyperexcitability and hyperalgesia in rats with dorsal root ganglia compression. J Neurophysiol. 2006;95:479-92.

104. Zheng JH, Walters ET, Song XJ. Dissociation of dorsal root ganglion neurons induces hyperexcitability that is maintained by increased responsiveness to cAMP and cGMP. J Neurophysiol. 2007;97:15-25.

105. Jensen TS, Gottrup H, Sindrup SH, Bach FW. The clinical picture of neuropathic pain. Eur J Pharmacol. 2001;429(1-3):1-11.

106. Burgess SE, Gardell LR, Ossipov MH, Malan TP Jr, Vanderah TW, Lai J, et al. Time-dependent descending facilitation from the rostral ventromedial medulla maintains, but not initiates, neuropathic pain. J Neurosci. 2002;22(12): 5129-36.

107. Lin Q, Palecek J, Paleckova V, Peng YB, Wu J, Cui ML, et al. Nitric oxide mediates the central sensitization of primate spinathalamic tract neurons. J Neurophysiol. 1999;81(3):1075-85.

108. Sanderkühler J, Liu XG. Induction of long-term potentiation at spinal synapses by noxious stimulation or nerve injury. Eur J Neurosci. 1998;10:2476-80.

109. Sotgiu ML, Beilla G. Contribution of central sensitization to the pain-related abnormal activity in neuropathic rats. Somatosens Mot Res. 2000;17(1):32-8.

110. Woolf CJ. Molecular signal responsible for the reorganization of the synaptic circuitry of the dorsal horn after peripheral nerve injury:the mechanisms of tactile allodynia. In: Borsook D, editor. Molecular neurobiology of pain, progress in pain research and management. Vol. 9. Seattle: International Association for the Study of Pain Press; 1997.

111. Mayer ML, Miller RJ. Excitatory amino acid receptors, second messengers and regulation of intracellular Ca^{2+} in mammalian neurons. Trends Pharmacol Sci. 1990;11(6):254-60.

112. Woolf CJ, Mannion RJ [review]. Neuropathic pain: aetiology, symptoms, mechanisms, and management. Lancet. 1999;353(9168):1959-64.

113. Rygh LJ, Kontinen VK, Suzuki R, Dickenson AH. Different increase in C-fibre evoked responses after nociceptive conditioning stimulation in sham-operated and neuropathic rats. Neurosci Lett. 2000;288(2):99-102.

114. Woolf CJ, Shortland P, Coggeshall RE. Peripheral nerve injury triggers central sprouting of myelinated afferents. Nature. 1992;355 (6355):75-8.

115. Woolf CJ, Shortland P, Reynolds M, Ridings J, Doubell T, Coggeshall RE. Reorganization of central terminals of myelinated primary afferents in the rat dorsal horn following peripheral axotomy. J Comp Neurol. 1995;360(1): 121-34.

116. Kohama I, Ishikawa K, Kocsis JD. Synaptic reorganization in the substantia gelatinosa after peripheral nerve neuroma formation: aberrant innervation of lamina II neurons by αβ afferents. J Neurosci. 2000;20(4):1538-49.

117. Okamoto M, Baba H, Goldstein PA, Higashi H, Shimoji K, Yoshimura M. Functional reorganization of sensory pathways in the rat spinal dorsal horn following peripheral nerve injury. J Physiol. 2001;532(Pt 1):241-50.

118. White FA, Kocsis JD. A-fiber sprouting in spinal cord dorsal horn is attenuated by proximal nerve stump encapsulation. Exp Neurol. 2002;177(2):385-95.

119. Hughes DI, Scott DT, Todd AJ, Riddell JS. Lack of evidence for sprouting of αβ afferents into the superficial laminas of the spinal cord dorsal horn after nerve section. J Neurosci. 2003;23(29):9491-9.

120. Battaglia AA, Sehayek K, Grist J, McMahon SB, Gavazzi I. EphB receptors and ephrin-B ligands regulate spinal sensory connectivity and modulate pain processing. Nat Neurosci. 2003;6(4):339-40.

121. Zheng JH, Cao JL, Song XJ. EphrinB activation of EphB receptors is critical for production and persistence of hyperalgesia and hyperexcitability of spinal dorsal horn neurons after peripheral nerve injury [abstract]. Presented at the Society for Neuroscience Meeting; 2005 Nov 12-16; Washington, DC.

122. Liu YB, Shi J, Lu CC, Wang ZB, Song XJ, Zou YM. Ryk-mediated Wnt repulsion regulates posterior-directed growth of corticospinal tract. Nat Neurosci. 2005;8(9):1151-9.

123. Tsuda T, Shigemoto-Mogami Y, Koizumi S, Mizokoshi A, Kohsaka S, Salter MW, et al. P2X4 receptor induced in spinal microglia gate tactile allodynia after nerve injury. Nature. 2003;424(6950):778-83.

124. Ma JY, Zhao ZQ. The involvement of glia in long-term plasticity in the spinal dorsal horn of the rat. Neuroreport. 2002;13(14): 1781-4.

125. Charlton JE, editor. Core curriculum for professional education in pain. 3rd ed. Seattle: International Association for the Study of Pain Press; 2005. p. 63-117.

126. Fuhr AW, Menke JM. Activator Methods chiropractic technique. Top Clin Chiropr. 2002;9(3): 30-43.

127. Osterbauer P, Fuhr AW, Keller TS. Description and analysis of Activator Methods chiropractic technique. Adv Chiropr. 1995;2:471-520.

128. Richard DR. The Activator story: development of a new concept in chiropractic. Chiropr J Austr. 1994;24(1):28-32.

129. Fuhr AW, Smith DB. Accuracy of piezoelectric accelerometers measuring displacement of a spinal adjusting instrument. J Manipulative Physiol Ther. 1986;9(1):15-21.

130. Smith DB, Fuhr AW, Davis BP. Skin accelerometer displacement and relative bone movement of adjacent vertebrae in response to chiropractic percussion thrusts. J Manipulative Physiol Ther. 1989;12(1):26-37.

SECTION II

CLINICAL OBSERVATIONS AND ADVANCED ASSESSMENT PROCEDURES

SECTION II

5

LEG LENGTH REACTIVITY

Rebecca S. Fischer

COMPONENTS AND THEORIES OF SPINAL STABILIZATION

We are, by nature, bipedal beings. Instinctively during infancy, neurological kinetic chains develop and mature and involve movements such as raising the head, rolling over, sitting up, crawling, standing, and eventually, walking (Figure 5-1). Our upright posture and walking is maintained by a unique neurological chain of reacting events. Every action, conscious or unconscious, is coordinated and is orchestrated through the neurological system. The nervous system applies constant checks and balances; this occurs through the feedback of mechanoreceptors when one is *preparing* to access and *during* the accessing of a biomechanical joint.

Mechanoreceptors, nociceptors, and proprioceptors communicate to the nervous system a stream of information from the muscles, ligaments, tendons, discs, cartilage, articular cartilage, synovial pressure, blood vessels, bone, and possibly, the myofascial connective tissue webbing system,[1] thereby coordinating the joints for just the right amount of mobility while stability for the action is maintained. This feedback loop, which is used to coordinate intended movements, takes into account the anticipated speed of movement and anticipated resistance.[2]

Stability and mobility must occur in the correct proportions if a healthy joint is to be maintained. A joint that is dysfunctional because of hypomobility or because of hypermobility causes problems and results in changes to the integrity and health of all related structures. The *repetition* of abnormal movement has compensating consequences and may result in disc degeneration, osteophyte formation, tightening of ligaments and muscles, or overstretching of tendons and ligaments, as well as the formation of myofascial adhesions. Abnormal neurobiomechanics outside of the neutral zone[3] creates an overall weakening at the joint, making it more susceptible to further injury and accelerating degeneration. A series

(cascade) of consequences are noted for joints associated with the malfunctioning joint, and learned patterns of neurological adaptation become imbedded in the nervous system. Even after correction of abnormal movement and the patient *appears* asymptomatic, the neurological effect can continue for months by remaining facilitated and therefore in a chronic state of subthreshold segmental excitation.[4]

Neuroarticular function can be assessed through the systematic evaluation of leg lengths and their reactivity throughout the course of ankle dorsiflexion and plantar flexion coupled with knee flexion and hip extension.[5] Feed forward mechanisms are activated from this passive movement via mechanoreceptors, proprioceptors, and nociceptors in the nervous system that have come from all involved structures. Neurological chains of information isolated within a malfunctioning biomechanical unit will feed back through the nervous system, creating an error in muscular activation; this can be visualized as a change in leg length. Leg length reactivity can then be assessed and incorporated into a system of analysis, so the need for adjustment can be determined and the aberrant neurobiomechanical unit can be measured post adjustment.

Biomechanical models of Keifer et al.[6,7] have defined spinal stability in terms of the compressive load-bearing capacity of the spine, and they have included pelvic rotation in the models of neutral posture. Previous beliefs and models of spinal stability considered that the spine is, by its structure alone, anatomically stable and capable of supporting gravity loads. However, through research this has been disputed and reveals the importance of the multifidus muscles as part of the local segmental control of the spine. The multifidus muscles are critical for spinal stability and for their role in decreasing the forces on global muscles. In addition, it was found that the compressive load-bearing capacity of the passive thoracolumbar spine (TLS) could be significantly enhanced through the use of varying amounts of pelvic rotation,

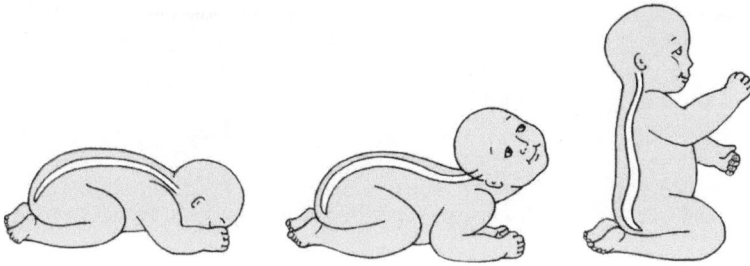

Figure 5-1 Neurological kinetic chains of developmental stages from infancy to walking. *(From Muscolino JE. Kinesiology: the skeletal system and muscle function. Enhanced edition. St. Louis: Mosby; 2006.)*

which allows for minimal muscular force. Research has been conducted to identify feasible mechanisms for maintaining spinal stability in neutral posture. This model was motivated by the observation of low levels of activity in the trunk muscles of live subjects when an upright posture was maintained.

Load-bearing capacity refers to the notion of stability in axial compression and the compressive strength of the system. Three different load centers were studied, and in all scenarios, pelvic rotation was seen to substantially stiffen the response of the TLS, so that physiologic loads could be carried with relatively small displacements to neutral posture. Pelvic rotations have been observed in neutral posture invivo and are affected by the magnitude of the compressive load and by spinal geometry.[7a,7b] Results point to the strong dependence of optimal pelvic rotation on spinal configuration. It appears that pelvic rotation stabilizes the TLS by increasing lordosis. Investigators determined that small muscle activation combined with pelvic rotation could fully exploit the passive load-bearing potential of the TLS by controlling spinal deformation, thus reducing movement from neutral postures. "The actions of muscles and pelvic rotation are postulated to be coordinated by a neural controller, with the horizontal translation at T1 being a likely feedback parameter."[6]

This research is significant in that pelvic rotation is the starting point for analysis and treatment in the Activator Method (AM). Functionally, pelvic leveling must be achieved or improved before one can progress to analysis and treatment of the spine. Pelvic distortion or rotation can be a factor in spinal stability throughout neutral postures, and this contributes to the appearance of Leg Length Inequality (LLI) reactivity. In maintaining spinal stability, the antigravity muscles serve as a support system that is integrated through the central and peripheral nervous systems, linking each segment together into a kinetic chain. This kinetic chain is part of the neurophysiological mechanisms of the joint protection system, which can be altered through injury, pain, and the deloading/decrease in proprioceptive input. Alterations in the kinetic chain include the development of impairments in the joint protection mechanisms and the creation of movement impairment syndromes and musculoskeletal pain syndromes. The three factors of deloading, injury, and pain all may lead to changes in motor control at a segmental level; this creates a unique neurological pathway or kinetic chain that is individualized.[4,8] This kinetic chain can lead to an adaptive vicious cycle that eventually causes progressive and increasing disability.[9]

Panjabi[10] has proposed that three systems contribute to lumbopelvic stability: a passive subsystem, an active subsystem, and a neural control subsystem. The passive structure of the spine and pelvis contributes to the control of all elements of stability, and it incorporates osseous and articular structures with spinal ligaments. The *passive musculoskeletal subsystem* includes the vertebrae, facet articulations, intervertebral discs, spinal ligaments, and joint capsules, as well as the passive mechanical properties of muscle. This passive subsystem offers the greatest restraint at the end range of movement.

The *active musculoskeletal subsystem* provides the mechanical ability to stabilize the spinal segments through force generated from the muscles. All the muscles and tendons surrounding the spinal column that can apply force to the spinal column constitute the active subsystem.

The *neural and feedback subsystem* consists of various force and motion transducers, located in ligaments, tendons, and muscles, and neural control centers. The nervous system senses the requirements of stability and plans strategies to meet the perceived demands through this feedback subsystem. The nerves and the central nervous system determine the requirements for spinal stability by monitoring the various transducer signals, and they direct the active subsystem to provide needed stability. The nervous system must coordinate the muscle activity in advance of perceived challenges to the inherent stability and must coordinate responses to afferent feedback from unpredictable challenges (Figure 5-2).[10]

Panjabi contends that the three subsystems are conceptually interdependent components of the spinal stabilization system, wherein one system is capable of compensating for deficits that may occur in the other and all are functionally interdependent[3,10]:

A dysfunction of a component of any one of the subsystems may lead to one or more of the following three possibilities:

a. An immediate response from other subsystems to successfully compensate

b. A long-term adaptation response of one or more subsystems

c. An injury to one or more components of any subsystem.

It is conceptualized that the first response results in normal function, the second results in normal function but with an altered spinal stabilizing system, and the third leads to overall system dysfunction, producing, for example, low back pain. In situations where additional loads or complex postures are anticipated, the neural control unit may alter the muscle recruitment strategy, with the temporary goal of enhancing the spine stability beyond the normal requirements.[10]

The segmental mechanical control between vertebrae results from the actions of the multifidus, intertransversarii, and interspinales muscles, but their role may be more proprioceptive of the forces exerted; therefore they may be more involved in the feedback mechanisms that occur in concert with mechanoreceptor action. Coordination of input by the nervous system incorporates all systems and controls the level of lumbopelvic stability in advance of the imposed forces—the feed forward mechanism. For example, activity of the lumbopelvic stabilizing muscles occurs before movement of the upper and lower limbs in a predictable manner.

The feed forward mechanism occurs when the central nervous system predicts the effects that movement will have on the body and plans a sequence of muscle activity to overcome the potential forces that will be imparted. This prediction involves a coordinated effort of local and global systems to stabilize the spine, allowing for extremity movement and incorporating the impending speed and resistant forces that may occur during limb movement.[11,12] Data suggest that the central nervous system uses feed forward nondirective specific activity of the intrinsic local muscles to control the movement of the intervertebral segments, in coordination with superficial global muscles, to control spinal orientation.[13] If sudden unpredictable forces occur, the nervous system uses feedback-mediated control that may be processed on a reflexive level.

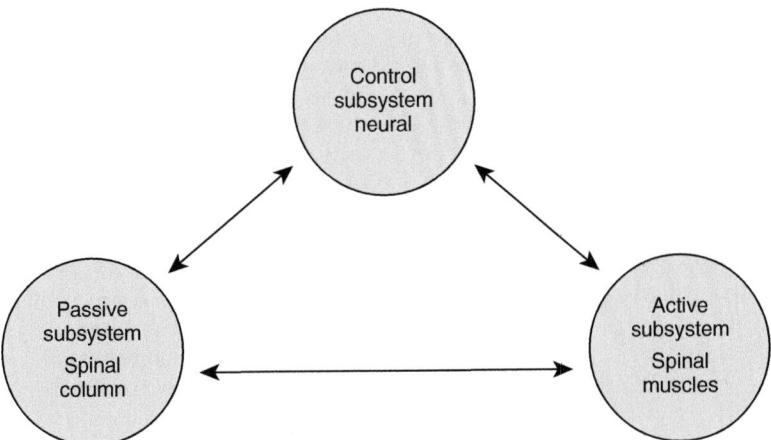

Figure 5-2 The stabilizing system of the spine. *(Modified from Panjabi MM. The stabilizing system of the spine. Part II. Neutral zone and stability hypothesis. J Spinal Disord. 1992;5[4]:390-7.)*

This is a long-loop reflex that involves information processed at higher levels of the central nervous system, including transcortical mechanisms. To maintain equilibrium and balance in the body, two strategies have been identified that involve ankle movement ("ankle strategy") or hip movement ("hip strategy").[14]

Through the feed forward mechanism, postural stability of the trunk may be controlled by stiffness in response to feedback from the mechanoreceptors and concurrent anticipated needs of the nervous system. The basic level of muscle stiffness occurs before the application of forces to the joint. Postural stability may be controlled by modulation of stiffness of the ankle muscles, which is a short reflex response.[15] Muscle stiffness is controlled through feedback from the mechanoreceptors of the muscle spindles and ligament afferents. The sensitivity of the sensory component of the muscle spindle results from the stretch reflex through gamma motoneurons. Feedback from mechanoreceptors in the lumbar disc and ligaments, along with the supraspinous ligament, contributes to control of stiffness in neutral posture, along with anticipated and *unexpected* forces that may occur.[16-19]

Evaluation of LLIs in a prone position, coupled with leg length reactivity or changes throughout varying degrees of ankle dorsiflexion, plantar flexion, knee flexion, hip extension, and sacroiliac and spinal movement, creates an avenue through which one can explore the neurology and biomechanical integrity of isolated joints throughout the anatomical chain. By combining feedback-mediated processes with feed forward mechanisms, using short-loop and long-loop reflexes, joint integrity is evaluated throughout the kinetic chain: stiffness, stability, translation, and rotation, along with soft tissue integration and motor control sequencing. These reactions involve processing in the central nervous system at the cortical level. This processing includes all of the compensating, chronic pain, and/or "spinal memory" learned patterns throughout the kinetic chain and may be part of the resultant leg length reactivity following Isolation, Pressure, and Stress Testing.

TERMS, DEFINITIONS, AND DIFFERENTIATION OF LEG LENGTH INEQUALITY

The AM uses Leg Length Analysis (LLA) in determining when, where, and when not to adjust. Debate has been ongoing for years regarding the importance of the degree or amount of LLI among the professions of chiropractic, osteopathic, orthopedic, and physical therapy. In standing postures alone, the gravitational effects of foot pronation coupled with pelvic rotation lead to multiple anatomical sites of reactive compensatory postures and muscular imbalances. Debate persists over the causes of LLI versus its consequences throughout the anatomical chain and the contribution of weight-bearing postures to LLI. A short leg, LLI, anatomical short leg, functional short leg, and the reactive leg are often used interchangeably, but they are indeed different entities. It is important to look at and define these conditions because clinically determination of cause guides treatment selection.

Within the chiropractic profession, the diagnostic approach involves looking at the overall kinetic chains relative to complaints and symptoms. From a holistic point of view, we are concerned with how the patient appears and functions in weight-bearing postures and activities. We take radiographs in weight bearing, versus the standard non–weight bearing in the medical field, because we are concerned not only equally about pathology, but chiropractically we evaluate postures and distortions, signs of dysfunction. A radiograph gives us a view into long-standing, chronic patterns of adaptation if they are present. This could appear as decreased disc space, spondylitic formation around the articular surfaces, wedging of vertebrae, and scoliosis. A basic starting point is an anterior-posterior radiographic view of the pelvis and lumbar spine obtained to evaluate LLI through measurement of femoral head heights. The next step is to determine whether pelvic rotation is a factor in the differences in femoral head height, or whether an anatomical short leg is involved.

True anatomical LLI can be measured through various techniques and by the incorporation of bilateral radiographs of the lower extremities. The most accurate determinant is an anterior-to-posterior view of the pelvis with the central ray at femoral head height. A true anatomical short leg is defined as a difference in the size and/or length of the structures between the ground and the head of the femur. Growth asymmetry of the lower limbs may be inherited. Most causes of anatomical LLI involve trauma or surgery. Other causes can be seen as processes that disrupt the growth plate, such as cysts, osteomyelitis, and polio. Clinical significance increases as the degree of inequality rises, leading to recommendations for heel lifts or the addition of height to the footwear worn on the short leg side. This is looked at as a "static" condition. For example, a patient experiences a fracture of the femur as a child; this disrupts the growth plate, and a leg shorter by one inch results. Treatment, if initiated before skeletal maturity, would most likely include a heel lift or a built-up shoe because of a significant residual discrepancy. Untreated, this condition will have an effect on standing posture. During movement, it may produce advanced degeneration in the joints from repetitive abnormal stresses, along with the potential development of scoliosis and vertebral rotation.

When weight-bearing postures are evaluated, it is noted that a large portion of LLI arises from foot pronation. This creates a cascade of rotational compensations at the tibia, femur, and pelvis (Figure 5-3).

When the foot/ankle complex is in pronation during standing and during gait, inward (medial) rotation of the entire lower extremity results. This twisting movement of the leg is accentuated in persons who have excessive or prolonged pronation. This alteration in gait can eventually cause specific degenerative changes that may be seen in the pelvis,[20] spine,[21] and hip joints.[22] Resultant increased rotational forces are transmitted up the leg into the pelvis and have a particular effect on the sacroiliac joint.[23]

"The most common biomechanical problem in the lower extremity is excessive pronation."[24] Overpronation leads to numerous other conditions.

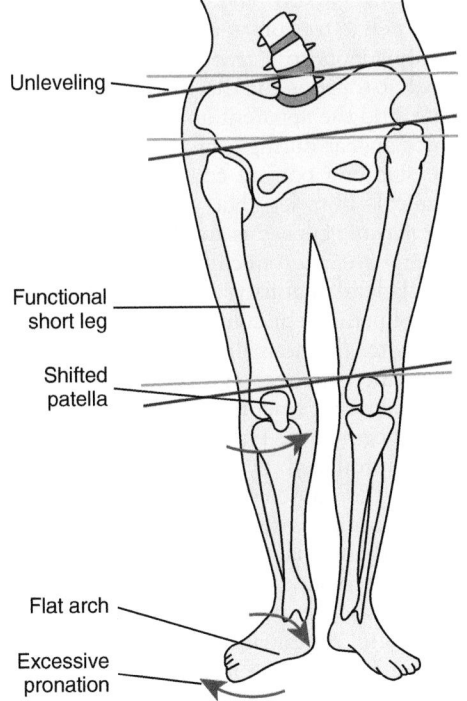

Unleveling

Functional
short leg

Shifted
patella

Flat arch

Excessive
pronation

Figure 5-3 Excessive pronation consequences.

Achilles tendonitis can occur as the result of overstressing forces at the Achilles tendon. Foot pronation greatly increases the probability of sustaining Achilles tendonitis, stress fractures of the tibia, tibial periostitis, and plantar fasciitis.[25] Tibial torsion (internal) rotation creates friction at the iliotibial band insertion on the lateral tibial plateau because of overstretching with resultant lateral knee pain and an iliotibial band syndrome. The extensor mechanism on the lateral aspect of the knee joint increases lateralization forces of the patella and increases the possibility of retropatellar pain, patellar tendonitis, and bursitis. A high risk for anterior cruciate ligament rupture has also been directly correlated with the amount and degree of observed pronation.[26] Patellofemoral instability and resultant anterior knee pain have been associated with external tibial rotation.[27] Overpronation can result in internal hip rotation, an anterior pelvic tilt, facet overload, and/or hamstring traction strain.

The traditional treatment of sprains and strains involves strengthening the damaged or weakened structure of the joint; however, the neurological aspect of rehabilitation is essential. Sprain produces altered proprioceptive input and predisposes the joint to recurring sprains.[28] To be beneficial, rehabilitation must include proprioceptive training to restore altered input to the muscles and structures that protect and stabilize the ankle.[29] Awareness and evaluation of the neurological control of the entire kinetic chain must therefore be performed as part of the treatment. If rehabilitation does not address proprioceptive training, neural control errors may become apparent through leg length reactivity.

Hyland recommends that when leg lengths are evaluated, the term *leg length discrepancy* (or *Leg Length Inequality* or *short leg*) should be used only when a patient's leg lengths are *asymmetrical while standing* and the spine is supported by the legs. In his opinion, a short leg can interfere with spinal/pelvic function only when the patient is standing upright and during gait.[30] Non–weight bearing measurements of leg length have been found to be unreliable.[31] Hyland states, "many variables (such as subluxations in the pelvis and spine, and muscle imbalances) affect the alignment and relative positioning of the legs and feet when a patient is prone or supine. In a relaxed, upright posture, these variables are no longer an issue." The only way to accurately assess for the possibility of a "true" anatomical short leg length discrepancy is to perform clinical and radiographic testing while the patient is in the standing, weight-bearing position.[32]

A functional short leg is defined as the difference in *alignment* of supporting structures between the ground and the femoral head. Unilateral excessive pronation can be a factor, along with knee valgus. In Hyland's opinion, a functional short leg cannot be caused by pelvic subluxations or lumbar muscle imbalances because these problems do not change the length of the leg (which ends at the femoral head) when the patient is standing. When a functional short leg is identified, the first goal of treatment is to improve the alignment of, and restore symmetry to, the lower extremities. Adjustments and exercises may be useful, but for long-term correction of excessive pronation, orthotic support is usually needed to balance functional leg lengths.[30] In the AM LLA, the Protocol begins at the knees and feet for most presentations of LLI in the prone position. The knees and feet are addressed before any pelvic distortions are treated, in keeping with Hyland's first goal of treatment.

Knutson recently reviewed the literature on and recommendations for clinical decision making in relation to anatomical and functional LLI.[33] Databases and library searches from 1970 through 2005 were conducted with the term "Leg Length Inequality." In this two-part publication, the first part reviewed the literature as it relates to the prevalence, magnitude, effects, and clinical significance of anatomical LLI. The prevalence of anatomical LLI obtained by accurate and reliable x-ray methods was found to be 90%; the mean was 5.2 mm (standard deviation [SD], 4.1). It was suggested by the evidence that for most people, anatomical LLI is not clinically significant until its magnitude reaches approximately 20 mm (approximately ¾ inch). Keep in mind, this is done with the patient in the weight-bearing, or upright, posture.

Knutson has described the functional "short leg," as we call it in AM, as unloaded leg length alignment asymmetry (LLAA), which is a "phenomenon much discussed and little understood." This phenomenon is also referred to as leg length reactivity. In reference to LLAA, Knutson proceeds to describe the LLA as used by the AM with the patient lying prone or supine; the pelvis is unloaded and the feet are examined for the presence of a "short leg," or alignment asymmetry. As he notes and agrees with Hyland, some believe that an anatomical short leg can be measured in this way, but the method is inadequate and unreliable.[33,34] The article continues to point out that examination of unloaded LLAA is a clinical test that is commonly used by chiropractors as a sign of "neuromuscular dysfunction."[33,35,36] The

authors raise the following questions: Can the unloaded leg check test be an indicator of an anatomic short leg? Is the test reliable and valid as an instrument to be used in measuring a functional "short leg"? Can LLAA findings be tainted by the presence of a true anatomical leg length discrepancy?

Some of the points in Knutson's article are important to consider. In the case of a "true anatomical short leg," long-term loading on the body can cause compensation that occurs through structural changes that become "normal" for that individual. The body adapts via Hueter Volkmann's law,[37] as the result of soft tissue changes,[38] and possibly through changes in lumbosacral facet angles.[21] Research was conducted to compare a device used to measure standing pelvic crest unleveling versus radiographs for anatomical LLI in asymptomatic patients. Intraexaminer and interexaminer reliability was found to be excellent, and validity was also determined.[39] However, when a low back pain group was assessed, the correlation between pelvic level and femoral head height was "substantially lower" in the low back pain group. "This indicates that some sort of functional pelvic tilt or torsion was present in the low back pain population that was unrelated to their anatomic LLI. While the decreased correlation between pelvic tilt and LLI in the back pain group was not examined relative to a functional short leg, the connection between back pain and the biomechanically unusual pelvic torsion stands out."[33] So it seems the body adapts to a true anatomical short leg with pelvic torsions and tilts that are used to compensate, and the apparent anatomically short leg may not appear during a prone LLA. A patient in the standing posture can appear to have an anatomical short leg, but upon prone LLA, it *may or may not* appear as an LLI.

When an anatomically short leg occurs before skeletal maturity, the body adapts with the use of permanent compensation. If a heel lift is added to the low iliac crest side in these patients, the body responds by increasing lateral lumbar flexion; it responds as if there was a level pelvis to begin with. These pre–skeletal maturity LLIs are produced by adaptive changes that occur in the muscles, ligaments, joints, and bones to compensate for imposed asymmetry. "Because these adaptive compensations to the LLI have become anatomic, they are not likely to change as the body moves from a loaded (standing) to an unloaded (supine, prone) position. The nervous system also appears to compensate, as was demonstrated in the study by Murrell et al.,[40] in which no loss of stability was observed in subjects with LLI, prompting investigators to point to 'long-term adaptation by the neuromuscular system.'"[33] If pre–skeletal maturity anatomical LLI adaptation or remodeling is considered normal when the patient is transitioning from standing to a prone position, patient leg lengths may appear to be even during the LLA.

Other studies show the persistence of pelvic torsion in subjects with anatomic LLI that occurred in both standing and sitting positions. In subjects with anatomic LLI in non–weight bearing positions, pelvic torsion persists, indicating that such torsion has been incorporated into the joints as the normal position.[41] Another study demonstrated that the side and magnitude of prone and especially supine "short legs" were not significantly correlated with radiographic anatomic LLI, indicating that they are separate phenomena.[42]

When the LLI is analyzed in non–weight bearing, the actual appearance of a short leg is thought to be due to hypertonicity of suprapelvic muscles.[38,43,44] Jemmett[45] believes that suprapelvic muscular hyperactivity is the result of "nervous system control errors" that cease to activate the small spinal stabilization muscles, principally the transverse abdominis and the multifidus. This leads to activation by the nervous system of the outer layer muscles (the large back and abdominal muscles) that provide primary movement to the trunk. Cooperstein has also stated that the short leg was "the consequence of ipsilateral suprapelvic muscular hyperactivity" because

> the sacrospinalis and quadratus lumborum muscles are hypertonic on the PI ilium side, but futile in their anti-gravitational attempt to pull up the pelvis and the sacral base in the standing position. Futility becomes triumphant as the patient is placed in the prone or supine position as these muscles are no longer trying to raise the pelvis against gravity, but only against the resistance afforded by the friction of the table exerted upon the recumbent patient. As a general rule, they succeed in laterally flexing the pelvis on the lumbar spine, raising the hip.[46]

A group of subjects were evaluated who did not have LLI but who did have LLAA. It was found that this group of subjects had significantly decreased endurance times for the erector and quadratus lumborum (QL) muscles.[47] This correlated with the side of LLAA being the side of the quadratus lumborum muscle that was quickest to fatigue; hypertonicity was a suspected cause of muscle fatigue. A study by Mincer et al.[48] found no correlation between anatomical LLI and altered muscle fatigue, providing further evidence that LLAA is a pathological process distinct from true LLI.

Further in Knutson,

> when standing, the actions of the QL depend on whether the spine or the pelvis is stabilized. If the pelvis is stabilized, QL contraction laterally flexes and extends the spine.[34,49,50] With the spine stable, QL contraction pulls cephalically through its attachment to the posterior aspect of the hemipelvis.[34,48] This load on the posterior aspect of the iliac crest could act to rotate the ipsilateral anterior hemipelvis lower—an AS ilium—causing the pelvis to torque and having the opposite effect on the contralateral hemipelvis—a PI ilium. The degree of torsion (if any) would be dependent on the tension in the QL and the freedom of movement of the pelvis, and any pre-existing pelvic torsion due to anatomic LLI. However, if the subject now adopts an unloaded posture—supine or prone—QL hypertonicity is freed from the load of the body and able to lift the ipsilateral hemipelvis, hip and leg in the cephalic direction, producing leg-length alignment asymmetry at the feet. This model is in agreement with Travell and Simons who write: "In recumbancy, active TrPs (trigger points) shorten the (quadratus lumborum) muscle and can thus distort pelvic alignment, elevating the pelvis on the side of the tense muscle."[34]

This is a possible explanation for the appearance of the PI ilium at the reactive short leg side in our AM analysis.

Slosberg completed a review of LLI.[51] He reviewed frequency, physiology, consequences, and reliability. A study of 376 children conducted at the Growth Study Center for Children's Hospital in Boston found that 95.5% of those tested had significant LLI. Investigators also cited another study of 830 children, 93% of whom had some degree of lateral hip asymmetry.[51] In a random sample of 50 freshman chiropractic students with no apparent pathology, 84% had LLI of 2 mm or more, and 46% had LLI greater than 5 mm.[52]

A study of 1157 subjects compared symptomatic and nonsymptomatic subjects with LLI. Seventy-five percent of the symptomatic subjects had an LLI of 5 mm or greater while in contrast, 43.5% of the controls had an LLI of 5 mm or greater. In this analysis, the unilateral symptoms of the sciatica and hip pain occurred significantly more frequently on the long leg side (78.5% vs. 21.5% in sciatica and 88.9% vs. 11.1% in hip pain).[22] Friberg went on to state that LLI has biomechanical, etiological, and clinical significance. "A major consequence of LLI is its contribution to a compensatory functional scoliosis. Such a postural anomaly results in a degree of lateral bending and rotation which compresses the concave side of the lower lumbar discs posterolaterally and may promote disc degeneration and bulging. Moreover, such functional scoliosis, if untreated, may result in structural, permanent scoliosis." He also states, "Morscher has shown that Leg Length Inequality leads to 'remarkable asymmetric increase in the activity of several muscle groups, making it impossible for the patient to maintain a resting standing position.'"[51]

A series of studies went on to report that LLI with its associated postural scoliosis results in pelvic obliquity, asymmetrical concavities of lumbar vertebral end plates, and wedging of the fifth lumbar vertebrae and traction spurs, as well as accelerated degeneration of the facet. This is due to an asymmetrical increase in loads carried by lumbar facets, which contributes to alterations in normal gliding movements.[21,53,54]

A different study plotted areas of lowered electrical skin resistance over the back. Once a subject had a stable pattern over a three-week period, a heel lift was inserted to produce a form of structural irritation. Korr et al. found that subjects had onset of pain within a few hours following insertion of the heel lifts, and these areas were associated with lowered skin resistance. Alterations in skin resistance are reportedly due to an increase in regional sympathetic pseudomotor activity.[55-57]

In another study noted by Slosberg, it was reported by Lawrence[58] that LLI is associated with asymmetrical distribution of weight. Even subjects with LLI of only 1 to 4 mm tend to bear more weight on the short leg; those with an LLI of 6 mm or greater bear more weight on the contralateral side. He believes that the difference in distribution of weight has to do with compensatory mechanisms involving the gluteus medius muscles. Earlier, as was noted in the study of literature by Knutson, evidence suggested that for most people, anatomical LLI is not clinically significant until the magnitude reaches approximately 20 mm. The literature noted by Slosberg is not in agreement with this assumption.

Thus the terminology and use of "Leg Length Inequality" can be looked at in two ways: as a "static" form in weight bearing, and in chiropractic, especially in the AM, as a means to evaluate a reactive, dynamic change. Leg length reactivity is a more accurate term when it is used as a tool of analysis because the lengths of the legs as a patient is lying prone are compared. In addition, we observe for changes in the relative length of the legs, at the feet, throughout different stages of ankle and knee flexion, and at times, with hip extension. We are observing the reactivity of the legs and are comparing them as they change following imposed forces and movements. Therefore leg length reactivity is a more accurate description when observing leg lengths after an Isolation Test, a Stress Test, and/or a Pressure Test. We are observing dynamic changes that occur throughout the AM Protocol. Although in the initial evaluation, we determined whether a "short leg" exists, and when that was decided, we labeled the short leg in Position #1 as the "functional short leg." This is not to be confused with previous definitions and discussions. An observable short leg is merely a description that indicates where to start the AM Protocol of evaluation; throughout the course of the Protocol, this is described as the Pelvic Deficient (PD) leg or PD side. Leg lengths are compared, and the amount of difference or shortness is used as a benchmark throughout other positions of analysis because leg lengths change relative to each other.

So the questions are as follows: How and why do leg lengths change? When leg lengths are observed, what creates the changes seen throughout the positions of analysis? What occurs during an Isolation Test that creates a change in prone leg length? The AM also uses Stress Tests and Pressure Tests, which may yield a dynamic reactivity in observable leg length. Leg length changes are also used to determine whether a beneficial adjustment was performed as a postadjustment analysis. The system of LLA used in the AM is based on prone, functional leg length inequalities and has been used for decades by thousands of practitioners. Even though the mechanisms that reveal how biomechanical or neurological dysfunction may manifest in changes in leg length reactivity are unclear, a large body of literature reports investigations of the significance and reproducibility of "Leg Length Inequality" as a reactive and dynamic change in comparative leg lengths.[59]

RELIABILITY AND USES OF LEG LENGTH ANALYSIS

Interexaminer and intraexaminer reliability when a prone[60] or supine[61] LLA is used to determine LLAA or a reactive leg has been shown in numerous studies. Cooperstein et al. investigated the accuracy of a compressive prone leg check in a controlled setting in subjects with specified amounts of artificially induced LLI.[62] They found that compressive prone leg checks were highly accurate in the detection of differences in LLI that were as small as ±1.87 mm, noting that "...compressive leg checking would be expected to identify the short or shortened leg side, irrespective of magnitude, 95.4% of the time."

A great summary of reliability was published by Fuhr and Menke.[63] "Several studies have investigated the reliability of the common denominator in Isolation, Pressure, and Stress Testing: relative leg-length observations. Most investigations have evaluated inter-examiner reliability in Position #1 and all have indicated good agreement for this type of observation."[64] (An excerpt of this publication can be found in Chapter 6, in the section on Related Research.)

Slosberg also cited DeBoer et al., who reported that prone leg length evaluation was "found to be a reliable clinical measure with statistically significant intra- and inter-examiner reliability. He concludes that the findings indicate that LLI represents a real phenomenon and that this method of evaluating LLI is clinically justified."[65] Slosberg suggests that the noted research indicates that LLI (leg length reactivity) is a frequent, significant, and reliable biomechanical finding that may contribute to back pain, hip pain, sciatica, and accelerated degeneration.

THE NERVOUS SYSTEM ERROR CALLED SUBLUXATION

In using AM, we are isolating nervous system and biomechanical errors through LLA. The actual "phenomenon" of leg length reactivity is a rather amazing, consistent, and reliable phenomenon, regardless of its ability to elucidate "how" this occurs. Philosophically, we are trying to reduce and eliminate neuroarticular dysfunction. Chiropractically, we use the term *subluxation*, not as a description of an "incomplete or partial dislocation"[66] but as a "complex." By definition, the word *subluxation*, outside of the chiropractic profession, is viewed as a somewhat "moderate to severe" condition when applied to a joint. Philosophically, it can be considered a "moderate to severe" condition within the field of chiropractic because subluxation consists of a neurological complex of consequences and symptoms.

Because of these different definitions and philosophical applications within the medical and research fields, chiropractic references are frequently prejudicial.[67,68] In the literature, this prejudice on the part of the medical research community has been documented in the reporting of spinal injury caused by spinal manipulative therapy and the assumption that spinal manipulative therapy is equivalent to chiropractic manipulative therapy (in particular, in a study titled "Vertebral Artery Dissections after Chiropractic Neck Manipulation..."), despite the fact that only 4 of the 36 reported cases (11%) were possibly performed by a chiropractor. Most of the spinal manipulative therapies that caused injury were provided by orthopedic surgeons (18/36; 50%). Actually, none of the four chiropractic-related injuries identified in this retrospective review was the result of care provided by qualified chiropractors.[69]

The chiropractic "subluxated" joint is considered a facilitated segment. In a spinal segment, this would respond to various stimuli in a more intense and prolonged manner than is normal. "The reason for such excessive responsiveness is due to the summation of subthreshold stimuli at an involved spinal segment. This brings the segmentally innervated paraspinal muscles closer to threshold."[4] Therefore the term *neuroarticular dysfunction* can be used as a more nonbiased term for a *subluxation complex*.

All practitioners in the health care industry are trying to evaluate areas of dysfunction and treat them with the goal of preventing and curing "dis-ease." Many different theories suggest explanations for what causes subluxation and ways to measure it, but the important thing to keep in mind is to view it as a complex. The subluxation complex can be created by acute processes such as trauma to the soft tissue structures, or by chronic, repetitive processes that result from occupational, congenital, or postural forces.

Recently, outside of the chiropractic profession, a shift in the focus of physical rehabilitation and research has occurred, away from the traditional "strengthen this muscle" approach to evaluation of the neuronal control system.[70-73] Stuart McGill, in *Ultimate Back Fitness and Performance*, states, "Train movement—not muscle." With this shift in concept, results reported in rehabilitation and their long-term benefits have substantially improved. From within these combined publications, considerable reproducible research has measured dysfunctional segmental control, or the subluxation complex. These studies are based on neurological control of the motor unit system with feed forward and feedback-mediated mechanisms. Theoretically, this approach looks at segmental control, starting with attainment of lumbopelvic stabilization before other anatomical structures are addressed. As was previously noted by Panjabi, three systems contribute to lumbopelvic stability: a passive subsystem, an active subsystem, and a neural control subsystem. In my opinion, leg length reactivity analysis involves the interaction between at least two of these systems—active and neural control—which in turn involves the passive subsystem and includes nociceptive pain sensors from inflamed passive structures.

Panjabi's theoretical spinal stability system model can also serve as a theoretical model proposed to explain neuroarticular dysfunction. However, the somatic-visceral component of the subluxation complex is not included in this model and can play a significant role. Let's look at two of Panjabi's figures. The first schematic represents the theoretical model for a normally functioning stabilizing system. The goal is to provide sufficient stability to the spine to match the instantaneous varying stability demands produced by changes in spinal posture and static and dynamic loads. The three subsystems work together to achieve the goal.

> As shown in [Figure 5-4], the information from the (1) passive subsystem sets up specific (2) spinal stability requirements. Consequently, requirements for (3) individual muscle tensions are determined by the neural control unit. The message is sent to the (4) force generators. Feedback is provided by the (5) force monitors by comparing the (6) "achieved" and (3) "required" individual muscle tensions.[10]

The passive (ligamentous) subsystem provides little stability to the spine when it is near the neutral position. It is at the end of the ranges of motion that the ligaments develop reactive forces to resist spinal motion. "The passive components probably function in the vicinity of the neutral position as transducers (signal-producing devices) for measuring vertebral positions and motions, similar to those proposed for knee ligaments,[74] and therefore are part of the neural control subsystem. Thus this subsystem is passive only in the sense that it by itself does not generate or produce spinal motions, but it is dynamically active in monitoring the transducer signals."[75]

As is shown in the schematic (see Figure 5-4), the active musculotendinous subsystem is the means through which the spinal system generates forces to provide stability to the spine. The magnitude of the force that is generated by each muscle is measured by the neural control subsystem through force transducers built into the tendons of the muscles. Information from the transducers is relayed to the neural control subsystem so that specific requirements for stability control can be determined. The tension of individual muscles is measured and adjusted and is dependent on dynamic posture and variation in lever arms and inertial loads of different masses and external loads. Deformation of ligaments throughout the neutral zone involves a large neuronal component. Soft tissues deform under spinal loads and are capable of providing a comprehensive set of signals from which stability requirements may be determined.

Panjabi's theory as illustrated above was confirmed in a study by Solomonow et al. (published in 1998).[19] It was confirmed that the supraspinal

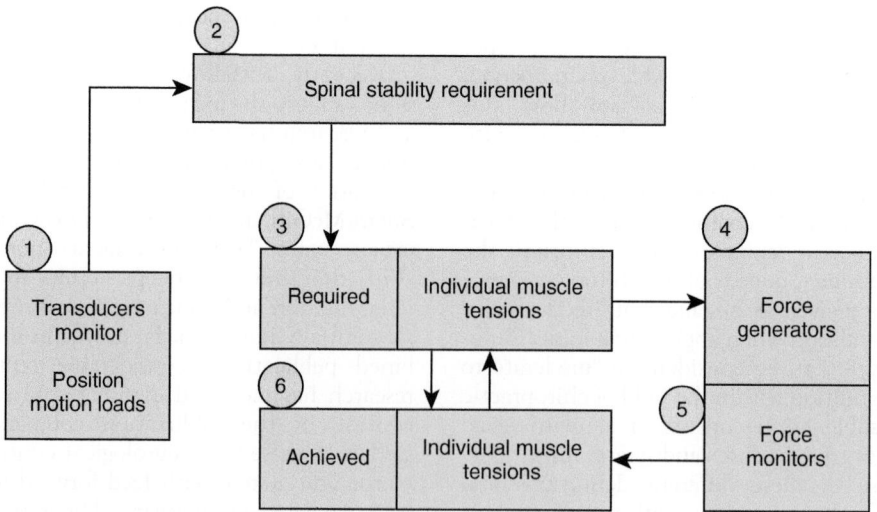

Figure 5-4 Factors and feedbacks in the stabilizing system. *(Modified from Panjabi MM. The stabilizing system of the spine. Part II. Neutral zone and stability hypothesis. J Spinal Disord. 1992;5[4]:390-7.)*

ligament that contains the mechanoreceptors (transducers) can indeed elicit, through the spinal interneurons and the motoneurons (control unit), muscular activity that tends to prevent distraction of at least two vertebrae from each other. In fact, this created stiffening in several rostral and caudal motion segments. Solomonow et al. confirmed the stabilization theory of Panjabi in two different cases. The authors noted, however, that much more work is required for assessment of the full details of this control system in different complex activities.

Through varying factors such as injury, degeneration, and disease, degradation of the spinal system may occur. Panjabi explains,

> The neural control subsystem perceives these deficiencies, which may develop suddenly or gradually, and attempts to compensate by initiating appropriate changes in the active subsystem. Although the necessary stability of the spine overall may be reestablished, the subsequent consequences may be deleterious to the individual component of the spinal system (e.g., accelerated degeneration of the various component of the spinal column, muscle spasm, injury, and fatigue). Over time, the consequences may be chronic dysfunction and pain.[75]

This is illustrated in Figure 5-5.

A dysfunction of the spinal stability system occurs through (1) injury, degeneration and/or disease which may decrease the (2) passive stability and/or (3) active stability. (4) The neural control unit attempts to remedy the stability loss by increasing the stabilizing function of the remaining spinal components: (5) passive

and (6) active. This may lead to (7) accelerated degeneration, abnormal muscle loading, and muscle fatigue. If these changes cannot adequately compensate for the stability loss, a (8) chronic dysfunction or pain may develop.[75]

NERVOUS SYSTEM REVIEW: THE RECEPTORS

A substantial amount of research has been conducted and published by Wada et al. Most of the 44 publications that were reviewed involve research on cats that sought to evaluate motoneurons, input afferents, synaptic relationships, and the resultant motor neuronal pathways. Studies primarily focused on the hind limb stimulus and resultant muscle activation mechanisms of the lumbar spine related to stiffness, stability, and the involvement of neuron pools. These abstracts (from 1989 to August 2006) describe the stimulus of cats' nociceptive reflex pathways to the foot extensors, which confirmed positive feedback mechanisms.[76] This is where the AM Protocol begins and utilizes its analysis, through the reactive leg. The neurology involved in leg reactivity is discussed in the following paragraphs.

Before we explore the nervous system neuron connections involved in the stability of the spine as related to leg length reactivity, some definitions and functions of the nervous system should be explained. An important consideration in neuroanatomy is that, compared with other species, the human cerebellum is *large* as the result of two major factors: the assumption of an erect position, and fine, learned activities made possible by the evolution of the hands.[77] "A function specific to the brain is integration, analysis, and storage of information for possible

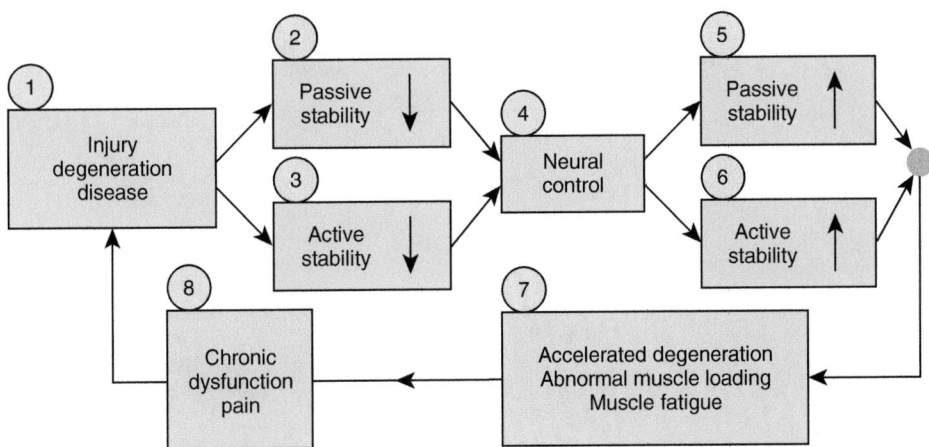

Figure 5-5 Compensating factors for spinal stability resulting from injury and degeneration. *(Modified from Panjabi MM. The stabilizing system of the spine. Part II. Neutral zone and stability hypothesis. J Spinal Disord. 1992;5[4]:390-7.)*

later use; this function is learning and memory."[78] Within the cerebral hemispheres of the brain are found reception centers for the following: (1) afferent impulses that are *perceived* and *interpreted* as pain, touch, sound, etc., (2) the storage of sensory information, which is the *learning* process, and (3) the retention of sensation-action patterns, which is *memory*.[77]

An upper motor neuron is found completely within the central nervous system that synapses with or regulates the actions of lower motor neurons. A lower motoneuron is a peripheral motoneuron that originates in the ventral horn of the gray matter of the spinal cord and terminates in skeletal muscle. An afferent nerve conducts *sensory* impulses *toward* the brain or spinal cord. An efferent nerve conducts *motor* impulses *away* from the brain and spinal cord (Figure 5-6).

The spinal cord carries out two main functions: (1) It connects the peripheral nervous system to the brain through the sensory neurons (afferents); and (2) it acts as a coordinating center and is responsible for simple reflexes. The spinal cord gives rise to 31 pairs of spinal nerves. These are mixed nerves because they contain both sensory and motor axons. All sensory axons pass into the dorsal root ganglion, where their cell bodies are located, and then into the spinal cord. All motor axons pass into the ventral roots before uniting with the sensory axons to form the mixed nerves. Interneurons carry impulses to and from specific receptors and effectors and are grouped together in spinal tracts.

A fasciculus is a bundle of muscles or nerves. A fasciculus of nerves is, more specifically, a division of the funiculus (a division of the white matter) of the spinal cord that comprises the fibers of one or more tracts. The term *fasciculus* is used by some to refer to a tract. The fibers within a fasciculus are held together by delicate connective tissue fibers that form the endoneurium (Henle's sheath). The entire fasciculus is surrounded by a sheath of connective tissue fibers referred to as the epineurium, which may contain numerous fat cells.[78]

A neuroganglion occurs outside of the central nervous system as a group of neuron cell bodies. A neuron is a nerve cell, the structural and functional unit of the nervous system. A neuron consists of a cell body and its processes, an axon, and one or more dendrites. Neurons function to initiate and conduct impulses. They transmit impulses to other neurons or cells by releasing neurotransmitters at synapses. Alternatively, a neuron may release neurohormones into the bloodstream.

At the basic level, an individual nerve consists of dendrites that connect with the cell body, nucleus, and myelinated axon and end in the axon terminals. Figure 5-7 is an illustration of an efferent (motor) neuron. The impulse moves from the dendrite toward the axon terminal.[79]

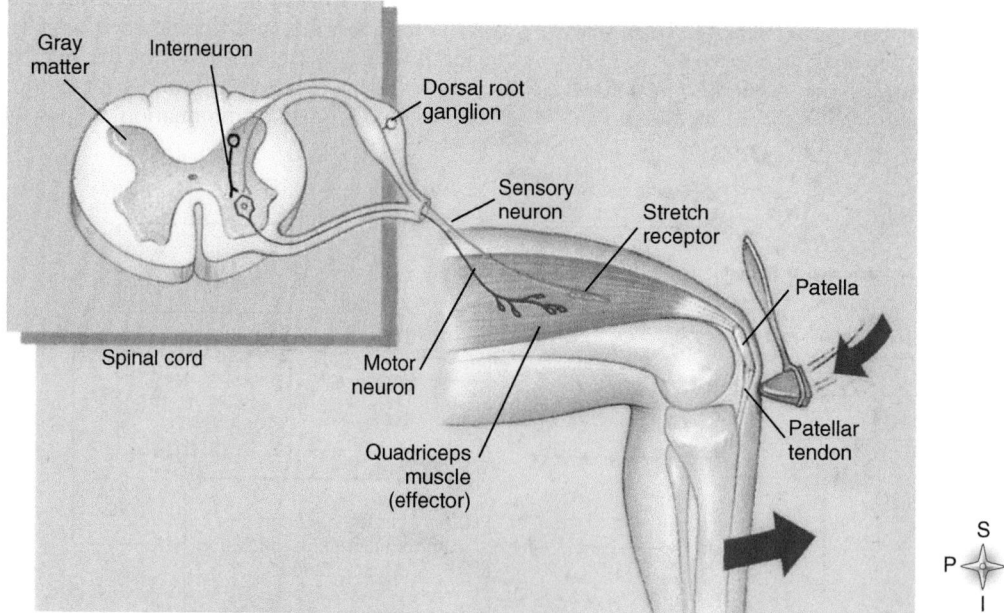

Figure 5-6 Neurological pathways from afferents through interneurons to the efferents. *(From Thibodeau GA, Patton KT. Anatomy & physiology. 6th ed. St. Louis: Mosby; 2007.)*

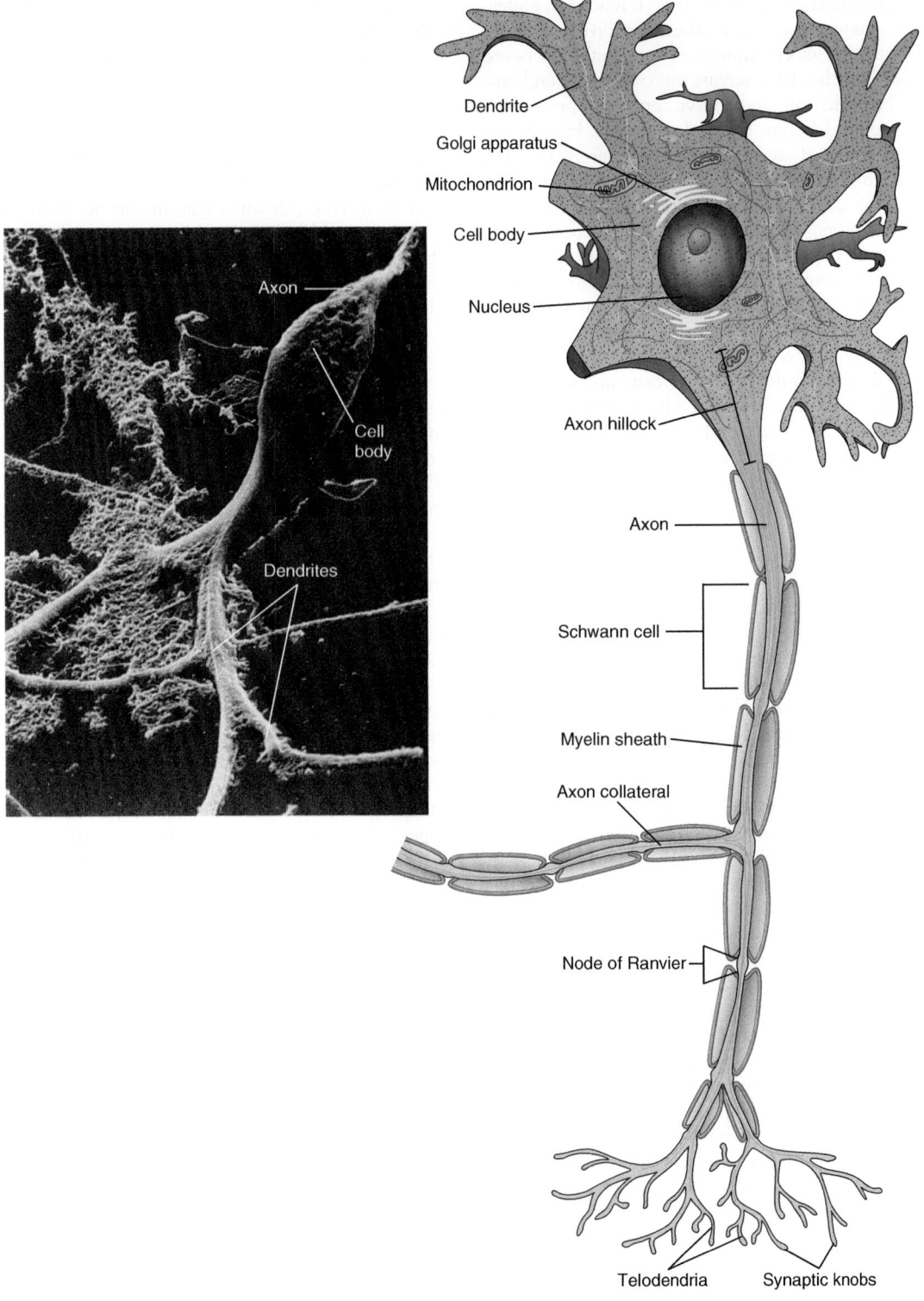

Figure 5-7 Efferent neuron components. *(From Thibodeau GA, Patton KT. Anatomy & physiology. 6th ed. St. Louis: Mosby; 2007.)*

An afferent (sensory) neuron is made up of afferent sensory receptors, and the direction of impulse is toward the axon terminal. A single afferent nerve fiber branches to innervate up to 90 nerve endings.

Nonencapsulated nerve endings provide a home for different types of receptors. Five different types of sensory receptors are classified according to the energy they transduce in creating the different senses. These include mechanoreceptors, chemoreceptors, photoreceptors, thermoreceptors, and electroreceptors.

- Mechanoreceptors transduce mechanical energy; this permits the hearing and feeling that are primarily involved in maintaining balance.
- Chemoreceptors transduce certain types of chemical compounds that enable taste and smelling.
- Photoreceptors transduce light energy through rods and cones, thereby generating light.
- Thermoreceptors transduce thermal energy.
- Electroreceptors respond to electrical stimuli.[80]

The sense of touch occurs primarily through Pacinian corpuscles, Meissner's corpuscles, Merkel's discs, Ruffini's endings, free nerve endings, and hair follicle receptors. Proprioception occurs primarily through the Golgi organs and the muscle spindles. Pain is received through the nociceptors, and temperature from thermoreceptors. Merkel's cells and Meissner's corpuscles occur in superficial skin layers. Pacinian corpuscles and Ruffini's endings are found primarily in subcutaneous tissue.

When leg length reactivity is evaluated, it is perhaps the mechanoreceptors that may be most involved. A mechanoreceptor is a sensory receptor that receives mechanical stimuli through touch, pressure, gravity, stretch, and movement. Mechanoreceptors allow us to detect and discern touch; through the sense of proprioception, they monitor the position of our muscles, bones, joints, and the motion of the body and detect sounds. Four main types of mechanoreceptors have been identified: Merkel's discs, Meissner's corpuscles, Pacinian corpuscles, and Ruffini's corpuscles.

Merkel's nerve endings are mechanoreceptors that are found in the epidermis and in the epithelial root sheath of a hair; they are involved in "tactile" sensations. Each ending consists of a Merkel's cell that appears in close apposition with an enlarged nerve terminal. This is sometimes referred to as a Merkel cell–neurite complex, or a Merkel's disc receptor, and is classified as a slowly adapting type I mechanoreceptor.

Merkel's nerve endings are extremely sensitive to tissue displacement, even up to less than 1 μm. Type I afferent fibers have smaller receptive fields than do type II fibers. Several studies indicate that type I fibers mediate high-resolution tactile

discrimination that is responsible for the ability of fingertips to feel fine, detailed surface patterns, as in the reading of Braille.[80,81] When two separate points in a single receptive field are stimulated, the person is unable to distinguish whether the touch is coming from two separate points. If the two points that are touched involve more than a single receptive field, then both contacts are felt. The degree to which detailed stimuli can be resolved is determined by the size of the receptive field of the mechanoreceptors. Thus Merkel's nerve endings and Meissner's corpuscles are most densely clustered in the highly sensitive fingertips.

Electrical recordings from single afferent nerve fibers in mammals have shown that responses of Merkel's nerve endings are characterized by a vigorous response to the onset of a mechanical ramp stimulus (dynamic); they then continue to fire during the plateau phase (static). The static phase of firing can last longer than 30 minutes. Sustained firing interspike intervals are irregular, in contrast to the highly regular pattern of interspike intervals attained with slowly adapting type II mechanoreceptors. They fire fastest when small points indent the skin, and they fire at a slow rate on slow curves or flat surfaces. Convexities further reduce their rate of firing.[80]

Merkel's discs are platelike expansions of sensory nerve endings in a somewhat rigid structure; because they are not encapsulated, these discs have a sustained response that can be seen in the form of an action potential or spikes to mechanical deflection of tissue. Of the four main types of mechanoreceptors, these are the most sensitive to vibrations at low frequencies, around 5 to 15 Hz. They have a sustained response to pressure, and Merkel's nerve endings are classified as slowly adapting. They occur in abundance around hair follicles. Corpuscles of Meissner are encapsulated and occur in the dermal papillae, particularly over the volar surface of the fingers and hand, as well as on the soles of the feet. Different receptors are activated at varying frequencies. Merkel's corpuscles are primarily stimulated at low frequencies (5 to 15 Hz), Meissner's at midrange frequencies (20 to 50 Hz); Pacinian corpuscles are stimulated at a low threshold but at high frequencies (60 to 400 Hz), and muscle spindles and Golgi tendons are stimulated primarily at high frequencies (100 Hz).[82]

Mechanoreceptors can be separated into categories on the basis of their rates of adaptivity. After mechanoreceptors receive a stimulus, they begin to fire impulses or action potentials at elevated frequency; the stronger the stimulus, the higher the frequency. Over time, the cell can adapt to a constant or static stimulus, and pulses subside to a normal rate. Phasic receptors are those that adapt quickly and return to a normal pulse rate. Tonic receptors are slow to return to their normal firing rate. Phasic mechanoreceptors are beneficial in sensing characteristics such as texture and vibrations, compared with tonic receptors, which are useful for temperature sense and proprioception.[79]

McLain and Pickar performed histologic analysis of normal human facet capsules to determine the density and distribution of encapsulated nerve endings in the thoracic and lumbar spine. In a summary of background data, they note, "Ongoing studies of spinal innervation have shown that human facet tissues contain mechanoreceptive endings capable of detecting motion and tissue distortion. The hypothesis has been advanced that signal proprioception may play a role in modulating protective muscular reflexes that prevent injury or facilitate healing."[83] Table 5-1 shows mechanoreceptor classifications from the harvested facet levels T3-T7 and T12-L4 from seven subjects. Encapsulated endings were classified according to the classification of Freeman and Wyke.[84]

Before the technical research is discussed, some other definitions should be considered. Each neuron can have thousands of other neurons that synapse on it. Some neurons release activating or depolarizing neurotransmitters; others release inhibitory or hyperpolarizing neurotransmitters. Neurotransmitters can inhibit the transmission of nerve impulses by opening chloride channels and/or potassium channels within the plasma membrane. Opening the membrane increases membrane potential by letting negatively charged chloride ions in, and positively charged potassium ions out. This hyperpolarizaion is called an inhibitory postsynaptic potential (IPSP).

Polarization is the electrical state that exists at the cell membrane of an excitable cell at rest; the inside is negatively charged in relation to the outside. Then, the inside of the cell is more positive in relation to the outside of the cell membrane; this is depolarization. When the polarized state at the cell membrane is restored (the cell is negative inside in relation to the outside) following depolarization, this is termed repolarization (Figure 5-8).[78]

See Chapter 4 for a more extensive and thorough neurology presentation. It is an excellent detailed view of the receptors, neurology pathways, and pain mechanisms.

CONNECTING THE RESEARCH OF THE HIND LIMB NEURONS

Recent neuroscience research, particularly over the past five years, has made great advancements that previously had been thought impossible. Most of the research efforts have focused on cats and rats. The genetic modification capabilities of rats have allowed greater specificity within the field of neurophysiology research that pertains to locomotion, lower limb neurologic tracts, and balance control. This has enabled and advanced more finite tracking of the neurological pathways and identification of neurons and their associated neurons. Genetic modification makes possible the targeting of classes of interneurons that form specific locomotor and reflex circuitry.[85] Pharmacological agents of neurotransmission[86] have advanced the capabilities of research levels, which has offered hope to those who have experienced spinal cord injury that walking may again be possible.

In the context of nervous system information provided earlier, a summary of several publications of Wada and colleagues is presented here. Most of these publications involve research on cats, and they have been published in brain research, biology, and veterinary medical science journals. This research looks primarily at neurons, motoneuron pools, and their reflexive connections in regard to locomotion.

The longissimus muscles were analyzed in the downslope walking of cats at 5 to 30 degrees. Bursts of electromyographic (EMG) activity did not become prominent until downslope walking reached an angle greater than 20 degrees. Specific segmental areas were involved in the different movements of the hind limbs. The tenth thoracic was found to facilitate inward movement. The first lumbar was involved in decreasing and controlling forward movement. The fifth lumbar decreased backward movement.[87]

During level and upslope cat walking, the three epaxial muscles—multifidus, iliocostalis, and longissimus—were measured. EMG bursts of these muscles increased stiffness and produced inward movement that decreased the lateral movement of the vertebral column. Results suggested that rhythmic EMG bursts in the epaxial muscles were produced by pattern generators, and the timing of EMG bursts among the different levels of epaxial muscles were altered by walking conditions and by input from the peripheral afferent and descending pathways.[88]

Another study looked at level and upslope treadmill walking of cats. As the grade of the upslope walking increased from horizontal, kinematic and EMG measurements were attained. During steep upslope walking, three EMG bursts became evident and were phase-locked to the outward, downward, and backward movements of the spinal column. Results suggest that the component of the locomotor pattern generator

Table 5-1	Types of Receptors Harvested from Thoracic and Lumbar Spine Facet Joints				
Type	Morphological Features	Average Size	Location	Probable Function	Eponymous or Descriptive Designations
1	Globular receptors; round, oval, or "bean" shaped, thinly encapsulated, and usually found in clusters	40-100 μm in diameter	Found in the fibrous capsule of joints and in periarticular ligaments and tendons; usually in superficial layers of dense connective tissue	Mechanoreceptor (slowly adapting, low-threshold afferent ending)	Ruffini's ending; Golgi-Mazzoni ending; Meissner's corpuscle; basket- or spray-type ending
2	Cylindrical corpuscles with thick lamellar encapsulations, and dense central axon core; parent axon may be bifid or trifid, entering at one terminal of the cylinder	250-350 μm in length, 100 μm in diameter	Found in deeper layers of fibrous capsule, at junctions of fibrous connective tissue and fat; often accompanied by vascular leash; oriented with connective tissue fibers of dense capsule or ligament	Mechanoreceptor (rapidly adapting, low-threshold afferent ending)	Pacinian corpuscle; Vater-Pacini corpuscle; Pacini-form corpuscle; Meissner's corpuscle; Golgi-Mazzoni body; bulbous corpuscle; clublike ending
3	Fusiform corpuscles with a thin capsule surrounding a densely arborizing neural meshwork; fine neuritis visible at higher magnification	Up to 600 μm in length, 100 μm in diameter	Found in ligaments and tendons, as well as in dense connective tissue of joint capsule	Mechanoreceptor (very slowly adapting, high-threshold afferent)	Golgi ending; Golgi-Mazzoni corpuscle
4	Unmyelinated free nerve endings and unencapsulated plexuses	0.5-1.5 μm in diameter	Found in all periarticular and intra-articular tissues except cartilage	Nociceptor (nonadapting)	

From McLain RF, Pickar JG. Mechanoreceptor endings in human thoracic and lumbar facet joints. Spine. 1998;23(2):168-73.

that produces rhythmical spinal column movements must generate a wide variety of EMG bursts within spinal column muscles and is dependent in part on sensory input from the spinal column and its musculature.[89] Later in this chapter, the research and significance of central pattern generators (locomotor pattern generator) in the spine are examined.

The relationship of longissimus lumborum muscle input resistance to the amplitude of monosynaptic and polysynaptic excitatory postsynaptic potentials (EPSPs) produced by electrical stimulation of group I muscle afferents was evaluated at different levels from the first to the fourth lumbar. Long motoneurons in the fourth lumbar spinal segment were examined in

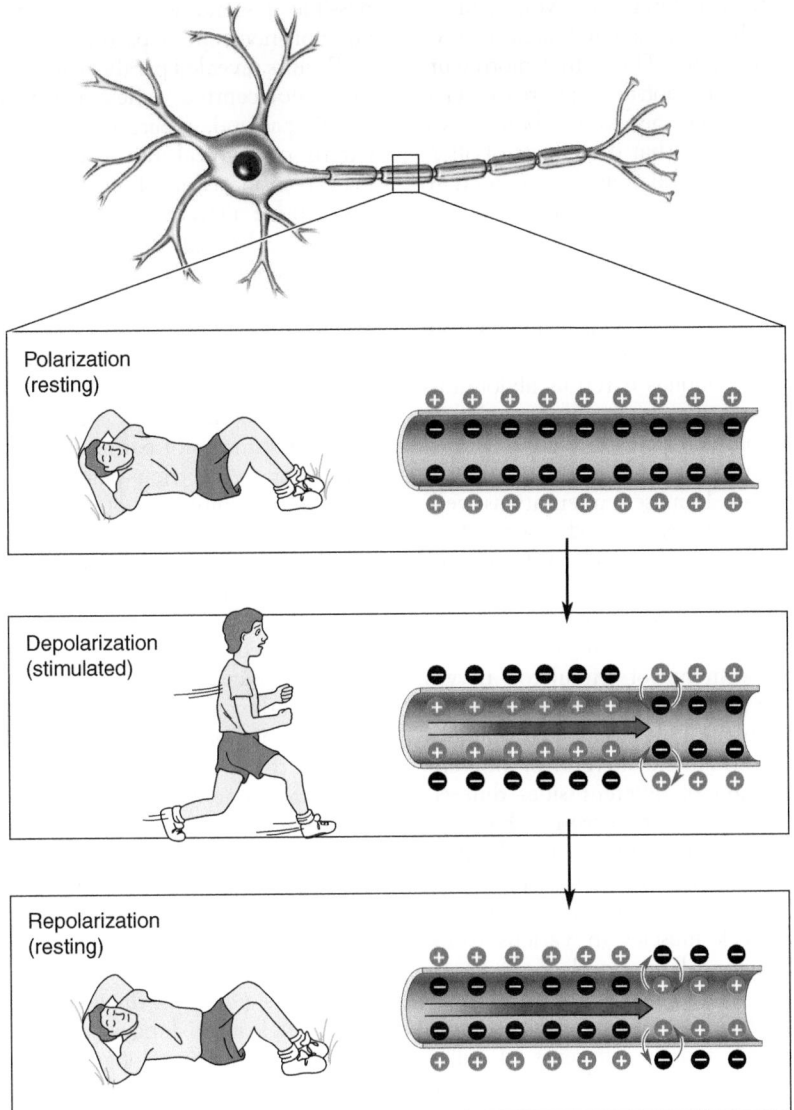

Figure 5-8 Polarization, depolarization, and repolarization. *(From Herlihy B, Maebius NK. The human body in health and illness. Philadelphia: Saunders; 2000.)*

an effort to gain insight into the neuronal control of trunk muscles. Research suggests *position-dependent control of motoneuron activity* by group I afferents. Motoneuron activities carried out by monosynaptic pathways and polysynaptic pathways from adjacent spinal segments are dependent on the "intrinsic properties of motoneurons" (e.g., input resistance); motoneuron activities carried out by polysynaptic pathways from far spinal segments have *independent* intrinsic properties.[90]

Previous studies have demonstrated that input patterns from hind limb muscles and cutaneous afferents vary among individual trunk muscle motoneurons.[91,92] This study was designed to examine the relationship between the synaptic pattern of hind limb afferents and the area innervated by motoneurons. Histological study of the longissimus lumborum indicated that the distribution of different fiber types—slow-twitch oxidative (SO), fast-twitch oxidative glycolytic (FOG), and fast-twitch glycolytic (FG)—depends on the area of the cross-section. Differentiation of the various fiber types can promote an understanding of essentially how long and how fast or fatigable their neurological control is. The ventromedial area and the dorsolateral areas possess a high content of SO and FG. The motoneurons that innervate the dorsolateral area receive muscle afferent inputs mainly from the ipsilateral side. Motoneurons that innervate the ventromedial area receive bilateral afferent inputs. The actual motoneurons that innervate the dorsolateral area receive EPSPs from cutaneous nerves on both sides. These findings indicate that the effects of afferent inputs from the hind limbs are related to motoneuron type, or the area innervated by the motoneurons.[93]

Another study looked at the reflex actions of group I and II afferents to longissimus lumborum motoneurons in the L1-L5 spinal segments from the epaxial muscle (longissimus) and the hypaxial muscle in the obliquus externus abdominus of the cat. Stimulation at an intensity below 1.5 times threshold activated only group I muscle afferents; stimulation of 2 to 5 times threshold activated group II muscle afferents as well. Longissimus motoneurons received group I afferent input mainly from the same and adjacent segments, and they received group II afferent inputs from a wider range of segments. The central latencies became longer as the distance between spinal segments of stimulated nerves and motoneurons increased. The patterns of convergence from the longissimus and obliquus externus abdominus muscle afferents of different spinal segments and of different sides differed considerably among motoneurons. Findings revealed various input patterns of individual motoneurons within the same motoneuron pool. This may reflect the complexity of neuronal control of the back muscles in various trunk movements, including lateral and dorsal bending, rotating, and fixation of the trunk.[94] Therefore different intensities of stimulation affect different types of muscle afferents. It also appears that integration of information from multiple areas and levels occurs during sharing of the same motoneuron pool.

A study published in 2001 mediated a positive feedback mechanism in the cat. Nociceptive reflex pathways to foot extensors were investigated, with particular attention given to those that do not follow a flexor reflex or withdrawal pattern. Nociceptive afferents of the footpad were activated by noxious radiant heat; for comparison, non-nociceptive afferents were activated by weak mechanical stimulation of the skin or by graded electrical nerve stimulation. During fictive locomotion, the reflex action of the afferents on hind limb motoneurons that innervated the plantaris and intrinsic foot extensors (tibial nerve) was investigated by intracellular recording, by monosynaptic reflex testing, and by the recording of neurograms. Pharmacological compounds were used to evaluate

possible descending control of the nociceptive and non-nociceptive pathways.

Results revealed parallel excitatory and inhibitory nociceptive reflex pathways from the central pad and, in part, from the toe pads to foot extensors. Typical flexor reflex patterns were evoked in most hind limb motoneuron pools by nociceptive afferents from different skin areas of the foot. Although the nociceptive flexor reflex pathways have a general nocifensive withdrawal function, the nociceptive excitatory nonflexor reflex to the foot extensors causes movement of the affected area toward the stimulus, or at least resistance against the stimulus, which mediates *positive feedback*.[76] This study revealed that a different stimulus of pain-sensing nociceptors as compared with non–pain-sensing receptors, along with stimulation of different skin areas of the foot (the toe pads vs. the footpads), created parallel nociceptive reflex pathways with negative and positive feedback functions to the foot extensors. Essentially, sensors from the foot are differentiated and have negative and positive feedback functions.

In another study, it was found that different postsynaptic potentials (PSPs) result from motoneurons that innervate the footpads to the hind limb. Experiments involved electrical stimulation of afferent nerves that innervate foot pads, and PSPs were recorded from hind limb motoneurons that innervate the following hind limb muscles of 16 cats: posterior biceps and semitendinosus, anterior biceps and semimembranosus, lateral gastrocnemius and soleus, medial gastrocnemius, plantaris, tibialis anterior, popliteus, flexor digitorum longus and flexor hallucis longus, and peroneus longus. The rate of occurrence of different types of PSPs (i.e., excitatory PSPs, inhibitory PSPs, mixed PSPs), the sizes of PSPs, and their central latencies were analyzed for each group of motoneurons, with the goal of identifying neural pathways from afferents that innervated footpads to hind limb motoneurons. In the posterior biceps and semitendinosus, anterior biceps and semimembranosus, and lateral gastrocnemius and soleus muscles, the rates of occurrence of different types of PSPs did not depend on the footpad stimulated.

But, the other groups of motoneurons' rates of occurrence depended on the foot pad stimulated. It was often noted that the size of the PSPs in the same motoneurons differed according to the foot pad stimulated. Measurements of the central latencies of the PSPs indicated that the shortest neural pathways for excitatory PSPs and inhibitory PSPs were disynaptic (central latencies < 1.8 ms). The functional role of neuronal pathways from afferent nerves innervating footpads to hind limb motoneurons could be to *maintain stability of the foot during different postural and motor activities.*[95]

It is amazing that this experiment studied so many different muscles and their responses to footpad stimulation. This study was an example of how extensively specialized and integrated the nervous system has to be to perform its numerous functions. Through the process of LLA, multiple neuronal pathways and their integration of function are stimulated.

Connection of the toe pads through the hind limbs to the lumbar spinal segments was studied. Research evaluated the effects in cats of electrical stimulation of the central pad in comparison with toe pads on the monosynaptic reflex in lumbar spinal segments. Various muscles and their monosynaptic reflexes were evaluated. When different toe pads were stimulated, the responses were recorded for different muscle actions in the knee and the low back. Remarkable differences were noted in the effects of toe pad conditioning stimulation on the flexor digitorum longus, extensor digitorum longus, peroneus brevis and tertius, and peroneus longus monosynaptic reflexes, depending on which toe pad was stimulated. Stimulation of the footpad inhibited monosynaptic reflexes to the lateral gastrocnemius, soleus, and medial gastrocnemius. When the central pad was stimulated, the plantaris was enhanced. Stimulation of the toe pads inhibited the plantaris. Results suggest that afferent inputs from the footpads modulate the activity of motoneurons, stabilize the foot, and help to maintain body balance.[96]

In other related research, investigators looked at different types of stimulation of the footpads. Monosynaptic reflexes were measured and evaluated for the effects of tonic pressure, phasic pressure, squeezing, and radiant heating at 50°C. Tonic pressure effects were very weak or were not detected. The pattern for the effects of phasic pressure was similar to that for squeezing, but the effects of squeezing were stronger than those of phasic pressure. Results indicated that the effects of mechanical stimulation were induced primarily by phasic afferent inputs. Monosynaptic reflex recordings revealed differential effects of mechanical stimulation and radiant heating. Overall, the results suggest differences in neuronal pathways caused by various types of receptors in the footpads.[97]

In our AM LLA with the use of Position #1, a quick pressure is applied to the bottom of the heel that mimics a weight-bearing stimulus. If motoneuron pools are at or near threshold because of dysfunction, this weight-bearing stimulus creates an exaggerated response because the patient is in a prone position, and the weight-bearing musculature response becomes more apparent. It is a phasic type of stimulus when performed correctly. This activity is enhanced by the addition of varying amounts of ankle dorsiflexion stimulus, and possibly some ankle inversion or eversion proprioceptive stimulus. Postural control mechanisms are centered around ankle movement, which is coupled with hip rotation and includes strategies for postural control.[14] The plantar aspect of the foot contains an abundance of mechanoreceptors of the corpuscles of Meissner because of sensation demands from the sole of the foot to maintain posture and balance. These are neurologically connected and parallel the nociceptive pathways; this creates feedback-mediated activity involving the feed forward mechanisms.

More research was conducted by Wada et al. to evaluate synaptic inputs to motoneurons that innervate the back and abdominal muscles in the lumbar part of the body through low-threshold hind limb muscle afferents. The connection between the back and abdominal motoneurons and low-threshold afferents from the hind limb muscles is monosynaptic. Input patterns of various hind limb muscles varied among individual motoneurons, even though they were within the same motoneuron pool, and synaptic organization seemed to differ from that for the leg motoneuron pool. Varying levels of threshold stimulus among the group I afferents affected different percentages of motoneurons by stimulating proximal muscle nerves versus distal muscle nerves when recorded for the iliocostalis lumborum and the obliquus externus abdominus. In this research, it was found that the overall projection pattern of low-threshold afferents from leg muscles to the lumbar spine, low back, and abdominal motoneurons suggests that group I afferent inputs are related to lateral and vertical movements, and that group II afferent inputs determine the stiffness of the trunk.[91]

Other studies looked at the spinal projections of afferent fibers that innervate the facet joints between the caudal vertebrae, again through examination of cats. Spinal dorsal roots below the second sacral segment were injected, and this gave rise to extensive craniocaudal distribution of a wheat germ agglutinin–horseradish peroxidase along the spinal cord. This indicated that many afferent fibers innervating unilateral facet joints terminate bilaterally in laminae I to II,

V to VI, and X of the thoracic, lumbar, sacral, and caudal spinal cord. These afferent fibers may convey a series of sensory information from the caudal facet joints to the spinal cord.[98]

Therefore the effects of stimuli to the hind limb feed into the stiffness and control of the lumbar spine and travel up the spinal cord. Additional research suggests that neuronal pathways perform different functions. Neuronal pathways from muscle afferents to back muscle motoneurons mainly increase the stiffness of the trunk to maintain its stability; pathways to the abdominal muscles help to extend the dorsal column by decreasing their activities.[99] Yet another study yielded findings that suggest that, within each motoneuron pool, some neurons act to increase stiffness of the trunk, or they move vertically in response to increased activity of cutaneous afferents, while the other motoneurons act to produce lateral bending of the trunk.[92]

CENTRAL PATTERN GENERATORS AND THE NEUROLOGY OF LOCOMOTION

With the research of Wada's group forming the basis, let's connect lower limb motoneurons to the low back and look at some neuronal pathway factors that contribute to stabilization, movement, locomotion, and balance control. It has been confirmed in many species, including humans, that coordinated flexor and extensor alternating movements can be produced in the absence of descending or afferent inputs to the lumbosacral spinal cord. The term *central pattern generator* (CPG) has been coined to refer to the network of neurons that produce patterned motor behavior in the absence of phasic inputs.[100] Networks within the spinal cord, even when isolated from the brain and sensory inputs, generate the basic pattern that underlies walking, as well as other motor behaviors that can be produced by spinal cord networks, such as hopping, walking, swimming, and scratching.[85,101] Many of the behaviors fundamental to animal life such as breathing, chewing, and locomotion, are rhythmic activities that are controlled by neuronal networks. New tools have emerged in the study of the mouse, in particular, that have made it possible to dissect the circuitry that underlies spinal locomotor networks. Advantages have combined genetic and electrophysiological techniques with the use of in vitro preparations. "Identifying neurons and connection within spinal networks is challenging because cells that comprise the locomotor network form part of a heterogeneous mix of interneurons within the ventral spinal cord."[85] This is important to

keep in mind: The CPGs are more complex than was first thought, and the cortical aspect of locomotion is more involved as well.

These advances allowed the dissecting away of all tissues, except for the spinal cord and the dorsal and ventral roots.[102] A signature of locomotor-like activity can be obtained by comparing the pattern produced in the ankle extensors and flexors with ventral root recordings from the left and right second lumbar with the fifth or sixth lumbar ventral roots in the mouse.[103] Populations of interneurons can be identified and other functions can be identified through a variety of pharmaceutical and electrical stimulation techniques. The exciting conclusion is an identified class of inhibitory interneurons contributes to the setting of the frequency of the rhythms during locomotor-like activity.

Other advances in techniques used to isolate the cellular mechanisms underlying left-right coordination in locomotor activities were made possible in the mouse by selectively exposing one half of the spinal cord to rhythm-inducing agonists. This technique separates the spinal cord into two halves by using a split bath of pharmaceuticals, creating the "hemi-CPG." EPSPs for the CPG were observed at the first through third lumbar motoneurons. These motoneurons typically receive a rhythmic inhibitory input that was found to be in phase with contralateral ventral root bursts in the contralateral ventral root. The neuron pools accessed were largely involved in the flexor activity of the lower limb. Observations revealed varying effects of antagonists between excitatory and inhibitory bursts; this suggests heterogeneity in the organization of contralateral rhythm-related potential pathways to different motoneurons. In these experiments, it was found that this crossed rhythmic inhibitory input "is typically mediated by pathways organized in a more complex way than in simpler vertebrates, although similarities in the organization of left-right coordinating pathways between these animals and the rat clearly exist."[104] This research was published in 1997.

A research project published in 1994 proposed the *half-center hypothesis*; this proposed that rhythmic motor activity is generated by reciprocal inhibition between two pools of interneurons located on each side of the spinal cord—an extensor half center that activates extensor motoneurons, and a flexor half center that excites flexor motoneurons.[105] Exactly where the CPGs are located in the spinal cord of a quadruped is unclear, but it appears that CPG networks that control hind limb

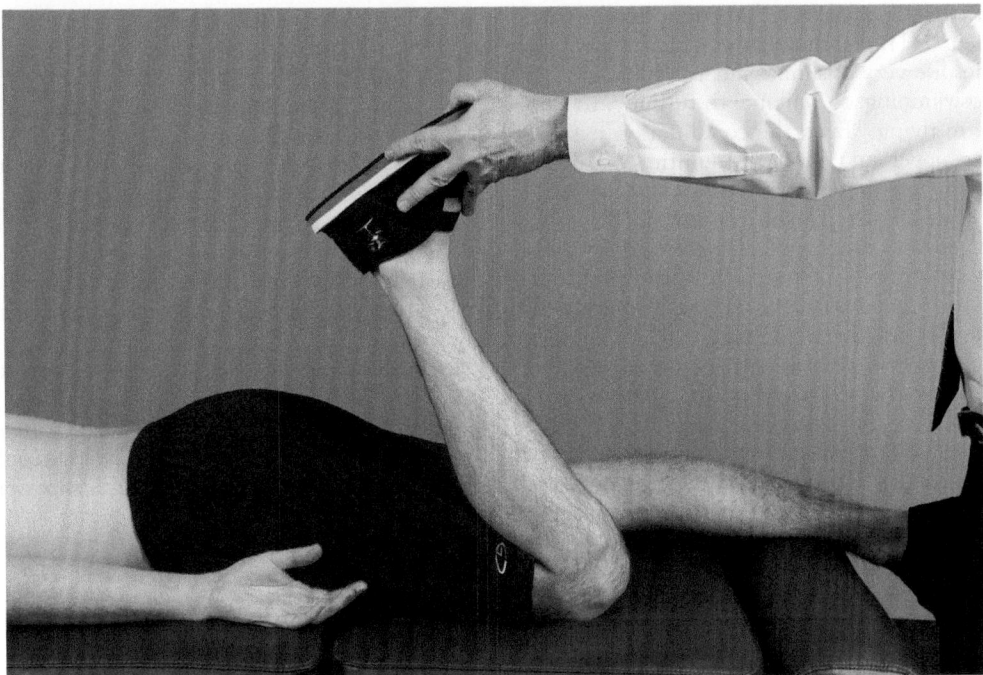

Figure 5-9 Unilateral knee flexion to resistance (Position #4).

movements are distributed throughout the hind limb enlargement and the lower thoracic cord.

Findings could help to explain the leg length reactivity that occurs through the utilization of Position #4 (Figure 5-9), which involves flexing the PD leg to resistance toward the buttocks following completion of an Isolation Test. Through unilateral flexion of the knee to resistance, the right-left mechanisms are singled out. This is coupled with neuronal pathways that are activated when both legs are evaluated in Position #1 and Position #2. This process of analysis can be used to evaluate side-specific pathways, and to investigate how they feed into and are coupled with bilateral movement.

Over the past 10 years, many research projects dissected the neurons of CPGs, with the assumption that neural networks within the spinal cord had a somewhat independent function. Some investigators held the belief that rhythmic movements such as walking, swimming, and hopping were performed by the CPGs in the spinal cord, and that the brain was involved only in telling it when to start, how fast to go, and when to stop. After transecting the spinal cords of rats, reattaching them, and adding embryonic neurological tissues, researchers were able to actually observe the rat "walking again." However, as many of you may have seen on television news video clips, this "quote-unquote" walking was *very* uncoordinated.

Nevertheless, and rightly so, this held out much promise and hope to the paraplegics and quadriplegics of the world.

The function of CPGs is further discussed in writings by Marilyn MacKay-Lyons in her review of the evidence.[101] She looks at other factors involved in the central pattern generation of locomotion, including supraspinal, sensory, and neuromodulatory influences that interact with CPGs to shape final motor output. CPGs are not that simple, especially in higher vertebrates. Inputs from beyond the spinal cord play a major role not only in initiating locomotion but also in adapting the locomotor pattern to environmental and motivational conditions. Most of the CPG research has focused on cats, rats, lampreys, and mice, but human studies have been reported as well. Contrary to previous findings, the sensory afferents are now known to be involved in muscle and cutaneous reflexes, and they have important regulatory functions in preserving balance and ensuring stable phase transitions during the locomotor cycle. Whether CPGs exists in humans is uncertain, and according to MacKay-Lyons, the "best guess" at this point is cautious affirmation.

One of the first points discussed in the review is the question of whether data obtained from one species of animals can be applied to another species. However, when applied to other species, the general neural organization of CPG function in locomotion appears to be similar in all species studied.[106] This is remarkable given that different species use very dissimilar modes of locomotion, from swimming, to walking, to running, to hopping, to flying. "Even the coordination patterns of the upper and lower extremities in human bipedal locomotion have features in common with those of quadrupedal locomotion."[107]

In research involving complete transection of the thoracic spine, adult cats placed on a treadmill can achieve alternating and coordinated movements of the hind limbs.[108,109] The term *fictive locomotion* is used for neural activity when these rhythmical patterns occur in the absence of movement. When deafferentation and paralysis are combined, studies have revealed that sensory input is not necessary during the generation of these stereotyped locomotor patterns.[110] As McKay-Lyons noted, "These findings do not imply, however, that, under normal conditions, sensory feedback is unimportant for functional locomotion."[101]

Motor behavior function is clearly thought of as part of a continuum scale. *Where* the behavior is on the continuum depends, at least in part, on the context within which it occurs. Previously, movements were considered to be voluntary or automatic. Now, it is the environment within the movement as it occurs that will determine the mix of supraspinal and spinal influences.[111] This could be related to the differences between walking on a paved path versus a rain-soaked steep mountain trail.

Supraspinal influences should be added to the picture of leg length reactivity; this is detailed within the subsequent research. Two points have been agreed upon regarding supraspinal influences and CPGs. (1) As was noted previously, supraspinal control of spinal locomotor CPGs appears to be similar for all classes of vertebrates.[112] Across classes of vertebrates, nuclei in the mesencephalon, referred to as the mesencephalic locomotor region (MLR), initiate locomotion through activation of lower brainstem reticulospinal neurons.[113] (2) Supraspinal-CPG interaction appears to be far more complex than was previously thought. Feed forward input from reticulospinal neurons through computer modeling reveals that neurons can have variable and unpredictable effects on spinal CPGs.[114] To stabilize locomotor rhythm, feedback via spinoreticular neurons and inputs from other regions of the brain appear to be necessary.[115] Additional support is provided by findings that the brainstem acts as a site of convergence for several inputs, and it appears to provide a locomotion-related gating function. This gating function involves spinoreticular input from the CPGs and from the visual and vestibular systems, which enables the motor control mechanisms to be more responsive to factors in the locomotion environment.[116]

Five functions in the control of locomotion from supraspinal areas have been identified:
1. Activating spinal locomotor CPGs
2. Controlling the intensity of CPG operation
3. Maintaining equilibrium during locomotion
4. Adapting limb movement to external conditions
5. Coordinating locomotion with other motor acts

The function of spinal CPGs is to generate the complex patterns of muscle activity required for actual locomotion. The main supraspinal centers include the following:
• Sensorimotor cortex
• Cerebellum
• Basal ganglia[117]

The basal ganglia have recently been considered an integral part of larger, distinct circuits that involve the cerebral cortex and the thalamus. They have been implicated in a wide variety of motor functions, including the planning, initiation, execution, and termination of motor programs and of motor learning.[118] The cerebellum receives efferent copies of CPG output to the motoneurons through the ventral spinocerebellar and spinoreticulocerebellar pathways, along with information about the activity of peripheral motor functions through the dorsal spinocerebellar tract. In turn, the cerebellum provides an indirect influence back to the motoneurons through the vestibulospinal, rubrospinal, reticulospinal, and corticospinal pathways.[117] The complete function of the cerebellum in locomotor control remains unclear. In research conducted on decerebrated animals, the result was reported as coarse, stereotyped movements with poor interlimb coordination and inaccurate foot placement, as well as equilibrium deficits.[119] The cerebellum's principal function may be the timing of muscle activation, "fine-tuning" the output by adapting each step cycle.[120]

Within the AM of analysis, different types of receptors are stimulated. This stimulation occurs not only within the CPGs of the lower extremities; it also travels up the spine, interacting with different neuronal pools along the way. Within the sensorimotor cortex, the cerebellum, and the basal ganglia, further processing of afferents is evaluated. Where learned memory patterns of nervous system errors are stored, I am not sure. It is theorized here that the nervous system errors can occur anywhere along the kinetic chain of activity that has been accessed. Because the main feedback for locomotion, balance, and standing starts at the receptors of the feet and around the ankle joint, the AM analysis starts in the right place. With the initial reading, large levels of reactivity may occur because when transitioning between Position #1 and Position #2, sensory afferent receptor activity is accumulating from the feet; through the legs, pelvis, and spine; and, finally, to the brain. Leg length reactivity can be dramatic. As each individual is uniquely analyzed and nervous system errors and biomechanical relationships restored and improved on functional feedback levels, the amount of leg length reactivity will lessen. However, for the individual being analyzed, the largest changes of reactivity can occur anywhere along the chain, kinetically and neurologically; this enables the practitioner to objectively determine where to focus treatment for each unique patient.

The following information may also explain, in part, what occurs during LLA that creates leg length reactivity. During locomotion, it was discovered there are two mechanisms involved during the phase shift of the termination of extension and the initiation of flexion. These are the mechanisms of hip extension and the unloading of hind-limb extensor muscles, and each has a different type of afferent input.[121,122] During hip extension, afferents of muscle spindles of the elongated hip flexor muscles are activated, triggering the monosynaptic stretch reflex, which initiates a flexor burst near the end of the stance phase.[123]

An emerging concept regarding the influence of Ib afferent feedback to locomotor CPGs is occurring. Stimulation of Ib afferents from the Golgi tendon organs of the ankle and knee extensors during fictive locomotion in cats with acutely transected spinal cords evokes excitation of extensor motoneurons, rather than anticipated Ib autogenic inhibition.[124] Subsequent research concluded that both Ia and Ib afferents from extensor muscles help to shape the amplitude, duration, and timing of ipsilateral extensor activity.[125] This unexpected finding in the research from spinalized cats of the effects of Ib afferents was hypothesized that in addition to the disynaptic inhibitory pathway from group Ib afferents to extensor motoneurons, there may be two additional pathways that open only during locomotor activity. This involves a disynaptic excitatory pathway from group Ib afferents to extensor motoneurons and an oligosynaptic pathway from group Ib afferents to extensor motoneurons via the CPG extensor half center.[122]

Extensive study has concentrated on the issue of phase-dependent modulation of muscle stretch receptor inputs in human locomotion. The degree of modulation involved is task dependent and is greater during walking than during quiet standing, and is even greater during running.[126] The phasic modulation of Ia input has been demonstrated by changes in magnitude of stretch reflexes and of H reflexes (the EMG analog of the stretch reflex) throughout the course of the gait cycle. The greatest activity occurs during flexion.[127] The principal source for presynaptic inhibition seems to be Ia afferents from hip and knee extensor muscles. From a functional perspective, it has been postulated that during quiet stance, activation of the soleus muscle stretch reflex helps to maintain anteroposterior stability, whereas during locomotion, decreasing the gain of these resistive reflexes prevents them from impeding lower extremity movements.[128]

During AM LLA transition between Position #1 and Position #2, plantar flexion at the ankle (Figure 5-10) applies a stretch to both hip flexors, knee extensors, and ankle dorsiflexors at the same time, and at the same speed. In the progression from Position #2 to Position #3 (Figure 5-11), movement is imparted into the hips in the form of hip extension, and into the pelvis and sacroiliac joints, with migrating movement into the sacrum, the lumbar spine, and upward cephalically. LLA involves stimulation of mechanoreceptors, proprioceptors, and nociceptors throughout different types of fictive weight-bearing activity. Plantar flexion of the ankles, performed as a fictive activity, can involve the kinetic chain in the transition between the stance phase of gait and the push-off stage. Nervous system errors can occur anywhere along the fictive chain of activity. The errors from the right and left centers coordinate the excitatory and inhibitory impulses from the afferents and create unequal contractions throughout the lumbar spine, pelvis, and lower limbs and thus be revealed as leg length reactivity.

In spite of studies that used deafferentation, nervous system isolation, paralysis, and, in humans, anesthetic blocks in the lower limbs, sensory feedback is an integral part of the overall motor control system. Studies prove that sensory feedback is critical in modifying CPG-generated motor programs to facilitate constant adaptations to the environment. "Without question, afferent input plays an important role in stabilizing the resulting motor behaviors. Many experiments have shown that sensory feedback can drive or terminate a rhythmic behavior without being necessary for the normal expression of the behavior."[129]

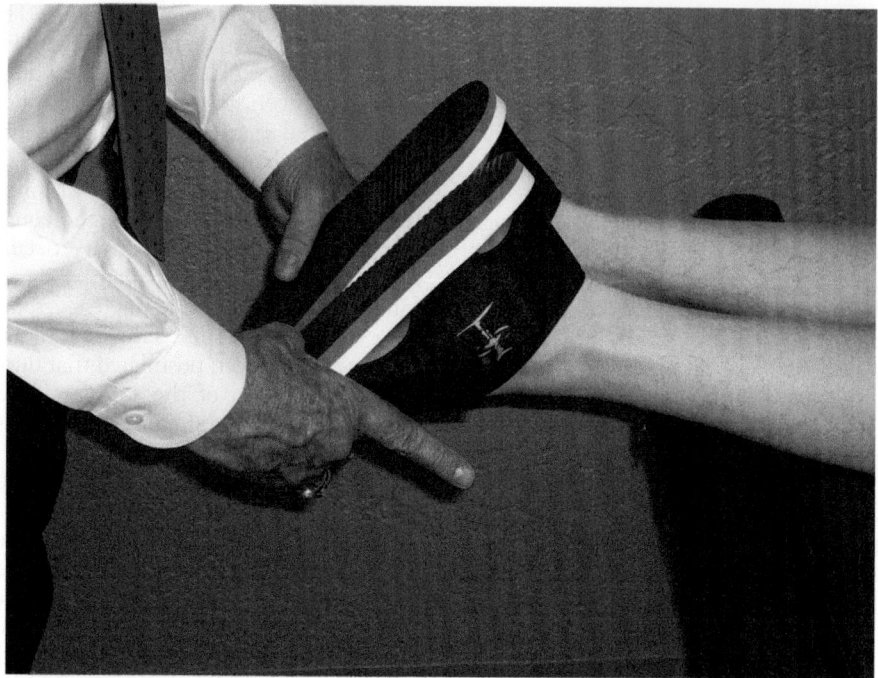

Figure 5-10   Plantar flexion to resistance transitioning from Position #1 to Position #2.

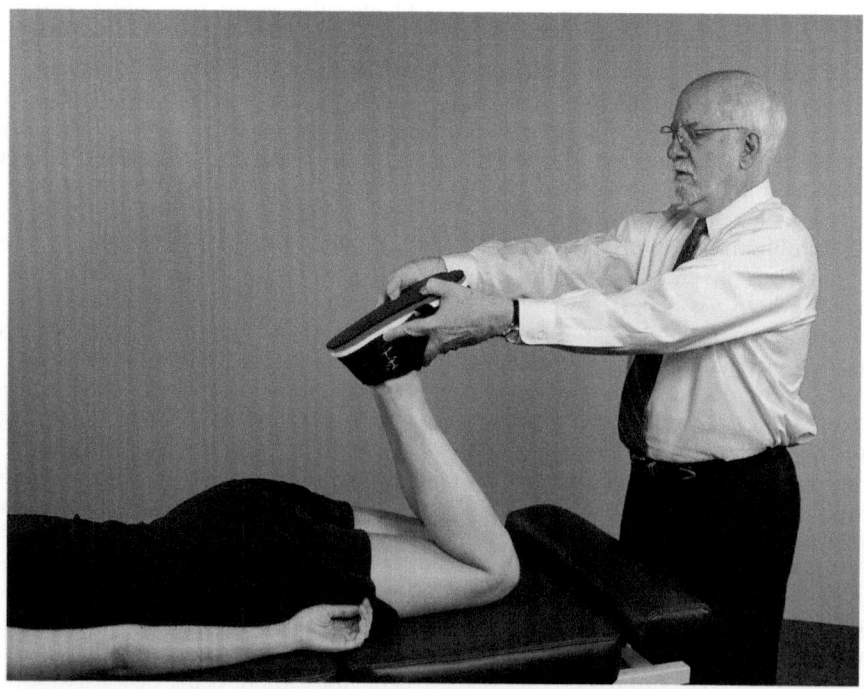

Figure 5-11   Bilateral knee flexion to resistance (Position #3).

Three potential roles have been identified for afferent feedback provided during the production of rhythmic movement; all three roles involve adapting movement to changes in the internal and external environments:

1. Reinforcement of CPG activities, particularly those involving load-bearing muscles such as the hind limb extensor muscles during the stance phase of gait
2. A timing function, whereby sensory feedback provides information to ensure that motor output is appropriate to the biomechanical state of the actual moving body part in terms of its position, direction of movement, and force
3. Facilitation during the phase transitions in rhythmic movements, in particular to ensure that a certain phase of the movement is not initiated until the appropriate biomechanical state of the moving part has been achieved[106]

Another hypothesis focuses on the theory of shared interneurons within CPG networks. Complex movements are configured from pools of multipotent interneurons. It was suggested that pattern generators should be "defined by the behaviors they produce rather than by anatomical boundaries."[111] Humans were observed while walking on a split-belt treadmill with different speeds between the limbs. While contralateral speed was maintained, ipsilateral speed was increased and was found to be associated with increases in ipsilateral gastrocnemius muscle and contralateral tibialis anterior muscle EMG activity. These findings were consistent with a model of flexible coupling involving separate locomotor centers of control for each limb.[130] This research lends additional support for the activation of mechanisms involved in Position #4 of AM analysis.

In a subsequent study in which a split-belt treadmill was used, adaptation to varying limb gaits was achieved within 12 to 15 strides. Over a short interval of walking at a common belt speed, readaptation to a different belt speed occurred within one to three strides.[131] However, when fast and slow sides were reversed, the motor learning effect was not transferred. Therefore in order for "CPG learning" to occur, an interaction between side-specific proprioceptors and spinal interneuronal circuits is necessary.

The pattern of infant stepping resembles that of tetrapods and other bipeds. However, with the maturation of human gait from infancy, determinants relative to humans have been identified. The identified differentiating determinants of human plantigrade gait include some of the following: during heel-strike at the initial contact, a loading response in early stance, pelvic-trunk rotations, and synchronized out-of-phase activity of lower-extremity extensor and flexor muscles. The maturation of human gait may involve reorganization in the spinal CPG circuitry and a more extensive supraspinal dependency on the regulation of locomotion.[132,133]

It has become evident that the nervous system has characteristics that involve a certain amount of plasticity. Treadmill training is being used increasingly to enhance the recovery of walking after transection of the spinal cord in animals, and in the treatment of spinal cord–injured humans. This implies some use-dependent plasticity in spinal pathways involved in locomotor generation. Seven subjects with incomplete spinal cord injury (SCI) underwent assisted treadmill walking with 40% of their body weight supported by an overhead frame. The effect was an immediate normalizing effect on both kinematic and kinetic aspects of gait pattern.[134] Another single subject with an incomplete C5-6 lesion of 7 months' duration with 32% of body weight support (BWS) found small but statistically significant (and purportedly clinically meaningful) improvements in walking speed and in some of the spatial variables of gait.[135]

In a significant study of 77 subjects with acute or chronic incomplete SCIs, 7 subjects with functionally complete paraplegia participated in acute rehabilitation using treadmill walking with BWS. It was reported that 92% (33 of 36) of subjects who initially were wheelchair dependent became able to walk independently, whereas the same level of mobility was achieved in 50% (12 of 24) of comparable subjects who underwent conventional therapy. Although it has been argued by some that the increase in muscle strength is the main consideration, alterations in actual muscle force did not occur. None of the subjects with complete paraplegia improved, and unfortunately, group assignments were not randomized.[136] In supported treadmill training, it is unclear whether improvements in mobility and EMG activity result from the relative contribution of plastic changes in neurologically preserved pathways, or whether they represent changes in the neural circuitry of spinal CPGs.

Marilyn MacKay-Lyons' concluding remarks exhibit receptivity and insight into the complexity of the nervous system:

> Accumulating physiological and behavioral evidence that adaptive processes can occur within the spinal cord has challenged the dogma that the spinal cord is a relatively nonplastic, hardwired conduit for relaying

supraspinal commands. It has become clear, however, that in the intact nervous system, CPGs do not operate in a vacuum but depend on the interplay of information between the brain and spinal cord, with the final motor output shaped by sensory feedback from peripheral receptors and reconfigured by neuromodulators. Further research at each level of interaction, from molecular, cellular, and intercellular to behavioral, will inform the other levels, and, one by one, the mysteries of animal and human locomotion will be solved.[137]

MECHANISMS OF BALANCE FROM THE ANKLE TO THE SPINE

In AM LLA, pressure is applied at the bottom of the calcaneus headward. This is coupled with small amounts of dorsiflexion and with inversion or eversion of the ankles, to start the analysis. This is referred to as Position #1 (Figure 5-12). Then, the feet are plantar-flexed to resistance (Figure 5-13) and are raised to Position #2, with the knees flexed to approximately 90 degrees (Figure 5-14). In the process of transitioning between Position #1 and Position #2, many neural control aspects are stimulated, creating a greater degree of observable leg length reactivity if a nervous system error occurs anywhere along the kinetic chain

of stimulation. Neural control processes of ankle, knee, hip, pelvis, and spinal propriocep-tors, mechanoreceptors, and nociceptors are stimulated, along with mechanisms of balance control. Plantar flexion of the ankle simulates the transition from stance to the push-off phase of gait. By plantarflexing to resistance, stretch reflexes are activated within lumbopelvic stabi-lizers, hip flexors, knee extensors, and ankle dorsiflexors (tibialis anterior). A Position #5 (Figure 5-15) is also included in the AM of analysis, which has been clinically observed and theorized to be related primarily to the pos-terior mechanical elements of the vertebrae, namely, focused around the facet joints. Subsequent research will attempt to explain this mechanism of analysis as well.

Published research illustrates the neurological connections noted in the previous paragraph. Genetically, we are programmed for bipedal locomotion. During standing and throughout locomotion, numerous neural pathways of control and stability are coupled with the constant assess-ment of environmental changes and feedback mechanisms to maintain balance and control that are fictively activated in AM LLA. Research has suggested that long-latency reflexes in the tibialis anterior muscle are evoked by activation of cutaneous afferents from the human foot, which is stimulated throughout LLA. It is also

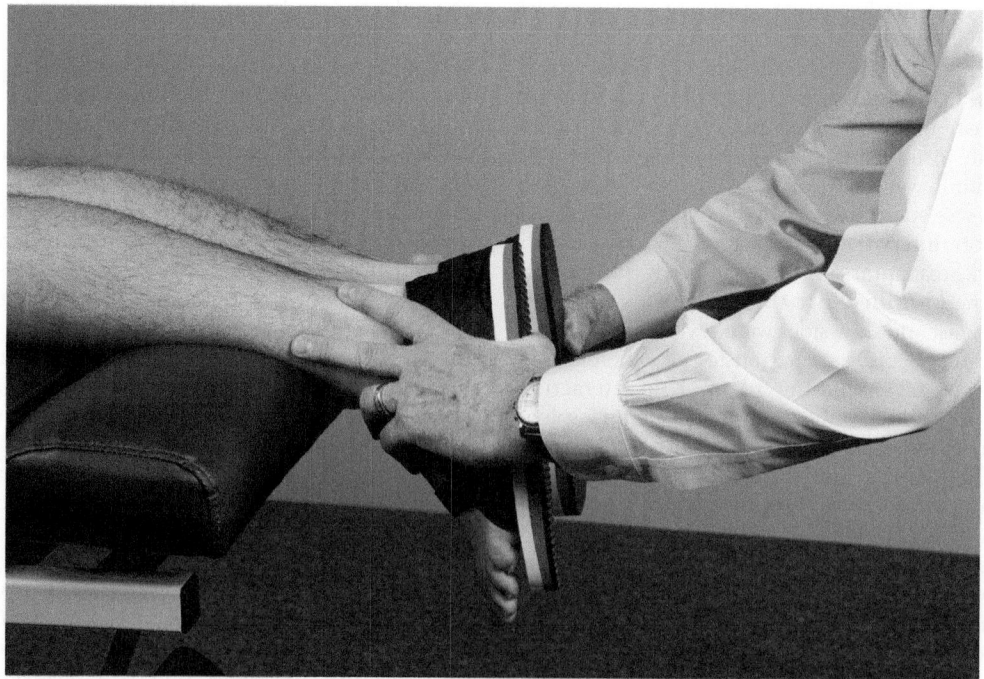

Figure 5-12 Bilateral fictive weight-bearing stimulus with Position #1.

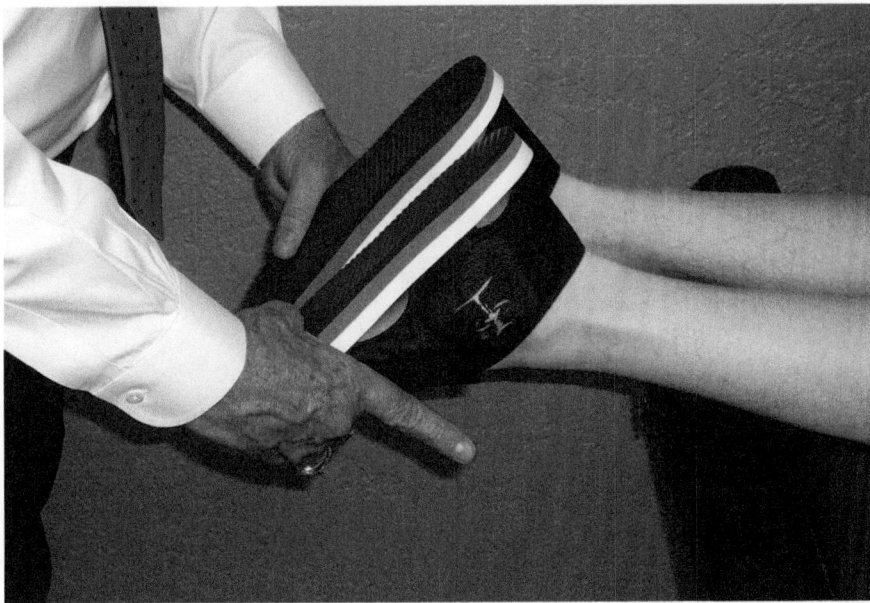

Figure 5-13 Activation of joint proprioceptors and stretch receptors of the hip flexors, knee extensors, and ankle dorsiflexors.

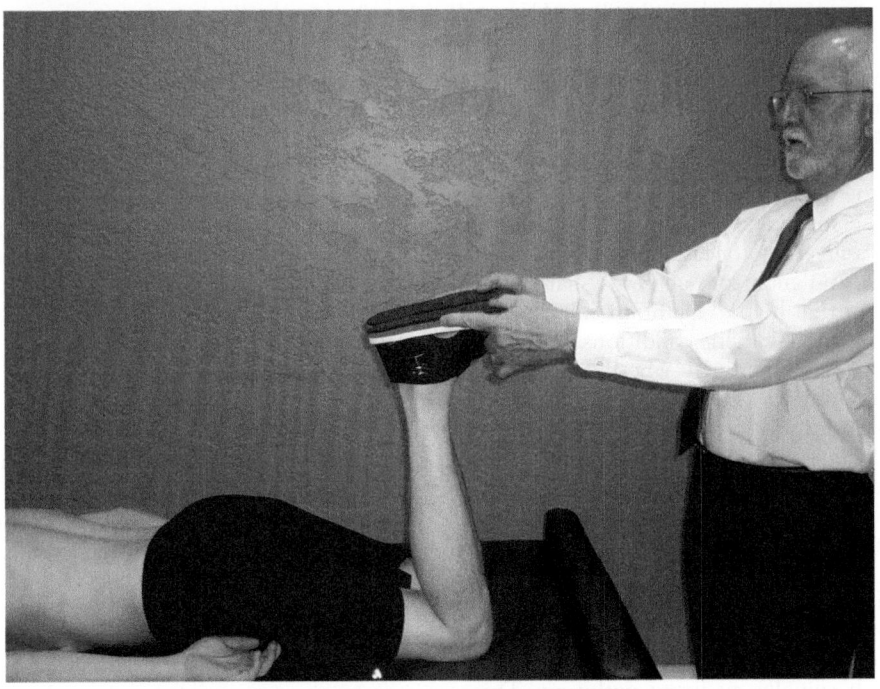

Figure 5-14 Position #2 to 90 degrees or before resistance.

suggested that this is mediated, at least in part, by a transcortical pathway.[138] Pathways from the foot and lower limb feed forward to activate the kinetic chain of a neural control system through the entire spine to the brain.

Findings raise the question as to the possibility of low-threshold *cutaneous* afferents sharing common interneurons with low-threshold *muscle* afferent reflexes that have identical onset latencies. Movements are influenced by complex

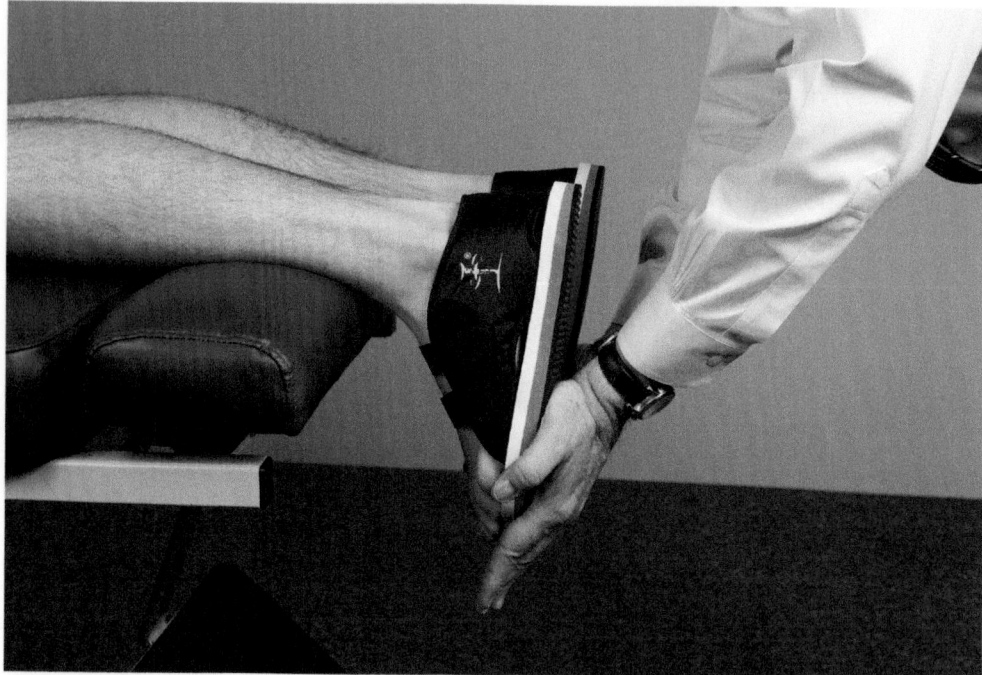

Figure 5-15   Dorsiflexion of both ankles to resistance (Position #5), stimulating balance mechanisms, proprioceptors, nociceptors, and mechanoreceptors, along with stretch reflexes of hip extensors, knee flexors, and ankle plantar flexors.

reflex effects that are associated with low-level stimulation of a cutaneous nerve, indicating a rich assortment of peripheral responses. The predominance of a specific effect is most likely determined by the interaction of this input with other peripheral signals and descending commands specific to a given motor task.[139] It makes sense that muscle and cutaneous afferents share common neurons that help to maintain balance and control throughout varying conditions.

Research has examined whether a strong synaptic coupling exists between tactile afferents in the sole of the foot and the motoneurons that supply muscles that act about the ankle. It has been known for some time that populations of cutaneous and muscle afferents can provide short-latency facilitation of motoneuron pools. Recently, it has been shown that input from individual low-threshold mechanoreceptors in the glabrous skin of the hand can modulate ongoing activity in muscles that act on the fingers through spinally mediated pathways. This research model for the hand was applied to the foot. A total of 53 low-threshold mechanoreceptors were recorded in the glabrous skin of the foot via microelectrodes inserted percutaneously into the tibial nerves of human subjects who were awake. Reflex modulation of ongoing whole muscle electromyography was observed for each of the four classes of low-threshold

cutaneous mechanoreceptors. Results indicate that strong synaptic coupling between tactile afferents and spinal motoneurons is not a specialization of the hand; the potential importance of cutaneous inputs from the sole of the foot in the control of gait and posture is emphasized.[140]

Previous research studies focused on responses to noxious stimulations of afferents. This is important in terms of leg length reactivity as it relates to phases of gait and cutaneous reflexes from the foot. The research revealed that

during human gait, transmission of cutaneous reflexes from the foot is controlled specifically according to the phase of the step cycle. These reflex responses can be evoked by non-nociceptive stimuli, and therefore it is thought that the large-myelinated and low-threshold $\alpha\beta$ afferent fibers mediate these reflexes. The sural nerve of both patients and healthy control subjects was stimulated electrically at a non-nociceptive intensity during the early and late swing phases while they walked on a treadmill. The responses were studied by recording electromyographic (EMG) activity of the biceps femoris (BF) and tibialis anterior (TA) of the stimulated leg. The TA responses for the healthy subjects were on average facilitatory during early swing and suppressive during end swing. It is concluded that low-threshold $\alpha\beta$

sensory fibers mediate these reflexes during human gait. The low threshold and the precise phase-dependent control of these responses suggest that these responses are important in the regulation of gait. The loss of such reflex activity may be related to the gait impairments of these patients.[141]

Another study examined human subjects in a supine position. Reflex responses were elicited in muscles that act at the ankle through electrical stimulation of low-threshold afferents from the foot in human subjects who were reclining supine. EMG recordings were made from the tibialis anterior (TA), peroneus longus (PL), soleus (SOL), medial gastrocnemius (MG), and lateral gastrocnemius (LG) muscles with the use of intramuscular wire electrodes. Subjects were then recorded in a standing posture without support and with their eyes closed. Reflex patterns were seen only in active muscles, and these patterns were similar to those in the reclining posture. "It is concluded that afferents from mechanoreceptors in the sole of the foot have multisynaptic reflex connections with the motoneuron pools innervating the muscles that act at the ankle. When the muscles are active in standing or walking, cutaneous feedback may play a role in modulating motoneuron output and thereby contribute to stabilization of stance and gait."[142]

Another study took six healthy subjects who were studied at rest and during different levels of steady voluntary contraction through the reflex responses of the TA muscle to stimulation of the cutaneous afferents arising from the plantar aspect of the foot. At rest, the threshold of response and the threshold of subjective pain sensation coincided. An interaction between nociceptive and non-nociceptive inputs was found at a premotoneuronal level during experiments of spatial summation. "It is therefore proposed that nociceptive and non-nociceptive cutaneous afferents arising from the foot sole use the same short-latency spinal pathway to contact TA MNs (motoneurons) and that their relative contribution to its segmental activation is contingent upon descending command."[143]

Another aspect proposed to be involved throughout AM LLA is the stimulation of stretch reflexes. Recently published studies have evaluated the effect of presynaptic versus postsynaptic mechanisms in decreasing spinal reflex response during passive muscle stretching. The change in EMG responses of two reflex pathways that shared a common pool of motoneurons, with (Hoffmann or H reflex)

or without (exteroceptive or E reflex) a presynaptic inhibitory mechanism, was compared. EMG activities were recorded in the soleus muscle in response to electrical stimulation of the tibial nerve at the popliteal fossa (H reflex) and at the ankle (E reflex) for different dorsiflexion angles of the ankle.

The results indicate that in the case of small-amplitude muscle stretching (10 degrees of dorsiflexion), a significant reduction (-25%; $P < 0.05$) in the Hmax/Mmax ratio was present without any significant change in the Emax/Mmax ratio. At a greater stretching amplitude (20 degrees of dorsiflexion), the E reflex was found to be reduced (-54.6%; $P < 0.001$) to a similar extent as the H reflex (-54.2%). As soon as the ankle joint returned to the neutral position (ankle at 90 degrees), the two reflex responses recovered their initial values. These results indicate that reduced motoneurone excitation during stretching is caused by pre- and postsynaptic mechanisms. Whereas premotoneuronal mechanisms are mainly involved in the case of small stretching amplitude, postsynaptic ones play a dominant role in the reflex inhibition when larger stretching amplitude is performed.[144]

With regard to Position #5 in the AM analysis, dorsiflexion of the ankles is brought to resistance in a quick manner (see Figure 5-15). As was noted in the research described earlier, activity was recorded at 10 and 20 degrees of dorsiflexion with varying responses: presynaptic and postsynaptic, reduced motoneuron excitation, and reflex inhibition. In the processes of AM LLA, varying degrees of ankle movement occur. Research described in the previous paragraph reveals that once the ankle joints were returned to neutral (90 degrees), the EMG recordings were quieted. After small amplitudes of muscle stretching (10 degrees of ankle dorsiflexion), the H reflex and the E reflex recovered their *initial* value. This could explain, in part, why threshold values return to normal levels as leg lengths become balanced. During LLA, normal movements create normal responses, and stimulation of neurons at subthreshold levels (i.e., neuroarticular dysfunction) (subluxation complex) produces an exaggerated response, as is seen in leg length reactivity.

In the AM, ideally, the patient is mechanically transitioned from a standing posture to a prone position with the use of a specially designed table (see Chapter 6, Figures 6-1 and 6-2). The patient is asked not to move or shift during this process. At rest, before any other stimulation is applied, the practitioner visually observes any signs of leg length reactivity. The first step of the analysis involves theoretically looking at the patient's preserved overall neurological patterns of upright, locomoting, weight-bearing posture. Further analysis and treatment are systematically designed to address and reduce nervous system errors from toes to head.

Other aspects of the previous study emphasize why it is important during AM LLA for the practitioner to keep his or her hands off the feet. Only 10 degrees of dorsiflexion creates EMG activity, and once the ankles have returned to the neutral position, this is quieted. By removing the hands from the patient, and eliminating any habitual contact between the practitioner and the patient, background noise per se can be reduced. The other aspect shows the neurological activity that occurs with passive stretching of the patient in non–weight bearing. Also, ankle dorsiflexion through utilization of Position #5 reveals activity at as early as 10 degrees of ankle dorsiflexion and activates more complex neuronal pathways and reflexes as the degree of dorsiflexion is increased.

The next couple of research projects presented will further the neurological connections, in humans, of the ankle to the hip. This next study was designed to investigate the influence of background EMG during changes in limb loading. Electrical stimulus intensity from the sural nerve evoked EMG responses in the proximal hip (ipsilateral gluteus medius and contralateral adductor longus) and in the distal ankle (ipsilateral soleus) muscles during quiet standing. An interesting phenomenon occurred: Reflex responses were consistently seen in the gluteus medius and soleus but not in the adductor longus. "The results demonstrate consistent sural nerve evoked EMG responses in both a hip (gluteus medius) and ankle (soleus) muscle. While the findings for soleus generally corroborate and extend previous studies, the responses observed for the lateral hip muscle have not been previously reported."[145] These connections can be related to some of the leg length reactivity correlation of pelvic rotation and hip movements, in addition to the following.

The objectives of this study were to identify the involved afferents and their relative contribution to soleus H-reflex modulation induced by changes in hip position, and to discuss how these effects relate to the activity of spinal interneuronal circuits. The study group included 11 subjects with incomplete SCI. The actions of group I synergistic and antagonistic muscle afferents (e.g., common peroneal nerve [CPN], medial gastrocnemius [MG]) and of tactile plantar cutaneous afferents on the soleus H reflex during controlled hip angle variations were evaluated. Plantar skin stimulation was performed with the hip extended at 10 degrees. Evidence emerged that in human chronic SCI, the classic key inhibitory reflex actions were switched to facilitory. Another important consideration for rehabilitation and leg length reactivity is that spinal processing of plantar cutaneous sensory input and the actions of synergistic/antagonistic muscle afferents interact with hip proprioceptive input.[146]

Another study involving SCI subjects concluded, "when changes in static hip joint position are imposed in SCI subjects, changes in afferent feedback from hip proprioceptors are capable of promoting a switch between excitatory and inhibitory pathways. Associated changes in H reflex (stretch reflex) latency and duration are consistent with the hypothesis that oligosynaptic inputs contribute to the hip angle-induced H reflex modulation."[147]

The next study was conducted with healthy human subjects, again for observation and evaluation of group I muscle afferents arising from the same spinal segments at the soleus innervation (e.g., CPN) or from more proximal spinal segments (femoral nerve; FN) on the soleus H reflex, and any modification that occurs as the result of changes in hip position: "These findings indicate that hip proprioceptors interact with spinal inhibitory interneurons to enhance spinal reflex excitability under static conditions. This neural switch might constitute an important feature of movement regulation in humans."[148]

Another connection between hip proprioceptors and plantar cutaneous mechanoreceptors was published. Investigators found that the effects of plantar skin stimulation on the flexion reflex were also dependent on the hip angle: "The results suggest that hip proprioceptors and plantar cutaneous mechanoreceptors strongly modulate flexion reflex pathways in chronic human SCI, verifying that this type of sensory afferent feedback interacts with spinal interneuronal circuits that have been considered as forerunners of stepping and locomotion."[149]

A related factor for consideration involves the feedback mechanisms and afferent receptors around and within the knee joint and cruciate ligaments. Throughout AM LLA, the knee is flexed at varying degrees, thereby stimulating knee joint proprioceptors. This, coupled with stretching of the quadriceps muscles, results in additional stimulation of afferents, which can result in changes in leg length reactivity. It is important to note that the cruciate ligaments contain many different sensory nerve endings: Ruffini's endings, Pacinian corpuscles, Golgi tendon organ–like endings, and free nerve endings. These nerve endings have different capabilities of providing the central nervous system with information about characteristics of movement, position-related stretches of the ligaments, and any noxious and chemical events that may be occurring. At relatively moderate loads, *not noxious*, the mechanoreceptor afferents are so potent that they may induce major changes in response to muscle spindle afferents. As researchers have pointed out, it is clearly unlikely that the ligaments are passive ropelike structures with a purely biomechanical function, and it is reasonable to assume that knee joint ligaments are capable of providing the central nervous system with a varied receptor inflow in all situations. Through application of tonically low traction force (5 to 40 N) to the cruciate ligaments, most of the observed effects on spindle afferent responses were caused by slowly adapting receptors with low thresholds to mechanical deformation.[150] This information is important to note because previous thought and research suggested that the mechanoreceptors are just located in the periarticular structures of the joint; therefore this research adds yet another dimension to the kinetic chains of information that are processed.

The sacroiliac joints have been theorized to have little movement capability, and thus little effect on maintaining stability or on locomotion. No test has been accepted for use in diagnosing sacroiliac joint pain, although several examination procedures have been developed in an attempt to relate pain to the sacroiliac joint. These are not considered to be validated.[151-153] However, the pelvis has an active role throughout gait or locomotion and clinically appears as a pain generator. The sacroiliac joint is richly innervated with thick, thin, and unmyelinated nerve fibers that are compatible with a broad range of sensory receptors, including encapsulated mechanoreceptors.[18,154,155]

Indahl et al.[18] studied 10 adolescent pigs and inserted EMG electrodes into the multifidus, gluteus medius, gluteus maximus, and quadratus lumborum muscles. Nerve elements of the sacroiliac joint were stimulated. The ventral area produced predominant contractions in the gluteus medius and quadratus lumborum muscles, and stimulation of the superficial dorsal layer of the sacroiliac joint capsule elicited responses predominantly in the medially located multifidus fascicles. Thus it appears that different areas of the sacroiliac joint play different roles in regulating the locomotive system.

Descending signals from the brainstem activate complex reflex systems in the spinal cord, where the myotactic units with their receptors and polysynaptic circuits are the building blocks. Afferent information is essential in the modification of muscle activation to make it well coordinated and functional. Mechanoreceptor responses due to loading and movements probably have a primary effect on modulation and modification of descending signals from higher levels of the central nervous system, which are responsible for initiation of movements.[156]

The findings from this study suggest that the sacroiliac joints are involved in activating muscles which are responsible for overall posture control and in the control of the lumbar spine on a segmental level.

One last important note by Indahl indicates that depending on how irritated or inflamed the structures of the sacroiliac joint may be, it may cause perturbation in the proprioceptive function of the different receptors and result in increased and prolonged muscle activation. This can activate nociceptors and cause pain. The irritation of low-threshold nerve endings in the sacroiliac joint tissue may trigger reflexive activation of the gluteal and paraspinal muscles that may become painful and also develop trigger points over time.

COORDINATION OF FEEDBACK MECHANISM FOR SPINAL STABILITY

This section builds on the previous section but focuses more on the spine and the body as a whole, including the coordinating feedback mechanisms and afferent inputs and strategies used for achieving stability and balance. We have examined research that connected the kinetic chain of afferent inputs from the toe pads, central pads, feet, ankles, knees, hips, sacroiliacs, and lumbar spine cephalically into the brain relative to their neurological effects on spinal stability in humans and animals. Recently published research reveals strategies that affect the body in maintaining balance in standing and during locomotion and what reacting mechanisms are involved when unstable surfaces are met during these activities.

In a study by Horak and Nashner,[14] subjects stood on a normal support surface and were exposed to brief forward and backward horizontal perturbations. Activity began in the ankle joint muscles and then radiated in sequence to the thigh and trunk muscles on the same dorsal or ventral aspect of the body. Compensatory torques within the activation pattern around the ankle joints restored equilibrium by moving the center of mass (COM) forward or backward. The term *ankle strategy* has been applied because this pattern restores equilibrium by moving the body primarily around the ankle joints. During corrective movements performed to maintain balance, the body rotated about the ankle joints as an approximately rigid mass.

In contrast, subjects stood on a support surface that was short in relation to foot length. To maintain balance while standing, subjects activated leg and trunk muscles at similar latencies but organized the activity differently. The trunk and thigh muscles antagonistic to those used in the ankle strategy were activated proximal-to-distal in sequence; this was opposite to the ankle strategy. Movements in this activation pattern produced a compensatory horizontal shear force against the support, but with little or no ankle torque. The term *hip strategy* has been used to refer to this pattern because resultant motion is focused primarily about the hip joints.

The results of this study show that subjects can synthesize a continuum of different postural movements by combining the two distinct strategies for ankle and hip at different magnitudes and temporal relations. The combination of strategies is influenced not only by the current support surface environment, but also by the subject's recent experiences. The two distinct strategies are influenced by prior experiences as well as by current feedback information. When a new surface condition is present, response patterns resemble those used under the previous condition. Additionally, changes in the biomechanical boundaries between the ankle and the hip can change as a result of pathology.[157,158]

An in-depth and well-engineered study by Winter et al.[15] observed mechanisms in the stiffness control of balance in quiet standing. This model assumed that muscles act as springs to cause the center of pressure (COP) to move in phase with the COM as the body sways about some desired position. Stiffness control provided by hip abductors/adductors is noted in the sagittal plane at the ankle plantar flexors and in the frontal plane.

These investigators cite many other studies that have shown that when various sensory systems are systematically manipulated, body sway is affected. One such study revealed that stimulation of the ankle muscle with vibration resulted in increased body sway that was directionally specific.[159] Investigators modeled and validated an inverted pendulum model to explain the anterior-to-posterior and medial-to-lateral accelerations of the COM during initiation and termination of gait, along with control mechanisms for maintaining balance that involved an ankle strategy and a hip strategy. The body's COM is regulated through movement of the COP under the feet. The COP is controlled by ankle plantarflexor/dorsiflexor torque in the sagittal plane and by hip abductor/adductor torque in the frontal plane. The authors propose that this restoration torque is set by the central nervous system setting of joint stiffness through appropriate muscle tone as a simple way of controlling body COM during quiet standing. Central nervous system control of balance at a wide stance is not as critical, whereas at a narrow width stance, joint stiffness must be more rigidly controlled. The ankle and hip strategies remained applicable and were unchanged in subjects between eyes open and eyes closed conditions.

Astronauts were observed and balance strategies in weight bearing and during long-term weightlessness of four months' duration were recorded in two subjects. Investigators analyzed the adaptation of dynamic movement-posture coordination during forward trunk bending. Evaluation of postural adjustments with trunk bending revealed that plantarflexion of the ankle joint angle remained close to preflight values. Researchers further concluded, "On the basis of experimental observation in normogravity and modeling studies, it was concluded that the postural adjustments cannot have a purely passive origin but must be produced by centrally controlled commands that are mainly focused on ankle flexor muscles. Comparable conclusions were drawn by Eng et al.[160] when they modeled the dynamic interactions between segments during arm raising."[161]

A well-designed study[162] examined the COM and lower limb dynamics and recovery response modulation of muscle activity during locomotion across unexpected compliant surfaces. Additionally, scaling behaviors (up and over the obstacle) of varying levels of compliance were observed. Eight young adults walked along a walkway and stepped on unexpected compliant surfaces in the middle of the travel path. These blocks within the walkway were able to be manipulated so that the surface was stable or would give way at different angles. Whole body kinematic information was collected, along with surface EMG details of selected bilateral lower limb and trunk muscles. Before this study was undertaken, it was largely unknown how the body controls the COM during walking when confronted with an abrupt change in surface compliance.

The first exposure to the unexpected compliant surface represents the true reactive response because no prior experience or knowledge about the surface was available[163] (the participants had not experienced nor had any knowledge that the surface could be depressed during their walking trial). These results were considered separately and were compared with baseline control trials for each measure. The first response was a stiffening response at the ankle, to stabilize the limb in contact with the unstable surface. Results were consistent with previous studies suggesting that the initial ankle extensor activity is preprogrammed for landing; more of a modulated reflex that is functionally appropriate for the type of perturbation encountered.

The biggest change between the first trial and subsequent trials was an increase in knee flexion after toe-off on the compliant surface for toe clearance. This action was performed to prevent tripping and to ensure safe forward progression. At first exposure to the unstable surface, peak COM was lower than in subsequent trials as seen by an increase in knee flexion that allowed toe clearance to be maintained in the early swing phase of the perturbed limb.

The central nervous system must not only maintain dynamic stability after the step onto an unstable surface, it also must manage step-off onto a more stable ground. The goal of the central nervous system appears to be to adjust lower limb dynamics for the subsequent step, rather than attempting to correct for the perturbation, thus *planning a feed forwarded strategy*. Another aspect is a postural control system designed to stabilize head movements during gait. Head stabilization is important during gait to stabilize visual input in the *goal-directed movement*[164] of the feed forwarded strategy. Overall results of the study suggest that the recovery response to a compliant surface perturbation is actively modulated by the central nervous system and is geared toward maintaining dynamic stability.[162]

The research presented in this section provides strong evidence about learned patterns of strategies used in previously encountered situations. These learned patterns are involved in current feedback mechanisms of control and in central nervous system preplanning and anticipating of the response to an unstable surface or condition. Significant changes in the first readings were observed and were considered the true reaction because the subject had no prior knowledge or experience about the surface. Upon additional courses over the walkway, with prior knowledge of footplate instability, different reactions were observed, showing evidence of learned pattern types of strategies in humans.

A recent publication (February 2007) compared healthy and low back pain subjects in terms of their ability to learn strategies during trunk flexion and extension. Participants underwent a learning phase during which feedback was provided; they then performed trials without feedback. Research suggested "that the observed changes in trunk motor control and trunk muscle recruitment strategies are not only mediated by a neurophysiologic adaptation to chronic pain but also by cognitive adaptations modulated by fear of movement and fear of reinjury."[165] In addition to cognitive involvement in learned strategies for these activities, and as shown in the learned patterns of recovery from an uneven surface previously experienced, this new publication provides further evidence of stored kinetic chain memory. These learned memory patterns include strategies used to avoid pain on the basis of feedback from nociception and are integrated with the conscious memory of what created the pain. This learned strategy is recalled and may be incorporated for future feed forwarded planning to avoid pain and reinjury, as motivated by the fear of repeating the experience of pain.

LEG LENGTH REACTIVITY CONNECTION IN ANALYSIS AND TREATMENT

The previous section's research showed the first response to an unstable surface is ankle stiffening. In order to maintain balance, the ankle and hip strategies revealed the body stiffens and moves about an inverted pendulum. Position #5 in the AM of analysis is connected to the evaluation of neuroarticular function of facet joints. In Figures 5-16 and 5-17, the subject is standing with a small block of wood under the balls of her feet to induce ankle dorsiflexion. As in the presented research from the previous section, she used ankle stiffness as her first noted response to maintain balance. In the figures, you can see a slight anterior lean and perhaps some mild tightening of the muscles around her knee joint, along with the posterior muscles of her thigh, hip, pelvis, and lower spine, designed to maintain her balance.

In Figure 5-18, I asked her to stand on a larger block of wood. This was the largest degree of ankle dorsiflexion that she was able to tolerate while maintaining her balance. Multiple factors were now added to the primary ankle stiffness response and were more apparent. I was able to easily observe the ankle and hip strategy as she balanced so we could take the photograph. In this position (Position #5 in weight bearing), the ankles stiffened and controlled the COM

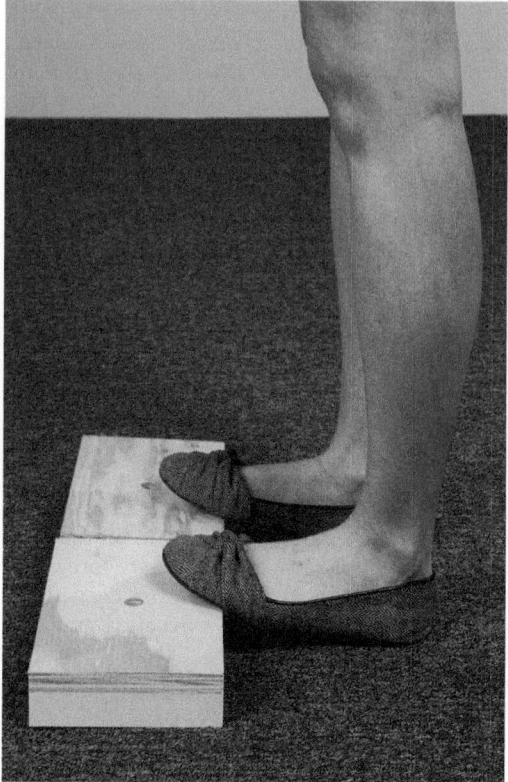

Figure 5-16 Model balancing with feet on a small block of wood.

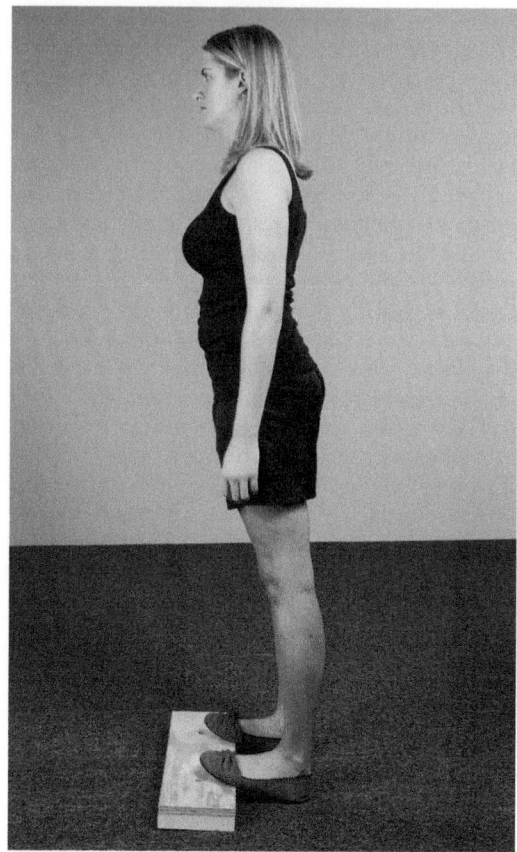

Figure 5-17 Maintaining balance: The model tightens muscles around her ankle and knee joints.

through feedback regarding the COP from the soles of her feet. The ankle plantar flexors, knee flexors, and hip extensors are undergoing a stretch stimulus. As observed in Figure 5-19, her body is stiff and she is leaning forward to maintain her balance. Her COM is now shifted anteriorly. To stiffen her body, the posterior elements of the spine are called into action. With the use of ankle and hip strategies as she leans forward, segmental control of the spine is activated by this stiffening process, primarily through contraction of the intersegmental muscles, namely, the multifidus muscles. As these illustrations crudely demonstrate (position of ankle dorsiflexion to resistance [Position #5]), it is primarily the integrity of the intervertebral facet joint's neurobiomechanical functions that are accessed to prevent the subject from falling forward.

To build on all previous research on additional areas of the spine, consider that during human locomotion, the arms are rhythmically set with the timing of gait (Figures 5-20 and 5-21). To achieve this activity, neurological pathways must exist that may be a preprogrammed type of feature and involve the learning capabilities of patterned strategies. Research in the neonatal mouse

involved electrical stimulation of the cauda equina, which evoked coordinated lumbar locomotor-like activity. Recordings from the second and fifth lumbar ventral roots (L2 and L5, respectively) displayed left-right and flexor-extensor alternation. This pattern is regarded as a signature of locomotor-like activity. The recording in the cervical roots (C8) revealed coupled patterns with those recorded from the L2 left and right neurograms.[85] This research reveals the rhythmic connections between lower limb activity and upper limb activity.

This research study along with studies presented in the previous section could lend support to involvement of AM Isolation Tests involving movements of the upper limbs and the head and resultant leg length reactivity. Coordinated activity occurs rhythmically between the upper and lower limbs without much conscious thought during walking on stable, consistent surfaces. Strategies of balance control are combined with ankle and hip strategies, along with head control, for visual input related to feed forward strategies. In the

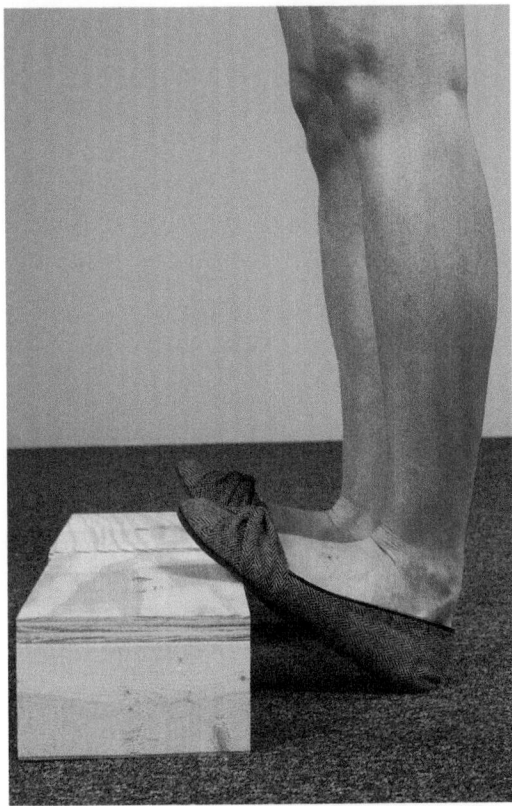

Figure 5-18 Model balancing on a large block of wood at maximum ankle dorsiflexion.

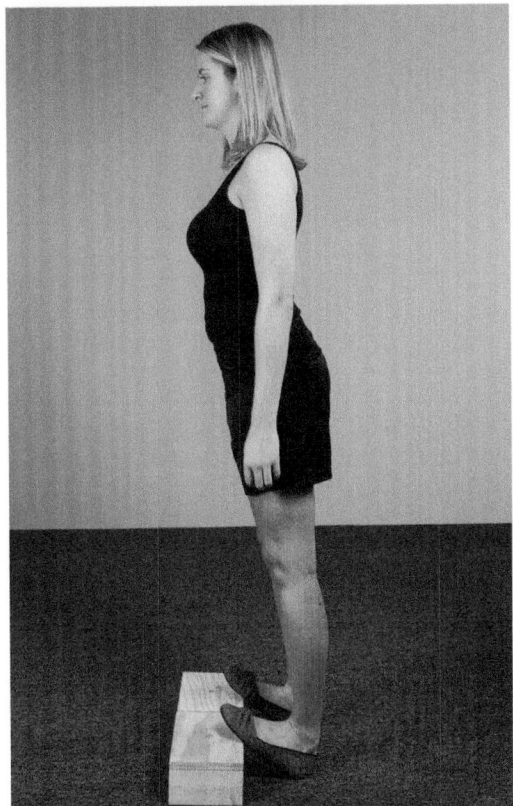

Figure 5-19 Maintaining balance requires anterior body lean, strong tightening of the ankle, knee, hip, pelvis, and lumbar muscles.

studies mentioned, to regain balance, only a small percentage of subjects used any substantial arm movements. When arm movements were observed, they did not contribute to overall balance outside of the ankle and hip strategies, nor did significant changes to the COM occur.

During LLA, fictive weight-bearing activity chains of neurological information are evaluated. Ankle stiffness was the starting point for reactive control of balance to varying conditions. In the AM Protocol, after initial evaluation of leg lengths when the legs become balanced, Isolation Testing begins. The patient starts to add positional postures while lying prone, such as placing the arm across the lower back and turning the head toward the PD side. Mechanisms of rhythmical input between the limbs (right to left and upper to lower) are entered into the kinetic chain of neurobiomechanical input. By adding these postural positions, different neurological chains of afferent input are influenced, and primary *segmental* interneuron pools of information and related biomechanical coupling mechanisms between the intervertebral segments are isolated for the movement performed. In the feed forward

mechanism, contractions to stabilize the spine occur before movement of the limb. This, combined with the position of the head as the visual input, is used in *goal-directed movement* as part of the planning process.

Research relative to leg length reactivity and Isolation Testing in subjects has compared those with symptoms and those without symptoms to show correlation with some limited validity.[166] Overall, Isolation Tests have been observed to yield consistent reproducibility before inclusion into the AM Protocol. The exact neuronal connections involved in a specific Isolation Test must be proven scientifically, but procedures included in the Isolation Tests have been proved over and over by repetition and through consensus of thousands of practitioners in the field. After the particular neuroarticular dysfunctional area is isolated and the nervous system error is corrected with use of the Activator Instrument, nervous input is normalized, muscle tone is recovered, and joint mobility is observed. Leg lengths appear balanced, and symptoms are reduced. Therefore leg length reactivity provides

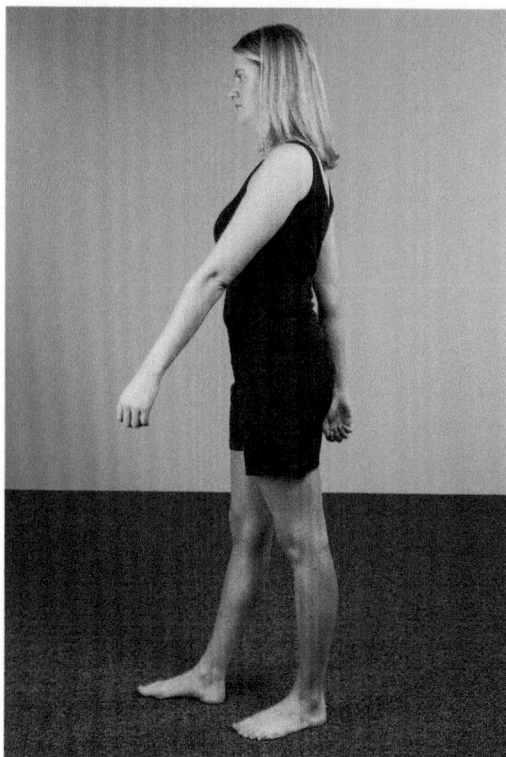

Figure 5-20   The arms swing in a natural rhythm to the gait of the lower limb.

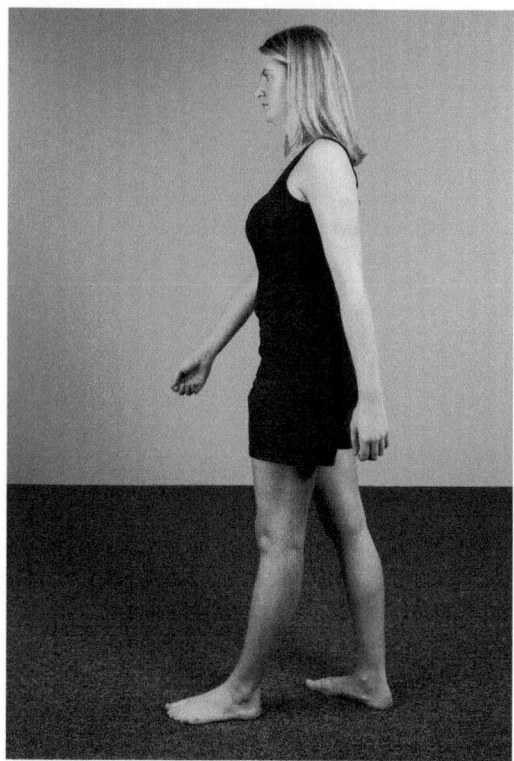

Figure 5-21   Walking involves coordinated input from central pattern generators, right to left interneurons, and upper to lower limb reflexes.

confirmation after the adjustment is provided to the validity of the isolation.

Neuronal connections between the lower limb and the lower spine are well documented in the pathways of leg length reactivity. The correlation of neuronal activity has also been shown between lower and upper limbs, along with the learned patterns in feed forward and feedback mechanisms involvement that are processed at the level of cortical involvement. AM includes Isolation Tests for each individual vertebra; these can be revealed as leg length reactivity if a neural component system error is present. Early in the chapter it was stated, "The segmental mechanical control between the vertebrae are from the actions of the multifidus, intertransversarii and interspinales muscles, but their role may be more proprioceptive of the forces exerted and therefore more involved in the feedback mechanisms which occurs in concert with the mechanoreceptors." Additionally, intervertebral segments may be found outside of the neutral zone and may have altered biomechanics as the result of processes such as disc degeneration, disc herniation, and spondylosis. These are some of the contributing factors to neuroarticular dysfunction that manifests as leg length reactivity.

Clinically, joint instability occurs as "nervous-system errors" and as the presence of "neuroarticular dysfunction." After analyzing the research in regard to neurological connections and muscular function, now the definitions of spinal instability causes and factors relative to leg length reactivity will be considered in the subsequent research. Definitions relevant to this have been addressed by Panjabi.[167] The neutral zone is "that part of the range of physiological intervertebral motion, measured from the neutral position, within which the spinal motion is produced with a minimal internal resistance. It is the zone of high flexibility or laxity." Neutral position is "the posture of the spine in which the overall internal stresses in the spinal column and the muscular effort to hold the posture are minimal." Range of motion is considered

the entire range of the physiological intervertebral motion, measured from the neutral position. It is divided into two parts: neutral and elastic zones. The elastic zone is that part of the physiological intervertebral motion, measured from the end of the neutral zone up to the physiological limit. Within the elastic zone, spinal motion is produced against a significant internal resistance. It is the zone of high stiffness. All of the above quantities exist for each one of the six degrees-of-freedom of motion, i.e., three rotations and three translations.[167]

Given these definitions, spinal movements in a healthy joint should be allowed near the neutral position with minimal expenditure of energy, yet should still provide significant resistance to prevent damaging motion beyond the ends of the physiological range of motion. "Clinical instability is defined as a significant decrease in the capacity of the stabilizing system of the spine to maintain the intervertebral neutral zones within the physiological limits so that there is no neurological dysfunction, no major deformity, and no incapacitation pain."[168] Panjabi summarizes his hypothesis as basically the size of the neutral zone is a better indicator of clinic spinal instability than the overall range of motion. Further, his theory would need to be supported by in vivo studies that were not possible at that time.

Kiefer et al.[169] (in a publication subsequent to Panjabi) explored an intricate model of the spine that consisted of passive components (the osteoligamentous spine) and active components (the spinal muscles). With a vertical load on the passive spine, little resistance is exhibited, but the load-bearing capacity in neutral posture is significantly enhanced by the muscles of the spine; this should be regarded as a *synergetic* system. Kiefer et al. found that relatively small muscle activations are sufficient to stabilize the spine in neutral posture under body weight. In addition, muscles that attach to the rib cage are important for control of overall spinal posture and maintenance of equilibrium. The muscles that attach to the lumbar vertebrae are primarily used to enhance the stability of the spine. Findings of in vivo studies on normal subjects[170] correlated with numerical modeling techniques. Results indicated that the passive spine and its accessory muscles in neutral posture exhibit synergy ("i.e., the behavior of the whole system is unpredicted by the behavior of its parts taken separately").[171] Keifer et al. also notes that the passive spine and the muscles are two physiologically distinct entities. In neutral posture, they function as a unique synergetic system and should not be decoupled into individual subsystems, but they represent a synergetic spinal system that combines the components.[169] This again illustrates how important the neural control system is to the coordination of the synergy of components.

Solomonow et al.[19] used electrical and mechanical stimulation in three patients and a feline model to determine whether mechanoreceptors in the human spine can reflexively recruit muscle force to stabilize the lumbar spine, and to demonstrate in the feline model that such ligamento-muscular synergy is elicited by mechanical deformation of the lumbar supraspinous ligament, the facet joint capsule, and the disc. The authors point out that the literature repeatedly and erroneously confirms ligaments have only a minor mechanical role; stability of the spine results from muscular co-contraction of the anterior and posterior muscles. Solomonow et al. confirmed that in humans, mechanoreceptors in the supraspinal ligament can reflexively elicit, upon mechanical deformation, activity of the paraspinal muscles within the two rostral and caudal motion segments.

Segmental instability in the lumbar spine has been associated with abnormal intervertebral motion. A study by Kaigle et al.[172] investigated alterations in segmental kinematics as a result of the interventions to the passive stabilizing components and to the lumbar musculature. Thirty-three pigs divided into four groups were subjected to various surgical injuries to the L3-L4 motion segment. Analysis included the evaluation of kinematic behavior in the neutral region. Their conclusions can be summarized as follows: Disc or facet injuries alone primarily alter the kinematic behavior of one of the range-of-motion variables. In the neutral region, where muscles are under reduced tension, the motion segment is highly susceptible to instability. Following injury, kinematic behavior on returning from full flexion or full extension is altered in the neutral region.

The intervertebral discs have been recognized as a source of pain, and the outer part of the annulus fibrosus has free nerve endings in the fetal state that develop into various types of receptors. In the adult, five types of nerve terminations can be found, and the complexity of the receptors increases with age.[173] Indahl et al.[16] in a porcine study found upon stimulation of the disc annulus fibrosus there were induced reactions in the multifidus on multiple levels and on the contralateral side. Stimulation of the facet joint capsule induced reactions predominantly on the same side and segmental level as the stimulation. In a more recent Indahl et al.[17] publication, the porcine experimental model revealed that a neuromuscular interaction exists between the intervertebral disc, the zygapophyseal joints, and the paraspinal longissimus muscles. This study also suggested the existence of a complex reflex system, which is responsible for the motion and stabilization of the lumbar spine.

Solomonow et al. received the 1999 Volvo Award in Biomechanical Studies for their work on the in vivo lumbar multifidus of the cat.[174] Biomechanical evidence indicates there is creep in the viscoelastic tissues of the spine that causes increased laxity in the intervertebral joints, and that cyclic occupational functions expose workers to a tenfold increase in episodes of low back injury and pain. The results of the study described for the first time the neurophysiologic process responsible for increased exposure of the spine to injury and pain during cyclic loading. Investigators concluded the following:

1. Laxity induced in the viscoelastic tissues of the spine (ligaments, disc, and joint capsule) by cyclic passive loading, as studied in the in vivo feline lumbar spine, desensitizes the mechanoreceptors within and causes significant decreases or complete elimination of reflexive muscular stabilizing forces in the multifidus muscles.
2. The decrease in activity of the multifidus muscle was most pronounced in the first 5 minutes of cyclic loading, with additional decreases observed over the 50-minute period. Overall activity was decreased by 85% in the first 5 minutes, and by additional subsequent 5% to 10% decreases.
3. During passive cyclic loading of the lumbar spine, a significant decrease in reflexive muscular activity of the multifidus muscles was linked directly to laxity in the viscoelastic structures but excluded muscle fatigue, neurologic habituation, or both.
4. "A 10-minute rest after a 50-minute cyclic passive loading of the lumbar spine results in a minor restoration of reflexive muscular activity, which diminishes at an accelerated rate.
5. The compound effect of increased intervertebral laxity caused by creep in the ligaments and disc together with the significant decrease or elimination of reflexive muscular forces from the paraspinal muscles during cyclic activity fully exposes the lumbar spine to instability and possible injury even when subjected to unloaded activity."[175]

A 2005 publication by DeVocht et al.[176] collected surface EMG data on 16 participants who were divided into two equal groups. One group received spinal manipulation following Diversified Protocol, and the other group Activator Protocol with the use of an Activator II Adjusting Instrument. The authors noted that chiropractors frequently will palpate for tight muscle bundles as an indication of where to adjust. It was

expected that through observation of preadjustment and postadjustment EMG recordings, the tight muscle bundles would be associated with a higher EMG level, which would diminish after appropriate spinal manipulation (SM). "It was presumed that elevated resting EMG levels would be indicative of some aberrant neuromuscular and/or biomechanical state that was correctable by SM. Most of the cases observed were consistent with our expectations."[177] Investigators note that in three out of four cases, a small increase in EMG activity from pretreatment was noted. They also reported that EMG recordings did not necessarily correlate with the level of symptoms the patient had claimed. This study had limitations, but the results support the notion that SM has a virtually immediate and presumable beneficial effect on at least some patients with low back pain; this resulted in lower EMG activity associated with hyperactive paraspinal muscles. It also supported findings consistent with the belief that tight muscle bundles are signs of spinal dysfunction that are correctable by SM.

Slosberg in three different publications[4,51] gives an excellent review of the literature and explanations of how leg length reactivity occurs within AM. He cites Denslow's work,[8,178,179] published in the 1940s, in which he described locating areas of hypertonicity by palpation and inserting needle electrodes into the areas of tight muscles. (In theory, some similarities may be noted to the previous study by DeVocht et al.) Denslow divided the areas of hypertonicity into "major" and "minor" lesions. During relaxation, normal areas exhibited no spontaneous electrical activity; however, in 20 of 25 areas of major lesions, spontaneous electrical activity was observed. He further noted factors that increased spontaneous activity; these included inhalation, painful stimuli, apprehension, and fatigue. Such stimuli in adjacent normal areas did not cause any activity. Slosberg noted that studies using EMG recordings confirm that in normal relaxed musculature, there is no electrical activity.[180-182]

Exaggerated reaction to minor stimuli or normal movement was postulated as an "enduring central excitatory state (C.E.S.) created by subthreshold stimuli." Slosberg noted in 1987 that today, "such a low threshold area would be identified as a 'facilitated segment.'"[4,183] The term defines a spinal segment that responds to various stimuli in a more intense and prolonged manner than is normal. "The reason for such excessive responsiveness is due to the summation of sub-threshold stimuli at an involved spinal segment. This brings the segmentally innervated paraspinal muscles closer to threshold."

Denslow's significant findings as summarized by Slosberg include the following:

- The threshold for a specific area, including facilitated segments, remains relatively constant for periods as long as several months.
- Each subject has his own unique pattern of low threshold (facilitated) areas.
- The right and left paraspinal muscles of the same segment may have markedly different thresholds.
- Major lesions are areas of rigidity and resistance to movement which are frequently associated with pain and spontaneous electrical activity.
- Minor lesions are areas of less rigidity and resistance which may be painless, exhibit no spontaneous activity, but may respond to minor stimuli with a prolonged and exaggerated reaction.[4]

Slosberg notes that the procedures of leg length analysis and Isolation Testing as developed by the AM are not based on clinical findings but "upon decades of scientific inquiry. Denslow's well known successor, Irvin Korr, demonstrated in a series of studies that there is a correlation between facilitated segments and altered segmental sympathetic tone."[55,56,184,185] Such findings suggest that after a corrective adjustment, not only are resultant localized areas of hypertonicity reduced, but their related autonomic and possibly visceral functions may be influenced as well.[186]

SUMMARIZING THE LEG LENGTH REACTIVITY PHENOMENON

Throughout this chapter, I have set forth evidence to support the phenomenon of leg length reactivity. In this lengthy chapter, only a small portion of supporting evidence on the contributing factors of the leg length phenomenon has been presented. In conclusion, the nervous system controls and coordinates all systems of the body. This involves constant monitoring and calculating and predicting of all human systems with the aim of homeostasis. The spinal stabilization system is complex, especially anatomically and neurologically. When short-loop ankle reflexes, long-loop reflexes, feed forward mechanisms, feedback-mediated responses, and the memory of learned patterns from multitudes of experiences are combined, cortical evaluation of function is observed through leg length reactivity. Leg length reactivity following Isolation Tests, Stress Tests, and Pressure Tests cannot be tied to a single feature anatomically, or neurologically. The integrity of the kinetic chain of activity is an integrated processing of all systems, which are evaluated and ultimately controlled by the central nervous system. The nervous system as the master controller is constantly evaluating and reevaluating the functions of the body, including blood supply, chemical compounds, and anatomical structures; these are integrated, remembered, and revealed as leg length reactivity changes when they are called upon for evaluation during LLA.

This chapter has revealed in depth the neurological connections that occur from and between the mechanoreceptors, proprioceptors, and nociceptors. Numerous research examples of animal and human kinetic chains of activities have been discussed. Neurological chains have been connected through research on the toe pads, central pads, sole of the foot, ankle joint movements, the knee and its ligaments, hip proprioceptors, sacroiliac, lumbar spine, lower limb right and left rhythmic patterns, rhythmic patterns between the lower and upper limbs, lumbar to cervical spine, and feed forwarded mechanisms of segmental control that progress from the lumbar spine throughout the rest of the spine to the brain. Research examples for the following kinetic chains of activities included spinal stability, spinal instability, locomotion, reflexive activity from cutaneous stimulations, strategies in balance control, recovery when unstable surfaces are encountered, and how the central nervous system is capable of learning and storing patterns of learned motor activities. These kinetic chains of information processed by the nervous system have been connected in various ways. The research presented in this chapter supports the AM system of analysis and treatment for Positions #1, #2, #3, #4, and #5, along with Isolation Testing.

Published research from more than sixty years ago regarding facilitated segments and leg length reactivity changes is being validated through the neurological relationships established by ongoing research and advanced technology. Leg length reactivity, as a diagnostic phenomenon, is a sensitive, reproducible, and specific tool the clinician can use to evaluate neuroarticular function and dysfunction throughout the axial skeleton and extremities. One day in the near future, I believe the technology may exist that will show all interneuronal connections that occur during AM analysis and the resultant leg length reactivity. Theoretically, I believe this could possibly involve glycolytic isotopes, specific electromagnetic elements, or a pharmacological agent allowing visualization of the entire neurological chain, as is possible with current technologies revealing the blood flow through heart valves out to the blood vessels, to the capillaries, and back through the veins. For now, leg length reactivity, even though it is a consistent, reliable, and reproducible phenomenon that has been used before and by the AM for more than four decades by thousands of practitioners, multiplied by the numbers of patients they benefit, leg length reactivity cannot *definitively* be explained or isolated by a *single* theory.

ACKNOWLEDGMENTS

I would like to thank Dr. Arlan W. Fuhr for the opportunities he has given me. His faith and trust in me to write this chapter without any of his personal influence over its contents is deeply appreciated. I am grateful to my family for all their love, understanding, and support over the past 2 years needed to dedicate to this project. I would like to thank Kelley L. Hunter for all her enthusiastic interest and encouragement. Her medical background and English skills throughout the writing and editing process were invaluable. Robert E. Snyders, Director of Learning Resources at Logan Chiropractic College, provided me with exceptional, accurate, and timely searches of the literature as requested. Also, editing input from Dr. Charlotte Watts and Dr. Lois Ward was an appreciated blessing.

REFERENCES

1. Vahl R, Vahl JB. The newer concept of the myofascial connective tissue webbing system. Chiropr Choice. 2006;5(5):13-6.
2. Richardson C, Hodges P, Hides J. Therapeutic exercise for lumbopelvic stabilization. 2nd ed. London: Churchill Livingstone; 2004. p. 20-2.
3. Panjabi MM. The stabilizing system of the spine. Part II. Neutral zone and stability hypothesis. J Spinal Disord. 1992;5(4):390-7.
4. Slosberg M. Special research report: Activator Methods isolation tests. Todays Chiro. 1987;16(3):16-43.
5. Fuhr AW, Colloca CJ, Green JR, Keller TS. Activator Methods chiropractic technique. St. Louis: Mosby; 1997.
6. Keifer A, Shirazi-Adl A, Parnianpour M. Stability of the human spine in neutral postures. Eur Spine J. 1997;6(1):45-53.
7. Keifer A, Shirazi-Adl A, Parnianpour M. Synergy of the human spine in neutral postures. Eur Spine J. 1998;7(6):471-9.
7a. Gracovetsky S. The spine engine. New York: Springer; 1988. p. 151-2.
7b. Parnianpour M, Shirazi-Adl A, Sparto P, Dariush B. The effect of compressive load on myoelectric activities of ten selected trunk muscles. Proceedings of the 12th TCIEA. Vol 3; 1994 August 15-19; Toronto, Ontario, Canada. p. 119-21.
8. Denslow JS. Analysis of the variability of spinal reflex thresholds. J Neurophysiol. 1944;7:207-15.
9. Richardson C, Hodges P, Hides J. Therapeutic exercise for lumbopelvic stabilization. 2nd ed. London: Churchill Livingstone; 2004. p. 6.
10. Panjabi MM. The stabilizing system of the spine. Part I. Function, dysfunction, adaption, and enhancement. J Spinal Disord. 1992;5(4): 383-9.
11. Hodges PW, Richardson CA. Relationship between limb movement speed and associated contraction of the trunk muscles. Ergonomics. 1997;40(11):1220-30.
12. Hodges PW, Richardson CA. Altered trunk muscle recruitment in people with low back pain with upper limb movement at different speeds. Arch Phys Med Rehabil. 1996;80(9):1005-12.
13. Hodges PW, Cresswell AG, Daggfeldt K, Thorstensson A. Preparatory trunk motion accompanies rapid upper limb movement. Exp Brain Res. 1999;124(1):69-79.
14. Horak F, Nashner LM. Central programming of postural movements: adaptation to altered support-surface configurations. J Neurophysiol. 1986;55(6):1369-81.
15. Winter DA, Patla AE, Prince F, Ishac MG, Gielo-Perczak K. Stiffness control of balance in quiet standing. J Neurophysiol. 1998;80(3): 1211-21.
16. Indahl A, Kaigle A, Reikeras O, Holm S. Electromyographic response of the porcine multifidus musculature after nerve stimulation. Spine. 1995;2(24):2652-8.
17. Indahl A, Kaigle A, Reikeras O, Holm S. Interaction between the porcine lumbar intervertebral disc, zygapophysial joints, and paraspinal muscles. Spine. 1997;22(24):2834-40.
18. Indahl A, Kaigle A, Reikeras O, Holm S. Sacroiliac joint involvement in activation of the porcine spinal and gluteal musculature. J Spinal Disord. 1999;12(4):325-30.
19. Solomonow M, Zhou B-H, Harris M, Lu Y, Baratta RV. The ligamento-muscular stabilizing system of the spine. Spine. 1998;23(23):2552-62.
20. Friberg O. The statics of postural pelvic tilt scoliosis: a radiographic study of 288 consecutive chronic LBP patients. Clin Biomech. 1987;2:212-9.
21. Giles LGF, Taylor JR. Lumbar spine structural changes associated with leg length inequality. Spine. 1982;7(2):159-62.
22. Friberg O. Clinical symptoms and biomechanics of lumbar spine and hip joint in leg length inequality. Spine. 1983;8(6):643-51.
23. Botte RR. An interpretation of the pronation syndrome and foot types of patients with low back pain. J Am Podiatry Assoc. 1981;71(5): 243-53.
24. Liebenson C. Rehabilitation of lower extremity disorders. Dyn Chiropr. January 1, 1997.

25. Busseuil C, Freychat P, Guedj EB, Lacour JR. Rearfoot-forefoot orientation and traumatic risk for runners. Foot Ankle Int. 1998;19(1):32-7.

26. Loudon JK, Jenkins W, Loudon KL. The relationship between static posture and ACL injury in female athletes. J Orthop Sports Phys Ther. 1996;24(2):91-7.

27. Turner MS. The association between tibial torsion and knee joint pathology. Clin Orthop Relat Res. 1994;(302):47-51.

28. Freeman MA, Dean MR, Hanham IW. The etiology and prevention of functional instability of the foot. J Bone Joint Surg Br. 1965;47(4):678-85.

29. Bassewitz H, Shapiro M. Persistent pain after ankle sprain: targeting the causes. Physician Sports Med. 1997;25.

30. Hyland JK. Functional leg length discrepancy. Roanoke (VA): Foot Levelers, Inc.; 1990. Orthopedic Notes AJ-0401-02ON; 2002.

31. Woerman AL, Binder-MacLeod SA. Leg length discrepancy assessment: accuracy and precision in five clinical methods of evaluation. J Orthop Sports Phys Ther. 1984;5:230-8.

32. Friberg O, Nurminen M, Korhonen K, Soinnen E, Mänttäri T. Accuracy and precision of clinical estimation of leg length inequality and lumbar scoliosis: comparison of clinical and radiological measurements. Int Disabil Stud. 1988;10(2):49-53.

33. Knutson GA. Anatomic and functional leg-length inequality: a review and recommendation for clinical decision-making. Part II. The functional or unloaded leg-length asymmetry. Chiropr Osteopat. 2005;13:12.

34. Travell JG, Simons DG. Quadratus lumborum muscle. In: Myofascial pain and dysfunction: the trigger point manual: the lower extremities. 2nd ed. Vol. 2. Baltimore: Williams & Wilkins; 1999. p. 35, 42, 107.

35. Mannello DM. Leg length inequality. J Manipulative Physiol Ther. 1992;15(9):576-90.

36. Walker BF, Buchbinder R. Most commonly used methods of detecting subluxation and the preferred term for its description: a survey of chiropractors in Victoria, Australia. J Manipulative Physiol Ther. 1997;20(9):583-8.

37. White A, Panjabi M.Clinical biomechanics of the spine. Philadelphia: JB Lippincott; 1987. p. 96, 352.

38. Gossman MR, Sahrmann SA, Rose SJ. Review of length-associated changes in muscle. Experimental evidence and clinical implications. Phys Ther. 1982;62(12):1799-808.

39. Petrone MR, Guinn J, Reddin A, Sutlive TG, Flynn TW, Garber WP. The accuracy of the Palpation Meter (PALM) for measuring pelvic crest height difference and leg length discrepancy. J Orthop Sports Phys Ther. 2003;33(6): 319-25.

40. Murrell P, Cornwall MW, Doucet SK. Leg-length discrepancy: effect on the amplitude of postural sway. Arch Phys Med Rehabil. 1991;72(9):646-8.

41. Klein KK, Redler I, Lowman CL. Asymmetries of growth in the pelvis and legs of children: a clinical and statistical study, 1964-1967. J Am Osteopath Assoc. 1968;68(2):105-8.

42. Rhodes DW, Mansfield ER, Bishop PA, Smith JF. Comparison of leg length inequality measurement methods as estimators of the femur head height difference in standing x-ray. J Manipulative Physiol Ther. 1995;18(7):448-52.

43. Cooperstein R, Lisi A. Pelvic torsion: anatomic considerations, construct validity, and chiropractic examination procedures. Top Clin Chiro. 2000;7(3):38-49.

44. Grostic JD. Dentate ligament—card distortion hypothesis. Chiropr Res J. 1988;1(1):47-55.

45. Jemmett R. Spinal stabilization: the new science of back pain. Halifax, Canada: Novont Health Publishing; 2003.

46. Cooperstein R. The reverse double whammy leg check. Dynam Chiropr. 1997;15(16):35-8.

47. Knutson GA, Owens E. Erector spinae and quadratus lumborum muscle endurance tests and supine leg-length alignment asymmetry: an observational study. J Manipulative Physiol Ther. 2005;28(8):575-81.

48. Mincer AE, Cummings GS, Andrew PD, Rau JL. Effect of leg length discrepancy on trunk muscle fatigue and unintended trunk movement. J Phys Ther Sci. 1997;9(1):1-6.

49. McGill SM, Childs A, Liebenson C. Endurance times for low back stabilization exercises: clinical targets for testing and training from a normal database. Arch Phys Med Rehabil. 1999;80:941-4.

50. Andersson EA, Oddsson LI, Grundstrom H, Nilsson J, Thorstensson A. EMG activities of the quadratus lumborum and erector spinae muscles during flexion-relaxation and other motor tasks. Clin Biomech. 1996;11(7):392-400.

51. Slosberg M. Activator Methods: an update and review (part two of two). Todays Chiro. 1988;17(4):17-9.

52. Lawrence D, Pugh J, Tasharaski C, Heinze W. Evaluation of a radiographic method determining short leg mensuration. ACA J Chiro. 1984; 8(6):49-51.

53. Giles LGF. Lumbosacral facetal "joint angles" associated with leg length instability. Rheumatol Rehabil. 1981;20(4):233-8.

54. Giles LGF, Taylor JR. Low back pain associated with leg length inequality. Spine. 1981;6(5): 510-21.

55. Korr IM, Thomas PE, Wright HM. Patterns of electrical skin resistance in man. Acta Neuroveg (Wien). 1958;17(1-2):77-98.

56. Korr IM, Wright HM, Thomas PE. Effects of experimental myofascial insults on cutaneous patterns of sympathetic activity in man. Acta Neuroveg (Wien). 1962;23:329-55.

57. Riley LH, Richter CP. Uses of the electrical skin resistance method in the study of patients with neck and upper extremity pain. Johns Hopkins Med J. 1975;137:69-74.

58. Lawrence D. Lateralization of weight in the presence of structural short leg: a preliminary report. J Manipulative Physiol Ther. 1984;7(2): 105-8.

59. Blustein SM, D'Amico JC. Limb length discrepancy identification, clinical significance and management. J Am Podiatr Med Assoc. 1985;75(4): 199-206.

60. Nguyen HT, Resnick DN, Caldwell SG, Elston EW, Bishop BB, Steinhouser JB, et al. Inter-examiner reliability of Activator Methods relative to leg length evaluation in the prone, extended position. J Manipulative Physiol Ther. 1999;22:565-9.

61. Hinson R, Brown SH. Supine leg length differential estimation: an inter- and intra-examiner reliability study. Chiropr Res J. 1998;5:17-22.

62. Cooperstein R, Morschhauser E, Lisi A, Nick TG. Validity of compressive leg checking in measuring artificial leg-length inequality. J Manipulative Physiol Ther. 2003;26(9):557-66.

63. Fuhr AW, Menke M. Status of Activator Methods chiropractic technique, theory, and practice. J Manipulative Physiol Ther. 2005;28(2):e1-e20.

64. Shambaugh P, Solafani L, Fanselow D. Reliability of the Derefield-Thompson test for leg-length inequality, and use of the test to demonstrate cervical adjusting efficacy. J Manipulative Physiol Ther. 1988;11(5):396-9.

65. DeBoer KF, Harmon RO, Savoie S, Tuttle CD. Inter- and intra-examiner reliability of leg-length differential measurement: a preliminary report. J Manipulative Physiol Ther. 1983;6(2): 61-5.

66. Dorland's illustrated medical dictionary. 25th ed. Philadelphia: Saunders; 1974.

67. Wenban AB. Inappropriate use of the title 'chiropractor' and term 'chiropractic manipulation' in the peer-reviewed biomedical literature. Chiropr Osteopat. 2006;14:16.

68. Terrett AGJ. Misuse of the literature by medical authors in discussing spinal manipulative therapy. J Manipulative Physiol Ther. 1995;18(4): 203-10.

69. Reuter U, Hämling M, Kavuk I, Einhäupl KM, Schielke E. Vertebral artery dissections after chiropractic neck manipulation in Germany over three years. J Neurol. 2006;253(6):724-30.

70. Jemmett R. Spinal stabilization: the new science of back pain. 2nd ed. Halifax, Canada: Novont Health Publishing; 2005.

71. Richardson C, Hodges PW, Hides J. Therapeutic exercise for lumbopelvic stabilization. 2nd ed. London: Churchill Livingstone; 2004.

72. McGill S. Low back disorders: evidence-based prevention and rehabilitation. Champaign (IL): Human Kinetics; 2002.

73. McGill S. Ultimate back fitness and performance. Waterloo, Canada: Wabuno Publishers; 2004.

74. Brand RA. Knee ligaments: a new view. J Biomech Eng. 1986;108(2):106-10.

75. Panjabi MM. The stabilizing system of the spine. Part I. Function, dysfunction, adaption, and enhancement. J Spinal Disord. 1992;5(4):385.

76. Schomburg ED, Steffens H, Wada N. Parallel nociceptive reflex pathways with negative and positive feedback functions to foot extensors in the cat. J Physiol. 2001;536(Pt 2):605-13.

77. House EL, Pansky B. A functional approach to neuroanatomy. 2nd ed. New York: McGraw-Hill; 1967.

78. Taber's cyclopedic medical dictionary. 20th ed. Philadelphia: FA Davis; 2005.

79. http://home.comcast.net/john.kimball./Biology Pages/E/Excitablecells.html.

80. Kandel ER, Schwartz JH, Jessell TM. Principles of neural science. 4th ed. New York: McGraw-Hill; 2000. p. 433.

81. Iggo A, Muir AR. The structure and function of a slowly adapting touch corpuscle in hairy skin. J Physiol (London). 1969;200(3):763-96.

82. AM research and development seminar lecture series, 2006-2007 copyright.

83. McLain RF, Pickar JG. Mechanorecptor endings in human thoracic and lumbar facet joints. Spine. 1998;23(2):168.

84. Wyke BD. The neurology of joints. Ann R Coll Surg Engl. 1967;41(1):25-50.

85. Gordon IT, Whelan PJ. Deciphering the organization and modulation of spinal locomotor central pattern generators. J Exp Biol. 2006;209(Pt 11): 2007-14.

86. Xu H, Whelan PJ, Wenner P. Development of an inhibitory interneuronal circuit in the embryonic spinal cord. J Neurophysiol. 2005;93(5): 2922-33.

87. Wada N, Miyajima N, Akatani J, Shimojo K, Kanda K. Electromyographic activity of M. longissimus and the kinematics of the vertebral column during level and downslope treadmill walking in cats. Brain Res. 2006;1103(1): 140-4.

88. Wada N, Akatani J, Miyajima N, Shimojo K, Kanda K. The role of vertebral column muscles in level versus upslope treadmill walking—an electromyographic and kinematic study. Brain Res. 2006;1090(1):99-109.

89. Wada N, Kanda K. Trunk movements and EMG activity in the cat: level versus upslope walking. Prog Brain Res. 2004;143:175-81.

90. Akatani J, Kanda K, Wada N. Synaptic input from homonymous group I afferents in the longissimus lumborum muscle motoneurons in the L4 spinal segment in cats. Exp Brain Res. 2004;156(3):396-8.

91. Wada N, Kanda K. Neuronal pathways from group-I and -II muscle afferents innervating hindlimb muscles to motoneurons innervating trunk muscles in low-spinal cats. Exp Brain Res. 2001;136(2):263-8.

92. Wada N, Shikaki N, Tokuriki M, Kanda K. Neuronal pathways from low-threshold hindlimb cutaneous afferents to motoneurons innervating trunk muscles in low-spinal cats. Exp Brain Res. 1999;128(4):543-9.

93. Akatani J, Miyata H, Kanda K, Wada N. Differential effects of hindlimb peripheral afferents on motoneurons innervating different parts of longissimus muscle in cats. Exp Brain Res. 2004;157(1):111-6.

94. Wada N, Takahashi K, Kanda K. Synaptic inputs from low threshold afferents of trunk muscles to motoneurons innervating the longissimus lumborum muscle in the spinal cat. Exp Brain Res. 2003;149(4):487-96.

95. Wada N, Kanda Y, Takayama R. Neuronal pathways from foot pad afferents to hindlimb motoneurons in the low spinalized cats. Arch Ital Biol. 1998;136(3):153-66.

96. Wada N. Differential effects of footpad stimulation on the monosynaptic reflex in the spinalized cat. J Vet Med Sci. 1993;55(2):247-9.

97. Wada N, Tokuridi M. Effects of afferent inputs from mechanical and nociceptive receptors in the footpads on the monosynaptic reflex in the spinalized cat. J Vet Med Sci. 1993;55(6):955-8.

98. Furukawa M, Wada N, Tokuriki M, Miyata H. Spinal projections of cat primary afferent fibers innervating caudal facet joints. J Vet Med Sci. 2000;62(9):1005-7.

99. Wada N, Kanda Y, Tokuriki M, Kanda K. Neuronal pathways from low-threshold muscle and cutaneous afferents innervating tail to trunk muscle motoneurons in the cat. J Comp Physiol [A]. 2000;186(7-8):771-9.

100. Grillner S. Control of locomotion in bipeds, tetrapods and fish. In: Brooks VB. Handbook of physiology: section 1: the nervous system. Volume II: motor control. Bethesda (MD): American Physiological Society, Waverly Press; 1981. p. 1179-236.

101. MacKay-Lyons M. Central pattern generation of locomotion: a review of the evidence. Phys Ther. 2002;82(1):69-83.

102. Jiang Z, Carlin KP, Brownstone RM. An in vitro functionally mature mouse spinal cord preparation for the study of spinal motor networks. Brain Res. 1999;93:1439-49.

103. Whelan P, Bonnot A, O'Donovan MJ. Properties of rhythmic activity generated by the isolated spinal cord of the neonatal mouse. J Neurophysiol. 2000;84(6):2821-33.

104. Kjaerulff O, Kiehn O. Crossed rhythmic synaptic input to motoneurons during selective activation of the contralateral spinal locomotor network. J Neurosci. 1997;17(24):9433-77.

105. Gossard JP, Brownstone RM, Barajon I, Hultborn H. Transmission in a locomotor-related group 1b pathway from hindlimb extensor muscles in the cat. Exp Brain Res. 1994;98: 213-28.

106. Pearson KG. Common principles of motor control in vertebrates and invertebrates. Annu Rev Neurosci. 1993;16:265-97.

107. Van Emmerik RE, Wagenaar RC, Van Wegen EE. Interlimb coupling patterns in human locomotion: are we bipeds or quadrupeds? Ann N Y Acad Sci. 1998;860:539-42.

108. Forrsberg H, Grillner S, Halberstain J. The locomotion of the low spinal cat. I. Coordination within a hindlimb. Acta Physiol Scand. 1980;108(3):269-81.

109. Barbeau H, Rossignol S. Recovery of locomotion after chronic spinalization in the adult cat. Brain Res. 1987;412(1):84-95.

110. Grillner S, Zangger P. The effect of dorsal root transection on the efferent motor pattern in the cat's hindlimb during locomotion. Acta Physiol Scand. 1984;120(3):393-405.

111. Dickinson PS. Interactions among neural networks for behavior. Curr Opin Neurobiol. 1995;5(6):792-8.

112. Grillner S. Ion channels and locomotion. Science. 1997;278(5340):1087-8.

113. Garcia-Rill E, Skinner RD. The mesencephalic locomotor region. II: Projections to reticulospinal neurons. Brain Res. 1987;411(1):13-20.

114. Jung R, Kiemel T, Cohen AG. Dynamic behavior of a neural network model of locomotor control in the lamprey. J Neurophysiol. 1996;75(3):1074-86.

115. Cohen AH, Guan L, Harris J, Jung R, Kiemel T. Interaction between the caudal brainstem and the lamprey central pattern generator for locomotion. Neuroscience. 1996;74(4):1161-73.

116. Grillner S, Matsushima T. The neural network underlying locomotion in lamprey: synaptic and cellular mechanisms. Neuron. 1991;7(1): 1-15.

117. Orlovsky GN. Cerebellum and locomotion. In: Shimamura M, Grillner S, Edgerton VR, editors. Neurobiological basis of human locomotion. Tokyo: Japan Scientific Societies Press; 1991. p. 187-99.

118. Wichmann T, DeLong MR. Functional and pathophysiological models of the basal ganglia. Curr Opin Neurobiol. 1996;6(6):751-8.

119. Arshavsky YIM, Gelfand GN, Orlovsky GN. The cerebellum and control of rhythmical movements. Trends Neurosci. 1983;6:417-22.

120. Lansner A, Ekeberg O. Neuronal network models of motor generation and control. Opin Neurobiol. 1994;4(6):903-8.

121. Rossignol S, Dubuc R. Spinal pattern generation. Curr Opin Neurobiol. 1994;4(6):894-902.

122. Pearson KG. Proprioceptive regulation of locomotion. Curr Opin Neurobiol. 1995;5(6): 786-91.

123. Andersson O, Forssberg H, Grillner S, Wallen P. Peripheral feedback mechanisms acting on the central pattern generators for locomotion in fish and cat. Can J Physiol Pharmacol. 1981;59(7):713-26.

124. Gossard JP, Floeter MK, Degtyarenko AM, Simon ES, Burke RE. Disynaptic vestibulospinal and reticulospinal excitation in cat lumbosacral motoneurons: modulation during fictive locomotion. Exp Brain Res. 1996;109(2):277-8.

125. Guertin P, Angel MJ, Perreault MC, McCrea DA. Ankle extensor group 1 afferents excite extensors throughout the hindlimb during fictive locomotion in the cat. J Physiol. 1995;487(Pt 1):197-209.

126. Stein RB, Capaday C. The modulation of human reflexes during functional motor tasks. Trends Neurosci. 1988;11(7):328-32.

127. Yang JF, Whelan PH. Neural mechanisms that contribute to cyclical modulation of the soleus H-reflex in walking humans. Exp Brain Res. 1993;95(3):547-56.

128. Brooke JD, Cheng J, Collins DF, MacIlroy WE, Misiaszek JE, Staines WR. Sensori-sensory afferent conditioning with leg movement: gain control in spinal reflex and ascending paths. Prog Neurobiol. 1997;51(4):393-421.

129. MacKay-Lyons M. Central pattern generation of locomotion: a review of the evidence. Phys Ther. 2002;82(1):73.

130. Dietz V, Zjilstra W, Duysens J. Human neuronal interlimb coordination during split-belt locomotion. Exp Brain Res. 1994;101(3):513-20.

131. Prokop T, Berger W, Zjilstra W, Dietz V. Adaptational and learning processes during human split-belt locomotion. Exp Brain Res. 1995;106(3):449-56.

132. Forrsberg H. Ontogeny of human locomotor control. I. Infant stepping, supported locomotion and transition to independent locomotion. Exp Brain Res. 1985;57(3):480-93.

133. Forrsberg H, Hirschfield H, Stokes VP. Development of human locomotor mechanisms. In: Shimamura M, Grillner S, Edgerton VR, editors. Neurobiolocial basis of human locomotion. Tokyo: Japan Scientific Societies Press; 1991. p. 259-73.

134. Visintin M, Barbeau H. The effects of body weight support on the locomotor pattern of spastic paretic patients. Can J Neurol Sci. 1989;16(3):315-25.

135. Gardner MB, Holden MK, Leikauskas JM, Richard RL. Partial body weight support with treadmill locomotion to improve gait after incomplete spinal cord injury: a single-subject experiment design. Phys Ther. 1998;78(4): 361-74.

136. Wernig A, Müller S, Nanassy A, Cagol E. Laufband therapy based on "rules of spinal locomotion" is effective in spinal cord injured persons. Eur J Neurosci. 1995;7(1):823-9.

137. MacKay-Lyons M. Central pattern generation of locomotion: a review of the evidence. Phys Ther. 2002;82(1):80.

138. Nielsen J, Petersen N, Fedirchuk B. Evidence suggesting a transcortical pathway from cutaneous foot afferents to tibialis anterior motoneurones in man. J Physiol. 1997;501(Pt 2):473-84.

139. Kukulka CG. The reflex effects of nonnoxious sural nerve stimulation on human triceps surae motor neurons. J Neurophysiol. 1994;71(5): 1897-906.

140. Fallon JB, Bent LR, McNulty PA, Macefield VG. Evidence for strong synaptic coupling between single tactile afferents from the sole of the foot and motoneurons supplying leg muscles. J Neurophysiol. 2005;94 (6):3795-804.

141. van Wezel BMH, van Engelen BGM, Gabreëls FJM, Gabreëls-Festen AA, Duysens J. αβ fibers mediate cutaneous reflexes during human walking. J Neurophysiol. 2000;83(5):2980-6.

142. Aniss AM, Gandevia SC, Burke D. Reflex responses in active muscles elicited by stimulation of low-threshold afferents from the human foot. J Neurophysiol. 1992;67(5):1375-84.

143. Rossi A, Zalaffi A, Decchi B. Interaction of nociceptive and non-nociceptive cutaneous afferents from foot sole in common reflex pathways to tibialis anterior motoneurones in humans. Brain Res. 1996;714(1-2):76-86.

144. Guissard N, Duchateau J, Hainaut K. Mechanisms of decreased motoneurone excitation during passive muscle stretching. Exp Brain Res. 2001;137(2):163-9.

145. Li S, Kukulka CG, Rogers MW, Brunt D, Bishop M. Sural nerve evoked response in human hip and ankle muscles while standing. Neurosci Lett. 2004;364(2):59-62.

146. Knikou M. Effects on hip joint angle changes on intersegmental spinal coupling in humans with spinal cord injury. Exp Brain Res. 2005; 167(3):381-93.

147. Knikou M, Rymer WZ. Hip angle induced modulation of H reflex amplitude, latency and duration in spinal cord injured humans. Clin Neurophysiol. 2002;113(11):1698-708.

148. Knikou M. Effects of changes in hip position on actions of spinal inhibitory interneurons in humans. Int J Neurosci. 2006;116(8):945-61.

149. Knikou M, Kay E, Rymer WZ. Modulation of flexion reflex induced by hip angle changes in human spinal cord injury. Exp Brain Res. 2006;168(4):577-86.

150. Johansson H, Sjolander P, Sojka P. A sensory role for the cruciate ligaments. Clin Orthop Rel Res. 1991;(268):161-78.

151. Bernard PN, Cassidy JD. Sacroiliac joint syndrome: pathophysiology, diagnosis and management. In: Frymoyer JW, editor. The adult spine: principles and practice. New York: Raven Press; 1991. p. 2107-31.

152. Laslett M, Williams M. The reliability of selected pain provocation tests for sacroiliac joint pathology. Spine. 1994;19(11):1243-9.

153. Potter NA, Rothstein JM. Intertester reliability for selected clinical tests of the sacroiliac joint. Phys Ther. 1985;65(11):1671-5.

154. Grob KR, Neuberger WL, Kisslig RO. Die innervation des sacroiliaclgelenkes beim menschen [German]. Z Rheumatol. 1995;54:117-22.

155. Ikeda R. [Innervation of the sacroiliac joint: macroscopical and histological studies.] Nippon Ika Daigaku Zasshi. 1991;58(5):587-97.

156. Indahl A, Kaigle A, Reikeras O, Holm S. Sacroiliac joint involvement in activation of the porcine spinal and gluteal musculature. J Spinal Disord. 1999;12(4):329-30.

157. Horak FB, Nashner LM, Nutt J. Postural instability in parkinsonian patients: sensory

organization and motor coordination. Soc Neurosci Abstr. 1984;(10):634.

158. Nashner LM, Horak FB, Diener HC. Selection of human postural synergies differ with peripheral somatosensory versus vestibular loss. Soc Neurosci Abstr. 1985;(11):704.

159. Fitzpatrick R, McCloskey DI. Task-dependent reflex responses and movement illusions evoked by galvanic vestibular stimulation in standing humans. J Physiol (Lond). 1994;(478):363-72.

160. Eng JJ, Winder DA, McMinnon CD, Patla AE. Interaction of the reactive moments and center of mass displacements for postural control during voluntary arm movements. Neurosci Res Commun. 1992;11:73-80.

161. Baroni G, Pedrocchi A, Ferrigno G, Massion J, Pedotti A. Static and dynamic postural control in long-term microgravity: evidence of a dual adaptation. J Appl Physiol. 2001;90 (1):205-15.

162. Marigold DS, Patla AE. Adapting locomotion to different surface compliances: neuromuscular responses and changes in movement dynamics. J Neurophysiol. 2005;94(3):1733-50.

163. Marigold DS, Patla AI. Strategies for dynamic stability during locomotion on a slippery surface: effects of prior experience and knowledge. J Neurophysiol. 2002;88:339-53.

164. Menz HB, Lord SR, Fitzpatrick RC. Acceleration patterns of the head and pelvis when walking on level and irregular surfaces. Gait Posture. 2003;18(1):35-46.

165. Descarreaux M, Lalonde C, Normand MC. Isometric force parameters and trunk muscle recruitment strategies in a population with low pack pain. J Manipulative Physiol Ther. 2007;30(2):91-7.

166. DeWitt JK, Osterbauer PJ, Stelmach GE, Fuhr AW. Optoelectric measurement of changes in leg length inequality resulting from isolation tests. J Manipulative Physiol Ther. 1994;17(8): 530-8.

167. Panjabi MM. The stabilizing system of the spine. Part II. Neutral zone and instability hypothesis. J Spinal Disord. 1992;5(4):391.

168. Panjabi MM. The stabilizing system of the spine. Part II. Neutral zone and instability hypothesis. J Spinal Disord. 1992;5(4):394.

169. Kiefer A, Shirazi-Adl A, Parnianpour M. Synergy of the human spine in neutral postures. Eur Spine J. 1998;7(6):471-9.

170. Parnianpour M, Shirazi-Adl A, Sparto P, Dariush B. The effect of compressive load on myoelectric activities of ten selected trunk muscles. Proceedings of the 12th TCIEA; 1994 Aug 15-19; Toronto, Ontario, Canada. p. 119-21.

171. Fuller RB. Synergetics. New York: Macmillan; 1975.

172. Kaigle AM, Holm SH, Hansson TH. Experimental instability in the lumbar spine. Spine. 1995;20(4):421-30.

173. Malinsky J. The ontogenetic development of nerve terminations in the intervertebral disc of man. Acta Anat (Basel). 1959;38:96-113.

174. Solomonow M, Zhou B-H, Baratta RV, Lu Y, Harris M. Biomechanics of increased exposure to lumbar injury caused by cyclic loading: Part I. Loss of reflexive muscular stabilization. Spine. 1999;24(23):2426-34.

175. Solomonow M, Zhou B-H, Baratta RV, Lu Y, Harris M. Biomechanics of increased exposure to lumbar injury caused by cyclic loading: Part I. Loss of reflexive muscular stabilization. Spine. 1999;24(23):2434.

176. DeVocht JW, Pickar JG, Wilder DG. Spinal manipulation alters electromyographic activity of paraspinal muscles: a descriptive study. J Manipulative Physiol Ther. 2005;28(7):465-71.

177. DeVocht JW, Pickar JG, Wilder DG. Spinal manipulation alters electromyographic activity of paraspinal muscles: a descriptive study. J Manipulative Physiol Ther. 2005;28(7):470.

178. Denslow JS, Hassett CC. The central excitatory state associated with postural abnormalities. J Neurophysiol. 1942;5:393-401.

179. Denslow JS, Korr IM, Krems AD. Quantitative studies of chronic facilitation in human motoneuron pools. Am J Phys. 1947;150(2): 229-38.

180. Plum F, Posner JB. Neurology: pathophysiology as an approach to neurologic diagnosis. In: Smith LH, Their SO, editors. Pathophysiology: the biological principles of disease. 2nd ed. Philadelphia: Saunders; 1985. p. 1092.

181. Basmajian JV. Muscles alive: their functions revealed by electromyography. 3rd ed. Baltimore: Williams & Wilkins; 1974.

182. Ortengren R, Andersson GB. Electromyographic studies of trunk muscles, with special reference to the functional anatomy of the lumbar spine. Spine. 1977;2(1):44-51.

183. Korr IM. The spinal cord as organizer of disease processes. III. Hyperactivity of the sympathetic innervation as a common factor in disease. J Am Osteopath Assoc. 1979;79(4):232-6.

184. Korr IM. Experimental alterations in segmental sympathetic (sweat glands) activity through myofascial and postural disturbances. Fed Proc. 1949;3:87.

185. Korr IM, Wright IM, Chace JA. Cutaneous patterns of sympathetic abnormalities of the musculoskeletal system. Acta Neuroveg (Wien). 1964;25:589-606.

186. Coote JH. Somatic sources of afferent input as factors in aberrant autonomic, sensory, and motor function. In: Korr IM, editor. Neurobiologic mechanisms of manipulative therapy New York: Plenum Press; 1977. p. 91-111.

LEG LENGTH ANALYSIS

A central feature of the Activator Method (AM) is Leg Length Analysis (LLA). AM assessment for neuroarticular dysfunction is based on the assumption that faulty biomechanical behavior of articulations is reflected by differences and changes in leg length. The assessment protocol consists of a series of prone leg length observations and provocative tests performed to evaluate the function of joints from the feet progressively upward throughout the axial skeleton.[1] When carefully and correctly performed, it is used to determine where to, when to, and when not to adjust. Furthermore, LLA developed as part of the clinical protocol of the AM generally enables the clinician to confidently and consistently identify neuroarticular dysfunction, even when the patient experiences atypical signs and symptoms.

This assessment involves repeated, systematic observations of relative leg lengths in the prone extended position and apparent changes in leg length when the knees are flexed to varying degrees. These multiple observations are used to interpret the results of a series of provocative maneuvers, including Pressure Testing, Isolation Testing, and Stress Testing for neuroarticular dysfunction at all levels of the axial skeleton and the extremities.[1] The functional short leg observed in the prone patient is critically important to establish with AM LLA because virtually all of the tests are based on reactions and relative changes observed in the length of the functional short leg. Traditionally, the short leg has been designated the Pelvic Deficient, or PD leg; this designation is used throughout the discussion and directions for leg testing provided in this text. The short leg is also sometimes referred to as the *reactive* leg because of its tendency to appear shorter or longer during different testing procedures. The PD leg tends to remain the reactive leg throughout the procedure for any given patient visit. Furthermore, if the PD leg has

been correctly identified at the outset, the same leg tends to be the patient's PD leg for subsequent visits. However, a significant injury, illness, or biomechanical or neurological stress may alter the pattern of Leg Length Inequality (LLI).

Because the PD leg is so important to the performance of all AM testing procedures, an accurate and consistent method of identifying the PD leg is critically important. The PD leg is visually observed during the initial leg check following placement of the patient in the prone position on the adjusting table. Therefore care with patient placement and meticulous observation of the feet and legs during the first LLA will have a very real impact on the success and accuracy of all subsequent AM procedures.

The following steps in patient placement and the initial leg check will help to ensure that leg length testing is accurate and consistent. If patient placement and the initial leg check are performed consistently and in accordance with the relatively rigorous procedure outlined subsequently, the AM practitioner obtains consistent baseline findings with each patient visit. Research and clinical experience show that proficiency-rated doctors of chiropractic who use the AM have good to very good intraexaminer reliability when evaluating a patient's PD or short leg. Clinically, the PD leg usually remains consistent throughout treatment, from the time of the initial LLA and throughout subsequent patient visits.

Furthermore, if different AM practitioners adhere to the LLA method described here, the quality of care for patients who may transfer from one practitioner to another is enhanced by the consistency of the technique. Research conducted to evaluate interexaminer reliability with the use of experienced chiropractors to measure the reproducibility of prone leg length assessment concludes that reliability of prone leg checks can be fair to good. Data suggest that radiographic evaluation has the highest level of reproducibility, followed by osseous pain evaluation; both were rated fair to excellent in interexaminer reliability, while static and motion palpation assessment procedures were rated fair to poor.[2] One study suggests that among clinicians with proper training in LLA, interexaminer reliability is as high as or higher than many other commonly practiced chiropractic analytical techniques.[3] Fuhr and Osterbauer[4] compared leg check results of four AM Advanced Proficiency rated doctors, who were also AM-certified instructors in a group of 30 subjects in the prone position and concluded that interexaminer reliability was fair to good. Andrew and Gemmell[5] observed four chiropractors who were experienced in AM LLA, while assessing 18 patients with unaltered gait. They found that observed agreement at 69% exceeded chance agreement at 52%.[5] Nguyen et al.[6] observed interexaminer reliability of two AM Advanced Proficiency rated and certified instructors in 34 subjects. They reported 85% agreement and concluded that there was good reproducibility between examiners who used the AM to detect LLI.[6] Prone LLA performed according to the AM has been favorable in these limited studies of interexaminer reliability. We acknowledge that further research is needed into the validity of the prone leg check as a neurobiomechanical assessment procedure, along with all other chiropractic assessment procedures.

Conducting the Initial Leg Check

Leg length testing and analysis is the primary method for determining the presence of neuroarticular dysfunction or misalignment in various regions of the body. Observation and interpretation of changes in apparent leg length guide analysis of the spine and extremities and are thought to enable the AM practitioner to do the following:

- Isolate neuroarticular dysfunction of axial skeleton articulations at the vertebral level.
- Determine the direction of misalignment in vertebral neuroarticular dysfunction.
- Identify or confirm neuroarticular dysfunction of extremity articulations.
- Confirm the direction of the adjustive force.
- Confirm postadjustment assessment.

To ensure an accurate and consistent LLA throughout the entire assessment protocol, it is critically important to perform an accurate initial leg check.

Some simple procedural guidelines help to ensure an accurate and consistent initial LLA.

Because virtually all leg length tests are performed with the patient in the prone position, patient placement on the adjusting table is crucially important from the beginning. Hydraulic tables are beneficial in preserving standing weight-bearing posture and dynamics by transferring the patient to the prone position without the need for movement on the patient's part. The electric lift mechanism is effective in transferring acute, elderly, and handicapped patients onto the table for care and returning them to the standing posture following treatment. The drop-away footboard, along with an elevation feature, reduces stress to the practitioner and enables proper ergonomics throughout testing.

With a hydraulic table in the vertical position, the patient steps onto the footboard, leans into the table surface, and passively rides down into the prone position as the table lift mechanism gently lowers the table from vertical to horizontal. Because no active positioning is required, the patient can be lowered into the prone position with minimal to no discomfort or pain (Figures 6-1 and 6-2). In addition, passive lowering to the prone position preserves and enhances the weight-bearing distortions and postural compensation characteristics of the patient's normal standing posture. When the footboard drops away, the patient's legs and feet are left unrestricted, so that LLI, inversion and eversion distortions, foot flare, and other asymmetries are readily observable.

Footwear. Before placing the patient on the adjusting table for the first time, inspect his or her footwear. Often, leg length discrepancies and changes in relative lengths are measurable but quite small. Worn and poorly fitted shoes or boots may obscure the more subtle observations required in an effective LLA. Proper footwear should fit the foot tightly and should have a back or a strap that maintains contact with the heel, especially with the knees flexed. High-top athletic shoes, Western boots, and lace-up work boots make the task of leg length evaluation difficult if not impossible and do not allow for visualization of or access around the malleoli. High-heeled pumps, sandals, slippers, and clogs also may defeat LLA because of the difficulty involved in finding points for comparison on each foot. If the patient is gripping his or her toes to keep the shoe on during analysis, or the doctor has to adjust the LLA technique to maintain the footwear against the heel, weight-bearing postural observations and testing procedures can become inaccurate.

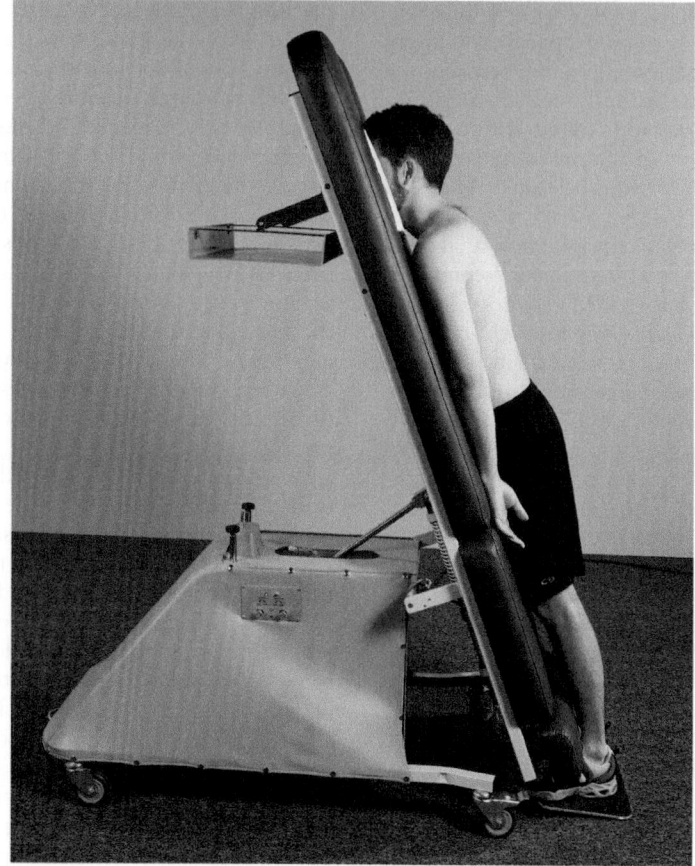

Figure 6-1 Patient on vertical table.

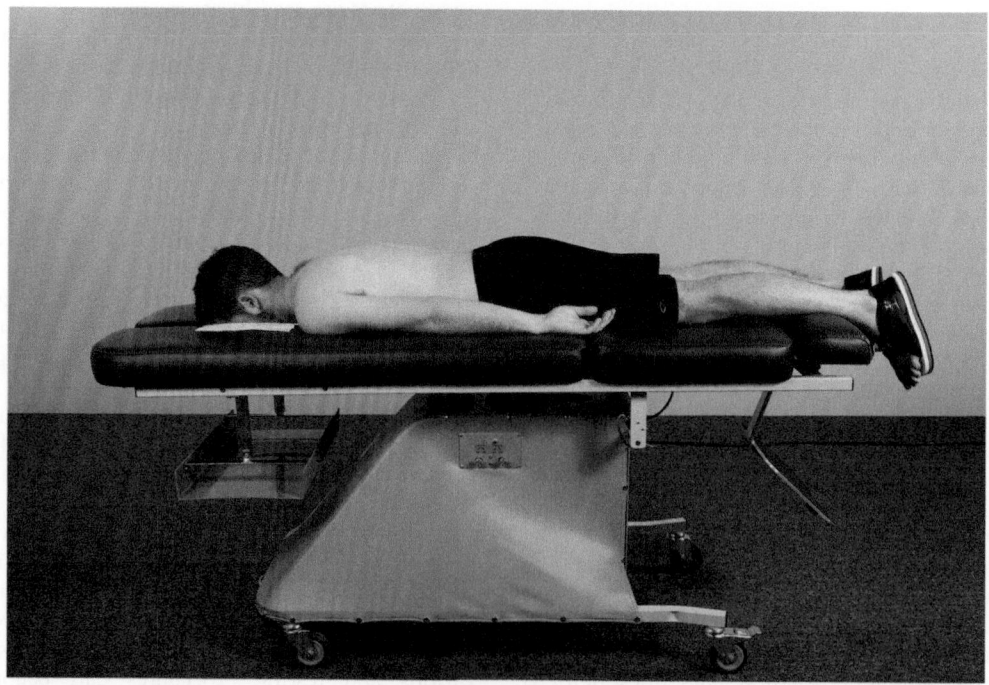

Figure 6-2 Patient on horizontal table.

Low-cut shoes that are not badly worn enable the clinician to observe the feet for LLI. Also, low-cut shoes or loafers are easier to slip on and off the patient's foot when adjustments of the foot and ankle are indicated. It may be useful to ask the patient to wear appropriate shoes for subsequent visits. An alternative is to use Activator shoes, also known as cast or surgical boots, with Velcro closures (Figure 6-3). These boots are not worn in standing posture and therefore would not be broken down or distorted as regular shoes may be. In addition, the Velcro closures make it simple to remove and replace the surgical boot when one is adjusting the foot and ankle.

Ask the patient to remove bulky clothing before getting onto the adjusting table. Heavy sweaters or jackets make it difficult to locate joints and other structures with consistency and accuracy and may obscure important visual indicators of patient problems. Also, have the patient remove bulky objects, keys, pens, billfolds, and so forth, from his or her pockets before getting onto the adjusting table. Emptying the pockets enhances patient comfort during treatment and helps to prevent distortions that result when a patient shifts weight or position to avoid discomfort from the contents of the pockets while lying prone.

Note that four essential steps are required for the initial LLA:

1. Patient placement—preserving postural distortions
2. Visual observation—noting leg length discrepancy
3. Position #1 procedure—identifying the PD leg
4. Position #2 procedure—specifically identifying the starting point for analysis and the side of adjustment during subsequent analysis

The order and thoroughness with which each step is performed predict the effectiveness and reliability of LLA for the AM. Remember, leg length findings and interpretations will help to guide you by indicating neurobiomechanical aberrancies as you proceed with evaluation and analysis of the patient's spine and extremities, thus affecting your adjusting protocol.

Patient Placement. In contrast to many other adjusting techniques, with the AM, placement of the patient on the adjusting table for the first time during each visit can be a major determinant in the accuracy of the leg check. Improper patient placement can result in diminished leg length discrepancies, reversal of the shorter and longer leg, and ambiguous or erroneous analysis of leg length during clinical procedures.

To avoid errors and to minimize ambiguous readings of leg length discrepancies, establish a consistent pattern of activities and procedures for performing the initial LLA. Be prepared to

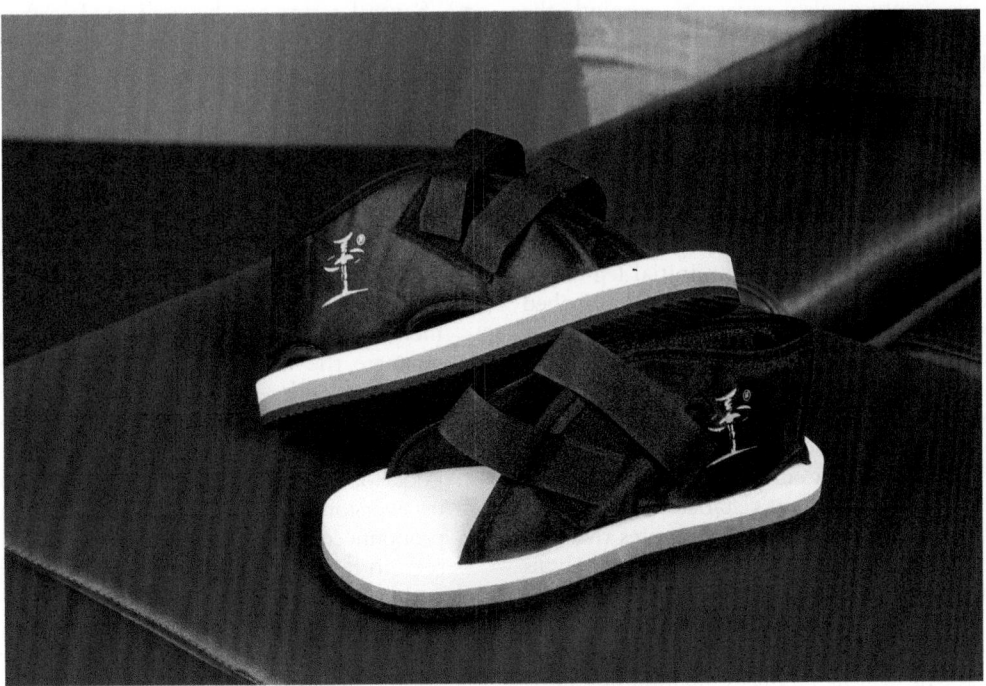

Figure 6-3 Activator adjusting shoes for analysis.

explain the procedures to the patient, and stress the importance of cooperation between patient and doctor.

Carefully position the patient on the adjusting table. For best results use the following step-by-step procedure:

1. Start with the table in the vertical position. If necessary, be sure the footboard is locked into a stable horizontal position (see Figure 6-1).
2. Instruct the patient to step onto the footboard. Guide the patient to ensure that the backs of the heels are even and parallel with the footboard, and that the stance is typical of the patient's normal standing posture. Ensure that the patient's shins are approximating the table.
3. Instruct the patient to lean forward against the table with the face centered in the face slot and with the arms at the sides, dorsum of the hands contacting and resting against the table.
4. Before lowering the table, ask the patient not to move or adjust his or her weight distribution while the table is descending, or once it is in the horizontal position. Next, inform the patient that you are going to lower the table.
5. Lower the table to the horizontal position. As the table descends, place a hand firmly over the patient's low back. Contact with the patient helps to offset feelings of nervousness or discomfort during positional changes. This contact also serves to remind the patient not to move or shift weight while the table is lowered.
6. Once the table is in the horizontal position, ask the patient to relax without moving until the initial leg test is complete. The patient's legs should extend past the bottom of the table far enough to allow the ankles and feet to move freely (see Figure 6-2).

Position the patient for the initial leg check with meticulous care. The procedure described here facilitates the most accurate and consistent LLA possible for identification of LLI as noted and to compare for subsequent visits.

Accuracy and consistency of the leg check are attained with the placement procedure described above for several reasons. First, consider the significance of the patient's stance on the footboard. Placing the feet parallel ensures that the patient's weight will be distributed as evenly as possible onto both feet. Attention to the standing posture helps to fix the gravitational distortions and subtle alterations to spinal curves that weight bearing produces, maintaining muscle imbalance, pelvic obliquity, and vertebral

subluxation complexes in the prone position. Asking the patient not to move during descent of the table until the initial leg check has been performed is also thought to preserve gravitational distortions. As a result, leg length inequalities and reactions in the PD leg tend to be more pronounced and more readily observable.

When an Activator portable table is used, steps should be provided at the foot of the table to assist the patient's placement on the table and to best preserve his or her standing, weight-bearing posture. The practitioner guides the patient's knees up onto the table, ensuring that the patellae are parallel to each other. The shins rest on the removable leg cushion, and the clinician ensures that there is adequate space between the dorsal aspect of the feet and the base of the table. The lateral malleoli should be readily accessible and cleared for analysis of leg lengths.

Visual Inspection: Observe Leg Length Discrepancy

Once the patient is in the prone position, stand at the foot of the table. Adopt a stance that permits a clear line of sight between the patient's feet, in line with the plantar surfaces of the feet. Ergonomically, the doctor should stand so that one foot is farther forward, or closer to the patient's feet (two-line stance). This stance allows the doctor to shift forward and backward between the feet when flexing the knees of the patient between Position #1 and Position #2. Several terms can be used to describe the doctor's stance. The most common of these are *scissor stance, fencing stance, in-line stance,* and *two-line stance.*

To ensure as accurate an LLA as possible, use the following step-by-step procedure:

1. Before touching the patient's feet, inspect them for LLI by comparing points on opposite feet. Bony landmarks such as the medial malleoli are useful points for identifying leg length discrepancy. However, it is recommended that while using the AM, one should compare the welt of the shoe at the heels. The welt is the point at which the leather upper of the shoe begins from the sole of the shoe.
2. Look for evidence of asymmetrical inversion or eversion. Most often, inversion is more pronounced on the short leg side, as can be seen in Figure 6-4. (Figure 6-4 illustrates this patient's natural inversion on the left—a possible sign of a left Pelvic Deficiency.) Inversion is thought to be a postural alteration that serves as an attempt to compensate for LLI.[7,8]

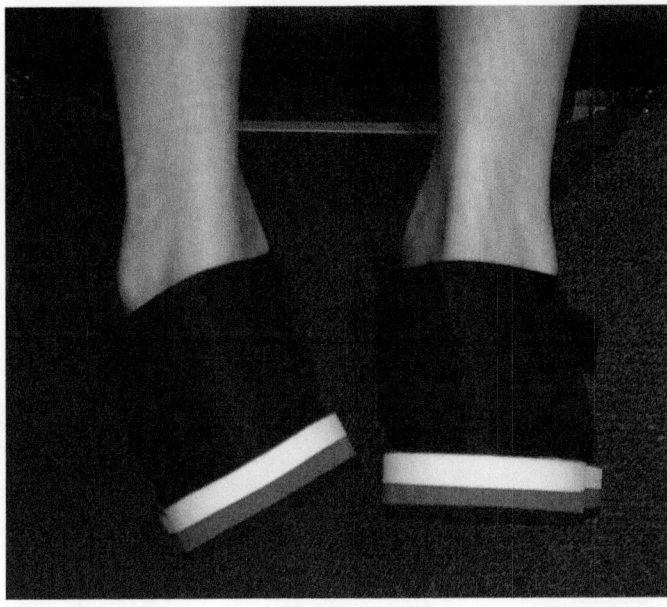

Figure 6-4 Inspecting feet for Leg Length Inequality.

3. Inspect the feet for excessive toe-out or toe-in foot flare. The feet will normally show moderate symmetrical toe-out flare of about 10 degrees. Asymmetrical foot flare may indicate ankle, knee, or hip misalignment.
4. Cup the palms of the hands over the lateral malleoli, and bring the legs together until the heels approximate, without forcing the heels together (Figure 6-5).
5. While cupping the heels, use gentle medial pressure, and avoid excessive force. It is more important to stop at soft tissue resistance than to completely approximate the heels. Soft tissue resistance may occur before heel approximation in those patients who are obese, or who have exceptionally large gastrocnemius muscles or inner thighs. Pushing the heels together past this point of initial resistance may lead to alterations in the patient's natural leg length discrepancy.

Position #1: Identifying the Pelvic Deficient Leg

Position #1 is the starting position for all AM LLAs. In Position #1, the patient's legs rest on an Activator table, allowing the knees to be in a slightly flexed position and the ankles and feet to be in a neutral, relaxed state.

In most cases, the short leg revealed by visual inspection is the PD or reactive leg. The previously stated procedure generally confirms the observation, but it is possible for the PD leg to appear longer with only visual observation, and its length is conclusively determined in Position #1. The following step-by-step procedure will reveal the true PD leg and will establish the starting point for AM analytical and adjusting procedures:

1. Place the thumbs in the approximate position of the heel on each shoe, position the index finger on the posterior aspect of the lateral malleolus, and position the middle finger just anterior to the lateral malleolus. AM-certified instructors and instructional materials sometimes refer to this hand placement as the "six-point landing" (Figure 6-6).
2. Using your thumbs, gently remove any inversion or eversion of the feet. Keep the heels and soles of the feet parallel with each other in an attempt to "mirror" the feet.
3. Using your thumbs, gently dorsiflex the feet. For some patients, it will be possible to dorsiflex the feet until each shoe heel and sole is vertical, and the feet form a right angle with the legs at the ankles. For many patients, however, calf muscle tension or biomechanical changes in the ankle joint may limit ankle dorsiflexion. Factors such as age, a history of ankle injuries, Achilles tendonitis, and the wearing of high-heeled shoes and boots can all contribute to restricted dorsiflexion of the ankle. When a patient

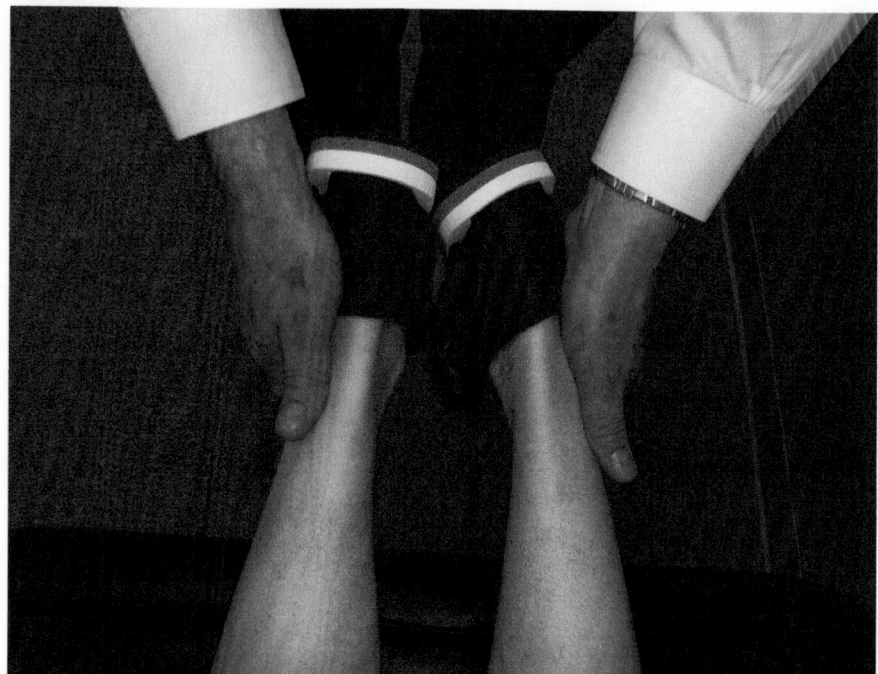

Figure 6-5   Cupping of the lateral malleoli.

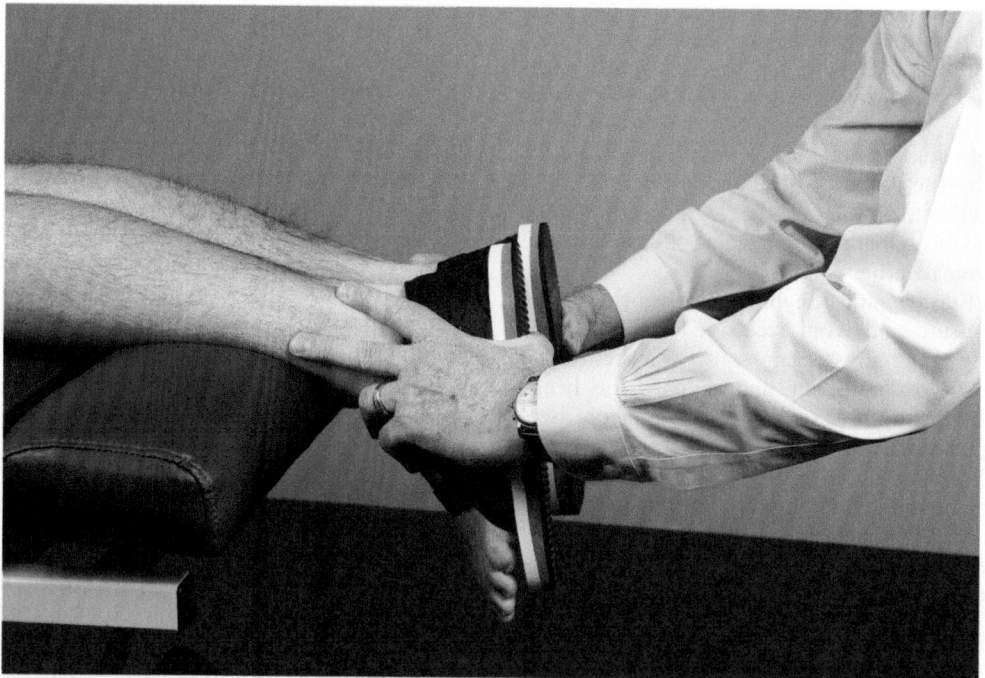

Figure 6-6   The "six-point landing": identifying the Pelvic Deficiency leg in Position #1. Illustrates a left Pelvic Deficiency.

demonstrates limited ankle range of motion, dorsiflex the feet only until the motion meets resistance.

4. Flare the feet (externally rotate) so the toes are abducted to a natural angle of 10 to 20 degrees. Flaring the feet tends to reduce

tension in ankle and calf musculature, preserving the natural posture, and allows more readily observable LLI.

5. Apply a gentle headward pressure with the thumbs pushing through the long axis (axes) of the legs.

6. The leg that shortens is the leg on the side of Pelvic Deficiency, or the PD leg. Figure 6-6 illustrates an example of left Pelvic Deficiency.

Identification of the PD leg is an essential component of the AM LLA because it is the foundation and starting point of the analysis. From this point onward, the short leg identified in the initial leg length test is considered the PD leg, or the reactive leg, and is the main indicator of neuroarticular dysfunction, subluxation, or facilitation, regardless of what level of the spine or articulation of the extremities is tested. Unless otherwise noted, we will use a left PD as our example in the book.

Position #2 Procedures: Specifying Neuroarticular Dysfunction Location

LLA in Position #1 indicates the presence of neuroarticular dysfunction or facilitation in the joint or structure tested, and Position #2 is thought to provide more precise information about the location and direction of the neuroarticular dysfunction. Specifically, Position #2 helps to reveal the *side of involvement* in the axial skeleton.

In its simplest sense, Position #2 is a leg length test that is performed with the legs flexed no more than 90 degrees at the knees or to resistance. If the best information possible is to be obtained from a Position #2 LLA, the test must be performed with precision and care. Use the following step-by-step procedure to perform a Position #2 LLA:

1. The doctor should stand in a two-line stance at the foot of the table within easy reach of the patient's feet, with one foot more forward than the other.
2. Contact the dorsal aspect of the patient's feet at the metatarsal-phalangeal junctions with the middle fingers of each hand. Flex the third, fourth, and fifth digits, if necessary, but keep the index fingers and thumbs extended and out of contact with the feet.
3. Using the middle fingers as fulcrums, plantar-flex the feet until slack is taken up, before lifting the legs off the table (Figure 6-7). Because the gastrocnemius muscle is a two-joint muscle that crosses both the knee and the ankle, plantar flexion of the ankle serves to make the muscle actively insufficient.[9] This avoids excessive proprioceptive input from the gastrocnemius muscle spindle's "stretch reflexes."
4. Site an imaginary line on the patient using the second sacral tubercle and the external occipital protuberance as reference points.
5. Lift the legs by raising the feet and flexing the knees. Keep the elbows tucked close to the body, and use the axial line on the patient as a reference to keep the legs and feet parallel and centered.
6. At about 30 to 40 degrees of knee flexion, or when the forearms are parallel to the floor,

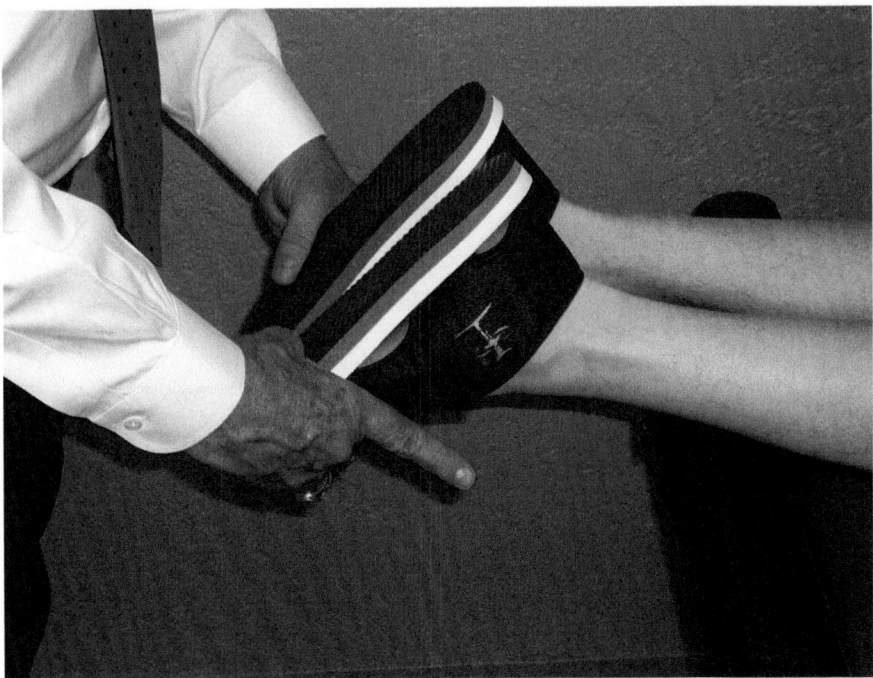

Figure 6-7   Plantar flexion of feet with middle fingers.

let the index fingers slide into the welt of the shoe, and position the thumbs on the soles of the shoes near the ball of each foot.

7. Using your thumbs as guides, abduct the feet into enough toe-out foot flare from relax tension in the legs and ankles. Attempt to preserve normal foot flare from the upright posture.

8. Continue to raise the feet until the knees are flexed to *no more than* 90 degrees, or until the change in the apparent length of the PD leg is noticeable (Figure 6-8).

9. With gentle thumb pressure on the balls of the feet, dorsiflex the feet to the point of resistance, or until the soles are horizontal.

Minimizing Error in the Leg Check

Following are some key reminders and tips for making LLA as accurate as possible:

1. *Remove inversion (supination) and plantar flexion with the legs extended in Position #1.*

Gentle removal of inversion and plantar flexion when the legs are in Position #1 enhances the accuracy of LLA in two ways. First, removal of inversion and plantar flexion minimizes error caused by inversion deformity produced by an ankle injury. In most cases, ankle inversion will be greater on the short leg, or the PD side. Removal of inversion and plantar flexion makes more obvious the apparent shortness of the PD leg, or reactivity.

Second, removal of inversion brings the welt of both shoes into close proximity and facilitates visual examination of each foot. As inversion and plantar flexion are removed, the shoes are pressed firmly against the patient's feet, and like points on the shoes therefore coincide with like anatomical points on the patient's feet.

2. *Be sure to keep the middle fingers on the metatarsal-phalangeal junctions, and plantarflex the ankles before raising the legs off the table into Position #2.*

Contact with the feet during elevation of the legs to Position #2 should be restricted to the metatarsal-phalangeal joints to minimize traction on the legs. By grasping the feet closer to the ankles, or by contacting the lower legs during elevation of the feet, it is easy to pull on the legs and distort or reverse true LLI.

3. *Keep the elbows tucked into the sides while raising the legs to Position #2.*

Accuracy of the Position #2 leg check analysis depends on symmetrical raising of the legs, in line with the longitudinal axis of the body. Keeping the elbows tucked into the sides helps to ensure that the legs will not drift to one side as they are raised. To help minimize examiner fatigue, keep the elbows tucked in toward the sides as the legs are raised, and lower them frequently during assessment of the pelvis and spine.

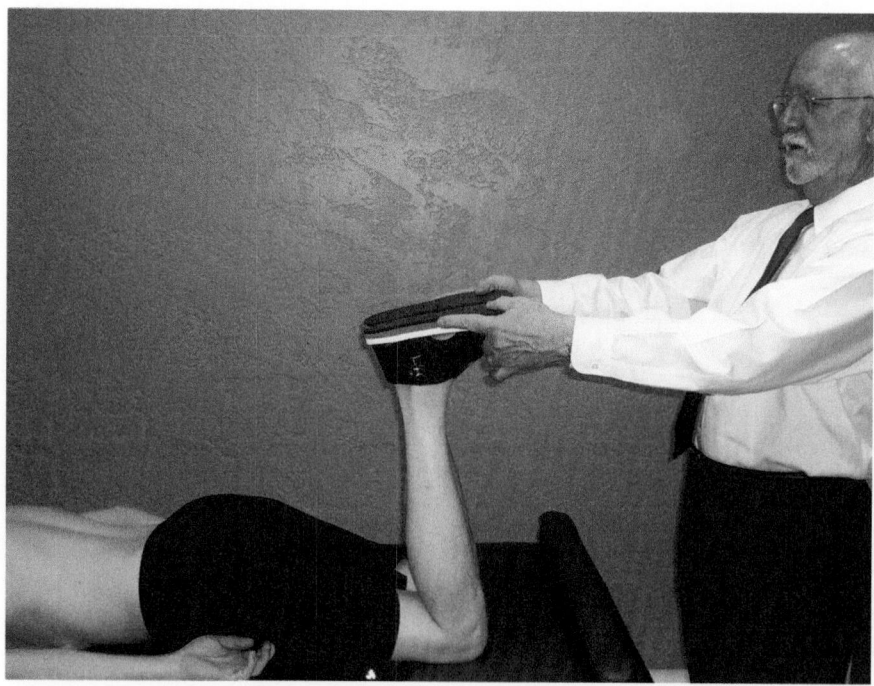

Figure 6-8   Raising the legs to Position #2.

4. *Let the feet form a "V" in Position #2, keeping the heels from touching, with the toes flared out.*

When the feet are allowed to flare out in Position #2, muscle tension in the legs and ankles is minimized. Furthermore, normal foot flare (external rotation) from the upright posture is preserved, as observed in Position #1.

5. *General considerations*

Because AM procedures are used to evaluate the mechanical and functional characteristics of the human frame, consistency in patient placement and leg testing ensures a more accurate appraisal of both upright and prone postures. Thus these postures can be monitored on subsequent visits for evaluation of improvement with regard to structural and functional outcomes.

Clinical Tips: The Finer Points of Leg Length Analysis

- Move the legs deliberately from Position #1 toward Position #2.
- Lower the legs slowly from Position #2 to Position #1.
- Do not drop the legs.
- Pay attention to the "feel" of the legs.
- Use a light touch.
- Do not wiggle or "play" with the feet or legs.
- Keep your index finger off of the Achilles tendon.
- Do not hold the feet while asking the patient to perform an Isolation Test.
- Do not dorsiflex feet in Position #2.

THE ACTIVATOR METHOD ANALYTICAL TECHNIQUE

Interpreting the Results of the Initial Leg Check

After identifying the PD leg in Position #1, raise the legs to Position #2, according to the procedure described in the previous section, and observe for relative changes in the PD leg. Specifically, in Position #2, observe for the PD leg to lengthen or shorten *relative* to its length in Position #1. The results of this initial leg check reveal the starting point for the AM assessment protocol.

Possibility One.   As the legs are raised into Position #2, inspection of leg lengths reveals that the PD leg *appears* to have lengthened (see Figures 6-6 through 6-9). Figure 6-9 represents a left PD leg that has lengthened in Position #2. When the PD leg lengthens in Position #2, the AM Protocol indicates that the testing procedure should start with the knees and the feet. Therefore proceed to testing and correction as indicated for the knees and the feet. Although the illustration for Possibility One in Figure 6-9 and our discussion here imply that the PD leg lengthens and appears longer than the other leg in Position #2, it is not actually necessary for the PD leg to "cross over." Remember, the change in leg length is a *relative* change, not an absolute change. For example, a PD leg might be observed to be 1 inch short in

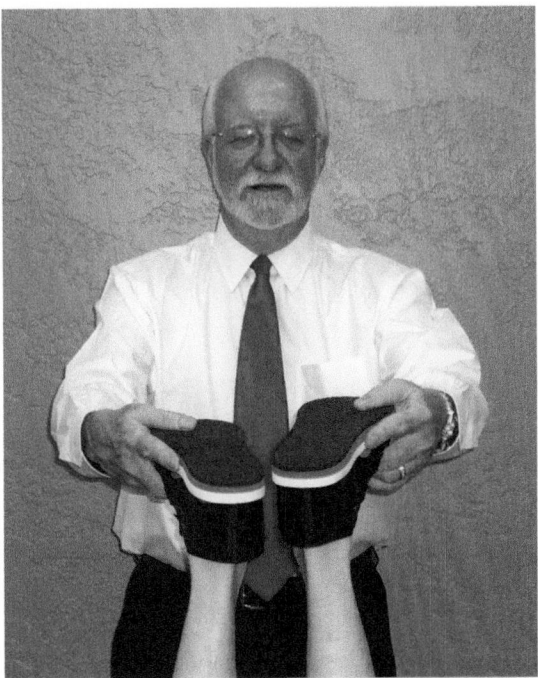

Figure 6-9 Possibility One: Pelvic Deficiency leg lengthens in Position #2.

Position #1 after initial prone placement of the patient. If, when the legs are raised into Position #2, the PD leg is now ¼ inch short, or just even in length with the opposite leg, this still represents a lengthening of the PD leg. Crossing over is more typical and would appear as follows: A PD leg might be observed to be 1 inch short in Position #1 following initial prone placement of the patient. If, when the feet are raised into Position #2, the PD leg is now ½ inch longer than the opposite leg. Both examples indicate relative lengthening—Possibility One. The AM Protocol calls for proceeding to evaluation of the knees and feet.

Possibility Two.   The second possibility occurs less frequently during the initial LLA. A small percentage of patients will present as a Possibility Two, and usually, their conditions are of a chronic nature. Following patient placement in a prone position, the short leg in the prone position—Position #1—is observed and determined to be the PD leg. The legs are then raised into Position #2, after which the PD leg *appears* to have stayed short or becomes shorter.

Figure 6-10 represents a left PD leg that has shortened in Position #2. An example of a Possibility Two patient would be as follows: Initial LLA reveals that the left PD leg is ½ inch short. When the legs are raised to Position #2, the left PD leg now appears 1 inch shorter

than the right leg. The AM Protocol indicates testing and adjustment of the fourth lumbar vertebra. Proceed to testing and correction as indicated for involvement of the fourth lumbar vertebra.

Possibility Three.   The third possibility occurs very rarely during the *initial* LLA. Even an asymptomatic patient typically has an identifiable PD leg, and it is usually the same leg at each visit. If the initial LLA still does not reveal a short or reactive leg in Position #1, and if there is still no lengthening or shortening of one of the legs in Position #2 (Figure 6-11), proceed to the pubic bone Isolation Test and adjustment.

Keep in mind, Possibility Three usually occurs during the *initial* LLA procedure. After the patient has received AM treatments and the patient has become balanced, the appearance of the legs as even in Position #1 and Position #2 can be a more common finding upon subsequent patient visits. If balanced legs are present, proceed to the pubic bone Isolation Testing procedure.

Types of Testing

The AM consists of three types of tests, all of which use LLA as part of their performance. These types of tests are:

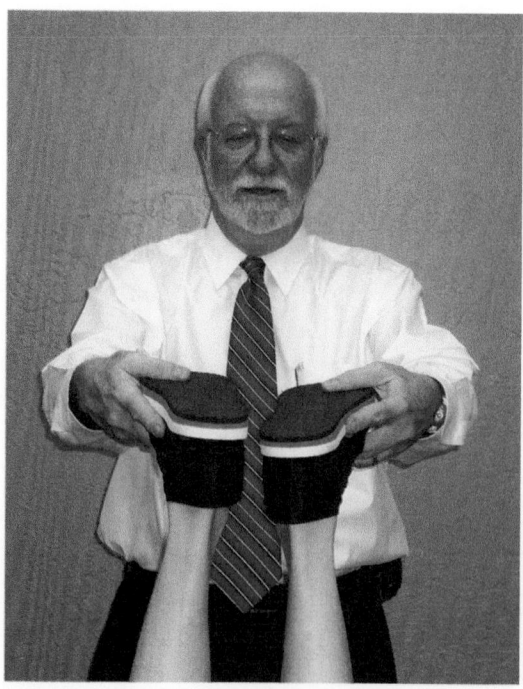

Figure 6-10   Possibility Two: Pelvic Deficiency leg shortens in Position #2.

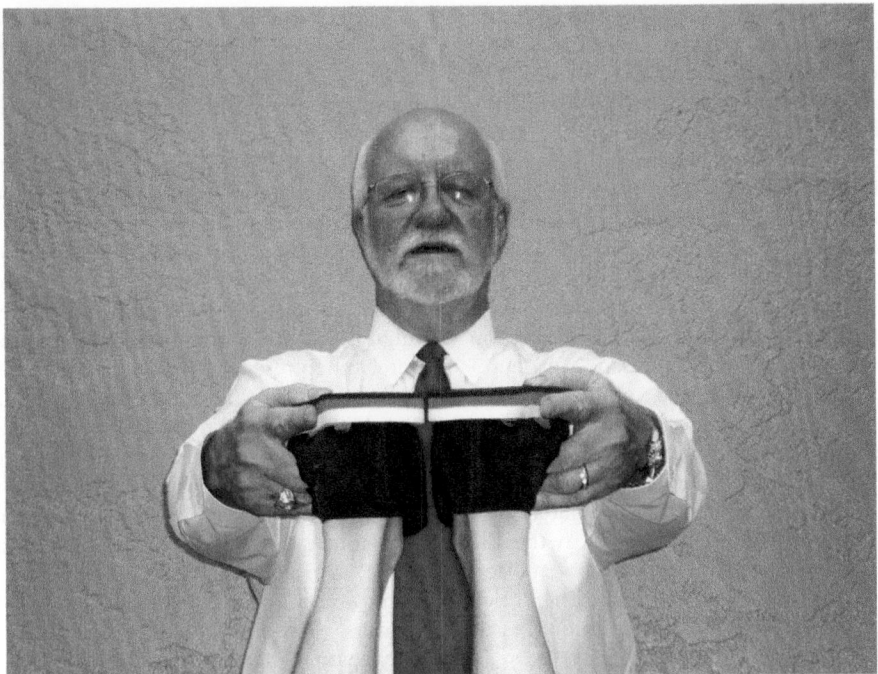

Figure 6-11 Possibility Three: Legs are of equal length in Positions #1 and #2.

- Pressure Tests
- Isolation Tests
- Stress Tests

Observation of reactivity in the PD leg when any of these tests is performed helps to guide the identification and assessment of neuroarticular dysfunction. These tests indicate when and where appropriate adjustment will improve joint neurology and biomechanics.

Pressure Tests. A Pressure Test involves the application of a gentle force on a vertebral segment or extremity joint into the direction of the adjustment, that is, the force is applied in a direction directly opposite to the direction of neuroarticular dysfunction. The force generally is provided as manual pressure that is applied to the vertebral motion segment or extremity articulation. Pressure Tests are performed only when the legs are imbalanced in Position #1, either upon initial LLA, or during the course of treatment in response to an Isolation or Stress Test that reveals neuroarticular dysfunction.

Pressure Tests are thought to be useful for confirming both the need for adjustment and the direction of the needed adjustment for axial or appendicular joint neuroarticular dysfunction. Interpreting the results of a Pressure Test still involves observation of the PD leg in Position #1. For example, the Isolation Test for fifth

lumbar vertebral involvement may cause reactivity of the PD leg, which shortens in Position #1. Reactivity or shortening of the PD leg indicates involvement or neuroarticular dysfunction of L5. If the PD leg lengthens in Position #2, the test indicates that L5 is involved on the side of Pelvic Deficiency, and it suggests that the fifth lumbar vertebra should be adjusted on the PD side. To confirm the findings of the Isolation Test, a Pressure Test may be used. Gentle pressure is applied to the inferior articular process of L5 on the side of Pelvic Deficiency in an anterior-to-superior direction through the joint plane line of the facet. If the legs become even or improve in Position #1, the Pressure Test may confirm the need for adjustment and the direction of the needed adjustment. Because preliminary investigation of Pressure Testing noted insufficient evidence for its effectiveness, further research is indicated.[10] However, on the basis of decades of clinical observations, Pressure Tests are included in the AM.

Isolation Tests. Isolation Tests are specific *active* movements performed by the patient that assist in the location and evaluation of neuroarticular dysfunctional motion segments of the spine and extremities. Before an Isolation Test is performed, appropriate corrections are made to balance the legs. The patient is then asked to perform a number of active motions that facilitate neurological pathways and increase tension in the musculature or other soft tissues of specific regions of the spine and appendicular skeleton. Isolation Tests also actively contract the muscles that stabilize vertebral segments in the spinal column, on the premise that these intersegmental muscles contract before active movements of the global muscles or main mobilizers of the extremities.[11-14] In general, when an Isolation Test is performed, reactivity of the PD leg in Position #1 is thought to indicate the presence of neuroarticular dysfunction. When a vertebral motion unit is tested by the specific AM Isolation Test for that level of the spine, the PD leg in Position #1 is observed for apparent length change. If the vertebral motion segment is not associated with dysfunction, no change or reactivity in the PD leg is noted in Position #1. If the vertebral motion segment is dysfunctional, shortening of the PD leg in Position #1 is seen when the Isolation Test is performed.

In summary, after an Isolation Test is performed, one of these three things occurs:
1. No reactivity in Position #1 or Position #2
2. Reactivity: The PD leg shortens in Position #1 and lengthens in Position #2.
3. Reactivity: The PD leg shortens in Position #1 and further shortens in Position #2.

On the basis of the findings described in numbers 2 and 3, you will then follow the Short/Long Rule, which is described subsequently. If the PD leg appears to lengthen in Position #2, the AM Protocol suggests the vertebrae being isolated should be adjusted on the PD side. If the PD leg appears to shorten in Position #2, the AM Protocol suggests the vertebra being isolated should be adjusted on the side Opposite Pelvic Deficiency.

After an Isolation Test is performed, changes in leg length resulting from neuroarticular dysfunction could possibly be explained as resultant dysfunction in neurological input and in physical contraction of the stabilization muscles, producing difficulty in activating the intersegmental muscles that would normally contract to stabilize the spine before extremity movement. Thus the central nervous system recruits the large global muscles of the back and trunk in an attempt to provide stabilization. This may range from activation of back extensors, quadratus lumborum, and psoas to hip muscles, such as rectus femoris. This creates a "stiffening" of the lumbar spine and pelvis as a unit, which affects normal, smooth movement.[15-17] As the examiner continues to flex

the knees bilaterally at the same rate of speed and the same degree of flexion, unilateral contraction of these muscles results in changes in leg length.

Anecdotal clinical observation and preliminary investigation support the notion that such protocol provides the optimum outcome in locating and reducing biomechanical aberrancies perceived as neuroarticular dysfunction through this method of analysis. Good reproducibility was found in a study of interexaminer reliability with Isolation Testing performed to detect the presence or absence of supposed joint dysfunction at C1.[18] Youngquist et al.[18] compared the results reported by two clinicians who performed leg length testing procedures and applied the Isolation Test in 72 subjects. Another study involved millimetric measurement of leg length differences by five clinicians while subjects' heads were centered, rotated right, and rotated left. Shambaugh and coinvestigators[19] reported, "All raters found highly significant differences in LLI when the head positions changed." Another laboratory evaluation of Isolation Testing involved optoelectrical measurement of heel position changes during cervical maneuvers, including resting, neck extensions, and chin tucks. In response to prone neck extension, significantly greater asymmetrical movement between legs was observed in subjects with chronic spinal complaints compared with asymptomatic controls.[20]

Stress Tests. Similar to Isolation Tests, Stress Tests are performed after the legs have been balanced. A Stress Test is the opposite of a Pressure Test. A Stress Test involves the application of a gentle force on a vertebral motion segment, joint, or other tissue in the direction of neuroarticular dysfunction. The applied force may result from direct manual pressure or traction on the anatomical structure being tested. A Stress Test can also be performed by means of passive movement of a structure, such as an extremity, toward its limit of motion in the direction of neuroarticular dysfunction. Stress Tests are most often used to identify and evaluate neuroarticular dysfunction in the upper and lower extremities.

When an extremity joint is tested by the specific AM Stress Test for that articulation, the PD leg is observed for apparent length change. If the joint is not associated with dysfunction, no change in the length of the PD leg is noted. If, however, the joint is dysfunctional, shortening of the PD leg in Position #1 will be seen when the Stress Test is performed.

The Short/Long Rule. The Short/Long Rule is used only after an Isolation Test has been performed. The Short/Long Rule is a general guideline used to determine the side of involvement of the neuroarticular dysfunction. When an affected vertebra is isolated by the specific Isolation Test for the vertebra, the PD leg shortens in Position #1. The legs are then raised to Position #2. According to the Short/Long Rule, Position #2 is used to determine side of involvement. If the PD leg relatively lengthens going to Position #2, this test indicates involvement on the PD side. If the PD leg relatively shortens going to Position #2, this test indicates involvement on the side Opposite Pelvic Deficiency. For example, a specific Isolation Test for the twelfth thoracic vertebra is performed. The left PD leg shortens in Position #1. The left PD leg then lengthens while going to Position #2. The AM Protocol suggests contact should be made on the left transverse process of T12 on the PD side. If, after the Isolation Test for T12 is performed, the left PD leg shortens in Position #1, and then gets shorter in Position #2, the Short/Long Rule of the AM Protocol suggests that contact should be made on the right transverse process of T12, on the Opposite PD (OPD) side. Of course, Pressure Testing T12, as described earlier, will help to confirm the side of correction.

ADDITIONAL LEG LENGTH ANALYSIS

In addition to the LLA using Position #1 and Position #2, the AM includes testing strategies designed to locate flexion (superior spinous) or extension (inferior spinous) of vertebral motion segments, segmental laterality (lateral listhesis) of vertebrae, and neuroarticular dysfunction of facets. These special tests involve Position #3, Position #4, and Position #5.

Position #3: Superior and Inferior Spinous Testing

A superior spinous (flexion) malposition or an inferior spinous (extension) malposition can occur anywhere in the spine. However, because of the support provided by the ribs and the natural posterior curvature of the thoracic spine, the thoracic vertebrae are less likely to be involved than are the lumbar and cervical motion segments.

To test for a superior or inferior spinous (flexion or extension) malposition at a given vertebral level, first perform the Isolation Test for the vertebra using Position #1 and Position #2. Pressure Test the vertebra, and adjust as indicated. Because no other Isolation Tests have been performed yet, that vertebra is still considered to be isolated. Raise the legs by flexing the knees in the same way that Position #2 is attained; however, continue to raise the legs *until the knees are flexed past 90 degrees* (Figure 6-12), or to the point of resistance

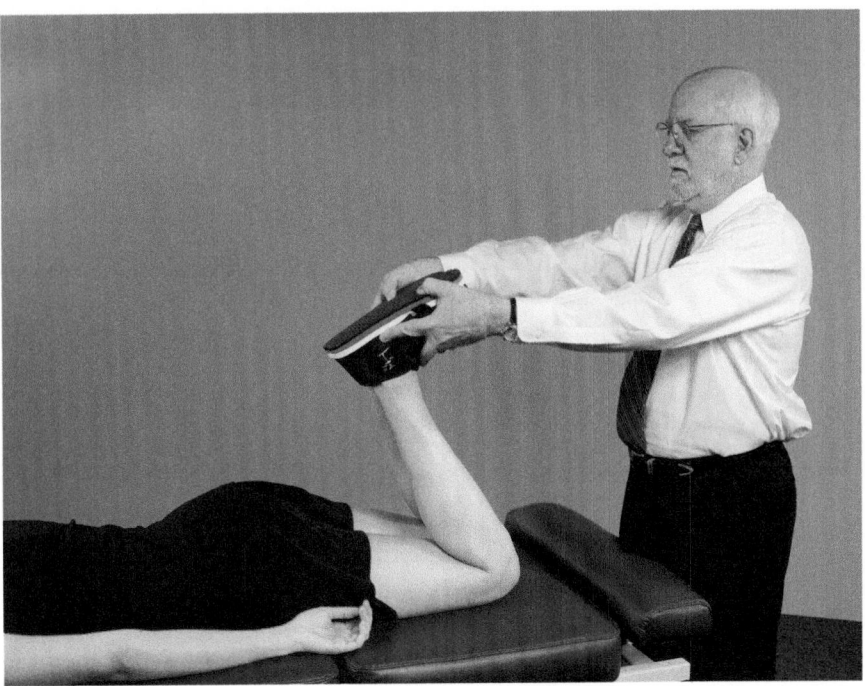

Figure 6-12 Position #3: Legs are flexed past 90 degrees to patient resistance.

of the patient. This is called Position #3. Observe the legs for relative changes in length in Position #3. As the result of nutation of the sacrum and pelvic girdle during this motion,[21,22] we hypothesize that leg reactivity in Position #3 results from stressing the pelvis and vertebral segments in the sagittal plane.

If the PD leg lengthens in Position #3, the spinous process of the segment tested has misaligned superiorly, or the vertebra is in a flexion malposition (Figure 6-13). If the PD leg shortens in Position #3, the spinous process of that tested segment has misaligned inferiorly, or the vertebra is in an extension malposition (Figure 6-14). Position #3 can also be used for the sacrum and the occiput.

Position #4: Segmental Laterality

Lateral listhesis (a lateral malposition) of a vertebral segment may occur at any level of the spine. Consider this as a "global" lateral malposition of the structure that is being isolated. To test for segmental laterality at a given vertebral level, first perform the Isolation Test for that vertebra using Positions #1 and #2. Pressure Test the vertebra, and adjust as indicated. Because no other Isolation Tests have been performed yet, that vertebra is considered to be isolated. Position #4 can also be used for the sacrum and the occiput.

Flex the knee on the PD side past 90 degrees while the leg Opposite Pelvic Deficiency remains on the table. This is known as Position #4 (Figure 6-15). Return the leg to Position #1, and look for shortening of the PD leg. If the PD leg shortens in Position #1, raise the legs to Position #2. Use the Short/Long Rule to interpret the test. If the PD leg lengthens in Position #2, the test suggests segmental laterality of the vertebra on the side of Pelvic Deficiency. If the PD leg shortens in Position #2, the test suggests segmental laterality of the vertebra on the side Opposite Pelvic Deficiency. Flexion of only one leg involves unilateral contraction of musculature, which creates a stress that is thought to initiate responses indicative of a lateral malposition.

Position #5: Neuroarticular Facet Dysfunction

After performing an Isolation Test for the involved segment and completing Positions #3 and #4, perform Position #5 for neuroarticular facet dysfunction. Position #5 is performed by the doctor who places the palms of the hands on the plantar aspect of the metatarsal-phalangeal junction of both feet and applies headward pressure in a quick manner, producing dorsiflexion of both ankles (Figure 6-16). Look for PD leg reactivity or shortening, and then raise the legs to Position #2 to determine the side of neuroarticular dysfunction of the facet, by following the Short/Long Rule. After the side of involvement has been determined, adjustment involves a two-step procedure. The contact points are the

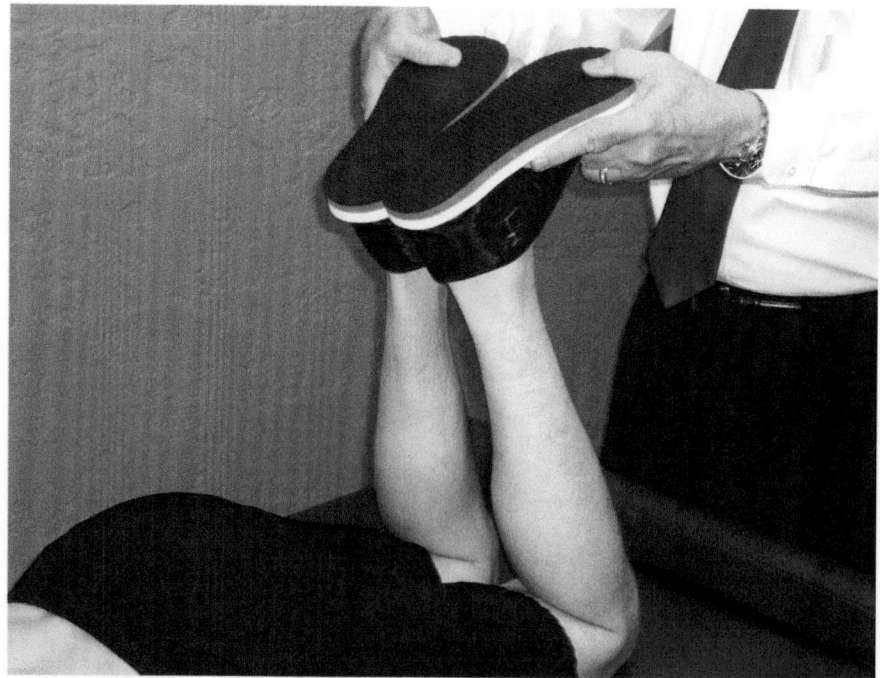

Figure 6-13   Superior spinous process (hyperflexion) in Position #3 with lengthening of Pelvic Deficiency leg.

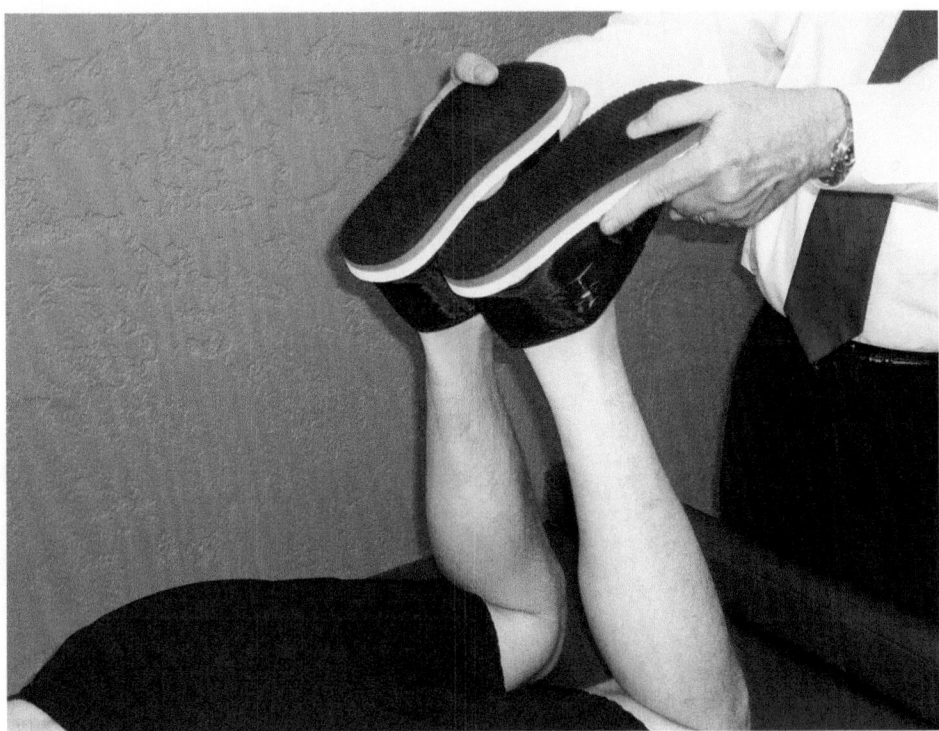

Figure 6-14 Inferior spinous process (hyperextension) in Position #3 with shortening of Pelvic Deficiency leg.

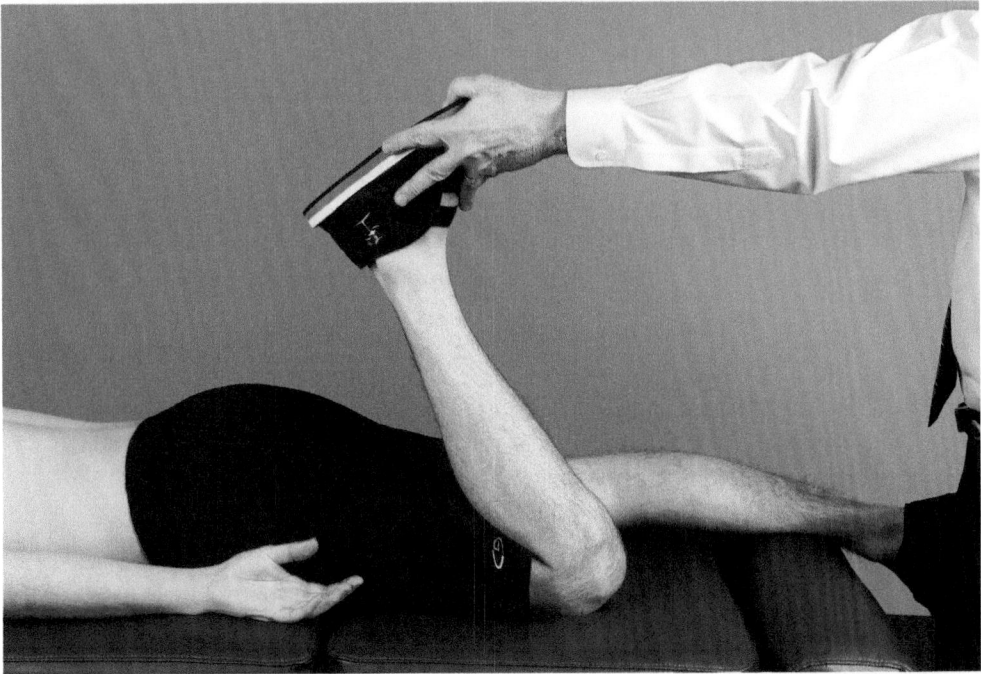

Figure 6-15 Position #4: segmental laterality.

anatomical structures closest to the superior and inferior aspects of the facet joint for the vertebra. In the lumbar spine, the first contact is made on the inferior articular process of the isolated vertebra and the side as indicated by the Short/Long Rule. The Line of Drive (LOD) is anterior, superior, and, if needed, medially directed through the facet joint plane (Figure 6-17). The second step in the adjustment involves contacting the superior articular process of the facet

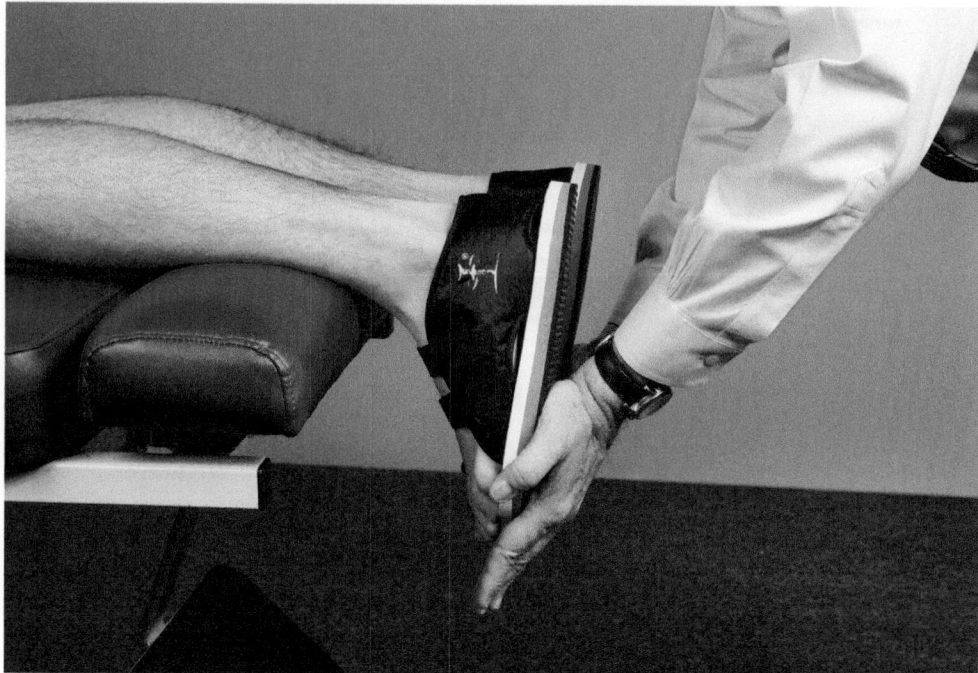

Figure 6-16   Position #5: facet involvement.

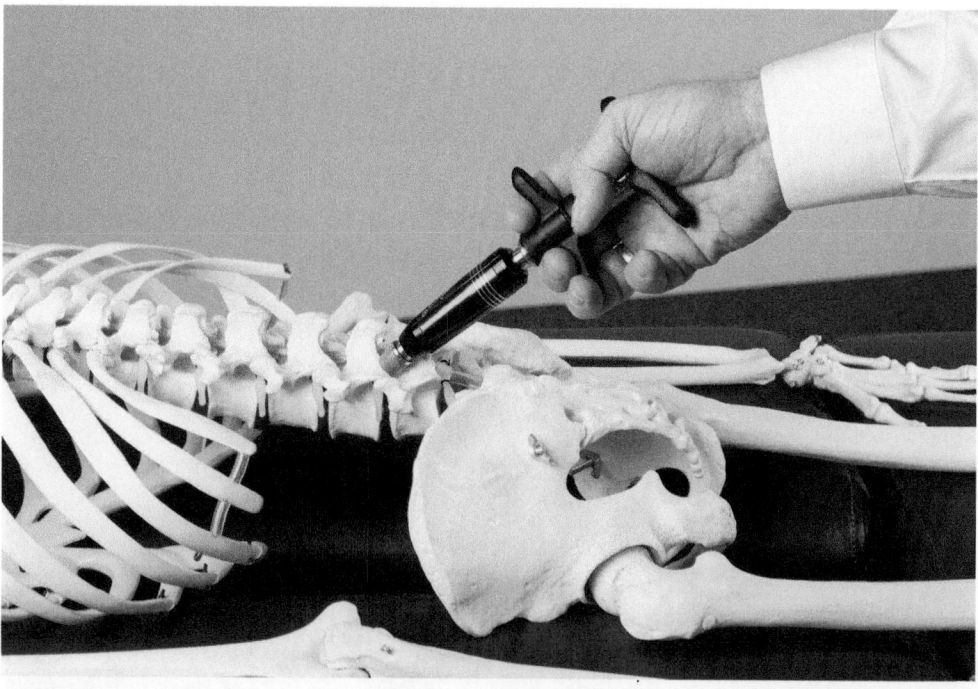

Figure 6-17   Adjustment of facet involvement. Step One: Line of Drive is anterior-superior and medial, if needed, through the joint plane of the facet.

joint on the segment below (Figure 6-18). The LOD is anterior, inferior, and, if needed, medially directed through the facet joint plane. The concept behind this adjustment is to "open up" or distract the facet joint.

With the utilization of Position #5, the specific contact point for involvement in the thoracic spine is as follows. The first contact point is the inferior aspect of the transverse process of the isolated vertebra and the side as indicated

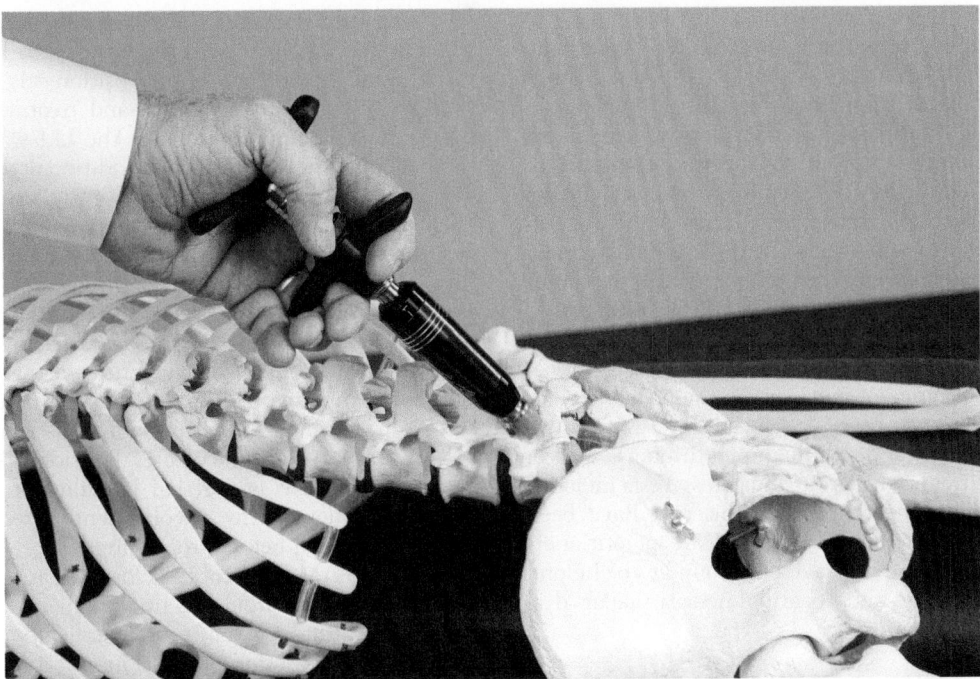

Figure 6-18 Adjustment of facet involvement. Step Two: Line of Drive is anterior-superior and medial, if needed, through the joint plane of the facet.

by the Short/Long Rule. The LOD is anterior, superior, and medial. The second contact is the superior aspect of the transverse process of the segment below. The LOD is anterior, inferior, and medial. For involvement of the cervical spine, the contact point is positioned on the superior or inferior aspect of the pedicle-lamina junction. LODs are anterior, superior or inferior, and medial.

An example of the Position #5 procedure would include the Isolation Test for L4. This would occur after completion of any findings in Position #3 and Position #4. The doctor places the OPD arm across the low back and dorsiflexes the ankles in a quick manner. If the patient has left Pelvic Deficiency, the left leg shortens in Position #1 and relatively shortens in Position #2, indicating a right L4-L5 neuroarticular facet dysfunction by following the Short/Long Rule. The first contact is made at the right L4 inferior articular process with an anterior and superior LOD. The second contact is made at the right L5 superior articular process with an anterior and inferior LOD.

Leg Test Analysis for the Extremities

Throughout AM analysis, the leg check is the primary method of determining the presence of neuroarticular dysfunction or facilitation. For most levels of the axial skeleton, reaction of the PD leg in Position #1 indicates involvement of the

motion segment or structure that is being isolated and tested. Then, Position #2 is used to indicate the side of involvement. Once the side of the neuroarticular dysfunction component has been corrected, the same vertebral level is tested for a flexion or extension malposition via Position #3, a lateral listhesis in Position #4, and a neuroarticular dysfunctional facet via Position #5.

LLA is also used for upper and lower extremity tests and isolations, but *only Position #1* is thought necessary to determine involvement. Position #2 is not necessary because the extremity Stress Test is a unilateral test; thus verification of the side of involvement is redundant. However, if the patient is not very reactive in Position #1, Position #2 can be used for increased sensitivity and as a sign of positive involvement. The essential four-step procedure for testing and adjusting extremity articulations is as follows:

1. Isolate and/or Stress Test the structure.
2. Look for shortening/reactivity of the PD leg in Position #1.
3. Adjust the structure using the appropriate contact point and LOD.
4. Look for the legs to become even again in Position #1.

Keep in mind, of course, that clinical judgment and experience are also critically important in assessing the structural and functional integrity of the spine and extremities.

Stress Testing Extremities

Most AM tests for neuroarticular dysfunction and misalignment of extremity joints are Stress Tests. For example, to Stress Test a "medial calcaneus" neuroarticular dysfunction, simply tap the lateral aspect of the heel in a lateral-to-medial direction. The name of the test indicates the direction of malposition; thus the Stress Test pushes the structure in the direction of the neuroarticular dysfunction, even farther to accentuate or exacerbate a reaction to that position.

Many of the Stress Tests used for the extremities are based on well-established orthopedic and range-of-motion assessment maneuvers. Others have been developed by AM clinical researchers and by field practitioners. All of the extremity Isolation and Stress Tests included in subsequent chapters of this text have been tested in field practice by AM practitioners and in many cases have been found to be helpful in detecting and locating neuroarticular dysfunction.

THE ACTIVATOR METHOD PROTOCOL AND IMPLEMENTATION PROCEDURES

A practitioner should become extremely proficient with the Basic Scan Protocol in Chapter 7 before progressing to any of the other chapters or advanced testing procedures. The remaining chapters are presented in the order the tests would be applied. This would be the utilization of the advanced tests for the sacrum, pelvis, and hip, then progressing through the spine with additional tests for the lumbar, thoracic, and cervical areas. The next incorporation would be the utilization of the temporomandibular joint tests, if indicated. Then the practitioner would use the knee, foot, and ankle tests if related to the area of chief complaint for the lower extremity. The next chapters present tests for the shoulder and clavicle, followed by the elbow, wrist, and hand for the upper extremity.

After completing Chapter 7 and the AM Basic Scan training, the practitioner will be able to begin applying the technique in the treatment of patients. The protocol of the AM requires every patient to receive the analysis and treatments as indicated by using the entire Basic Scan Protocol as presented in Chapter 7. Using the AM Basic Scan Protocol will allow the practitioner to effectively treat most patient complaints and problems. Any additional complaints, especially for the extremities, can be addressed with the utilization of Stress Tests and Pressure Tests.

With completion of the remaining chapters of Advanced AM tests and adjustments, the following protocol would apply. Every patient will first be evaluated with the Basic Scan Protocol. After assessment using Position #1 and Position #2, any involvements and treatments that did not completely balance the LLI would then require the utilization of additional tests. The AM Protocol calls for the use of Position #3 to determine superiority (hyperflexion malposition) or inferiority (hyperextension malposition). Position #3 can be used throughout the axial skeleton, from the sacrum up through the occiput, after the Isolation Test has been performed and the adjustment given for a specific segment. Any involvement should be treated before progressing to other tests or adjustments.

Next, the AM Protocol uses Position #4 to determine if there is a global laterality of the isolated segment. Any involvement detected should be treated before progressing.

Then the AM Protocol calls for evaluation of facet involvement from the fifth lumbar vertebra cephalad through the second cervical vertebra with the utilization of Position #5.

The AM Advanced Protocol therefore calls for the additional analysis and treatment of any segment found to be involved and treated with the utilization of Positions #3, #4, and #5 found throughout the Basic Scan Analysis. Additional tests, along with the use of Positions #3, #4, and #5, are then added relative to the patient's area of chief complaint. The physical location of the related chief complaint structures and any neurological association to the area of chief complaint determines which additional tests are used. Other considerations relative to the thoracic spine are the utilizations of the Inhalation (costovertebral) and Exhalation (costosternal) Tests. These are performed after an Isolation Test throughout the thoracic spine.

Keep in mind when using the AM Protocol, the indications for adjustments are a significant change observed in leg length reactivity. If, for example, you have performed the Isolation Test for the fifth lumbar and there is only a small amount of leg length change in Position #1 and Position #2, advance to the next Isolation Test for the segment above, or the next segment in the Basic Scan. In this example, perform the Isolation Test for fourth lumbar involvement, and typically a significant change will be observed in leg length reactivity. The fourth lumbar would be indicated for adjustment because a *significant* change in leg length occurred. Keep in mind that segments and structures are coupled, both physically and neurologically. The AM Protocol calls for adjusting fewer involvements that create larger leg length changes than trying to discern a small amount of change and performing larger numbers of adjustments. Thus the terminology used is *relative* changes in leg length or reactivity.

Instrument Patient Contact

It is advisable to maintain a firm contact with the instrument to the patient. Preliminary studies in Belgium showed there were more electrical responses with changes in the LOD, or placement of the instrument in relation to the

patient. At the time of publication, recent follow-up studies question the importance of those findings. Within the AM, we are very precise with our contact points and the LODs for each adjustment. At this time, we advise it is better to hold the Activator Adjusting Instrument more perpendicular to the patient, especially in the curvatures of the spine, to maintain a firm, steady contact than being as particular to the *exact* recommended LOD.

RELATED RESEARCH

Boxes 6-1 to 6-4 provide related research on leg length evaluations.

Box 6-1

RELIABILITY OF LEG LENGTH EVALUATIONS

Several studies have investigated the reliability of the common denominator found in Isolation Tests, Pressure Tests, and Stress Tests, which are the relative leg length observations. Most investigations have evaluated interexaminer reliability in Position #1 (Table 6-1), and all have indicated good agreement for this type of observation. However, two studies reported data that do not permit judgments about agreement beyond chance.[19,27] DeBoer et al.[24] studied 40 chiropractic freshmen who were "free of any known neurological or musculoskeletal defects." The students found good to excellent intraexaminer and weaker interexaminer reliability among experienced clinicians who measured prone, extended leg length differences at the heel-sole interface in millimeters. Rhudy and Burke[25] found "poor" to "substantial" concordance beyond chance in a trial involving three nonexpert examiners who used Thompson Technique procedures, and "moderate" to "substantial" agreement beyond chance when three expert examiners observed for leg length discrepancy. All subjects were identified as patients. However, inadequate description of procedures and units of analysis in this report limits its interpretability.

Three studies have explored the interexaminer reliability of leg length evaluations as performed through the Activator Method (AM). Andrew and Gemmell[5] supervised four chiropractors who were experienced in AM leg checks who examined 18 patients with "normal gait," ages 7 to 70 years. They found that observed agreement (69%) exceeded chance agreement (52%); the κ statistic for concordance may be estimated from these figures as κ = 0.35 (i.e., "fair" agreement). Fuhr and Osterbauer[4] used four AM instructors to examine the leg lengths

of 30 other AM instructors. They found marginal to excellent concordance beyond chance for trichotomous observations (left short, right short, or even leg lengths) and weaker inferential coefficients of agreement for millimetric recordings of the differences between right versus left heel-sole interfaces. Unfortunately, methodological problems hamper interpretation of these findings. These weaknesses include lack of randomization of the order of examiners and the vocal report of the short-leg side in the presence of the subject.

Nguyen et al.[6] used two AM instructors to examine 34 patients for relative leg lengths; the order of examiners was randomly assigned, and the recording process was silent. Inferential analysis (unweighted κ = 0.66; $P < .001$) revealed good agreement beyond chance, and findings were in the midrange of the concordance coefficients reported by Fuhr and Osterbauer.[4] Once again, findings of even legs were uncommon, and no agreement was reported between examiners for this category of observation.

With the exception of DeBoer et al.,[24] all of these investigators evaluated the interexaminer reliability of leg checks in the prone, extended position only; the reliability of AM leg length evaluations in Position #2 (flexed knee) has yet to be studied. However, DeBoer et al. found that strong intraexaminer reliability (intraclass correlation coefficients [ICCs]) varied from 0.64 to 0.69 ($P < .05$ in all instances) among clinicians who measured apparent leg length differences with knees flexed. Weaker coefficients were found for pairwise interexaminer concordance in Position #2 (ICC = 0.06 [not significant {ns}], 0.30 [$P < .05$], and 0.34 [$P < .05$]). These findings involved ratio scale data (millimeters). It should also be noted that

Continued

Box 6-1—cont'd

AM leg length evaluations in Position #2 are not merely judgments of relative leg lengths, but rather are intended to judge change in the apparent length of the Pelvic Deficient leg from Position #1 to Position #2. Although such information might be extrapolated from the raw data of DeBoer et al. (e.g., by converting millimetric data to a dichotomous scale, and looking for change in the side of the relative short-leg length from Position #1 to Position #2), the observation task itself differs from that used in the AM Protocol.

Youngquist et al.[18] studied examiners' ability to agree on a segmental level of a presumed lesion (subluxation) on the basis of Isolation Testing. Although it was not an assessment of Position #2 leg check reliability, this study offers indirect support of the idea that examiners can agree on this component of the AM assessment procedure.

The reliability of AM leg lengths in Position #1 appears to be adequate. The most methodologically sound leg length reliability study[6] involved a patient sample and found agreement beyond chance that paralleled findings of other studies involving weaker methods and nonpatient samples.[4,5] Findings for the AM method of leg length evaluation also parallel those for other non-AM leg check procedures.[24,25] However, the reliability of AM leg checks made in Position #2 has yet to be directly evaluated.

PRESSURE TESTING

The only studies conducted to directly address the reactivity of leg length changes in response to articular Pressure Testing and adjusting (at various segmental levels) did not find consistent changes in leg length.[10,26] Haas et al.[10,26] used 42 symptomatic and asymptomatic students, faculty, and staff members of a chiropractic college as subjects. They concluded that leg length changes in response to Pressure Testing and adjusting constitute a "diagnostic illusion." However, several design limitations may inhibit full interpretation. These included the small number of subjects who "met the eligibility criterion for adjustment" (n = 6), the unevenness that random assignment may have produced across groups, and an unusual lack of "stability" (i.e., test-retest reliability) observed in several phases of the studies. Nonetheless, these papers challenge the usefulness of articular Pressure Testing and merit further investigation.

ISOLATION TESTING

Good reproducibility was found in a study of the interexaminer reliability of Isolation Testing conducted to detect the presence or absence of joint dysfunction at C1.[18] Youngquist et al.[18] recruited patients with (n = 34) and without (n = 38) histories of adjustment at C1, who were examined by two clinicians "experienced in leg length testing procedures and the application of the Isolation Test." Although experienced with this method, the clinicians did not rehearse the Isolation Tests together in unblended fashion before the trial. Evaluation and intervention at all indicated segments below the atlas were conducted in each patient before designated examiners conducted the isolation maneuver (i.e., chin tuck) for the first cervical segment. Two examination sessions on separate days yielded two samples (n = 24 and n = 48); concordance beyond chance for the dichotomous decision was κ = 0.52 (P < .01) for the first sample and κ = 0.55 (P < .001) for the second, indicating better than chance agreement between clinicians for this assessment procedure.

Another study involved millimetric measurement of leg length differences by five clinicians while subjects' heads were centered, rotated right, and rotated left. Shambaugh et al.[19] reported, "All raters found highly significant differences in LLI [Leg Length Inequality] when the head positions changed (P < .001)." Unfortunately, the nature of the inferential statistical test they used was unclear. Whether these findings are comparable to the trichotomous (short, long, or even leg lengths) observations made by clinicians is also uncertain.

Falltrick and Pierson[27] studied the responsiveness of leg lengths to several provocations. They found no changes in leg lengths when subjects were asked to rotate their heads while a blinded examiner measured leg lengths in millimeters. These recordings were produced by noting distances along a meter stick extending from a pedestal placed on the subject's midlumbar regions to the ankles. Neither were there any significant differences in LLI among subjects identified as "cervically lesioned" (by independent methods, palpation, etc.) versus those without these presumed dysfunctions. Although subjects were able to produce observable changes in leg length when requested to voluntarily "hip hike," unilateral electromuscular stimulation of the midthoracic and midlumbar regions did not produce significantly

Box 6-1—cont'd

different leg lengths, despite observable titanic contractions in the stimulated areas.

Another laboratory evaluation of Isolation Testing[20] involved "opto-electrical" measurement of heel position changes during cervical maneuvers, including resting, neck extensions, and chin tucks. In response to prone neck extension, more asymmetrical movements between legs were observed in subjects with chronic spinal complaints compared with asymptomatic controls. Whether the recorded phenomenon is comparable or related to that observed by clinicians is unclear but merits further scrutiny.

Rhudy and Burke[25] found "fair" to no concordance beyond chance among three nonexpert examiners who observed for leg length discrepancies according to Thompson Technique procedures in 19 patients during right and left head rotations. A second sample of 22 patients were evaluated for leg length discrepancy by three "expert" examiners during the same isolation maneuvers; "poor" to "moderate" agreement beyond chance was reported. Unfortunately, the units of analysis (e.g., two-choice vs. three-choice observations) were not given. Exact κ values and associated probabilities were not stated; instead, adjectives were applied to κ values according to the schedule shown in Table 6-2.

Taken together, these five studies[18-20,25,27] are still insufficient to substantiate the validity of AM Isolation Testing. However, several additional comments are in order. The report of Shambaugh et al.,[19] which suggests the responsiveness of relative leg lengths to head positioning, must be challenged for lack of clarity of the data analysis. The investigation of Rhudy and Burke[25] did not consider reactivity of leg lengths to head motions but explored variations in reliability as a function of head position. As well, their project[25] made use of both instrumental and Thompson Technique methods of assessment and did not indicate the units of analysis used (e.g., dichotomous vs. trichotomous leg length findings). DeWitt et al.[20] found that prone leg lengths did change in response to various neck and head movements, as measured by opto-electrical equipment. Further investigation is required to verify whether the clinicians' prone leg check can be equated to the laboratory measuring procedure.

Similarly, considerable procedural variations were noted between the methods of Falltrick and Pierson[27] and those used in the AM (e.g., ratio data vs. AM dichotomous observations, lack of cephalad pressure applied to the feet before measurement, no adjustments below the cervical spine before cervical maneuvers were conducted).

Although Youngquist et al.[18] showed moderate levels of agreement beyond chance among observers for cervical segmental dysfunction, this paper should be considered provocative rather than conclusive. This report experimentally addresses the responsiveness of leg length to isolation maneuvers. As the only example of a direct evaluation of the isolation methods of the AM, it may provide a model for further investigation.

FUTURE INQUIRY INTO ACTIVATOR METHOD ASSESSMENT

Available data do not permit assertions concerning the validity of AM assessment procedures for the detection of supposed joint lesions or targets for adjustive intervention. Even so, the analysis system continues to be taught and used because it is said to be a clinically useful aid in directing AM treatment provided by AM-trained practitioners. Even so, the subtle clinical assessment performed by AM analysis remains an area for future research. As with any chiropractic technique, today's evidence-based climate requires investigation with regard to safety, efficacy, patient satisfaction, and cost. The contribution of AM analysis could be explored by two general linear models: (1) a factorial design, with AM analysis included as one level of independent variables, and (2) multiple regression, with AM analysis included as a predictor variable that contributes to clinical cost and outcome as criterion variables. Either or both of these research strategies can be added as a treatment arm in future research into any chiropractic technique.

From Fuhr AW, Menke JM. Status of Activator Methods chiropractic technique, theory, and practice. J Manipulative Physiol Ther. 2005:28(2);e1-e20.

Table 6-1	Characteristics of Several Studies of the Intraexaminer and Interexaminer Reliability of Leg Length Evaluations in the Prone Extended Position (Position #1)			
Authors, Date	**Subjects**	**Examiners**	**Design and Statistics**	**Findings and Limitations**
Venn et al.[23] (1983)	30 Nonacute patients	20 Chiropractic interns and clinic tutors	3 Repeated leg length observations reported as number of examiners who found right short, left short, or even legs; % agreement and X^2 values combined	Concordance beyond chance among observers cannot be determined from raw data reported nor from inferential statistics provided
DeBoer et al.[24] (1983)	40 Chiropractic freshmen, age 21-35 yr	3 Chiropractic clinic faculty members	Each subject measured twice by each examiner for leg length difference in millimeters; concordance evaluated by ICCs	ICCs for interexaminer reliability were 0.23 (ns), 0.32 ($P < .05$), and 0.37 ($P < .05$); ICCs for intraexaminer concordance were 0.52, 0.70, and 0.77 ($P < .05$ in all cases); measurement system differs from the Activator Method
Andrew and Gemmell[5] (1987)	18 Patients with normal gait, age 7-70 yr	4 Chiropractors experienced in leg checks	Each patient examined by 4 blinded examiners; "mean pairwise agreement" and "mean chance agreement" computed for trichotomous choice	Mean pairwise agreement was 69%; mean chance agreement was 52%; κ not reported but can be estimated as κ = 0.35
Shambaugh et al.[19] (1988)	26 Chiropractic freshmen; 10 with no prior adjustments	5 Chiropractors	5 Repeated recordings of millimetric differences in prone leg lengths recorded with head positioned center, right rotated, and left rotated	Concordance beyond chance among observers cannot be determined from raw data reported nor from inferential statistics provided
Fuhr and Osterbauer[4] (1989)	30 Activator instructors	4 Activator instructors, with approximately 10-yr experience each; all AAPR	Interexaminer concordance for trichotomous findings (left short, even, or right short leg) assessed by unweighted κ in 6 pairwise comparisons; interexaminer concordance for absolute differences in leg lengths assessed by pairwise and 4-examiner ICC	κ Pairwise values ranged from 0.31-0.75 (all significant at $P < .05$ or better); no agreement on "even" legs; ICC overall concordance was 0.59 ($P < .05$); pairwise ICC comparisons were generally weaker, ranging from 0.14-0.71; order of examiners was not randomized, and examiners were familiar with subjects

Authors, Date	Subjects	Examiners	Design and Statistics	Findings and Limitations
Rhudy and Burke[25] (1990)	Study 1: 19 patients	3 Nonexpert examiners	Interexaminer concordance for "discrepancy in leg length" according to Thompson Technique, assessed by κ coefficient	"Poor" to "substantial" concordance, but unit of analysis is unclear
	Study 2: 22 patients	3 Expert examiners	Interexaminer concordance for "discrepancy in leg length" according to Thompson Technique, assessed by κ coefficient	"Moderate" to "substantial" concordance, but unit of analysis is unclear
Nguyen et al.[6] (1999)	34 Patients: 23 women and 11 men, age 28-88 (mean 58) yr	2 Activator instructors, both AAPR	Interexaminer concordance for trichotomous findings (left short, even, or right short leg) assessed by unweighted κ; reanalysis of dichotomous findings (excluding 2 cases where "even" legs observed) by unweighted κ	3×3 Unweighted $\kappa = 0.66$ ($P < .001$); no agreement on "even" legs; reanalysis by 2×2 κ produced similarly strong agreement beyond chance

From Fuhr AW, Menke JM. Status of Activator Methods chiropractic technique, theory, and practice. J Manipulative Physiol Ther. 2005;28(2);e1-e20.
The study of reliability of Isolation Testing by Youngquist et al.[18] is excluded from this table because it involved testing leg lengths in Position #2.
AAPR, Activator Advanced Proficiency Rated; *ICC,* intraclass correlation coefficient.

Table 6-2 Values of κ Coefficients and Corresponding Adjectives Used by Rhudy and Burke[25]

κ Value	Adjective	κ Value	Adjective	κ Value	Adjective
<0	None	0.21-0.40	Fair	0.61-0.80	Substantial
0.00-0.20	Poor	0.41-0.60	Moderate	0.81-1.00	Almost perfect

From Fuhr AW, Menke JM. Status of Activator Methods chiropractic technique, theory, and practice. J Manipulative Physiol Ther. 2005;28(2);e1-e20.

Box 6-2

Reference: Fuhr AW, Osterbauer PJ. Interexaminer reliability of relative leg length evaluations in the prone extended position. Chiropr Tech. 1989; 1(1):13-8.

ABSTRACT

The interexaminer reliability of relative leg length evaluation was studied by examiners on a sample of 30 subjects. Prone leg length was examined categorically, whether heels were even, or whether there was a relative shortness to either side. Relative leg length differences were estimated with the use of a ruler. Concordance was computed using κ and intraclass correlation coefficients. The κ statistic yielded "fair" to "good" concordance (ranges, 0.31 to 0.75) among the six combinations of examiner pairs. Results support the reliability of observing and measuring relative Leg Length Inequality in the prone position and are intended to establish a baseline for future investigation.

Box 6-3

Reference: Nguyen HT, Resnick DN, Caldwell SG, Elston EW, Bishop BB, Steinhouser JB, et al. Inter-examiner reliability of Activator Methods: relative leg length evaluation in the prone, extended position. J Manipulative Physiol Ther. 1999; 22(9):565-9.

ABSTRACT

To investigate the interexaminer reliability of the prone extended relative leg length check as described by Activator Methods, Inc., Nguyen et al. employed two Activator instructors to examine 34 patients for relative leg lengths; the order of examiners was randomly assigned, and the recording process was silent. Inferential analysis (unweighted $\kappa = 0.66$; p < .001) revealed good agreement beyond chance.

Box 6-4

Reference: Schneider M, Homonai R, Moreland B, Delitto A. Interexaminer reliability of the prone leg length analysis procedure. J Manipulative Physiol Ther. 2007;30(7):514-21.

OBJECTIVE

The purpose of this study was to perform an interexaminer reliability evaluation of the prone leg length analysis procedure.

METHODS

Two chiropractors each examined a series of 45 patients with a history of low back pain. Patients were in the prone position, with the knees in both extended and flexed positions, and with the head rotated right and left. The clinicians were asked to determine the side of the short leg with knees extended and if a change in leg length occurred with head rotation or when the knees were flexed. They were also asked to visually judge the amount of leg length differential by categorizing the difference as either less than 0.25, 0.25 to 0.5, 0.5 to 0.75, or more than 0.75 in. The head rotation portion of the test was performed only with patients (n = 22) in whom the leg length differential was determined to be less than 0.25 in.

RESULTS

κ statistics and frequency distributions were calculated for each of the respective observations. Reliability of determining the side of the short leg with knees extended was good at 82% agreement ($\kappa = 0.65$) but fair for determining the amount of leg length difference at 67% agreement ($\kappa = 0.28$). Reliability of the head rotation testing procedure was extremely poor, with only 50% and 45% agreement about the observed change in leg length with the head rotated left and right, respectively ($\kappa = 0.04$, $\kappa = -0.195$). There was no significant correlation found between the side of reported pain by the patient and the side of the short leg as noted by either clinician ($\chi = 0.55$, P = .91, and $\chi = 1.55$, P = .67). All of the patients (100%) were judged to have a leg length difference by both clinicians. When the knees were flexed, there was 93% agreement that the short leg became longer (43/45 cases), with no reported cases of the short leg getting shorter. Calculation of κ statistics was confounded for these last 2 observations because of extremely high prevalence bias.

CONCLUSIONS

The results indicate that two clinicians show good reliability in determining the side of the short leg in the prone position with knees extended but show poor reliability when determining the precise amount of that leg length difference. The head rotation test for assessing changes in leg length was unreliable in this sample of patients. There does not appear to be any correlation between the side of pain noted by the patient and the side of the short leg as observed by the clinicians; all 45 patients in this sample were found to have a short leg by both clinicians.

REFERENCES

1. Fuhr AW, Menke JM. Status of Activator Methods chiropractic technique, theory, and practice. J Manipulative Physiol Ther. 2005;28(2):e1-e20.
2. Osterbauer PJ, Fuhr AW, Keller TS. Description and analysis of AMCT. In: Lawrence DJ, Cassidy JD, McGregor M, Meeker WC, Vernon HT, editors. Advances in chiropractic. Vol 2. St. Louis: Mosby; 1995. p. 471-520.
3. Fuhr AW, Menke JM. Activator Methods chiropractic technique. Top Clin Chiropr. 2003;(3): 30-43.
4. Fuhr AW, Osterbauer PJ. Inter-examiner reliability of relative leg length evaluations in the prone extended position. Chiropr Tech. 1989;2(1):13-8.
5. Andrew S, Gemmell H. Inter-examiner agreement in determining side of functional short leg using the Activator Methods test for short leg. J Chiropr Assoc Okla. 1987;5:8-9.
6. Nguyen HT, Resnick DN, Caldwell SG, Elston EW, Bishop BB, Steinhouser JB, et al. Interexaminer reliability of Activator Methods: relative leg length evaluation in the prone extended position. J Manipulative Physiol Ther. 1999;22(9): 565-9.
7. McCaw ST. Leg length inequality: implications for running prevention. Sports Med. 1992;14(6):422-9.
8. McCaw ST, Bates BT. Biomechanical implications of mild leg length inequality. Br J Sports Med. 1991;25(1):10-3.
9. Peters LM. Manual muscle testing: a visual guide. Atlanta: Susan Hunter Publishing; 1986.
10. Haas M, Peterson D, Panzer D, Rothman E, Solomon S, Krein R, et al. Reactivity of leg alignment to articular pressure testing: evaluation of a diagnostic test using a randomized crossover clinical trial approach. J Manipulative Physiol Ther. 1993;16(4):220-7.
11. Hodges P, Richardson C. Feed forward contraction of transverse abdominis is not influenced by the direction of arm movement. Exp Brain Res. 1997;114(2):362-70.
12. Bouisset S, Zattara M. A sequence of postural adjustments precedes voluntary movement. Neurosci Lett. 1981;22:263-70.
13. Aruin A, Latash M. Directional specificity of postural muscles in feed-forward postural reactions during fast voluntary arm movements. Exp Brain Res. 1995;103(2):323-32.
14. Belen'kii V, Gurfinkel' VS, Pal'tsev Y. [Control elements of voluntary movements.]. Biofizika. 1967;12(1):135-41.
15. Panjabi M. The stabilizing system of the spine. Part I. Function, dysfunction, adaption, and enhancement. J Spinal Disord. 1992;5(4):383-9.
16. Gardner-Morse M, Stokes IA, Laible JP. Role of muscles in lumbar spine stability in maximum extension efforts. J Orthop Res. 1995;13(5): 802-8.
17. Cholewicki J, McGill S. Mechanical stability of the in vivo lumbar spine: implications for injury and chronic low back pain. Clin Biomech (Bristol, Avon). 1996;11(1):1-15.
18. Youngquist MW, Fuhr AW, Osterbauer PJ. Interexaminer reliability of an isolation test for the identification of an upper cervical subluxation. J Manipulative Physiol Ther. 1989;12(2): 93-7.
19. Shambaugh P, Solafani L, Fanselow D. Reliability of the Derefield-Thompson test for leg-length inequality, and use of the test to demonstrate cervical adjusting efficacy. J Manipulative Physiol Ther. 1988;11(5):396-9.
20. DeWitt JK, Osterbauer PJ, Stelmach GE, Fuhr AW. Optoelectric measurement of changes in leg length inequality resulting from isolation tests. J Manipulative Physiol Ther. 1994;17(8): 530-8.
21. Magee DJ. Orthopedic physical assessment. Philadelphia: Saunders; 1987.
22. Kapandji IA. The physiology of the joints. New York: Churchill Livingstone; 1974.
23. Venn EK, Wakefield KA, Thompson PR. A comparative study of leg-length checks. Euro J Chiropr. 1983;31(2):68-80.
24. DeBoer KF, Harmon RO, Savoie S, Tuttle CD. Inter- and intra-examiner reliability of leg length differential measurements: a preliminary study. J Manipulative Physiol Ther. 1983;6(2): 61-6.
25. Rhudy TR, Burke JM. Inter-examiner reliability of functional leg-length assessment. Am J Chiropr Med. 1990;3(2):63-6.
26. Haas M, Peterson D, Rothman EH, Panzer D, Krein R, Johansen R, et al. Responsiveness of leg alignment changes associated with articular pressure testing to spinal manipulation: the use of a randomized clinical trial design to evaluate a diagnostic test with a dichotomous outcome. J Manipulative Physiol Ther. 1993; 16 (5):306-11.
27. Falltrick DR, Pierson SD. Precise measurement of functional leg-length inequality and changes due to cervical spine rotation in pain-free students. J Manipulative Physiol Ther. 1989;12(5): 364-8.

SECTION III

ACTIVATOR METHOD ANALYSIS

7

THE ACTIVATOR METHOD BASIC SCAN PROTOCOL

The Activator Method (AM) provides a systematic clinical approach to neuroarticular dysfunctions in the form of protocols for identifying and treating a wide variety of common complaints of neuromusculoskeletal origin. The AM originated as a chiropractic technique that addressed the spine. However, the core of the AM Basic Scan Protocol consists of tests and adjustments that address select segmental levels of the axial skeleton, as well as areas of the feet, knees, pelvis and shoulders. The reason for the relatively restricted scope of the AM Basic Scan Protocol is that clinical experience has shown that most often, neuroarticular dysfunctions of consequence tend to occur at stress points, often located at the transitional vertebrae of the spine and at select areas in the feet, knees, pelvis, and shoulders. The AM Basic Scan Protocol addresses the "majors" of the spine (neuroarticular dysfunctions) that are involved in high concentrations of neurological coordination and feedback mechanisms.

Part of the chiropractic approach to conservative clinical care consists of avoidance of overadjusting. One way to limit excessive adjusting is to differentiate between major complexes and minor compensations. Clinical experience suggests that major complexes tend to occur at stress and transition points in the spine. Dysfunction or misalignment of other vertebrae may occur secondarily or as compensations to the stresses induced in the dynamic structure of the spine by fixation or aberrant motion at the major stress areas of transitional vertebrae. Therefore adjustment of majors frequently eliminates compensatory or minor dysfunctions.[1] In the experience of many practitioners, assessment and adjustment when indicated of just those areas listed in the Basic Scan will reduce neuroarticular dysfunction, normalize posture and Leg Length Inequality, and provide symptomatic relief of musculoskeletal complaints. At the same time, use of the Protocol avoids "chasing symptoms"

of the patient with a mixed or ambiguous clinical presentation. The AM Basic Scan Protocol consists of the sequence of Isolation Tests and adjustments most frequently seen during the first two or three visits for a new patient and at routine maintenance visits by returning patients.

The vertebral motor units and other articulations included in the AM Basic Scan Protocol are listed in Table 7-1. Note that only a few vertebrae are listed for each region of the spine.

INITIAL LEG CHECK

As was observed in the previous chapter, the Leg Length Analysis is a guide to clinical decision making throughout the AM. Changes observed in the Pelvic Deficient (PD) or reactive leg help the practitioner to identify misalignment and neuroarticular dysfunction at all levels of the spinal column and at articulations of the extremities. As central and important as the leg test is in the AM, it still is only one parameter. Sound clinical judgment and information from a thorough history and appropriate physical examination form the basis for a legitimate and effective treatment plan.

From the initial prone placement of the patient, determine the side of Pelvic Deficiency. The short leg in the prone extended position, Position #1, is the PD leg (Figure 7-1). Next, raise the legs to Position #2. If the short leg lengthens in Position #2 (Figure 7-2) (Possibility One), proceed to the knees and feet (Figure 7-5 and Table 7-2). If the short leg stays short or gets shorter in Position #2 (Figure 7-3) (Possibility Two), proceed to the Fourth Lumbar Isolation Test (Figure 7-25 and Table 7-2). If the legs are even in Position #1 and Position #2 (Figure 7-4) (Possibility Three), proceed to the pubic bone Isolation Test (Figure 7-19 and Table 7-4).

When performing adjustments, it is advisable to maintain a firm contact with the instrument

Table 7-1	The Activator Method Basic Scan Protocol
Lower Extremities	Medial knee
	Lateral knee
Pelvis	Anterior-Superior ilium
	Posterior-Inferior ilium
Symphysis Pubis	
Lumbar Spine	L5
	L4
	L2
Lower Thoracic Spine	T12
	T8 and corresponding rib
Upper Thoracic Spine	T6 and corresponding rib
	T4 and corresponding rib
	T1
	First ribs
Upper Extremities	Medial scapula
	Lateral scapula
Cervical Spine	C7
	C5
	C2/C1
Occiput	

to the patient. Preliminary studies in Belgium showed there were more electrical responses with changes in the Line of Drive (LOD), or placement of the instrument in relationship to the patient. Recent follow-up studies at the time of publication are questioning the importance of those findings. Within the AM, we are very precise with our contact points and the LODs for each adjustment. We are advising at this time that it is better to hold the Activator Adjusting Instrument more perpendicular to the patient, especially in the curvatures of the spine, in order to maintain a firm, steady contact than being as particular to the *exact* recommended LOD.

BASIC SCAN PROTOCOL–IN-DEPTH

If the PD leg lengthens while going to Position #2, when the patient is initially examined, begin with Pressure Testing and adjusting of the knees and feet. Use the following four-step sequence to test for knee and foot involvement:

Knees and Feet
1. Pressure Test the medial knee joint on the PD side, and adjust the talus and knee if indicated.
2. Pressure Test the medial knee joint on the side Opposite Pelvic Deficiency, and adjust the talus and knee if indicated.

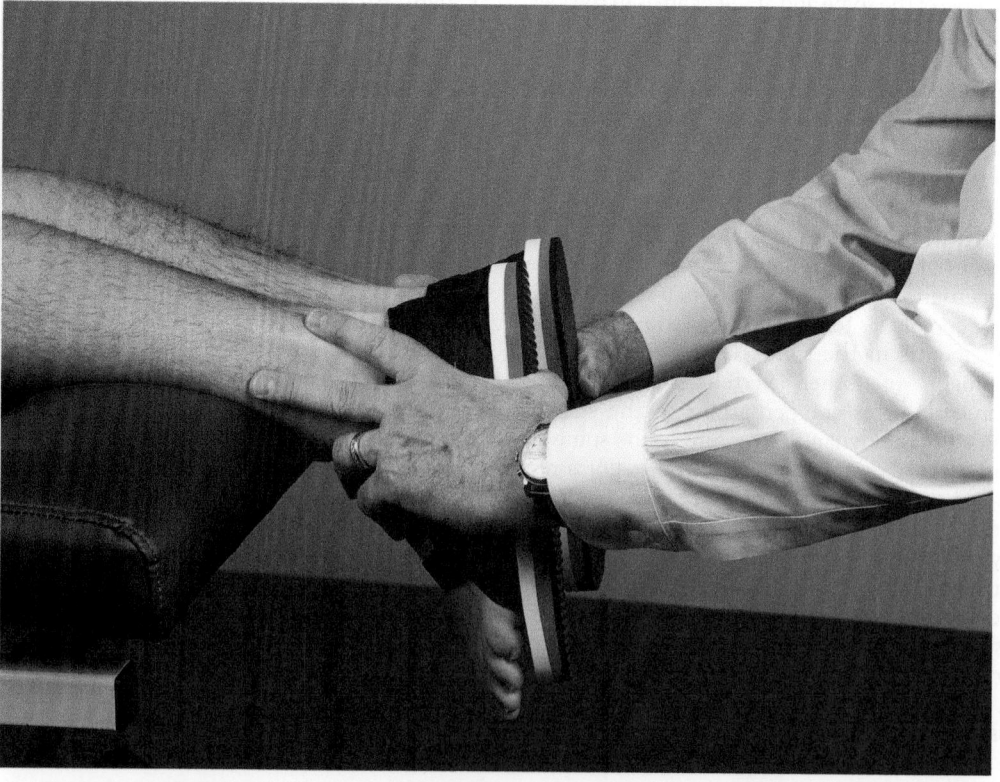

Figure 7-1 The short leg is observed in the prone position–Position #1.

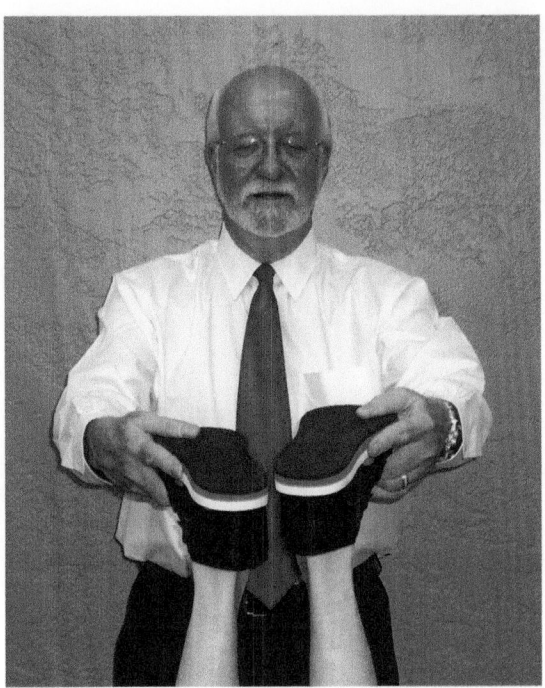

Figure 7-2 Possibility One—Pelvic Deficiency leg lengthens in Position #2.

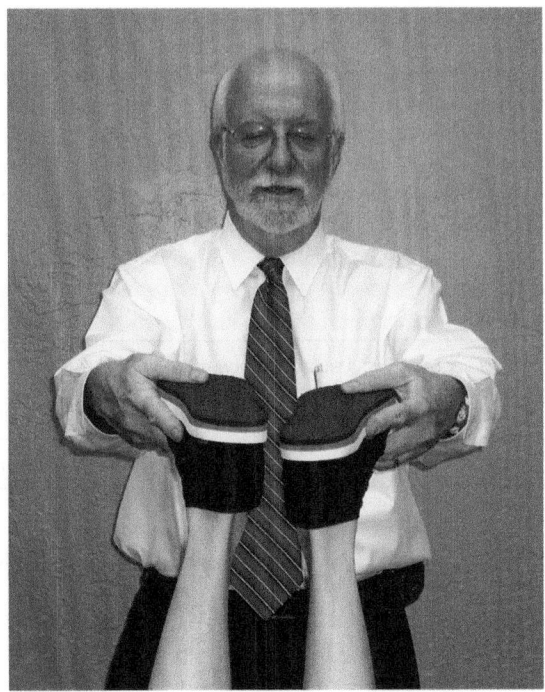

Figure 7-3 Possibility Two—Pelvic Deficiency leg shortens in Position #2.

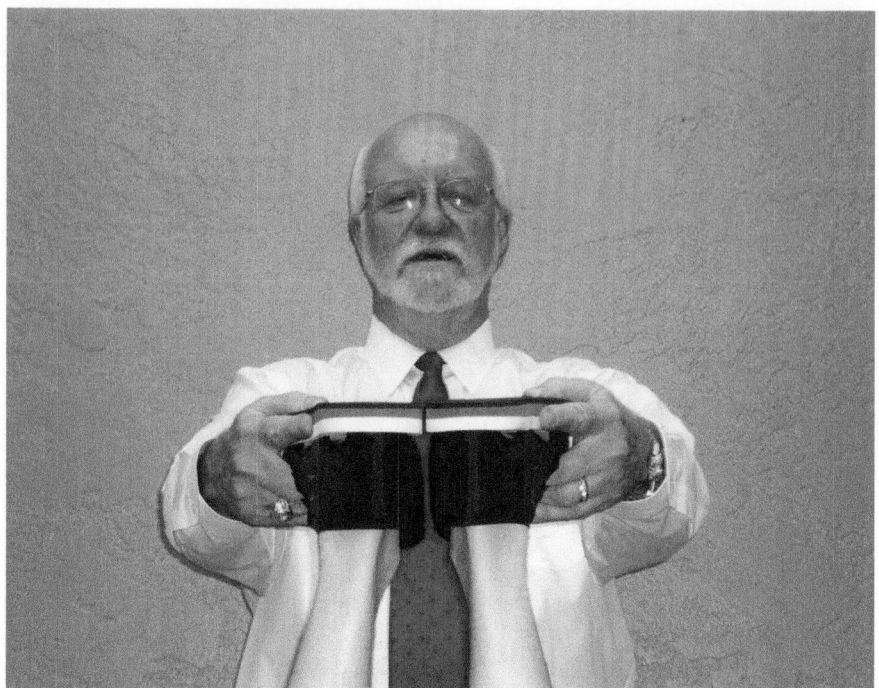

Figure 7-4 Possibility Three—legs are of equal lengths in Positions #1 and #2.

3. Pressure Test the lateral knee joint on the PD side, and adjust the cuboid and knee if indicated.
4. Pressure Test the lateral knee joint on the side Opposite Pelvic Deficiency, and adjust the cuboid and knee if indicated.

A *Pressure Test* involves a firm but gentle force applied to a joint or other structure in the direction of adjustment. If the legs become even, or if the difference between them decreases following a Pressure Test, the need for correction is indicated.

For most patients, a PD leg that lengthens going to Position #2 from the initial leg check is more likely to be associated with pelvic involvement than with the knees and feet. Knee and foot involvement does tend to be encountered frequently in athletes involved in running and jumping sports[2-4] and to some extent in body contact sports, so it is important to rule out neuroarticular dysfunction and instability of the lower extremity[5] before you proceed to the assessment of the pelvis and the rest of the axial skeleton.

Table 7-2 **Summary—Tests and Adjustments: The Activator Method Basic Scan Protocol**			
POSSIBILITY ONE: RAISE LEGS TO POSITION #2—PD LEG LENGTHENS			
		ADJUSTMENT	
Articular Dysfunction	**Test**	**Segmental Contact Point**	**Line of Drive**
KNEE			
Medial Knee Joint	Pressure Test medial collateral ligament lateral and inferior	*Step One*: Medial border of talus	Posterior-superior and lateral
		Step Two: Medial knee joint space	Lateral and inferior

Table 7-2 Summary—Tests and Adjustments: The Activator Method Basic Scan Protocol—cont'd

POSSIBILITY ONE: RAISE LEGS TO POSITION #2—PD LEG LENGTHENS

Articular Dysfunction	Test	Segmental Contact Point	Line of Drive
		ADJUSTMENT	
Lateral Knee Joint	Pressure Test lateral collateral ligament medial and inferior	*Step One*: Inferior lateral aspect of cuboid	Posterior-superior and medial
		Step Two: Lateral knee joint space	Medial and inferior
PELVIS			
Anterior-Superior Ilium	Pressure Test crest of ilium inferior-medial	*Step One*: Base of sacrum on side OPD	Anterior-inferior
		Step Two: Crest of ilium	Inferior-medial
		Step Three: Ischial tuberosity	Anterior-inferior
Posterior-Inferior Ilium	Pressure Test under sacrotuberous ligament posterior-superior and lateral	*Step One*: Spine of ischium	Posterior, superior, and lateral
		Step Two: Sacrotuberous ligament	Posterior, superior, and lateral
		Step Three: Lateral aspect of ilium	Anterior-superior
SYMPHYSIS PUBIS			
Superior Pube	Instruct patient to squeeze knees together. PD leg lengthens going to Position #2	Superior aspect of pubic bone on side of PD	Inferior
Inferior Pube	Instruct patient to squeeze knees together. PD leg shortens going to Position #2	Inferior aspect of pubic bone on side OPD	Superior

Note: Continue the rest of the Activator Method Basic Scan Protocol by next testing L5 and the rest of the vertebrae and shoulders as indicated.

POSSIBILITY TWO: RAISE LEGS TO POSITION #2—PD LEG STAYS SHORT OR GETS SHORTER

Articular Dysfunction	Test	Segmental Contact Point	Line of Drive
		ADJUSTMENT	
L4	OPD arm across the low back		
L4—OPD	PD leg goes short on raising legs to Position #2	Inferior articular process on L4 on side OPD	Anterior-superior
L4—PD side	PD leg lengthens in Position #2	Inferior articular process on L4 side of PD	Anterior-superior

Note: Continue the rest of the Activator Method Basic Scan Protocol by next testing L2 and the rest of the vertebrae and shoulders as indicated.
For a patient who presents with even legs in Position #1 that have no relative change and thus remain even in Position #2 (Possibility Three), begin the Protocol with the symphysis pubis assessment and the rest of the vertebrae and shoulders as indicated.
OPD, Opposite Pelvic Deficency; *PD*, Pelvic Deficency.

Medial Knee. Always start assessing the knees and feet by Pressure Testing for medial knee dysfunction on the side of Pelvic Deficiency.

Pressure Test. To Pressure Test the medial knee, apply a firm but gentle pressure by stroking over the medial collateral ligament. Apply the pressure in a lateral and inferior direction (Figure 7-5). Be sure that the stroking motion crosses the knee joint. If leg lengths balance or become more even in Position #1, proceed to the adjustment for medial knee involvement.

Adjustment. When medial knee involvement is indicated by Pressure Testing, the AM Protocol calls for adjustment of the talus on the side of involvement, before the medial knee is addressed. Step One is the adjustment of an anterior, inferior, and medial talus misalignment. Contact the medial border of the talus, anterior-inferior to the medial malleolus. To adjust the talus, a posterior, superior, and lateral LOD is used (Figure 7-6). Step Two is to adjust the medial knee. The knee joint can subluxate medially and superiorly.[6] To ensure proper placement of the tip of the instrument, flex and extend the knee while palpating for the joint space. Locate the bony prominence of the medial aspect of the tibial plateau. The contact point is just slightly above the tibial plateau on the medial collateral ligament in the medial knee joint space. The LOD is lateral and inferior (Figure 7-7).

If Pressure Testing for a medial knee on the PD side does not balance the legs or cause them to become more even, or if the legs are still uneven after the talus and medial knee on the side of Pelvic Deficiency are adjusted, proceed by Pressure Testing for a medial knee on the side Opposite Pelvic Deficiency. If Pressure Testing balances the legs, or if they are improved in Position #1, adjust the talus and the medial knee on the side Opposite Pelvic Deficiency. The procedure for correcting medial knee neuroarticular dysfunction on the side Opposite Pelvic Deficiency is the same as that described previously on the PD side.

Lateral Knee. If, after Pressure Testing and adjustment as indicated for medial knees, the legs still are not balanced, perform Pressure Tests and adjustments as indicated for lateral knee dysfunction. Start by Pressure Testing for lateral knee dysfunction on the side of Pelvic Deficiency.

Pressure Test. To Pressure Test a lateral knee, apply a firm but gentle pressure by stroking over the lateral collateral ligament. Be careful not to involve the fibula in the Pressure Test. Apply pressure in a medial and inferior direction

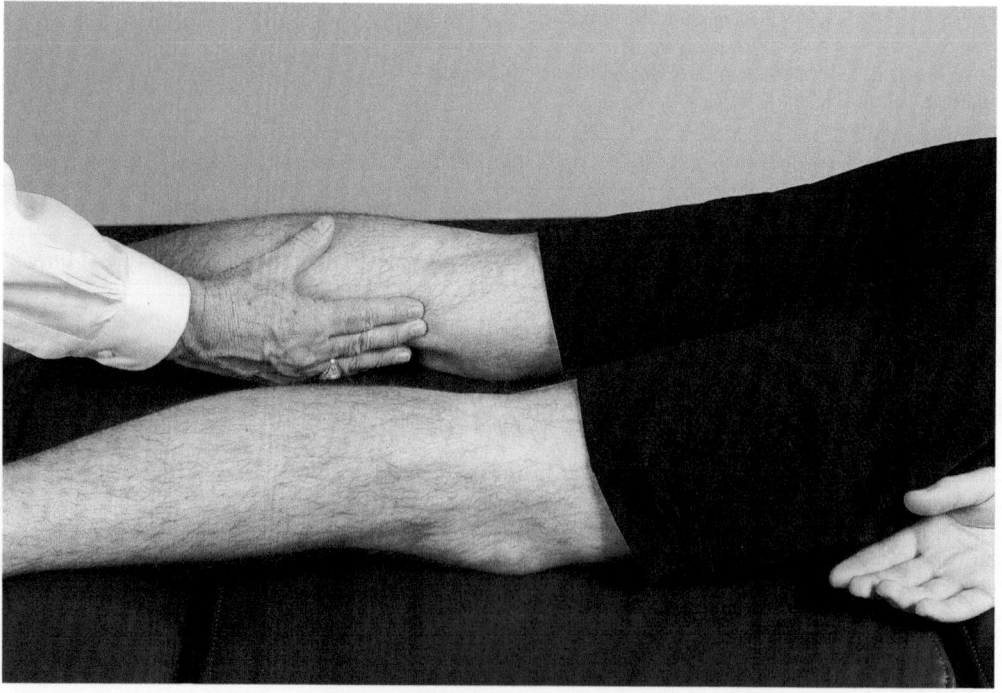

Figure 7-5 Pressure Test for medial knee.

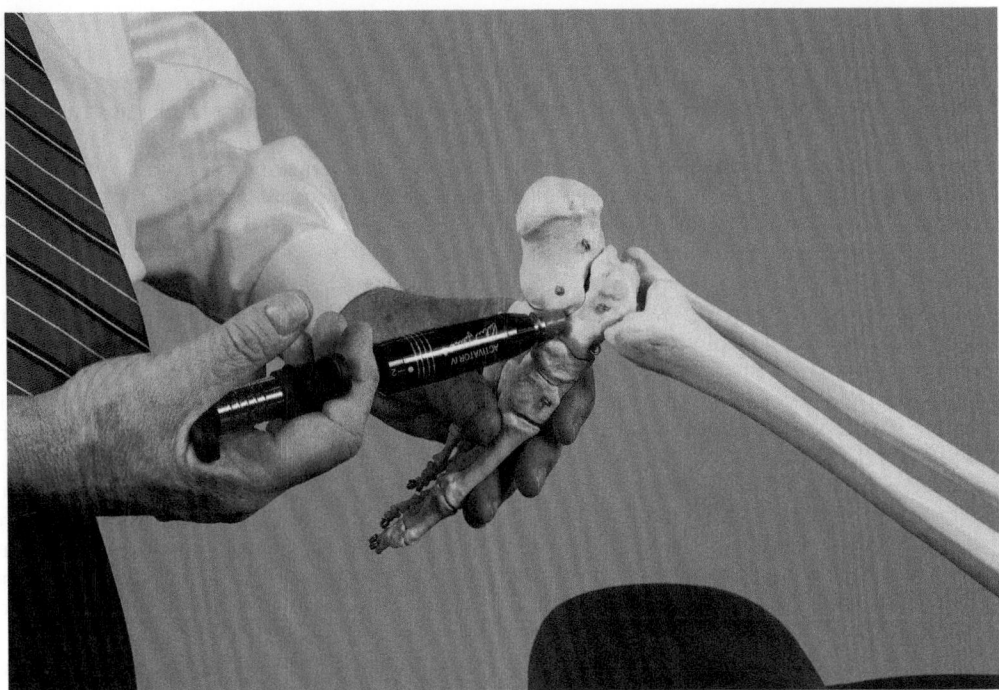

Figure 7-6 Step One adjustment for medial knee—medial border of talus. Line of Drive is posterior-superior and lateral.

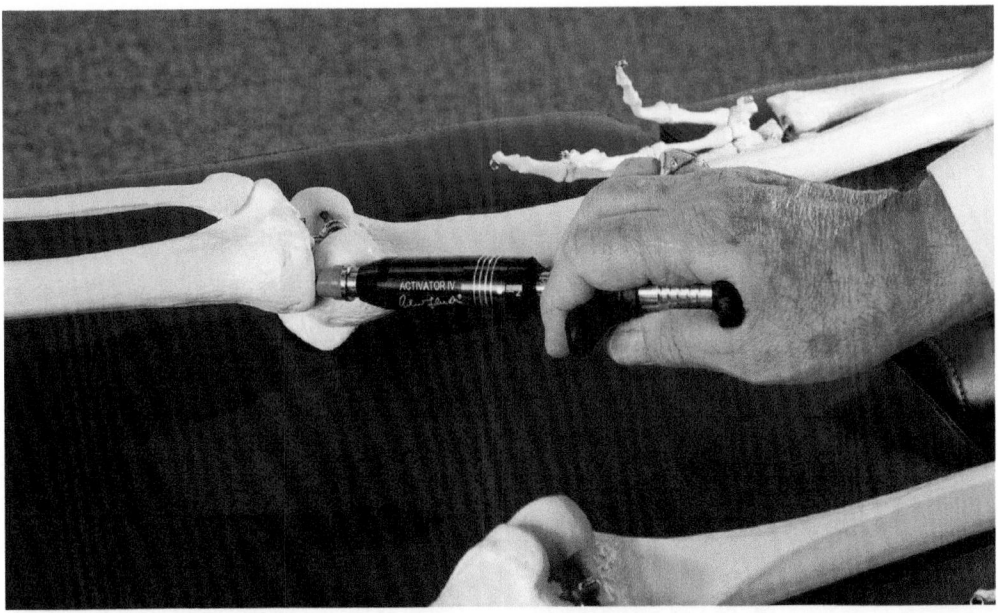

Figure 7-7 Step Two adjustment for medial knee—medial knee joint space. Line of Drive is lateral and inferior.

(Figure 7-8). Be sure that the stroking motion crosses the knee joint. If the leg lengths balance or become more even in Position #1, proceed to the adjustment for lateral knee involvement.

Adjustment. When lateral knee involvement is indicated by Pressure Testing, the AM Protocol calls for adjustment of the cuboid on the side of involvement before adjustment of the lateral knee. The cuboid is the most commonly subluxated bone in the foot and is usually noted in an anterior, inferior, and lateral involvement.[7,8] To adjust the cuboid, contact its inferior and lateral aspect, just posterior to the articulation between the cuboid and the fifth metatarsal. The LOD is posterior, superior, and medial (Figure 7-9). The second step is to adjust the lateral knee misalignment, which involves a lateral and superior tibia.[6] To ensure proper placement of the tip of the instrument, flex and extend the knee while palpating for the joint space. Locate the bony prominence of the superior-lateral aspect of the tibial plateau. The contact point is just slightly above the tibial plateau on the lateral collateral ligament, within the knee joint space. Make sure

to avoid contact with the fibula. The LOD is medial and inferior (Figure 7-10).

If Pressure Testing for a lateral knee on the PD side does not balance the legs or cause them to become more even, or if the legs are still uneven after adjustments are made for the lateral knee on the side of Pelvic Deficiency, proceed by Pressure Testing for a lateral knee on the side Opposite Pelvic Deficiency. If Pressure Testing balances the legs, or if they are improved in Position #1, adjust the cuboid and the lateral knee on the side Opposite Pelvic Deficiency. The procedure for correcting lateral knee neuroarticular dysfunction on the side Opposite Pelvic Deficiency is the same as that described previously.

Once the knees and feet have been tested and adjusted as indicated, proceed to the Stress Tests and Isolation Tests for the pelvis, including the sacroiliac joints and pubic bones. If upon the first two or three visits, you observe that the knees and feet are not involved, it is not necessary to continue assessing them upon subsequent visits for that patient. A summary for medial and lateral knee joint tests and adjusments is noted in Table 7-3.

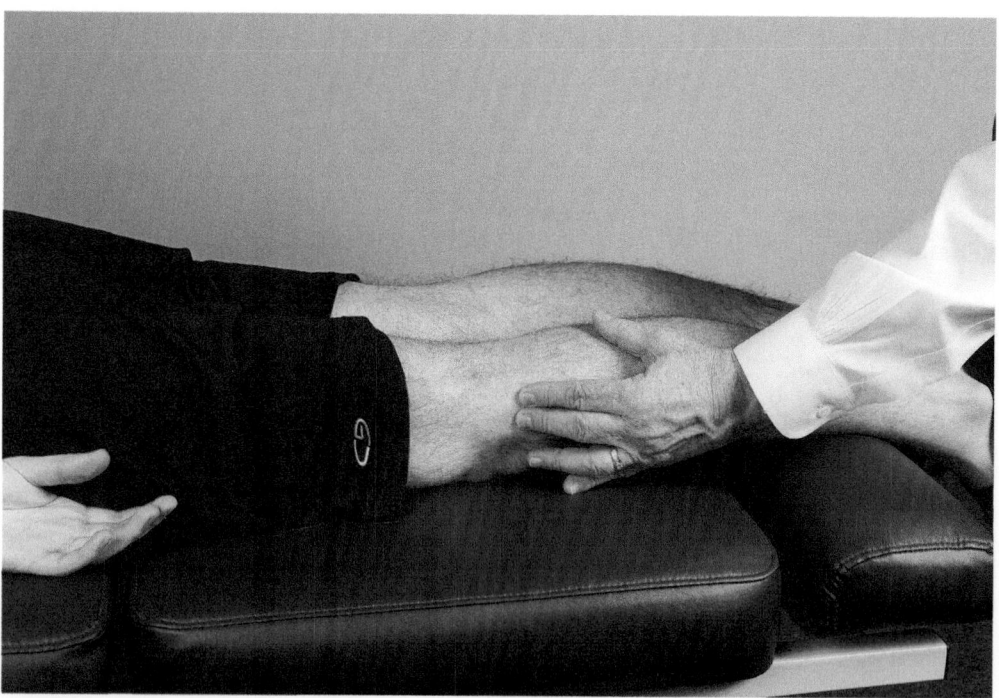

Figure 7-8 Pressure Test for lateral knee.

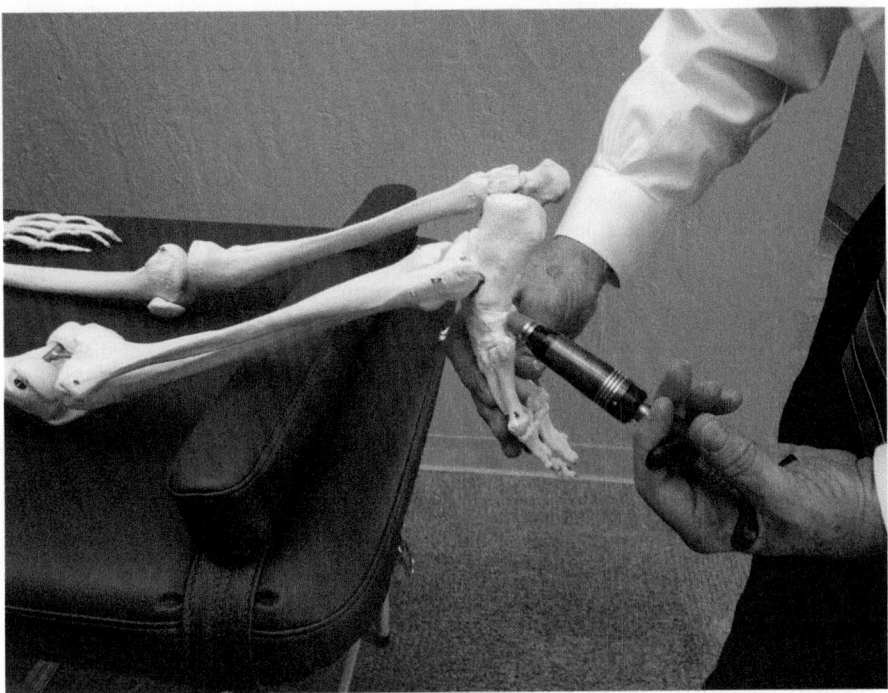

Figure 7-9 Step One adjustment for lateral knee—inferior lateral aspect of cuboid. Line of Drive is posterior-superior and medial.

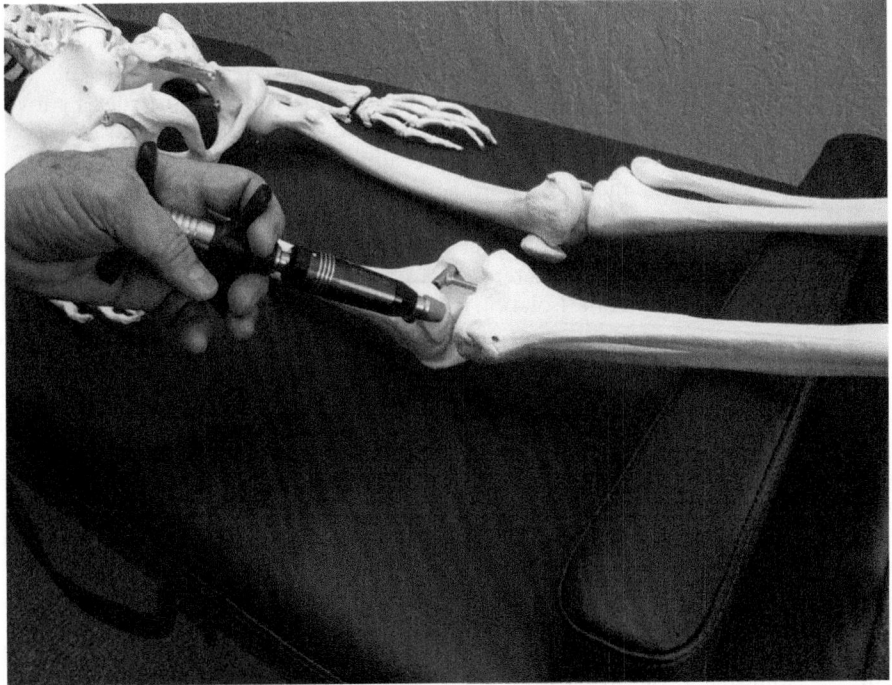

Figure 7-10 Step Two adjustment for lateral knee—lateral knee joint space. Line of Drive is medial-inferior.

Table 7-3	**The Activator Method Basic Scan Protocol: Knees and Feet**		
		ADJUSTMENT	
Articular Dysfunction	**Test**	**Segmental Contact Point**	**Line of Drive**
Medial Knee Joint	Pressure Test medial collateral ligament lateral and inferior	*Step One*: Medial border of talus	Posterior-superior and lateral
		Step Two: Medial knee joint space	Medial-inferior
Lateral Knee Joint	Pressure Test lateral collateral ligament lateral and inferior	*Step One*: Inferior later aspect of the cuboid	Posterior-superior and medial
		Step Two: Lateral knee joint space	Medial-inferior

CLINICAL TIP: When Pressure Testing for medial or lateral knee involvement, apply gentle pressure over the knee joint, and do not use long strokes down the thigh or calf. This is a common mistake, especially for novice Activator practitioners. Long strokes activate multiple levels of proprioceptive input, causing false-positive knee involvement findings.

If the legs are still not balanced in Position #1 after testing and adjusting of the knees and feet as described in the Basic Scan Protocol, proceed to the first of the pelvic tests. The tests of the pelvis, the first for an anterior-superior (AS) ilium and the second for a posterior-inferior (PI) ilium, are Pressure Tests, that is, the joints are tested by the application of a gentle force into *the direction of adjustment*. A positive Pressure Test indicates the presence of neuroarticular dysfunction or involvement as observed by the leg lengths balancing or becoming more even in Position #1.

If legs are balanced in Position #1 and Position #2, after any or all of the above medial and lateral knee tests, proceed to the pubic bone Isolation Test.

Pelvis

Anterior-Superior Ilium

Pressure Test.   To Pressure Test for an AS ilium, contact the iliac crest and apply a gentle inferior and medial pressure to the crest of the ilium on the side Opposite Pelvic Deficiency in a plane parallel to the plane line of the sacroiliac joint (Figure 7-11). Look for the legs to balance or become more even in Position #1; this indicates that correction of an AS ilium is necessary.
Adjustment.   Adjustment of an AS ilium requires a single thrust on each of the three

contact points with the Activator Adjusting Instrument as follows:

1. Contact the base of the sacrum on the side Opposite Pelvic Deficiency about one-half inch lateral to the first sacral tubercle. The LOD is anterior and inferior (Figure 7-12).
2. Contact the crest of the ilium about one inch superior to the posterior superior iliac spine. The LOD is inferior and medial parallel to the plane line of the sacroiliac articulation (Figure 7-13).
3. Contact the superior aspect of the ischial tuberosity. The LOD is anterior and inferior (Figure 7-14).

Posterior-Inferior Ilium.   Following adjustment of an AS ilium, or if the Pressure Test for an AS ilium is negative, consider PI involvement of the ilium *on the side of Pelvic Deficiency*. The PI ilium is most commonly involved.
Pressure Test.   To Pressure Test for a PI ilium, make a firm thumb contact under the sacrotuberous ligament on the side of Pelvic Deficiency. Apply firm pressure in a superior, lateral, and posterior direction parallel to the plane line of the sacroiliac joint (Figure 7-15). Look for the legs to balance in Position #1; this indicates the necessity for PI ilium adjustment.
Adjustment.   Adjustment of a PI ilium requires a single thrust on each of the three contact points with the Activator Adjusting Instrument as follows:

1. First, direct the tip of the instrument toward the spine of the ischium on the side of Pelvic Deficiency. Position the tip of the instrument in the soft tissue of the gluteus maximus just medial to the ischial tuberosity. The LOD is posterior, superior, and lateral (Figure 7-16).

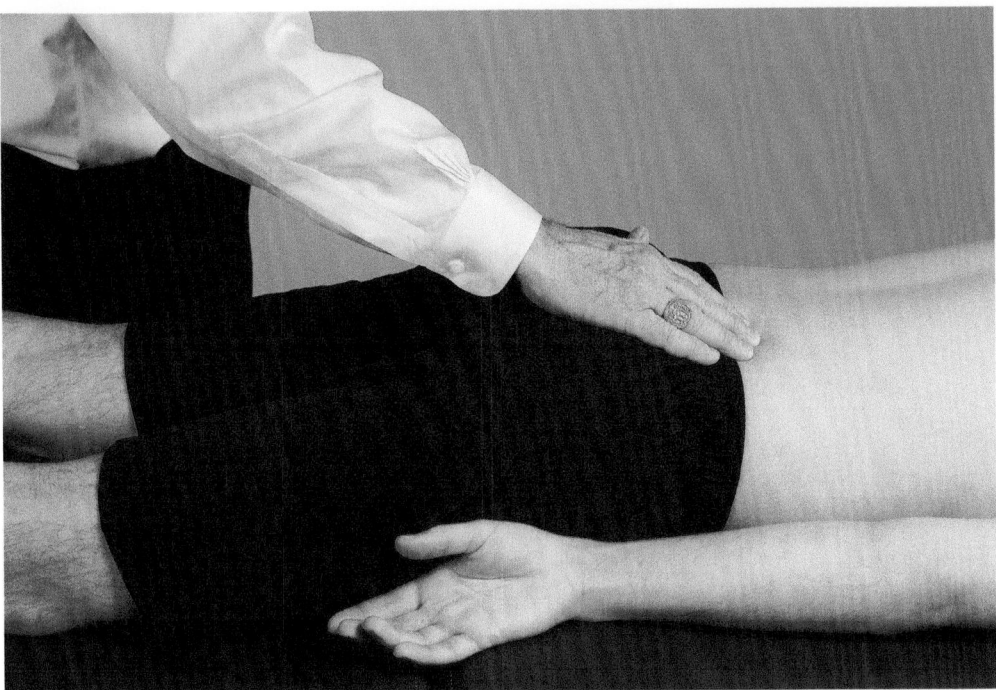

Figure 7-11   Pressure Test for anterior-superior ilium.

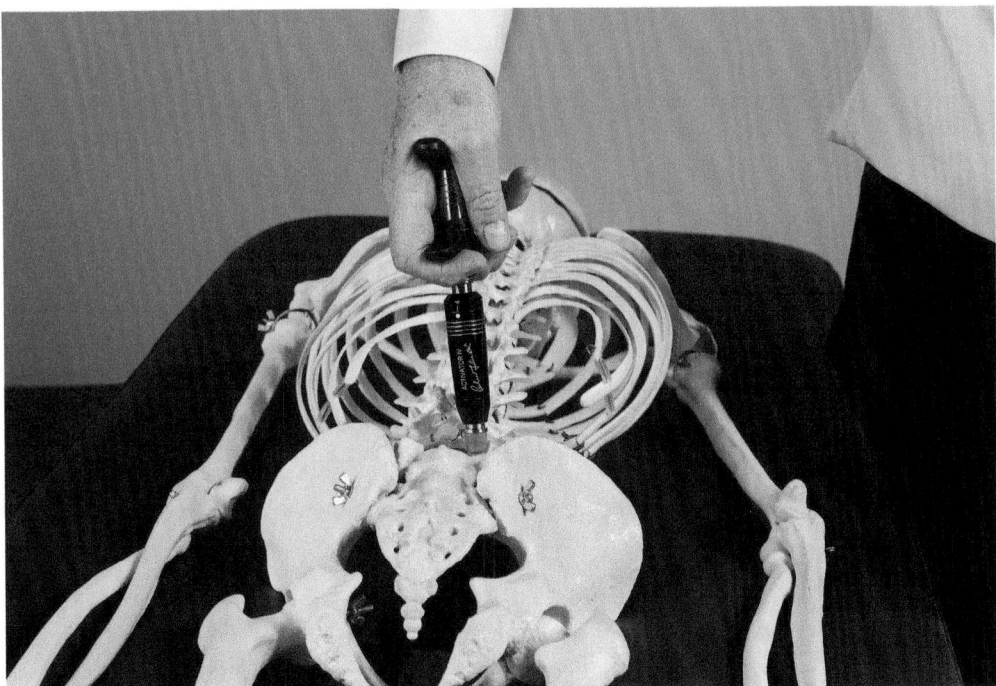

Figure 7-12   Adjustment for anterior-superior ilium. Step One: Contact base of sacrum on side Opposite Pelvic Deficiency. Line of Drive is anterior-inferior.

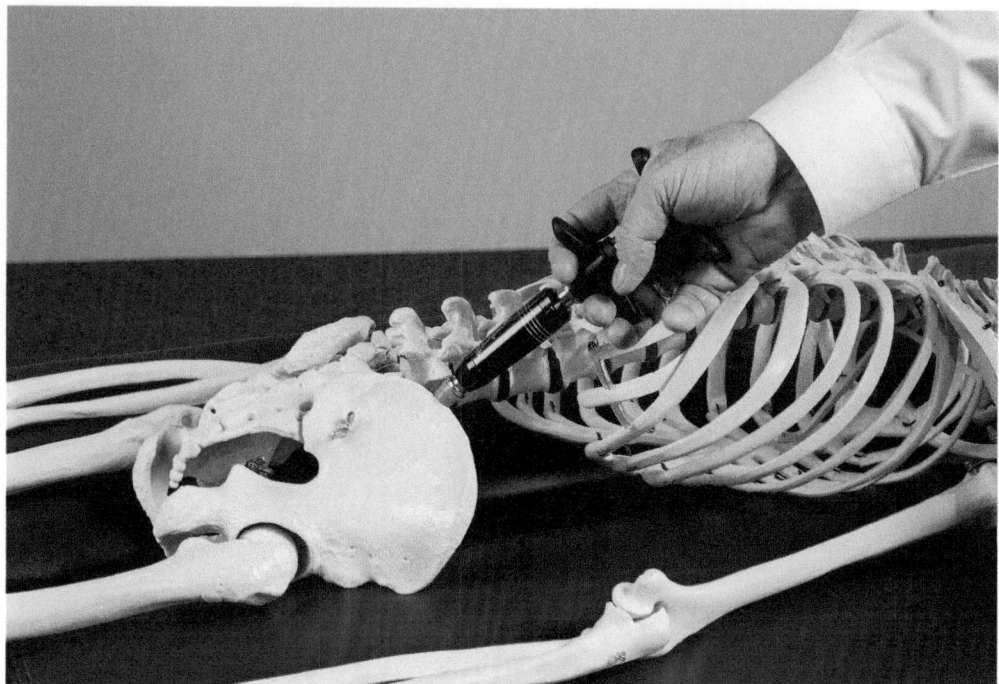

Figure 7-13 Adjustment for anterior-superior ilium. Step Two: Contact crest of ilium. Line of Drive is inferior-medial.

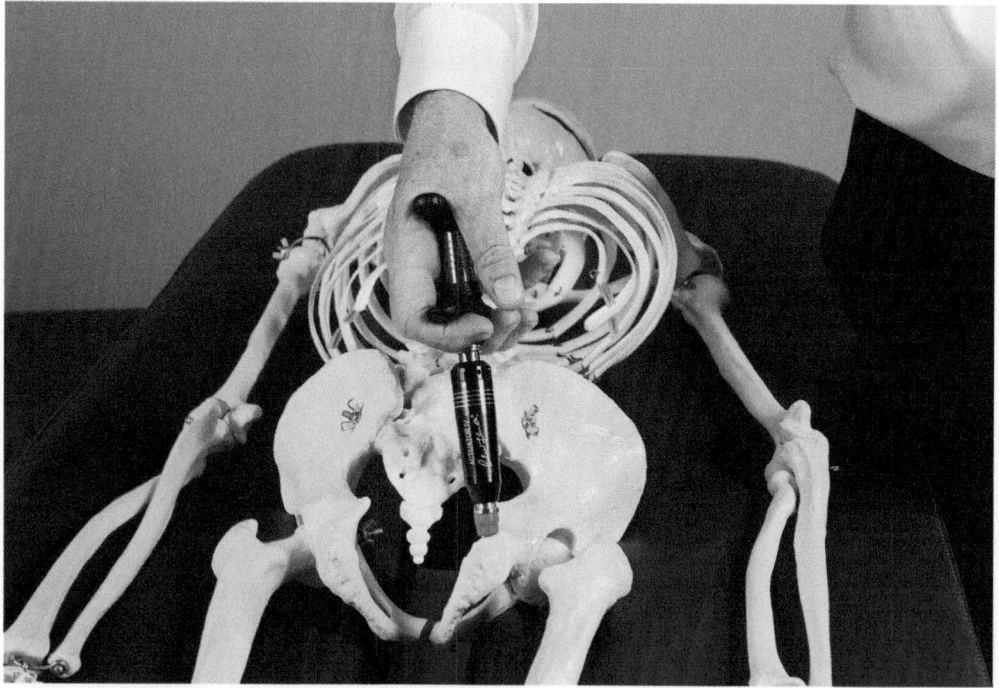

Figure 7-14 Adjustment for anterior-superior ilium. Step Three: Contact superior aspect of ischial tuberosity. Line of Drive is anterior-inferior.

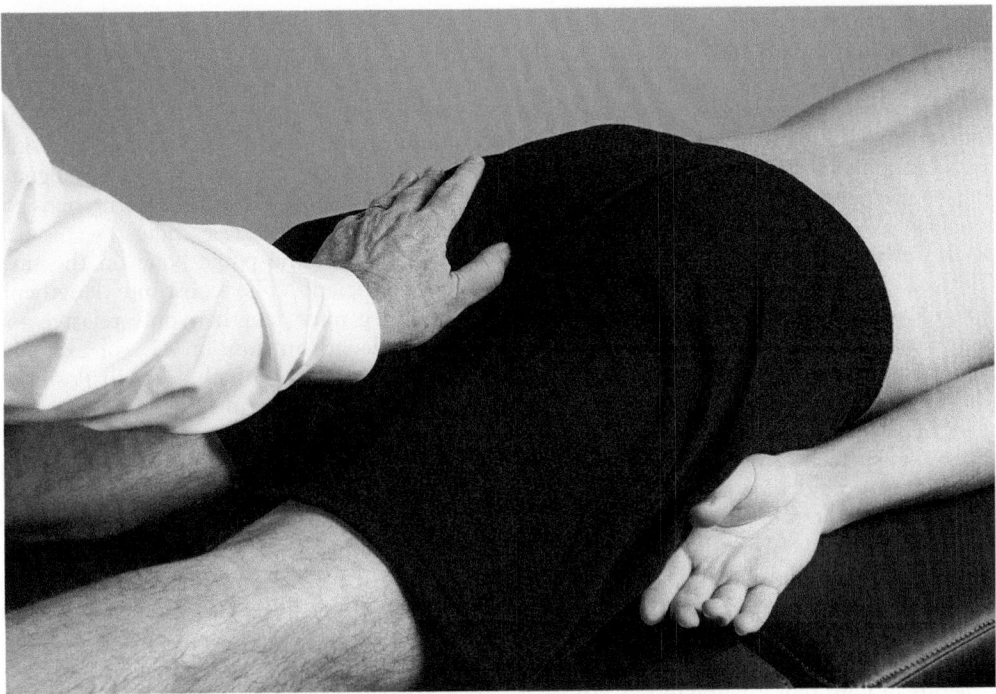

Figure 7-15 Pressure Test for posterior-inferior ilium.

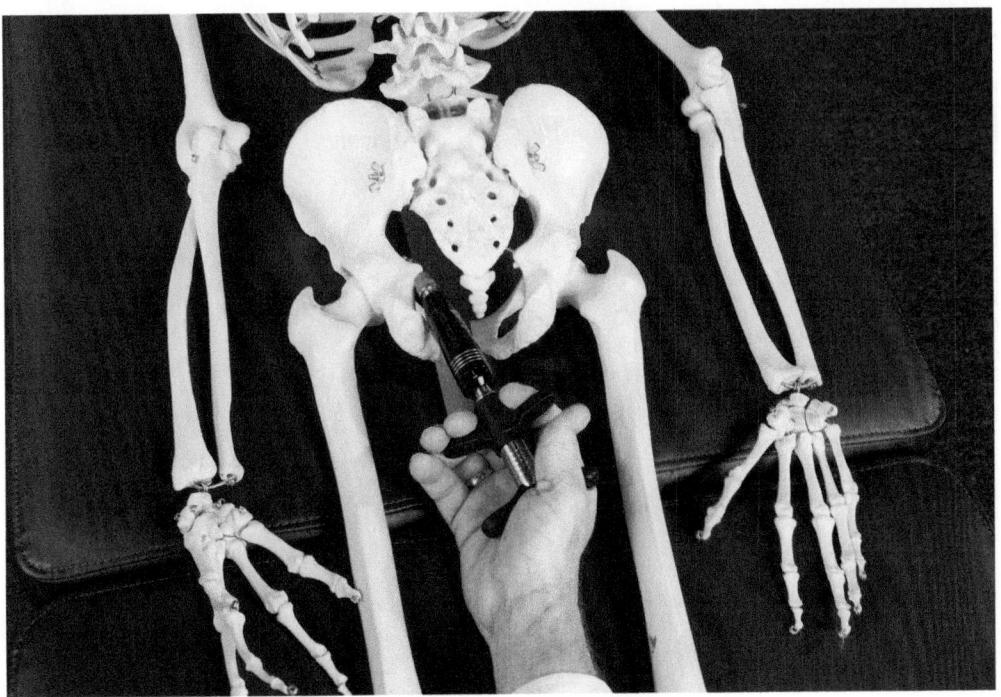

Figure 7-16 Adjustment for posterior-inferior ilium. Step One: Contact spine of ischium on side of Pelvic Deficiency. Line of Drive is posterior, superior, and lateral.

2. Next, place the tip of the instrument under the sacrotuberous ligament in the sciatic notch on the side of Pelvic Deficiency. The LOD is posterior, superior, and lateral (Figure 7-17).
3. Contact the iliac fossa just lateral to the sacroiliac joint in the soft tissue of the gluteus medius. The LOD is anterior and superior (Figure 7-18).

Symphysis Pubis. After testing and adjusting as indicated of the knees and feet and the AS and PI iliums, leg lengths typically will be balanced in Position #1 and Position #2. If in the initial Leg Length Analysis the patient presented as a Possibility Three, this is the starting point for the Basic Scan Protocol. The final pelvic test and adjustment is used for the symphysis pubis. As proposed by Hildebrant,[9] considerable torsion is possible at the symphysis pubis; this has been verified by the work of Frigerio et al.[10]

Because of previous leveling of the pelvis and leg lengths, the symphysis pubis test is an *Isolation Test*. In an Isolation Test, the patient usually performs a motion or assumes a position that affects the structure or joint that is being tested. An Isolation Test is positive when reactivity or shortening of the PD leg is noted in Position #1.

Isolation Test. To isolate the symphysis pubis, instruct the patient to squeeze the knees together (Figure 7-19). Look for reactivity or shortening of the PD leg in Position #1, and raise the legs to Position #2 to inspect for leg length changes.

Position #2 is used to determine the side of involvement and the direction of misalignment of the pubic bones. If the PD leg lengthens going to Position #2, the test indicates a superior involvement of the pubic bone on the side of Pelvic Deficiency. To constitute lengthening, the PD leg must lengthen only relative to its apparent length in Position #1. For example, if the PD leg were one inch short in Position #1 and only one-quarter inch short in Position #2, it would be relatively longer in Position #2.

If the PD leg becomes shorter in Position #2, the test indicates inferior involvement of the pubic bone on the side Opposite Pelvic Deficiency.

Adjustment for Superior Pubic Bone. First, raise the table and place the patient in the supine position. Next, inform the patient of the involvement and your intent to adjust the pubic bone. Keep in mind issues of sensitivity and sexual boundaries. It is recommended that the doctor have an assistant in the room when examining or adjusting a patient. Thoroughly explain the procedure of the adjustment to the

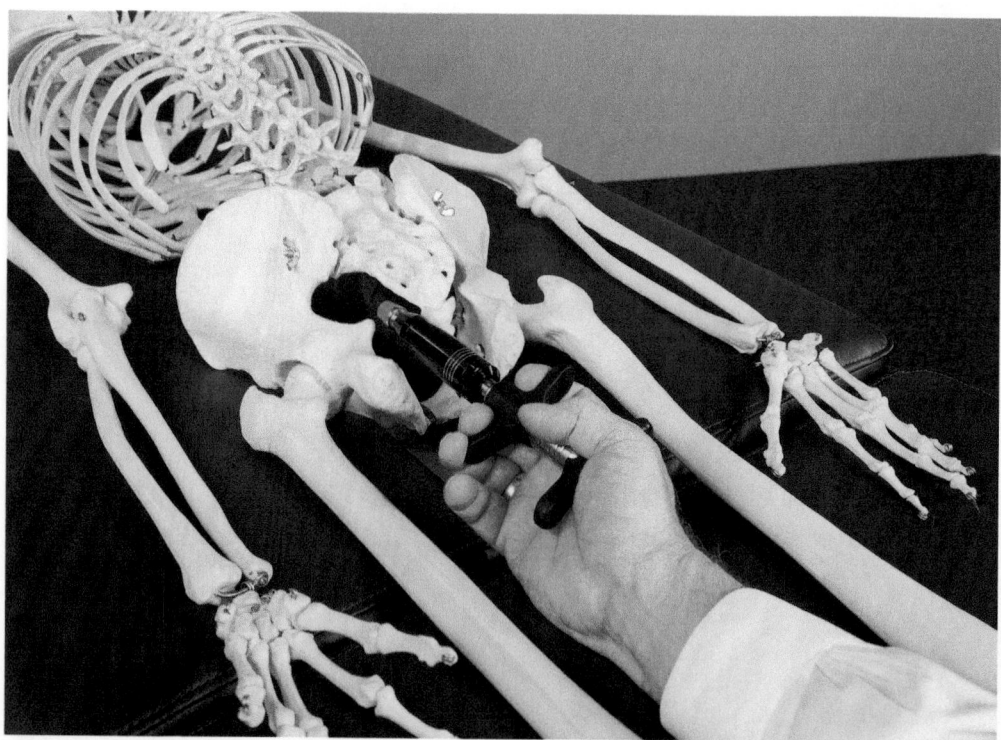

Figure 7-17 Adjustment for posterior-inferior ilium. Step Two: Contact under sacrotuberous ligament in sciatic notch on side of Pelvic Deficiency. Line of Drive is posterior, superior, and lateral.

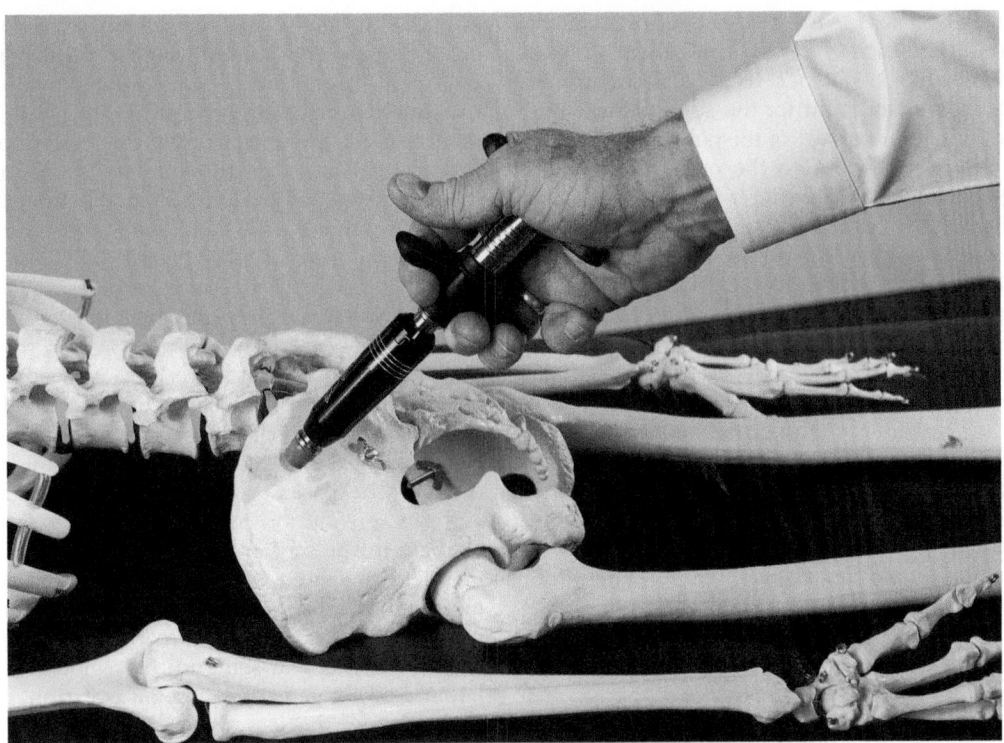

Figure 7-18   Adjustment for posterior-inferior ilium. Step Three: Contact the iliac fossa. Line of Drive is anterior-superior.

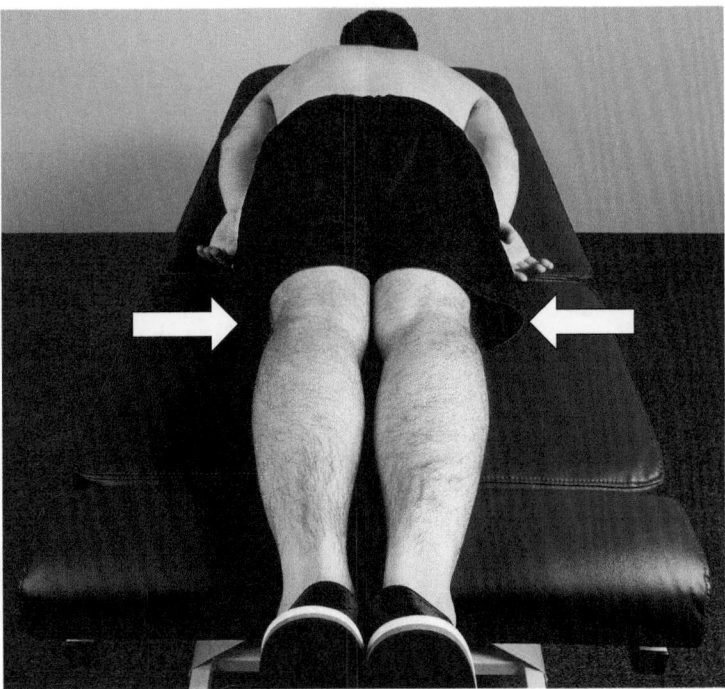

Figure 7-19   Isolation Test for symphysis pubis; patient squeezes knees together.

patient, perhaps with the use of a skeletal model. Desensitize by using the patient's hand, underneath the doctor's hand if necessary, to find the contact point for the adjustment. Contact the superior aspect of the pubic bone on the PD side just superior to the pubic tubercle. A palpable and sensitive trigger point may also be located in the belly of the rectus abdominis muscle about one inch superior to the pubic tubercle with superior involvement of the pubic bone. Depending on the build of the patient, it may be helpful to take a tissue pull by drawing the thumb of the free hand superiorly and lateral over the pubic tubercle. Use the thumb to stabilize the instrument during the adjustment. The LOD is straight inferior (Figure 7-20).

Adjustment for Inferior Pubic Bone.   First raise the table and place the patient in the supine position. Next, inform the patient of the involvement and your intent to adjust the pubic bone. On the OPD side, contact the inferior aspect of the pubic arch just lateral to the pubic symphysis. The LOD is straight superior (Figure 7-21 and Table 7-4).

Lumbar Spine

After testing and adjustment of the pelvis, with the legs balanced in Position #1 and Position #2, the AM Basic Scan Protocol calls for evaluation of the lumbar spine. In the Basic Scan Protocol,

only L5, L4, and L2 are routinely tested, and the procedure for adjusting all lumbar vertebrae is essentially the same. The contact point is the inferior articular process on the side of involvement as indicated by the Short/Long Rule as per Leg Length Analysis in Position #2. The zygapophyseal joints of lumbar vertebral motion segments have a predominantly sagittal orientation of 90 degrees.[11] The LOD for all standard lumbar corrections is anterior and superior through the plane line of the facet (Figure 7-22).

Because leg lengths have already been balanced, the tests for lumbar neuroarticular dysfunction are primarily Isolation Tests. An Isolation Test is a specific motion or maneuver used by the patient to localize an individual vertebra or motion unit, often by creating changes in the tension of a muscle or group of muscles associated with the vertebra. These movements are thought to facilitate the paraspinal muscles and the neuroarticular components of the lumbar spine in the regions of L5, L4, and L2. In general, before an Isolation Test is performed, the legs are even in Position #1 and in Position #2. When the Isolation Test for a specific vertebral motor unit is performed, if the PD leg reacts, typically shortening in Position #1, this indicates involvement of the vertebral level tested. However, not all patients will

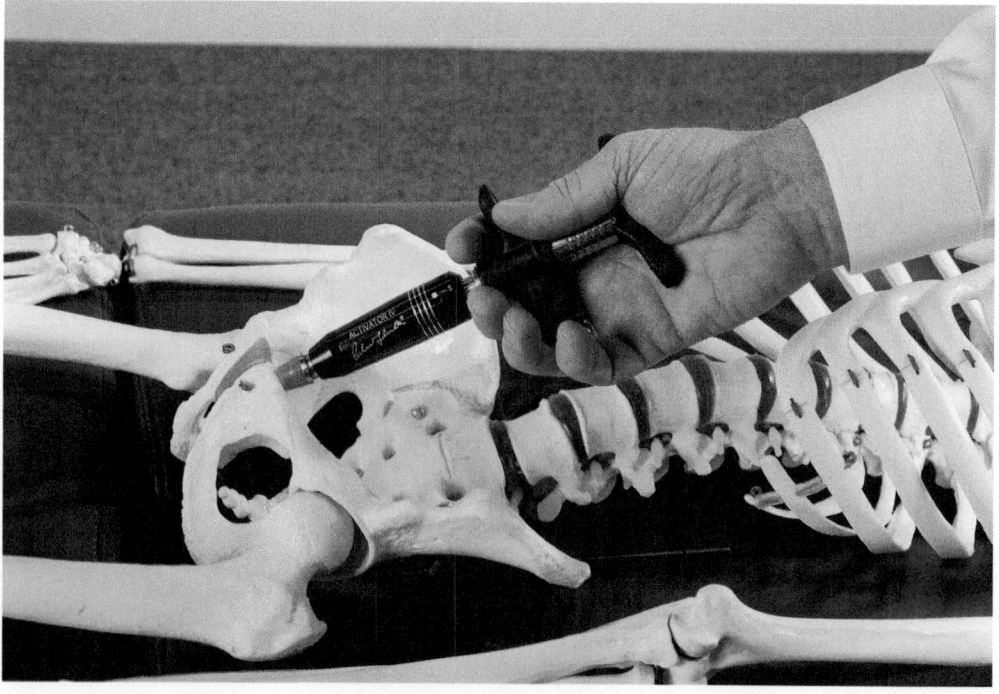

Figure 7-20   Adjustment for superior pubic bone. Line of Drive is inferior.

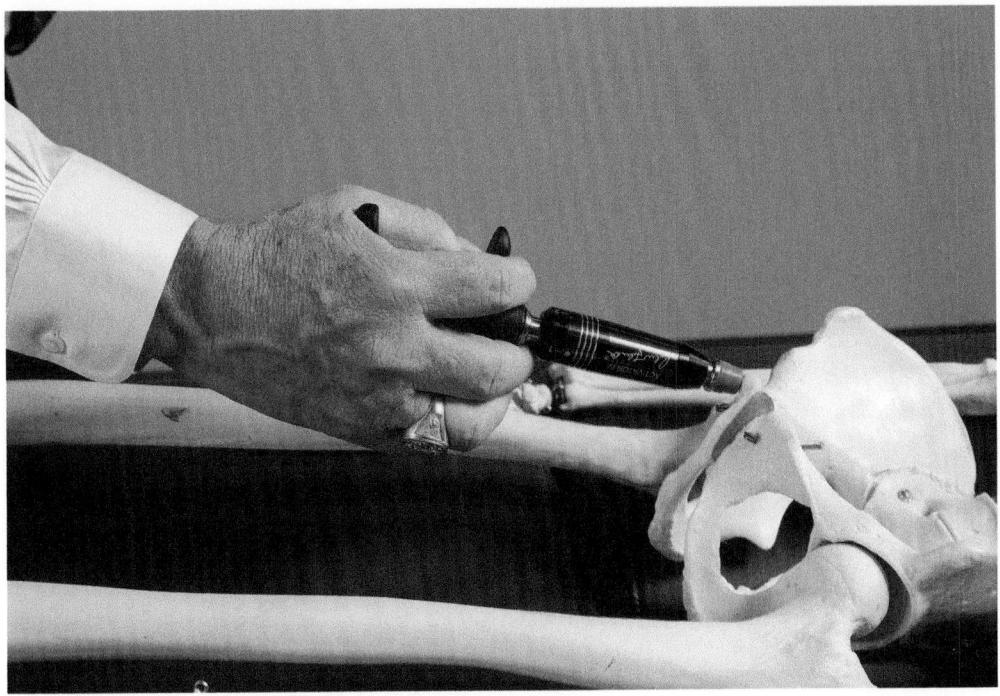

Figure 7-21   Adjustment for inferior pubic bone. Line of Drive is superior.

Table 7-4   The Activator Method Basic Scan Protocol: Pelvis

		ADJUSTMENT	
Articular Dysfunction	Test	Segmental Contact Point	Line of Drive
Anterior-Superior Ilium	Pressure Test inferior and medial at the crest of the ilium on the side OPD	*Step One*: Base of sacrum on side OPD	Anterior-inferior
		Step Two: Crest of ilium	Inferior-medial
		Step Three: Ischial tuberosity	Anterior-inferior
Posterior-Inferior Ilium	Pressure Test superior, lateral, and posterior with a firm thumb contact under the sacrotuberous ligament on the side of PD	*Step One*: Spine of ischium	Posterior, superior and lateral
		Step Two: Sacrotuberous ligament	Posterior, superior and lateral
		Step Three: Iliac fossa	Anterior-superior
Superior Pubic Bone	Instruct the patient to squeeze the knees together. PD leg lengthens in Position #2.	Superior aspect of PD pubic bone	Inferior
Inferior Pubic Bone	Instruct the patient to squeeze the knees together. PD leg shortens in Position #2.	Inferior aspect of OPD pubic bone	Superior

OPD, Opposite Pelvic Deficiency; *PD*, Pelvic Deficiency.

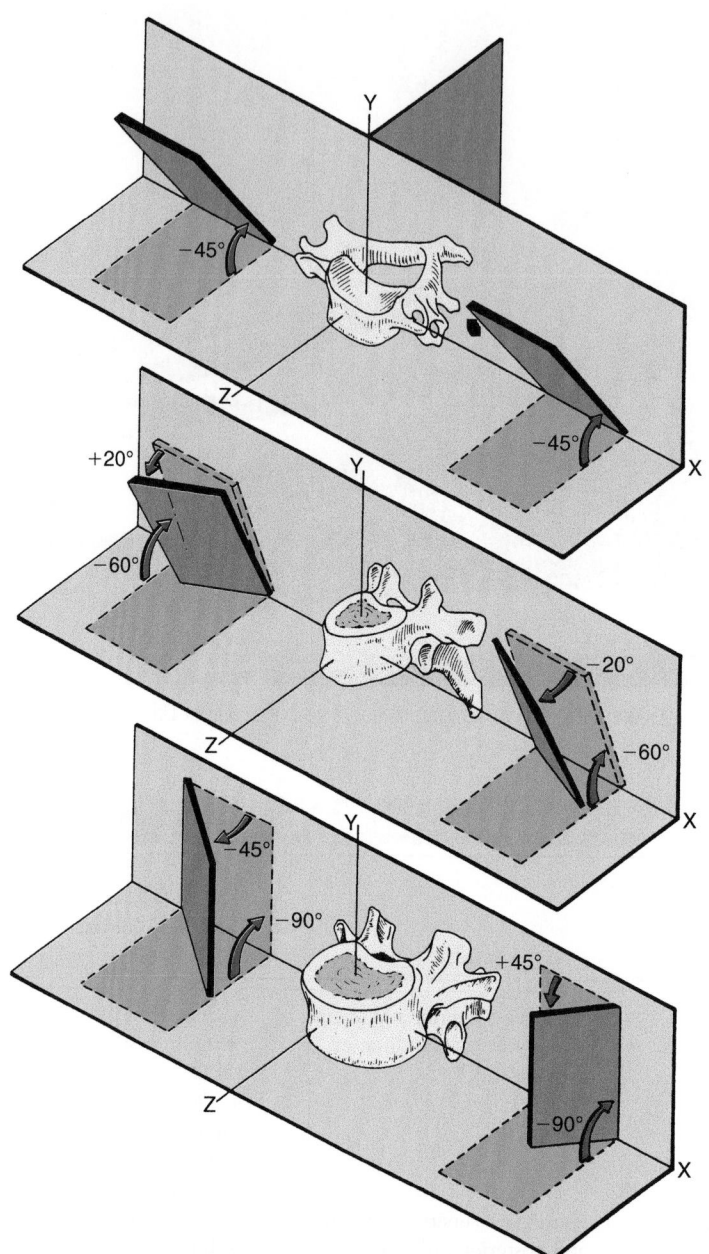

Figure 7-22 Orientation of the facet joints. (See rest of description on p. 240 of *Activator Methods Chiropractic Technique.*) (*Modified from White AA, Panjabi MM. Clinical biomechanics of the spine. Philadelphia: JB Lippincott; 1978.*)

react as strongly in Position #1 as they do in Position #2. Routinely go to Position #2 after performing an Isolation Test to confirm positive involvement or noninvolvement. Use the Short/Long Rule to determine the side of involvement.

A *Pressure Test* may be used to clarify the results of an Isolation Test. A Pressure Test, by definition, involves gentle but firm pressure on an affected joint or other structure in the direction of adjustment.

If an Isolation Test is positive, indicating neuroarticular dysfunction of a vertebral motor unit, the PD leg will shorten in Position #1. Raising the legs to Position #2 and noting the relative lengthening or shortening suggests the side of involvement. A correctly applied Pressure Test in an anterior and superior direction on the side of involvement of the vertebra will cause the legs to balance or to become even in Position #1 and Position #2. If the legs balance or significantly improve toward balancing, after performance of the Pressure Test, the AM Protocol calls for adjustment of the involved vertebral motor unit on the side as indicated by the Short/Long Rule.

Lumbar Vertebrae

Fifth Lumbar (L5). The knees, feet, and pelvis have been tested and adjusted. At this point, the leg lengths should be more even or balanced in Position #1 and Position #2. The AM Basic Scan Protocol then calls for Isolation Testing and adjusting if necessary of the fifth lumbar vertebra.

Isolation Test. To isolate the fifth lumbar, instruct the patient to place the forearm on the side of Pelvic Deficiency on the low back (Figure 7-23). The arm should rest lightly and comfortably on the low back at the lumbosacral level, palm facing upward toward the ceiling, and the dorsal aspect of the hand should lie over the fifth lumbar vertebra. Look for PD leg reactivity in Position #1. Then proceed to Position #2, observing relative changes in the PD leg. Follow the Short/Long Rule. If the PD leg lengthens in Position #2, fifth lumbar motor unit involvement is on the side of Pelvic Deficiency. If the PD leg shortens in Position #2, fifth lumbar motor unit involvement is on the side Opposite Pelvic Deficiency. Pressure Test

to confirm by applying a gentle, firm anterior and superior pressure on the inferior articular process, and observe for balancing of the legs in Position #1 and/or Position #2.

Adjustment. To adjust fifth lumbar involvement, contact the inferior articular process on the side indicated by the Short/Long Rule. The LOD is anterior and superior through the plane line of the facet (Figure 7-24).

Fourth Lumbar (L4). After testing and adjusting the fifth lumbar vertebra, proceed to isolation of the fourth lumbar vertebra.

Isolation Test. To isolate a fourth lumbar vertebra, instruct the patient to place the forearm on the side Opposite Pelvic Deficiency on the low back (Figure 7-25). The arm should rest lightly and comfortably on the low back at the lumbosacral level, palm facing upward toward the ceiling, and the dorsal aspect of the hand should lie over the fourth lumbar vertebra. Look for PD leg reactivity in Position #1. Then proceed to Position #2, observing relative changes in the PD leg. Follow the Short/Long Rule.

If the PD leg lengthens in Position #2, fourth lumbar motor unit involvement is on the side of Pelvic Deficiency. If the PD leg undergoes relative shortening in Position #2, fourth lumbar motor unit involvement is on the side Opposite Pelvic Deficiency. Pressure Test to confirm by applying a gentle, firm anterior and superior

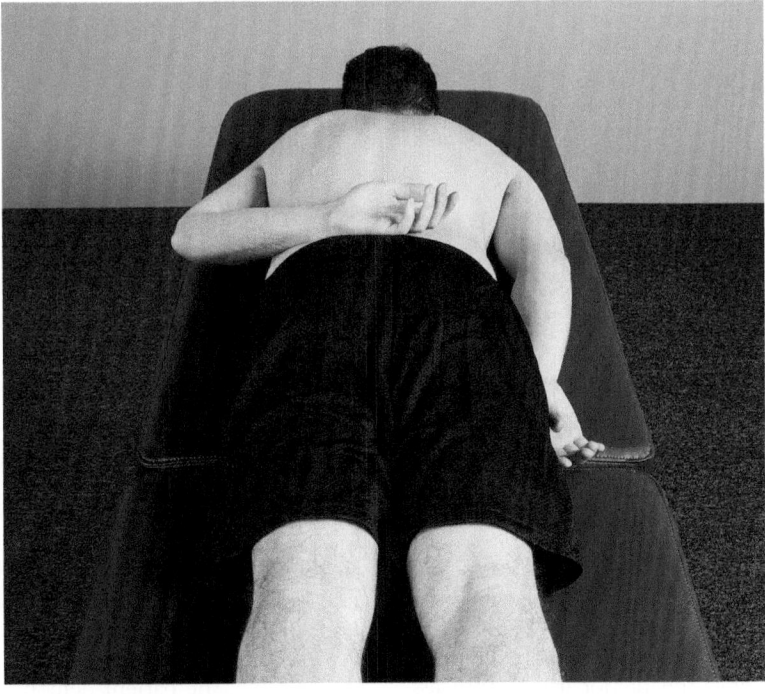

Figure 7-23 Isolation Test for fifth lumbar.

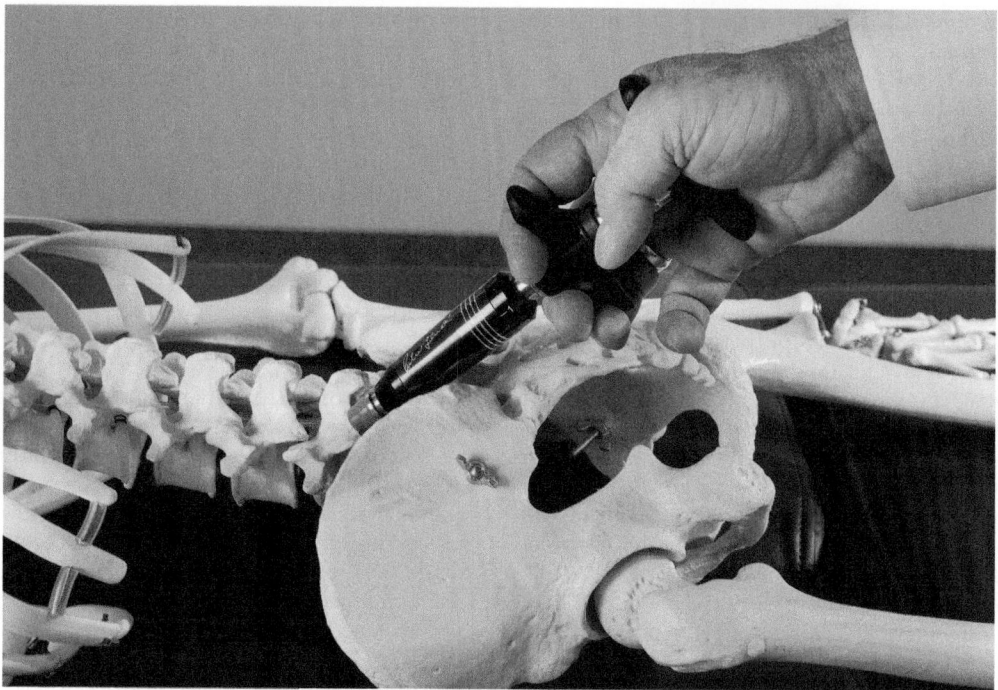

Figure 7-24   Adjustment for fifth lumbar. Line of Drive is anterior-superior.

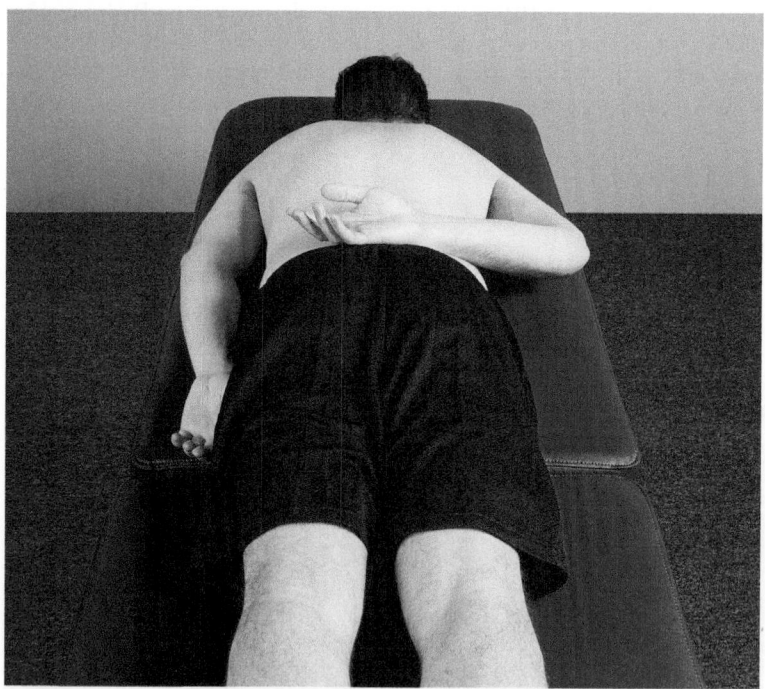

Figure 7-25   Isolation Test for fourth lumbar.

pressure on the inferior articular process, and observe for balancing of the legs in Position #1 and/or Position #2.

Adjustment.   To adjust fourth lumbar involvement, contact the inferior articular process

on the side indicated by the Short/Long Rule. The LOD is anterior and superior through the plane line of the facet (Figure 7-26).

Note: If, after initial placement of the patient on the table, the patient demonstrates a PD leg

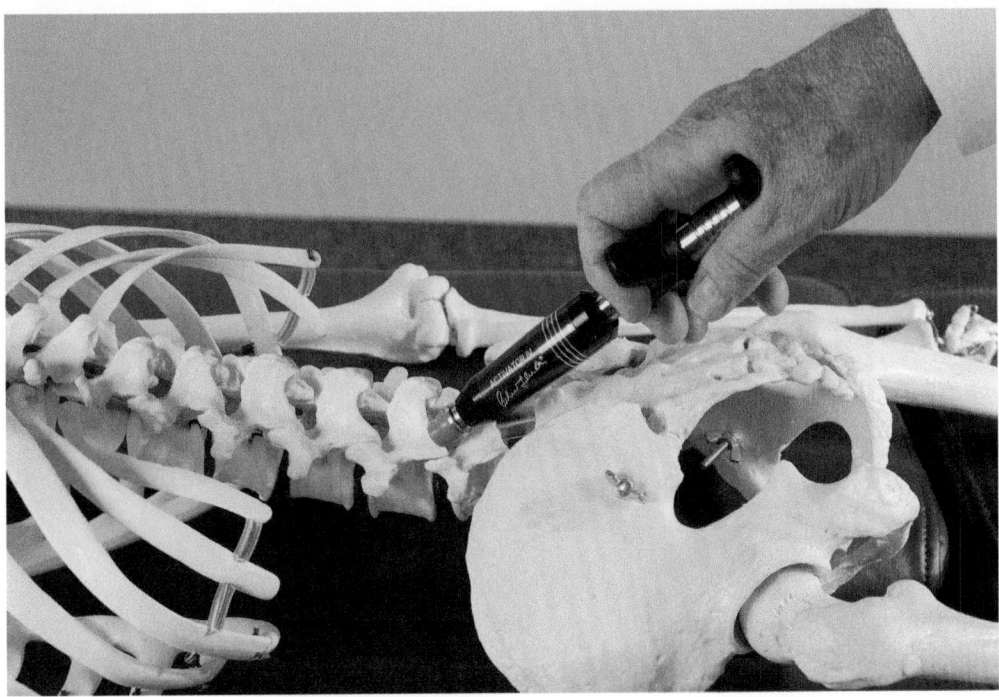

Figure 7-26   Adjustment for fourth lumbar. Line of Drive is anterior-superior.

that shortens in Position #2, Possibility Two, the Basic Scan Protocol calls for testing and adjustment of the fourth lumbar first. This procedure bypasses the knees, feet, and pelvis and proceeds directly to the fourth lumbar. From the fourth lumbar vertebra onward, all procedures for remaining vertebrae are the same.

Second Lumbar (L2).   After testing and adjusting the fourth lumbar vertebra, proceed to isolation of the second lumbar vertebra.

Isolation Test.   To isolate a second lumbar vertebra, instruct the patient to place the forearms of both arms on the low back (Figure 7-27). The arms should rest lightly and comfortably on the low back at the lumbosacral level, palms facing upward toward the ceiling. Look for PD leg reactivity in Position #1. Then proceed to Position #2, observing relative changes in the PD leg. Follow the Short/Long Rule. If the PD leg undergoes relative lengthening in Position #2, second lumbar motor unit involvement is on the side of Pelvic Deficiency. If the PD leg shortens in Position #2, second lumbar motor unit involvement is on the side Opposite Pelvic Deficiency. Pressure Test to confirm by applying a gentle, firm anterior and superior pressure on the inferior articular process, and observe for balancing of the legs in Position #1 and/or Position #2.

Adjustment.   To adjust for second lumbar involvement, contact the inferior articular process

on the side indicated by the Short/Long Rule. The LOD is anterior and superior through the plane line of the facet (Figure 7-28 and Table 7-5).

Thoracic Vertebrae and Ribs

After testing and adjustment of the lumbar spine, the AM Basic Scan Protocol calls for evaluation of T12 and T8 in the lower thoracic spine; T6, T4, and T1 in the upper thoracic spine; and the first ribs. In addition to the vertebral segments, the corresponding rib of each segment is adjusted from T10 through T2.

The procedure for adjustment of all thoracic vertebrae is essentially the same. The contact point is the transverse process on the side of involvement as indicated by the Short/Long Rule or Leg Length Analysis in Position #2. The zygapophyseal joints of thoracic vertebral motion segments have an anterior, superior (60 degrees), and slightly medial orientation (20 degrees) (see Figure 7-22).[11] The LOD for all standard thoracic corrections therefore is anterior, superior, and slightly medial through the joint plane line of the facet.

The tests for thoracic neuroarticular dysfunction are mainly Isolation Tests. In an Isolation Test, a specific motion or maneuver by the patient is used to localize an individual vertebra or motion unit by creating articular changes and increasing tension in a muscle or group of

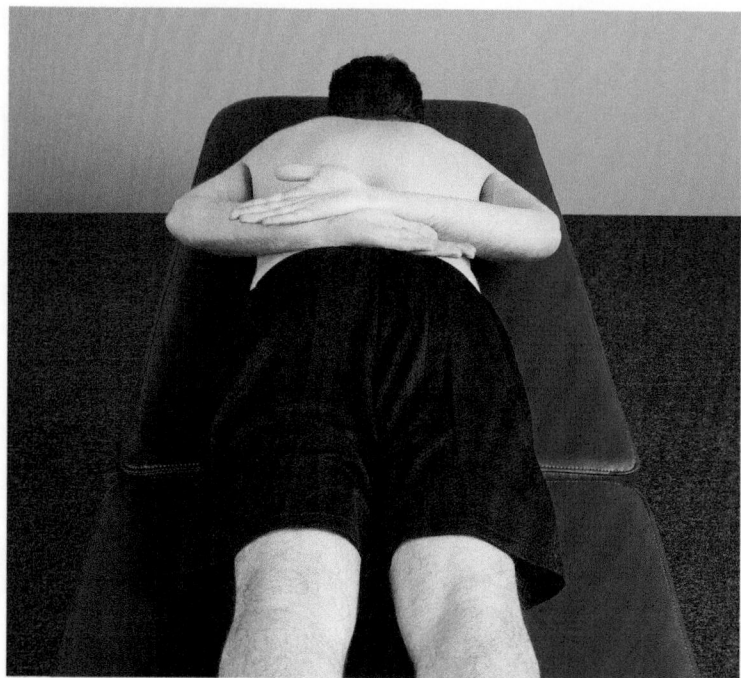

Figure 7-27   Isolation Test for second lumbar.

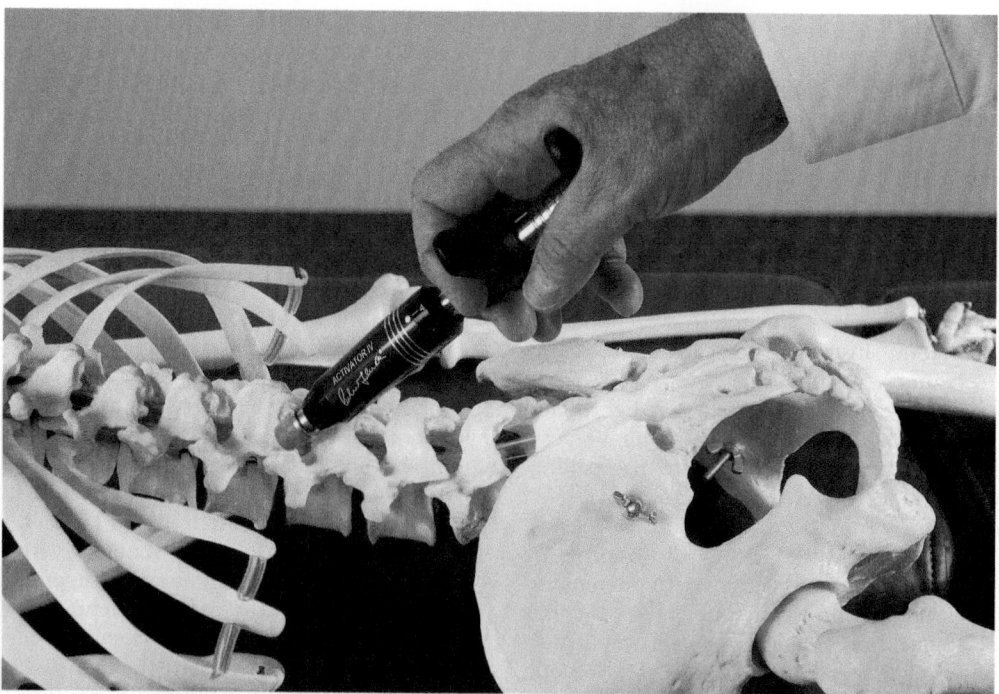

Figure 7-28   Adjustment for second lumbar. Line of Drive is anterior-superior.

muscles associated with the vertebra. These motions are thought to facilitate paraspinal muscle and neuroarticular components of the region of the thoracic spine that is being tested. In general, before an Isolation Test is performed, the

legs are even in Position #1 and Position #2. If, when the Isolation Test or maneuver for a specific vertebral motor unit is performed, the PD leg exhibits reactivity in Position #1 and/or Position #2, this indicates involvement of the

Table 7-5 The Activator Method Basic Scan Protocol: Lumbar Spine

Articular Dysfunction	Test	ADJUSTMENT	
		Segmental Contact Point	Line of Drive
Fifth Lumbar (L5)	Instruct patient to place forearm on side of Pelvic Deficiency on low back with palm up	Inferior articular process on side indicated by Short/Long Rule	Anterior-superior
Fourth Lumbar (L4)	Instruct patient to place forearm on side Opposite Pelvic Deficiency on low back with palm up	Inferior articular process on side indicated by Short/Long Rule	Anterior-superior
Second Lumbar (L2)	Instruct patient to place both forearms on low back with palms up	Inferior articular process on side indicated by Short/Long Rule	Anterior-superior

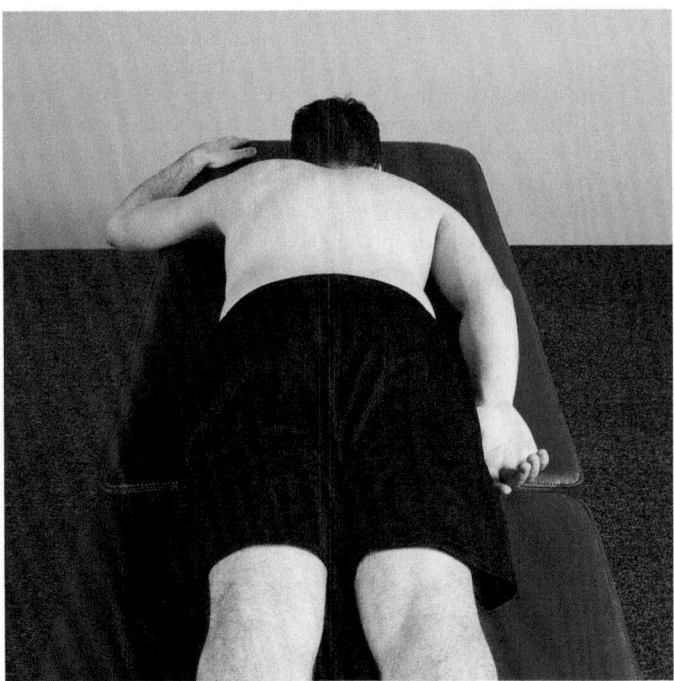

Figure 7-29 Isolation Test for twelfth thoracic.

vertebral level tested. Use the Short/Long Rule in Position #2 to determine the side of involvement.

Lower Thoracic Vertebrae and Ribs

Twelfth Thoracic (T12). After testing and adjusting of all lumbar vertebrae, proceed to assessment of the lower thoracic spine, beginning with the twelfth thoracic vertebra. Before testing

of T12, the legs should be even or close to even in Position #1 and Position #2.

Isolation Test. To isolate the twelfth thoracic vertebra, instruct the patient to abduct the shoulder on the side of Pelvic Deficiency and to rest that forearm on the table superior and lateral to the head (Figure 7-29). Look for PD leg reactivity in Position #1. Then proceed to Position #2, observing relative changes in the PD leg. Follow the Short/Long Rule. If the PD leg undergoes relative lengthening in Position #2, adjustment is performed on the side of Pelvic Deficiency. If the PD leg shortens in Position #2, adjustment is performed on the side Opposite Pelvic Deficiency. Pressure Test to confirm by applying a gentle, firm anterior and superior pressure on the transverse process of the involved side, and observe for balancing of the legs in Position #1 and/or Position #2.

Adjustment. To adjust twelfth thoracic vertebral involvement, contact the transverse process on the side indicated by the Short/Long Rule. The LOD is anterior, superior, and slightly medial through the 60 degree plane line of the facet (Figure 7-30). Note that in the example shown in Figure 7-30, the adjustment is being performed on the right transverse process of the twelfth thoracic vertebra. In keeping with the Short/Long Rule, this indicated that a relative shortening occurred in Position #2.

Twelfth Rib Involvement

Isolation Test. To test the twelfth rib, repeat the T12 Isolation Test by instructing the patient to raise the arm on the side of Pelvic Deficiency and rest the forearm on the table superior and lateral to the head. (Refer to Figure 7-29.) Next ask the patient to inhale deeply and hold briefly. This is thought to stress the costovertebral junction. Look for reactivity of the PD leg in Position #1, and ask the patient to exhale and breathe normally at this time.

Raise the legs to Position #2 and use the Short/Long Rule to determine the side of involvement. If the PD leg lengthens in Position #2, the test suggests twelfth rib involvement on the side of Pelvic Deficiency. If the PD leg shortens in Position #2, the test suggests twelfth rib involvement on the side Opposite Pelvic Deficiency. Pressure Test to confirm rib involvement by applying a firm but gentle thumb pressure on the body of the rib, directing the pressure laterally and inferiorly along the longitudinal axis of the rib. Observe for balancing of the legs in Position #1 and/or Position #2.

Adjustment. To adjust twelfth rib involvement, contact the body of the rib about one-half inch lateral to the transverse process on the side of rib involvement. The LOD is lateral and inferior along the longitudinal axis of the rib (Figure 7-31).

Although the tenth through second ribs are routinely adjusted whenever the corresponding vertebral segment is adjusted, the eleventh and twelfth ribs are tested on the basis of patient complaints. The twelfth and eleventh ribs, possibly because they are floating ribs, may be symptomatic independent of the eleventh and

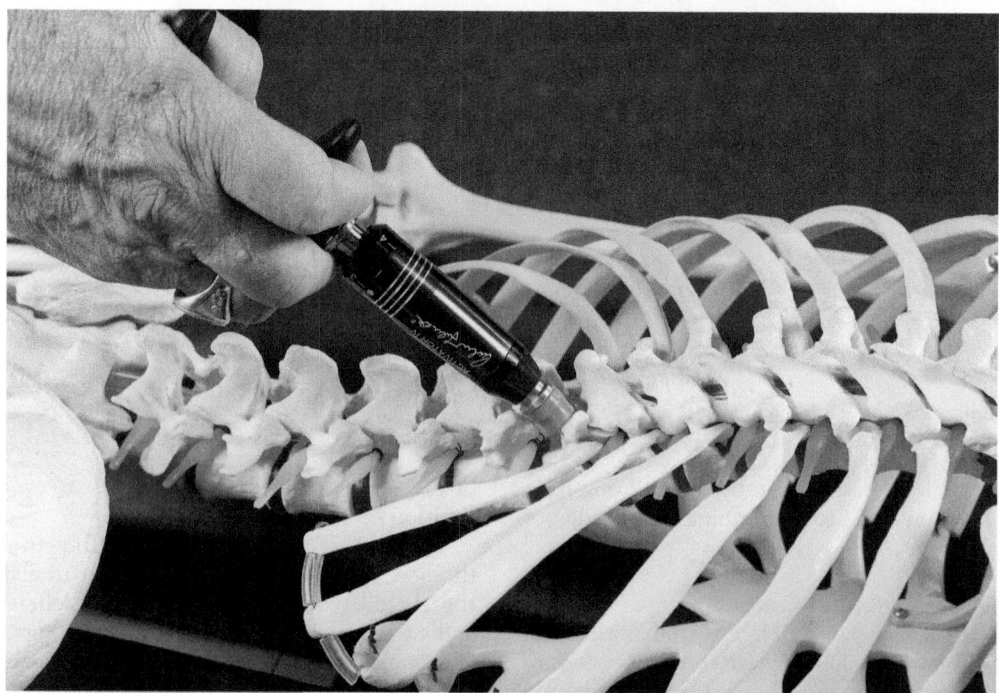

Figure 7-30 Adjustment for twelfth thoracic. Line of Drive is anterior-superior and slightly medial.

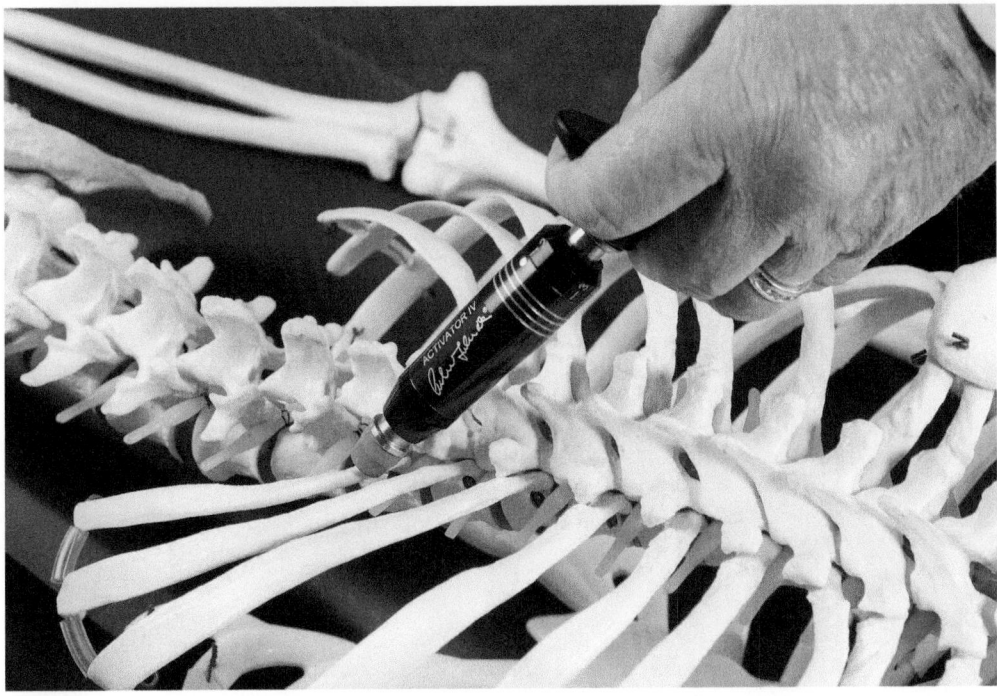

Figure 7-31   Adjustment for twelfth rib. Line of Drive is lateral and inferior along the longitudinal axis of the rib.

twelfth thoracic vertebral motion segments. When a patient experiences costovertebral pain that radiates out over the flank, consider involvement of the eleventh or twelfth rib.

Eighth Thoracic (T8).   The only other segment in the lower thoracic spine region tested in the Basic Scan Protocol is the eighth thoracic vertebra. After testing and adjustment as indicated of T12, and before proceeding to T8, the legs should be even or close to even in Position #1 and Position #2.

Isolation Test.   To isolate the eighth thoracic vertebra, instruct the patient to abduct both arms at the shoulders, and to rest the forearms on the table superior and lateral to the head (Figure 7-32). Look for PD leg reactivity in Position #1. Then proceed to Position #2, observing relative changes in the PD leg. Follow the Short/Long Rule. If the PD leg undergoes relative lengthening in Position #2, the adjustment is performed on the side of Pelvic Deficiency. If the PD leg shortens in Position #2, the adjustment is performed on the side Opposite Pelvic Deficiency. Pressure Test to confirm by applying a gentle, firm anterior and superior pressure on the transverse process of the involved side, and observe for balancing of the legs in Position #1 and/or Position #2.

Adjustment.   To adjust eighth thoracic vertebral involvement, contact the transverse

process on the side indicated by the Short/Long Rule. The LOD is anterior, superior, and slightly medial through the plane line of the facet (Figure 7-33).

Eighth Rib Involvement.   After adjustment of the eighth thoracic vertebra, adjust the eighth rib on the side opposite the vertebral adjustment.

Adjustment.   To adjust an eighth rib involvement, contact the body of the rib about one-half inch lateral to the transverse process on the side of rib involvement (Figure 7-34). The LOD is lateral and inferior along the longitudinal axis of the rib.

To ensure an effective adjustment and to minimize discomfort for the patient, use the thumb of the free hand to take a lateral and inferior tissue pull over the contact point on the rib. Use the thumb to stabilize the tip of the instrument on the body of the rib during the adjustment.

Upper Thoracic Vertebrae and Ribs
Sixth Thoracic (T6).   After testing and adjustment of the eighth thoracic vertebra and corresponding rib, ask the patient to bring the arms back down to the sides, and proceed to the Isolation Test for the sixth thoracic vertebra.

Isolation Test.   To isolate the sixth thoracic vertebra, instruct the patient to turn the

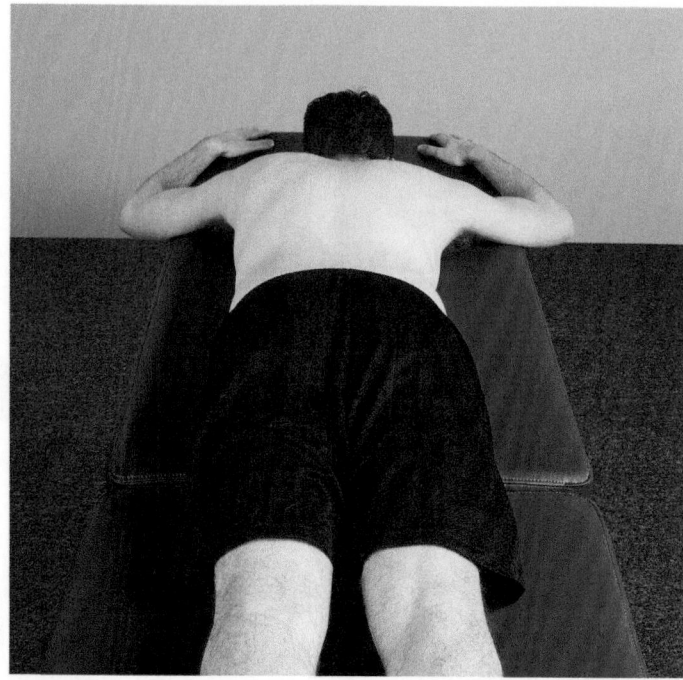

Figure 7-32 Isolation Test for eighth thoracic.

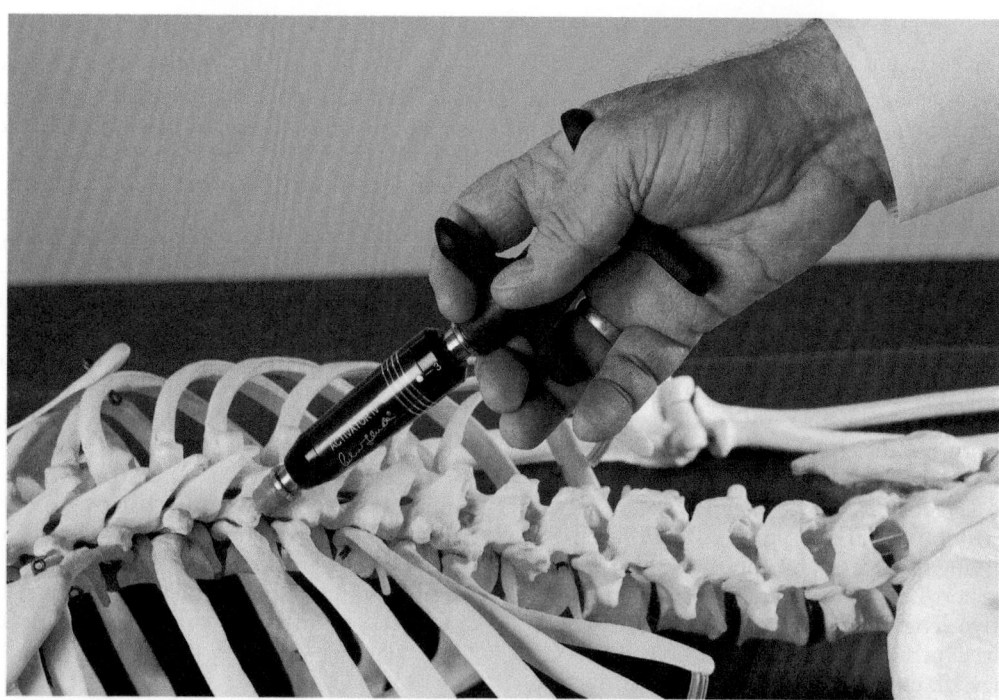

Figure 7-33 Adjustment for eighth thoracic. Line of Drive is anterior-superior and slightly medial.

face to the side of Pelvic Deficiency and rest the head on the table (Figure 7-35). Look for PD leg reactivity in Position #1. Then proceed to Position #2, observing relative changes in the PD leg. Follow the Short/Long Rule. If the PD leg undergoes relative lengthening in Position #2, adjustment is performed on the side of Pelvic Deficiency. If the PD leg shortens in Position #2, adjustment is performed on the side Opposite Pelvic Deficiency. Pressure Test to confirm

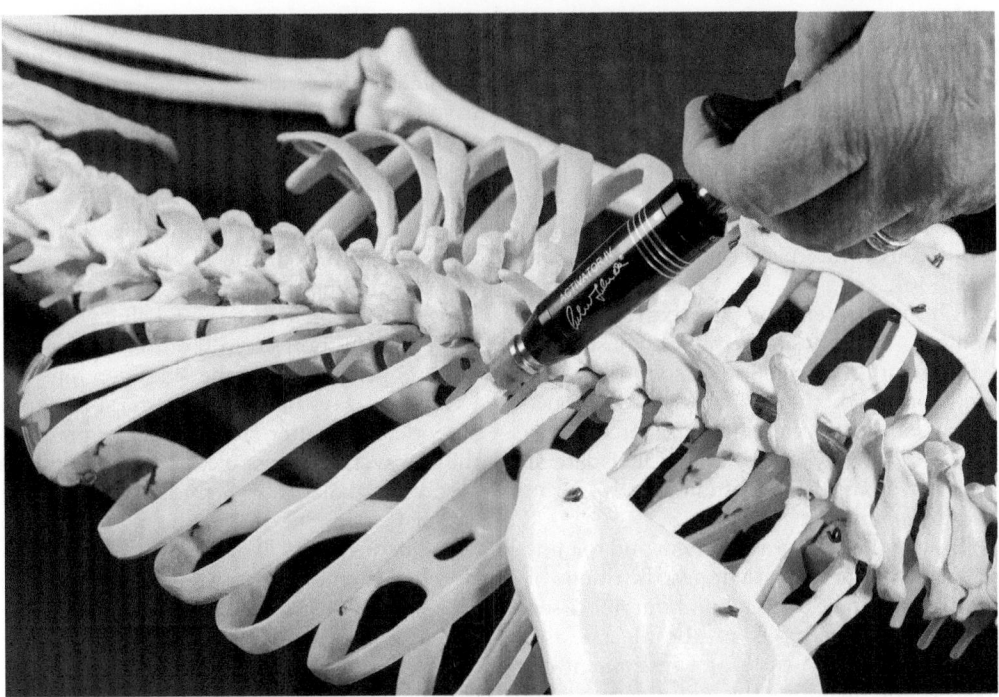

Figure 7-34 Adjustment for eighth rib. Line of Drive is lateral and inferior along the longitudinal axis of the rib.

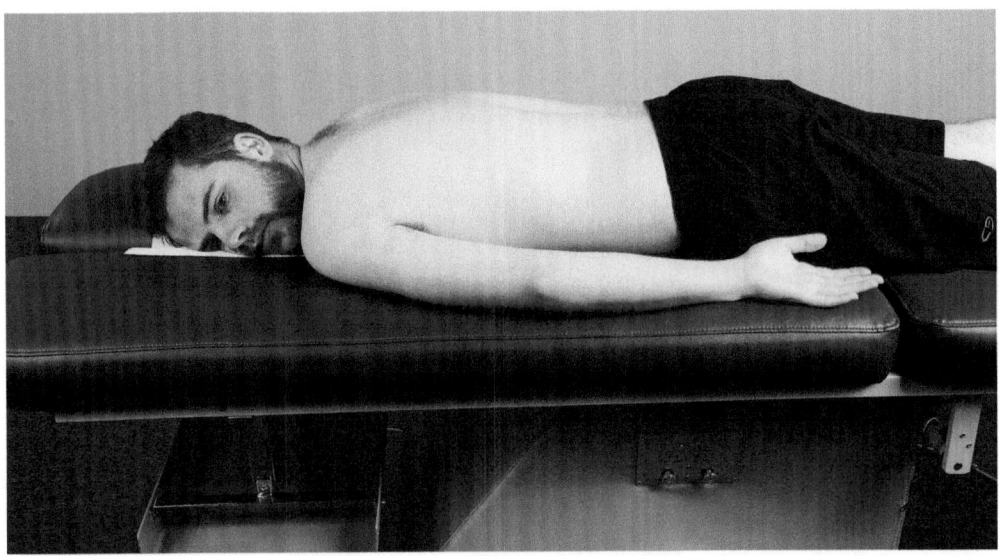

Figure 7-35 Isolation Test for sixth thoracic.

by applying a gentle, firm anterior and superior pressure on the transverse process of the involved side, and observe for balancing of the legs in Position #1 and/or Position #2.

Adjustment.   To adjust sixth thoracic vertebral involvement, contact the transverse process on the side indicated by the Short/Long Rule. The LOD is anterior, superior, and slightly medial through the plane line of the facet (Figure 7-36).

Sixth Rib Involvement.   The sixth rib is adjusted on the side opposite vertebral adjustment.

Adjustment.   To adjust for sixth rib involvement, contact the body of the rib about one-half inch lateral to the transverse process on the side of rib involvement. The LOD is lateral and inferior along the longitudinal axis of the rib (Figure 7-37).

To ensure an effective adjustment and to minimize discomfort for the patient, use the thumb of the free hand to take a lateral and inferior tissue pull over the contact point on the rib. Use the thumb to stabilize the tip of the instrument on the body of the rib during the adjustment.

Fourth Thoracic (T4).   After testing and adjustment of the sixth thoracic vertebra and corresponding rib, ask the patient to keep the arms at the sides with the head turned to the PD side. Proceed to the Isolation Test for the fourth thoracic vertebra.

Isolation Test.   To isolate the fourth thoracic vertebra, instruct the patient to lift the shoulder on the side of Pelvic Deficiency away from the table in a posterior movement (toward the ceiling) and then to put it back down (Figure 7-38). Look for PD leg reactivity in Position #1. Then proceed to Position #2, observing relative changes in the PD leg. Follow the Short/Long Rule. If the PD leg undergoes relative lengthening in Position #2, the adjustment is performed on the side of Pelvic Deficiency. If the PD leg shortens in Position #2, the adjustment is performed on the side Opposite Pelvic Deficiency. Pressure Test to confirm by applying a gentle, firm anterior and superior pressure on the transverse process of the involved side, and observe for balancing of the legs in Position #1 and/or Position #2.

Adjustment.   To adjust fourth thoracic vertebral involvement, contact the transverse process on the side indicated by the Short/Long Rule. The LOD is anterior, superior, and slightly medial through the plane line of the facet (Figure 7-39).

Fourth Rib Involvement.   The fourth rib is adjusted on the side opposite vertebral adjustment.

Adjustment.   To adjust for fourth rib involvement, contact the body of the rib about one-half inch lateral to the transverse process on the side of rib involvement. The LOD

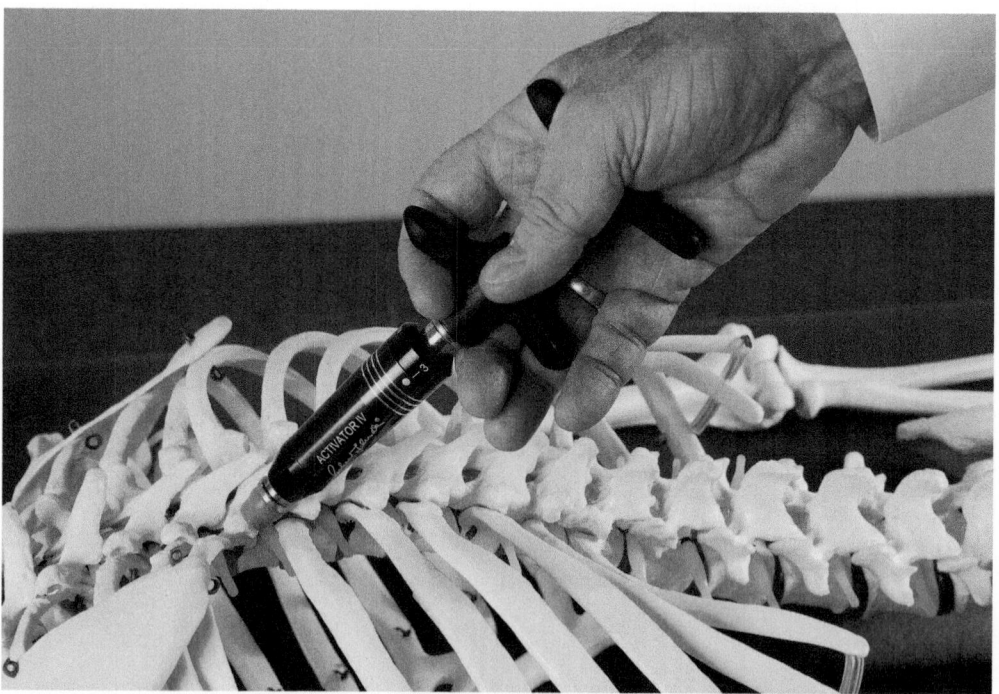

Figure 7-36   Adjustment for sixth thoracic. Line of Drive is anterior-superior and slightly medial.

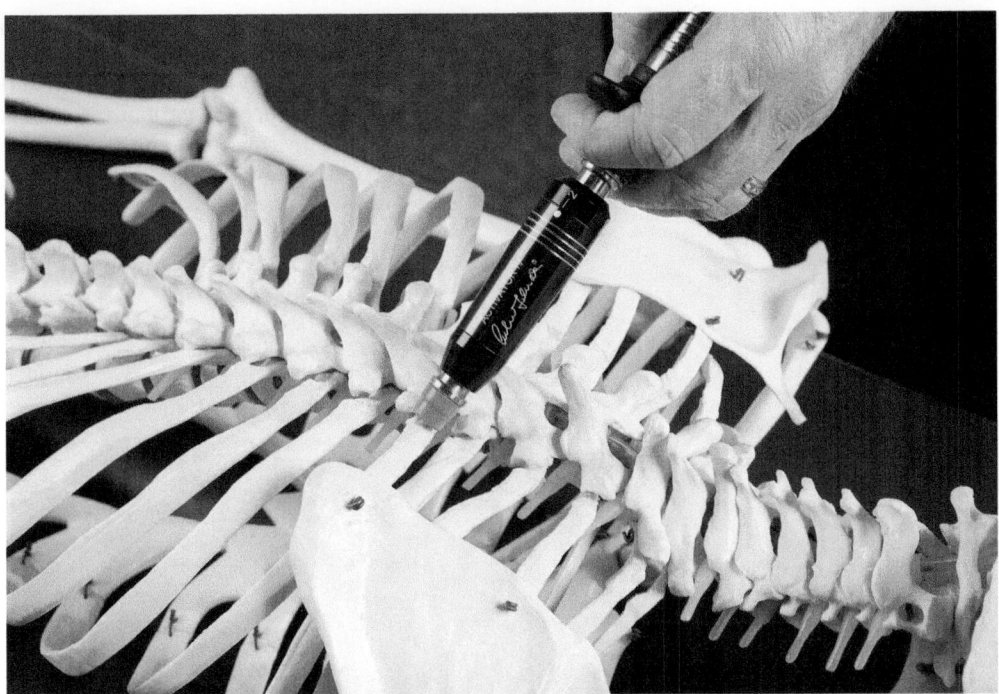

Figure 7-37   Adjustment for sixth rib. Line of Drive is lateral and inferior along the longitudinal axis of the rib.

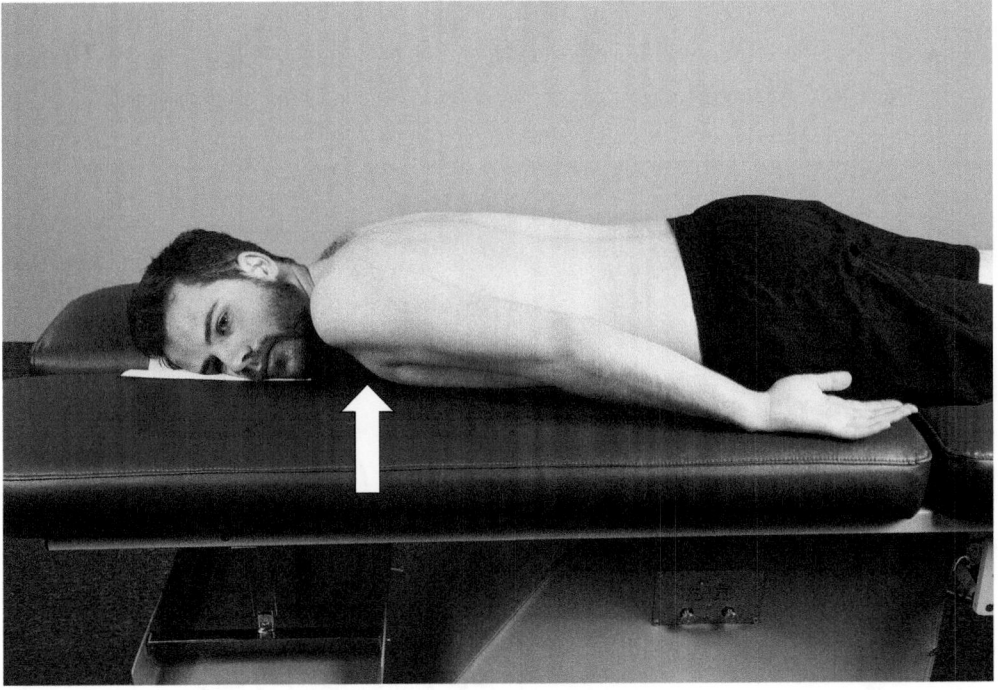

Figure 7-38   Isolation Test for fourth thoracic.

is lateral and inferior along the longitudinal axis of the rib (Figure 7-40).

To ensure effective adjustment and to minimize discomfort for the patient, use the thumb of the free hand to take a lateral and inferior tissue pull over the contact point on the rib. Use the thumb to stabilize the tip of the instrument on the body of the rib during the adjustment.

First Thoracic (T1). After testing and adjustment as indicated of the fourth thoracic vertebra and corresponding rib, ask the patient to keep the arms at the sides with the head turned to the PD side. Proceed to an Isolation Test for the first thoracic vertebra.

Isolation Test. To isolate the first thoracic vertebra, instruct the patient to shrug both

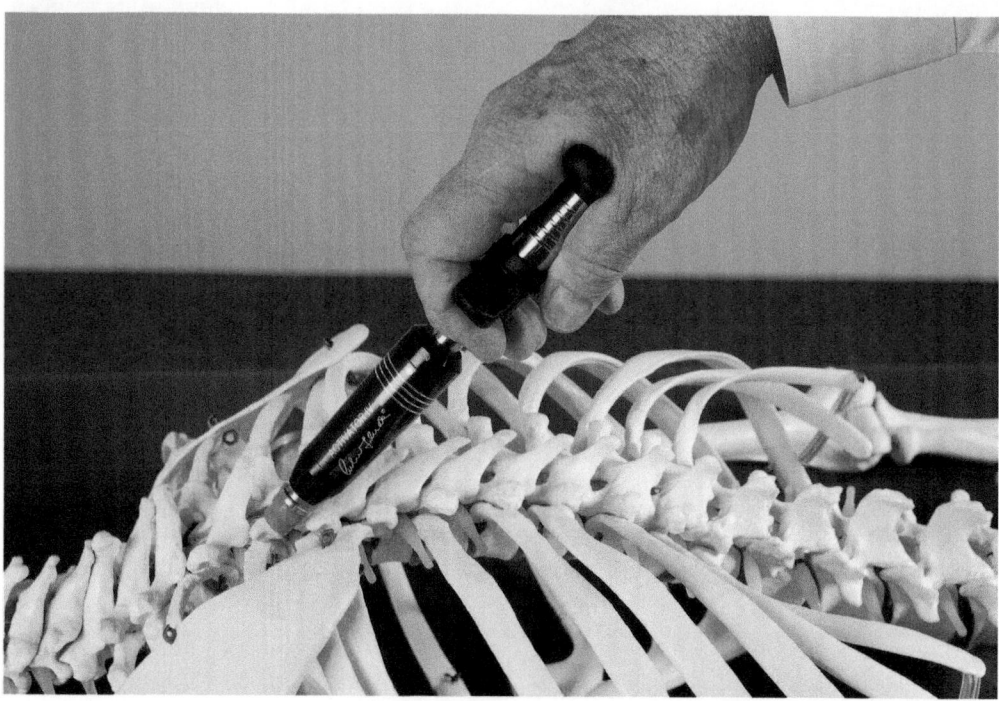

Figure 7-39 Adjustment for fourth thoracic. Line of Drive is anterior-superior and slightly medial.

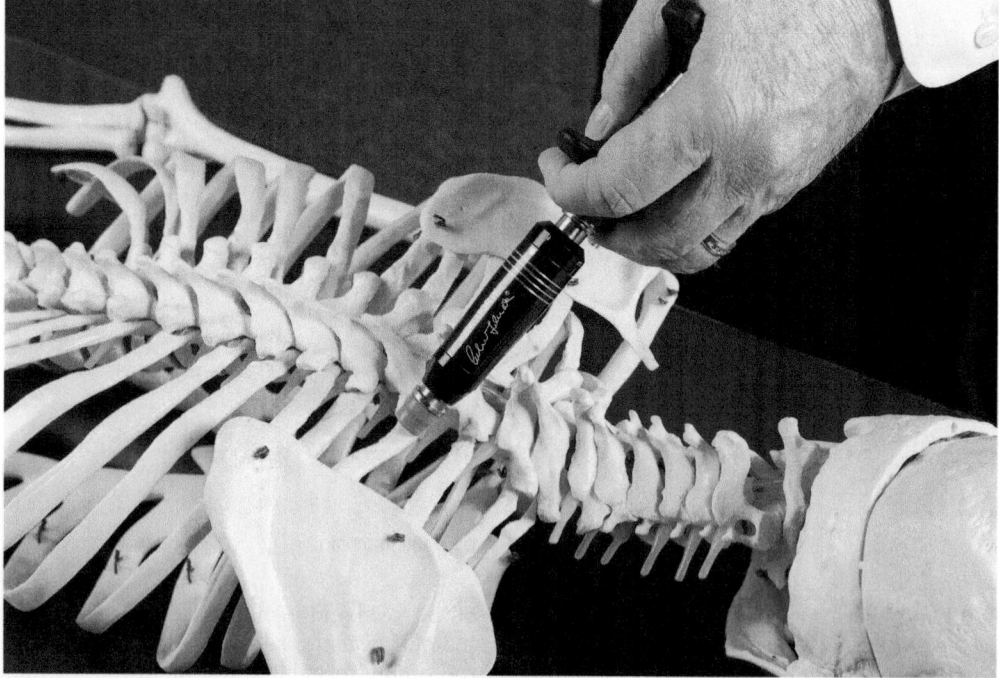

Figure 7-40 Adjustment for fourth thoracic rib. Line of Drive is lateral and inferior along the longitudinal axis of the rib.

shoulders toward the ears and then relax (Figure 7-41). Look for PD leg reactivity in Position #1. Then proceed to Position #2, observing relative changes in the PD leg. Follow the Short/Long Rule. If the PD leg relatively lengthens in Position #2, first thoracic vertebral involvement is on the side of Pelvic Deficiency. If the PD leg relatively shortens in Position #2, first thoracic involvement is on the side Opposite Pelvic Deficiency. Pressure Test to confirm by applying a gentle, firm anterior and superior pressure on the transverse process of the involved side, and observe for balancing of the legs in Position #1 and/or Position #2.

Adjustment. To adjust first thoracic vertebral involvement, contact the transverse process on the side indicated by the Short/Long Rule. The LOD is anterior and slightly medial through the plane line of the facet (Figure 7-42).

To ensure an effective contact and LOD, ask the patient to turn the face back to a neutral, face-down position during adjustment of the first thoracic vertebra. Depending on the build of the patient, it may be advisable to draw back the superior portion of the upper trapezius muscle on the side of involvement to facilitate a good contact with the transverse of T1. After T1 has been adjusted, be sure to instruct the patient

to turn the face back to the side of Pelvic Deficiency before proceeding to isolating the first ribs and the scapular pattern.

First Rib Involvement. After completion of the adjustment of the first thoracic vertebra as indicated, test for an elevation involvement of the first rib.

Isolation Test. To test the first rib after adjusting a first thoracic vertebra, ask the patient to keep the face turned to the side of Pelvic Deficiency. Next, instruct the patient to roll both shoulders superiorly, posteriorly, and inferiorly in a circular motion, and then to relax (Figure 7-43). This motion is similar to Eden's costoclavicular test for neurovascular entrapment in thoracic outlet syndrome and is meant to stress the first ribs.[12] As the patient relaxes after performing the test, look for PD leg reactivity in Position #1. Then proceed to Position #2, while observing relative changes in the PD leg. Follow the Short/Long Rule. If the PD leg relatively lengthens in Position #2, the test suggests first rib involvement on the side of Pelvic Deficiency. If the PD leg relatively shortens in Position #2, the test suggests first rib involvement on the side Opposite Pelvic Deficiency. Pressure Test to confirm rib involvement by applying a firm but gentle thumb pressure on the body of the rib, directing the pressure inferiorly.

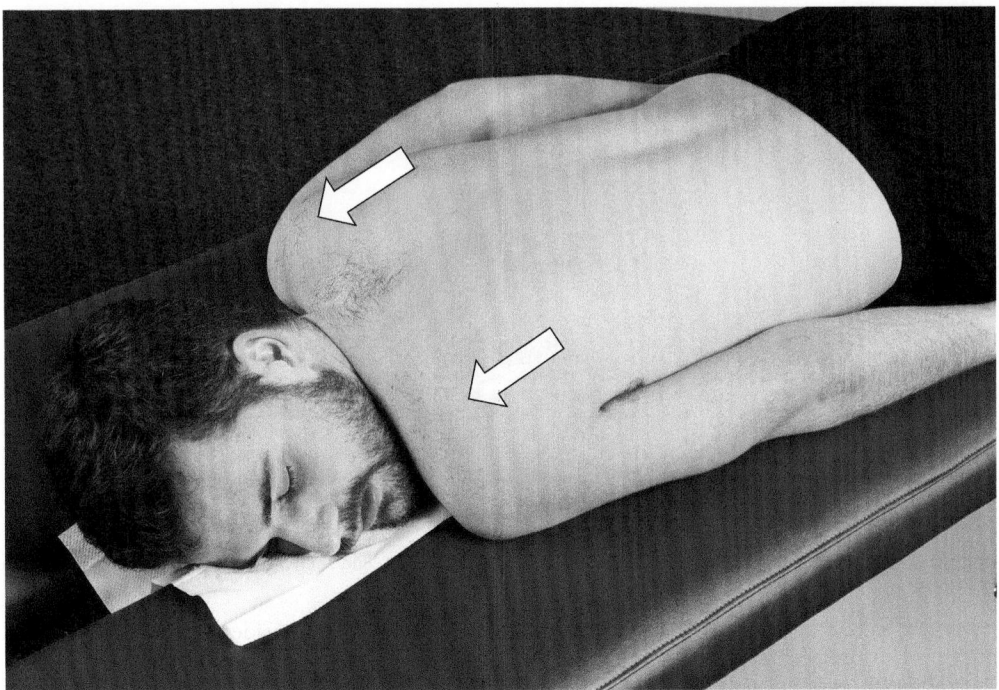

Figure 7-41   Isolation Test for first thoracic.

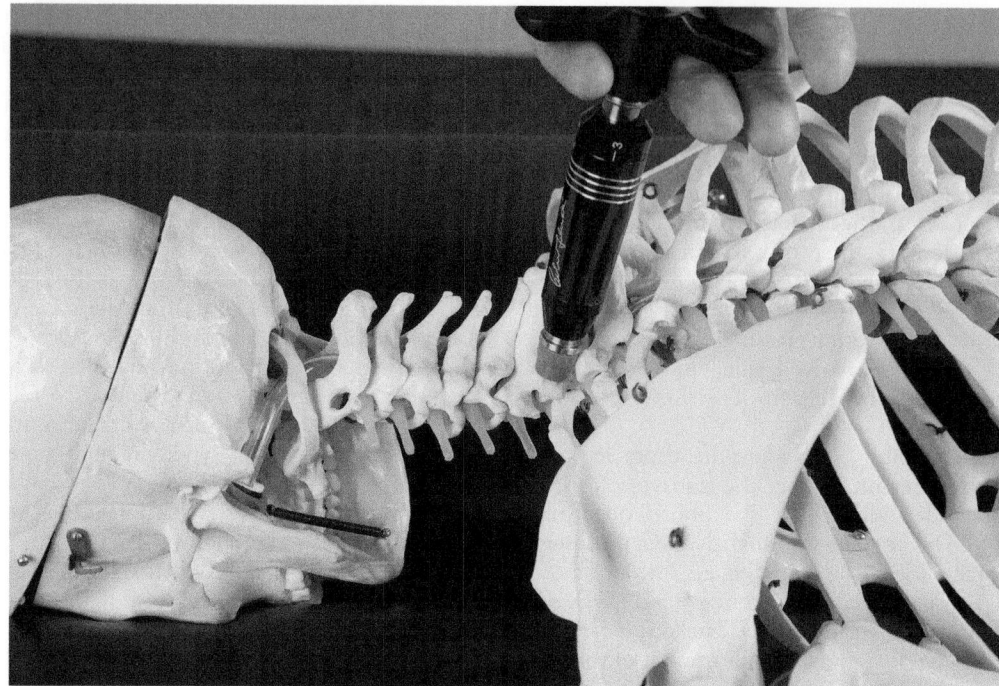

Figure 7-42   Adjustment for first thoracic. Line of Drive is anterior and slightly medial.

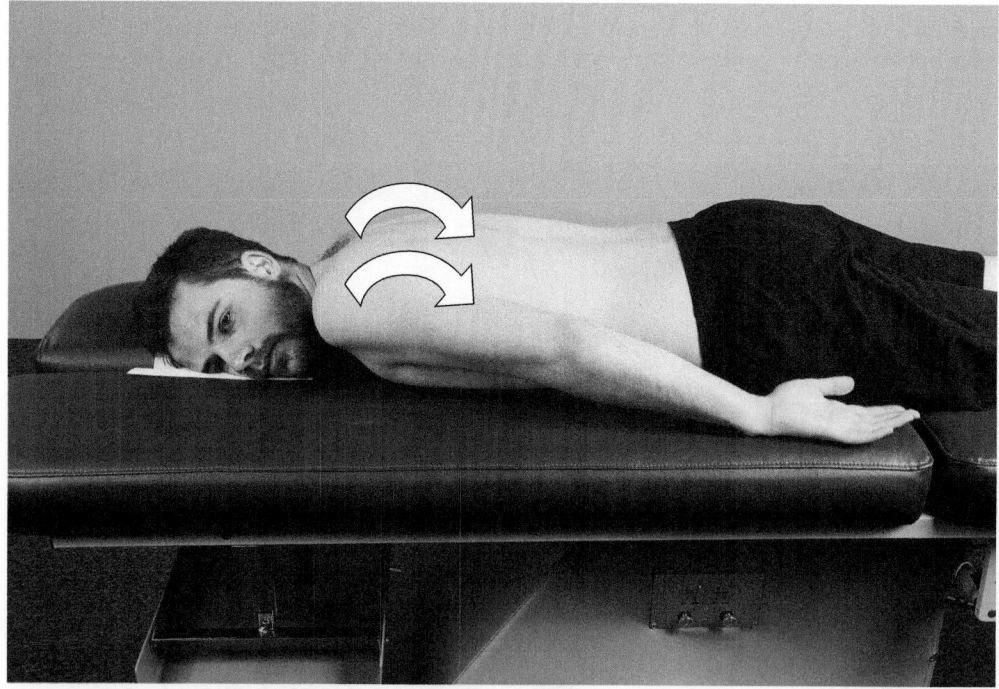

Figure 7-43   Isolation Test for first rib: Roll both shoulders superiorly, posterior, and inferiorly in a circular motion, and then relax.

Observe for balancing of the legs in Position #1 and/or Position #2.

Occasionally, patients will experience bilateral first rib involvement. If the leg lengths are not even or are considerably improved after Isolation Testing and adjustment of the first rib on one side, Pressure Test the first rib on the other side. Apply a firm but gentle thumb pressure on

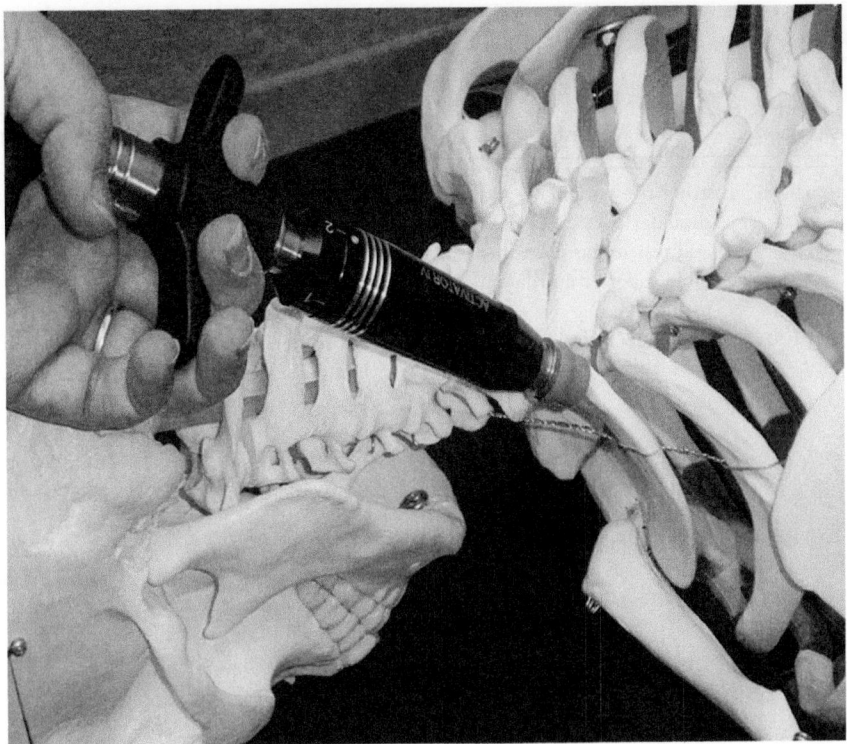

Figure 7-44   Adjustment for first rib. Line of Drive is inferior.

the body of the rib. Direct the pressure inferiorly. If the leg lengths become even in Position
#1 and Position #2, the Pressure Test indicates
facilitation of the first rib on the other side.

Adjustment.   To adjust a superior first
rib, contact the body of the rib about one-half
inch lateral to the transverse process on the
side of rib involvement. The LOD is inferior
(Figure 7-44). In some patients, the angle of
the first rib may be even closer to horizontal
and the LOD; therefore would be anterior and
inferior.

Have the patient turn the head to the neutral, face-down position while you are adjusting
the first rib. To ensure an effective adjustment
and to minimize discomfort for the patient, use
the thumb of the free hand to take a posterior
and inferior tissue pull over the contact point
on the rib. It may be advisable to draw back
the superior portion of the upper trapezius to
facilitate good contact with the body of the
rib. Use the thumb to stabilize the tip of the
instrument on the body of the rib during the
adjustment.

Be sure to have the patient turn the head
back to the side of Pelvic Deficiency before
you proceed to the scapular pattern assessment
(Table 7-6).

Clinical Observations

When a patient tests positive for first rib involvement, be alert for any indications of neurovascular
compression and thoracic outlet syndrome.
Patient complaints of numbness or tingling in
the hands or fingers, altered pulses in the upper
extremity, atrophic changes to the hand or arm,
or coldness of the extremities may indicate neurological and/or vascular compromise.

Perform the Wright hyperabduction test,
Eden's costoclavicular test, and Adson's test for
radial pulse compromise when thoracic outlet
syndrome is suspected. Also perform the Activator Method Stress Tests and adjustments as indicated for shoulder and clavicle involvement (see
Chapter 16).

Scapulae

The Basic Scan Protocol requires assessment of
two common scapular involvements as part of
the routine thoracic spine screening. Inclusion
of the scapular pattern as part of the thoracic
spine evaluation takes into consideration the
anatomical and functional relationship between
the shoulder and the spine. The scapulothoracic
articulation plays a significant role in shoulder

Table 7-6   The Activator Method Basic Scan Protocol: Thoracic Spine and Ribs

Articular Dysfunction	Test	ADJUSTMENT	
		Segmental Contact Point	Line of Drive
Twelfth Thoracic (T12)	Instruct the patient to abduct shoulder on side of PD and rest forearm on the table superior and lateral to the head	Transverse process according to the Short/Long Rule	Anterior-superior, slightly medial
Twelfth (T12) Rib Involvement	Repeat T12 Isolation Test and have patient inhale	Body of rib one-half inch lateral to transverse process on side of rib involvement	Lateral and inferior along the longitudinal axis of the rib
Eighth Thoracic (T8)	Instruct the patient to abduct both arms at the shoulders and rest the forearms on the table superior and lateral to the head	*Step One:* Contact the transverse process according to the Short/Long Rule	Anterior-superior, slightly medial
		Step Two: Body of corresponding rib	Lateral-inferior along the longitudinal axis of the rib
Sixth Thoracic (T6)	Instruct the patient to turn face toward side of PD and rest head on table	*Step One:* Contact the transverse process according to the Short/Long Rule	Anterior-superior, slightly medial
		Step Two: Body of corresponding rib	Lateral-inferior along the longitudinal axis of the rib
Fourth Thoracic (T4)	Instruct the patient to keep face to PD side and lift shoulder on side of PD in a posterior motion	*Step One:* Contact the transverse process according to the Short/Long Rule	Anterior-superior, slightly medial
		Step Two: Body of corresponding rib	Lateral-inferior along the longitudinal axis of the rib
First Thoracic (T1)	Instruct the patient to keep face to PD side and shrug both shoulders headward, then relax	Transverse process according to the Short/Long Rule	Anterior-medial
First (T1) Rib Involvement	Instruct the patient to keep the face turned toward side of PD and roll both shoulders superiorly, posteriorly, and inferiorly in circular motion. Follow Short/Long Rule for side. Repeat for bilateral involvement.	Posterior trapezius tissue pull: body of rib	Inferior

PD, Pelvic Deficiency.

movement, and impairment of its motion or anatomical malposition is likely to affect the thoracic spine. As part of the Basic Scan Protocol, perform Isolation Tests and adjustments for the following scapular patterns:

• Medial/Lateral scapula on the side of Pelvic Deficiency

• Medial/Lateral scapula on the side Opposite Pelvic Deficiency

The recommended procedure for the AM is to confine testing and adjustment to the above scapular involvements for the first two or three patient encounters before proceeding to the advanced shoulder tests discussed in Chapter 16.

Shoulder Involvement—Medial and Lateral Scapulae.
Because of associated variations in the shoulder girdle that occur in response to postural alterations of the thoracic spine, such as a postural "high" shoulder, neuroarticular dysfunction of the shoulder merits further discussion. After testing and adjusting the first thoracic vertebra and/or first rib, perform Isolation Tests and adjustments as indicated for the scapulae. Before testing the scapulae, however, make sure that the patient's head is once again turned to the side of Pelvic Deficiency. Test the scapula on the side of Pelvic Deficiency first; then perform adjustments as indicated before the scapula was tested and adjusted on the side Opposite Pelvic Deficiency.

As interpreted in other AM Isolation Tests, reactivity of the PD leg in Position #1 indicates scapular involvement on the side tested. The shoulder Isolation Test uses a variation in the interpretation of Position #2. The *long* leg in Position #2 indicates the *direction of involvement* of the scapula that is being tested. The reference point for shoulder testing is the inferior angle of the scapula. The inferior angle of the scapula moves toward the long leg side in Position #2. For example, if the left shoulder is tested for scapular dysfunction and the right leg is the apparent long leg in Position #2, the left scapula is considered to have rotated medially in reference to the inferior angle, that is, the inferior angle of the left scapula has moved toward the midline; this is referred to as medial scapular involvement.

CLINICAL TIP: Frequently, the testing and interpretation for shoulder involvement can be difficult to grasp. An alternative way to approach the shoulder Isolation Test is as follows:
Step One: Ask the patient to squeeze the PD elbow into his or her side.
Step Two: Look for reactivity, such as shortening of the PD leg in Position #1.
One of the next two Pressure Tests will balance the legs.
Step Three: If Position #1 is reactive, Pressure Test the PD scapula on the inferior fossa in a medial-to-lateral direction.
Step Four: If balancing occurs, proceed to the adjustment for a medial scapular pattern.
Step Five (if necessary): If balancing did not occur, Pressure Test the PD scapula on the inferior fossa in a lateral-to-medial direction.
Step Six: If balancing occurs, proceed to the adjustment for a lateral scapular pattern.
Repeat the above steps after the shoulder adjustment, if it was indicated, for the Opposite PD shoulder.

CLINICAL TIP: Shoulders seem to fall into a particular pattern. The medial scapula is usually found on the side of Pelvic Deficiency. The lateral scapula is usually found on the side Opposite Pelvic Deficiency. When a deviation to this pattern occurs, trauma is usually involved.

The AM includes one additional factor in the pattern of scapular dysfunction. Because the scapulothoracic articulation is the primary site of interaction between the upper extremity and the torso, rotation of the scapula may involve the whole kinetic chain of the upper extremity. Consequently, the AM Basic Scan Protocol calls for adjustment of four different elements of the upper extremity kinetic chain when one is adjusting a medial or a lateral scapular pattern. Therefore when Isolation and Pressure Testing indicates medial rotation of the scapula, adjust for each of the following upper extremity neuroarticular dysfunctions:
• Medial ala of the scapula
• Inferior humerus
• Posterior-superior radius
• Anterior lunate
Similarly, when Pressure Testing indicates lateral rotation of the scapula, adjust for each of the following neuroarticular dysfunctions:
• Lateral ala of the scapula
• Superior humerus
• Inferior-lateral ulna
• Posterior distal carpals, avoiding the lunate
Both shoulders may show scapular patterns, and the direction of scapular rotation may be the same or different from side to side. Therefore it is important to perform shoulder Isolation Tests and adjustments to the scapulae before proceeding with the Basic Scan Protocol for the cervical spine.
Isolation Test. Perform shoulder Isolation Tests by testing the shoulder on the side of Pelvic Deficiency first, then by testing the shoulder on the side Opposite Pelvic Deficiency. After testing and adjustment of the first rib, have the patient turn his or her head to the side of Pelvic Deficiency and keep the arms resting on the table at the sides—the same position that is used for testing of all upper thoracic segments from T6 and above. Instruct the patient to squeeze the elbow of the arm on the side of Pelvic Deficiency against the trunk; this stresses the shoulder girdle (Figure 7-45). Look for reactivity of the PD leg in Position #1, and raise the legs to Position #2 to determine the direction of scapular involvement. After completion of testing and adjustment of the shoulder on the side of Pelvic Deficiency, instruct the patient to

squeeze the elbow on the side Opposite Pelvic Deficiency against the trunk; this stresses the shoulder girdle. Look for reactivity of the PD leg in Position #1 and raise the legs to Position #2 to determine the direction of scapular involvement.

If the left shoulder is being tested and the left PD leg shortens in Position #1, take the legs to

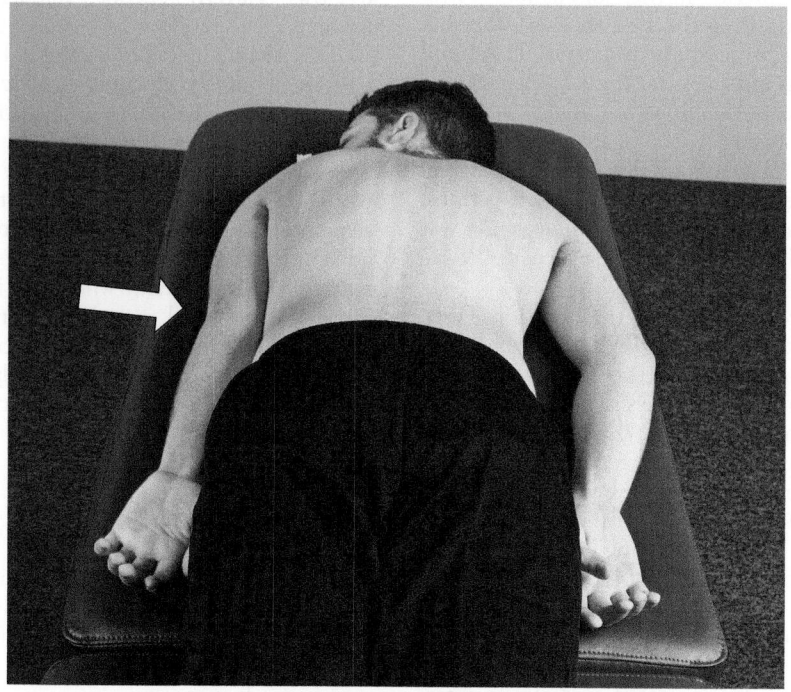

Figure 7-45 Isolation Test for medial or lateral scapular Pelvic Deficiency side.

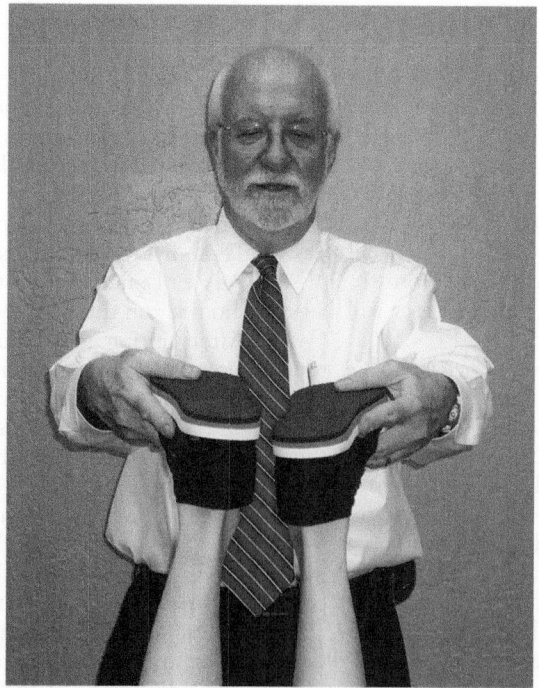

Figure 7-46 Medial scapula: Inferior border of scapula rotates toward the long leg in Position #2.

Position #2. If the left leg is long in Position #2, the test indicates that the inferior angle of the left scapula has deviated to the left, long leg, and the scapula is in a lateral involvement. Pressure Test to confirm by contacting the ala of the scapula with the palm of the hand or the fingers, and rotate the scapula by pushing the inferior angle toward the midline of the body. A lateral scapula is indicated if Pressure Testing causes the legs to balance in Position #1 and Position #2.

If the left shoulder is being tested and the left PD leg shortens, take the legs to Position #2. In Position #2, the right leg appears as the long leg; the test then indicates that the inferior angle of the scapula being tested has deviated to the right, or the midline, and the scapula is in a medial involvement. Pressure Test to confirm by contacting the ala of the scapula with the palm of the hand or the fingers, and rotate the scapula by pushing the inferior angle away from the midline of the body. A medial scapula is indicated if Pressure Testing causes the legs to balance in Position #1 and Position #2.

If the right shoulder is being tested and the left PD leg shortens in Position #1, take the legs to Position #2. If the right leg is long in Position #2, the test indicates that the inferior angle of the right scapula has deviated to the right, long leg, and the scapula is in a lateral involvement. Pressure Test to confirm by contacting the ala of the scapula with the palm of the hand or the fingers, and rotate the scapula by pushing the inferior angle toward the midline of the body. A lateral scapula is indicated if Pressure Testing causes the legs to balance in Position #1 and Position #2.

If the right shoulder is being tested and the left PD leg shortens, take the legs to Position #2. In Position #2, the left leg appears as the long leg; then the test indicates that the inferior angle of the scapula being tested has deviated to the left, or the midline, and the scapula is in a medial involvement. Pressure Test to confirm by contacting the ala of the scapula with the palm of the hand or the fingers, and rotate the scapula by pushing the inferior angle away from the midline of the body. A medial scapula is indicated if Pressure Testing causes the legs to balance in Position #1 and Position #2.

Adjustment for Medial Scapula. As was noted earlier, adjustment of a medial scapula involves adjustment of four elements of the kinetic chain of the upper extremity: scapula, humerus, radius, and lunate. For this example, see Figures 7-45 and 7-46, which indicate a medial scapula pattern. Therefore four contacts and thrusts occur:

- First, adjust for a medial scapula by contacting the medial border of the ala of the scapula. The LOD is straight lateral (Figure 7-47).
- Second, adjust for an inferior humerus by contacting the proximal third, lateral aspect of the shaft of the humerus on the deltoid muscle. The LOD is superior (proximal) toward the glenohumeral articulation of the shoulder (Figure 7-48).
- Third, contact the posterior, superior (proximal) aspect of the head of the radius. The LOD is anterior and inferior (distal) along the longitudinal axis of the radius (Figure 7-49).
- Finally, contact the anterior (volar) aspect of the lunate just distal to the wrist crease. The LOD is straight posterior (Figure 7-50).

To ensure an effective line of adjustment and to minimize patient discomfort when adjusting the scapula, take a firm medial-to-lateral soft tissue pull over the wing of the scapula with the thumb of the free hand. Keep the thumb in position on the scapula and use it to stabilize the tip of the instrument during the adjustment. Avoid repetitive strain injury by standing on the side opposite the medial scapula. In this manner, the instrument may be used without putting the hand into extreme flexion or extension while adjusting the scapula.

For adjustment of the humerus, use the thumb of the free hand to take an inferior-to-superior (distal-to-proximal) tissue pull over the lateral humerus. Use the thumb to stabilize the tip of the instrument during the adjustment.

To facilitate adjustment of the radius, swing the patient's arm up alongside of the head, and rest the forearm, palm down, on the table. During active or passive pronation and supination of the forearm, palpate for the head of the radius as it rotates in the annular ligament. Take a proximal-to-distal tissue pull over the head of the radius with the thumb of the free hand. Use the thumb to stabilize the tip of the instrument during the adjustment.

To adjust the anterior lunate, place the patient's arm back down beside the body so that the forearm rests with the palm of the hand facing toward the ceiling. Palpate for the lunate by creating motion in the radiocarpal joint or by having the patient oppose the thumb and the fifth phalanx. The distal aspect of the lunate is generally at the level of the wrist crease on the volar aspect of the wrist.

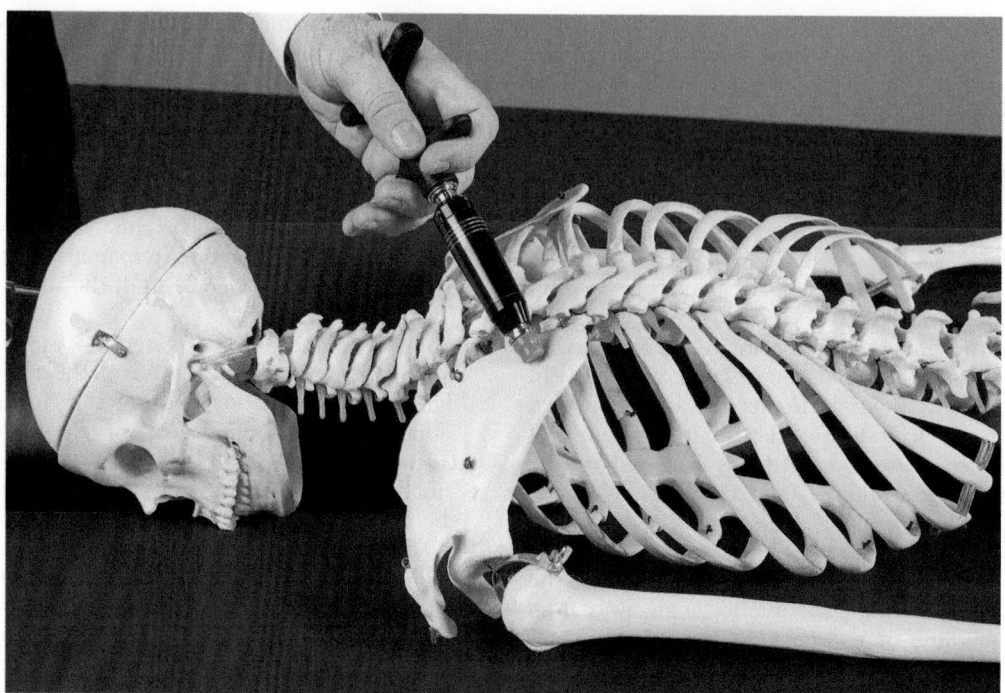

Figure 7-47   Medial scapula. Step One: ala of scapula. Line of Drive is lateral.

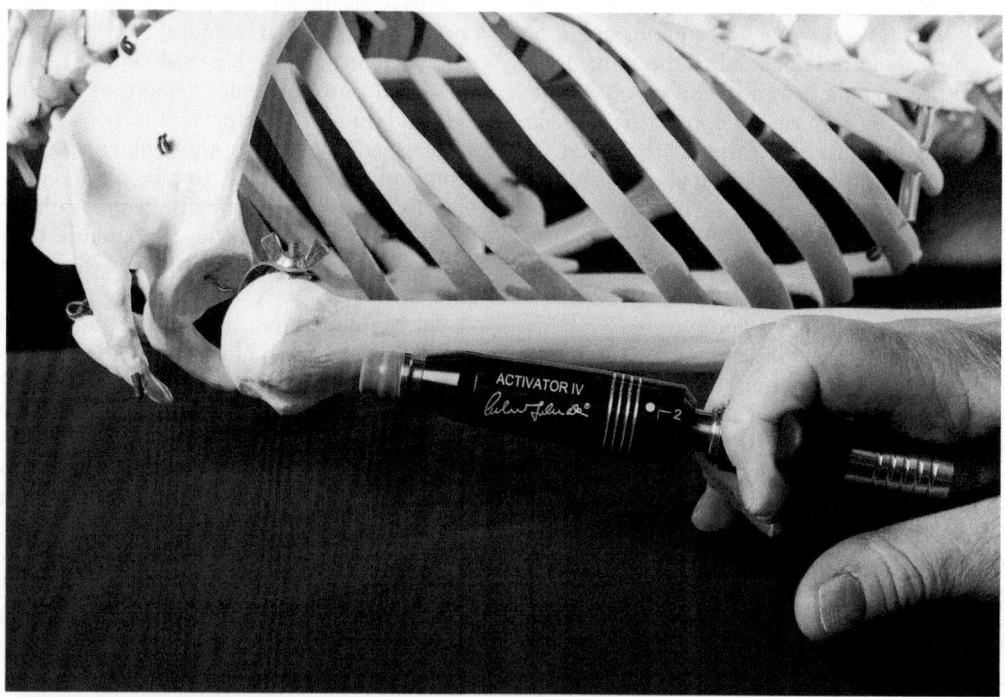

Figure 7-48   Medial scapula. Step Two: proximal, lateral third of humerus. Line of Drive is superior.

Adjustment for Lateral Scapula.   For this example, see Figures 7-51 and 7-52, which indicate lateral scapular involvement. As with the medial scapula, the lateral scapular adjustment requires adjustment of four elements of the kinetic chain of the upper extremity: scapula, humerus, ulna, and distal carpals. Four sets of contacts and thrusts occur:

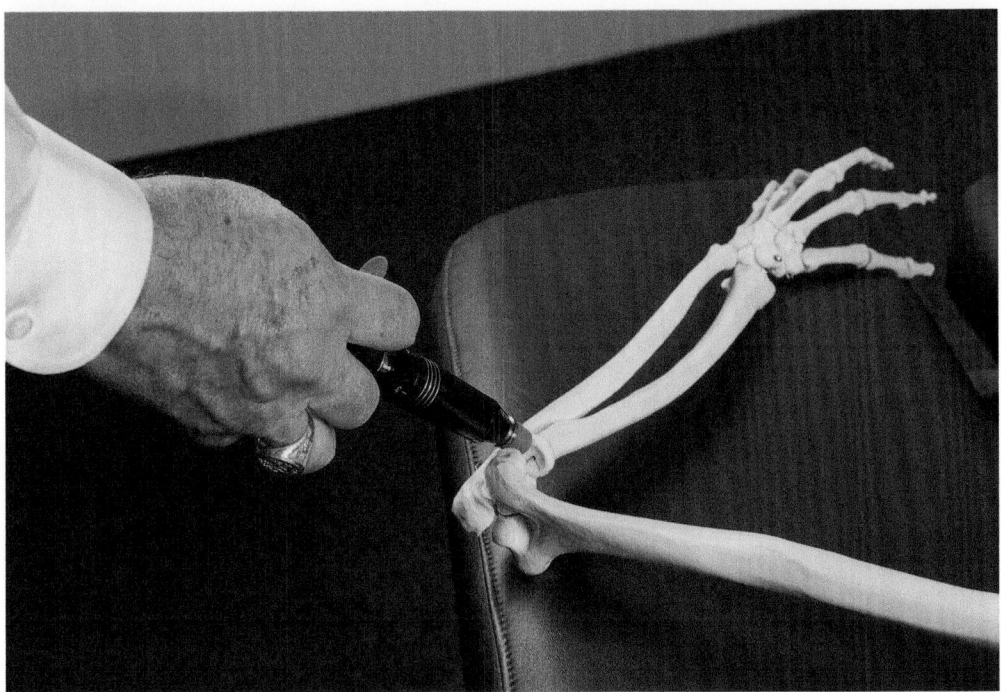

Figure 7-49 Medial scapula. Step Three: proximal radius inferior. Line of Drive is anterior and inferior (distal).

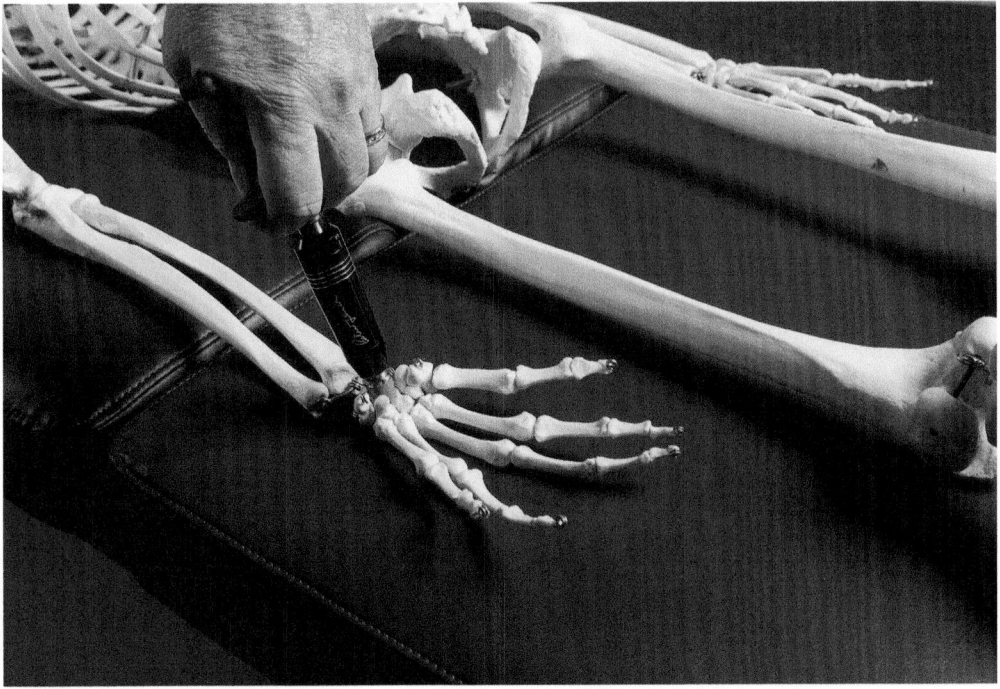

Figure 7-50 Medial scapula. Step Four: anterior lunate. Line of Drive is posterior.

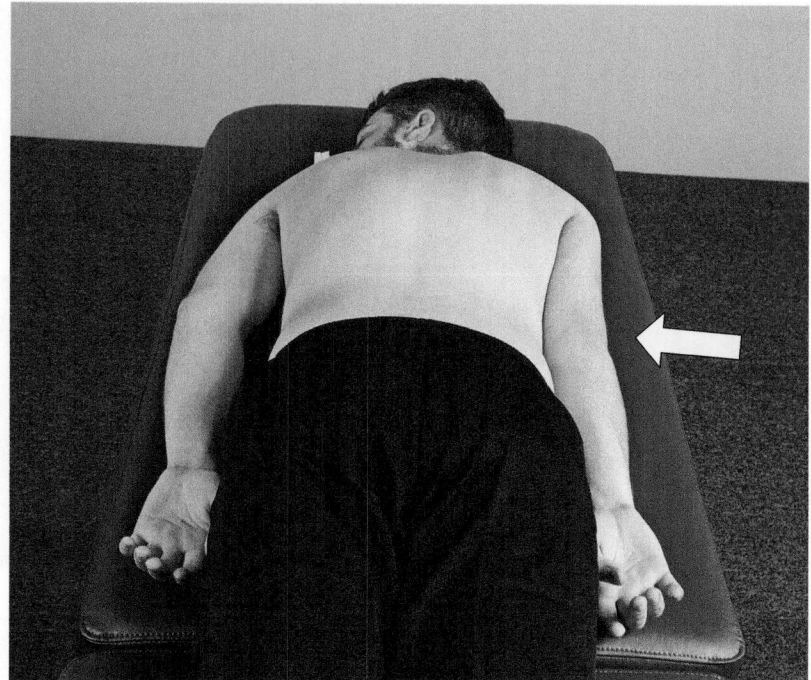

Figure 7-51   Isolation Test for medial or lateral scapular Opposite Pelvic Deficiency side.

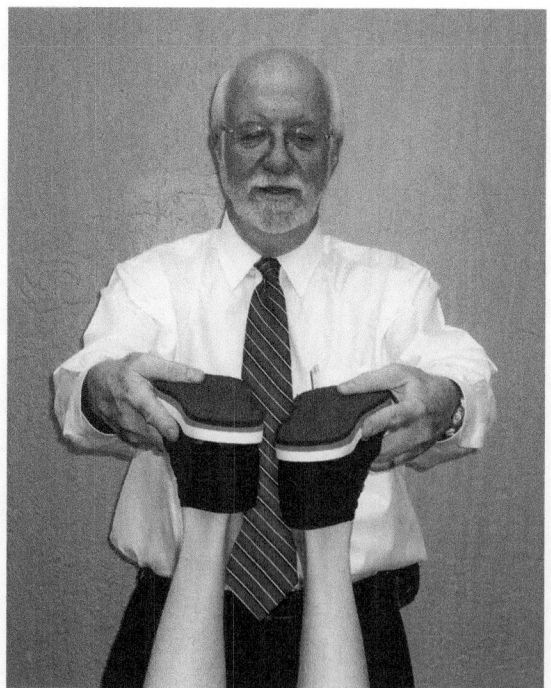

Figure 7-52   Lateral scapula: Inferior border of scapula rotates toward the long leg in Position #2.

- First, adjust for a lateral scapula by contacting the lateral border of the ala of the scapula. The LOD is straight medial (Figure 7-53).
- Second, adjust for a superior humerus by contacting the proximal third, lateral aspect of the shaft of the humerus on the deltoid muscle. The LOD is inferior (distal) toward the elbow (Figure 7-54).
- Third, adjust for an inferior-lateral ulna by contacting the anterior aspect of the proximal ulna. The LOD is superior (proximal) and anatomically medial (Figure 7-55).
- Finally, adjust for the posterior distal carpal row by contacting the dorsal aspect of the hand at the level of the distal carpals. The LOD is straight anterior (Figures 7-56 and 7-57). Make two thrusts on the distal carpal row with the instrument for most patients, but use three thrusts for the patient with large hands. Avoid contact of the lunate.

To ensure an effective LOD and to minimize patient discomfort when adjusting the scapula, take a firm lateral-to-medial soft tissue pull over the wing of the scapula with the thumb of the free hand. Keep the thumb in position on the scapula, and use it to stabilize the tip of the instrument during the adjustment. Avoid repetitive strain injury by standing on the same side of the lateral scapula. In this manner, the instrument may be used without putting the hand into extreme flexion or extension while adjusting the scapula.

For adjustment of the humerus, use the thumb of the free hand to take a superior-to-inferior (proximal to distal) tissue pull over the proximal end of the humerus. Use the thumb to stabilize the tip of the instrument during the adjustment.

To facilitate adjustment of the ulna, flex the patient's elbow and move the arm out to the side of the table. Locate the olecranon process and palpate inferiorly along the ulnar border, contacting approximately one inch below the olecranon. The LOD is superior (proximal) and anatomically medial. It will be toward the olecranon process with the arm positioned as stated above. Directing the thrust toward the olecranon process of the ulna in a superior-to-lateral direction helps to ensure an accurate LOD. Depending on the build of the patient, it may be useful to use the thumb of the free hand to stabilize the tip of the instrument during the adjustment.

To adjust posterior distal carpals, have the patient turn the hand so the palm is resting flat on the table. Palpate for the distal row of carpal bones by creating motion in the radiocarpal joint. The distal carpals are generally nearly one inch distal to the radiocarpal joint (Table 7-7).

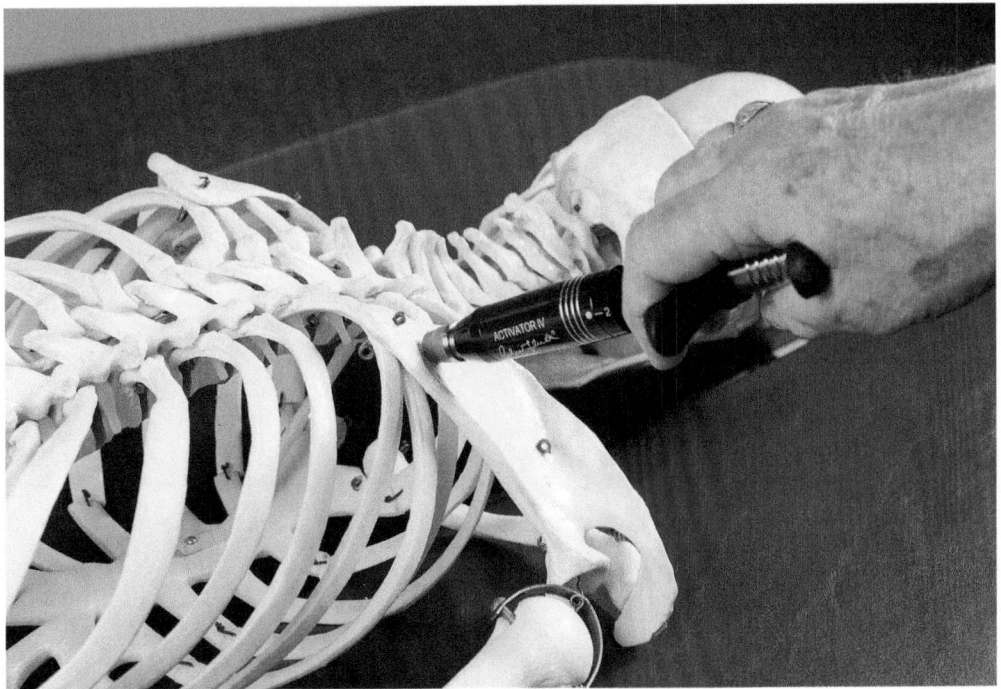

Figure 7-53 Lateral scapula. Step One: ala of scapula. Line of Drive is medial.

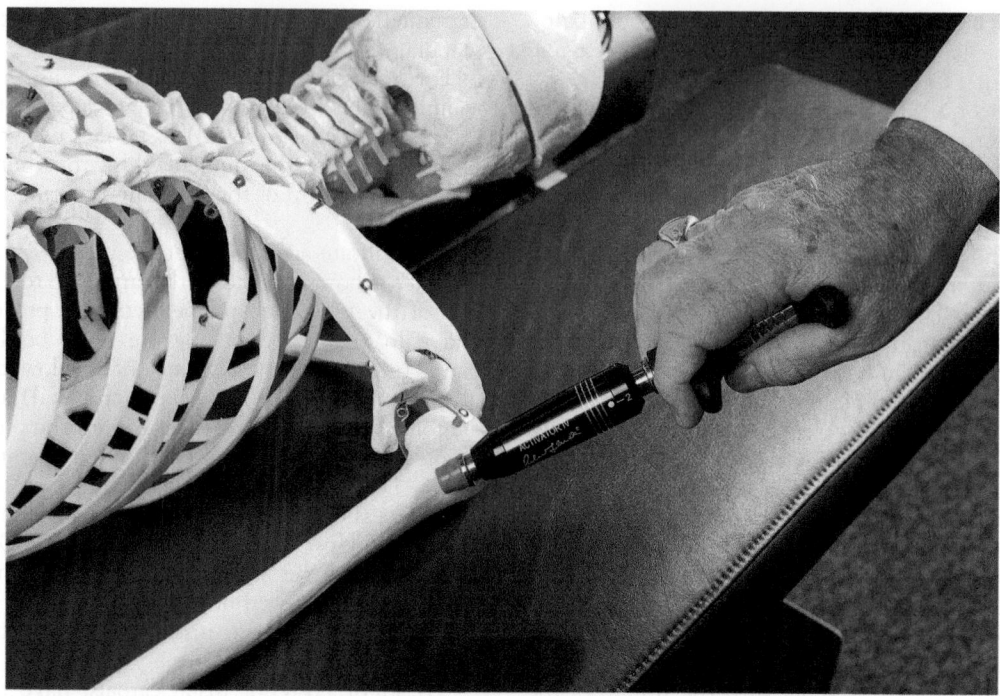

Figure 7-54   Lateral scapula. Step Two: proximal, lateral third of humerus. Line of Drive is inferior.

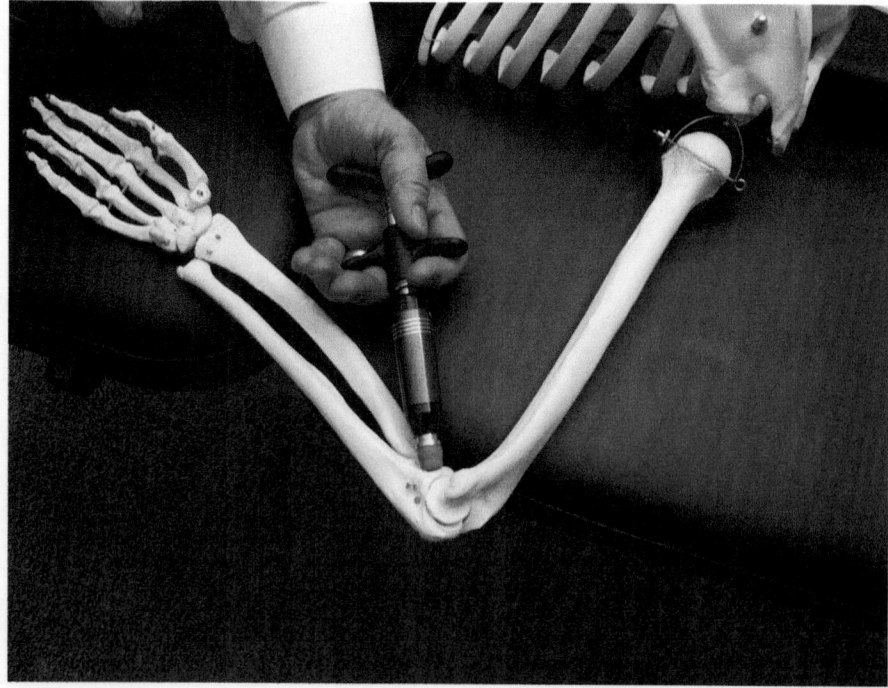

Figure 7-55   Lateral scapula. Step Three: proximal ulna. Line of Drive is superior (proximal) and anatomically medial.

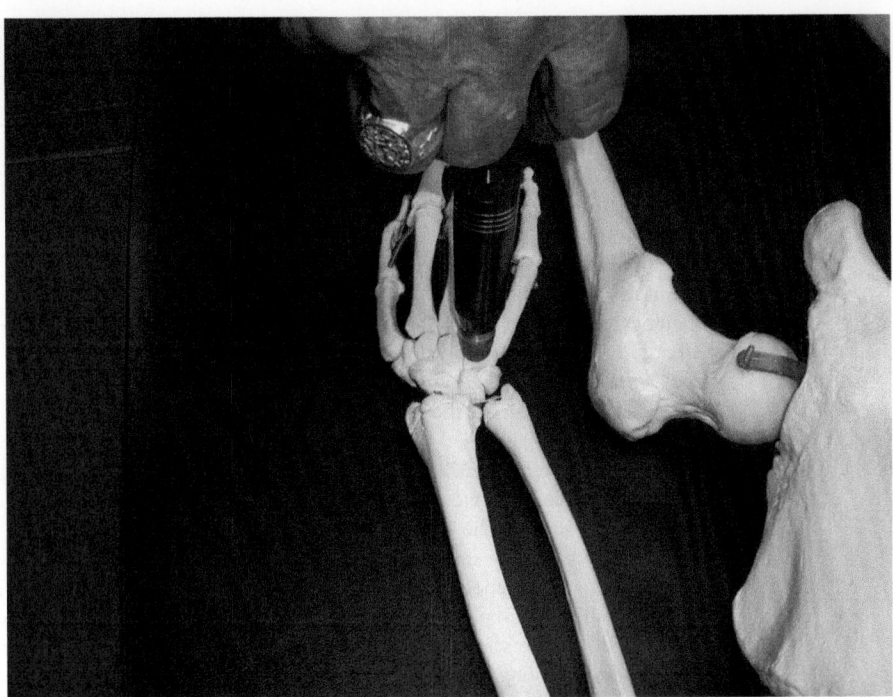

Figure 7-56 Lateral scapula. Step Four: posterior distal carpals. Line of Drive is anterior.

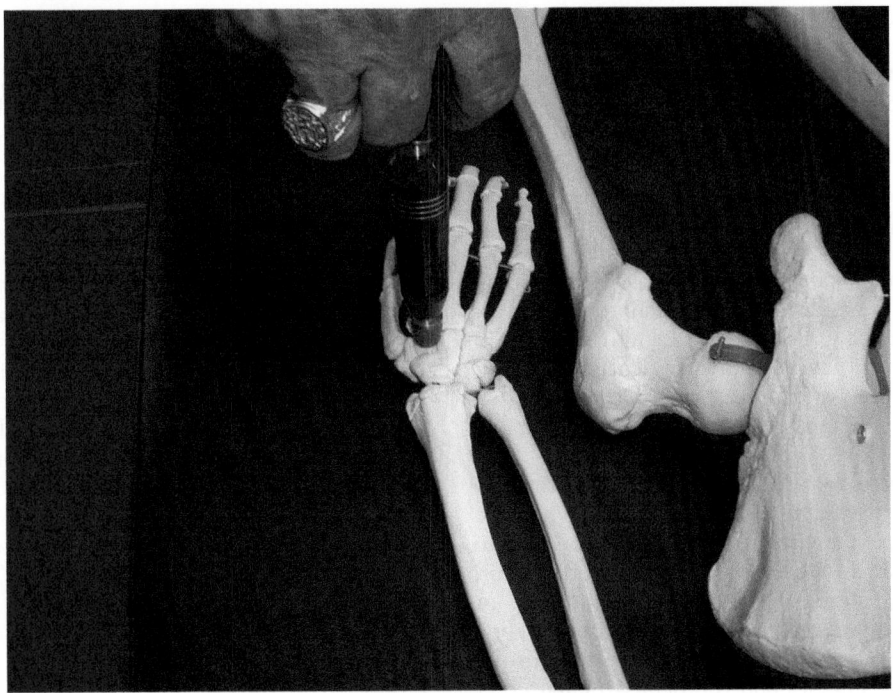

Figure 7-57 Lateral scapula. Step Four: posterior distal carpals. Line of Drive is anterior.

Table 7-7 The Activator Method Basic Scan Protocol: Scapular Patterns			
		ADJUSTMENT	
Articular Dysfunction	**Test**	**Segmental Contact Point**	**Line of Drive**
Medial Scapula	Instruct the patient to keep face turned toward side of Pelvic Deficiency and squeeze elbow of the arm on the side of Pelvic Deficiency against the side of the body. Inferior border of the scapula rotates toward the long leg in Position #2 (toward the midline).	1. Scapula ala 2. Proximal, lateral third of humerus 3. Proximal radius 4. Anterior lunate	Lateral Superior Anterior Posterior
Lateral Scapula	Instruct the patient to keep face turned toward side of Pelvic Deficiency and squeeze the elbow of the arm on the side Opposite Pelvic Deficiency against the side of the body. Inferior border of the scapula rotates toward the long leg in Position #2 (away from the midline).	1. Scapula ala 2. Proximal, lateral third of humerus 3. Proximal ulna 4. Posterior carpals	Medial Inferior Superior (proximal) and medial Anterior

Cervical Vertebrae

After testing and adjusting as indicated of the thoracic spine and scapulae, the AM calls for evaluation of the cervical spine. In the Basic Scan Protocol, the following vertebrae are routinely tested and adjusted as indicated:

- Seventh cervical vertebra (C7)
- Fifth cervical vertebra (C5)
- Axis (C2)
- Atlas (C1)
- Posterior occiput

The procedure for adjustment of each of the typical cervical vertebrae is essentially the same. The contact point is the pedicle-lamina junction on the side of involvement indicated by the Short/Long Rule or Leg Length Analysis in Position #2. The LOD for cervical segment C7 through C2 is anterior, superior, and medial through the plane line of the facets at 45 degrees.

The tests for cervical vertebrae are primarily Isolation Tests. In an Isolation Test, a specific motion or maneuver by the patient is used to localize an individual vertebra or motion unit, often by increasing tension in a muscle or group of muscles associated with that vertebra. These movements are thought to facilitate the paraspinal muscles and the neuroarticular components of the cervical spine in the C7, C5,

and upper cervical regions. In general, before an Isolation Test is performed, the legs are even and balanced in Position #1 and Position #2. If, when the Isolation Test or the maneuver for a specific vertebral motor unit is performed, the PD leg shortens in Position #1, the test is positive; this indicates involvement of the vertebral level that is being tested. By taking the legs into Position #2, involvement can be confirmed because some patients will react more strongly in Position #2. Application of the Short/Long Rule is used to determine the side of involvement. If an Isolation Test is positive, indicating neuroarticular dysfunction, the legs will become uneven in Position #1 as the PD leg reacts and shortens. Follow the Short/Long Rule. If relative lengthening occurs in the PD leg in Position #2, involvement of the vertebra on the side of Pelvic Deficiency is indicated. If the PD leg relatively shortens in Position #2, involvement of the vertebra on the side Opposite Pelvic Deficiency is indicated.

A *Pressure Test* may be used to clarify the results of an Isolation Test. A Pressure Test, by definition, involves a gentle but firm pressure on an affected joint or other structure into the direction of adjustment. A correctly applied Pressure Test on the side of involvement over the pedicle-lamina junction of the affected vertebrae will cause the legs to balance or become even in Position #1 and Position #2. If the legs balance after the Pressure Test is performed, the AM Protocol calls for adjustment of the involved vertebra indicated by the Isolation Test, on the side indicated by the Short/Long Rule in Position #2 and in the direction of the force applied during the Pressure Test.

Cervical Vertebrae and Occiput

Seventh Cervical (C7).   The AM Basic Scan Protocol calls for Isolation Testing and adjusting as indicated for the seventh cervical vertebra following adjustment of the upper thoracic spine and scapulae. When the thoracic spine and the scapulae have been tested and adjusted as indicated, the legs are typically even and balanced in Position #1 and Position #2.

Isolation Test.   During testing of the upper thoracic spine and scapulae, the head is turned to the side of Pelvic Deficiency. To isolate the seventh cervical vertebra, instruct the patient to turn the head back to a face-down neutral position (Figure 7-58). As the patient turns the head back to the neutral position, look for PD leg reactivity in Position #1. Then proceed to Position #2, observing relative changes in the PD leg. Follow the Short/Long Rule. If the PD leg lengthens in Position #2, seventh cervical vertebral involvement is on the side of Pelvic Deficiency. If the PD leg shortens in Position #2, seventh cervical vertebral involvement is on the side Opposite Pelvic Deficiency.

Pressure Test to confirm by applying a gentle but firm anterior-to-superior pressure on the pedicle-lamina junction through the plane line of the facets on the side of involvement indicated by the Short/Long Rule.

Adjustment.   To adjust seventh cervical vertebral involvement, contact the pedicle-lamina junction on the side of involvement. The LOD is anterior, superior, and slightly medial through the plane line of the facets (Figure 7-59).

Fifth Cervical (C5).   After Isolation Testing and adjustment as indicated for C7, proceed to testing the fifth cervical vertebra.

Isolation Test.   After testing of C7, the head is in the neutral, face-down position. Instruct the patient to extend the neck slightly by raising the head from the table (Figure 7-60). It is not necessary for the patient to lift the head into exaggerated extension. Simply have the patient look up and break contact with the table by raising the head about one inch and then return the head to the neutral, face-down position. Look for PD leg reactivity in Position #1. Then proceed to Position #2, observing relative changes in the PD leg. Follow the Short/Long Rule. If the PD leg lengthens in Position #2, fifth cervical vertebral involvement is on the side of Pelvic Deficiency. If the PD leg shortens in Position #2, fifth cervical vertebral involvement is on the side Opposite Pelvic Deficiency. Pressure Test to confirm by applying a gentle but firm anterior-to-superior pressure on

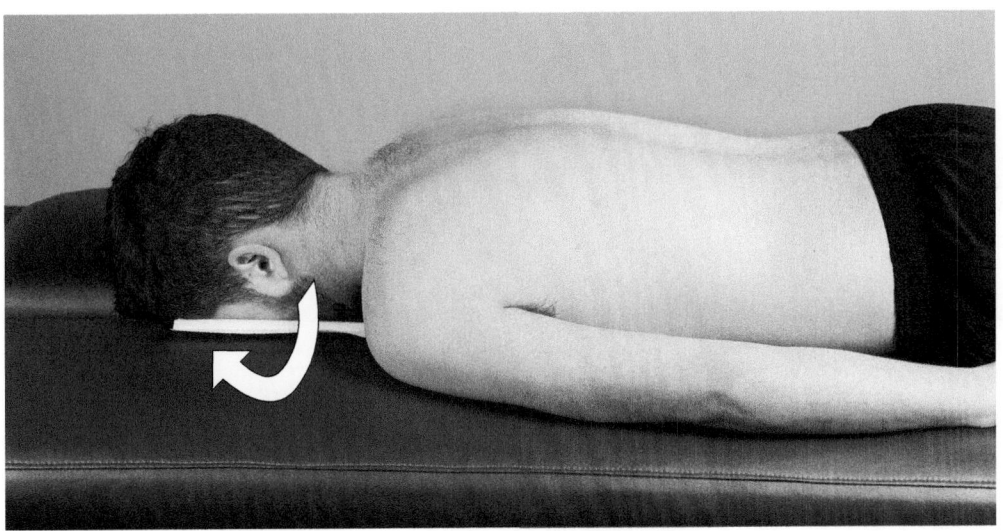

Figure 7-58   Isolation Test for seventh cervical.

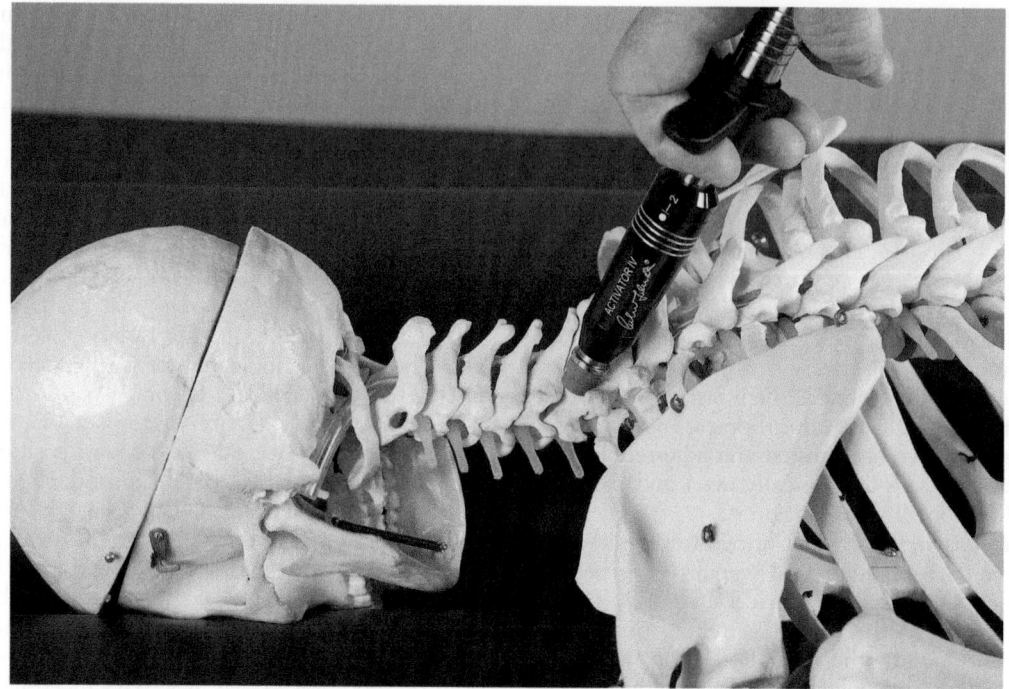

Figure 7-59   Adjustment for seventh cervical. Line of Drive is anterior-superior and slightly medial.

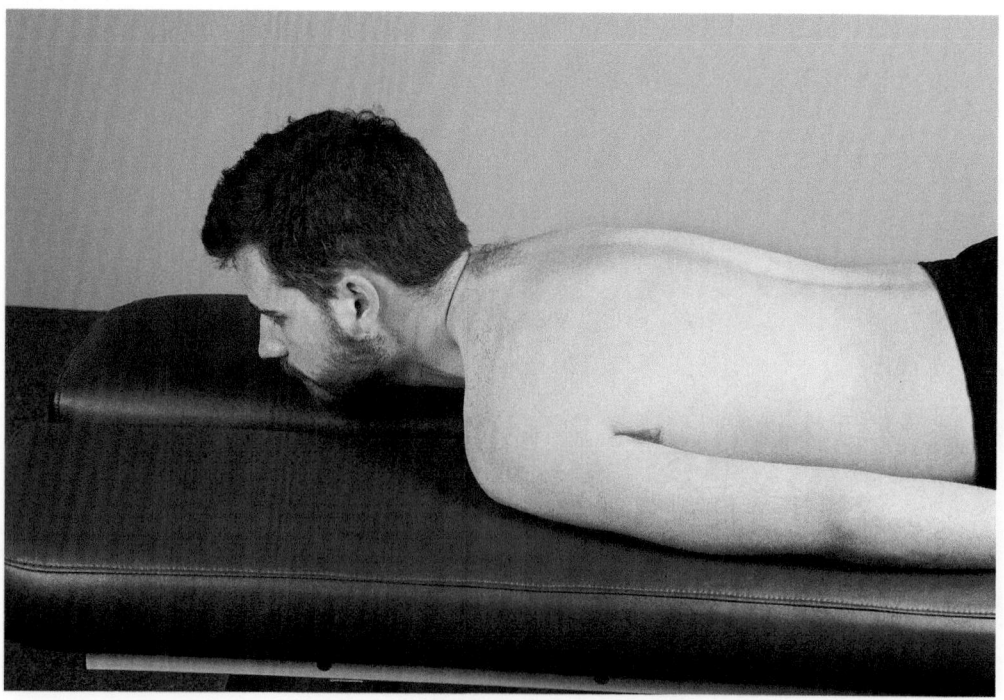

Figure 7-60   Isolation Test for fifth cervical.

the pedicle-lamina junction through the plane line of the facets on the side of involvement indicated by the Short/Long Rule, and observe for balancing of the legs in Position #1 and/or Position #2.

Adjustment. To adjust fifth cervical vertebral involvement, contact the pedicle-lamina junction on the side of involvement. The LOD is anterior, superior, and slightly medial through the plane line of the facets (Figure 7-61).

Axis-Atlas (C2-C1) Involvement. Following Isolation Testing and adjustment as indicated for C5, proceed to testing of the second and first cervical vertebrae.

Isolation Test. After testing of C5, the head is once again in the neutral, face-down position. Instruct the patient to slightly tuck the chin toward the chest and then relax (Figure 7-62). The neck flexion need not be exaggerated. Look for PD leg reactivity in Position #1. Then proceed to Position #2, observing relative changes in the PD leg. If the PD leg lengthens in Position #2, the first cervical vertebra (atlas) is involved on the side of Pelvic Deficiency. If the PD leg shortens in Position #2, the second cervical vertebra (axis) is involved on the side Opposite Pelvic Deficiency. Pressure Test the axis to confirm by applying an anterior and superior pressure on the pedicle-lamina junction of axis on the side Opposite Pelvic Deficiency; observe for balancing of the legs in Position #1 and/or Position #2.

Pressure Test the atlas to confirm by applying a gentle but firm lateral-to-medial pressure on the transverse of the atlas on the side of Pelvic Deficiency; observe for balancing of the legs in Position #1 and/or Position #2.

Adjustment for Axis (C2). To adjust second cervical (axis) vertebral involvement, contact the pedicle-lamina junction on the side Opposite Pelvic Deficiency. The LOD is anterior, superior, and slightly medial through the plane line of the facets (Figure 7-63).

Adjustment for Atlas (C1). To adjust a first cervical (atlas) involvement or lateral translation, contact the most lateral aspect of the transverse process. The LOD is straight medial (Figure 7-64). Use the thumb to stabilize the tip of the instrument during adjustment of the atlas.

Posterior Occiput. The last segment included in the AM Basic Scan Protocol for the cervical spine is the atlanto-occipital joint.

Isolation Test. Following isolation and adjustment of the C2-C1 segments, the patient's head will be in the neutral, face-down position. Instruct the patient to gently push his or her face into the table (Figure 7-65); this stresses the atlanto-occipital region. Look for PD leg reactivity in Position #1. Then proceed to Position #2, observing relative changes in the PD leg. Follow the Short/Long Rule. If the PD leg lengthens in Position #2, occiput involvement

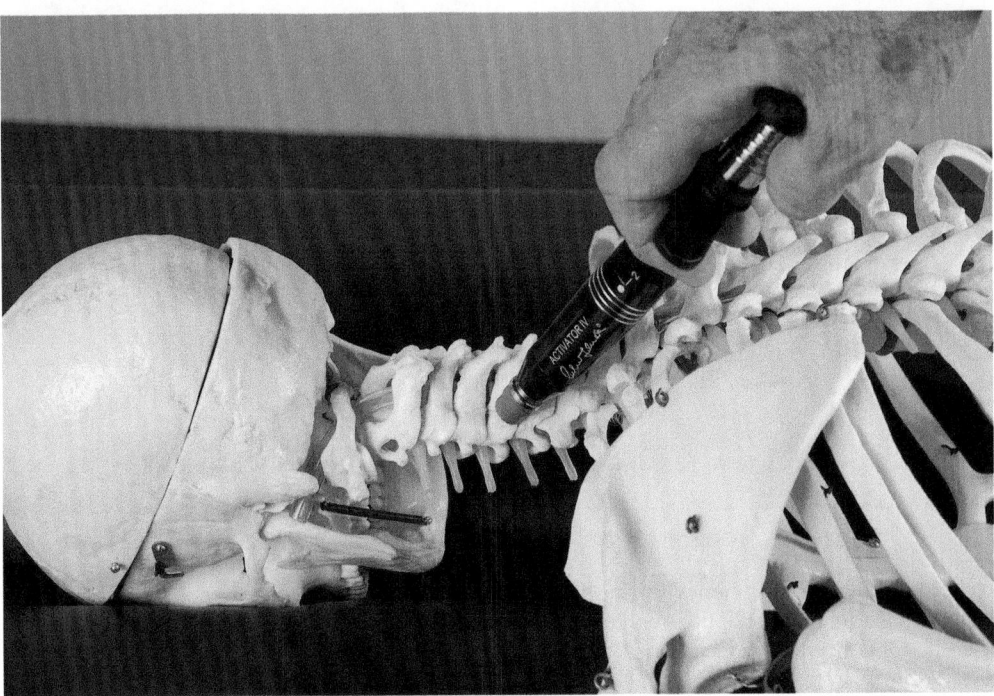

Figure 7-61 Adjustment for fifth cervical. Line of Drive is anterior-superior and slightly medial.

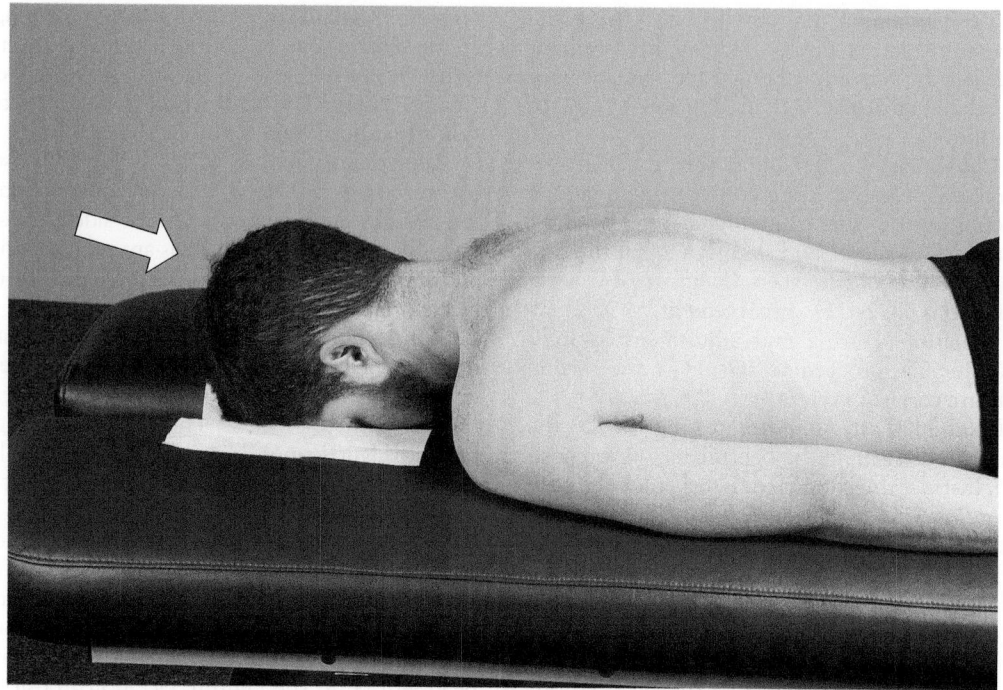

Figure 7-62   Isolation Test for axis (C2) and atlas (C1); slightly tuck chin toward the chest.

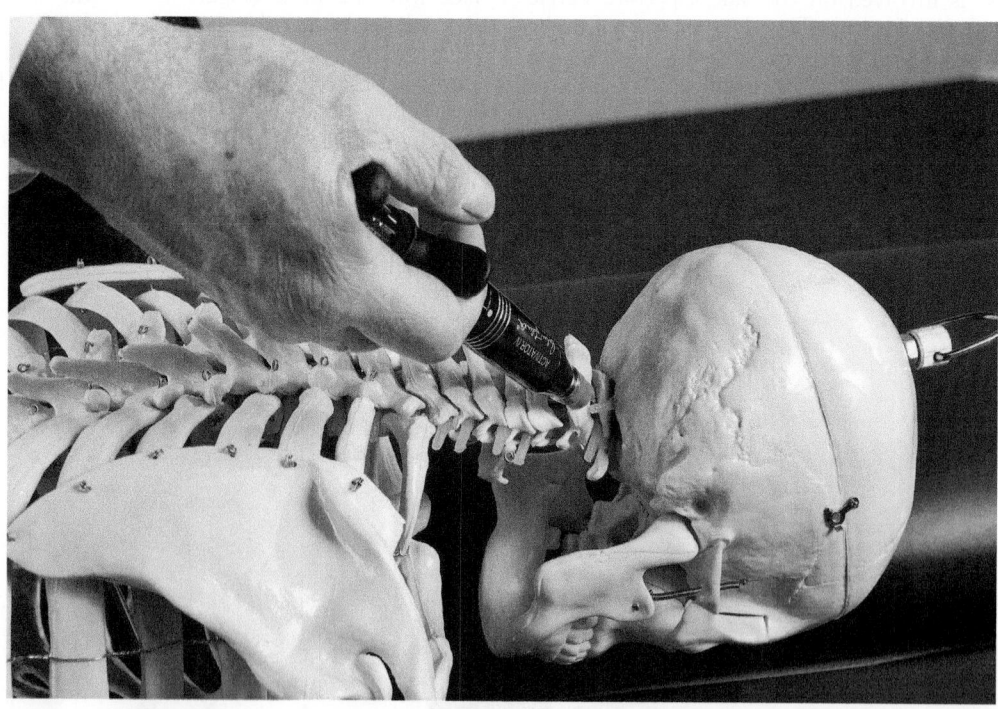

Figure 7-63   Adjustment for axis. Line of Drive is anterior-superior and slightly medial.

is on the side of Pelvic Deficiency. If the PD leg shortens in Position #2, occiput involvement is on the side Opposite Pelvic Deficiency. Pressure Test to confirm by applying a firm but gentle anterior pressure to the occiput on the side of involvement indicated by the Short/Long Rule,

and observe for balancing of the legs in Position #1 and/or Position #2.

Adjustment.   To adjust a posterior occiput, contact the posterior aspect of the occiput at the inferior nuchal line. The LOD is anterior (Figure 7-66).

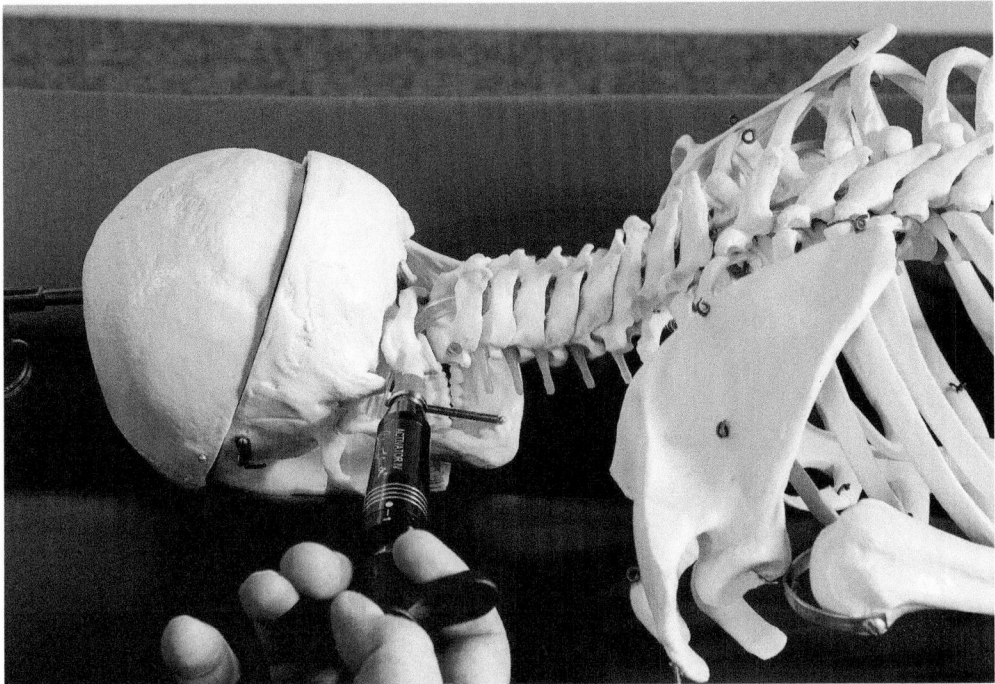

Figure 7-64 Adjustment for atlas. Line of Drive is straight medial.

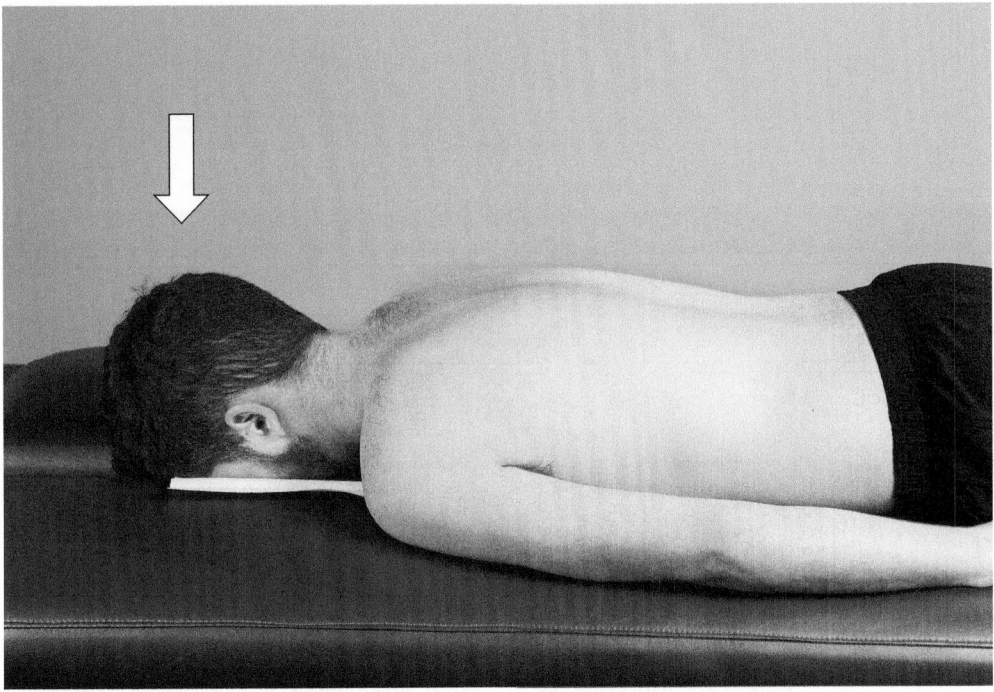

Figure 7-65 Isolation Test for occiput; gently push the face into the table.

To ensure patient protection and an effective LOD, place the thumb and thumb web of the free hand over the posterior arch of the atlas. Use the thumb of the free hand to stabilize the instrument during the adjustment. After an occiput adjustment is performed, repeat the Isolation Test to discern whether a bilateral posterior occiput involvement is present; if so, adjust the other side (Table 7-8).

Box 7-1 is a summary of published research relative to Isolation Testing and resultant leg length reactivity for the fifth cervical and the atlas/axis.

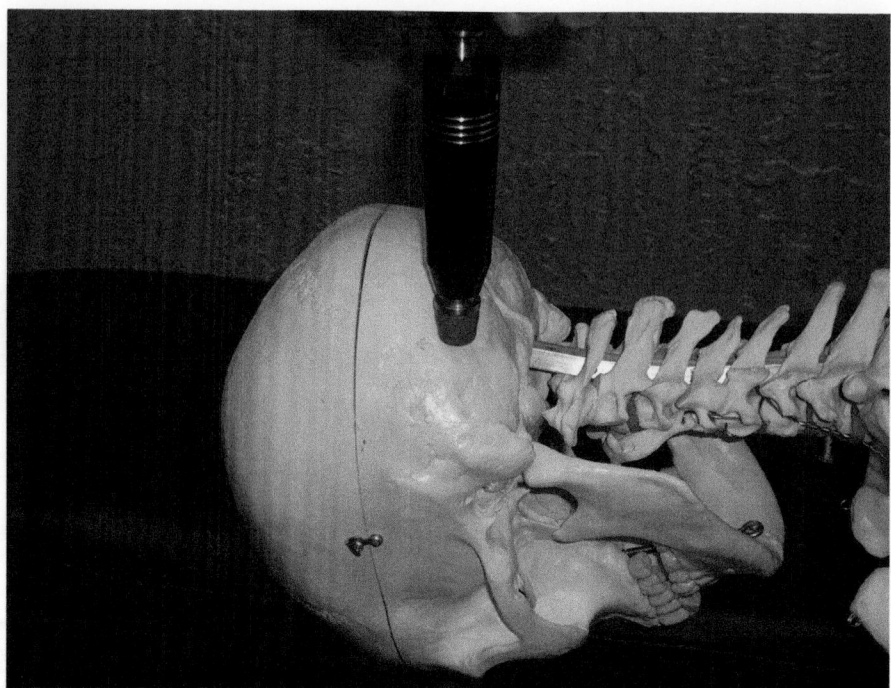

Figure 7-66 Adjustment for occiput. Line of Drive is anterior.

Table 7-8 **The Activator Method Basic Scan Protocol: Cervical Spine and Ribs**

Articular Dysfunction	Test	ADJUSTMENT	
		Segmental Contact Point	Line of Drive
Seventh Cervical (C7)	Instruct the patient to turn head to face-down neutral position	Pedicle-lamina junction on side of involvement	Anterior-superior and slightly medial
Fifth Cervical (C5)	Instruct the patient to extend neck by raising head slightly	Pedicle-lamina junction on side of involvement	Anterior-superior and slightly medial
Axis (C2)	Instruct the patient to flex neck by tucking chin toward chest (shortening in Position #2)	Pedicle-lamina junction on side Opposite Pelvic Deficiency	Anterior-superior and slightly medial
Atlas (C1) Translation	Instruct the patient to flex neck by tucking chin toward chest (lengthening in Position #2)	Most lateral aspect of transverse process on Pelvic Deficiency side	Straight medial
Posterior Occiput	Instruct the patient to push face gently into table	Posterior aspect of occiput at inferior nuchal line	Anterior

RELATED RESEARCH

Box 7-1

Reference: DeWitt JK, Osterbauer PJ, Stelmach GE, Fuhr AW. Optoelectric measurement of changes in leg length inequality resulting from isolation tests. J Manipulative Physiol Ther. 1994;17(8):530–8.

ABSTRACT
OBJECTIVES
(a) Establish a precise, standardized method to assess prone leg alignment changes (functional "Leg Length Inequality") that have, until now, been reported to occur clinically as a result of putative chiropractic subluxation Isolation Tests (neck flexion [C1-C2] and extension [C5]); and (b) describe differences in leg alignment changes in a group of healthy subjects and patients with chronic spinal complaints.

INTERVENTIONS AND OUTCOMES
Five subjects who exhibited involuntary leg reactions were tested with the use of an opto-electrical motion analysis system. During each testing session, the subject lay prone on an adjusting table while infrared light-emitting diodes (IREDs) were affixed to the heels of fracture boots. In the rest position, the neck was in neutral flexion so the face rested on the surface of the table. Before testing was begun, the examination area was in neutral flexion, so the face rested on the surface of the table. Also before testing, the examination area was calibrated, which resulted in root mean square (RMS) errors of less than 0.3 mm. Data were collected for ten seconds by three cameras that were positioned to record movement of the IREDs. During each testing session, each subject preformed two movements: a head-up movement, during which the subject extended the neck and then returned to a resting position; and a chin-tuck movement, in which the subject flexed the neck and then returned to a resting position. A testing session consisted of three no-movement baseline trials, followed by three head-up trials and three chin-tuck trials. Examination of output displacement histories showed that during all trials, movement occurred at the heels in the direction of the subject's longitudinal axis. During the head-up trials, most cases showed a net shortening in heel position during head movement.

REFERENCES

1. Plaugher G. Textbook of clinical chiropractic. Baltimore: Williams & Wilkins; 1993.
2. Armstrong TJ. Mechanical stressors. In: Rosenstock L, Cullen MR, editors. Textbook of clinical occupational and environmental medicine. Philadelphia: Saunders; 1994.
3. Bottomley MB. Risks and injuries in athletics and running. In: McLatchie GR, Lennox CME, editors. The soft tissues: trauma and sports injuries. London: Butterworth-Heinemann; 1993.
4. McCaw ST. Leg length inequality—implications for running prevention. Sports Med. 1992;14(6): 422-9.
5. Davis DG. Manipulation of the lower extremity. In: Subotnick SI, editor. Sports medicine of the lower extremity. London: Churchill Livingstone; 1989.
6. Magee DJ. Orthopedic physical assessment. Philadelphia: Saunders; 1987. p. 266-313.
7. Schafer RC. Clinical biomechanics: musculo-skeletal actions and reactions. Baltimore: Williams & Wilkins; 1983. p. 596.
8. Marshall P, Hamilton WG. Cuboid subluxations in ballet dancers. Am J Sports Med. 1992;20(2): 169-75.
9. Hildebrandt RW. Chiropractic spinography: a manual of technology and interpretation. 2nd ed. Baltimore: Williams & Wilkins; 1985.
10. Frigerio NA, Stowe RS, Howe JW. Movement of the sacroiliac joint. Clin Orthop. 1974;(100): 370-7.
11. White AA, Panjabi MM. Clinical biomechanics of the spine. Philadelphia: Lippincott; 1990.
12. Cipriano JJ. Photographic manual of regional orthopaedic tests. Baltimore: Williams & Wilkins; 1985.

8

ADDITIONAL TESTS FOR THE SACRUM, PELVIS, AND RELATED STRUCTURES

Neuroarticular dysfunction of pelvic articulations, especially of the sacroiliac (SI) joints, is a common finding in patients with musculoskeletal complaints and especially low back pain. Pelvic shear dysfunction of the SI joints, observed in the posterior-inferior (PI) ilium and in the anterior-superior (AS) ilium, has been clinically observed to produce hypertonicity in the pelvic musculature,[1-3] and, as was discussed in the section on Leg Length Analysis in Chapter 6, it may also be a factor in the development of Pelvic Deficiency. In addition to local effects on musculature that have an impact on gait and posture, neuroarticular dysfunction of the pelvis may affect stability and function in the rest of the spine by altering normal curves and restricting motion.

The biomechanics of the pelvis have been studied with regard to Leg Length Inequality (LLI).[4] Although it is now accepted that only a small amount of movement occurs at the SI joints,[5] global motion of the pelvis (i.e., pelvic rotation and translation) is significant movement that is related to LLI. Upon examining the effects of varying degrees of imposed leg length difference on symmetry of the innominate bones in healthy women, Cummings et al.[4] showed that posterior innominate bone rotation occurs on the side of an imposed short leg, and anterior rotation occurs on the side opposite. They further noted that the amount of pelvic obliquity increased in an approximately linear fashion as the leg length difference increased from two eighths of an inch to seven eighths of an inch. As was noted by Lawrence,[6] when the innominate is anterior, a long leg is noted on mensuration; conversely, a posterior innominate presents a short leg on mensuration. Hildebrandt[7] has discussed the term "innominate cleave," which refers to the normal interpelvic biomechanical action in which the bilaterally opposed ilia of the innominate bones move in an anterolateral-posteromedial direction, relative to each other and to the sacrum. Such discussion is consistent with general listing determinations of AS and PI in terms of pelvic rotation, shear, and translation. Alterations of the pelvic girdle are thought to be responsible for alterations of hip and knee flexors and extensors; this has been noted by Cooperstein as a theory that may explain apparent leg length changes from Position #1 to Position #2.[8] SI joint adjustment/manipulation has been found to create reflexogenic changes that are likely to be mediated by joint and/or muscle afferents.[9] These findings will be significant in the application of the Activator Method (AM) Protocols.

It must be noted that the pelvis is able to rotate and translate in eight simple movements and four degrees of freedom.[10] Subsequently, at times, additional tests and adjusting procedures are required to normalize the Pelvic Deficiency and to relieve the symptoms.

Pelvic involvement, in addition to involvement of the AS and PI ilium and the symphysis pubis of the AM Basic Scan Protocol, is indicated when Basic Scan Protocol adjustments of AS and PI ilium fail to significantly normalize the Pelvic Deficiency. Further testing is also indicated when a patient reports low back pain that radiates to the buttock and hip, reduction or alteration of SI or lumbosacral range of motion, or pain in the coccyx. Be alert also to patient reports of pain in the following lumbosacral or SI articulations during performance of Leg Length Analysis (LLA) tests:

- Anterior or Posterior Sacral Base
- Lateral Sacral Base
- Sacral Rotation (Clockwise or Counter-Clockwise)
- Internal Ilium or Anterior-Inferior Sacrum
- External Ilium or Posterior-Superior Sacrum
- Lateral Iliums
- Lateral Ischial Tuberosities
- Medial Ischial Tuberosity
- Lateral Coccyx
- Anterior or Posterior Base of Coccyx
- Anterior Pubic Bone
- Lateral Pubic Bone

For most patients who experience low back pain or pelvic problems, assessment and adjustment of the most frequently encountered pelvic neuroarticular dysfunctions—AS and PI ilium and pubic bone superiority or inferiority—are effective.

COMMON COMPLAINTS

Nearly everyone will experience low back pain at some time, and men and women are affected equally. Low back pain occurs most often between the ages of 30 and 50, in part because of the aging process but also as a result of sedentary lifestyles with too little (sometimes punctuated by too much) exercise. Back pain is the second most common neurological ailment in the United States.[11] Of course, low back complaints have traditionally been a major cause of time lost from work and a significant factor in workers' compensation and other insurance claims.[12] The relationship of pelvic dysfunction to low back pain is believed to involve both neuromuscular and biomechanical components.[12]

The role of the pelvis has a profound effect on the biomechanics of the SI joints and on LLI. LLI has been identified as a predisposing factor for acute and chronic injuries to the SI joints.[4] Authors have ascribed pain arising from the SI joints to strain on the SI ligaments, which in many cases results from LLI.[13,14] The SI joint has been implicated as a source of chronic low back pain[15] that has been described as localized to the buttock region.[16] SI joint dysfunction has been further identified in both symptomatic and asymptomatic populations.[17]

All patients should receive a complete and thorough evaluation from history taking to examination. When a patient reports low back and pelvic complaints, he or she should be observed for postural and gait abnormalities. With pelvic complaints, a patient frequently adopts an antalgic gait to avoid a painful component of motion and mobility.[18] Common gait abnormalities include the "hip-hiking" gait, the "vaulting" gait, and the "flexion" gait.[19] With the hip-hiking gait, the patient exhibits a unilateral high iliac crest, usually on the side of involvement. (The high hip is frequently, but not always, on the Pelvic Deficient [PD] side.) As the patient walks, the pelvis appears to rise up higher on the side of involvement, especially during the toe-off portion of gait. The asymmetrical elevation of the hip and pelvis is most likely caused by compensation that results from chronic loss of mobility at the SI joint. The vaulting gait is often very pronounced with an acute SI sprain

or strain injury. It is characterized by an alternating fast-slow gait asymmetry or a limp, with which the patient avoids pain by putting as little weight as possible for as short a time as possible on the leg of the involved side. A patient with a flexion gait may find it difficult to stand up straight, especially after just getting up from a chair. The patient may also raise the upper body into as erect a posture as is comfortable by walking the hands up the thighs when getting up from a sitting position. Many of the same features of gait that are related to pelvic joint involvement may accompany problems in the lumbar spine, and care must be taken to differentiate pelvic from lumbar involvement.

In addition to observation of gait, several orthopedic examinations can be performed to help the practitioner assess pelvic joint dysfunction. Most of these tests involve some stress applied to the SI joints, and the positive finding is pain. Disc lesions may be ruled out by having the patient perform a Valsalva maneuver. The test is performed by having the patient seated comfortably, with the arms slightly flexed at the elbows. The patient is instructed to take a deep breath and hold it. While holding the deep breath, the patient is asked to bear down to create greater intra-abdominal pressue. Reproduction of radicular pain is indicative of nerve root compression by a space-occupying mass in the spine.[20] This can result from nerve root entrapment at an intervertebral foramen or within the neural canal, and it may indicate a herniated intervertebral disc. The straight leg raise or Lasegue's test should be used to assess the patient for nerve entrapment syndrome or sciatic neuralgia because it has been found to be the most reliable and strongly recommended objective test.[21,22]

Specific maneuvers and signs used to assess the function of SI joints include Gaenslen's test, the Lewin-Gaenslen test, Goldthwait's test, and SI compression tests.[23] With Gaenslen's test, which should be avoided with pregnant, pediatric, and geriatric patients, the patient is positioned supine at the edge of the table. The examiner acutely flexes the knee and thigh of the unaffected leg to the patient's abdomen. This moves the lumbar spine firmly into the table and fixes both the pelvis and the lumbar spine. With the other hand of the examiner on top of the knee of the affected side, pressure is gradually increased to hyperextend the affected thigh. The test is positive if pain is felt in the SI area or is referred down the thigh. The test should be performed bilaterally.[24]

A much less stressful variant of Gaenslen's test is the Lewin-Gaenslen maneuver. The patient lies in the side posture position with the affected SI joint up. The leg and hip are passively extended to rotate the ilium relative to the sacrum. Once again, a finding of pain in the region of the SI joint indicates joint disease. Problems with the SI joint may be of a chronic degenerative nature or may be related to an acute sprain or strain injury.

Goldthwait's test helps the practitioner to differentiate between signs and symptoms of pelvic (SI) origin and manifestations of lumbar vertebral involvement. With Goldthwait's test, the patient is placed in the supine position with the knee straight and relaxed. The hip of the affected side is passively flexed while the examiner palpates the lumbosacral junction. Reproduction or exacerbation of low back pain *before* the lumbosacral articulation moves suggests involvement at the SI joints. If the patient experiences low back pain *after* movement of the lower lumbar spine, lumbar vertebral involvement is indicated.

Finally, the iliac compression test may be used to confirm SI involvement, especially when acute sacroiliitis is present. The patient is placed laterally recumbent, and manual pressure is applied at the iliac fossa just lateral to the SI joint. The pressure must be firm and sustained for thirty seconds or longer. Reproduction or exacerbation of pain in the SI joint is indicative of active, acute inflammation of the joint. The SI compression test is contraindicated for pregnant patients because of the ligamentous laxity typically associated with late-stage pregnancy.

CONCURRENT CONDITIONS

Low back pain with apparent involvement of the pelvis infrequently can be a manifestation of concurrent visceral or other diseases.[25] An example is the pain of cystitis, which may refer to the suprapubic region[26] and may imitate misalignment of the symphysis pubis. Urinary tract infections with inflammation of the urinary bladder occur more frequently in female patients. These infections are highly resistant to treatment. Frequently, dysmenorrhea or premenstrual tension syndrome also may manifest with low back and pelvic pain and must be differentiated from pain of musculoskeletal or biomechanical origin. Investigation into the effectiveness of spinal manipulation with such disorders is being conducted and has shown positive results, although such conditions must be monitored closely.[27-29]

A frequent underlying cause of pelvic region pain in older males is prostate involvement. Acute prostatitis is of sudden onset and is characterized by urinary urgency with scant volume output. Frequently, acute prostatitis manifests with pain over the thigh transmitted via the lateral femoral cutaneous nerve. Benign prostatic enlargement is an almost inevitable phenomenon in elderly males and must be monitored via periodic prostate examination. Low back pain and pelvic involvement of insidious onset also may be indicators of prostate malignancy. Prostate cancer, if it metastasizes, spreads to the bones of the lumbar spine and pelvis. Suspicious findings from appropriate physical examination and laboratory evaluation may indicate the need for a urological consult.[30] Patients with colorectal disease, inflammatory bowel disorders, diverticulitis, and regional ileitis (Crohn's disease) also may experience low back and pelvic pain as a result of viscerosomatic referral.[31] When low back pain appears to originate from causes other than biomechanical or neuromuscular dysfunction, referral is indicated.

TESTING AND ADJUSTING THE SACRUM, PELVIS, AND RELATED STRUCTURES

Anterior or Posterior Sacral Base

When a patient suffers with low back pain and reduced SI range of motion, consider an anterior or posterior sacral base. An anterior sacral base is nutation of the sacrum, when the sacral base has moved anterior and inferior, or is in a flexed malposition. This results in an increase in the sacral base angle (Ferguson's angle). A posterior sacral base is counter nutation of the sacrum, when the sacral base has moved posterior and superior, or is in an extension malposition. This results in a decrease in the sacral base angle. When bringing the patient's legs to Position #2 or Position #3 is difficult because of patient complaints of exquisite pain at the lumbosacral junction, consider testing for an anterior or posterior sacral base.

Isolation Test. To test for an anterior or posterior sacral base, flex the legs past Position #2 to Position #3 (knees flexed past 90 degrees) until you meet resistance. If the PD leg lengthens in Position #3 (Figure 8-1), the test indicates an anterior sacral base (nutation-flexion malposition).

If the PD leg shortens in Position #3 (Figure 8-2), the test indicates a posterior sacral base (counternutation-extension malposition).

Adjustment for Anterior Sacral Base. To adjust an anterior sacral base, position the tip of the instrument on the superior aspect of the third sacral tubercle for the contact point. The Line of Drive (LOD) is inferior and anterior (Figure 8-3).

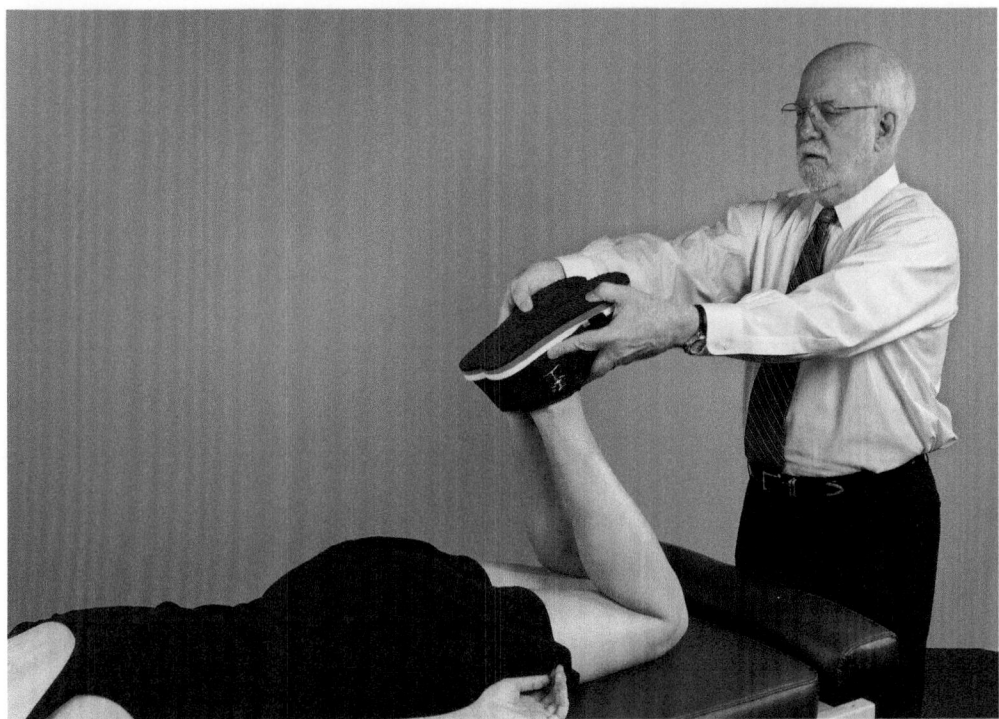

Figure 8-1 Lengthening of Pelvic Deficiency leg in Position #3 indicates superior sacrum.

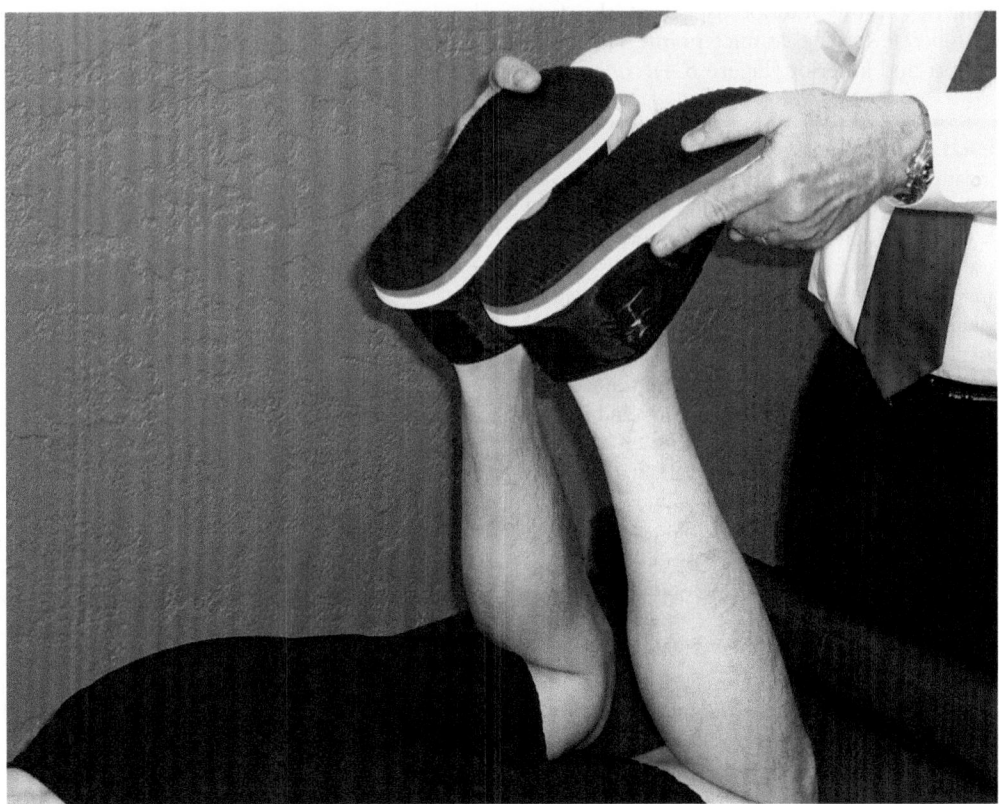

Figure 8-2 Shortening of Pelvic Deficiency leg in Position #3 indicates inferior sacrum.

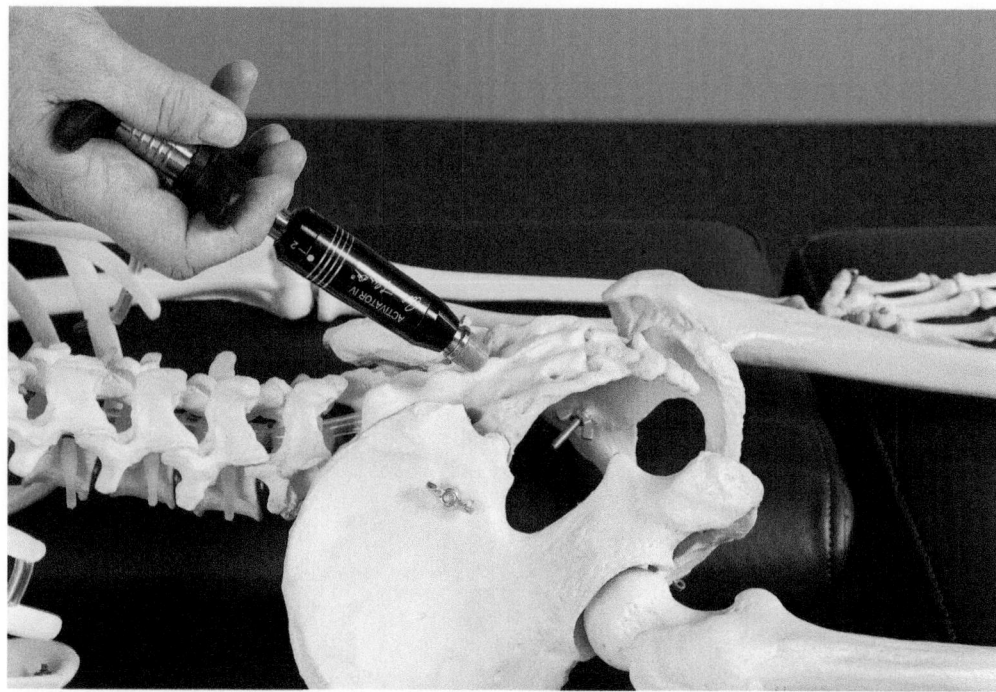

Figure 8-3   Adjustment for superior sacrum. Line of Drive is anterior-inferior.

Adjustment for Posterior Sacral Base.   To adjust a posterior sacral base, position the tip of the instrument on the inferior aspect of the first sacral tubercle for the contact point. The LOD is superior and anterior (Figure 8-4).

Clinical Observations

A relatively reliable indicator of sacral rotational malposition is the patient's gait and standing posture. With an anterior sacral base, nutation may cause hyperlordosis of the patient's lumbar spine. It may be difficult for the patient to stand upright, and any attempt to extend the low back may be extremely painful. The patient may demonstrate positive Kemp's test results with pain at the sacroiliac or lumbosacral joints on extension and rotation. Getting up from a sitting position is also likely to be very painful for the patient with an anterior sacral base.

When a patient has a posterior sacral base (counternutation-extension malposition), antalgic posture and gait may involve flattening of the lumbar spine into hypolordosis. The patient may also stand and walk with the buttocks tucked under the torso in a "pelvic tilt" position.

Lateral Sacral Base

When a patient presents with low back pain that radiates to the hip, or when previous procedures have failed to normalize the Pelvic Deficiency, consider lateralization of the sacral base.

Isolation Test.   After performing and completing the pelvis test, use the Position #4 test for laterality of the sacral base. Flex the PD leg toward the buttocks until you meet resistance. Look for PD leg reactivity in Position #1. Then proceed to Position #2, while observing relative changes in the PD leg. Follow the Short/Long Rule. Relative lengthening of the PD leg in Position #2 indicates a global, lateral shift of the sacrum to the side of Pelvic Deficiency. Relative shortening of the PD leg in Position #2 indicates a global, lateral shift of the sacrum toward the side of Opposite Pelvic Deficiency.

Alternative Lateral Sacral Base.   This test is a little more involved than the previous test for lateral sacral base, but it provides a great patient education opportunity. Test for a lateral sacral base by instructing the patient to raise the PD leg off the table by extending the hip without bending the knee. Apply a firm posterior-to-anterior pressure to the base of the sacrum to prevent the patient from raising the anterior superior iliac spine off the table. Note the height to which the patient is able to extend the leg, and then ask the patient to lower the leg. Next, instruct the patient to raise the leg Opposite Pelvic Deficiency by extending the hip without bending the knee. Again apply a firm

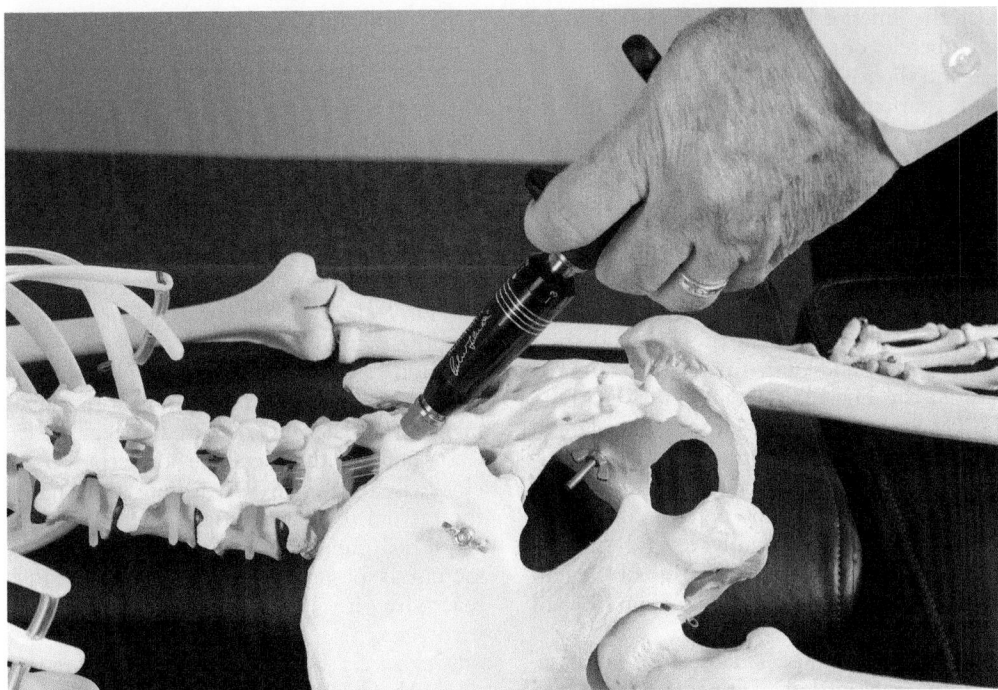

Figure 8-4 Adjustment for inferior sacrum. Line of Drive is anterior-superior.

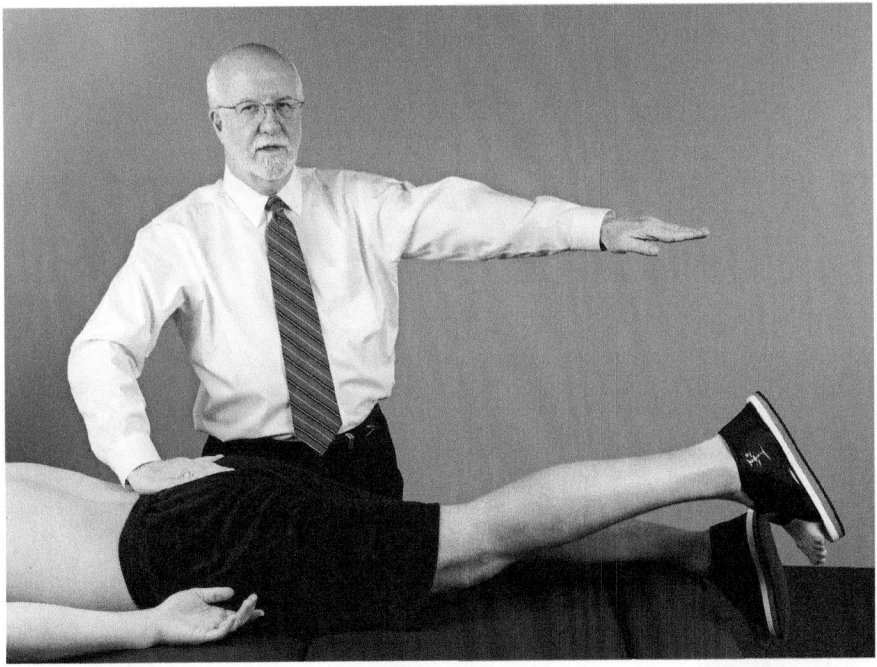

Figure 8-5 Straight leg Isolation Test for lateral sacral base; compare heights of active straight leg hip extension. Sacral base is lateral to restricted extension side.

posterior-to-anterior pressure to the base of the sacrum to prevent the anterior superior iliac spine from being lifted off the table (Figure 8-5). Note the height to which the patient is able to extend the leg, and then ask the patient to lower the leg. The sacral base tends to subluxate laterally to the lower leg side or the side of limited hip extension. In the example illustrated, the left hip extension is on the restricted side. To adjust this left lateral sacral base, as in Figure 8-5, contact the inferior-lateral aspect of the third sacral tubercle on the left side. The LOD is medial and slightly superior.

For a patient in acute pain or an elderly patient with limited hip and pelvic range of motion, it may be difficult to perform the Isolation Test for lateral sacral base in the way described previously. Another alternate method of performing the Isolation Test involves passive rather than active ranges of motion for the hip and SI joints. Use a Stress Test by placing the index and middle fingers on the first and third sacral tubercles, and push the sacrum laterally away from the PD side (Figure 8-6). Reactivity of the PD leg in Position #1 indicates a lateral sacrum toward the side Opposite Pelvic Deficiency. If no reactivity occurs, perform the Stress Test again, but in the opposite direction, and push the sacrum laterally toward the PD side (Figure 8-7). Reactivity of the PD leg in Position #1 indicates a lateral sacrum toward the PD side.

Adjustment. To adjust a lateral sacral base, contact the inferior-lateral aspect of the third sacral tubercle on the side of sacral base laterality. The LOD is medial and slightly superior (Figure 8-8).

Sacral Rotation–Clockwise–Counter-Clockwise

After pelvis tests and adjustments are performed as indicated, if the patient persists with pain in the lumbosacral region, consider Stress Testing for sacral rotation.

Stress Test. The doctor makes a firm contact on the sacrum with the palm of the hand, with the fingers pointed cephalad, parallel and over the sacral tubercles. Push anteriorly to maintain a firm contact, and then rotate your hand in a clockwise direction (Figure 8-9), stressing the sacrum inferiorly on the right side and superiorly on the left side. Look for PD leg reactivity in Position #1, indicating involvement. If no reactivity occurred, repeat the Stress Test but in the opposite direction–counterclockwise (Figure 8-10). Rotate your hand on the sacrum so that the right side of the sacrum is pushed superiorly and the left side of the sacrum is pushed inferiorly. Look for PD leg reactivity in Position #1, which indicates involvement.

Adjustment. Both adjustments will require a single thrust on two contact points. For clockwise sacral rotation involvement, the first contact is found just lateral to the first sacral tubercle on the right side. The LOD is anterior,

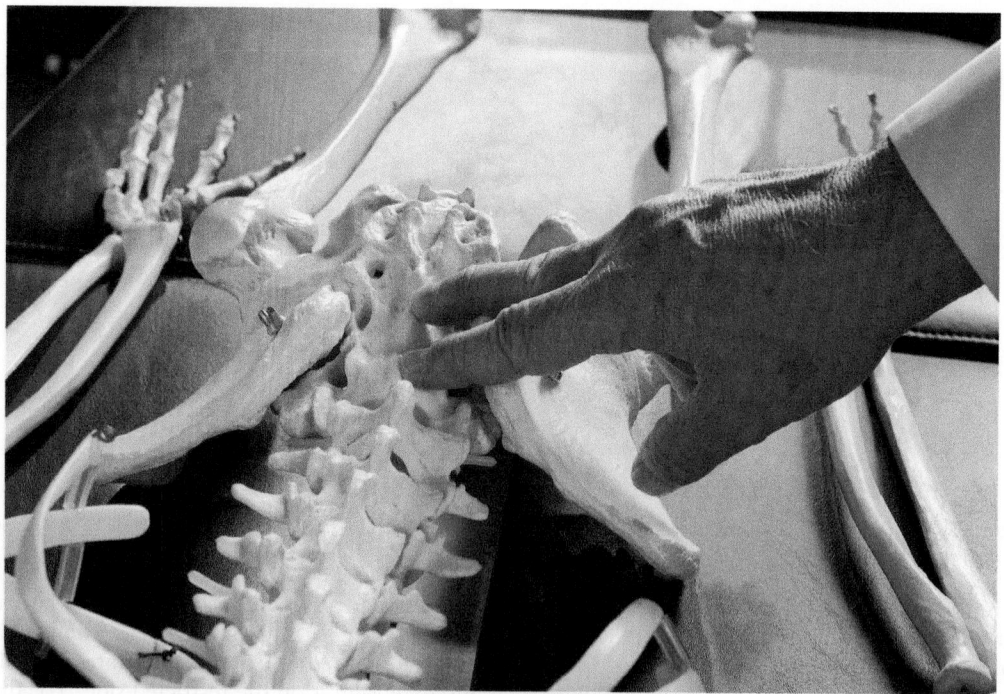

Figure 8-6 Alternative Stress Test for right lateral sacral base.

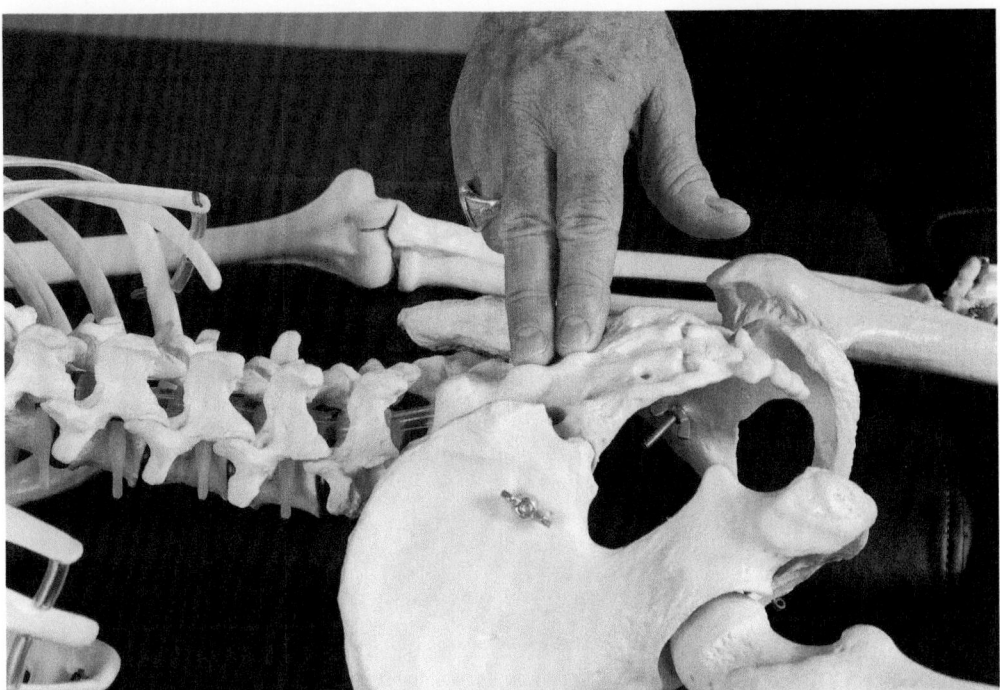

Figure 8-7 Alternative Stress Test for left lateral sacral base.

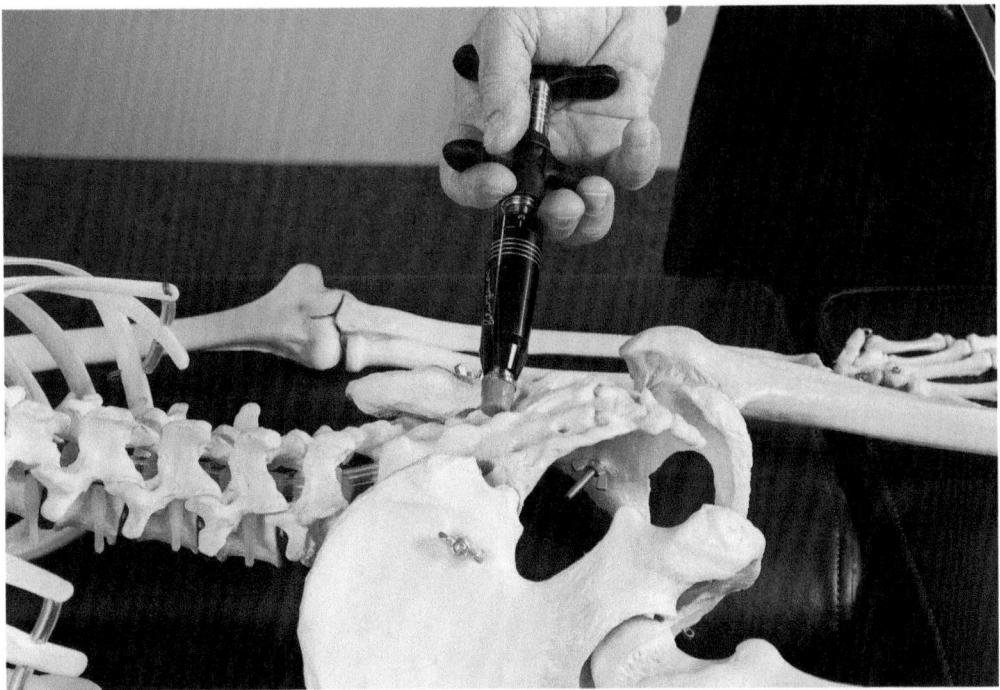

Figure 8-8 Adjustment for lateral sacral base. Line of Drive is medial and slightly superior.

superior, and slightly medial (Figure 8-11). The second contact point is found just lateral to the third sacral tubercle on the left side. The LOD is anterior, inferior, and slightly medial (Figure 8-12).

For counter-clockwise sacral rotation involvement, the first contact is found just lateral to the first sacral tubercle on the left side (Figure 8-13). The LOD is anterior, superior, and slightly medial. The second contact point

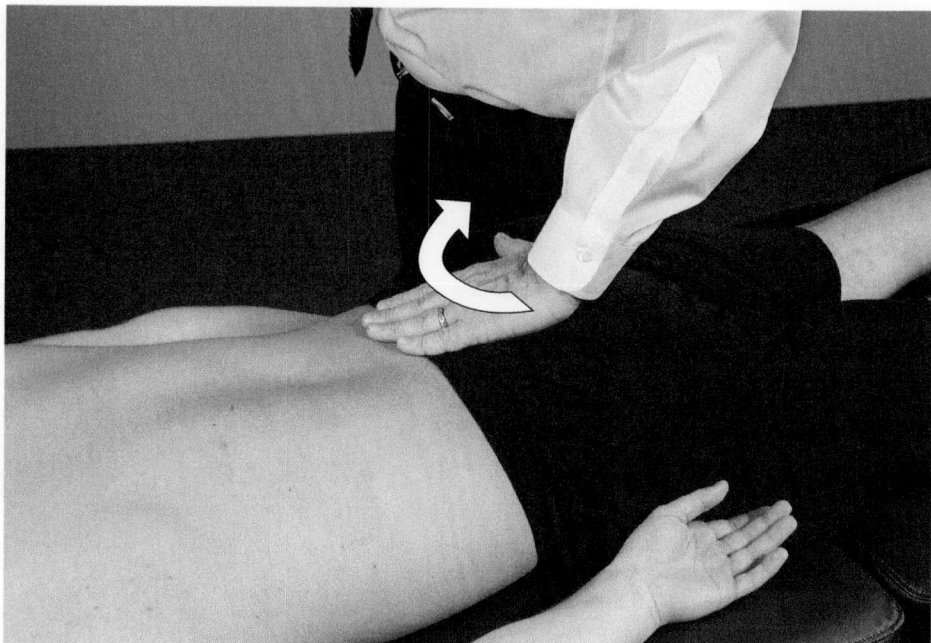

Figure 8-9 Stress Test for clockwise sacrum; firm contact on sacrum with the palm of the hand, fingers pointed cephalad, parallel and over the sacral tubercles. Push anteriorly to maintain a firm contact, and then rotate your hand in a clockwise direction, stressing the sacrum inferiorly on the right side and superiorly on the left side.

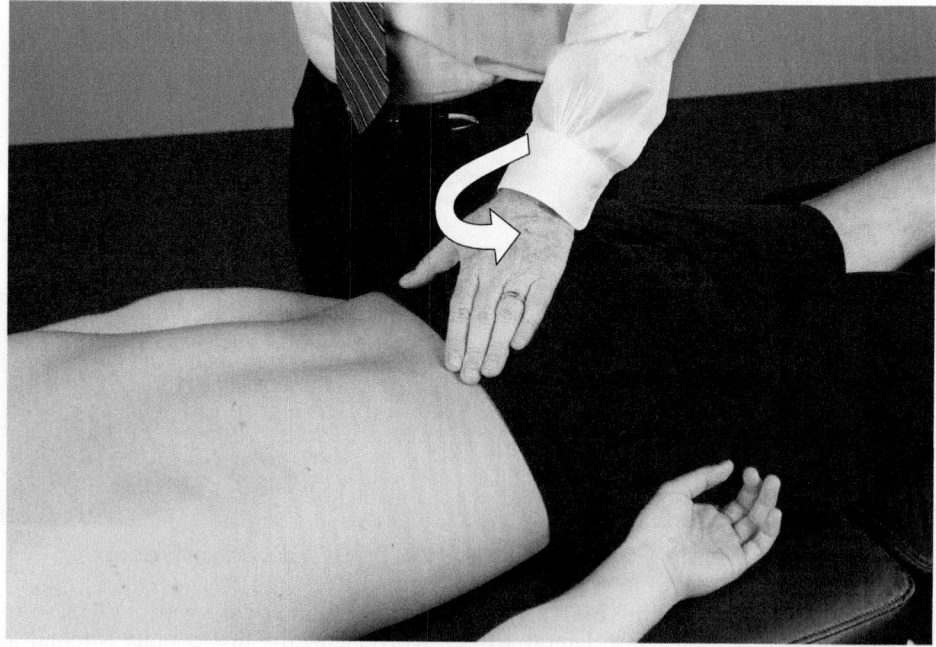

Figure 8-10 Stress Test for counter-clockwise sacrum; firm contact on sacrum with the palm of the hand, fingers pointed cephalad, parallel and over the sacral tubercles. Rotate your hand on the sacrum so that the right side of the sacrum is pushed superiorly, and the left side of the sacrum is pushed inferiorly.

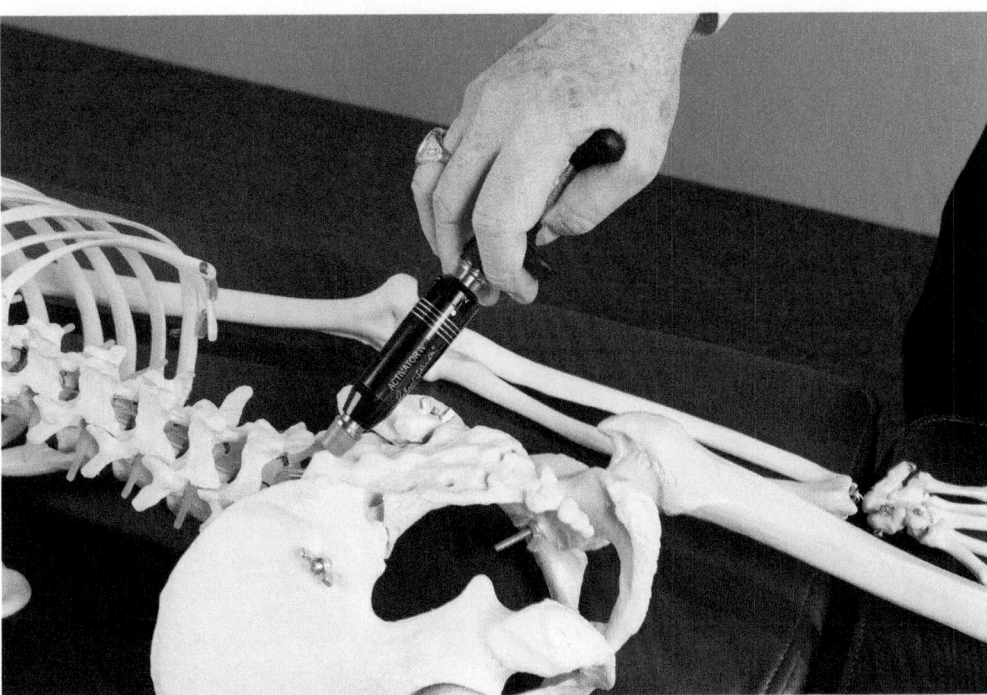

Figure 8-11 Adjustment clockwise sacrum. Step One: Contact just lateral to the first sacral tubercle on the right side. Line of Drive is anterior, medial, and slightly superior.

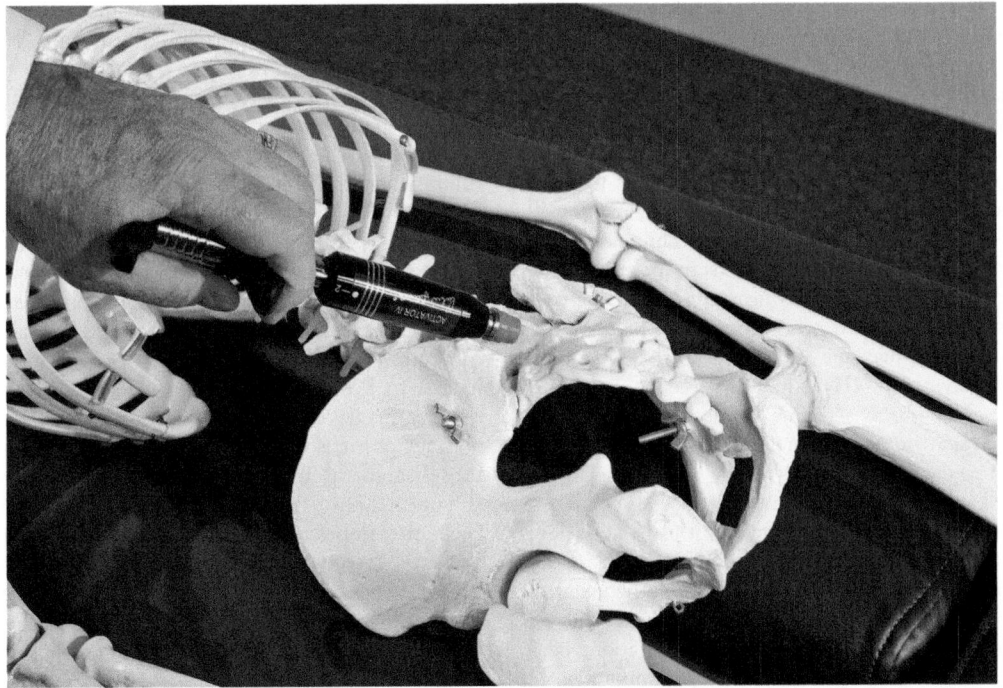

Figure 8-12 Adjustment clockwise sacrum. Step Two: Contact just lateral to the third sacral tubercle on the left side. Line of Drive is anterior, inferior, and slightly medial.

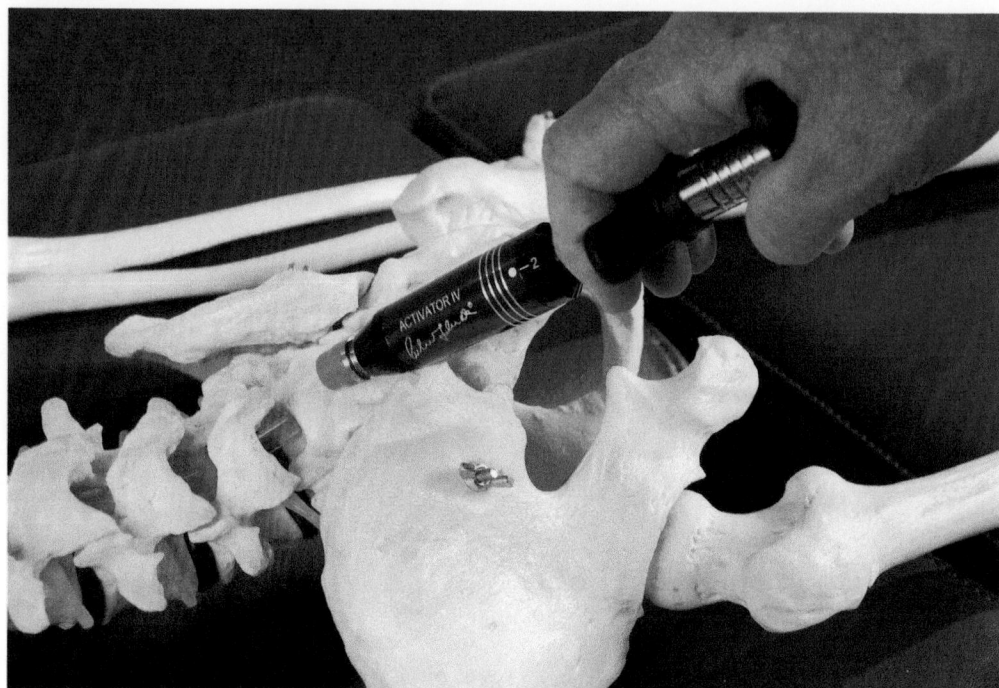

Figure 8-13   Adjustment counter-clockwise sacrum. Step One: Contact lateral to the first sacral tubercle on the left side. Line of Drive is anterior medial and slightly superior.

is found just lateral to the third sacral tubercle on the right side. The LOD is anterior, inferior, and slightly medial (Figure 8-14).

Clinical Observations

A patient with a lateral sacral base subluxation may be especially tender to deep palpation in the gluteal region. As the sacral base misaligns laterally, the apex tends to deviate to the opposite side. In fact, the malposition is analogous to the sacral apex right and sacral apex left subluxations of the Diversified and Thompson techniques.

Deviation of the sacrum tends to increase tension in the sacrotuberous ligament and may give rise to the painful trigger points often observed in the gluteus maximus of patients with low back and pelvic pain.[33] Hypertonicity of pelvic extensor muscles probably accounts for the restricted thigh extension noted on the side of sacral laterality during the Isolation Test.

Lateral sacral base subluxation may also underlie piriformis muscle contracture or spasm. The piriformis muscle, which originates on the sacrum and inserts on the greater trochanter of the femur, is a major external rotator of the hip. For the patient with lateral sacral base subluxation, be sure to evaluate hip function and perform an Isolation Test and adjustment as indicated for greater trochanter subluxations.

SIDE NOTE: INDIVIDUAL SACRAL SEGMENT If the pelvis has been cleared with the AM Basic Scan Protocol and additional advanced sacrum and pelvis adjustments have been made, but the patient continues to report "pinpoint" pain "right here," as the patient points to a particular spot on the sacrum, consider testing for individual sacral segment involvement. First, contact the PD side of the sacral base just lateral to the first sacral tubercle. Stress Test anteriorly while pulling your fingers inferiorly down the PD side of the sacrum (Figure 8-15). Look for reactivity in Position #1. If reactivity occurred, then Pressure Test the individual sacral segments on the Opposite PD (OPD) side, starting just lateral to the first sacral tubercle (Figure 8-16), and look for improvement in LLI in Position #1. If improvement is noted, this is a positive finding for the adjustment. The contact point is on the OPD side, just lateral to the first sacral tubercle. The LOD is anterior (Figure 8-17).

If no improvement in LLI occurred with Pressure Testing at the first sacral tubercle, then Pressure Test just lateral to the second sacral tubercle on the OPD side, observing for balance in Position #1. Continue Pressure Testing each sacral segment on the OPD side and looking for improvement in LLI in Position #1 to determine the individual sacral segment that may need adjustment.

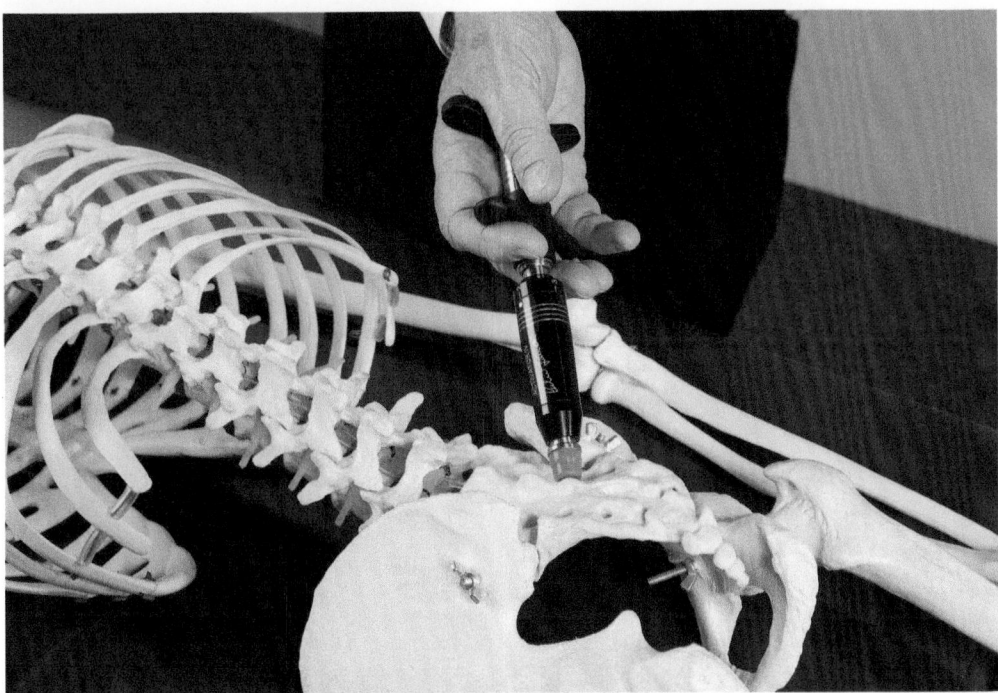

Figure 8-14 Adjustment counter-clockwise sacrum. Step Two: Contact just lateral to the third sacral tubercle on the right side. Line of Drive is anterior, inferior, and slightly medial.

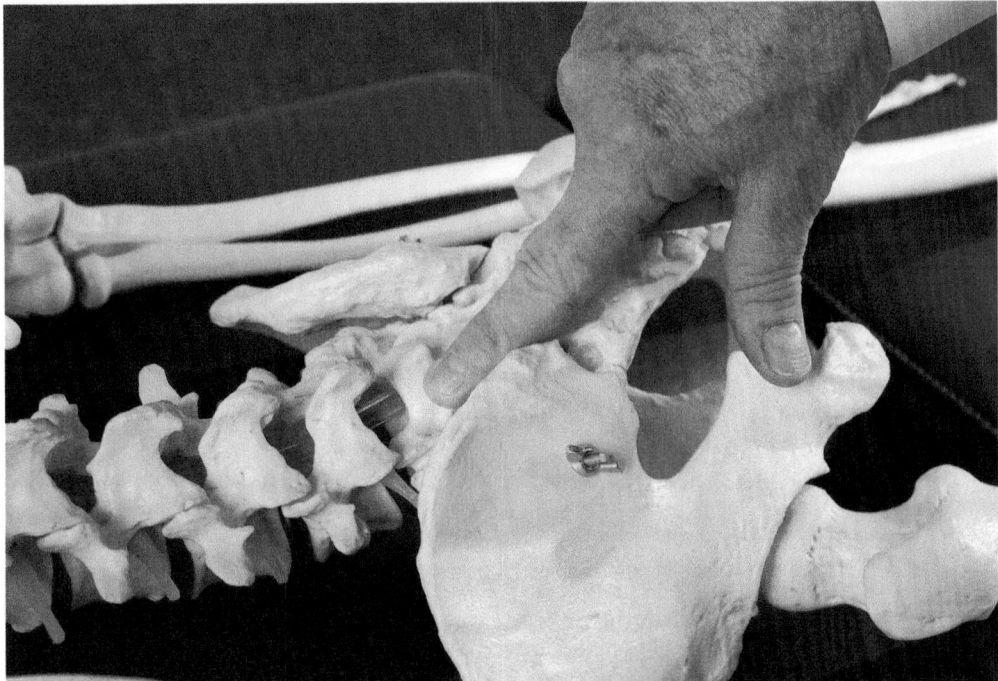

Figure 8-15 Stress Test Pelvic Deficiency (PD) side for individual sacral segments. First, contact the PD side of the sacral base just lateral to the first sacral tubercle. Stress Test anterior while pulling your fingers inferiorly down the PD side of the sacrum.

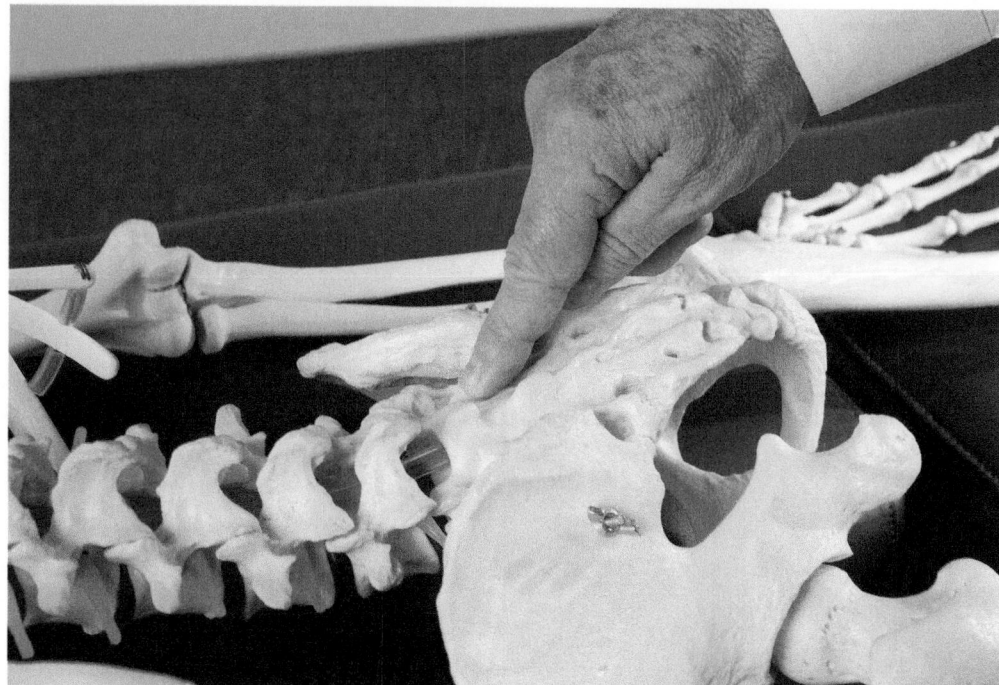

Figure 8-16 Pressure Test Opposite Pelvic Deficiency (OPD) side for individual sacral segments on the OPD side starting just lateral to the first sacral tubercle.

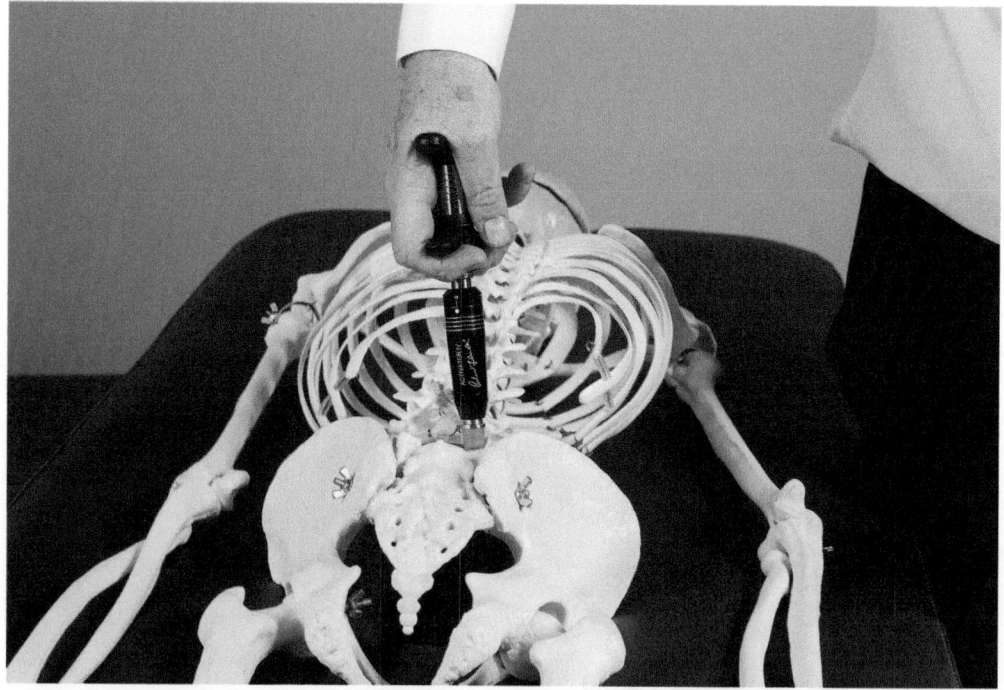

Figure 8-17 Adjustment for individual sacral segments. Line of Drive is anterior.

If no reactivity was observed when the Stress Test was used on the side of Pelvic Deficiency, consider Stress Testing on the OPD side. Contact just lateral to the first sacral tubercle on the OPD side. Stress Test in an anterior direction while pulling your fingers inferiorly down the OPD side of the sacrum. Look for reactivity in Position #1. Next, Pressure Test the individual sacral segments on the PD side, starting just lateral to the S1 tubercle, and look for improvement in LLI in Position #1 (Figure 8-18). If improvement is noted, adjustment is applied to the PD side, lateral to the first sacral tubercle, with an anterior LOD. If no improvement in LLI is seen with the Pressure Test at the first sacral tubercle, then Pressure Test just lateral to the second sacral tubercle on the PD side. Continue Pressure Testing each sacral segment on the PD side and looking for improvement in LLI in Position #1.

Most of the time, only one or two individualized sacral segments are involved. These can be found on the ipsilateral side or on the contralateral side from each other. Test to locate the sacral segment(s) that need to be adjusted. If the PD side was adjusted lateral to the first sacral tubercle, then the Stress Test on the OPD side would be used for the remaining sacral segments, and so forth.

Lateral Coccyx

Persistent pain in the sacrococcygeal region may result from misalignment of the coccyx. Coccydynia may be the consequence of a "fall on the tail bone" or cycling accidents.[18] With (1) patient complaints of hemorrhoids, (2) pain that occurs especially during sitting that localizes to the sacrococcygeal region, (3) women throughout pregnancy, labor, and delivery, and

(4) patient symptoms in the coccygeal region when sacral adjustments do not relieve symptoms, consider coccyx neuroarticular dysfunction.

Isolation Test. To test for a lateral coccyx, instruct the patient to squeeze the buttocks together (Figure 8-19). Look for PD leg reactivity in Position #1. Then proceed to Position #2, observing relative changes in the PD leg. Follow the Short/Long Rule to determine the side of adjustment. If the PD leg lengthens in Position #2, the base of the coccyx is malpositioned laterally toward the PD side. If the Pelvic Deficiency shortens in Position #2, the base of the coccyx is malpositioned laterally toward the OPD side.

Adjustment. To adjust a lateral coccyx malposition, contact is directed into the fibers of the sacrococcygeal ligament. Never directly contact the apex of the coccyx. Position the tip of the instrument just lateral to the base of the coccyx at the sacrococcygeal joint on the side indicated by the Short/Long Rule. The LOD is superior, lateral, and posterior (Figure 8-20).

To ensure an effective contact and a correct LOD, take a medial-to-lateral and inferior-to-superior tissue pull over the coccyx with the thumb of the free hand. The contact occurs in the soft tissue just lateral to the coccyx, and the force of the thrust is directed into the fibers of the sacrococcygeal ligament.

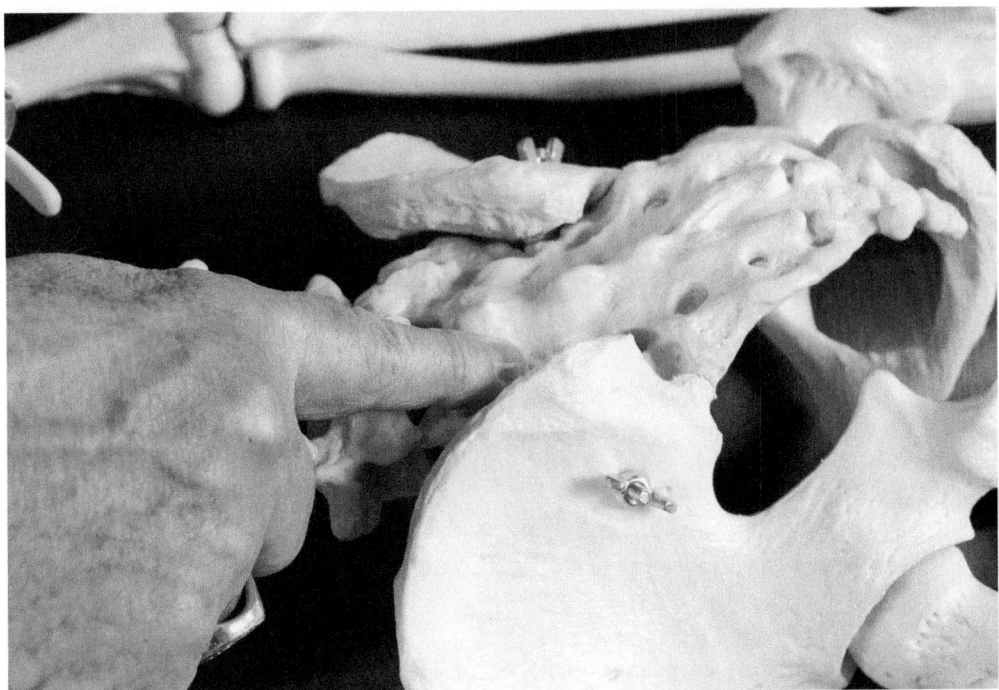

Figure 8-18 Pressure Test Pelvic Deficiency side for individual sacral segments starting just lateral to S1 tubercle. Look for improvement of the Leg Length Inequality in Position #1.

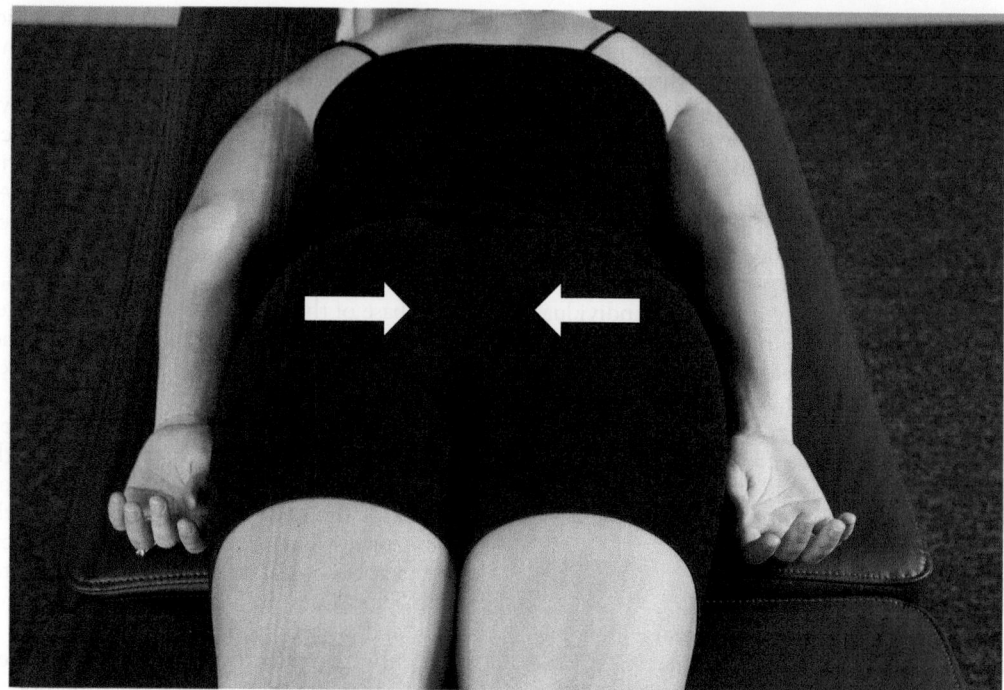

Figure 8-19 Isolation Test for coccyx; squeeze the buttocks together.

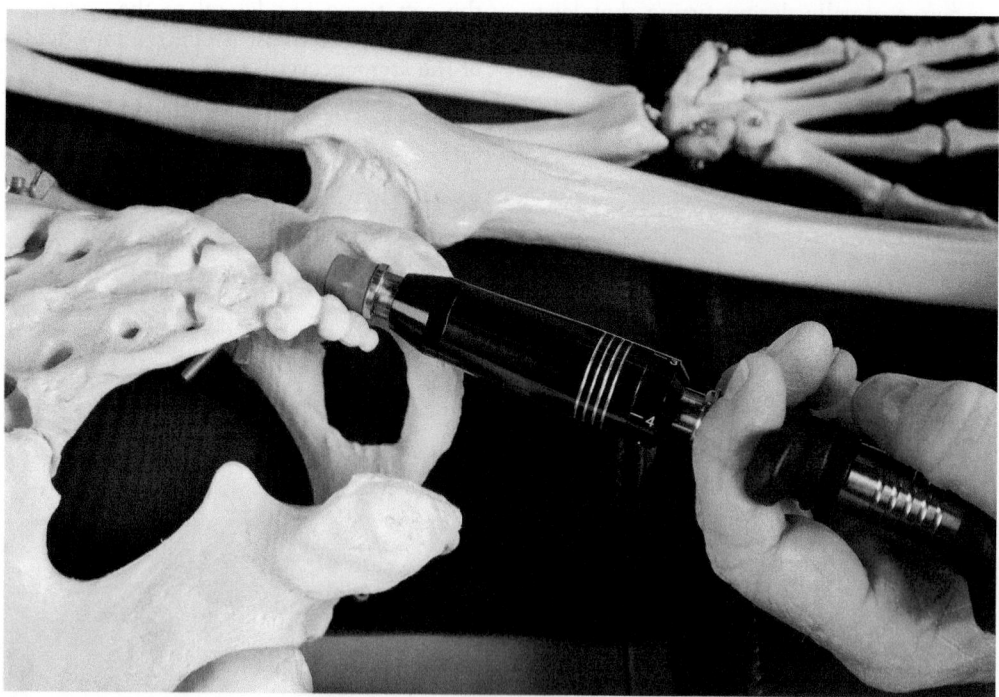

Figure 8-20 Adjustment for coccyx. Line of Drive is superior, lateral, and posterior.

Anterior or Posterior Base of the Coccyx

This involvement occurs frequently after a fall, after a slip involving the "splits" with contralateral hip flexion and hip extension, during late stages of pregnancy, and after childbirth. Also, consider whether symptoms are still present or LLI did not improve after adjustments were made for a lateral coccyx.

Stress Test. When involved, this is usually exquisitely tender, so apply the Stress Test with a light amount of pressure. First, contact the base of the coccyx and apply a gentle superior and anterior pressure (Figure 8-21). Look for PD leg reactivity in Position #1, indicating involvement of an anterior coccygeal base. If no reactivity occurred, contact the base of the coccyx and apply a very gentle inferior and anterior pressure (Figure 8-22). Look for PD leg reactivity in Position #1, indicating involvement of a posterior coccygeal base.

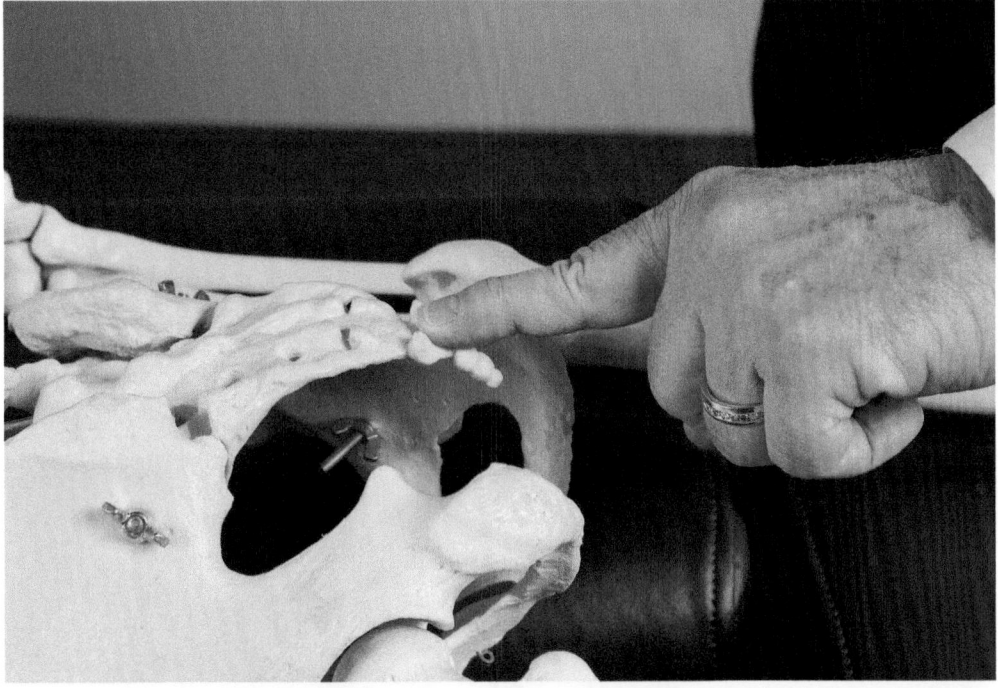

Figure 8-21   Stress Test for anterior coccyx base.

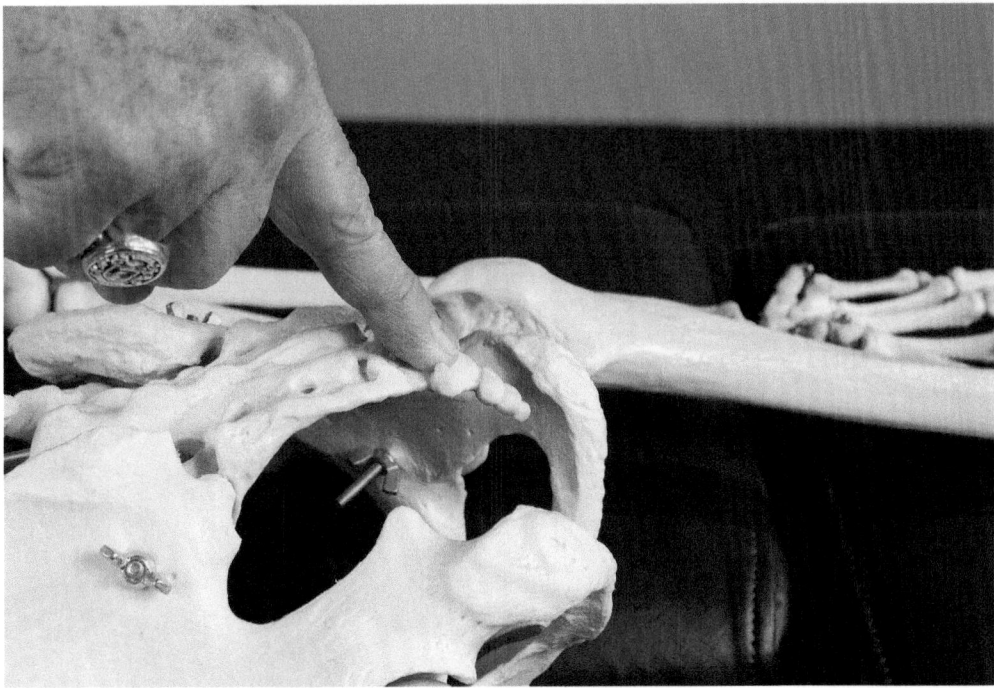

Figure 8-22   Stress Test for posterior coccyx base.

Adjustment.   Anatomically, a sacrococcygeal disc may be deranged, and/or a coccyx dislocation or fracture may have occurred. The integrity of the sacrococcygeal joint should be thoroughly evaluated before adjustments are made. All adjustments are made through the thumb or a digit on the lowest Activator Instrument setting.

For an anterior coccygeal base, contact the base of the coccyx with the thumb. Adjust through the thumb with an inferior and anterior LOD (Figure 8-23). For a posterior coccygeal base, contact the base of the coccyx. Adjust through the thumb with a superior and anterior LOD (Figure 8-24).

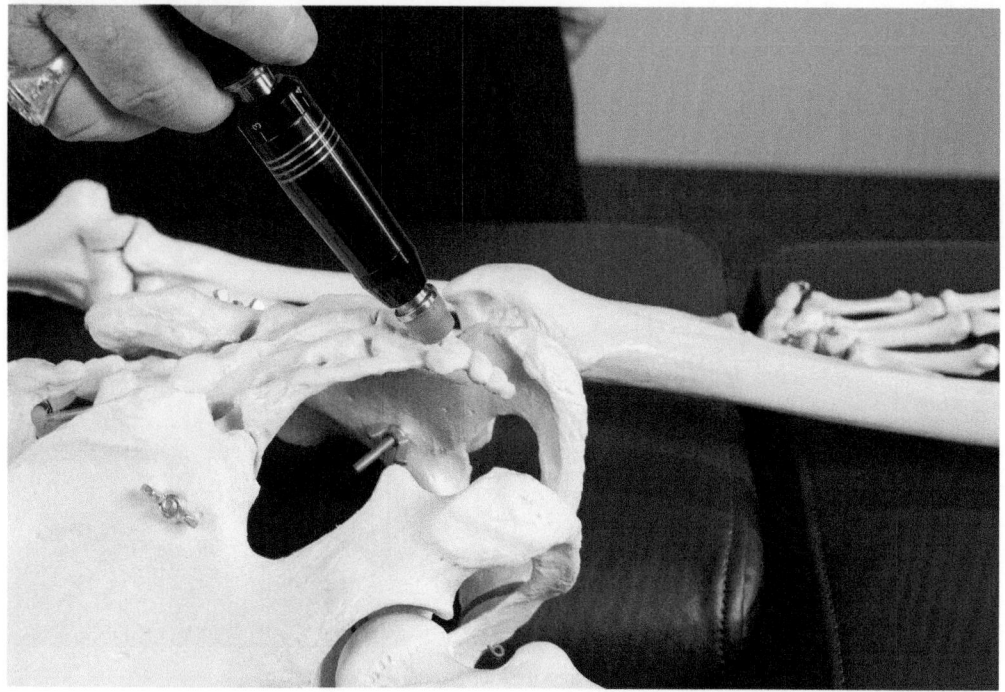

Figure 8-23   Adjustment for anterior coccyx base. Adjust through thumb. Line of Drive is inferior and anterior.

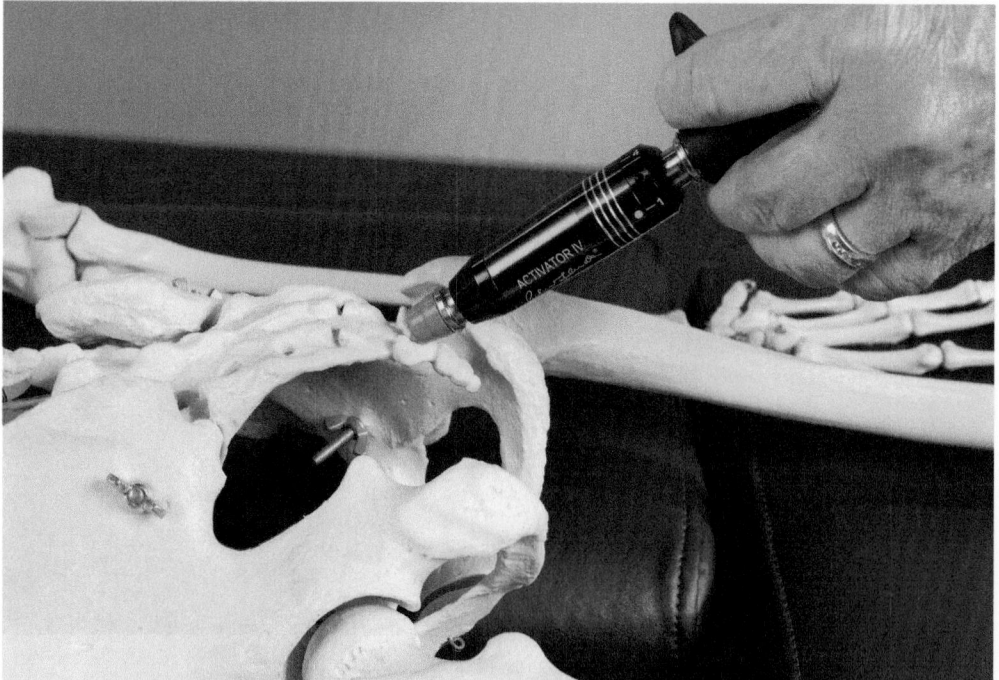

Figure 8-24   Adjustment for posterior coccyx base. Adjust through thumb. Line of Drive is superior and anterior.

Internal Ilium or Anterior-Inferior Sacrum

Rotation or torsion of the pelvic ring can cause a relatively internally rotated ilium or an anterior-inferior sacrum at the SI joint.[32] When a patient exhibits a flattening of the buttock on the PD side, possibly accompanied by an asymmetrical unilateral foot flare on the PD side, consider an internally rotated ilium or an anterior-inferior sacrum.

Stress Test. To test for an internal ilium or an anterior-inferior sacrum, passively extend the patient's PD hip to the point of tension to test for involvement of the SI joint on the PD side. The doctor places one hand under the anterior distal thigh above the knee of the PD side. Then perform the Stress Test by inducing hip extension, raising the patient's thigh off the table and extending the hip just to the point of tension (Figure 8-25). Lower the leg, and immediately look for PD leg reactivity in Position #1. Then proceed to Position #2, observing relative changes in the PD leg. If the PD leg lengthens in Position #2, the test indicates internal rotation of the ilium on the side of Pelvic Deficiency. If the PD leg shortens in Position #2, the test indicates an anterior-inferior sacrum on the side of Pelvic Deficiency.

Adjustment for Internal Ilium. To adjust an internally rotated ilium, contact the medial border of the posterior-superior iliac spine on the side of Pelvic Deficiency. The LOD is straight lateral (Figure 8-26).

Adjustment for Anterior-Inferior Sacrum. To adjust an anterior-inferior sacrum, position the tip of the instrument in the soft tissue mass of the gluteal muscles under the sacrotuberous ligament on the side of Pelvic Deficiency. The LOD is posterior, superior, and lateral (Figure 8-27) (same as second contact for a PI ilium in the Basic Scan).

> ### Clinical Observations
> Sudden onset of coccydynia may be related to trauma such as a fall or a cycling accident. However, trauma to the coccyx is not the only cause. Insidious onset of coccygeal pain has also been linked to clothing that fits too tight. Jeans appear to be the main culprit because denim is generally heavy, durable, and stretch resistant. Furthermore, denim jeans have a strong midline seam that provides very little give when the wearer is in a sitting position. Coccydynia is very common during pregnancy and in the postpartum period.

External Ilium or Posterior-Superior Sacrum

Rotation or torsion of the pelvic ring can also cause external rotation of the ilium or of a posterior-superior sacrum relative to the SI joint on the side Opposite Pelvic Deficiency.[30] External rotation of the ilium may result in bunching of the buttock musculature on the side of involvement, as well as an asymmetrical toe-in

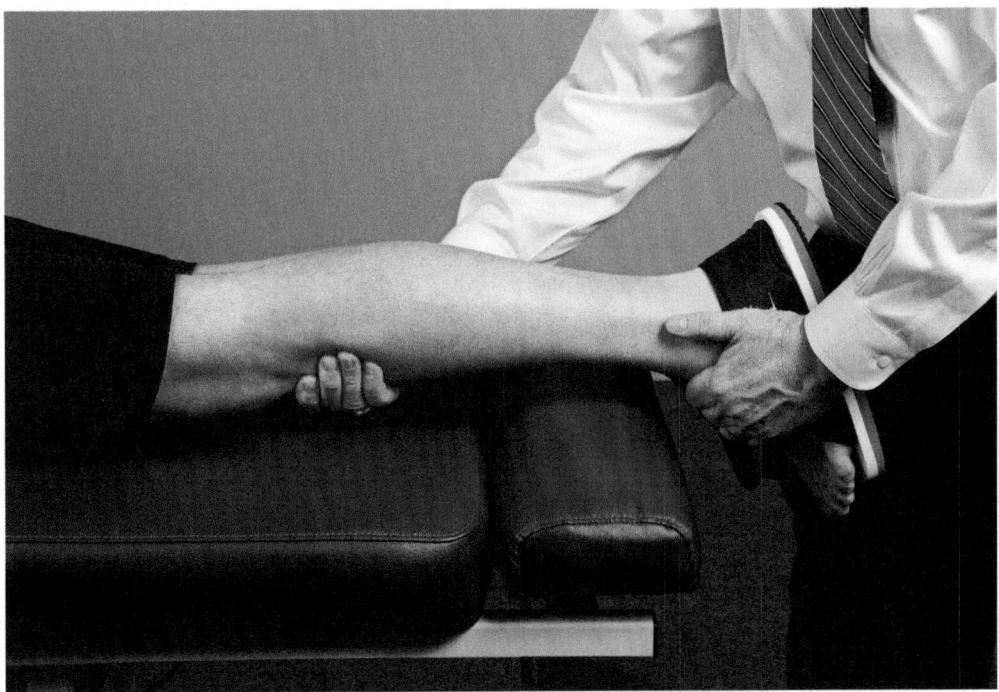

Figure 8-25 Stress Test on Pelvic Deficiency side for internal ilium or anterior-inferior sacrum.

deformity of the foot on the side Opposite Pelvic Deficiency.

Stress Test. To test for an external ilium or posterior-superior sacrum, passively extend the patient's leg at the hip on the side Opposite Pelvic Deficiency. The doctor places one hand under the anterior distal thigh above the knee of the OPD side. Then perform the Stress Test

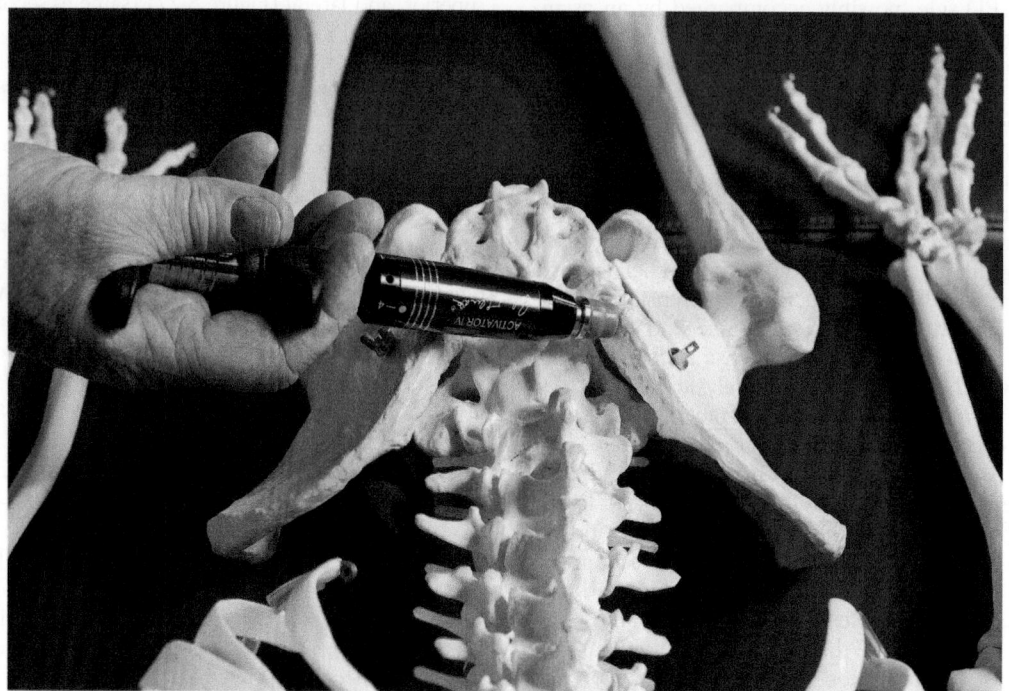

Figure 8-26 Adjustment for internal ilium. Line of Drive is lateral.

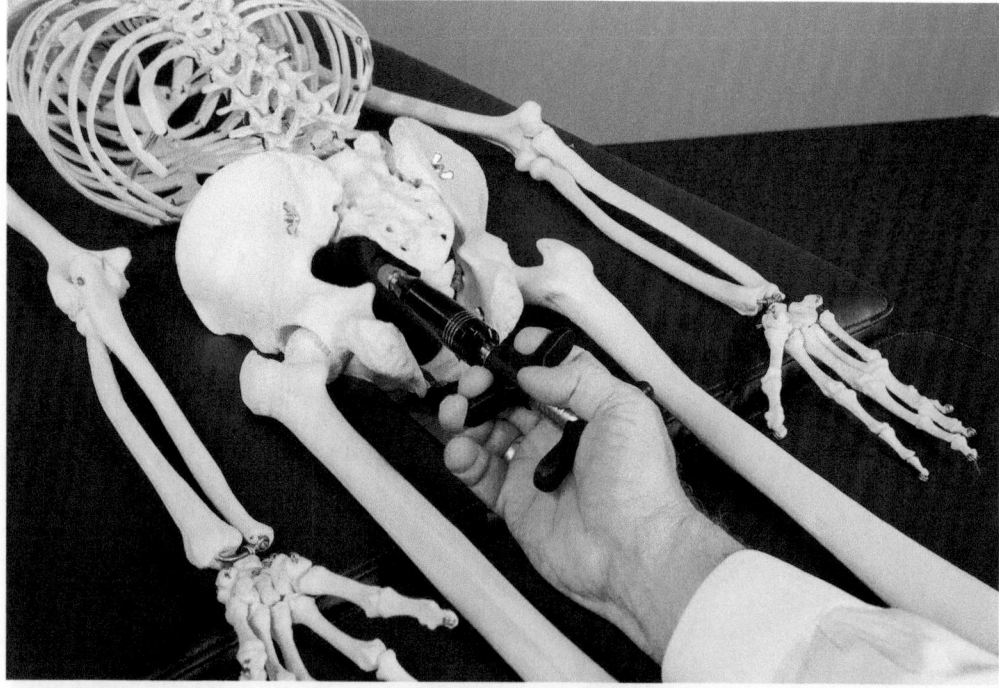

Figure 8-27 Adjustment for anterior-inferior sacrum. Line of Drive is posterior, superior, and lateral.

by inducing hip extension, raising the patient's thigh off the table, and extending the hip just to the point of tension (Figure 8-28). Lower the leg, and immediately look for PD leg reactivity in Position #1. Then proceed to Position #2, observing relative changes in the PD leg. If the PD leg lengthens in Position #2, the test indicates an external ilium on the side Opposite Pelvic Deficiency. If the PD leg shortens in Position #2, the test indicates a posterior-superior sacrum on the side Opposite Pelvic Deficiency.

Adjustment for External Ilium. To adjust an externally rotated ilium, contact the lateral aspect of the posterior-superior iliac spine on the side Opposite Pelvic Deficiency. The LOD is straight medial (Figure 8-29).

Adjustment for Posterior-Superior Sacrum. To adjust a posterior-superior sacrum, position the tip of the instrument one-half inch lateral to the first sacral tubercle on the side Opposite Pelvic Deficiency. The LOD is anterior and inferior (Figure 8-30).

CLINICAL TIP: To help remember the test findings, Lengthening is iLium involvement, and Shortening is Sacral involvement. Keep the *L*'s and the *S*'s together. Raising the PD leg is an internal iLium with Lengthening in Position #2. Raising the PD leg is an AI Sacrum (the second contact of the PI ilium) with Shortening in Position #2. When raising the OPD leg, Lengthening

in Position #2 is an external iLium. Raising the OPD leg is a PS Sacrum (first contact of an AS ilium) with Shortening in Position #2.

Bilateral Lateral Iliums

For the elderly patient with a sedentary lifestyle, it is frequently difficult and uncomfortable to get up from a sitting position. The patient may have vague low back pain and stiffness without a specific history of trauma or concurrent illness. Consider bilateral lateral iliums.

Stress Test. To test bilateral lateral iliums, contact the medial aspect of both posterior-superior iliac spines. Simultaneously push straight laterally across both posterior-superior iliac spines as if to open the SI articulations (Figure 8-31). Look for reactivity of the PD leg in Position #1. Because this is a Stress Test for bilateral involvement of the iliums at the SI joints, it is not necessary to raise the legs to Position #2.

Adjustment. To adjust bilateral lateral iliums, use two instruments simultaneously if possible. Apply the tip of the instruments to the lateral aspect of each posterior-superior iliac spine. The LODs are straight medial (Figures 8-32 and 8-33).

Bilateral Lateral Ischial Tuberosities

Bilateral dysfunction of the SI joints may result from repetitive motion injury to the pelvis. Truck drivers, farmers, and other heavy

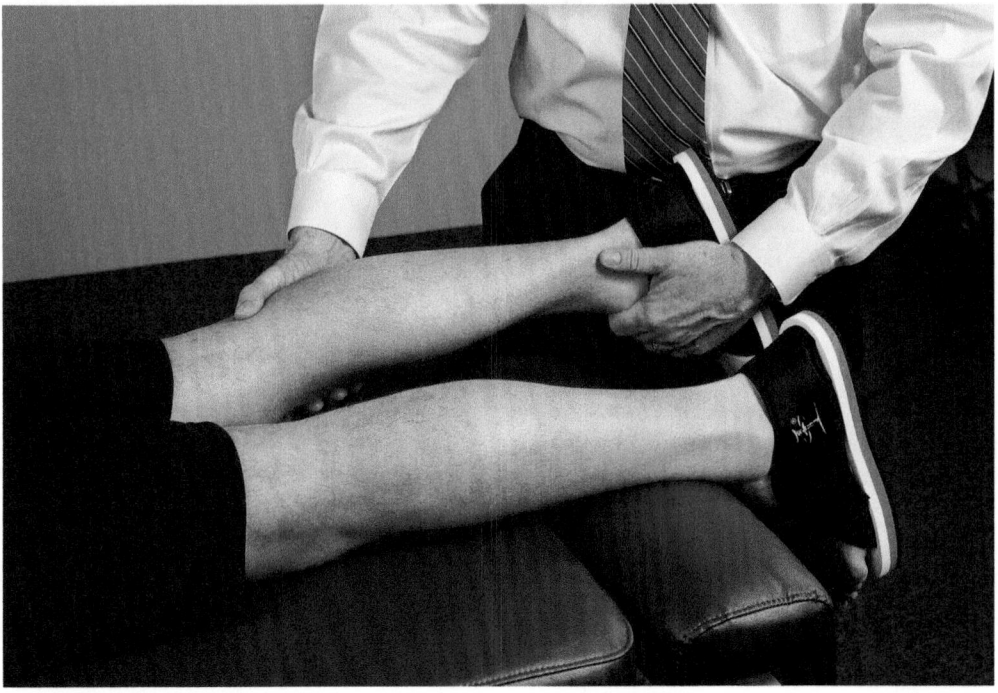

Figure 8-28 Stress Test on Opposite Pelvic Deficiency side for external ilium or posterior-superior sacrum.

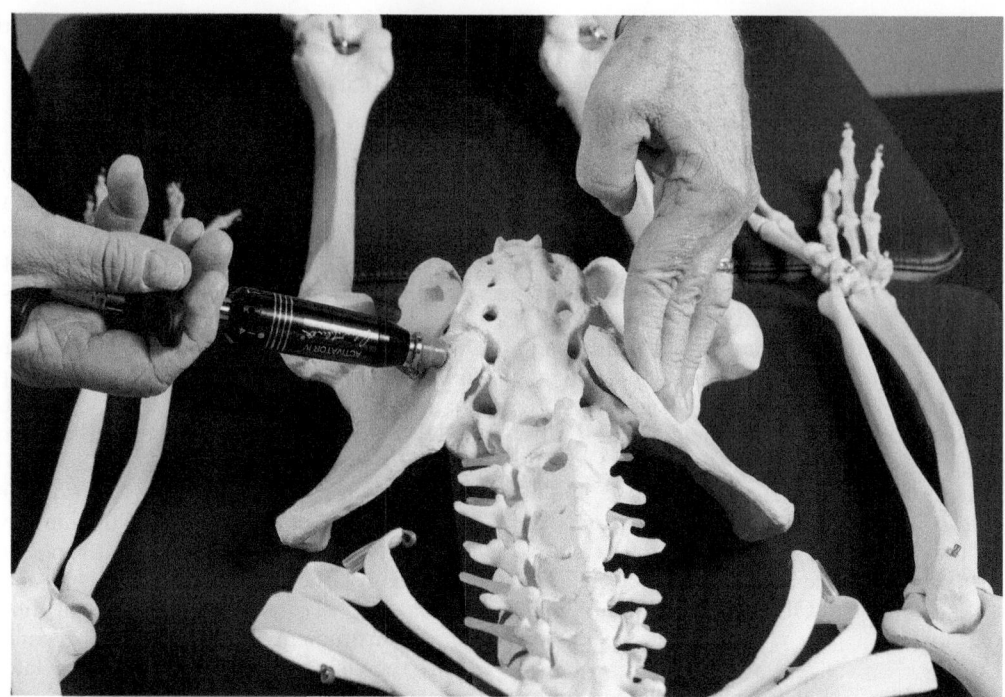

Figure 8-29 Adjustment for external ilium. Line of Drive is medial.

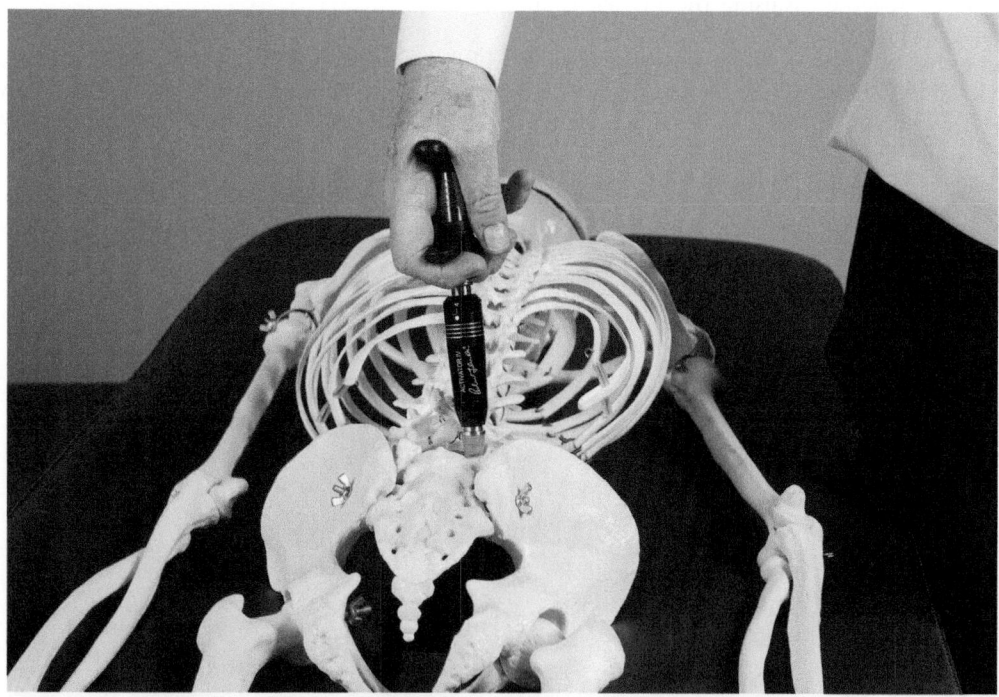

Figure 8-30 Adjustment for posterior-superior sacrum. Line of Drive is anterior-inferior.

equipment operators may be at increased risk of developing bilateral lateral iliums because of the vibratory impact on the low back and pelvis associated with truck and tractor seats. Other factors may include sitting on narrow seats or stools, bicycling, and motorcycle riding, especially when the activity is done in an extraordinary way. This could involve the "weekend warrior" who goes out for a long ride on a Saturday, having not participated in this activity for

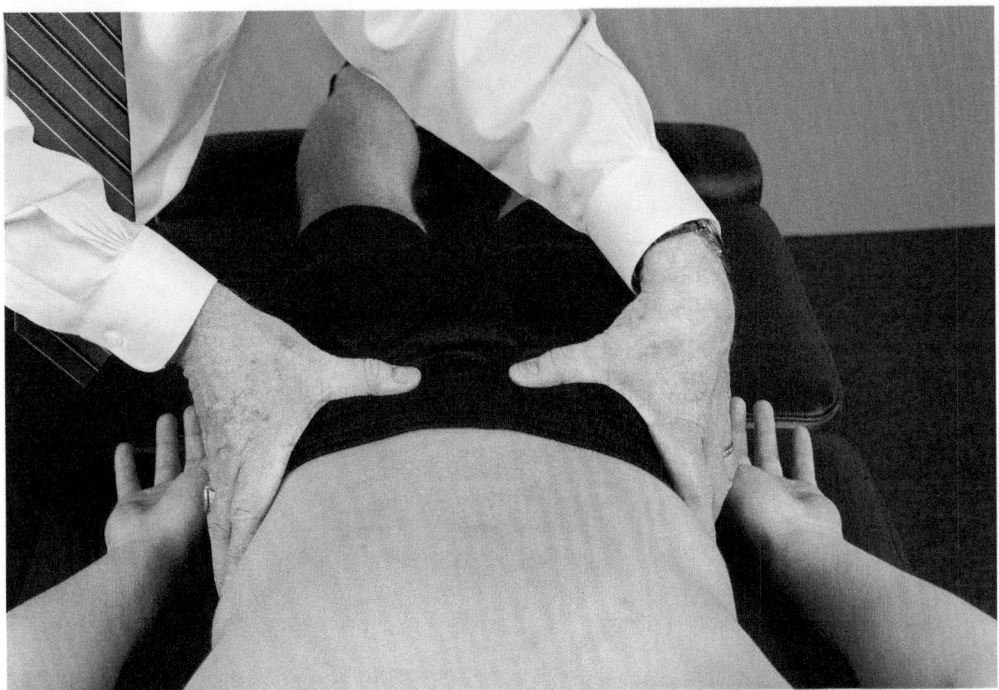

Figure 8-31 Stress Test for bilateral lateral iliums.

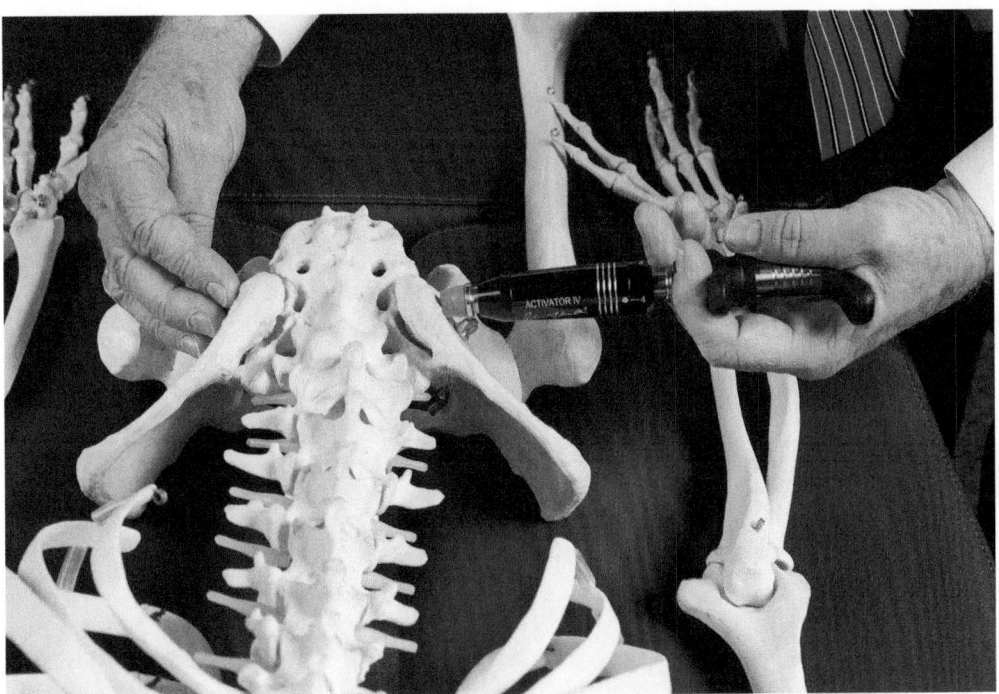

Figure 8-32 Adjustment for bilateral lateral iliums, one of two. Line of Drive is medial.

days or weeks. The patient typically complains of pain, a deep ache, or a "muscle pull" and points directly to the ischial tuberosity.

Stress Test. To test for bilateral lateral ischial tuberosities, place a thumb on the medial aspect of each tuberosity. Apply a firm, gentle pressure simultaneously on the tuberosities in a straight lateral direction (Figures 8-34 and 8-35). Look for reactivity of the PD leg in Position #1. Because this is a test for bilateral involvement of the ischial tuberosities, it is not necessary to raise the legs to Position #2.

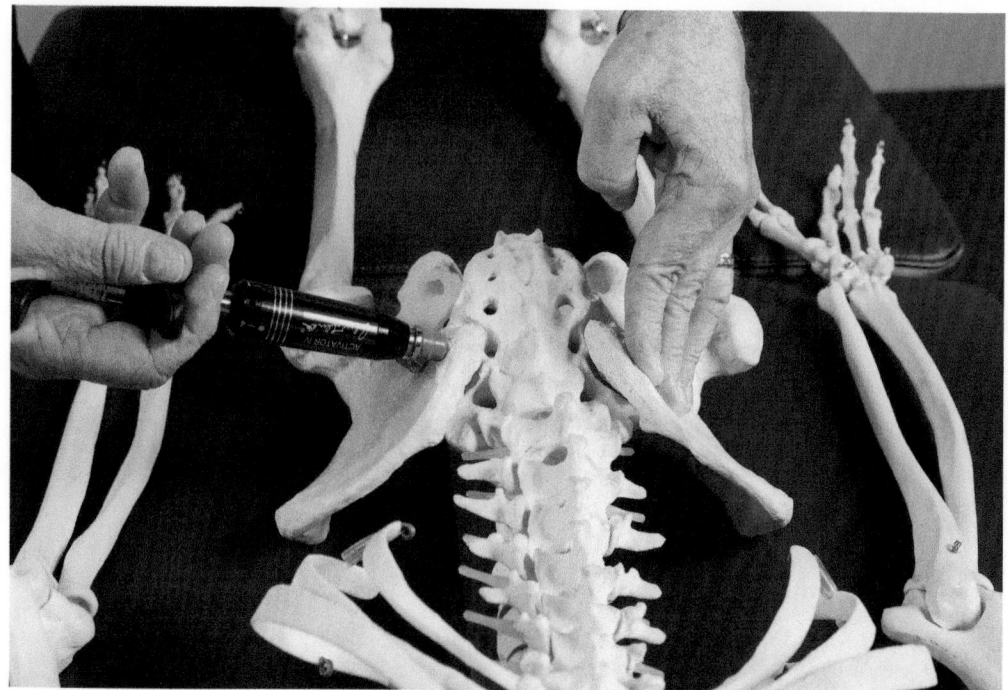

Figure 8-33   Adjustment for bilateral lateral iliums, two of two. Line of Drive is medial.

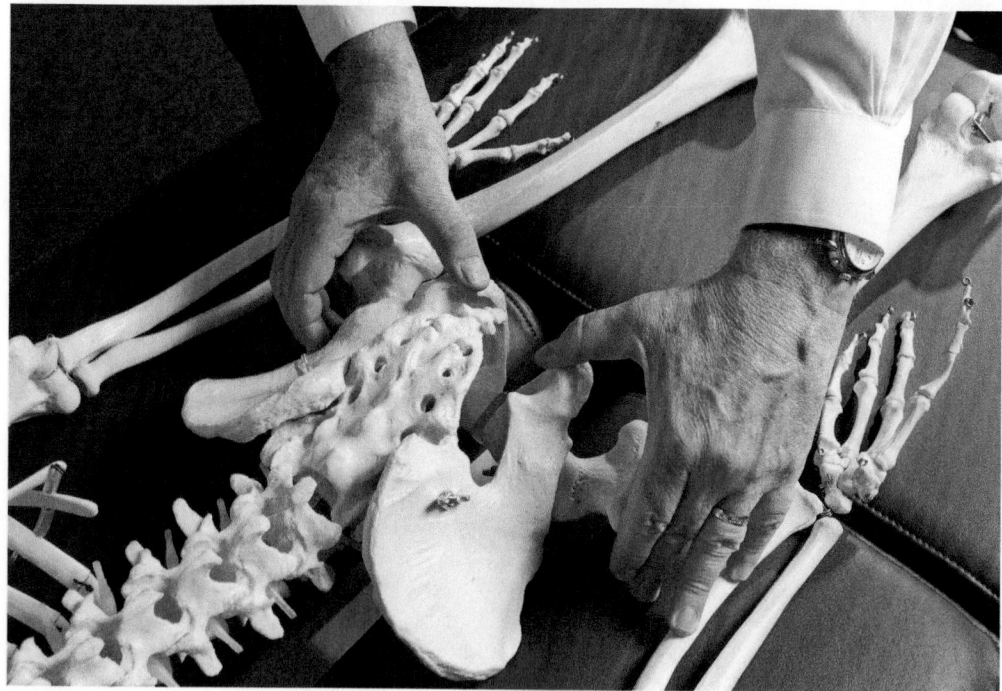

Figure 8-34   Stress Test for bilateral lateral ischial tuberosities.

Adjustment.   To adjust bilateral lateral ischial tuberosities, use two instruments if possible. Contact the lateral aspect of each ischial tuberosity with the tips of the instruments. The LOD for each instrument is straight medial. If only one instrument is used, block the opposite ischial tuberosity when performing the adjustment (Figures 8-36 and 8-37).

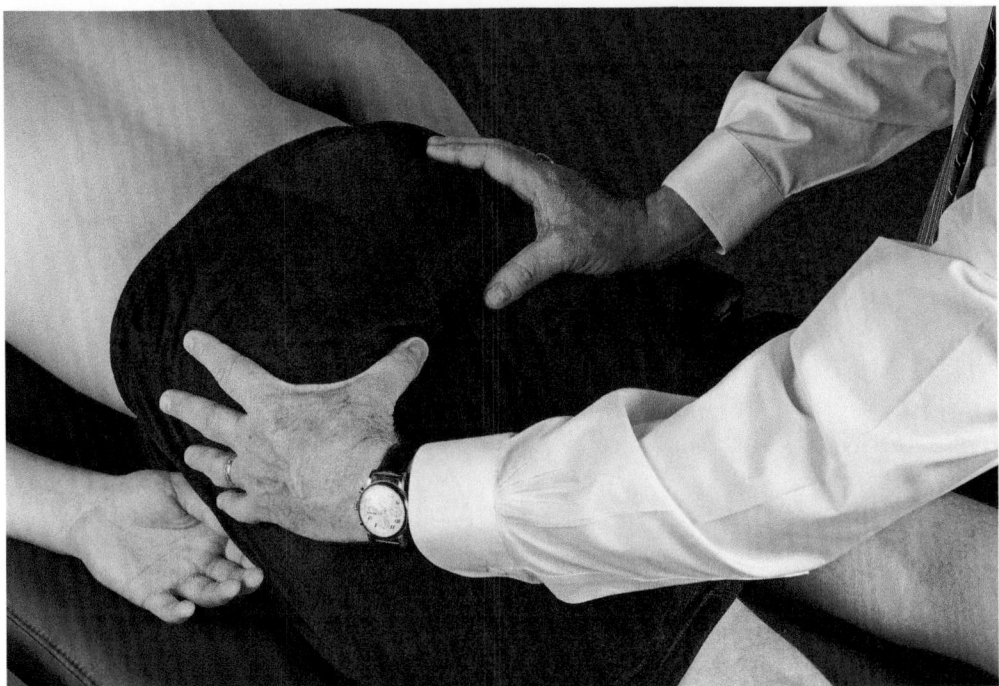

Figure 8-35 Stress Test for bilateral lateral ischial tuberosities.

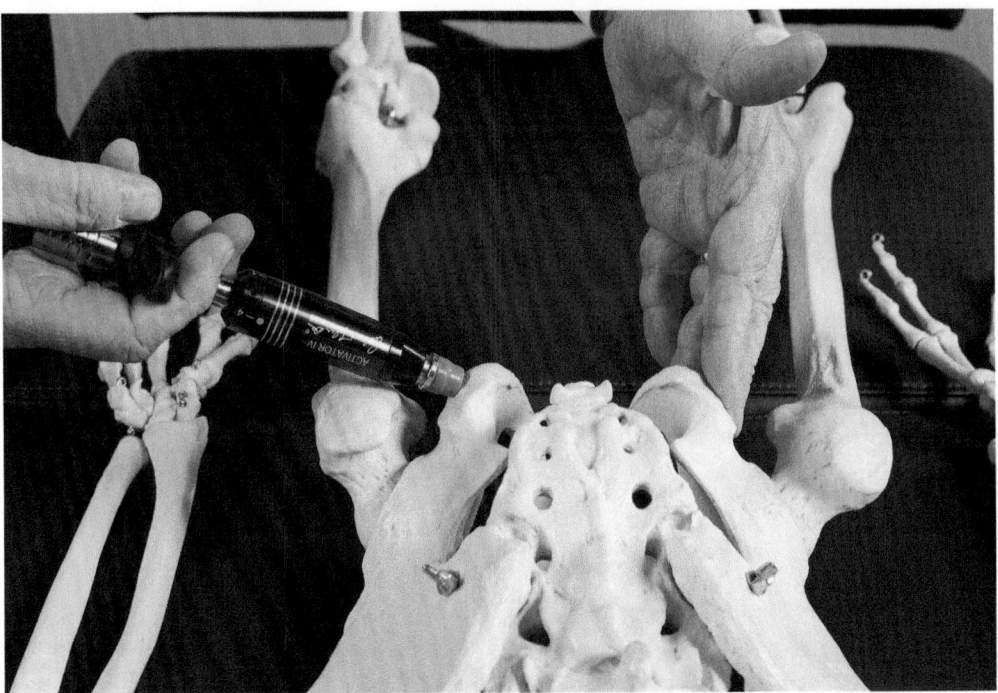

Figure 8-36 Adjustment for bilateral lateral ischial tuberosities, one of two. Line of Drive is medial.

Medial Ischial Tuberosity

In those patients who complain of pain upon sitting, pain in the posterior thigh, hamstring tightness, or difficulty standing for long periods because of tension in the hamstrings, consider testing for a medial ischial tuberosity on the involved side.

Stress Test. To Stress Test for a medial ischial tuberosity, push the ischial tuberosity on the involved side in a lateral-to-medial direction

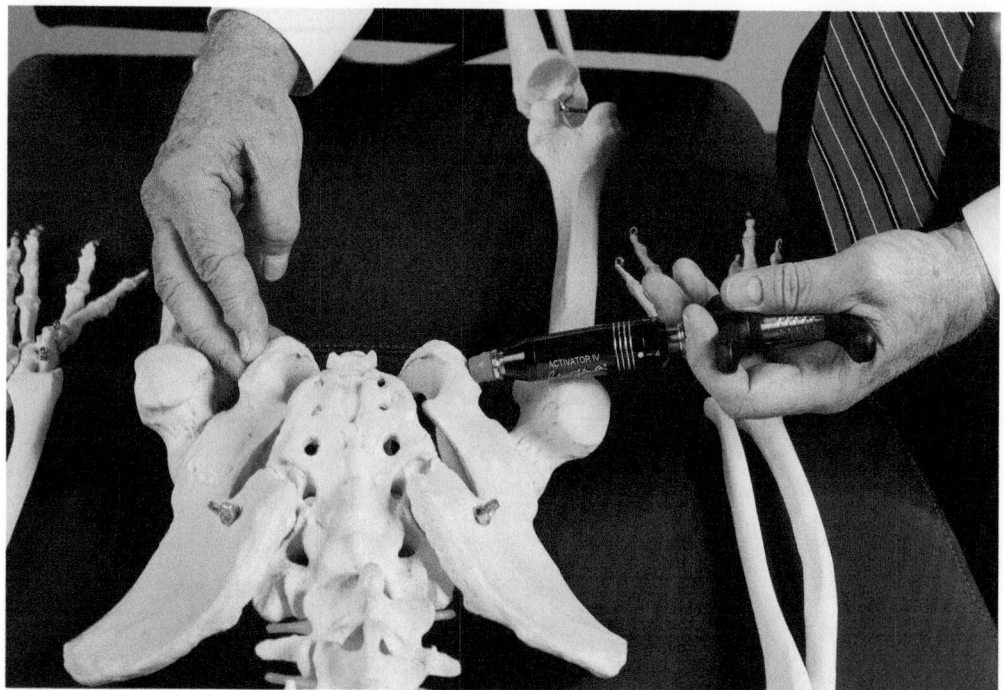

Figure 8-37 Adjustment for bilateral lateral ischial tuberosities, two of two. Line of Drive is medial.

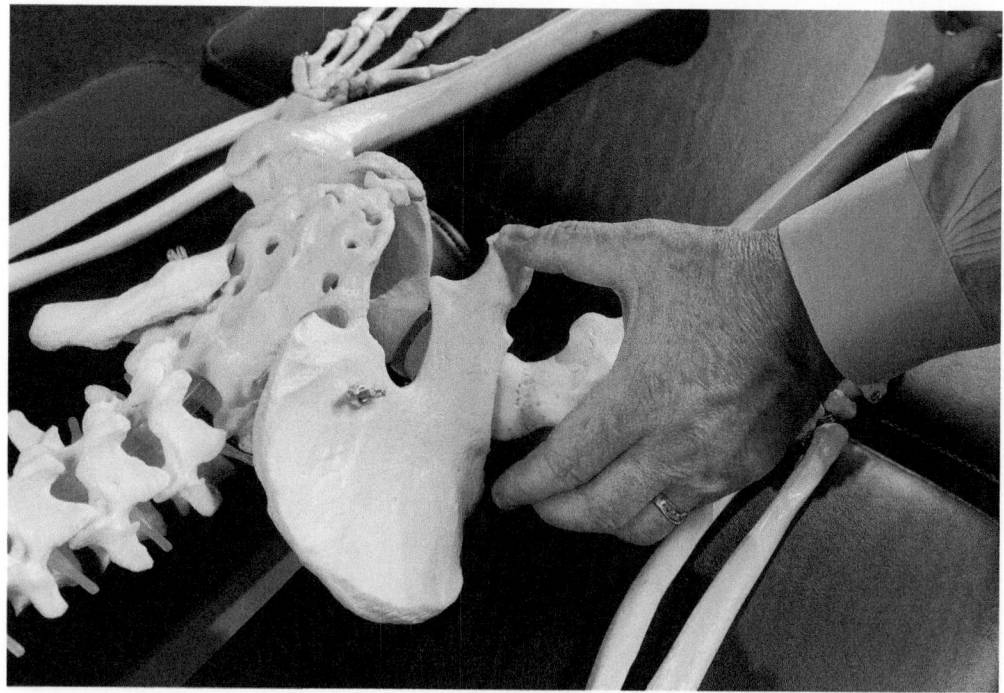

Figure 8-38 Stress Test for medial ischium.

(Figure 8-38). Look for reactivity of the PD leg in Position #1.

Adjustment. To adjust a medial ischial tuberosity, contact the medial border of the ischial tuberosity. The LOD is lateral (Figure 8-39).

Anterior Pubic Bone

When hip or SI dysfunctions recur, or when adjustments are not maintained, consider the third component of the pelvic girdle—the symphysis pubis. Stability of the bony ring of the

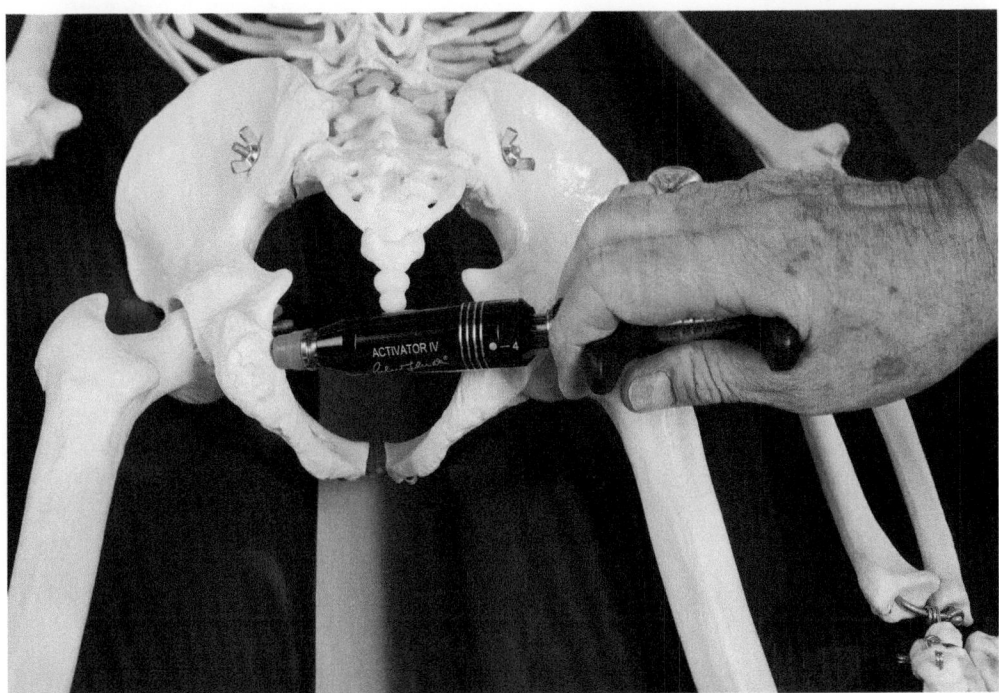

Figure 8-39   Adjustment for medial ischium. Line of Drive is lateral.

pelvis is only as strong as its weakest component, and if the symphysis pubis is misaligned, the SI and hip joints may not be able to maintain their full functional integrity. Superior and inferior pubic bone Stress Tests are part of the AM Basic Scan Protocol, but adjustment of inferior or superior pubic bones may not completely resolve dysfunction of the pelvic girdle. Therefore consider an anterior malposition of the pubic bone.

Isolation Test.   To isolate an anterior pubic bone, ask the patient to press the hip on the side of the PD leg against the surface of the table (Figure 8-40). Look for reactivity of the PD leg in Position #1. If no reaction is detected in the PD leg, ask the patient to press the hip on the side Opposite Pelvic Deficiency against the surface of the table. Again, look for reactivity of the PD leg in Position #1.

Adjustment.   To adjust an anterior pubic bone, raise the table and reposition the patient in the supine position. Contact the anterior aspect of the pubic bone just lateral to the symphysis pubis. The LOD is straight posterior (Figure 8-41).

SIDE NOTE: After doing the Isolation Test for superior or inferior pubes in the Basic Scan Protocol and determining the malposition that needs to be adjusted, begin testing for an anterior pube and then proceed with testing for the lateral pube before raising the table and placing the patient in the supine position. This maximizes the patient's and the doctor's time and avoids repositioning of the patient numerous times.

SIDE NOTE: PRONE PUBIC ADJUSTING During the Basic Scan Protocol, the pubes are isolated when the patient is instructed to squeeze the knees together. Look for PD leg reactivity in Position #1. Then proceed to Position #2, while observing relative changes in the PD leg. A modification is used by following the Short/Long Rule. In Position #2, lengthening indicates a superior pube on the PD side, and shortening indicates an inferior pube on the OPD side. The adjustment requires the patient to be in the supine position. Instead of changing the patient's position in the middle of the Basic Scan assessment, many experienced AM practitioners will wait until they have finished testing and adjusting the patient prone before they reposition the patient supine. When you are using this procedure, before you reposition the patient to a supine position to adjust for pubic bone involvement, it is wise to perform the pubic bone Isolation Test again.

An alternative is to use a prone pube adjustment if the test reveals a superior pube on the PD side. Contact the opposite ischial tuberosity on the posterior aspect. The LOD is straight anterior (Figure 8-42). Re-perform the Isolation Test, after the adjustment is made, by instructing the patient to squeeze the knees together while you look in Position #1 for reactivity.

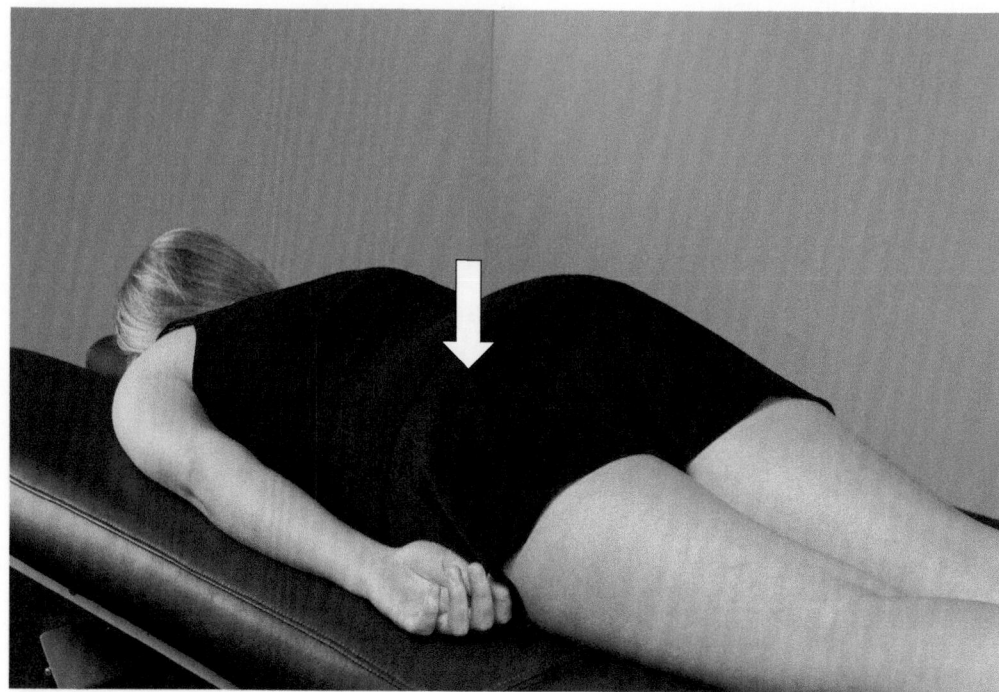

Figure 8-40   Isolation Test for anterior pubic bone; press the hip against the surface of the table.

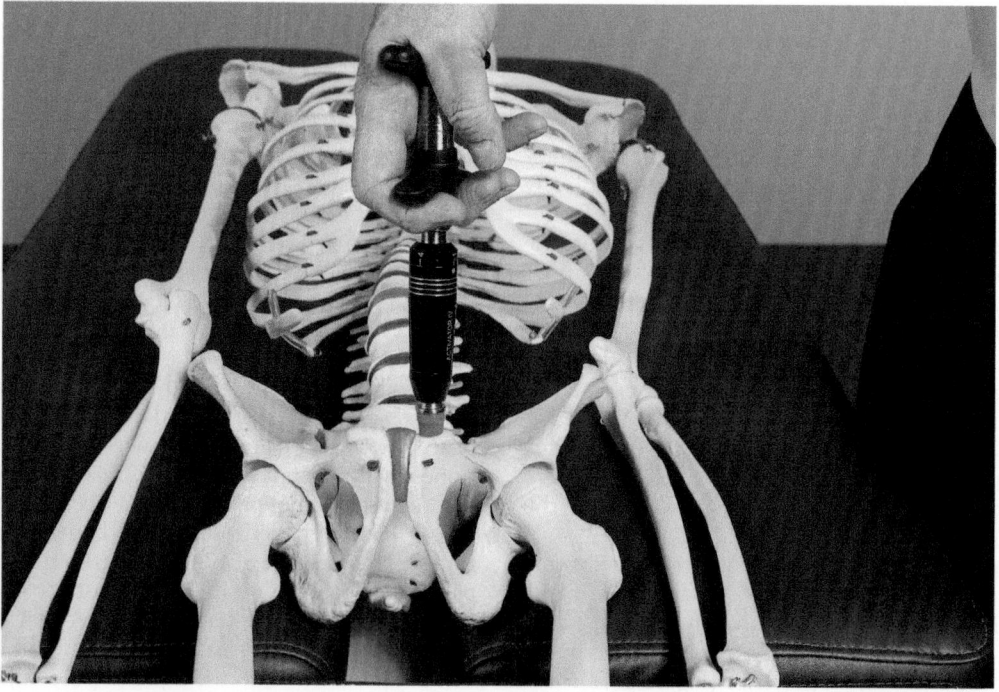

Figure 8-41   Adjustment for anterior pubic bone. Line of Drive is posterior.

This is a good procedure to use to make sure the adjustment was corrective. If reactivity is noted in Position #1, the correction was not made, and the traditional adjustment on the anterior aspect of the pubic bone will have to be performed with the patient in the supine position (Figure 8-43).

SIDE NOTE: LATERAL PUBE When a patient experiences severe groin pain or is unable to ambulate without pain, consider testing for a lateral pube.

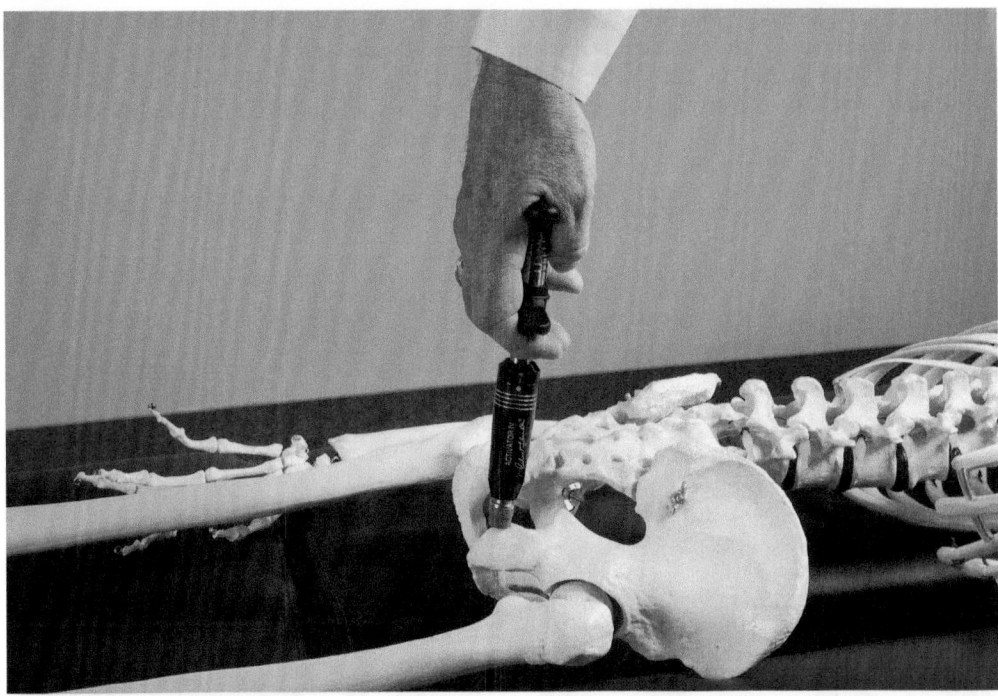

Figure 8-42 Prone adjustment for a superior Pelvic Deficiency pubic bone.

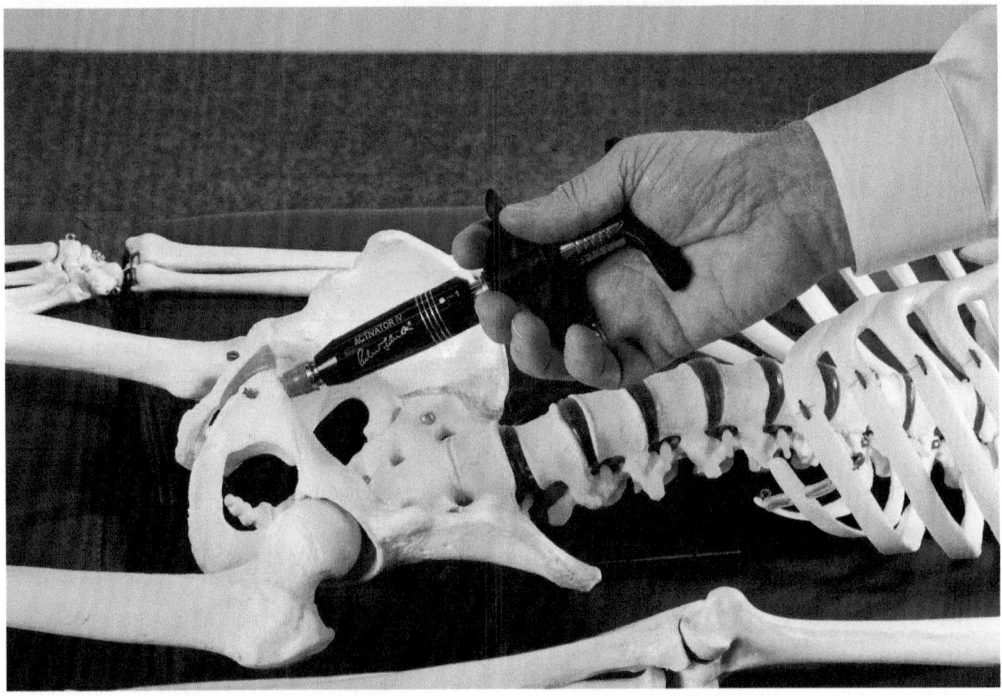

Figure 8-43 Adjustment for superior pubic bone. Line of Drive is inferior.

Isolation Test. Before stressing, all pelvic and trochanteric tests should have been completed and adjusted as indicated. After isolating the pubes, as per Basic Scan Protocol, use Position #4 with the PD leg flexed past 90 degrees, until you meet resistance. Look for PD leg reactivity in Position #1. Then proceed to Position #2, while observing relative changes in the PD leg. The side of lengthening in Position #2 is the side of laterality of the involved pubic bone.

Adjustment.   To adjust for a lateral pube, contact the involved pubic bone, which is three quarters of an inch lateral to the pubic symphysis, while the LOD is directly medial (Figure 8-44).

Mechanical force, manually assisted chiropractic adjusting (AM) for the pelvis and sacrum are summarized in Table 8-1. See also Boxes 8-1, 8-2, and 8-3 for summaries of related research.

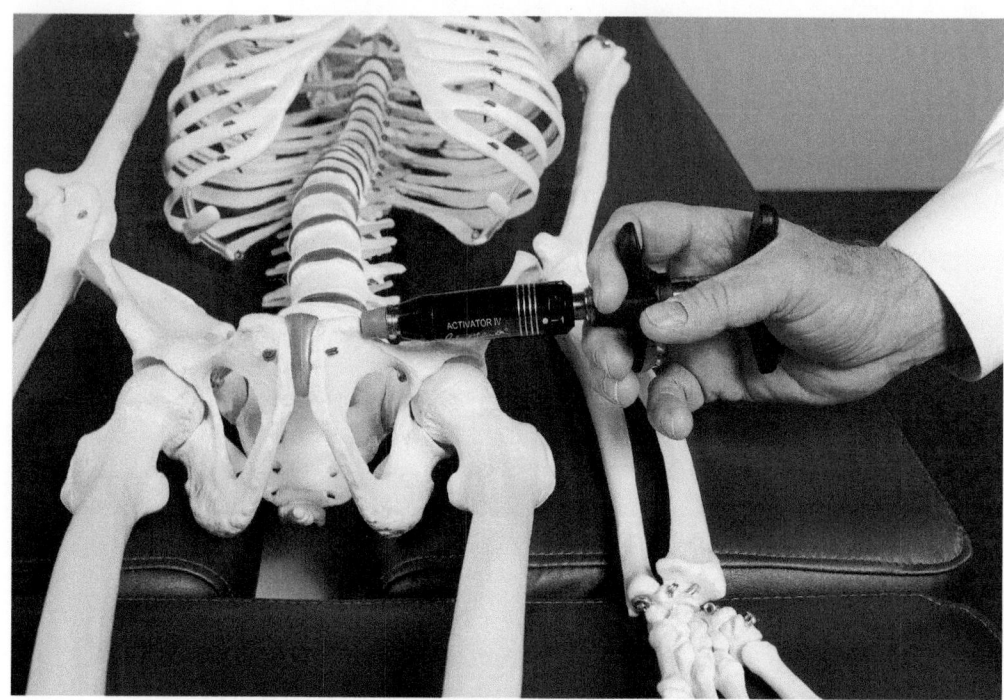

Figure 8-44   Adjustment for lateral pubic bone. Line of Drive is medial.

Table 8-1   Summary Table of Tests and Adjustments for the Sacrum, Pelvis, and Related Structures

Articular Dysfunction	Test	Segmental Contact Point	Line of Drive
		ADJUSTMENT	
Anterior Sacral Base	Flex legs to Position #3—PD leg lengthens	Superior aspect of third sacral tubercle	Anterior-inferior
Posterior Sacral Base	Flex legs to Position #3—PD leg shortens	Inferior aspect of first sacral tubercle	Anterior-superior
Lateral Sacral Base	Position #4	Inferior-lateral aspect of third sacral tubercle on the side indicated by the Short/Long Rule	Medial and slightly superior
Alternative Lateral Sacral Base	Instruct patient to lift each leg off table without bending at the knee. The sacrum is lateral toward restricted leg side, usually away from Pelvic Deficiency.	Inferior-lateral aspect of third sacral tubercle on the restricted hip extension side	Medial and slightly superior

Table 8-1	**Summary Table of Tests and Adjustments for the Sacrum, Pelvis, and Related Structures—cont'd**		

| Articular Dysfunction | Test | ADJUSTMENT | |
		Segmental Contact Point	Line of Drive
Internal Ilium	Lift and extend patient's leg on PD side. Lengthening in Position #2.	Medial border of PSIS	Lateral
or Anterior-Inferior Sacrum	Shortening in Position #2	Under sacrotuberous ligament on PD side	Posterior, superior, and lateral
External Ilium	Lift and extend patient's leg on side OPD. Lengthening in Position #2.	Lateral border of PSIS on OPD	Medial
or Posterior-Superior Sacrum	Shortening in Position #2	Posterior sacrum one-half inch lateral to first sacral tubercle on OPD	Anterior-inferior
Sacral Clockwise Rotation	Doctor places palm on sacrum, with firm contact rotating in clockwise direction	*Step One*: Lateral to first sacral tubercle on the right side	Anterior, superior, and slightly medial
		Step Two: Lateral to third sacral tubercle on the left side	Anterior, inferior, and slightly medial
Sacral Counter-Clockwise Rotation	Doctor places palm on sacrum, with firm contact rotating in counter-clockwise direction	*Step One*: Lateral to first sacral tubercle on the left side	Anterior, superior, and slightly medial
		Step Two: Lateral to third sacral tubercle on the right side	Anterior, inferior, and slightly medial
Bilateral Lateral Iliums	Push lateral on both PSIS	Lateral aspect of each PSIS with the use of two instruments simultaneously	Medial
Bilateral Lateral Ischial Tuberosities	Push lateral on both ischial tuberosities simultaneously	Lateral aspect of the ischial tuberosity with the use of two instruments simultaneously	Medial
Medial Ischial Tuberosity	Push medial on involved ischial tuberosity	Medial ischial tuberosity	Lateral
Lateral Coccyx	Instruct patient to squeeze buttocks together	Sacrococcygeal ligament lateral to the base of the coccyx on the side indicated by the Short/Long Rule	Superior, lateral, and posterior

Continued

Table 8-1	**Summary Table of Tests and Adjustments for the Sacrum, Pelvis, and Related Structures—cont'd**		
		ADJUSTMENT	
Articular Dysfunction	**Test**	**Segmental Contact Point**	**Line of Drive**
Anterior Base of Coccyx	Stress Test base of coccyx; push lightly with stroking motion superior and anterior	Contact base of coccyx with thumb	Through thumb, inferior and anterior
Posterior Base of Coccyx	Stress Test base of coccyx; push lightly with stroking motion inferior and anterior	Contact base of coccyx with thumb	Through thumb, superior and anterior
Anterior Pubic Bone	Instruct patient to push pubes one at a time into surface of table	Anterior aspect of pubic bone	Posterior
Lateral Pubic Bone	Instruct the patient to squeeze the knees together. After checking Positions #1 and #2, use Position #4. Follow Short/Long Rule.	Contact the involved pube on the lengthening side, three quarters of an inch lateral to the pubic symphysis	Medial
Sacral Segments	Stress downward on PD side of sacrum just lateral to sacral tubercles	Pressure Test individual OPD sacral segments, starting just lateral to first sacral tubercle. If balancing does not occur, continue Pressure Testing second, then third sacral tubercle.	Anterior
	Stress downward on OPD side of sacrum just lateral to sacral tubercles	Pressure Test individual PD sacral segments, starting just lateral to first sacral tubercle. If balancing does not occur, continue Pressure Testing second, then third sacral tubercle.	Anterior

OPD, Opposite Pelvic Deficiency; *PD,* Pelvic Deficiency; *PSIS,* posterior superior iliac spine.

RELATED RESEARCH

Box 8-1

Reference: Osterbauer PJ, DeBoer KF, Widmaier RS, Petermann EA, Fuhr AW. Treatment and biomechanical assessment of patients with chronic sacroiliac joint syndrome. J Manipulative Physiol Ther. 1993;16(2):82–90.

ABSTRACT
OBJECTIVE
To evaluate diagnostic and biomechanical correlates and treatment outcomes of manipulative/adjustive care in patients highly selected for sacroiliac joint syndrome (SIJS)

DESIGN
Descriptive case series, 1-week baseline, 1-year follow-up

SETTING
Private practice of chiropractic

PATIENTS
Ten of 153 consecutive new patients (4 male and 6 female) with "primary," chronic, uncomplicated SIJS were selected over an 11-month period on the basis of painful SIJ and provocation tests.

OUTCOME MEASURES
Back pain (visual analog scale), Oswestry disability index, lumbar provocation tests, and biomechanical measures of gait and postural sway

INTERVENTION
Six-week regimen of mechanical force, manually assisted (MFMA), short lever adjustments with an Activator instrument

RESULTS
Pain decreased significantly from a mean baseline value of 25 to 12 (t = 2.28; p < .05). Likewise, average disability scores diminished from 28% to 13% (t = 2.3; p < .05), and a reduction in the number of positive provocation tests was noted (Fisher's exact probability range, Z = 0.025 to 0.045). Gait and sway parameters were indistinguishable from those without pain, before or after treatment. Response to the 1-year follow-up questionnaire (6/10) revealed stability of symptoms at a low level.

CONCLUSIONS
Although most subjects recorded some degree of positive outcome, we conclude that (1) discrete SIJS remains difficult to diagnose, but diagnosis may be possible through judicious choice of screening tests; (2) MFMA may benefit some patients with chronic SIJ pain; and (3) gait and sway measurement yielded no correlation with clinical condition.

Box 8-2

Reference: Polkinghorn BS, Colloca CJ. Chiropractic treatment of coccygodynia via external instrumental adjusting procedures utilizing Activator Methods Chiropractic Technique. J Manipulative Physiol Ther. 1999;22(6):411–6.

ABSTRACT
OBJECTIVE
To discuss a case of coccygodynia that responded favorably to conservative chiropractic adjusting procedures with the Activator Method technique and the Activator II Adjusting Instrument (AAI-II).

CLINICAL FEATURES
A 29-year-old woman had unremitting coccygeal pain of 3 weeks' duration. The problem began after she had moved heavy boxes while at work. The pain was characterized by a continual dull ache in the coccygeal region, accompanied by intermittent sharp pain, particularly upon sitting or rising from a seated position. She had been taking self-prescribed over-the-counter analgesics (aspirin and ibuprofen) for 3 weeks without obtaining relief.

INTERVENTION AND OUTCOME
Treatment consisted of mechanical force, manually assisted short-lever chiropractic adjusting procedures to the coccygeal area, primarily the sacrococcygeal ligament. The AAI-II was used to deliver the adjustment according to diagnostic and treatment protocols as specified for the Activator Method. The patient experienced complete resolution of her pain after the first treatment.

Continued

Box 8-2—cont'd

CONCLUSION

Chiropractic coccygeal manipulation may be effectively delivered via instrumental adjustment in certain cases of coccygodynia. The use of an AAI-II in administering the coccygeal adjustment has the benefit of ensuring a gentle, noninvasive procedure that is comfortably tolerated by the patient. This method of coccygeal adjustment may warrant consideration in certain cases of coccygodynia.

Box 8-3

Reference: Shearar K, Colloca C, White H. A randomized clinical trial of manual versus mechanical force manipulation in the treatment of sacroiliac joint syndrome. J Manipulative Physiol Ther. 2004;28(1):493–501.

ABSTRACT

This study was submitted as a dissertation to the Faculty of Health, in compliance with the requirements for the Master's Degree in Technology from the Chiropractic Department, Durban Institute of Technology, Durban, South Africa. Sacroiliac joint (SIJ) syndrome is a common presenting disorder among patients with back pain. Previous research has demonstrated a benefit of spinal manipulation in patients with SIJ syndrome. However, no study has compared the relative effectiveness of different forms of spinal manipulation or chiropractic adjustments in its management. The purpose of this study was to determine the relative effect of instrument-delivered as compared with traditional, manually delivered thrust chiropractic adjustments in the treatment of SIJ syndrome.

METHODS

A prospective, randomized, comparative clinical trial was conducted at the outpatient chiropractic clinic, Durban Institute of Technology, Durban, South Africa. Sixty patients (31 male, 29 female, ages 18 to 59 years) in whom SIJ syndrome was diagnosed were randomly assigned to two groups of 30 subjects. Each subject received four chiropractic adjustments over a 2-week period and was subsequently evaluated at 1-week follow-up. The subjects in one group (group 1) received side posture, high-velocity, low-amplitude (HVLA) chiropractic adjustments for symptomatic SIJ via the National-Diversified technique. Subjects in the other group (group 2) received mechanical force, manually assisted (MFMA) chiropractic adjustments for symptomatic SIJ with the use of an Activator Adjusting Instrument. Both groups received only chiropractic adjustment as treatment intervention, and no other treatment modalities or interventions, including medications, were used. Outcomes included the Numerical Pain Rating Scale (NRS)-101, the Revised Oswestry Low Back Pain Disability Questionnaire (Oswestry), algometry, and the Orthopedic Rating Scale (ORS). Outcomes were statistically analyzed with the Mann-Whitney U test (for intergroup analysis) and Friedman's t test (for intragroup analysis) to assess differences from the first to the third and final consultations within and between groups.

RESULTS

No significant differences between groups were noted at the initial consultation for any of the subjective and objective variables. Statistically significant improvements in subjective and objective outcomes were observed in both groups from the first to third, third to fifth, and first to fifth consultations for all measures except pain pressure threshold. Specifically, statistically significant improvements ($p < .001$) in mean NRS (group 1 = 49.1 to 23.4; group 2 = 48.9 to 22.5), Oswestry (group 1 = 37.4 to 18.5; group 2 = 36.6 to 15.1), ORS (group 1 = 7.6 to 0.6; group 2 = 7.5 to 0.8), and algometry measures (group 1 = 4.8 to 6.5; group 2 = 5.0 to 6.8) were observed from the first to the last visit for both groups. Statistical analysis of subjective and objective data showed equal improvement for both groups. Intergroup analysis showed a slight difference between the two groups, favoring MFMA (group 2). However, these observations were not statistically significant for all outcome measures.

CONCLUSION

The results of this clinical trial indicate that a relatively short regimen of both MFMA and HVLA chiropractic adjustments provides a beneficial effect associated with reducing pain and disability in patients with SIJ syndrome. Neither MFMA nor HVLA adjustments were found to be more effective than the other in the treatment of this patient population.

REFERENCES

1. Vink P, Kamphuisen HAC. Leg length inequality, pelvic tilt and lumbar back muscle activity during standing. Clin Biomech. 1989;4:115-7.
2. Strong R, Thomas PE. Patterns of muscle activity in the leg, hip, and torso associated with anomalous fifth lumbar conditions. J Am Osteopath Assoc. 1968;67(9):1039-41.
3. D'Amico JC, Dinowitz HD, Polchaninoff M. Limb length discrepancy: an electrodynographic analysis. J Am Podiatr Med Assoc. 1985;75(12):639-43.
4. Cummings G, Scholz JP, Barnes K. The effect of imposed leg length difference on pelvic bone symmetry. Spine. 1993;18(3):368-73.
5. Jacob HAC, Kissling RO. The mobility of the sacroiliac joints in healthy volunteers between 20 and 50 years of age. Clin Biomech. 1995;10(7):352-61.
6. Lawrence DJ. Sacroiliac joint—part two: clinical considerations. In: Cox JM, editor. Low back pain mechanism, diagnosis and treatment. 5th ed. Baltimore: Williams & Wilkins; 1990. p. 229-42.
7. Hildebrandt RW. Chiropractic spinography: a manual of technology and interpretation. 2nd ed. Baltimore: Williams & Wilkins; 1985.
8. Cooperstein R. The Derefield pelvic leg check: a kinesiological interpretation. Chiro Tech. 1991;3(2):60-5.
9. Murphy BA, Dawson NJ, Slack JR. Sacroiliac joint manipulation decreases the H-reflex. Electromyogr Clin Neurophysiol. 1995;35(2):87-94.
10. Harrison DD. Spinal biomechanics: a chiropractic perspective. Self-published, 1992.
11. National Institutes of Health (NIH). Low back pain fact sheet. Bethesda (MD): NIH; November 8, 2006.
12. Nachemson AL. Newest knowledge of low back pain. A critical look. Clin Orthop. 1992;(279):8-20.
13. Pitkin HC, Pheasant HC. Sacrarthrogenetic telalgia. J Bone Joint Surg Am. 1936;18:365-74.
14. Fortin JD, Aprill CN, Ponthieux B, Pier J. Sacroiliac joint: pain referral maps upon applying a new injection/arthrography technique. Part II: clinical evaluation. Spine. 1994;19(13):1483-9.
15. Schwarzer AC, Aprill CN, Bogduk N. The sacroiliac joint in chronic low back pain. Spine. 1995;20(1):31-7.
16. Fortin JD, Dwyer AP, West S, Pier J. Sacroiliac joint: pain referral maps upon applying a new injection/arthrography technique. Part I: symptomatic volunteers. Spine. 1994;19(13):1475-82.
17. Dreyfuss P, Dryer S, Griffin J, Hoffman J, Walsh N. Positive sacroiliac screening tests in asymptomatic adults. Spine. 1994;19(10):1138-43.
18. Magee DJ. Orthopedic physical assessment. Philadelphia: Saunders; 1987. p. 266-313.
19. Whittle MW. Gait analysis. In: McLatchie GR, Lennox CME, editors. The soft tissues: trauma and sports injuries. London: Butterworth-Heinemann; 1993.
20. Evans RC. Illustrated orthopedic physical assessment. 2nd ed. St. Louis: Mosby; 2001. p. 149-51.
21. Hoehler FK, Tobis JS. Low back pain and its treatment by spinal manipulation: measures of flexibility and asymmetry. Rheumatol Rehabil. 1982;21(1):21-6.
22. Miller B, Leo K, Clarke WR, Fairchild ML, Stultz M, Hanson L. Reliability of neurological testing in patients with low back pain. Phys Ther. 1986;66(5):1-11.
23. Hoppenfeld S. Physical examination of the spine and extremities. Norwalk (CT): Appleton-Century-Crofts; 1976.
24. Evans RC. Illustrated orthopedic physical assessment. 2nd ed. St. Louis: Mosby; 2001. p. 640-1.
25. Nansel D, Szlazak M. Somatic dysfunction and the phenomenon of visceral disease simulation: a probable explanation for the apparent effectiveness of somatic therapy in patients presumed to be suffering from true visceral disease. J Manipulative Physiol Ther. 1995;18(6):379-97.
26. Keating JC, McCarron K, James J, Gruenberg J, Lonczak RS. Urobehavioral intervention in the rehabilitation of lower urinary tract dysfunction: a case report. J Manipulative Physiol Ther. 1985;8(3):185-9.
27. Kokjohn K, Schmid DM, Triano JJ, Brenan PC. The effect of spinal manipulation on pain and prostaglandin levels in women with primary dysmenorrhea. J Manipulative Physiol Ther. 1992;15(5):279-85.
28. Boesler D, Warner M, Alpers A, Finnerty EP, Kilmore MA. Efficacy of high-velocity low-amplitude manipulative technique in subjects with low-back pain during menstrual cramping. J Am Osteopath Assoc. 1993;93(2):203-14.
29. Stude DE. The management of symptoms associated with premenstrual syndrome. J Manipulative Physiol Ther. 1991;14(3):209-16.
30. Wickes D. Laboratory evaluation. In: Cox JM, editor. Low back pain mechanism, diagnosis and treatment. 5th ed. Baltimore: Williams & Wilkins; 1990. p. 420-36.
31. Cox JM. Low back pain mechanism, diagnosis and treatment. 5th ed. Baltimore: Williams & Wilkins; 1990.
32. Plaugher G. Textbook of clinical chiropractic. Baltimore: Williams & Wilkins; 1993.
33. Travell JG, Simons DG. Myofascial pain and dysfunction: the trigger point manual. Baltimore: Williams & Wilkins; 1983.

9

ADDITIONAL TESTS FOR THE HIP AND RELATED STRUCTURES

Attention to hip, pubic bone, and psoas muscle contracture or spasm is indicated when a patient experiences any of the following:

- Reduction or alteration of hip joint range of motion
- Piriformis syndrome
- Trochanteric bursitis
- Groin pain (psoas syndrome)
- Instability of the pelvis, sacroiliac joints, and low back
- Iliotibial band syndrome

Symptoms can be intermittent and variable and may be relieved by testing and adjusting according to the Activator Method (AM) Basic Scan Protocol.

COMMON HIP COMPLAINTS

The hip joint is one of the largest and most stable joints in the body.[1] The orientation of the hip articulation is such that weight bearing and mobility generate large stresses on the neck of the femur, the femoral head, and the acetabular fossa in the innominate bone of the pelvis. Consequently, pain from the hip can be referred to other areas. Alterations to the osseous structures of the hip articulations or to the muscle groups that control the hip, especially the extensors and flexors, will have an immediate impact on posture and gait.[2] Many of the conditions described below may be related to correctable neuroarticular dysfunctions of the hip joint and related structures. Restoration of hip range of motion, as well as relief of pain, can help to prevent degenerative changes to the joint and periarticular soft tissue and also may prevent pelvic unleveling and compensations in the spine.[3]

Reduction or Alteration of Hip Joint Range of Motion

The hip is a multiaxial ball-and-socket joint that is anatomically classified as an *enarthrodial diarthrosis*. One of the most important joints in mobility, the hip, is capable of seven standard motions: flexion, extension, abduction, adduction, internal rotation, external rotation, and circumduction. Average range of motion values for the hip are listed in Box 9-1.[4-6]

Because fluid motion of the hip is an essential component of walking, any reduction or alteration of hip range of motion can affect gait. Be alert to abnormal gaits in patients with hip joint complaints. If range of motion in the hip is limited by pain, the patient may exhibit one of several types of antalgic gaits or limps. *Vaulting, lurching, and hip-hiking* gaits all may be related to hip joint dysfunction with altered range of motion.[6,7]

The vaulting gait is probably the most common of the antalgic gaits; it generally occurs with acute onset of hip discomfort. Here, the patient puts weight on the affected leg but quickly swings the other leg through to minimize the intensity and duration of pain in the affected hip. The vaulting gait is easily recognized because its rhythm is asymmetrical with a *fast-pace, slow-pace* tempo as the patient alternates from affected leg to well leg.

The other two gaits tend to serve as compensations for chronic hip dysfunctions. The lurching gait, in which the patient leans into abduction or extension as the affected leg takes the weight, is not only a sign of altered hip mobility and function, but it suggests impairment of the gluteal muscle group, especially the gluteus maximus and the gluteus medius. Often, the arms are held out to the sides or the rear to assist with balance.

The hip-hiking gait develops with a fused joint or hypomobile joint. With fusion of the hip, degenerative joint disease (osteoarthritis), muscle contracture or spasm of extensor and flexor muscles, and trochanteric bursitis, the patient may raise the pelvis so that the foot may clear the ground as it swings through in the forward gait.[8] In addition to hiking the pelvis up, the patient may swing the affected leg out through a lateral arc. As a result, the hip-hiking gait causes

Box 9-1	**Hip Ranges of Motion**
Flexion	135 degrees
Extension	30 degrees
Abduction	45 degrees
Adduction	20 degrees
Internal rotation	45 degrees
External rotation	45 degrees
Circumduction	360 degrees

The range-of-motion values listed here and elsewhere in *The Activator Method* are averages of values published in various sources and should not be interpreted as "normal" for a given patient. Ranges of motion may be influenced by factors such as age, gender, weight, build, and general physical activity.[4-6]

rotational and shear stresses to the hip on the well side, resulting in the potential for bilateral hip dysfunction.

Not all abnormal gaits are antalgic, and they do not all manifest with asymmetry. Be alert to the excessive unilateral *toe-in* or *toe-out* foot flare that can occur with internal and external rotation misalignment or dysfunction of the hip joint.

When a patient experiences altered range of motion of the hip, gait abnormalities, or point tenderness in and around the joint, perform Isolation Tests and adjustments as necessary for at least the following misalignments:
- Internal (Anterior-Inferior Greater Trochanter) Hip Rotation
- External (Posterior-Superior Greater Trochanter) Hip Rotation
- Lateral Proximal Femur
- Superior Femur

Piriformis Syndrome

The piriformis muscle, which is located deep to the gluteal group, is a major external (lateral) rotator of the thigh. Originating on the anterior aspect of the sacrum and inserting on the greater trochanter of the femur, the piriformis is also a synergist for abduction and extension of the thigh.[9]

Piriformis muscle contracture can present with a gnawing pain deep in the buttock of the affected side. The muscle, especially at the musculotendinous junction near its insertion on the greater trochanter, is frequently tender to palpation.[10] It is not uncommon for piriformis syndrome to present with pain and paresthesias in the buttock, hip, posterior thigh, and leg to the foot. This is aggravated by prolonged sitting or activity.[11]

Because of the approximation of the sciatic nerve and the belly of the piriformis, a spasm of the piriformis may occur with apparent sciatic neuralgia.[12] The piriformis when inflamed has also been found to release a biochemical agent that irritates the sciatic nerve, possibly causing sciatic neuritis.[13] Consequently, orthopedic tests like the straight leg raise test (Lasegue's test) and Braggard's test may be positive. However, with piriformis syndrome affecting the sciatic nerve, the well leg raising test and Fajersztajn's test (contralateral Braggard's) will not elicit a pain response.

With piriformis syndrome, the greater trochanter tends to be pulled posteriorly, which is designated in the AM as external hip rotation, and a toe-out foot flare is typically observable in the patient's gait. The prone patient on the adjusting table may also exhibit pronounced toe-out foot flare.

When a patient describes symptoms that resemble sciatic neuralgia, hypertonicity of the hip extensors and rotators, and point tenderness over the greater trochanter, perform Stress Tests and adjustments as necessary for at least the following misalignments of the hip:
- External (Posterior-Superior Greater Trochanter) Hip Rotation
- Piriformis
- Superior Femur

Trochanteric Bursitis

The trochanteric bursae are deep to the soft tissues and muscles of the hip. Several small bursae are associated with the tendons of all three gluteal muscles, as well as the piriformis muscle. In trochanteric bursitis, tight fascia lata and hamstrings, as well as Leg Length Inequality (LLI), are frequently observed.[14] Pain on deep palpation of tissues posterior and slightly medial to the greater trochanter may indicate trochanteric bursitis. Also, extreme hip flexion as in a squatting position can increase tension in the gluteal muscles, creating pressure and pain in even mildly inflamed trochanteric bursae.

Flexion and extension maneuvers of the hip can exacerbate trochanteric bursitis. Some of the AM Stress Tests in this chapter may trigger a mild to moderate pain response, for example, tests for rotation malposition of the hip and for lateral proximal femur malposition.

When a patient reports symptoms of trochanteric bursitis, perform Stress Tests and adjustments as necessary for the following misalignments of the hip:
- External (Posterior-Superior Greater Trochanter) Hip Rotation

- Internal (Anterior-Inferior Greater Trochanter) Hip Rotation
- Lateral Proximal Femur

Groin Pain

The greater psoas muscle originates on T12 and the first through fourth lumbar vertebrae, passes deep through the abdomen and pelvis, and inserts on the lesser trochanter of the femur.[9] It is the principal flexor muscle of the hip. The psoas major is also a synergist for both internal and external rotation of the hip. Pain in the groin that resembles that of an inguinal hernia but that shows no clinical evidence of herniation may indicate psoas muscle spasm or contracture.

When the patient has been sitting for an extended period, "truck driver's syndrome," that is, pain in the inguinal region or low back, may occur when a standing position is resumed. The patient may also exhibit a version of Minor's sign by "walking the hands" up the thighs when getting up from a sitting position as tension in a contracted psoas muscle increases.

A positive Thomas' test, in which the thigh on the uninvolved side is passively flexed against the patient's abdomen, causing the hip of the affected side to flex, indicates psoas muscle contracture.[6] Hip extension during Gaenslen's test or the Lewin-Gaenslen test may also be limited and may exacerbate groin, pelvic cavity, or abdominal discomfort with psoas muscle involvement.

A bursa is also located deep to the insertion tendon of the psoas muscle as it passes medial to the lesser trochanter of the femur. Patrick's test, sometimes known by the acronym FABERE, with passive *f*lexion, *ab*duction, *e*xternal *r*otation, and *e*xtension of the hip, may provoke a pain response deep in the hip joint if this bursa is inflamed.

When a patient experiences inguinal pain, perform Isolation Tests and adjustments as necessary for the following involvements:
- Internal (Anterior-Inferior Greater Trochanter) Hip Rotation
- Inferior Femur
- Psoas Muscle Imbalance (see Chapter 10)

Unstable Pelvis, Sacroiliac Joints, and Low Back

Recurrent dysfunction in the pelvic articulations, especially the sacroiliac joints, can be an indication of hip joint involvement, even when the hip itself is asymptomatic. The hip is the most mobile part of the pelvic girdle; therefore any alteration to its function can affect normal function of the sacroiliac joints, symphysis pubis, and lumbar vertebrae by way of the psoas muscle.

Painless but limited range of motion, as already noted, may cause an antalgic or asymmetrical gait with an elevated iliac crest and resultant pelvic imbalance. A vaulting or arching gait can also contribute to pelvic shear dysfunction of the sacroiliac joints, presenting as an anterior-superior (AS) ilium or a posterior-inferior (PI) ilium. The AS and PI iliums are an essential part of testing and adjusting in the AM Basic Scan Protocol. Their recurrence or persistence after standard adjusting procedures are performed can indicate silent hip involvement.

Furthermore, pubic bone involvement can affect the stability of the other pelvic and lumbopelvic articulations, as well as the hip. The symphysis pubis, even though it is not a very mobile joint, is part of the ring structure of the bony pelvis, and any alteration to joint integrity within the ring affects the stability of the whole ring.[15]

When a patient experiences pain resulting from instability of the pelvis, sacroiliac joints, or low back, especially when the pain does not respond well to adjustments provided through the AM Basic Scan Protocol, perform Isolation Tests and adjustments as necessary for the following involvements:
- Anterior Pubic Bone (see Chapter 8)
- Psoas Muscle Imbalance (see Chapter 10)
- Internal (Anterior-Inferior Greater Trochanter) Hip Rotation
- External (Posterior-Superior Greater Trochanter) Hip Rotation
- Internal or External Ilium
- Piriformis

Iliotibial Band Syndrome

The iliotibial band (ITB) is a fascial sheath that extends from the tensor fascia lata (TFL) muscle at the greater trochanter along the lateral aspect of the thigh and inserts into the lateral tibial condyle. The TFL muscle attaches from the anterior superior iliac spine and inserts into the ITB at the greater trochanter. Most commonly, ITB syndrome affects runners who train on uneven ground. Hypertonicity of the TFL muscle causes tension in the fascia of the ITB and leads to biomechanical dysfunction of the hip and knee. The TFL is an internal rotator of the hip, and prolonged tension leads to malposition of the hip in internal rotation. Pain may extend down the lateral thigh and upward over the buttocks if the gluteal fascia becomes involved as well.[11] An additional malposition of the tibia in external rotation may result from tension of the ITB on the insertion to the tibia. If the tight fascia produces traction over the fibular head, compression of the common peroneal nerve results in neurological symptoms in the foot. Thus a patient who presents with buttock pain, lateral thigh pain, and pain and/or numbness in the foot requires a workup for differentiating lumbar radiculopathy from various biomechanical disorders of the pelvis and hip, including ITB syndrome.

Ober's test is a differential for ITB contracture. With the patient lying involved side up, abduct, flex, and extend the involved hip while palpating the greater trochanter for the ITB to glide smoothly over it during these ranges of motion. If the fascia is tight, the hip will get locked up as you slowly adduct the leg back to neutral. This is a positive sign for ITB contracture.

When a patient experiences lateral thigh pain due to ITB syndrome, perform Isolation Tests and adjustments as necessary for the following involvements:

- Internal (Anterior-Inferior Greater Trochanter) Hip Rotation
- Superior Femur
- Lateral Femur
- Inferior Femur
- Piriformis

CONCURRENT CONDITIONS

Both developmental and acquired disorders can contribute to hip symptoms and altered biomechanics. Osteoarthritis or degenerative joint disease (DJD) is, of course, one of the most common conditions that impair hip function. DJD of the hip may occur as the consequence of a genetic predisposition that develops in the absence of a well-defined predisposing disease or other injury to the joint. LLI has also been implicated as a major contributing factor in the development of unilateral degenerative disease of the hip.[16]

Congenital hip dysplasia, if unrecognized at birth or during early development, can also predispose one to developing DJD of the hip. A routine part of neonatal assessment is the performance of Ortolani's "click" test, in which the infant's thighs are flexed, abducted, and externally rotated. An audible or palpable "click" within the joint suggests malposition of the femoral head within the acetabular fossa. Visual observation of asymmetrical fat folds on the baby's thighs can also be an indicator of congenital hip dysplasia.

Problems with the hip can develop as the child matures and begins walking. Because of the malposition of the femur, neither the femoral head nor the acetabulum may ossify correctly. When the condition is recognized early, noninvasive interventions such as bracing or casting may be used effectively. Rarely, surgical interventions performed to reposition the femoral head are used in a child. If dysplasia is not recognized early, the femur may develop a pseudoarticulation with the innominate bone usually superior and posterior to the acetabulum, and the patient will have an anatomically short leg, pelvic obliquity, and gait abnormalities.[17]

Trauma to the hip that results from a motor vehicle collision, a sports injury, or a fall can also lead to DJD of the hip. If the femoral neck is fractured, the blood supply to the femoral head may be impaired. As a result, the femoral head may undergo avascular necrosis. Weight bearing on the demineralized bone tends to flatten the head and alter the biomechanics of the joint.

Ischemic necrosis of the femoral head can occur without a history of significant trauma to the hip. Legg-Calvé-Perthe's disease, also known as *coxa plana*, appears to be a familial and perhaps a genetic condition that primarily affects boys ages 4 to 10 years.[16] The same flattening of the femoral head occurs and can predispose the patient to developing DJD of the hip later in life.

In advanced osteoporosis, the hip is especially vulnerable to injury. Perhaps the reality behind the sad but not uncommon event in which "Grandma fell and broke her hip" is that "Grandma broke her hip and fell." The neck of the femur becomes thin and brittle and is subject to spontaneous fracture. Of course, the fracture is not really spontaneous, but the force required to break the neck of an osteoporotic femur is often minimal. In many cases, the hip fracture has occurred when the patient steps off a curb or a kitchen step stool. For an elderly patient, a hip fracture can have devastating consequences because of its impact on mobility and independence.

When a patient suffers from hip complaints of acute or chronic onset, be sure to conduct a thorough history and examination of the region, including range-of-motion testing and standard orthopedic and neurological examinations. Radiographic examination can rule out fracture or necrosis of the femoral head and can be used to evaluate the hip joint for the typical changes of DJD.

TESTING AND ADJUSTING THE HIP AND RELATED STRUCTURES

When the patient's complaints or examination findings indicate involvement of the hip and its related structures, the following Stress Tests and adjustments of the hip are performed:

- Internal (Anterior-Inferior Greater Trochanter) Hip Rotation

- External (Posterior-Superior Greater Trochanter) Hip Rotation
- Lateral Proximal Femur
- Superior Femur
- Inferior Femur

In addition to testing and adjustment of the femor-acetabular joint, three related structures should be tested and adjusted if necessary:

- Piriformis
- Anterior pubic bone (see Chapter 8)
- Psoas muscle imbalance (see Chapter 10)

Internal (Anterior-Inferior Greater Trochanter) Hip Rotation

Internal hip rotation should be considered when the patient demonstrates unilateral "toe-in." A normal gait and resting stance show slight "toe-out" foot flare that is symmetrical and balanced. Normally, visual inspection of the feet of a patient on the adjusting table typically reveals moderate toe-out foot flare of both feet when the legs are in Position #1. When the legs are raised to Position #2, the feet normally flare out to a neutral, relaxed position, forming an angle of 10 to 20 degrees from the midline (median sagittal plane) of the body.

When the hip is rotated internally, the foot on the affected side rarely shows true malposition, but it is noticeably less flared out during walking or standing, or when the patient is on the adjusting table with the legs in Position #1.

Stress Test.   Use the patient's leg to Stress Test for neuroarticular dysfunction of an internally rotated hip. With the patient in Position #1, flex the knee on the side of involvement to 90 degrees. Then rotate the leg below the knee away from the midline of the body (Figure 9-1).

Because the knee is locked into position with the knee in flexion, rotation of the lower leg away from the midline simultaneously rotates the femur internally and moves the greater trochanter anteriorly. After returning the leg to Position #1, look for Pelvic Deficient (PD) leg reactivity.

Adjustment.   To adjust an internally rotated hip, contact the anterior aspect of the greater trochanter. The Line of Drive (LOD) is posterior and slightly superior (Figure 9-2). During internal hip rotation, the greater trochanter is moved in an anterior direction, and because of the neck of the femur, it shifts slightly inferiorly as well. Therefore superiority is added to achieve a better LOD via the angle of the neck of the femur. In most cases, it is relatively easy to position the instrument without moving the patient. Simply locate the anterior aspect of the greater trochanter by palpating for the point at which the lateral thigh flares out at the level of the hip joint.

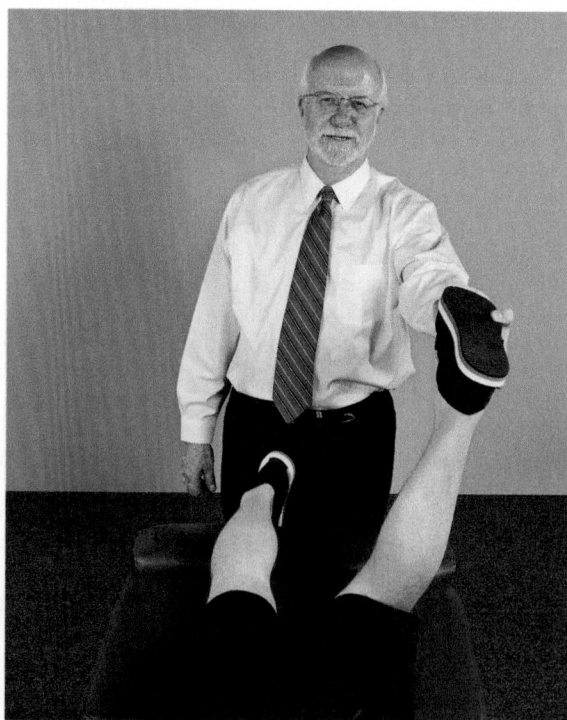

Figure 9-1   Stress Test for internal (anterior-inferior greater trochanter) hip rotation.

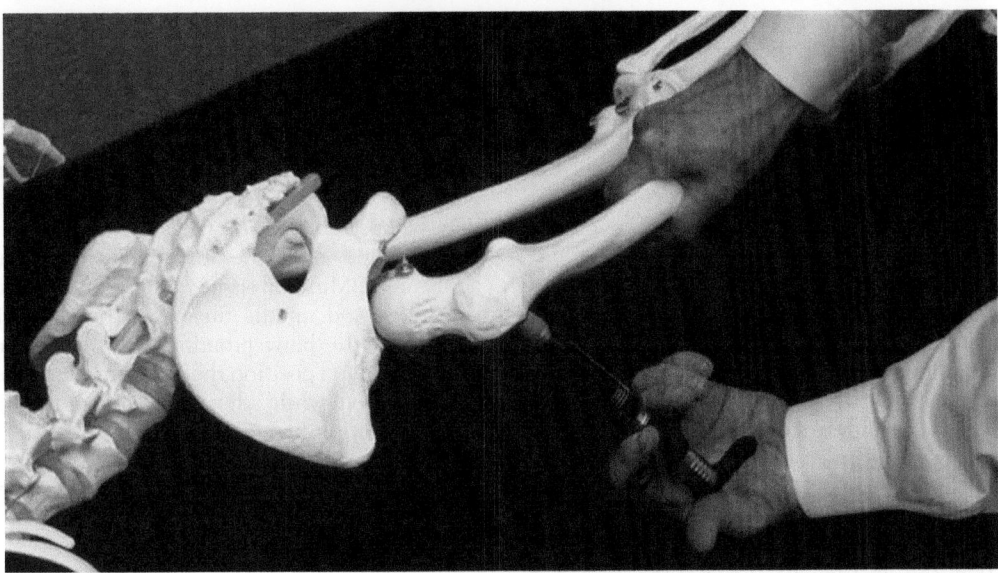

Figure 9-2 Adjustment for internal hip rotation. Line of Drive is posterior and slightly superior.

For the patient with large thighs, it may be difficult to get the best LOD without making some accommodation. To ensure an accurate adjustment, use the stabilization (free) hand to roll the patient's hip back and away from the table. With the index and middle fingers of the stabilizing hand over the greater trochanter, take a tissue pull over the bony prominence. Keep the fingers slightly apart, and position the tip of the instrument between them. The LOD remains posterior and slightly superior.

For a small framed patient or a child, the hip may be too far from the edge of the table to attain the correct LOD. One way to adjust the patient is to use the stabilizing hand to roll the hip back and away from the table, as is suggested for the heavy patient.

Clinical Observations

Consider internal hip rotation when a patient reports hip joint pain or pain that radiates back from the greater trochanter to the sacroiliac joint.

Be sure to rule out neuromuscular disease that can weaken external rotators of the hip. Limb girdle muscular dystrophy, a history of polio, and the progressive neurogenic atrophy of multiple sclerosis and amyotrophic lateral sclerosis can all contribute to weak hip muscles.

External (Posterior-Superior Greater Trochanter) Hip Rotation

External rotation of the hip should be considered when the patient exhibits unilateral "toe-out" foot flare. A normal gait and resting stance reveal slight toe-out flare, but it is symmetrical and balanced. Visual inspection of the feet of a patient on the adjusting table normally reveals moderate bilateral toe-out foot flare when the legs are in Position #1. When the legs are raised to Position #2, the feet normally flare out to a neutral, relaxed position, forming an angle of 10 to 20 degrees from the midline of the body.

When the hip is externally rotated, the foot on the affected side exhibits pronounced toe-out foot flare during walking, although the patient may not show readily observable gait abnormality. When the patient is in Position #1 on the adjusting table, the foot on the side of external hip rotation flares out more than on the other side, and the buttock on the side of involvement may appear flared because of the contracture of the gluteal muscles and the external rotators of the hip. If the hip has been in external rotation for an extended time, the patient's shoes are likely to show excessive and asymmetrical wear on the posterior and lateral aspects of the heel on the side of involvement.

Stress Test. Use the patient's leg to Stress Test for neuroarticular dysfunction of an externally rotated hip. With the patient in Position #1, flex the knee on the side of involvement to 90 degrees. Then rotate the leg below the knee across the midline of the body (Figure 9-3).

Because the knee is locked into position when it is flexed, rotation of the lower leg toward the midline simultaneously rotates the femur externally, and the greater trochanter moves posteriorly. Look for reactivity of the PD leg in Position #1.

Adjustment. To adjust an externally rotated hip, contact the posterior aspect of the greater trochanter. During external hip rotation, the greater trochanter is moved into a posterior direction; because of the neck of the femur, this movement shifts it slightly superior as well. Therefore inferiority is added to attain a better LOD via the angle of the neck of the femur. The LOD is anterior and slightly inferior (Figure 9-4).

With most patients, it is relatively easy to position the instrument. Locate the posterior aspect of the greater trochanter by palpating for the point at which the lateral thigh flares out at the level of the hip joint.

For the overweight or obese patient, it may be necessary to palpate deeply for the bony structure of the greater trochanter. It is also advisable to take a medial-to-lateral soft tissue pull over the greater trochanter with the stabilization (free) hand to ensure specificity of the adjustment. With the index and middle fingers of the stabilizing hand over the greater trochanter, take a tissue pull over the bony prominence. Keep the fingers slightly apart, and position the tip of the instrument between them. The LOD remains anterior and slightly inferior.

For the small framed patient or a child, the greater trochanter is very easy to locate, but it still may be advisable to use the stabilizing hand to position and hold the instrument during the adjustment. Minimal tissue pull is required. Place the index and middle fingers of the stabilizing hand over the bony prominence of the greater trochanter, and position the tip of the instrument between them while adjusting in an anterior and slightly inferior direction.

Clinical Observations

Consider external hip rotation when a patient experiences piriformis syndrome, anterior groin pain, or psoas spasm. Complaints of hip, hamstring, or calf pain that cannot be related to concurrent sacroiliac involvement may also suggest external (posterior-superior) rotation of the greater trochanter.

A sprain injury of the Y-shaped ligament of Bigelow may cause adaptive external (posterior-superior) rotation of the greater trochanter. In such a case, the patient should be evaluated for malposition of the femoral head in the acetabulum.

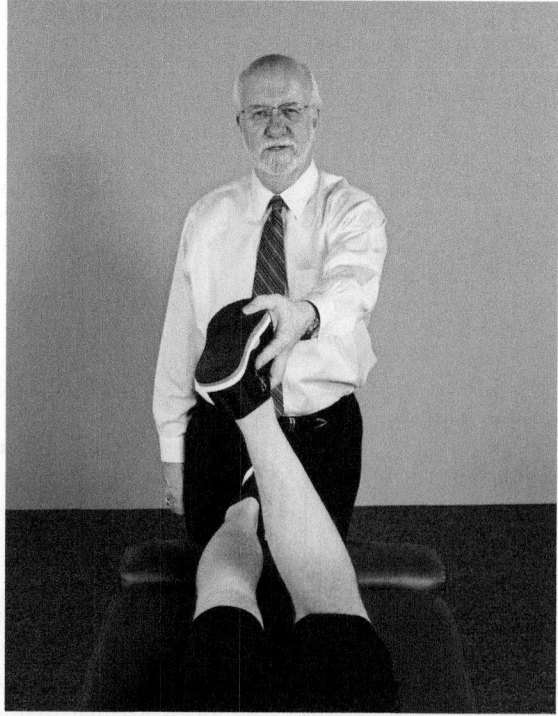

Figure 9-3   Stress Test for external (posterior-superior greater trochanter) hip rotation.

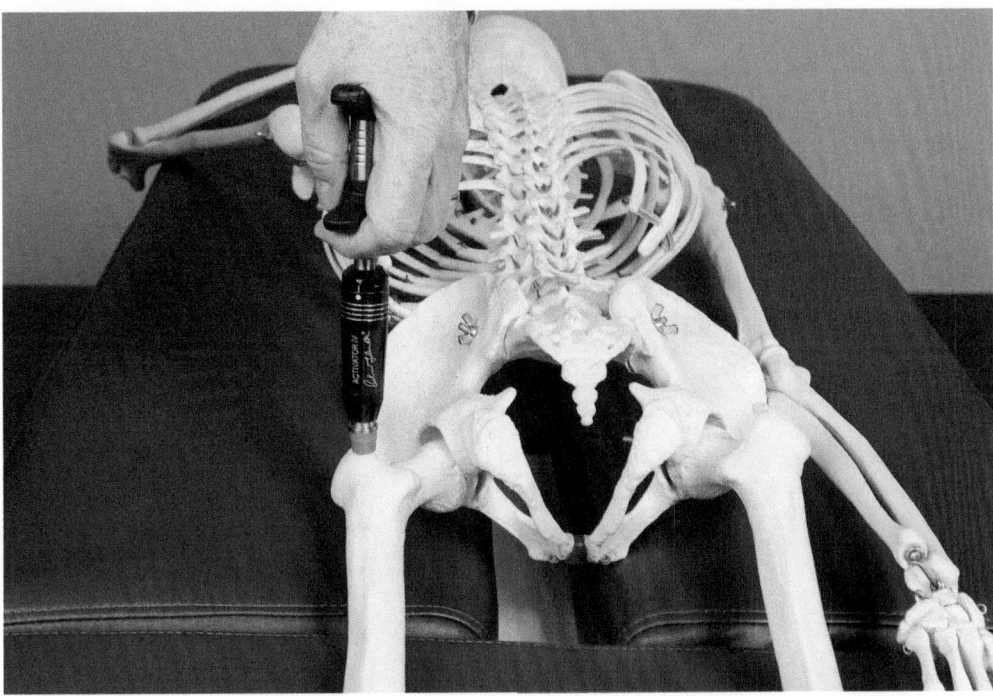

Figure 9-4 Adjustment for external hip rotation. Line of Drive is anterior and slightly inferior.

Lateral Proximal Femur

Consider a lateral neuroarticular dysfunction of the proximal femur when a patient reports pain deep in the hip joint, along the line of the femoral neck, or at the head of the femur. This pain may be exacerbated during Patrick's test for flexion, abduction, external rotation, and extension of the hip.

Stress Test.   To Stress Test for a lateral proximal femur, take a firm tissue pull over the greater trochanter. Grasp the soft tissue anterior and posterior to the trochanter between the thumb and fingers, and pull it straight laterally (Figure 9-5). Look for reactivity of the PD leg in Position #1.

Adjustment.   To adjust a lateral proximal femur, contact the lateral aspect of the trochanter. The LOD is medial and superior along the axis of the femoral neck at an angle of 30 to 40 degrees (Figure 9-6).

The greater trochanter tends to be close to the surface in most patients and is readily palpable through the subcutaneous tissue. For the patient with heavy thighs, however, it may be useful to compress the tissue over the lateral aspect of the trochanter with the index and middle fingers. Spread the fingers apart enough to accommodate the tip of the instrument, and use the split-finger position to stabilize the instrument and to maintain soft tissue compression during the adjustment.

Clinical Observations

For the osteoporotic patient who presents with pain deep in the hip, be sure to rule out fracture.

Also, when a patient reports pain after a blow to the hip region sustained in an athletic activity, auto collision, or fall, assess the joint for fracture or for complications of avascular necrosis of the femoral head.

Superior Femur

When a patient experiences hip pain that is exacerbated by walking or that began after he or she jumped from a height such as a platform, a truck bed, or a loading dock, for example, consider a superior malposition of the femur. Also, patients with a history of DJD of the hip tend to develop a lurching gait or a gluteus medius limp. Contracture or weakening of the gluteus medius develops gradually as compensation for gaits that are adapted to loss of hip range of motion, and the involuntary shortening of the muscle can pull the femur superiorly.

Stress Test.   To Stress Test for neuroarticular dysfunction involvement of a superior femur,

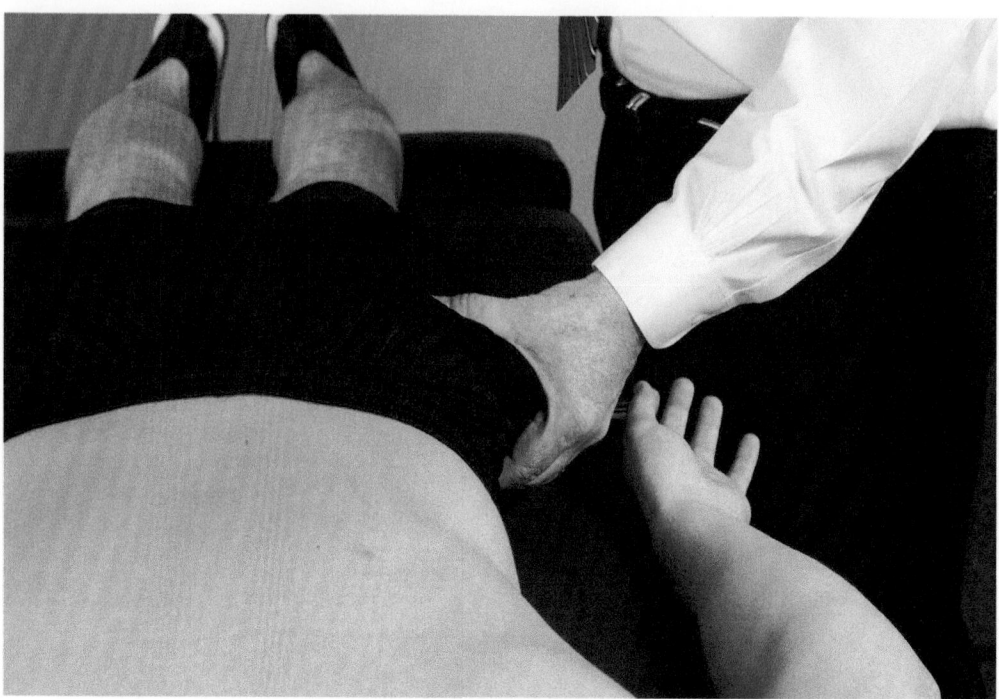

Figure 9-5 Stress Test for lateral proximal hip.

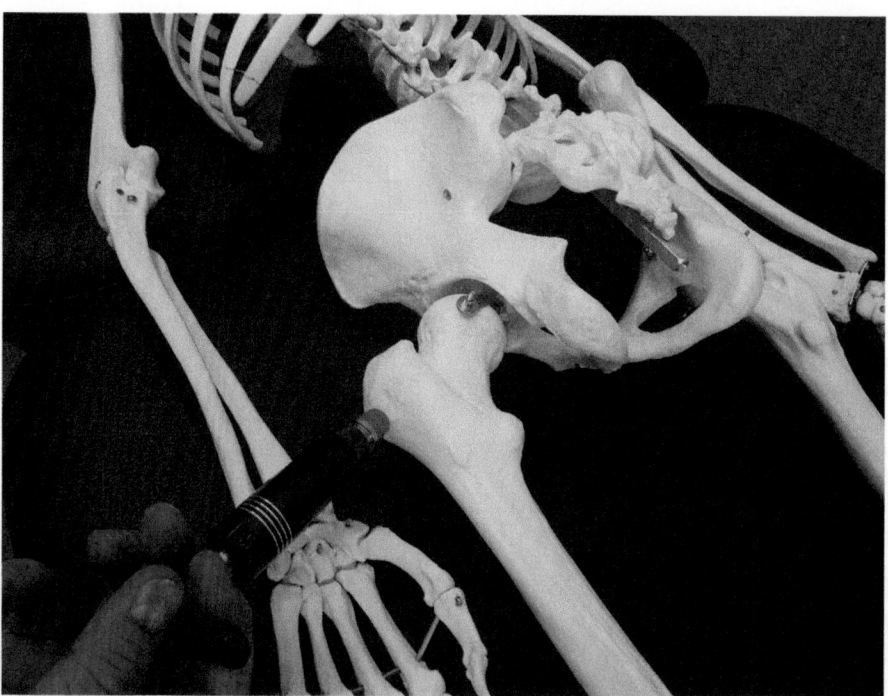

Figure 9-6 Adjustment for lateral proximal hip. Line of Drive is medial and superior.

contact the inferior aspect of the greater trochanter and Stress Test the femur in a superior (cephalad) direction (Figure 9-7). Look for reactivity of the PD leg in Position #1.

Adjustment. To adjust a superior femur, place the tip of the instrument at the superior aspect of the bony prominence of the trochanter at the insertion point of the gluteus medius

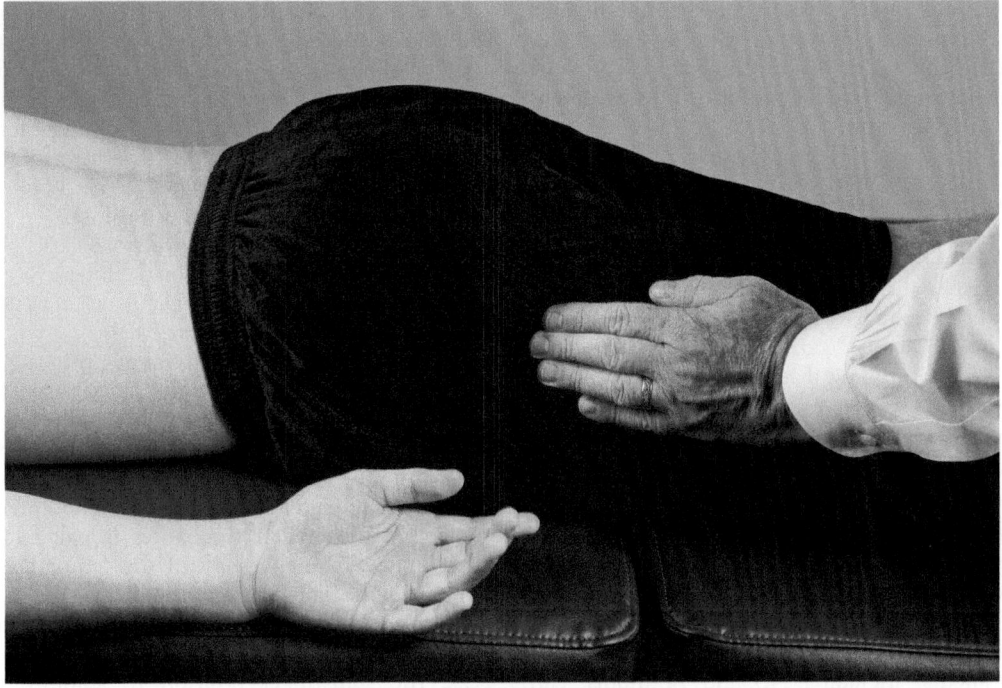

Figure 9-7 Stress Test for superior hip.

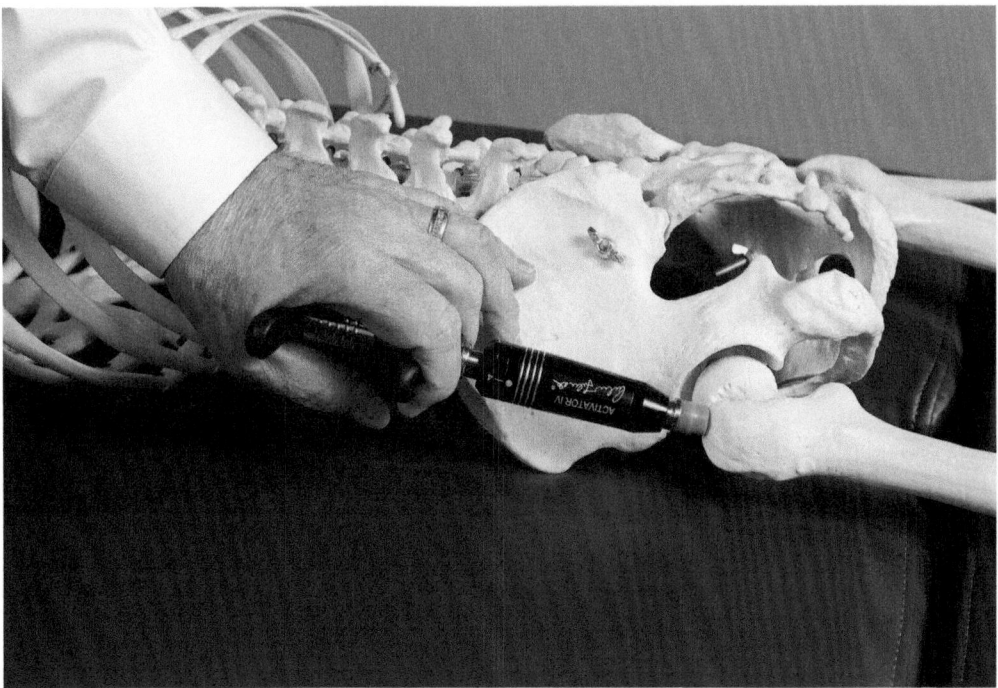

Figure 9-8 Adjustment for superior hip. Line of Drive is inferior and slightly medial.

muscle. The LOD is inferior and slightly medial (Figure 9-8).

The superior aspect of the greater trochanter is generally easily accessible for positioning the instrument. Depending on the build of the patient, taking a tissue pull inferiorly over the trochanter may help to ensure accuracy of the adjustment. Take the tissue pull with the index and middle fingers of the stabilization hand, spread the fingers apart enough to accommodate the tip of the instrument, and use the split-finger position to stabilize the instrument during adjustment.

Clinical Observations

When a patient has a persistent superior femur, the probability is great that degenerative changes to the hip joint have already started. Make a point of monitoring the "good hip" because the antalgic or asymmetrical gait that develops with degenerative joint disease of the hip often increases stresses to the asymptomatic leg.

Inferior Femur

A patient with a recent history of knee injury, especially to the medial collateral ligament, may develop spasms or contractures of the adductor muscles of the thigh. Similarly, pelvic misalignments, including AS and PI iliums, can produce hypertonicity in the adductor muscles of the thigh. When a patient experiences tight adductors and describes deep, achy pain in the region of the ischial tuberosity and the medial thigh, consider malposition of an inferior femur.

Stress Test. To Stress Test for an inferior femur, push inferiorly on the superior aspect of the greater trochanter (Figure 9-9). Look for reactivity of the PD leg in Position #1.

Adjustment. To adjust an inferior femur, position the tip of the instrument on the inferior aspect of the bony prominence. The LOD is straight superior and slightly medial (Figure 9-10).

To ensure effective instrument position and a correct LOD, palpate for the lateral aspect of the femur. Using the index and middle fingers of the stabilization hand, take a firm tissue pull from inferior to superior over the bony prominence of the greater trochanter. The inferior aspect of the greater trochanter is palpable at the point where the shaft of the femur begins to angle medially toward the knee. Maintain the tissue pull with the fingers apart enough to accommodate the tip of the instrument. Use the split-finger position to stabilize the instrument during the adjustment.

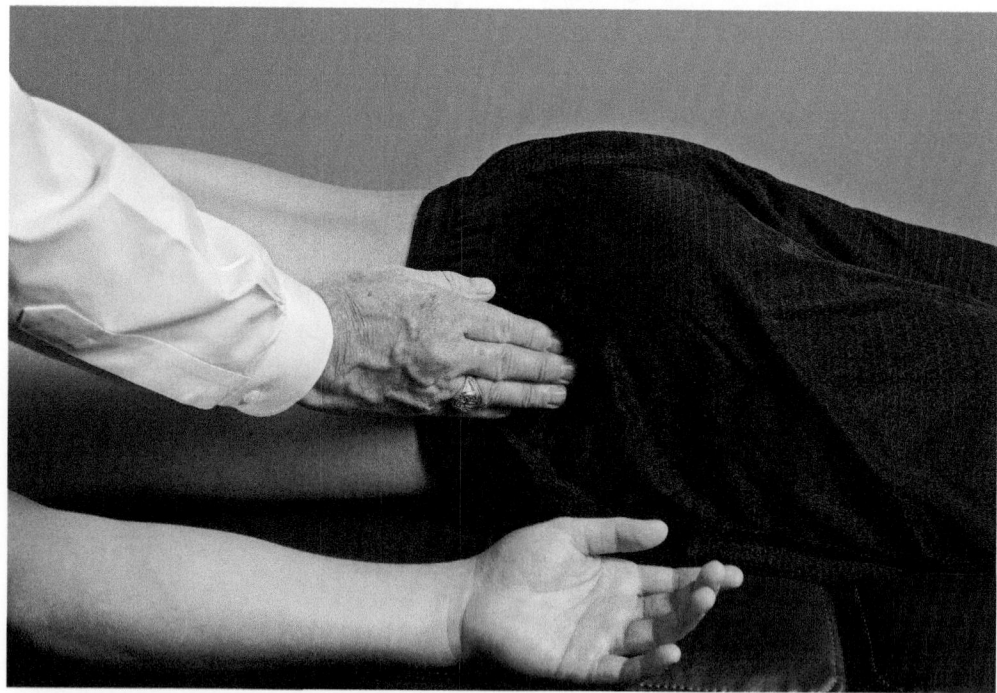

Figure 9-9   Stress Test for inferior hip.

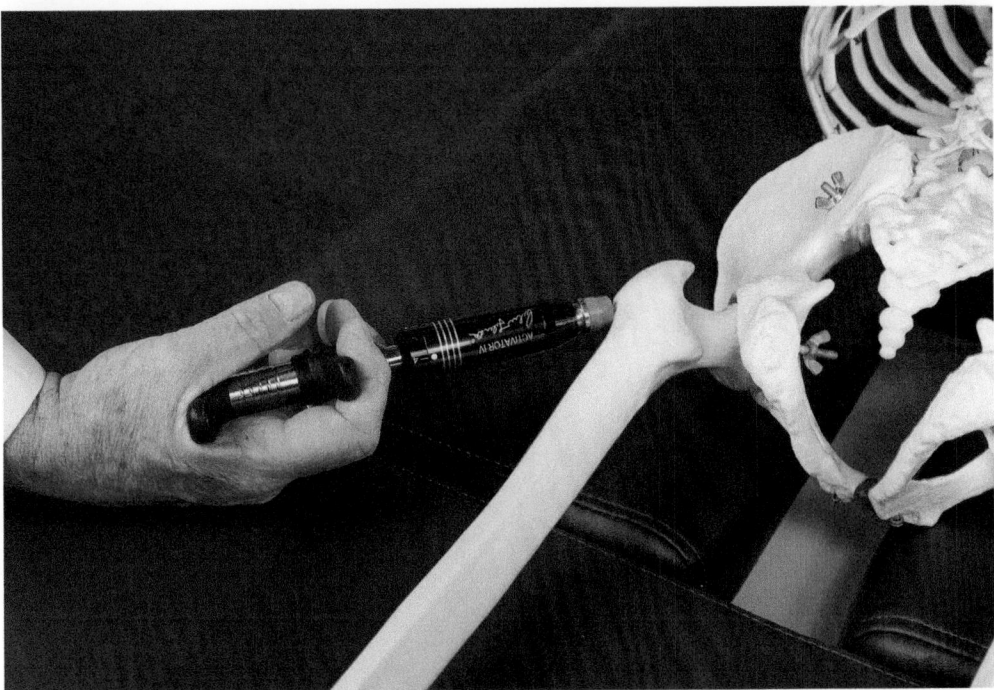

Figure 9-10 Adjustment for inferior hip. Line of Drive is superior and slightly medial.

Clinical Observations

Contracture of the thigh adductors may develop gradually with onset of degenerative joint disease of the knee, even though the knee is not necessarily symptomatic. When a patient demonstrates a persistent or chronic inferior femur, be sure to perform full hip and knee range-of-motion testing.

Activities that might contribute to acute onset of an inferior greater trochanter include horseback riding and off-road motorcycle and all-terrain vehicle riding.

Piriformis

When a patient experiences pain in the sacroiliac joint, buttock, and/or posterior thigh or sciatica, consider testing the piriformis muscle. If the reactive leg or PD leg is on the involved side, pain may be due to increased tension in the piriformis muscle. Before evaluation to explore piriformis involvement is initiated, the pelvis and the hip should be tested and adjusted for all neuroarticular dysfunctions, in particular, performance of the external rotation of the hip Stress Test.

Stress Test. To Stress Test for involvement of the piriformis, use an active resistive muscle test by taking the involved leg to 90 degrees of knee flexion with the doctor's hand on the medial aspect of the distal tibia. The patient is asked to resist the doctor's pressure by bringing the leg across the midline of the body, resisting external hip rotation (Figure 9-11). Look for PD leg reactivity in Position #1.

Adjustment. To adjust piriformis involvement, use one thrust on each of the three contact points. First, make contact one-half inch lateral to the sacral border. The second contact should be made one-half inch medial to the greater trochanter, and the third contact should be made on the attachment of the piriformis at the greater trochanter. The LODs are anterior-inferior-lateral (Figures 9-12 through 9-14; Table 9-1).

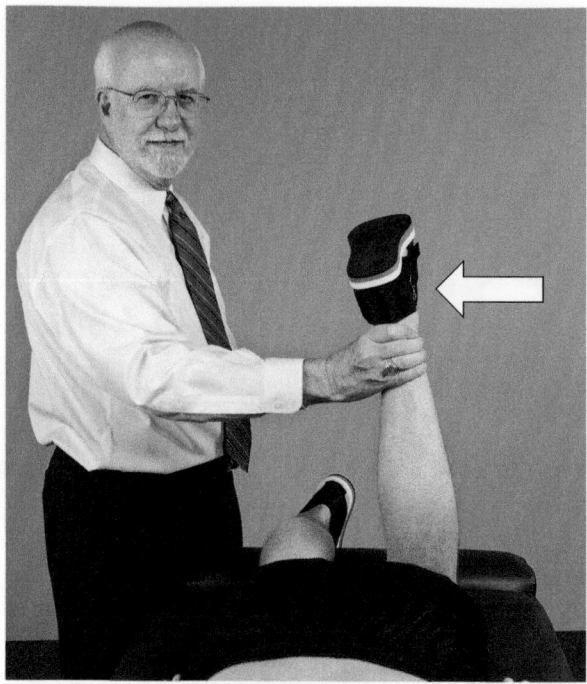

Figure 9-11   Stress Test for piriformis.

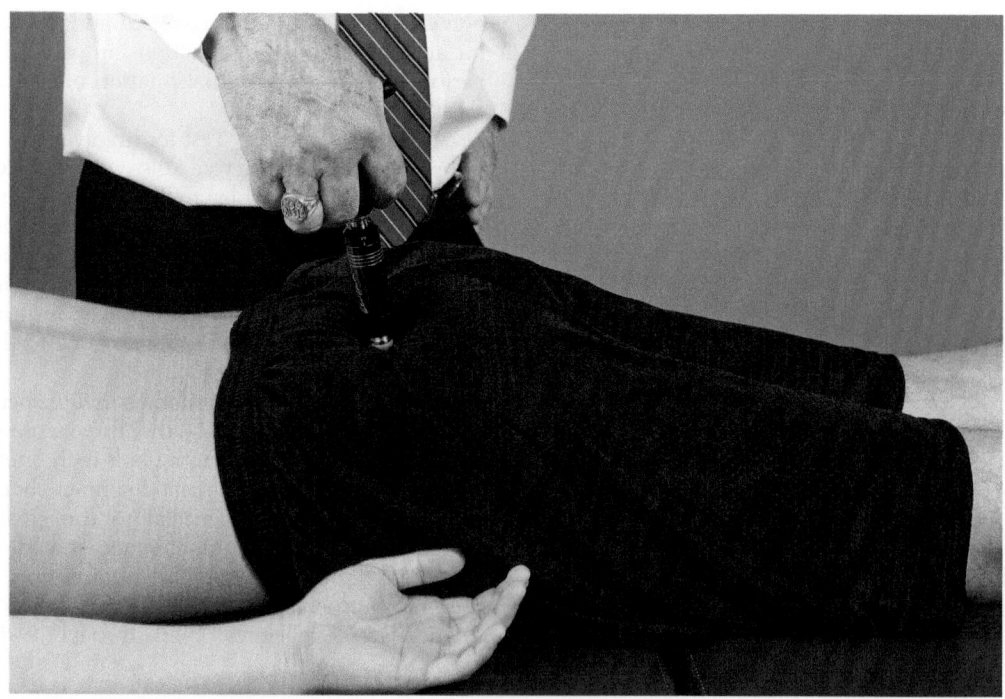

Figure 9-12   Adjustment for piriformis. Step One: Line of Drive is anterior, inferior, and lateral.

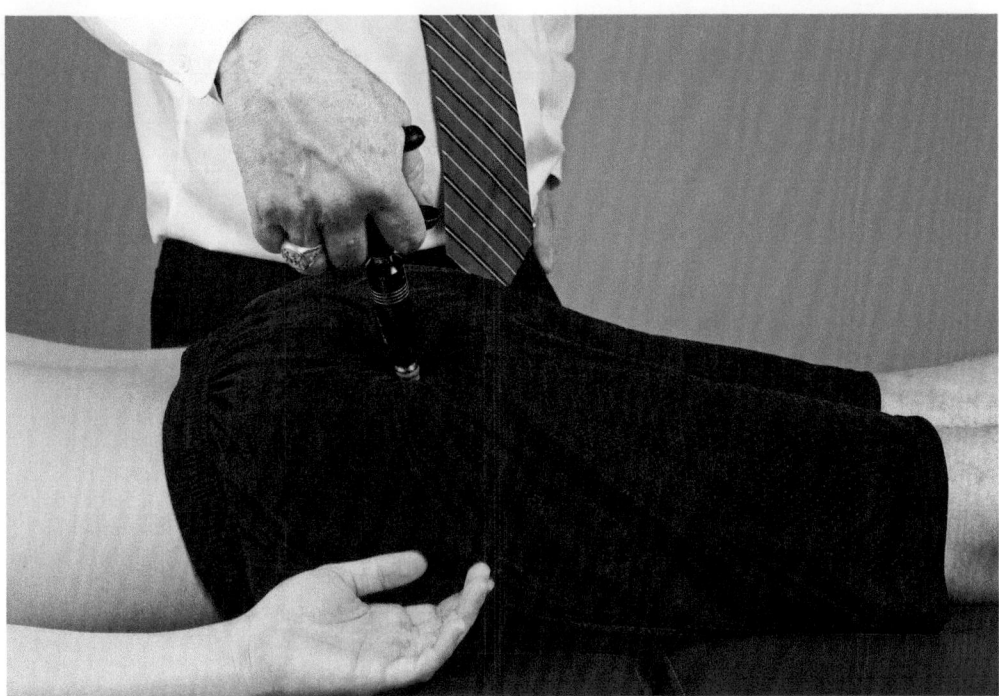

Figure 9-13 Adjustment for piriformis. Step Two: Line of Drive is anterior, inferior, and lateral.

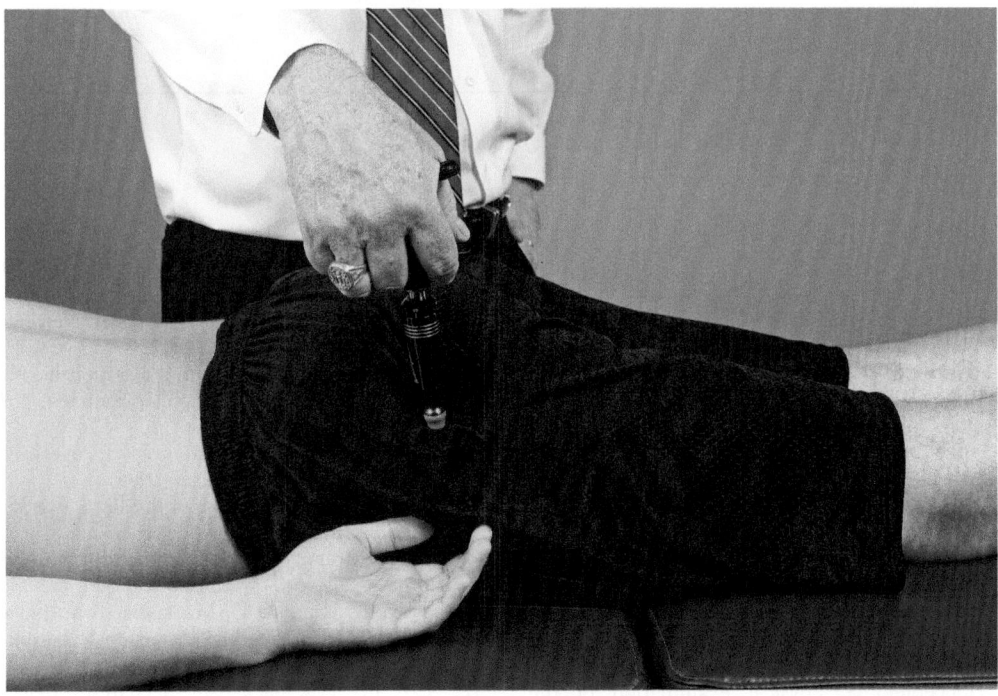

Figure 9-14 Adjustment for piriformis. Step Three: Line of Drive is anterior, inferior, and lateral.

Table 9-1   Summary Table of Tests and Adjustments for the Hip and Related Structures

| Neuroarticular Dysfunction | Test | Adjustment | |
		Segmental Contact Point	Line of Drive
Internal (Anterior-Inferior) Hip Rotation	Flex knee to 90 degrees. Rotate leg below knee away from midline of the body.	Anterior aspect of greater trochanter	Posterior and superior
External (Posterior-Superior) Hip Rotation	Flex knee to 90 degrees. Rotate leg below knee toward midline of the body.	Posterior aspect of greater trochanter	Anterior and inferior
Lateral Proximal Femur	Grasp tissue over greater trochanter, and pull straight laterally	Lateral greater trochanter	Medial and superior
Superior Femur	Push superior on inferior aspect of the greater trochanter	Superior aspect of greater trochanter	Inferior and slightly medial
Inferior Femur	Push inferior on superior aspect of greater trochanter	Inferior aspect of greater trochanter	Superior and slightly medial
Piriformis	Flex knee to 90 degrees. Doctor places hand on medial distal tibia and asks patient to resist toward the midline, externally rotating the hip.	*Step One*: One-half inch lateral to the sacral border	Anterior-inferior-lateral
		Step Two: One-half inch medial to the greater trochanter	Anterior-inferior-lateral
		Step Three: On attachment of the piriformis to the greater trochanter	Anterior-inferior-lateral

REFERENCES

1. Magee DJ. The hip. In: Orthopedic physical assessment. Philadelphia: Saunders; 1987. p. 239-65.
2. Whittle MW. Gait analysis. In: McLatchie GR, Lennox CME, editors. The soft tissues: trauma and sports injuries. London: Butterworth-Heinemann; 1993.
3. Friberg O. Clinical symptoms and biomechanics of lumbar spine and hip joint in leg length inequality. Spine. 1983;8(6):643-51.
4. Cipriano JJ. Photographic manual of regional orthopaedic tests. Baltimore: Williams & Wilkins; 1985.
5. Evans RC. Illustrated essentials in orthopedic physical assessment. St. Louis: Mosby; 1994.
6. Hoppenfeld S. Physical examination of the spine and extremities. Norwalk (CT): Appleton-Century-Crofts; 1976.
7. Callaghan JJ. Examination of the hip. In: Clark CR, Bonfiglio M, editors. Orthopaedics: essentials of diagnosis and treatment. New York: Churchill Livingstone; 1994.
8. Magee DJ. Gait assessment. In: Orthopedic physical assessment. Philadelphia: Saunders; 1987. p. 362-76.
9. Clemente CD. Gray's anatomy. 30th American ed. Philadelphia: Lea & Febiger; 1985.
10. Davis DG. Manipulation of the lower extremity. In: Subotnick SI, editor. Sports medicine of the lower extremity. London: Churchill Livingstone; 1989.
11. Travell J, Simons D. Myofascial pain and dysfunction: the trigger point manual. Baltimore: Williams & Wilkins; 1992.
12. Cox JM. Low back pain mechanism, diagnosis and treatment. 5th ed. Baltimore: Williams & Wilkins; 1990.

13. Steiner C, Staubs C, Ganon M, Buhlinger CD. Piriformis syndrome: pathogenesis, diagnosis, and treatment. J Am Osteopath Assoc. 1987; 87(4): 318-22.

14. O'Neill DB, Micheli LJ. Overuse injury in the young athlete. Clin Sports Med. 1988;7: 591-610.

15. Hildebrandt RW. Chiropractic spinography: a manual of technology and interpretation. 2nd ed. Baltimore: Williams & Wilkins; 1985.

16. Gofton JP. Studies in osteoarthritis of the hip. IV. Biomechanics and clinical considerations. Can Med Assoc J. 1971;104(11):1007-11.

17. Yochum TR, Rowe LJ. Essentials of skeletal radiology. 2nd ed. Baltimore: Williams & Wilkins; 1995.

10 ADDITIONAL LUMBAR TESTS AND ADJUSTMENTS

Although low back pain frequently involves pelvic articulations, especially the sacroiliac joints, the lumbar intervertebral and lumbosacral joints also play a significant role in this common patient complaint. In most instances, the L5 assessment follows routine examination and adjustment of the anterior-superior (AS) and posterior-inferior (PI) ilium and symphysis pubis sequence of the Basic Scan Protocol. If on initial examination, the Pelvic Deficient (PD) leg shortens in Position #2, the leg length test indicates that the knees, feet, pelvis, and L5 should be bypassed, and testing should begin at the fourth lumbar.

After examination and adjustment of the AS and PI iliums and the symphysis pubis, perform Isolation Tests and adjustments as indicated for neuroarticular dysfunctions of the following lumbar vertebrae included in the Basic Scan Protocol:

- Fifth Lumbar (L5)
- Fourth Lumbar (L4)
- Second Lumbar (L2)

When patient complaints and examination findings indicate the need, perform Isolation and Stress Tests to look for additional lumbar neuroarticular dysfunctions:

- Third Lumbar (L3)
- First Lumbar (L1)
- Unilateral Lumbosacral Facet Syndrome
- Superior or Inferior Spinous (Flexion or Extension Malposition)
- Segmental Laterality
- Quadratus Lumborum

Clinicians familiar with the Activator Method (AM) report that most patients with low back pain related to neuroarticular dysfunction of the lumbar vertebrae do not require more than testing and adjustment of the fifth, fourth, and second lumbars as indicated. Nevertheless, it is important for the practitioner to monitor low back complaints closely because of their frequency and serious impact on a patient's mobility, productivity, and quality of life.

COMMON COMPLAINTS

Nearly everyone has low back pain at some time, and men and women are affected equally. At some point, back pain interferes with work, routine daily activities, or recreation. Low back pain occurs most often between the ages of 30 and 50 years, in part because of the aging process but also as a result of sedentary lifestyles with too little (sometimes punctuated by too much) exercise. Americans spend at least $50 billion each year on low back pain, which is the most common cause of job-related disability and a leading contributor to missed work. Back pain is the second most common neurological ailment in the United States—only headache is more common.[1] Spinal complaints present a major challenge in health care. The prevalence of spinal symptoms for which patients seek the expertise of a physician is the fourth highest, behind throat symptoms, cough, and earache or ear infection.[2] Next to the common cold, low back symptoms are the most common reason for visits to primary care physicians.[3] Internationally conducted epidemiological studies have revealed the enormous societal impact of low back disorders that cause worker absenteeism.[4] In 1989, the direct annual cost of personal medical care for back pain was six times higher than that for AIDS ($17.9 billion for back pain vs. $3.3 billion for AIDS).[5]

Acute or short-term low back pain generally can last from a few days to a few weeks. Most *acute* back pain appears to be mechanical in nature.[1] Chiropractic has become a major provider of services for those who report lumbar spine complaints.[6] Several studies have indicated that chiropractic is more beneficial,[7] more satisfactory with patients,[7] and more cost-effective[8-11] than medical management of low back pain. It has been reported that only 0.25% of patients with low back pain may require surgery[12]; this has sparked investigation into the effectiveness of other treatment methods, including spinal manipulation.[7,13-15] Spinal manipulation has proved effective in several studies of low back pain. After a comprehensive literature review of more than 15,000 articles was completed, the U.S. Agency for Health Care Policy and Research recently suggested that conservative care, including spinal manipulation as performed by chiropractors, is one of the most efficacious clinical responses to acute low back pain complaints.[10] The investigation into the effectiveness of spinal manipulation for chronic low back pain has begun to be proven worthy in the literature.[16]

When a patient experiences low back pain, it is important to rule out conditions and complicating factors that might contraindicate spinal manipulation/adjustment by which the patient would benefit from concurrent care or referral. Therefore a thorough history and examination, including range-of-motion testing and appropriate orthopedic and neurological assessment and instrumentation, is standard clinical procedure when a patient reports low back pain. Additional special tests such as diagnostic imaging may be indicated by examination findings and clinical judgment.

Similar to pelvic complaints, abnormalities of gait and posture are significant indicators of low back pain related to the lumbar spine. A common antalgic adaptation to lumbar neuroarticular dysfunction and other injury is the flexion posture. If disc wedging occurs as part of the lumbar vertebral subluxation complex, the patient may show variations in flexion posture.[17] For example, a rotational or anterior-lateral antalgic stance has been related to the tortipelvis phenomenon.[18] In tortipelvis, the torso rotates and leans to the side opposite the disc wedging. It is painful and difficult for the patient to assume a fully erect posture with acute tortipelvis. Functional scoliotic variations of the lumbar spine have been associated with Leg Length Inequality[19,20]; often, these respond favorably to chiropractic care.

Acute lumbar involvement in low back pain is frequently accompanied by painful paraspinal muscle spasm and contracture. Musculature and other soft tissue feel rigid and warm to the touch. Paraspinal muscle contracture can severely limit lumbar range of motion during an acute low back pain event. Evaluation of the lumbar spine should be performed in its six standard ranges of motion: flexion, extension, lateral flexion (bending) to the right and left, and rotation to the right and left. Average values for lumbar ranges of motion are listed in Box 10-1.[21,22]

Lumbar ranges of motion, which are extremely variable because of the wide range of available

Box 10-1 **Lumbar Ranges of Motion**[20,21]	
Flexion	45 to 60 degrees
Extension	15 to 20 degrees
Lateral flexion	25 to 30 degrees
Rotation	10 to 15 degrees

The average range-of-motion values listed here and elsewhere in *The Activator Method* are averages of values published in various sources and should not be interpreted as "normal for a given patient." Ranges of motion may be influenced by such factors as age, gender, weight, build, and general physical activity.

evaluative techniques, depend on factors such as age, weight, segmental orientation, muscular control, facet orientation, and degenerative changes.[23] Recently, the Back Range of Motion Instrument (BROM II) was found to be reliable in the measurement of lumbar mobility.[24] This instrument was shown to reflect very similar data to the double inclinometer method, with concurrent validity partially supported (intraclass correlation coefficient in all planes ranges from 0.27 to 0.75).

Baseline measures of range of motion of the lumbar spine are useful standards against which to compare and assess patient progress and treatment outcomes. However, qualitative assessment of motion may be clinically more valuable than quantitative assessment. Instruct the patient to perform active ranges of motion of the lumbar spine. Observe for smooth, fluid motion, bilateral symmetry, and evidence of pain-restricted motion.

Provide support for the patient who is in pain during range-of-motion testing. Support the patient by holding the pelvis firmly during performance of range-of-motion activities. A firm grasp on the pelvis not only gives the patient support, it also restricts motion in the pelvis and helps to eliminate compensatory motions of the hips when lumbar movement is restricted by pain, muscle spasm, or joint dysfunction.

Several orthopedic and neurological tests are performed to identify lumbar and lumbosacral involvement.[25] Tests like Lasegue's test, or the straight leg raise test, are useful for identifying nerve root entrapment syndrome, especially from a disc lesion.[26,27] The straight leg raise test is designed to traction the sciatic nerve. The test is performed on the supine patient by passively flexing the leg at the hip with the knee in an extended position. Reproduction or exacerbation of neuralgic pain along the course of the sciatic nerve may be an indication of nerve root or peripheral nerve entrapment. If the pain is localized to the low back, hip, or posterior thigh, tight hamstring muscles are indicated.

A second test, Braggard's test, is typically performed after a positive straight leg raise is done.[28] In Braggard's test, the leg used to elicit a positive straight leg raise test is raised to the point of pain and then is lowered by 5 degrees. The foot and ankle are then forcibly dorsiflexed. If dorsiflexion reproduces or exacerbates pain by tractioning the sciatic nerve, a disc lesion or a space-occupying lesion is suggested.[29]

The well leg raise test, or contralateral Lasegue's test, is a third test that may be used to evaluate the possibility of a space-occupying lesion, usually a disc herniation or prolapse. To perform the well leg raise, raise the leg on the side opposite the side of involvement. Reproduction of neuralgic pain on the affected side suggests a midline space-occupying lesion in the lumbar region of the spine.[29]

Fajersztajn's test, which is sometimes known as contralateral Braggard's test, is a fourth test that is used to assess the possibility of lumbar disc involvement. In this test, the well leg is raised to the point of pain and is lowered by 5 degrees, and the foot and ankle are forcibly dorsiflexed. Once again, reproduction or exacerbation of pain in the sciatic nerve on the side of involvement suggests a midline space-occupying lesion or disc protrusion.[29] Motor strength, dermatomal testing, and reflex assessment further aid in the diagnosis of lumbar spinal disorders.[29,30]

Three other tests can help to rule out serious disease of the lumbar spine and of neurological structures. The Valsalva maneuver is performed by having the patient seated comfortably, with the arms slightly flexed at the elbows. The patient is instructed to take a deep breath and hold it. While holding the deep breath, the patient is asked to bear down to create greater intra-abdominal pressure. Reproduction of radicular pain is indicative of nerve root compression by a space-occupying mass in the spine.[31] This can result from nerve root entrapment at an intervertebral foramen or within the neural canal, and it may indicate a herniated intervertebral disc.[32]

Two tests are used to assess meningeal irritation caused by infectious or toxic meningitis.[30,33] In Kernig's test, the head and neck of the supine patient are passively flexed. Sudden radiating pain and buckling of the hips and knees suggest meningeal involvement. Brudzinski's sign is a variant of the straight leg raise. The patient lies supine while the examiner flexes the hip and knee. Then the knee is extended. Sudden radiating pain suggests meningeal irritation.

Additional clinical signs are likely to be present to confirm an impression of meningeal involvement. With most forms of meningitis, the patient is febrile, usually has a moderate irregular fever, demonstrates nuchal rigidity (stiff neck), may be photophobic, and has a severe headache. Of course, any form of meningitis is a clear, life-threatening emergency.

Two other orthopedic tests are very useful for a chiropractic assessment of patients with a low back pain complaint.[33] Goldthwait's test helps the practitioner to differentiate sacroiliac, lumbosacral and lumbar articulations as origins of low pain. The patient is placed in the supine position. The examiner palpates the low back and positions the fingers of one hand at the lumbosacral junction on the spinous processes of as many lumbar vertebrae as possible. With the other hand, the examiner flexes the patient's hip. If low back pain is reproduced or exacerbated before movement is palpated at the lumbosacral articulation, pain most likely originates at the sacroiliac joints. If low back pain is reproduced or exacerbated when movement is palpated at the lumbosacral articulation, the L5-S1 joint is likely involved. If low back pain is reproduced or exacerbated after the lumbosacral joint is set into motion, then a higher lumbar motor unit is most likely the source of low back pain. Often, the patient and the examiner can localize the source of lumbar pain when Goldthwait's test is properly performed.

A relatively common component of low back pain is lumbar facet syndrome.[29] With facet syndrome, the patient is likely to demonstrate pain-restricted range of motion on extension. Also, when lumbar ranges of motion are examined, the patient may be able to exhibit normal or nearly normal lumbar flexion. However, when the patient tries to stand upright, pain from lumbar facet impingement may restrict and slow the patient's return to an upright posture.

As has been noted by Panjabi,[34] functional changes in a spinal motor unit lead to progression of degenerative changes. Asymmetrical disc injury at one level creates disturbed joint kinematics above and below, causing asymmetrical movements at the facet joints. This disturbance causes unequal shearing of facet loads, resulting in intra-articular cartilage degeneration, joint space narrowing, and facet arthrosis.[34] Radiographs of the lumbar spine may well reveal an L5 retrolisthesis or degenerative alteration of the facets, which progresses after onset of degenerative disc disease. Macnab's lines drawn along the superior aspect of the sacrum and along the inferior L5 vertebral plate may allow for visualization of facet imbrications. If Macnab's lines intersect the region of the intervertebral foramen, this indicates possible facet imbrications. This radiographic finding coupled with localized groin, buttock, and/or thigh pain constitutes the facet syndrome.[29] Posterior joint complex pain rarely extends beyond the calf and into the foot; however, in cases of advanced nerve root compression, this situation may occur.[35]

Kemp's test is a useful procedure for evaluating passive range of motion of the lumbar spine and for screening the patient for lumbar facet syndrome.[29] To perform Kemp's test, one should stand behind and lateral to the patient. Place one hand on the patient's iliac crest to prevent it from moving. Grasp the patient's shoulder on the opposite side. Passively rotate, laterally flex, and extend the lumbar spine. Reproduction or exacerbation of low back pain on the side of lateral rotation suggests lumbar facet syndrome.

CONCURRENT CONDITIONS

Visceral disorders may cause pain referral to the pelvis and low back. When a patient has an atypical low back pain complaint, examine the health history to rule out viscerosomatic disease.

Genitourinary and colorectal disorders can underlie low back pain of insidious onset. Radiating flank pain that originates at the thoracolumbar junction, for example, may result from a vertebral or costovertebral subluxation complex, or it may occur as the early manifestation of kidney disease such as pyelonephritis, glomerulonephritis, or nephrolithiasis. The cardinal signs of urolithiasis are radiating flank pain and blood in the urine.[36] An abdominal aortic aneurysm may also mimic low back pain. Appropriate physical and radiological examinations assist in the identification of such disorders.[35]

Inflammatory and noninflammatory arthritides may also cause low back pain.[29] Degenerative disc disease or osteoarthritis of the spine is probably the most common form of arthritis. Although it is a chronic condition, osteoarthritis of the lumbar spine may be associated with intermittent acute exacerbations of low back pain. Ankylosing spondylitis is a progressive inflammatory arthritis that affects the pelvis and spine in adolescent and young adult males. The progression of ankylosing spondylitis, also known as Marie-Strumpell disease, is characterized, as are many autoimmune diseases, by unpredictable, intermittent periods of acute exacerbation and remission. Both osteoarthritis and ankylosing spondylitis can cause significant restriction to lumbar range of motion, as well as significant soft tissue pain and swelling during acute phases. The low force and specificity of the AM may be particularly effective in restoring and maintaining mobility while minimizing patient discomfort after acute exacerbation of either condition.

ADDITIONAL LUMBAR TESTING AND ADJUSTING

In addition to the L5, L4, and L2 tests and adjustments included in the Basic Scan Protocol, further lumbar involvement is suggested when the patient describes point tenderness at specific vertebral levels, when leg lengths do not balance after testing and adjustment, or when examination findings indicate. This testing begins with L3.

Third Lumbar (L3)

Consider neuroarticular dysfunction of the third lumbar vertebra when the patient has a concurrent knee complaint, or when examination findings reveal tenderness, restricted motion, or dermatomal involvement.

Isolation Test. Perform the Isolation Test for the third lumbar vertebra after testing and adjusting L4. Once the fourth lumbar vertebra has been tested and adjusted, instruct the patient to place the arm back on the table.

To isolate the third lumbar vertebra, instruct the patient to lift the hip on the side of Pelvic Deficiency off the table. The motion need not be very pronounced. Simply have the patient roll the hip on the side of Pelvic Deficiency up far enough to break contact between the anterior superior iliac spine and the surface of the table (Figure 10-1). This movement is thought to facilitate the movement of paraspinal muscles and neuroarticular components in the midlumbar spine in the region of L3. Look for PD leg reactivity in Position #1. Then proceed to Position #2, while observing relative changes in the PD leg. Follow the Short/Long Rule. If the PD leg lengthens in Position #2, the third lumbar motor unit involvement can be found on the side of Pelvic Deficiency. If the PD leg shortens in Position #2, the third lumbar motor unit involvement is on the side Opposite Pelvic Deficiency.

Pressure Test to confirm by applying a gentle, firm anterior and superior pressure on the inferior articular process, and observe for balancing of the legs in Position #1 and/or Position #2.

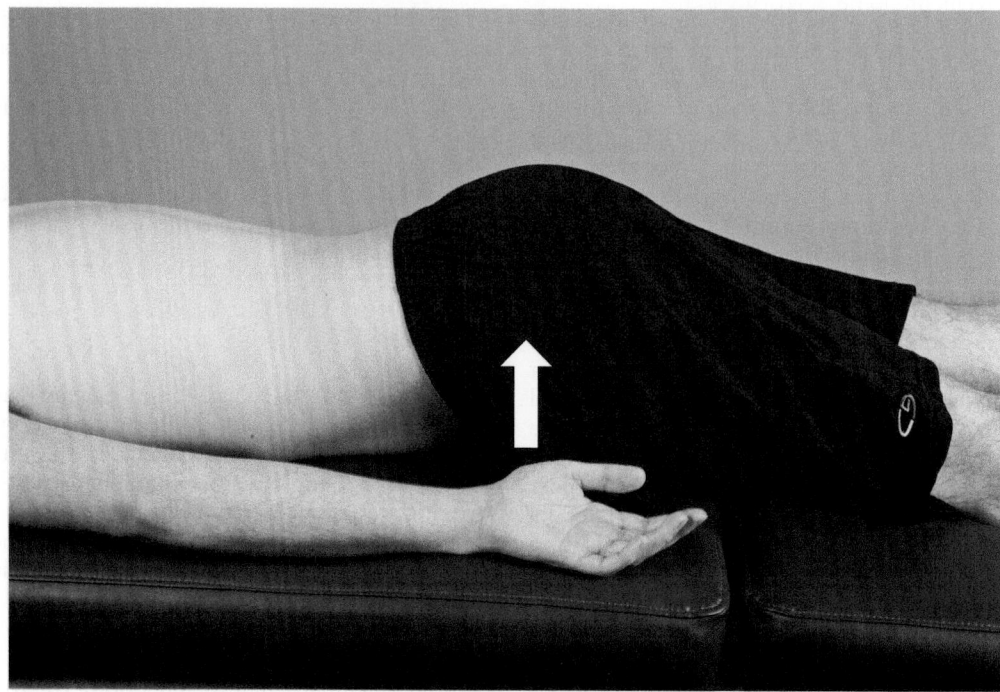

Figure 10-1   Isolation Test for third lumbar.

Adjustment.   To adjust for third lumbar involvement, contact the inferior articular process on the side indicated by the Short/Long Rule. The Line of Drive (LOD) is anterior and superior through the plane line of the facet (Figure 10-2). In this example, the adjustment is performed on the PD side. This would indicate that following the Short/Long Rule results in a relative lengthening in Position #2.

Alternative Third Lumbar Test.   A complaint of knee pain on the Opposite PD (OPD) side may not cause a reaction when the PD side of the hip is lifted off of the table. Isolation for third lumbar involvement can occur by lifting the OPD hip off of the table. Follow the AM Protocol after isolation to look for a relative leg length change in Position #1, and to follow the Short/Long Rule in Position #2 to determine the appropriate side for adjustment.

First Lumbar (L1)

After testing and adjustment of L2 have been performed, The AM Basic Scan Protocol normally proceeds to the twelfth thoracic vertebra. If patient complaints and examination findings warrant, it may be necessary to assess the first lumbar vertebra.

Isolation Test.   To isolate the first lumbar vertebra after the second lumbar vertebra has been tested and adjusted, instruct the patient to keep

the forearm on the OPD side on the low back. Ask the patient to raise and place the forearm of the PD side on the table superior and lateral to the head (Figure 10-3). This movement and position are thought to assist the paraspinal muscles and neuroarticular components in the region of the upper lumbar spine or L1. Look for PD leg reactivity in Position #1. Then proceed to Position #2, while observing relative changes in the PD leg. Follow the Short/Long Rule.

If the PD leg lengthens in Position #2, the first lumbar motor unit involvement is noted on the side of Pelvic Deficiency. If the PD leg shortens in Position #2, first lumbar motor unit involvement can be observed on the OPD side. Pressure Test to confirm by applying a gentle, firm anterior and superior pressure on the inferior articular process, as indicated by the Short/Long Rule, and observe for balance of the legs in Position #1 and/or Position #2.

Adjustment.   To adjust first lumbar motor unit involvement, contact the inferior articular process on the side indicated by the Short/Long Rule. The LOD is found anterior and superior through the plane line of the facet (Figure 10-4). In this example, the adjustment is performed on the OPD side. This indicates that following the Short/Long Rule resulted in a relative shortening in Position #2.

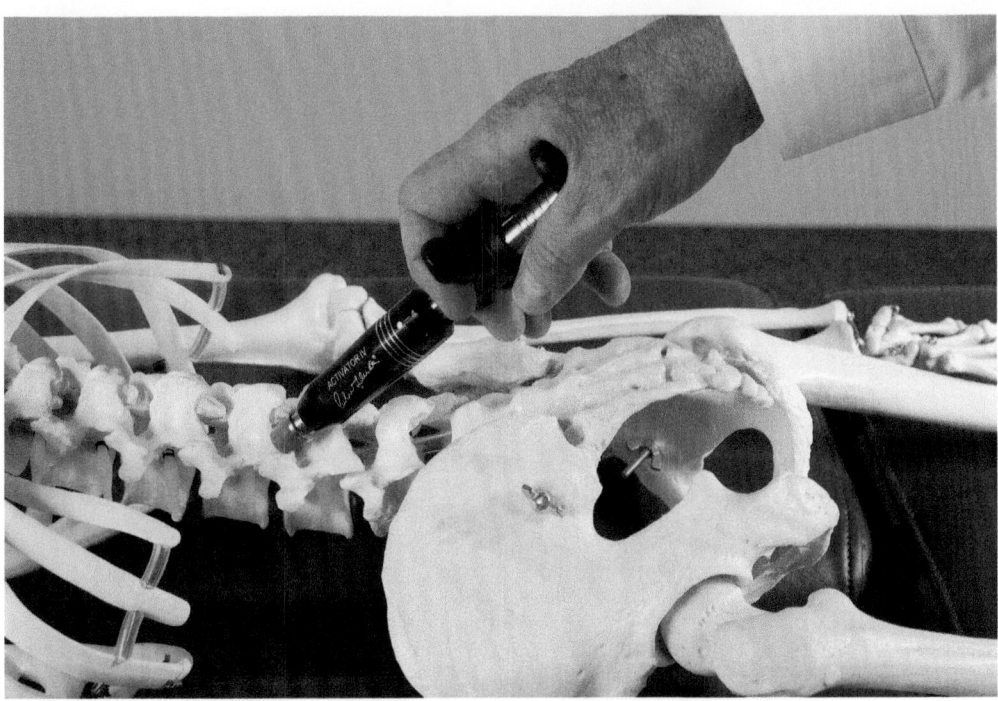

Figure 10-2 Adjustment for third lumbar. Line of Drive is anterior and superior.

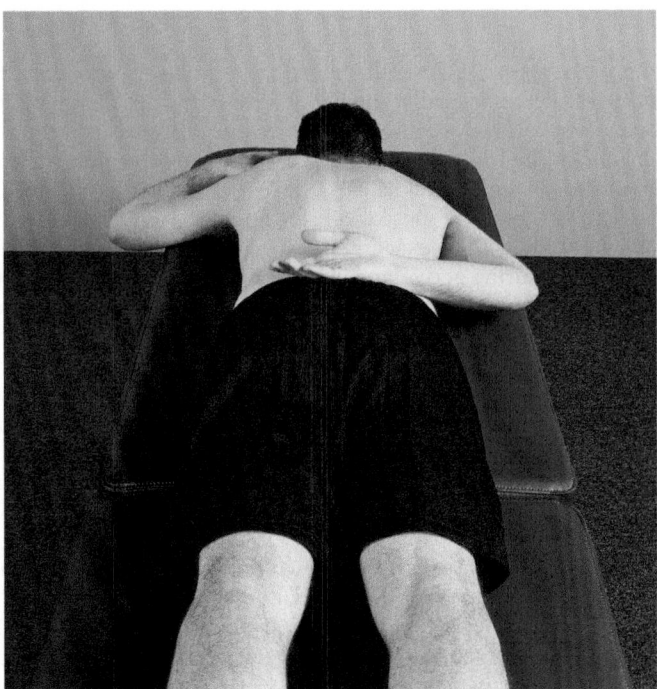

Figure 10-3 Isolation Test for first lumbar.

Facet Syndromes

When a patient experiences low back pain that is exacerbated by extension and rotation of the lumbar vertebrae or lumbosacral joints or by radiological evidence, consider facet syndrome.

Facet syndrome is generally a unilateral phenomenon that consists of rotation and extension malposition of a vertebra, shifting weight bearing posteriorly and laterally onto the zygapophyseal joint on the side of involvement. The two

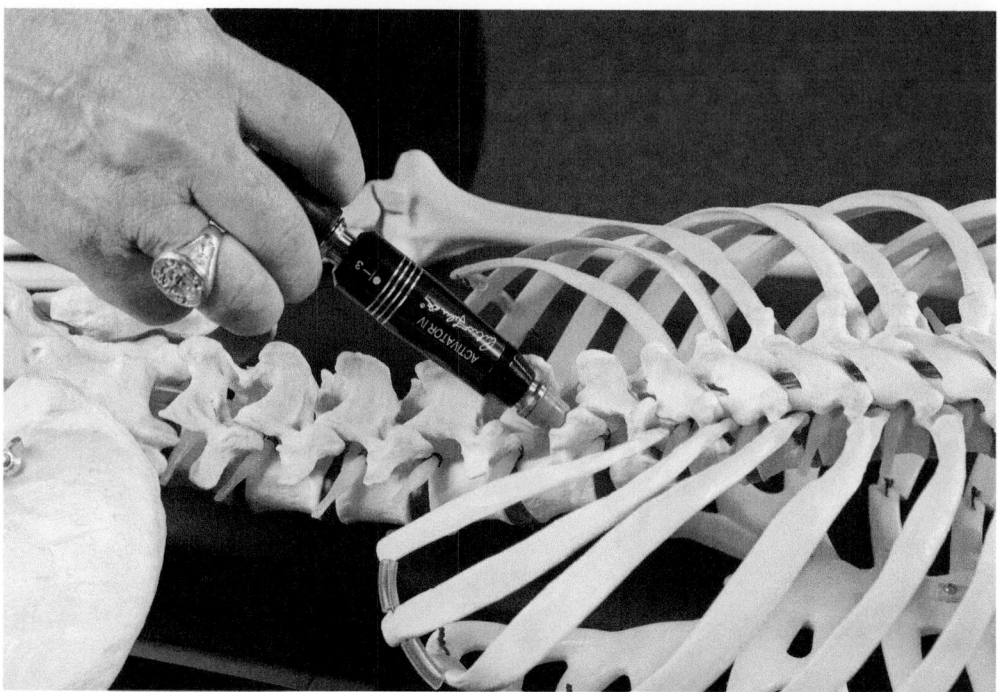

Figure 10-4   Adjustment for first lumbar. Line of Drive is anterior and superior.

most caudal motor units of the spine—L5-S1 (the lumbosacral joint) and L4-L5—are, logically, the most likely to develop facet syndrome because of their transitional and stress-prone locations.

Unilateral L5-S1 Facet Syndrome.   Unilateral pain localized at the lumbosacral articulation suggests L5-S1 facet syndrome. Pain is likely to be exacerbated by extension maneuvers during active and passive lumbar range-of-motion testing. The patient may experience sharp, localized pain when Kemp's test is performed. With Kemp's test, which may be performed with the patient standing or seated, the lumbar spine is passively rotated, laterally flexed, and extended. Radiating pain to the lower extremities indicates a disc or other space-occupying lesion of the lumbar region.[33] Although sharp, localized pain on extension and rotation is not strictly a positive Kemp's test, it may indicate facet involvement at the lumbosacral articulation.[29,33]

Before you attempt to isolate and adjust for a unilateral lumbosacral facet syndrome, complete testing and adjustment for pelvic misalignments (e.g., AS and PI iliums, superior or inferior pubic bone, superior or inferior sacrum). Perform the Isolation Test and adjustment as indicated for the standard L5 motor unit involvement. Also, evaluate L5 for superior or inferior spinous malposition by using Position #3. An inferior

spinous subluxation or an extension malposition of L5 is the misalignment that is more likely to be encountered in conjunction with lumbosacral facet involvement. Once L5 involvements have been cleared, proceed to Stress Testing for unilateral L5-S1 facet syndrome.

Stress Test.   To Stress Test for L5-S1 facet syndrome, instruct the patient to perform the Isolation Test for the fifth lumbar by placing the forearm on the side of Pelvic Deficiency on the low back (Figure 10-5). Firmly dorsiflex both feet simultaneously, as is done when Position #5 is attained (Figure 10-6). This movement is thought to stress the L5-S1 facets and involves the neurological feed forward mechanism that simulates the push-off phase of gait. Look for PD leg reactivity in Position #1. Then proceed to Position #2, while observing relative changes in the PD leg. Follow the Short/Long Rule.

If the PD leg lengthens in Position #2, the test suggests L5-S1 facet involvement on the side of Pelvic Deficiency. If the PD leg shortens in Position #2, the test suggests L5-S1 facet involvement on the OPD side. Pressure Test to confirm involvement by applying gentle but firm superior pressure on the inferior articular process of L5 and simultaneously inferior pressure on the ala of the sacrum on the side of involvement. Look for the legs to balance in Position #1 and/or Position #2.

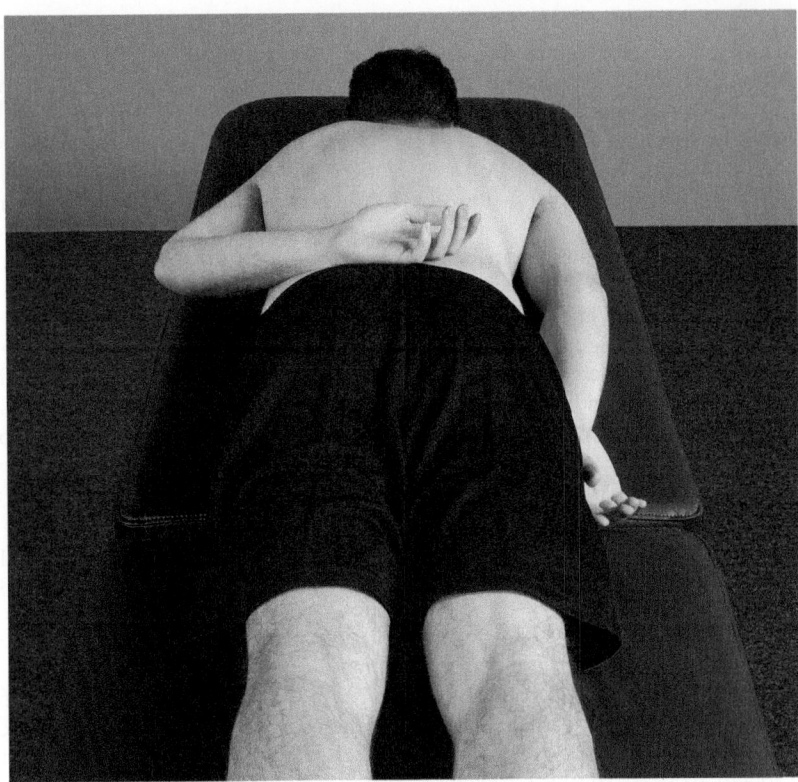

Figure 10-5 Isolation Test for fifth lumbar.

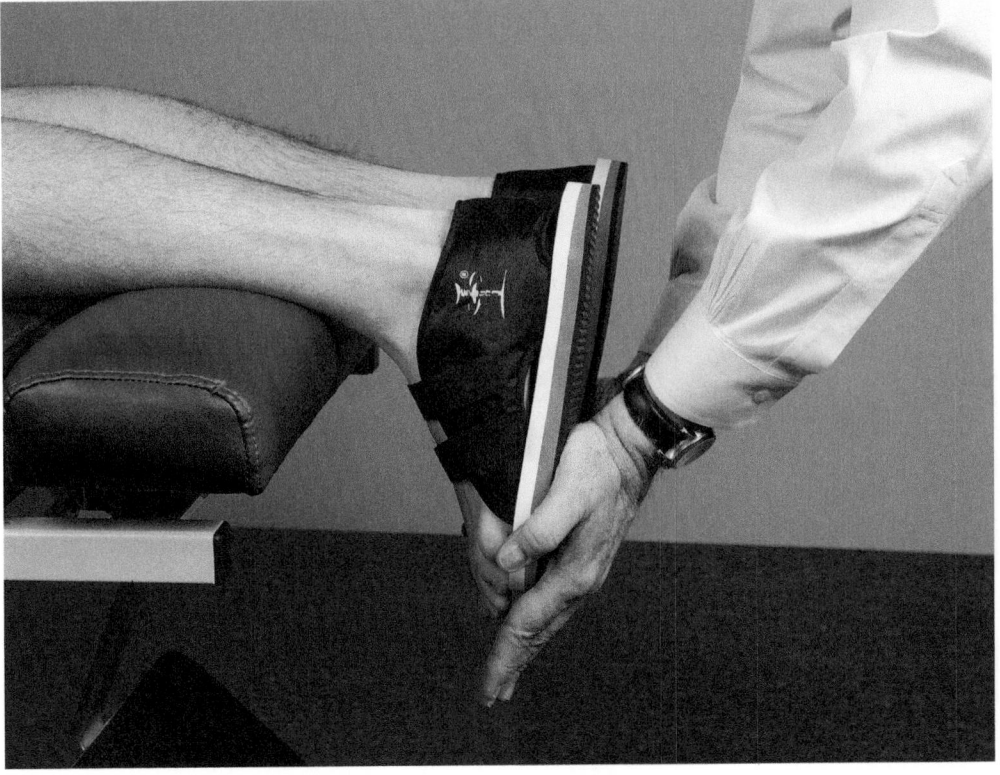

Figure 10-6 Stress Test for L5-S1 facet.

Adjustment. The adjustment for L5-S1 facet involvement consists of two contacts and thrusts. For the first part of the adjustment, contact the inferior articular process of the fifth lumbar vertebra on the side of involvement, as indicated by the Short/Long Rule. The LOD is anterior and superior through the plane line of the facet (Figure 10-7).

For the second part of the adjustment, contact the ala of the sacrum on the side of involvement, as indicated by the Short/Long Rule. The LOD is anterior and inferior (Figure 10-8).

Unilateral L4-L5 Facet Syndrome. Unilateral pain at the level of the fourth and fifth lumbars may also suggest facet involvement. The pain of facet syndrome is likely to be exacerbated by extension, lateral flexion, and rotation of the lumbar spine during active or passive range-of-motion testing. Similar to lumbosacral facet syndrome, L4-L5 facet syndrome is likely to be exacerbated by performance of Kemp's test.

Stress Test. To Stress Test for L4-L5 facet syndrome, instruct the patient to place the forearm on the OPD side of the low back (Figure 10-9). Perform Position #5 by firmly dorsiflexing both feet simultaneously (see Figure 10-6). This movement is thought to stress the L4-L5 facets. Look for PD leg reactivity in Position #1. Then proceed to Position #2, while observing relative

changes in the PD leg. Follow the Short/Long Rule. If the PD leg lengthens in Position #2, the test suggests L4-L5 facet involvement on the side of Pelvic Deficiency. If the PD leg shortens in Position #2, the test suggests L4-L5 facet involvement on the OPD side.

Adjustment. The adjustment for L4-L5 facet involvement consists of two contacts and thrusts. For the first part of the adjustment, contact the inferior articular process of L4 on the side of involvement, as indicated by the Short/Long Rule. The LOD is anterior and superior through the plane line of the facet (Figure 10-10).

For the second part of the adjustment, contact the superior articular process of L5 on the side of involvement, as indicated by the Short/Long Rule. The LOD is anterior and inferior (Figure 10-11).

SIDE NOTE: The AM Protocol requires testing of the isolated vertebra in Position #3 after motor unit involvement has been found, and/or if the vertebra is in the area of the chief complaint. Association of an inferior L5 spinous with an L5-S1 facet syndrome or an inferior L4 spinous with an L4-L5 facet syndrome is common. The AM Protocol uses Position #3 for Superiority/Flexion or Inferiority/Extension of the vertebra. Always test for one involvement when the other one is found.

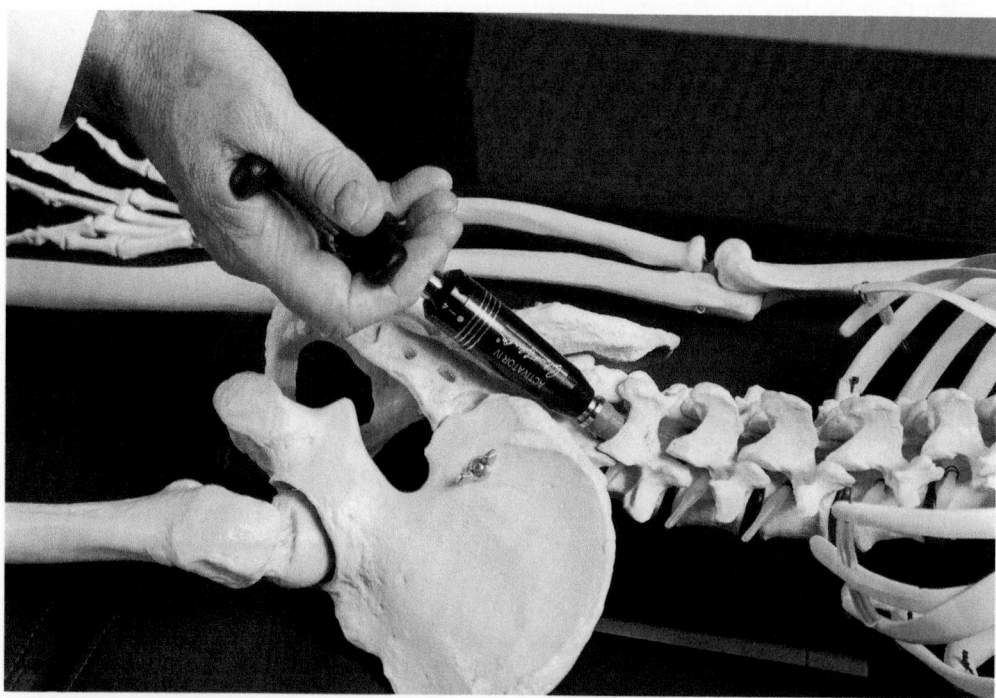

Figure 10-7   Adjustment for Opposite Pelvic Deficiency L5-S1 facet, Step One. Line of Drive is anterior and superior.

Position #3—Superior/Flexion or Inferior/ Extension of the Lumbar Spinous

If lumbar symptoms persist, or if adjustments of typical lumbar motor unit involvements do not stabilize, consider a superior or inferior spinous misalignment at the level of involvement. In the AM, the term *superior spinous* refers to a vertebra in flexion malposition, in which the spinous process has deviated superiorly. The term *inferior spinous* refers to a vertebra in extension

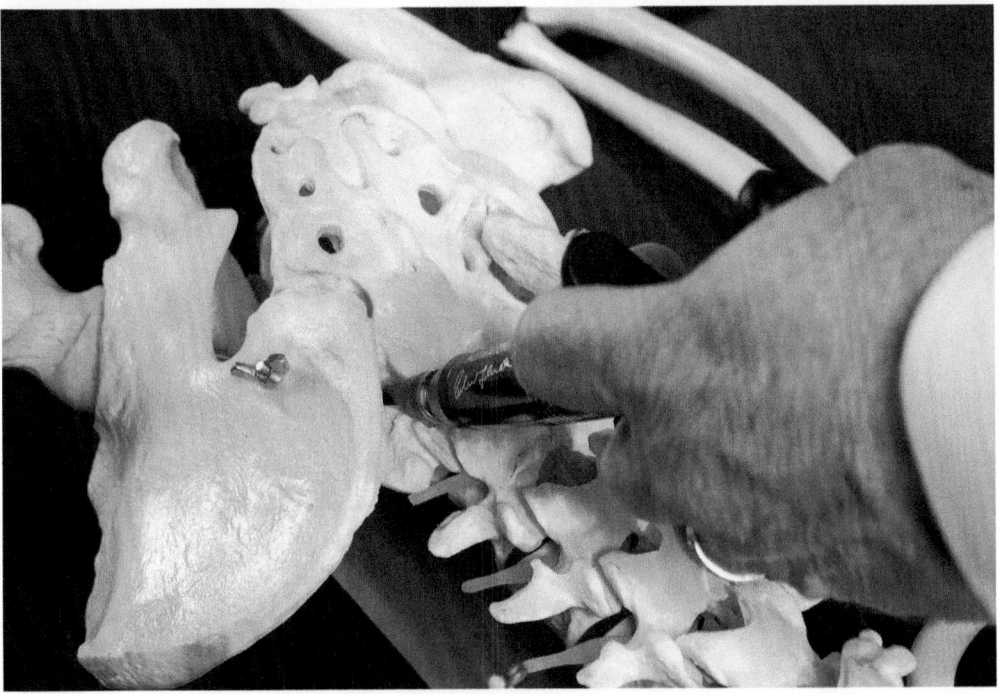

Figure 10-8   Adjustment for Opposite Pelvic Deficiency L5-S1 facet, Step Two. Line of Drive is anterior and inferior.

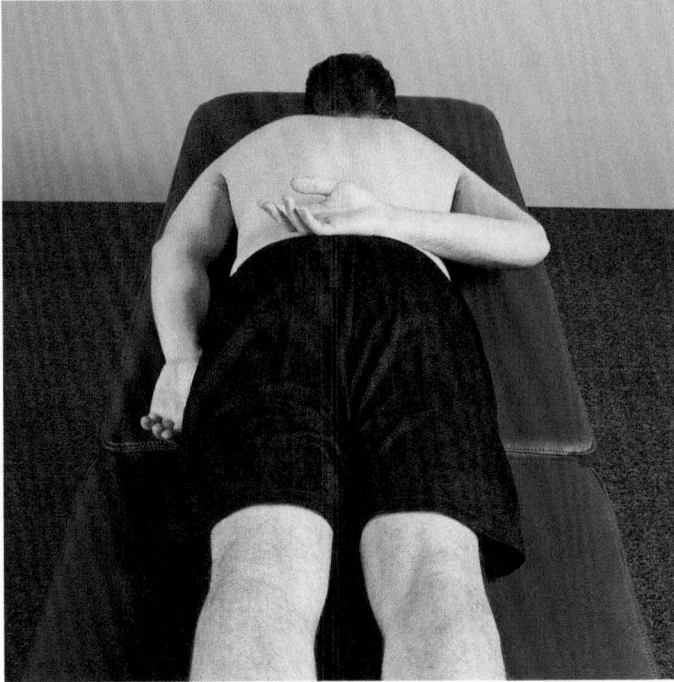

Figure 10-9   Isolation Test for fourth lumbar.

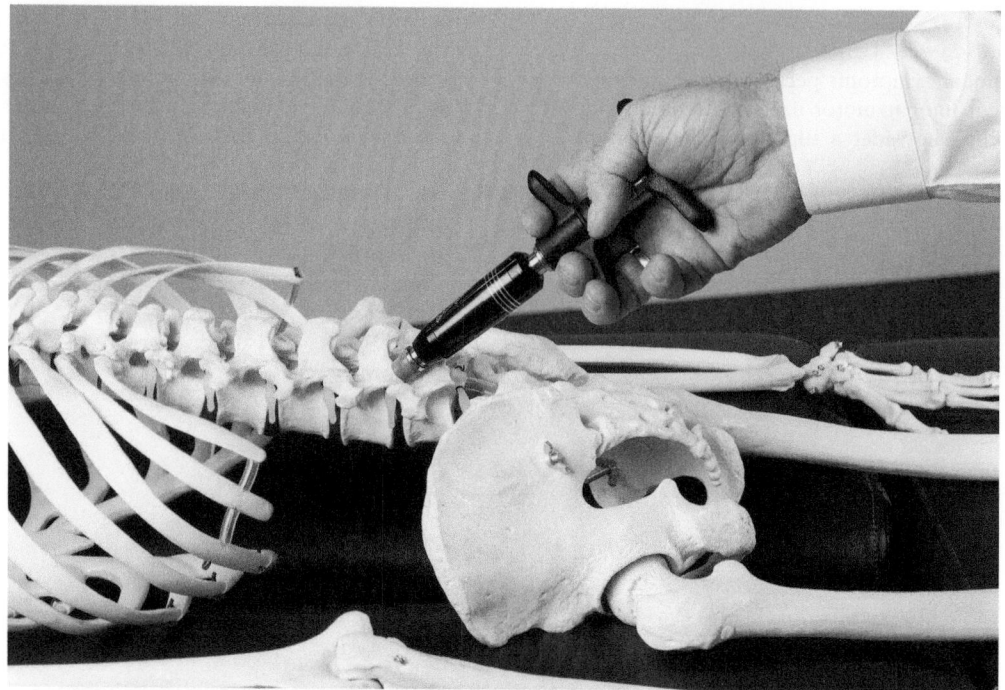

Figure 10-10 Adjustment for Pelvic Deficiency L4-L5 facet, Step One. Line of Drive is anterior and superior.

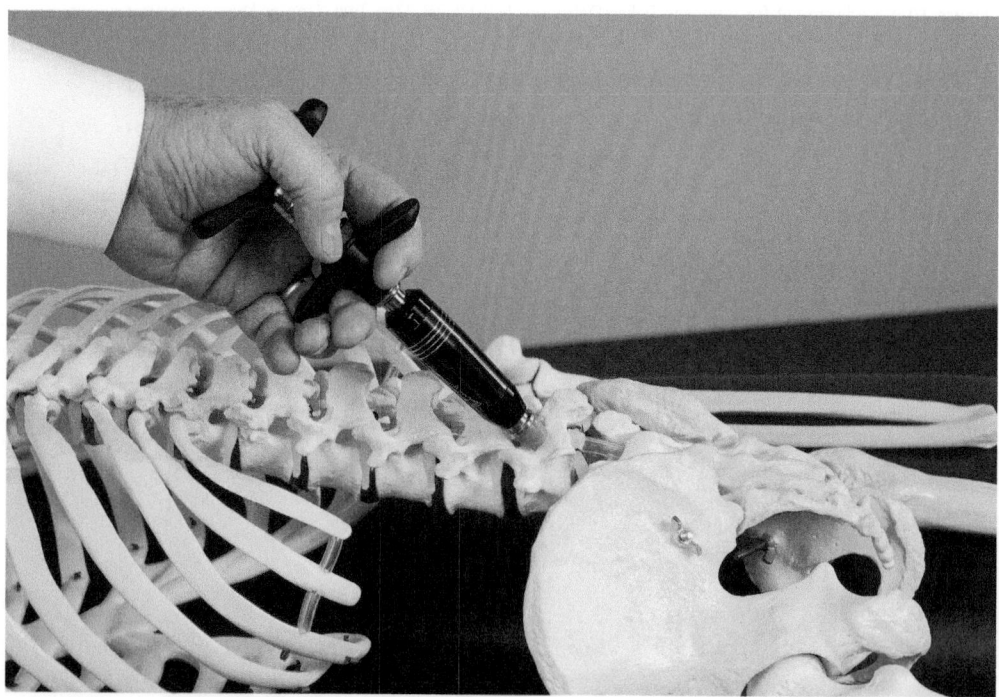

Figure 10-11 Adjustment for Pelvic Deficiency L4-L5 facet, Step Two. Line of Drive is anterior and inferior.

malposition in a place where the spinous process has deviated inferiorly.

Isolation Test. To test for a superior or inferior spinous of a lumbar vertebra, instruct the patient to perform the Isolation Test maneuver for the specific vertebral level. For example, to isolate L4, ask the patient to place the forearm of the OPD side on the low back (see Figure 10-9). After the patient has performed the isolation maneuver for a given lumbar vertebral level, Stress Test the vertebra further by raising the legs to Position #3. In Position #3, the legs are flexed past the 90 degrees of Position #2, or to resistance (Figure 10-12). This action is thought to further stress the isolated area in the sagittal plane.

If the PD leg lengthens in Position #3 (see Figure 10-12), the test indicates a flexion malposition or a superior spinous of the involved lumbar vertebra. If the PD leg shortens in Position #3 (Figure 10-13), the test indicates extension malposition or an inferior spinous of the involved lumbar vertebra.

Adjustment for an Inferior Spinous or Extension Malposition. To adjust an inferior spinous (extension malposition) of a lumbar vertebra, contact the inferior aspect of the spinous process. The LOD is superior and slightly anterior to maintain contact (Figure 10-14).

To facilitate the LOD and to ensure as effective an adjustment as possible, use the thumb of the free hand to take an inferior-to-superior tissue pull over the spinous process of the vertebra to be adjusted. Use the thumb to stabilize the tip of the instrument during the adjustment.

Adjustment for a Superior Spinous of Flexion Malposition. To adjust a superior spinous (flexion malposition) of a lumbar vertebra, contact the superior aspect of the spinous process. The LOD is inferior and slightly anterior to maintain contact (Figure 10-15).

To facilitate the LOD and to ensure as effective an adjustment as possible, use the thumb of the free hand to take a superior-to-inferior tissue pull over the spinous process of the vertebra to be adjusted. Use the thumb to stabilize the tip of the instrument during the adjustment.

Position #4—Segmental Laterality

For patients who experience pain at the apex of scoliosis in the lumbar region, usually at the level of L2 or L1, it is advised to use testing step Position #4 to locate segmental laterality. Also, segmental laterality may be found in patients with pain down the anterior area of the thigh and involvement in near-side or far-side vehicle collisions.

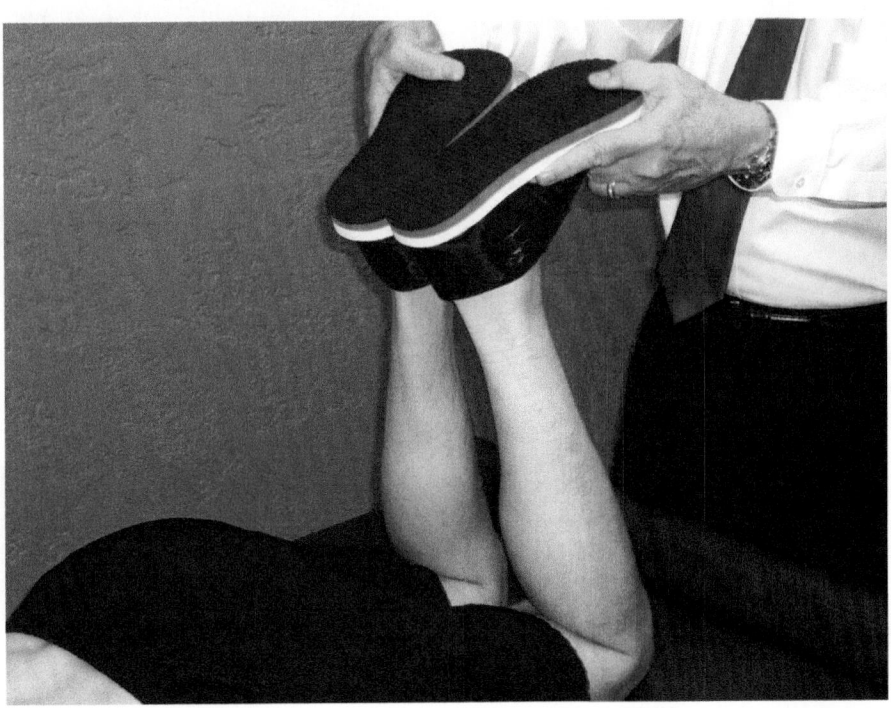

Figure 10-12 The Pelvic Deficiency leg lengthens in Position #3, indicating superior spinous.

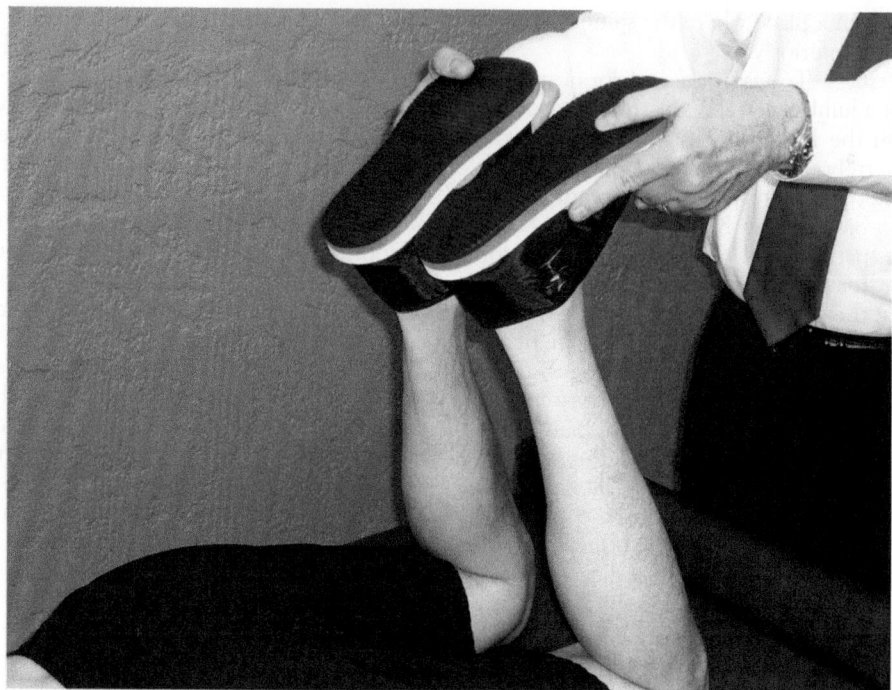

Figure 10-13 The Pelvic Deficiency leg shortens in Position #3, indicating inferior spinous.

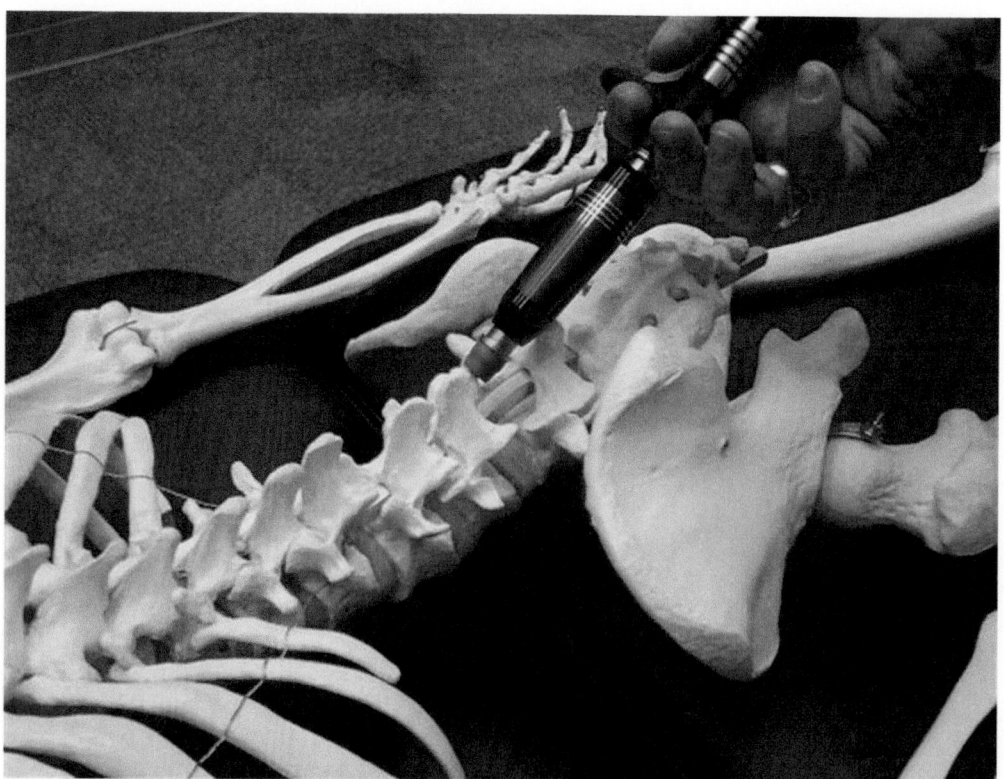

Figure 10-14 Adjustment for inferior spinous. Line of Drive is superior and slightly anterior.

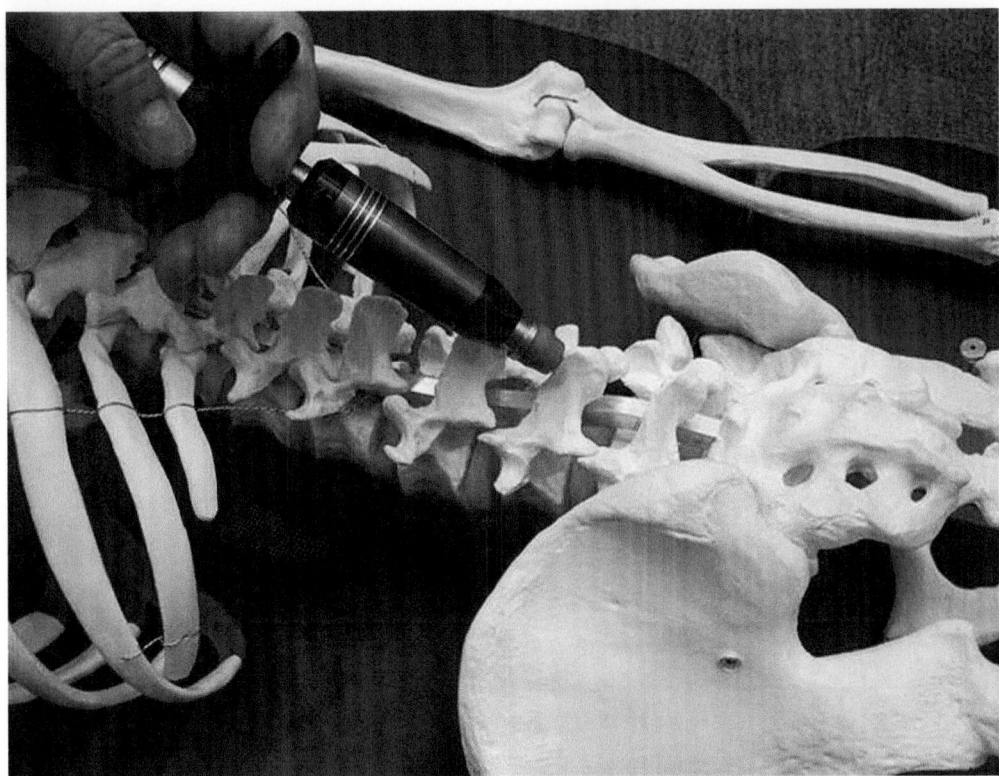

Figure 10-15 Adjustment for superior spinous. Line of Drive is inferior and slightly anterior.

Isolation Test. To test for segmental laterality at a given vertebral level, first perform the Isolation Test for that vertebra using Positions #1 and Position #2. Pressure Test the vertebra, and adjust as indicated. Our example for this test is the second lumbar vertebra (both forearms resting on the low back; see Chapter 7, Figure 7-27). Because no other Isolation Tests have been performed to this point, that vertebra is still considered to be isolated. Flex the knee on the PD side past 90 degrees and/or to resistance while the OPD leg remains on the table. This is known as Position #4 (Figure 10-16). Look for PD leg reactivity in Position #1. Then proceed to Position #2, while observing relative changes in the PD leg. Follow the Short/Long Rule.

Adjustment. To adjust for segmental laterality, use the thumb to brace the spinous process and stop rotation during the adjustment. Contact the pedicle-lamina junction on the side as indicated by the Short/Long Rule. The LOD is straight medial (Figure 10-17).

Note: Position #3 and Position #4 can be used throughout the axial skeletal system from the sacrum through the occiput. Also, the Facet Stress Test, known as Position #5, may be used from the fifth lumbar superiorly through the second cervical vertebra.

SIDE NOTE: QUADRATUS LUMBORUM If a patient experiences pain over the posterior superior iliac spine and/or pain into the greater trochanter region, or pain between the twelfth rib and the iliac crest and/or into the lower quadrant of the abdominals, consider testing for and adjusting the tendinous junctions of the quadratus lumborum. Quadratus lumborum complaints often arise in those patients who stand for long periods of time or experience acute low back spasms and active disk syndromes with compensating antalgic postures.

The quadratus lumborum is generally composed of two major components.[37] The lateral portion of the muscle arises from the iliolumbar ligament at the iliac crest and inserts into the lower border of the twelfth rib. The medial portion arises from the iliac crest and attaches by four small tendons to the apices of the adjacent transverse processes of the upper lumbar vertebrae. Additional fibers, anterior to the superiormedially directed fibers, pass superiorlaterally from the lower three to four transverse processes of the lumbar vertebra, to the lower margin of the twelfth rib. The quadratus lumborum passes through the lateral lumbosacral arch of the diaphragm.[38] The quadratus lumborum muscle is a hip elevator when the lumbar spine is stabilized,

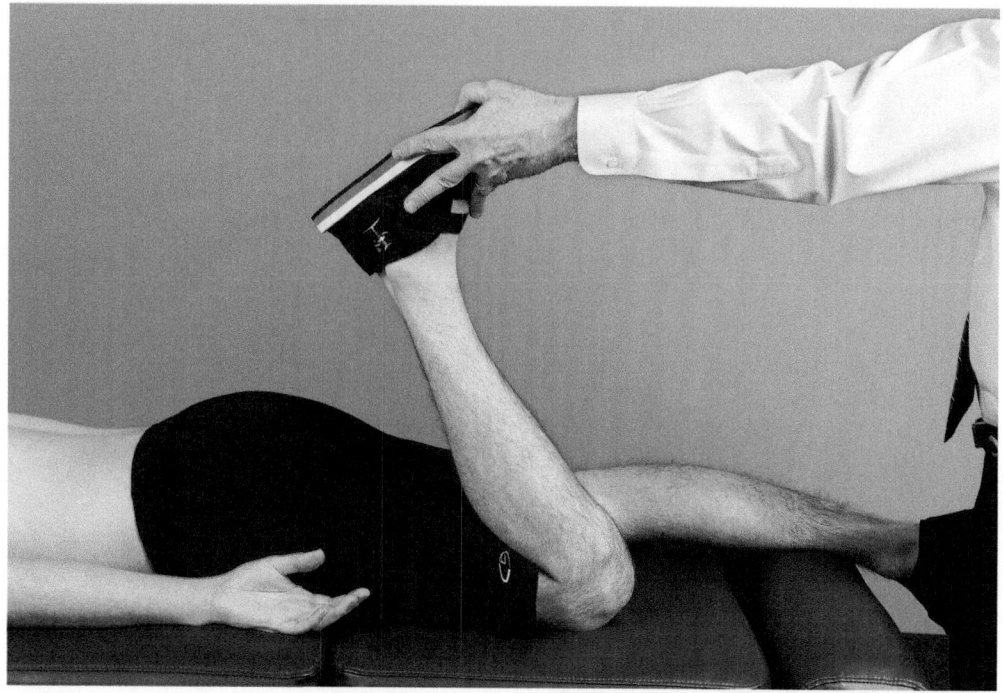

Figure 10-16 Position #4: segmental laterality.

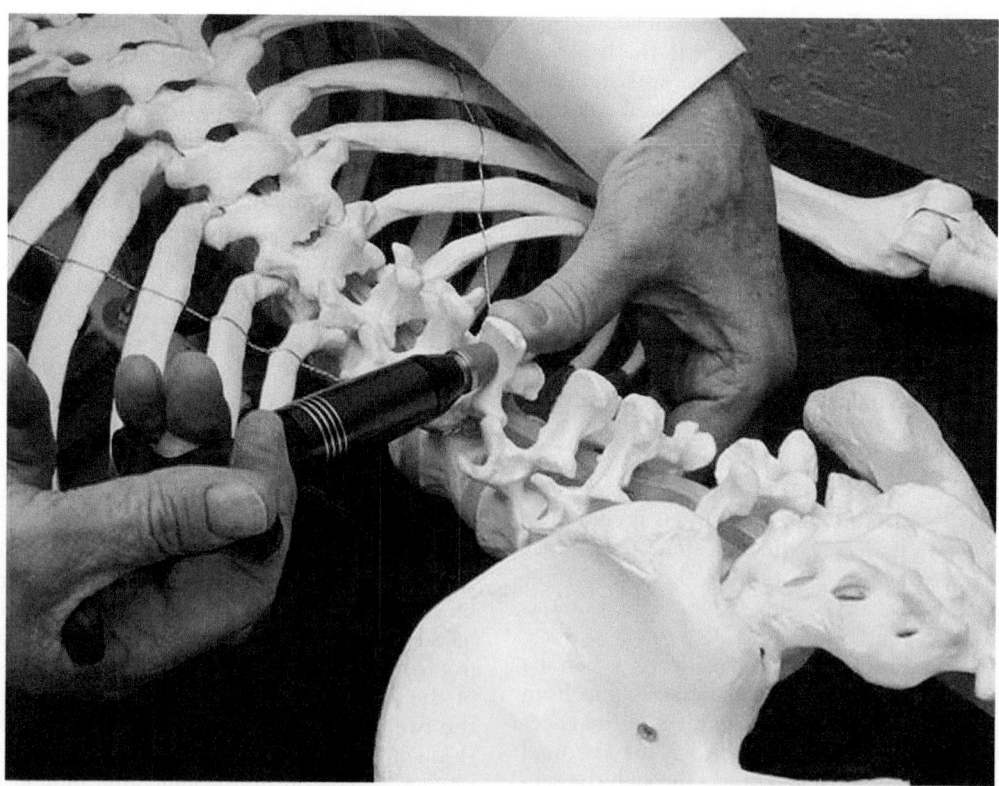

Figure 10-17 Adjustment for segmental laterality. Line of Drive is medial.

and it is a lateral flexor of the lumbar spine when the hip is stabilized. It can also elevate the pelvis or depress the thorax.[37]

Isolation Test.   Ask the patient to reach with the hand toward the knee on the affected side, thus laterally flexing the lumbar spine. This movement should be just sufficient to contract the quadratus lumborum without affecting the lower half of the body (Figure 10-18). Look for PD leg reactivity in Position #1. You may also choose to test the opposite side for involvement by following the same procedure on the OPD side and then looking for PD leg reactivity in Position #1. Involvement may be bilateral.

Adjustment.   To adjust the attachments of the quadratus lumborum, contact the superior attachment at the twelfth rib. The LOD is superior and slightly medial (Figure 10-19). The second contact is found on the inferior attachment at the iliac crest. The LOD is inferior and slightly lateral (Figure 10-20).

Psoas Muscle Imbalance

When a patient experiences groin pain, pubic bone pain, or low back pain or exhibits large Leg Length Inequalities, consider psoas muscle imbalance. Also, evaluate for psoas asymmetry when a patient suffers from functional scoliosis of the lumbar spine. Unilateral psoas contracture is relatively common in association with the lumbar subluxation complex. Facilitation and contracture of the iliopsoas muscle complex can alter hip range of motion because of the muscle's role in hip flexion. In addition, a contracture of the psoas muscle may produce a positive Thomas' test. Often low back pain, groin complaints, and inner thigh symptoms may be caused by pain that is referred from the psoas muscle. Paresthesias and dysesthesias in the anterior thigh can be due to entrapment of the anterior femoral cutaneous nerve between the quadratus lumborum and the iliopsoas.[39] In these cases, testing and correcting the quadratus lumborum and the psoas muscle on the affected side may offer the patient some relief.

Isolation Test.   To isolate for involvement of the psoas muscle, lift the patient's legs to induce slight flexion of the knees, and hold them while you ask the patient to press both knees into the table top (Figure 10-21). Look for PD leg reactivity in Position #1. Then proceed to Position #2, while observing relative changes in the PD leg. Follow the Short/Long Rule. If the PD leg lengthens in Position #2, adjust on the PD side. If the PD leg shortens in Position #2, adjust on the side Opposite Pelvic Deficiency.

Adjustment.   To adjust for psoas muscle imbalance, first raise the table and reposition the patient in the supine position. Contact the

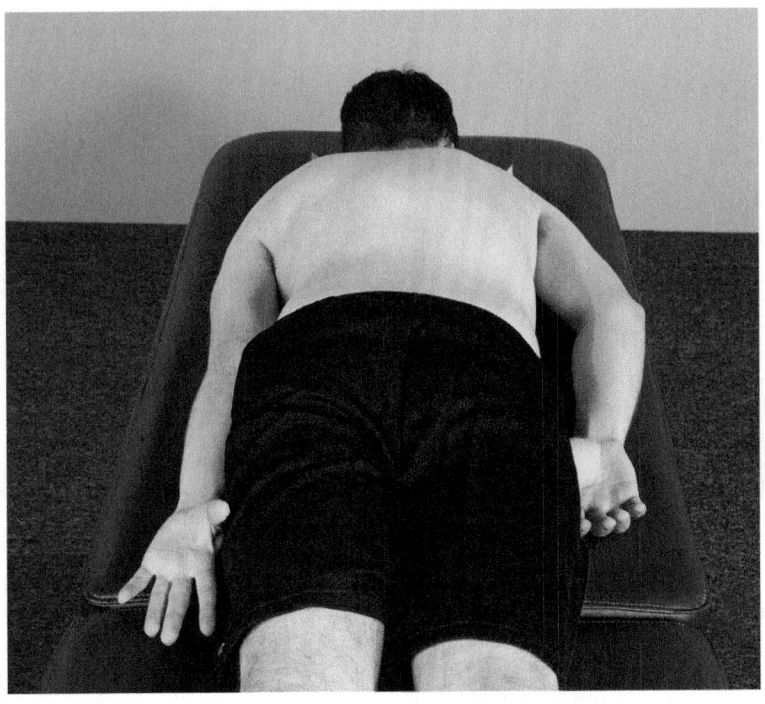

Figure 10-18   Isolation Test for quadratus lumborum.

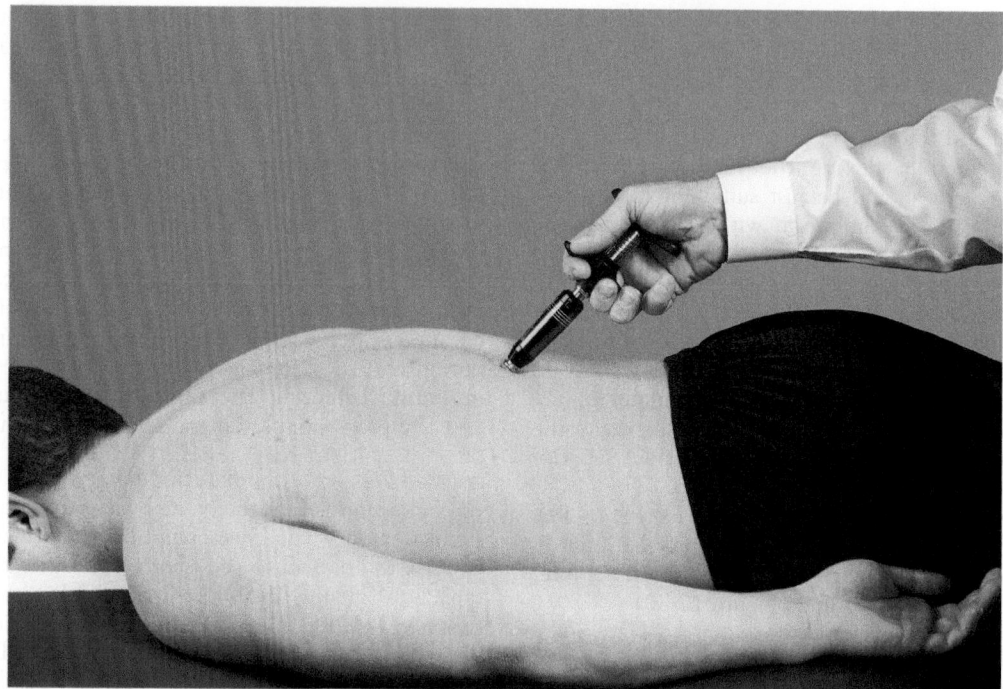

Figure 10-19   Adjustment for quadratus lumborum, Step One. Line of Drive is superior and slightly medial.

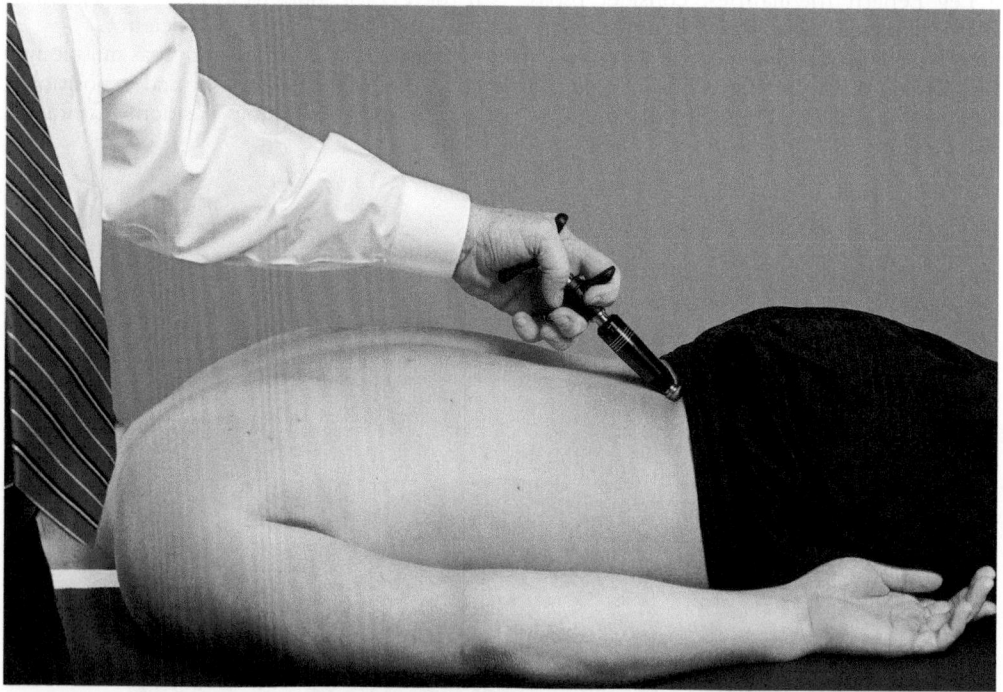

Figure 10-20   Adjustment for quadratus lumborum, Step Two. Line of Drive is inferior and slightly lateral.

abdomen over the belly of the psoas muscle about three inches superior to the inguinal ligament and at the lateral border of the rectus abdominus. The LOD is inferior, slightly posterior, and slightly lateral in line with the fibers of the psoas muscle (Figure 10-22).

For the patient with a pendulous abdomen, it may be advisable to compress tissue over the psoas muscle before positioning the tip of the instrument.

Mechanical force, manually assisted chiropractic adjusting for the lumbar spine is summarized in Table 10-1. Related research is summarized and presented in Boxes 10-2 through 10-8.

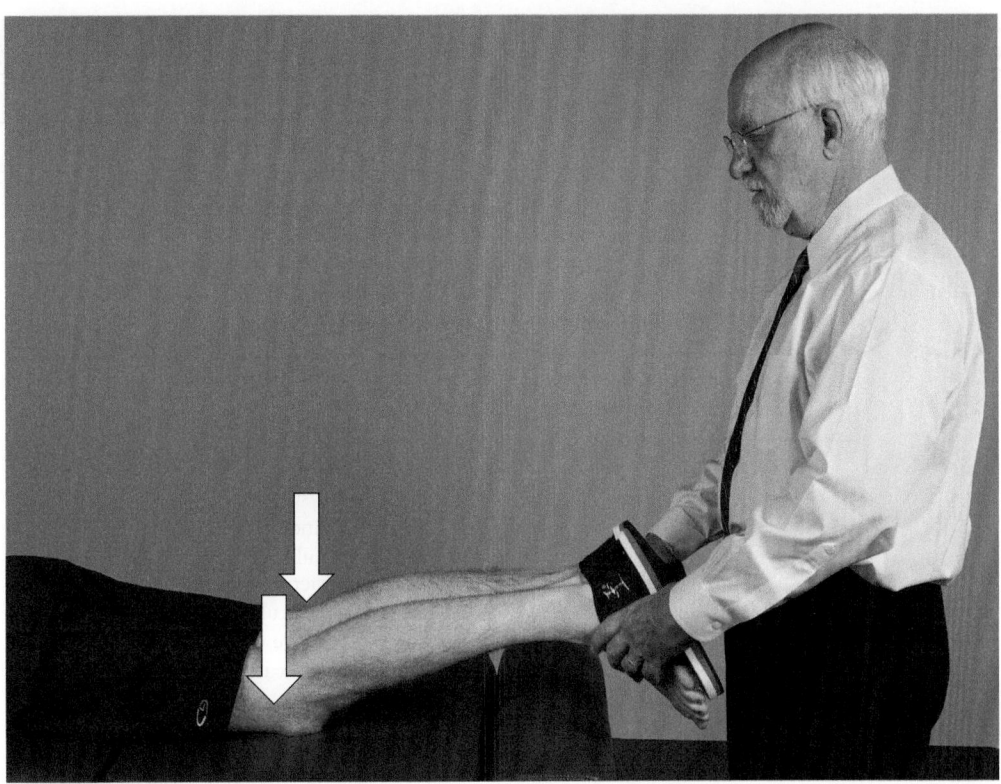

Figure 10-21   Isolation Test for psoas muscle imbalance; patient pushes knees into table.

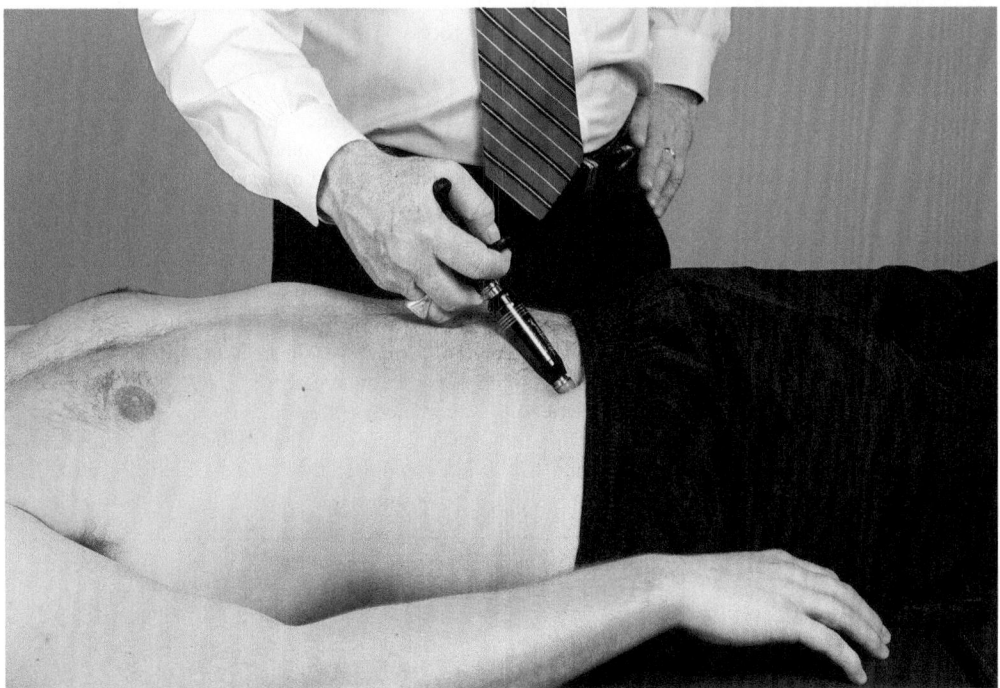

Figure 10-22   Adjustment for psoas muscle imbalance. Line of Drive is inferior, slightly posterior, and slightly lateral.

Table 10-1 Summary Table—Additional Tests and Adjustments for the Lumbar Spine

Articular Dysfunction	Test	ADJUSTMENT	
		Segmental Contact Point	Line of Drive
Third Lumbar	Instruct patient to lift hip on side of PD off the table	Inferior articular process on side indicated by Short/Long Rule	Anterior-superior
First Lumbar	Instruct patient to place and rest the OPD forearm on the low back and then place the forearm of the PD side on the table superior and lateral next to head	Inferior articular process on side indicated by Short/Long Rule	Anterior-superior
Unilateral L5-S1 Facet Syndrome	Instruct patient to place forearm on side of PD on low back with palm up. Dorsiflex both feet simultaneously.	*Step One*: Inferior articular process of L5 on side of involvement as indicated by Short/Long Rule	Anterior-superior
		Step Two: Ala of sacrum	Anterior-inferior
Unilateral L4-L5 Facet Syndrome	Instruct patient to place OPD forearm on low back with palm up. Dorsiflex both feet simultaneously.	*Step One*: Inferior articular process of L4 on side of involvement as indicated by Short/Long Rule	Anterior-superior
		Step Two: Superior articular process of L5 on side of involvement as indicated by Short/Long Rule	Anterior-inferior
Inferior Spinous/ Extension Malposition	Raise legs past 90 degrees to Position #3. If PD leg shortens, indicates inferior spinous.	Inferior aspect of the spinous process	Superior
Superior Spinous/ Flexion Malposition	Raise legs past 90 degrees to Position #3. If PD leg lengthens, indicates superior spinous.	Superior aspect of the spinous process	Inferior
Segmental Laterality	Flex the knee on the PD side past 90 degrees to Position #4. Follow the Short/Long Rule in Position #2.	Pedicle-lamina junction. Use thumb to brace spinous process, stopping rotation.	Medial
Quadratus Lumborum	Ask the patient to reach toward the knee on the involved side	*Step One*: Superior attachment to twelfth rib	Superior and medial
		Step Two: Inferior attachment to iliac crest	Inferior and lateral
Psoas Imbalance	Doctor grasps proximal to ankle, flex knees to 30 degrees, instructs patient to push knees into table. Follow the Short/Long Rule.	The abdomen over the belly of the psoas muscle about three inches superior to the inguinal ligament and at the lateral border of the rectus abdominis	Inferior, slightly posterior, and slightly lateral in line with the fibers of the psoas muscle

OPD, Opposite Pelvic Deficiency; *PD*, Pelvic Deficiency.

RELATED RESEARCH

Box 10-2

Reference: Gemmell HA, Jacobson BH. The immediate effect of Activator vs. Meric adjustment on acute low back pain: a randomized controlled trial. J Manipulative Physiol Ther. 1995;18(7):453-6.

ABSTRACT

OBJECTIVE

To compare the immediate effects on pain of Meric and Activator adjustments in patients with acute low back pain (LBP)

DESIGN

Adjustments were compared using a randomized, controlled clinical trial for relative effectiveness.

SETTING

The study was conducted at a private chiropractic clinic in Tulsa, Oklahoma.

PATIENTS

Thirty consecutive established patients who presented with acute LBP were studied. Sixteen subjects were randomly assigned to the Meric group and 14 to an Activator group. The mean (standard deviation [SD]) age was 53.5 years (9.5) for the Activator group and 51.8 years (10.3) for the Meric group.

INTERVENTION

Subjects received a single Meric or Activator adjustment to the posterior joints involved.

OUTCOME MEASURES

Before and immediately after adjustments were made, subjects rated their pain intensity on a visual analog pain scale.

RESULTS

The mean reduction in pain for the Activator group was means = 22.2, SD = 21.7; for the Meric group means = 21.8, SD = 21.5. The results reveal no significant difference between Meric and Activator adjustments in reducing acute LBP (F = .005; df = 2, 27; p = .941).

CONCLUSION

This study demonstrated no advantage of one procedure over the other for the reduction of pain.

Box 10-3

Reference: Richards GL, Thompson JS, Osterbauer PJ, Fuhr AW. Low force chiropractic care of two patients with sciatic neuropathy and lumbar disc herniation. Am J Chiropractic Med. 1990;3(1): 25-32.

ABSTRACT

Two patients with sciatic neuropathy and confirmed disc herniation were treated with a low-force treatment regimen that consisted of Activator Instrument adjusting, pelvic blocking, high-voltage galvanic current, and exercise. Computed tomography (CT) scans with multiplanar data imaging and clinical observation were used to monitor patients both during diagnosis and as treatment progressed. Results of follow-up CT scans in the first case revealed complete absence of disc herniation. A follow-up scan in the second case revealed the continued presence of a silent disc bulge at the L3-L4 level and a partial decrease in herniation at the L4-L5 level. The bulge appeared to have shifted away from the nerve root. Pain levels in both patients decreased from severe to minimal. Patients gained the ability to stand, sit, and walk for longer periods without discomfort; lifting tasks also became easier. Patients were able to return to full work capacity at three and nine months, respectively. This case study is unique to the literature because it documents the use of a treatment regimen that included low-force adjustments. Although no conclusion may be made concerning efficacy of any one type of treatment, favorable patient outcomes are somewhat encouraging.

Box 10-4

Reference: Colloca CJ, Keller TS, Gunzburg R. Biomechanical and neurophysiological responses to spinal manipulation in patients with lumbar radiculopathy. J Manipulative Physiol Ther. 2004;27(1):1-15.

ABSTRACT
OBJECTIVE

The purpose of this study was to quantify in vivo vertebral motions and neurophysiological responses during spinal manipulation.

METHODS

Nine patients who were undergoing lumbar decompression surgery participated in this study. Spinal manipulative thrusts (SMTs) ($\approx$5 ms; 30 N [Sham], 88 N, 117 N, and 150 N [max]) were administered treatment to lumbar spine facet joints (FJs) and spinous processes (SPs) adjacent to an intraosseous pin with an attached triaxial accelerometer and bipolar electrodes cradled around the S1 spinal nerve roots. Peak baseline amplitude compound action potential (CAP) response and peak-peak amplitude axial (AX), posterior-anterior (PA), and medial-lateral (ML) acceleration time and displacement time responses were computed for each SMT. Within-subject statistical analyses of the effects of contact point and force magnitude on vertebral displacements and CAP responses were performed.

RESULTS

SMTs ($\approx$88 N) resulted in significantly greater peak-to-peak ML, PA, and AX vertebral displacements compared with sham thrusts (p < .002). SMTs delivered to the FJs resulted in approximately threefold greater ML motions compared with SPs (p < .001). SMTs over the SPs resulted in significantly greater AX displacements compared with SMTs applied to the FJs (p < .05). Seventy-five percent of SMTs resulted in positive CAP responses with a mean latency of 12.0 ms. Collectively, the magnitude of the CAP responses was significantly greater for max setting SMTs compared with sham (p < .01).

CONCLUSIONS

Impulsive SMTs in human subjects were found to stimulate spinal nerve root responses that were temporally related to the onset of vertebral motion. Further work, including examination of the frequency and force duration dependency of SMT, is necessary to elucidate the clinical relevance of enhanced or absent CAP responses in patients.

Box 10-5

Reference: Polkinghorn BS, Colloca CJ. Treatment of symptomatic lumbar disc herniation using Activator Methods chiropractic technique. J Manipulative Physiol Ther. 1998;21(3):187-96.

ABSTRACT
OBJECTIVE

To describe a case of symptomatic lumbar disc herniation successfully treated via the Activator Method

CLINICAL FEATURES

A 26-year-old man suffered from a chronic multisymptom complex composed of low back pain and left lower extremity symptoms, including footdrop and associated muscle weakness with atrophy for 2 years after an athletic injury. Magnetic resonance imaging revealed a 6-mm focal central disc protrusion with accompanying deformation of the thecal sac.

INTERVENTION AND OUTCOME

Chiropractic intervention consisted of mechanical force, manually assisted short-lever adjusting procedures via an Activator Adjusting Instrument (AAI). The patient responded favorably and the multisystem complex resolved within 90 days of treatment. No residuals or recurrences were noted at examination more than 1 year later.

CONCLUSION

This suggests that chiropractic treatment of lumbar disc disorders may be effective in certain cases, via mechanical force, manually assisted adjusting procedures using an AAI. It is speculated that use of an AAI may provide definitive benefits over side-posture manipulation in treatment of resistive disc lesions because of a lack of torsional stress imposed upon the disc during instrumental spinal adjustment.

Box 10-6

Reference: Song X-J, Qiang G, Cao G, Wang J-L, Zheng B, Rupert RL. Spinal manipulation reduces pain and hyperalgesia after lumbar intervertebral foramen inflammation in the rat. J Manipulative Physiol Ther. 2006;29(1):5213.

ABSTRACT
OBJECTIVE

To document potential mediating effects of Activator-Assisted Spinal Manipulative Therapy (ASMT) on pain and hyperalgesia after acute intervertebral foramen (IVF) inflammation

METHODS

IVF inflammation was mimicked by in vivo delivery of inflammatory soup directly into the L5 IVF in adult male Sprague-Dawley rats. Thermal hyperalgesia and mechanical allodynia were determined by the shortened latency of foot withdrawal to radiant heat and von Frey filament stimulation to the hind paw, respectively. Intracellular recordings were obtained in vitro from L5 dorsal root ganglion (DRG) somata. DRG inflammation was examined by observation of the appearance and hematoxylin and eosin staining. ASMT was applied to the spinous process of L4, L5, and L6. A series of 10 adjustments was initiated 24 hours after surgery and subsequently were applied daily for 7 consecutive days and every other day during the second week.

RESULTS

(1) ASMT applied to L5-L6 or L5 and L6 spinous processes significantly reduced the severity and duration of thermal and mechanical hyperalgesia produced by IVF inflammation. However, ASMT applied to L4 did not affect the response in rats with IVF inflammation or in controls.
(2) Electrophysiological studies showed that hyperexcitability of the DRG neurons produced by IVF inflammation was significantly reduced by ASMT. (3) Pathological studies showed that manifestations of DRG inflammation, such as increased vascularization and satellitosis, were significantly reduced 2 to 3 weeks after ASMT.

CONCLUSIONS

These studies show that ASMT can significantly reduce the severity and shorten the duration of pain and hyperalgesia caused by lumbar IVF inflammation. This effect may result from ASMT-induced faster elimination of inflammation and recovery of excitability of the inflamed DRG neurons by improving blood and nutrition supplement to the DRG within the affected IVF. Manipulation of a specific spinal segment may play an important role in optimizing recovery from lesions involving IVF inflammation.

Box 10-7

Reference: Keller TS, Colloca CJ. Mechanical force spinal manipulation increases trunk muscle strength assessed by electromyography: a comparative clinical trial. J Manipulative Physiol Ther. 2000;23(9):585-95.

ABSTRACT
OBJECTIVE

The objective of this study was to determine whether mechanical force, manually assisted (MFMA) spinal manipulative therapy (SMT) affects paraspinal muscle strength as assessed through use of surface electromyography (sEMG).

DESIGN

Prospective clinical trial comparing sEMG output in 1 active treatment group and 2 control groups

SETTING

Outpatient chiropractic clinic, Phoenix, Arizona

SUBJECTS

Forty subjects with low back pain (LBP) participated in the study. Twenty patients with LBP (9 females and 11 males with a mean age of 35 years and 51 years, respectively) and 20 age- and sex-matched sham-SMT/control LBP subjects (10 females and 10 males with a mean age of 40 years and 52 years, respectively) were assessed.

METHODS

Twenty consecutive patients with LBP (SMT treatment group) performed maximum voluntary contraction (MVC) isometric trunk extensions while lying prone on a treatment table. Surface,

Continued

Box 10-7—cont'd

linear-enveloped sEMG was recorded from the erector spinae musculature at L3 and L5 during a trunk extension procedure. Patients were then assessed through use of the Activator Method Protocol, during which time they were treated through use of MFMA SMT. MFMA SMT treatment was followed by a dynamic stiffness and algometry assessment, after which a second or post-MVC isometric trunk extension and sEMG assessment were performed. Another 20 consecutive subjects with LBP were assigned to one of two other groups: a sham-SMT group and a control group. The sham-SMT group underwent the same experimental protocol with the exception that subjects received a sham-MFMA SMT and dynamic stiffness assessment. Control group subjects received no SMT treatment, stiffness assessment, or algometry assessment intervention. Within-group analysis of MVC sEMG output (pre-SMT vs. post-SMT sEMG output) and across-group analysis of MVC sEMG output ratio (post-SMT sEMG/pre-SMT sEMG output) during MVC was performed through use of a paired observations t test (POTT) and a robust analysis of variance (RANOVA), respectively.

MAIN OUTCOME MEASURES

Surface, linear-enveloped EMG recordings during isometric MVC trunk extension were used as the primary outcome measure.

RESULTS

Nineteen of 20 patients in the SMT treatment group showed a positive increase in sEMG output during MVC (range, −9.7% to 66.8%) after active MFMA SMT treatment and stiffness assessment. The SMT treatment group showed a significant (POTT, $p < .001$) increase in erector spinae muscle sEMG output (21% increase in comparison with pre-SMT levels) during MVC isometric trunk extension trials. No significant changes were noted in pre-SMT versus post-SMT MVC sEMG output for the sham-SMT (5.8% increase) and control (3.9% increase) groups. Moreover, the sEMG output ratio of the SMT treatment group was significantly greater (robust analysis of variance, $p = .05$) than that of the sham-SMT group or that of the control group.

CONCLUSIONS

Results of this preliminary clinical trial demonstrated that MFMA SMT results in a significant increase in sEMG erector spinae isometric MVC muscle output. These findings indicate that altered muscle function may be a potential short-term therapeutic effect of MFMA SMT, and they form a basis for a randomized, controlled clinical trial to further investigate acute and long-term changes in low back function.

Box 10-8

OTHER REPORTS RELATED TO THE LUMBAR SPINE
- Nathan M, Keller TS. Measurement and analysis of the in vivo posteroanterior impulse response of the human thoracolumbar spine: a feasibility study. J Manipulative Physiol Ther. 1994;17(7):431-41.
- Smith DB, Fuhr AW, Davis BP. Skin accelerometer displacement and relative bone movement of adjacent vertebrae in response to chiropractic percussion thrusts. J Manipulative Physiol Ther. 1989;12(1):26-37.

Clinical Observations
In patients who have radicular symptoms, particularly into their lower limbs, the relationship of the Pelvic Deficiency side can be predictive of how long or complicated the case may be. Radicular symptoms that occur on the side Opposite Pelvic Deficiency indicate a more common or typical case. However, radicular symptoms that occur on the same side of the Pelvic Deficiency are not as common and will usually be a sign of a more complicated case that may require more treatments then most cases.

REFERENCES

1. National Institutes of Health (NIH). Low back pain fact sheet. Bethesda (MD): NIH; November 8, 2006.
2. Deyo RA, Cherkin D, Conrad D, Volinn E. Cost, controversy, crisis: low back pain and the health of the public. Annu Rev Public Health. 1991;12:141-56.
3. Cypress BK. Characteristics of patient visits for back symptoms: a national perspective. Am J Public Health. 1983;73(4):389-95.
4. Nachemson AL. Newest knowledge of low back pain. A critical look. Clin Orthop. (279):8-20.

5. Lee C. Challenges of the spine specialists North American Spine Society Presidential Address. Minneapolis, Minnesota, October 1994. Spine. 1995;20(16):1749-52.
6. Shekelle PG, Brook RH. A community-based study of the use of chiropractic services. Am J Public Health. 1991;81(4):439-42.
7. Meade TW, Dyer S, Browne W, Frank AO. Randomized comparison of chiropractic and hospital outpatient management for low back pain: results from extended follow up. BMJ. 1995;311 (7001):349-51.
8. Kukurin GW. Chiropractic vs. medical management of work-related back injuries: cost comparison studies of workers compensation cases. Dig Chiropr Econ. 1995;37(4):28-34.
9. Stano M. Further analysis of health care costs for chiropractic and medical patients. J Manipulative Physiol Ther. 1994;17(7):442-6.
10. Bigos S, Bowyer O, Braen G et al. Acute low back problems in adults. Rockville (MD): Agency for Health Care Policy and Research, Public Health Service, U.S Department of Health and Human Services; December 1994. Clinical Practice Guideline No. 14. AHCPR Publication No. 95–0642.
11. Jarvis KB, Phillips RB, Morris EK. Cost per case comparison of back injury claims of chiropractic versus medical management for conditions with identical diagnostic codes. J Occip Med. 1991; 33(8):847-52.
12. Kraemer J. Presidential address natural course and prognosis of intervertebral disc diseases: International Society for the Study of the Lumbar Spine Seattle, Washington, June 1994. Spine 1995; 20:635-9.
13. Koes BW, Bouter LM, van Mameren H, Essers AH, Verstegen GM, Hofhuizen DM et al. Randomized clinical trial of manipulative therapy and physiotherapy for persistent back and neck complaints: results of one year follow up. BMJ. 1992;304(6827):601-5.
14. Shekelle PG. Spine update: spinal manipulation. Spine. 1994;19(7):858-61.
15. Twomey L, Taylor J. Spine update: exercise and spinal manipulation in the treatment of low back pain. Spine. 1995;20(5):615-9.
16. Triano JJ, McGregor M, Hondras MA, Brennan PC. Manipulative therapy versus education programs in chronic low back pain. Spine. 1995;20 (8):948-55.
17. Plaugher G. Textbook of clinical chiropractic. Baltimore: William & Wilkins; 1993.
18. Barge F. Tortipelvis. Vol 1. Amherst: Palmer Publications; 1994.
19. Friberg O. Clinical symptoms and biomechanics of lumbar spine and hip joint in leg length inequality. Spine. 1983;8(6):643-51.
20. Giles LGF, Taylor JR. Lumbar spine structural changes associated with leg length inequality. Spine. 1982;7(2):159-62.
21. Bogduk N, Twomey LT. Clinical anatomy of the lumbar spine. London: Churchill Livingstone; 1991.
22. Cramer GD, Darby SA. Basic and clinical anatomy of the spine, spinal cord, and ANS. St. Louis: Mosby; 1995.
23. Blunt KL, Gatterman MI, Bereznick DE. Kinesiology: an essential approach toward understanding the chiropractic subluxation. In: Gatterman MI, editor. Foundations of chiropractic: subluxation, St. Louis: Mosby; 1995. p. 190-224.
24. Breum J, Wiberg J, Bolton JE. Reliability and concurrent validity of the BROM II for measuring lumbar mobility. J Manipulative Physiol Ther. 1995;18(8):497-502.
25. Souza T. Which orthopedic tests are really necessary? In: Lawrence DJ, Cassidy JD, McGregor M, Meeker WC, Vernon HT, editors. Advances in chiropractic. vol 1. St. Louis: Mosby; 1994. p. 101-158.
26. Hakelius A. Prognosis in sciatica. Acta Orthop Scand Suppl. 1970;129:1-76.
27. Hirsch C. Efficiency of surgery in low back disorders. Pathoanatomical, experimental, and clinical studies. J Bone Joint Surg Am. 1965;47:991-1004.
28. Troup JDG. Straight-leg raising (SLR) and the qualifying tests for increased root tension: their predictive value after back and sciatic pain. Spine. 1981;6(5):526-7.
29. Cox JM. Low back pain mechanism, diagnosis and treatment. 5th ed. Baltimore: Williams & Wilkins; 1990.
30. Hoppenfeld S. Physical examination of the spine and extremities. Norwalk (CT): Appleton-Century-Crofts; 1976.
31. Evans RC. Illustrated orthopedic physical assessment. 2nd ed. St. Louis: Mosby; 1996. p. 149-151.
32. Raney RL. The effects of flexion, extension, Valsalva maneuver, and abdominal compression on the larger volume myelographic column. Paper presented at the International Symposium for Study of the Lumbar Spine; June 8, 1978; San Francisco.
33. Mazion JM. Illustrated manual of neurological reflexes/signs/tests and orthopedic signs/tests/maneuvers for office procedures. Arizona City: Mazion; 1980.
34. Panjabi MM, Drag MH, Chung TQ. Effects of disc injury on mechanical behavior of the human spine. Spine. 1984;9(7):707-13.
35. Schofferman J, Zucherman J. History and physical examination: state of the art reviews. Spine. 1986;1:14.
36. Moore KL. Clinically oriented anatomy. 3rd ed. Baltimore: Williams & Wilkins; 1992.
37. Williams PL, Warwick R, Dyson M, Bannister LH, editors. Gray's anatomy. 37th ed. Edinburgh: Churchill Livingstone; 1989. p. 592-604.
38. Richardson C, Hodges P, Hides J. Therapeutic exercise for lumbopelvic stabilization. 2nd ed. London: Churchill Livingstone; 2004. p. 39.
39. Travell J, Simons D. Myofascial pain and dysfunction the trigger point manual. Baltimore: Williams & Wilkins; 1992.

11

ADDITIONAL TESTS AND ADJUSTMENTS FOR THE THORACIC VERTEBRAE, RIBS, AND ANTERIOR THORAX

Thoracic spine complaints and associated rib neuroarticular dysfunctions are frequently related to postural stresses produced by prolonged periods of sitting, by inadequate workstations, or by inadequate back supports in chairs or vehicles.[1] Pain between the shoulder blades, known as "driver's back," is a commonly reported musculoskeletal complaint.

The Activator Method Protocol calls for assessment of the thoracic spine and the scapulae after testing and adjustment for the lumbar spine have been performed. Regardless of whether the procedure was initiated with the knees and feet or with the fourth lumbar vertebra, the procedure for the thoracic spine and cervical region is the same.

If testing and adjustments during the Basic Scan Protocol for the thoracic region do not improve the thoracic spine as expected through the care plan, or if patient complaints and examination findings so indicate, perform Isolation Tests and adjustments as indicated for the following additional involvements of the thoracic spine region:

- Tenth Thoracic (T10) and corresponding rib
- Eleventh Thoracic (T11)
- Eleventh Rib Involvement
- Ninth Thoracic (T9) and corresponding rib
- Seventh Thoracic (T7) and corresponding rib
- Fifth Thoracic (T5) and corresponding rib
- Third Thoracic (T3) and corresponding rib
- Second Thoracic (T2) and corresponding rib
- Rib Involvement Costovertebral/Costosternal
- Fourth Rib Involvement
- Third Rib Involvement
- Superior/Inferior Rib Involvement
- Lateral Rib Involvement
- Scalenus Anticus Involvement
- Hiatal Hernia Symptoms
- Xiphoid Involvement
- Superior Manubrium of the Sternum

It is not likely that all or even most of these involvements of the thoracic spine will require testing or adjustment for any one patient.

On the other hand, it is not unusual for several vertebrae within a region of the thoracic spine to be simultaneously involved, in part because of the nature of their facet orientations and the interconnections of the costovertebral articulations. For example, examination and Isolation Testing may indicate involvement of three or four of the midthoracic (T5-T8) vertebrae at the same time.

COMMON COMPLAINTS

Thoracic spine pain and neuroarticular dysfunction have been related to postural faults that resulted from abnormal stresses and strains on the human frame. Lifestyle adaptations in the workplace and habitual repetitive tasks have been related to an ergonomically unsound workstation.[1] A computer keyboard that is placed too high for the operator or a chair that is too low or too high for a desk can cause both direct and indirect stresses to the thoracic spine. When a work surface is too high for the worker, the tendency is to extend or "arch" the back to raise the arms and hands to a more comfortable working position. Arching the back may exaggerate or enhance the anterior curvature or lordosis of the lumbar spine, but it also tends to flatten the thoracic spine by reducing the normal posterior curvature or kyphosis. Prolonged periods of sitting with the back in an unnaturally arched position may induce soft tissue strain in the paraspinal muscles and may contribute to neuroarticular dysfunction of the thoracic spine and consequent pain and dysfunction.

When a work surface is too low for the worker, there is a tendency to flex the spine and to lower the arms and hands to a more comfortable working position. Sitting with the spine in constant flexion may exaggerate or enhance the normal kyphosis or posterior curvature of the thoracic spine. The ribs, however, may play a role in preventing excessive exaggeration of the anterior curvature of a healthy thoracic spine. Still, prolonged periods of sitting in a slouched flexion posture are likely to stress paraspinal muscles and other soft tissues, with possible impact on the stability of the thoracic spine and rib articulations. Furthermore, prolonged flexion of the spine may contribute to a reduction in lumbar lordosis, with increased risk of low back pain and injury.

Thoracic spine complaints may also result from compensatory and antalgic postural adaptations to an inadequate workstation, especially one at which a worker is required to do data entry or other computer work as part of the job. Ideally, a computer keyboard should be positioned so that the operator can sit in a comfortable, neutral position and reach the keyboard without extending or flexing the wrists. The forearms should be parallel with the floor with the elbows flexed to 90 degrees and the shoulders adducted in the neutral position.[1]

When a keyboard is positioned too high, as it would be on the surface of a desk or table of standard height, the operator typically must make a number of compensations. The operator may start typing with the wrists in extension. As the wrists begin to fatigue, the shoulders may be adducted to bring the forearms parallel with the floor. This compensation actually creates two problems. As the shoulders abduct, the worker may have to bend the wrists into ulnar deviation to maintain the home position on the keyboard. At the same time, the constant static load from holding the shoulders and arms in abduction may stress muscles of the scapulothoracic articulation. Motion of the scapulothoracic articulation contributes to about one third of the motion of shoulder abduction.[2,3] As a result, hypertonicity of the rhomboids and other muscles of the thoracic spine region may contribute to burning pain "between the shoulder blades" caused by vertebral and rib head articular dysfunctions in the midthoracic region.

Chest wall pain associated with thoracic vertebral or rib neuroarticular dysfunction may occur after trauma to the rib cage or extreme exertion. Body contact sports provide opportunities for blunt trauma to the rib cage with the potential for bruising, straining of intercostal muscles, and frank subluxation of costotransverse and costovertebral joints. Rib head neuroarticular dysfunction may be accompanied by exquisitely sharp pain that radiates along the course of the intercostal nerve at the level of involvement, or intercostal radiculitis.

Thoracic outlet syndrome may be diagnosed in the patient who experiences pain and/or numbness down the arm, forearm, and hand. Several neurovascular tests can be used to differentiate thoracic outlet syndromes from simple trigger point pain referral or radiculopathy. Adson's and Reverse Adson's tests will be positive for entrapment of the upper cords of the brachial plexus if scalene anticus and medius are hypertonic. The Wright test will be positive if pectoralis minor hypertonicity is resulting in entrapment of the lower cords of the plexus. The Roos test, Halstead's maneuver, and Reverse Bakody's tests are also differential tests for this condition.

The patient may experience pain-limited breathing with thoracic vertebral or rib head neuroarticular dysfunction. Of course, it is important to rule out fracture and chest disease when a patient is experiencing thoracic spine pain. One feature of the biomechanical disturbance associated with thoracic neuroarticular dysfunction is that the vertebra and the rib involved tend to be tender to palpation and percussion. Nevertheless, it is sound clinical procedure to collect a thorough history and perform a regional examination, including special tests and radiologic examination where indicated, when a patient experiences thoracic spine or chest wall pain.

CONCURRENT CONDITIONS

Several conditions may underlie complaints of thoracic spine pain or rib involvement, and these must be ruled out by careful and thorough examination of the patient. The normal thoracic curve is a kyphosis that extends from T2 to T12. Absence of this kyphosis is known as the straight back syndrome, which has been associated with systolic heart murmurs and other heart diseases.[4,5] Advanced osteoporosis with the characteristic "dowager hump" associated with anterior wedging compression of thoracic vertebrae is a common phenomenon. Osteoporotic changes may affect at least half of the adult population older than 50 years of age,[6] and contributing factors include inadequate dietary calcium intake, corticosteroid therapy, and immobility. Postmenopausal women demonstrate a significant rise in the incidence of advanced osteoporosis or Gibbus deformity.[2] Alteration of the thoracic kyphosis typical of osteoporosis may be accompanied by thoracic vertebral and rib pain as the standard orientation of articular surfaces changes with the increasing posterior curvature. Always use the lowest setting for the Activator Adjusting Instrument when you are adjusting an osteoporotic patient. Lung disease such as infectious disorders, chronic inflammatory conditions, chronic obstructive pulmonary disease (COPD), and neoplastic diseases may underlie complaints of thoracic vertebral and chest wall pain.[7] When a patient describes thoracic pain that is not of readily identifiable neurobiomechanical origin, make a point of ruling out serious chest disease with appropriate history, examination, and special tests as indicated.

A respiratory infection frequently manifests with coughing and sneezing. The explosive force of air leaving the respiratory tract during a sneeze may create enough intrathoracic pressure to subluxate rib heads and thoracic vertebrae. Consequently, it is not unusual for a patient with a cold or flu to feel some thoracic and chest wall discomfort. However, it is sound clinical procedure to examine a patient with coldlike or flulike symptoms for signs of acute bronchitis, pleurisy, or pneumonia. In many cases, the patient may be febrile. A low-grade fever tends to be associated with a viral infection; a high-grade fever is more suggestive of a bacterial infection and should be monitored closely.

Acute bronchitis is typically accompanied by a persistent, productive cough.[7] Auscultation reveals coarse rales, especially on inspiration, and the patient may exhibit increased inspiratory effort. Pleurisy is suggested by pain-limited inspiration, dull percussion sounds over the lung fields, and auscultation of a pleural friction rub. Radiographic examination may reveal a fluid meniscus at one or both costophrenic angles. Pneumonia may present with the coughing typical of bronchitis and with pleuritic chest pain. In addition, consolidation of one or more lobes of the lungs may occur as alveolar spaces fill with fluid. A patient with acute bronchitis, pleurisy, or pneumonia should be under concurrent care until resolution of the respiratory illness.

Chronic respiratory conditions may also contribute to chest wall and thoracic spine complaints. With COPD, chronic asthma, emphysema, and fibrotic lung disease (pneumoconiosis), biomechanical stresses and changes to the thoracic spine and rib articulations are characteristic.[8,9] A common change is an increase in the anterior-to-posterior (AP) diameter of the thoracic cavity. The "barrel chest" of chronic pulmonary disease is likely to create stresses on thoracic and costovertebral articulations and may predispose the joints to many of the neuroarticular dysfunctions described in the following pages.

Scheuermann's disease is a relatively common cause of exaggerated thoracic kyphosis in children and adolescents.[10] Axial loading of the spine in activities like horseback riding and ski jumping[11] may cause wedging of thoracic and lumbar vertebrae by compressing the vertebral bodies, causing damage to the epiphyseal growth plates. Scheuermann's disease is a spinal deformity with an autosomal dominant inheritance. It occurs primarily during early adolescence, and the exaggerated thoracic kyphosis is sometimes referred to as "round back." Incidence is 0.4% with no gender preference. About 50% of patients report back pain in the affected area; others complain of poor posture or fatigue. Adults with Scheuermann's disease will have involvement of three or more segments, with wedging at greater than 5 degrees; 25% will have associated spondylolisthesis.[12] Diagnosis is usually made through clinical presentation and weight-bearing radiographic examination. The altered thoracic curvature may cause clinical signs and symptoms by provoking muscle contractures and spasms and by altering the orientation of thoracic vertebral facets and costovertebral joints. Radiographic examination may be used to rule out Scheuermann's disease. If the condition is present, a lateral view of the spine reveals wedging defects and end plate irregularities.[13] Treatment is symptomatic and consists of rest, moderation of activity, and the use of anti-inflammatories. Severe cases may involve plaster casts and braces, such as the Milwaukee brace. Operative treatment is reserved for severe cases after the patient has stopped growing.[14]

Thirty percent of youth involved in soccer and gymnastics develop Schmorl's nodes. Schmorl's nodes are formed by the intercalary infusion of cartilaginous tissue in the end plates. Herniation of the nucleus pulposus occurs through a cracked vertebral end plate into the vertebral body. Resultant bone necrosis is detectable on radiographs as Schmorl's nodes.[12,14]

Lateral curvature or lateral deviation of the spine is known as scoliosis.[4] It usually consists of two curves—the original abnormal curve and a compensatory curve in the opposite direction.[14] Scoliosis can be located in any region of the spine; however, it is more commonly found in the thoracic spine because of its length and central location. Scoliotic deformities can result in paraspinal muscle imbalance,[15] decreased dorsolumbar range of motion, dorsolumbar pain syndromes, and, in severe cases, impaired lung capacity and cardiac output.[4] Causes of scoliosis have ranged from developmental and anatomical (as seen with hemivertebra) to unknown causes (idiopathic). Biomechanical, genetic, metabolic, growth, and neurological factors have all been implicated as causes of scoliosis.[4] Dixson[16] reported that approximately 40% of the curves detected on school screening may be attributed to Leg Length Inequality during adolescence. Others too have noted the relationship of Leg Length Inequality to scoliotic curvatures.[17-19] The degree of curvature may be ascertained with use of the Cobb method. In this method, lines are drawn on the superior and inferior end plates of the maximally tilted vertebral bodies of a curvature in the AP or posterior-to-anterior projection, perpendicular lines are dropped, and an intersecting angle is formed.[20] The presence of a long C curve is indicative of myopathic scoliosis, which is due to weakening of the spinal muscles. Structural scoliosis can be distinguished from functional scoliosis by having the patient bend forward at the waist (Adam's test).[21] Straightening of the scoliotic curvature in the flexed position is indicative of a functional scoliosis. The presence and elevation of muscles on one side of the thorax in the upright and flexed position has been used as an indicator of structural scoliosis.[15]

ADDITIONAL TESTS AND ADJUSTMENTS FOR THE THORACIC VERTEBRAE AND RIBS

In addition to the findings of tests and adjustments included in the Basic Scan Protocol, thoracic spine involvement is suggested when the patient reports point tenderness at specific vertebral levels, when leg lengths do not balance after testing and adjustment, or when examination findings so indicate. Because many ribs articulate with two vertebrae, it is also possible for adjacent vertebrae to be involved in the same neuroarticular complex.

Tenth Thoracic (T10)

If adjusting the twelfth thoracic vertebra does not cause the legs to remain even in Position #1 and Position #2, if signs and symptoms persist, or if examination findings so indicate, consider other neuroarticular dysfunctions of the lower thoracic spine. Note that the testing sequence for the four lower thoracic segments is T12, T10, T11, and T9. Isolation Test maneuvers are coordinated more effectively if this patterned approach to testing the lower thoracic vertebrae is used. Therefore, after testing and adjusting of T12 as indicated, proceed to Isolation Testing of T10.

Isolation Test. After testing of T12 has been performed, the patient's arm on the side of Pelvic Deficiency will still be raised with the

forearm resting on the table superior and lateral to the head. To isolate the tenth thoracic vertebra, instruct the patient to lower the arm on the side of Pelvic Deficiency back down to the side and rest it on the table (Figure 11-1). This movement and position are thought to facilitate the paraspinal muscles and neuroarticular components of the lower thoracic spine in the region of T10. Look for Pelvic Deficient (PD) leg reactivity in Position #1. Then proceed to Position #2, while observing relative changes in the PD leg. Follow the Short/Long Rule.

If the PD leg lengthens in Position #2, tenth thoracic motor unit involvement is on the side of Pelvic Deficiency. If the PD leg shortens in Position #2, tenth thoracic motor unit involvement is on the side Opposite Pelvic Deficiency. Pressure Test to confirm by applying a firm but gentle anterior and superior pressure on the transverse process of the involved side.

Adjustment. To adjust a tenth thoracic vertebra, contact the transverse process on the side indicated by the Short/Long Rule. The Line of Drive (LOD) is anterior, superior, and slightly medial through the plane line of the facet (Figure 11-2).

After you have adjusted the tenth thoracic vertebra, adjust the tenth rib on the side opposite the vertebral adjustment.

Corresponding Tenth Rib Adjustment. The tenth rib is adjusted on the side opposite vertebral adjustment. To adjust the tenth rib, contact the body of the rib about one-half inch lateral to the transverse process on the side of rib involvement. The LOD is lateral and inferior along the longitudinal axis of the rib (Figure 11-3).

To ensure an effective adjustment and to minimize discomfort for the patient, use the thumb of the free hand to take a lateral and inferior tissue pull over the contact point on the rib. Use the thumb to stabilize the tip of the instrument on the body of the rib during the adjustment.

Eleventh Thoracic (T11)

If Isolation Testing indicates involvement of both T12 and T10, consider concurrent involvement of T11 and T9. Shared neurology and coupling of intervening rib heads, as well as patterns of hypertonicity of paraspinal muscles, suggest that adjacent segments misalign in the same direction. However, contralateral involvement is possible, and the vertebrae should be tested independently with specific Isolation Tests.

Isolation Test. After testing and adjustment of T10, the patient's arms will be down at the sides

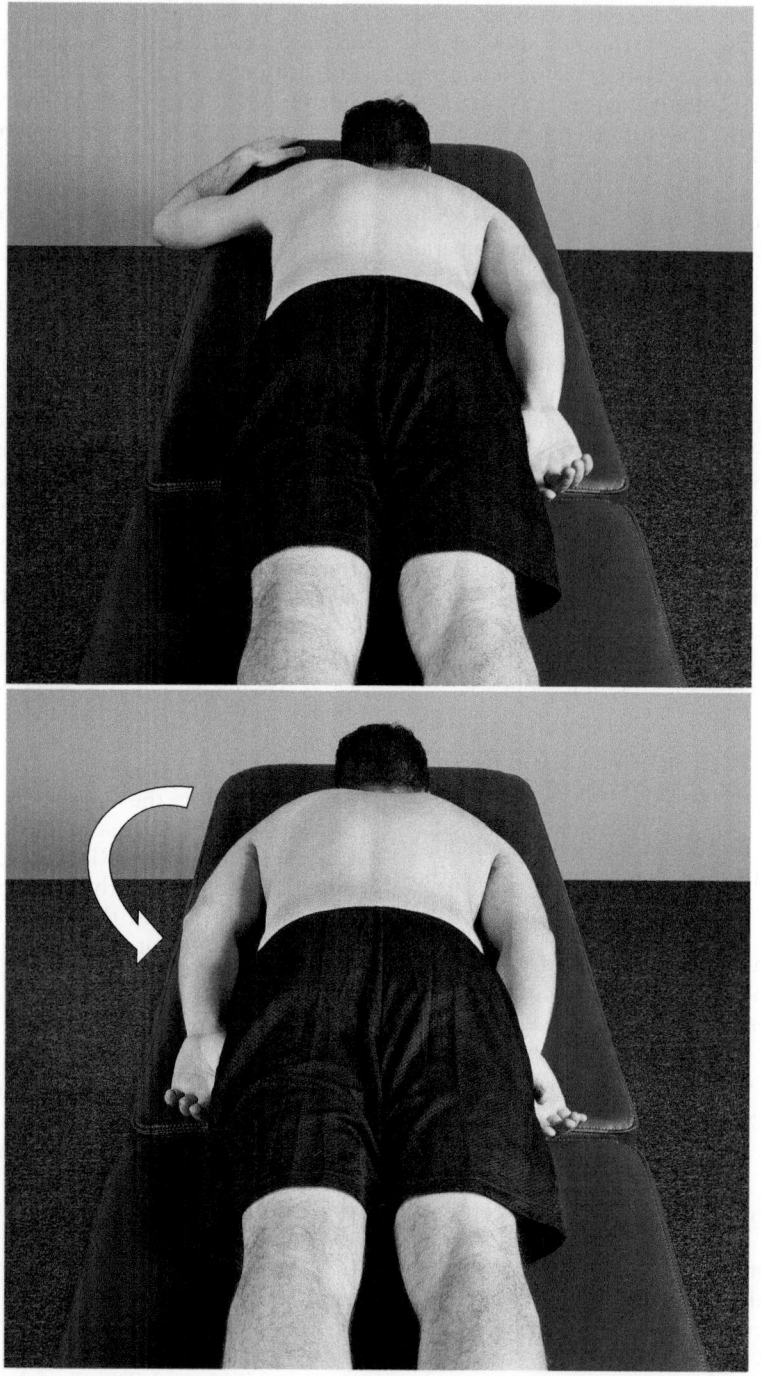

Figure 11-1   Isolation Test for tenth thoracic; patient returns arm to side after twelfth thoracic test.

and resting on the table. To isolate the eleventh thoracic vertebra, instruct the patient to raise his or her arm on the side Opposite Pelvic Deficiency and rest the forearm on the table superior and lateral to the head (Figure 11-4). This movement and position are thought to facilitate the paraspinal muscles and neuroarticular components of the lower thoracic spine in the region of T11. Look for PD leg reactivity in Position #1. Then proceed to Position #2, while observing relative changes in the PD leg. Follow the Short/Long Rule.

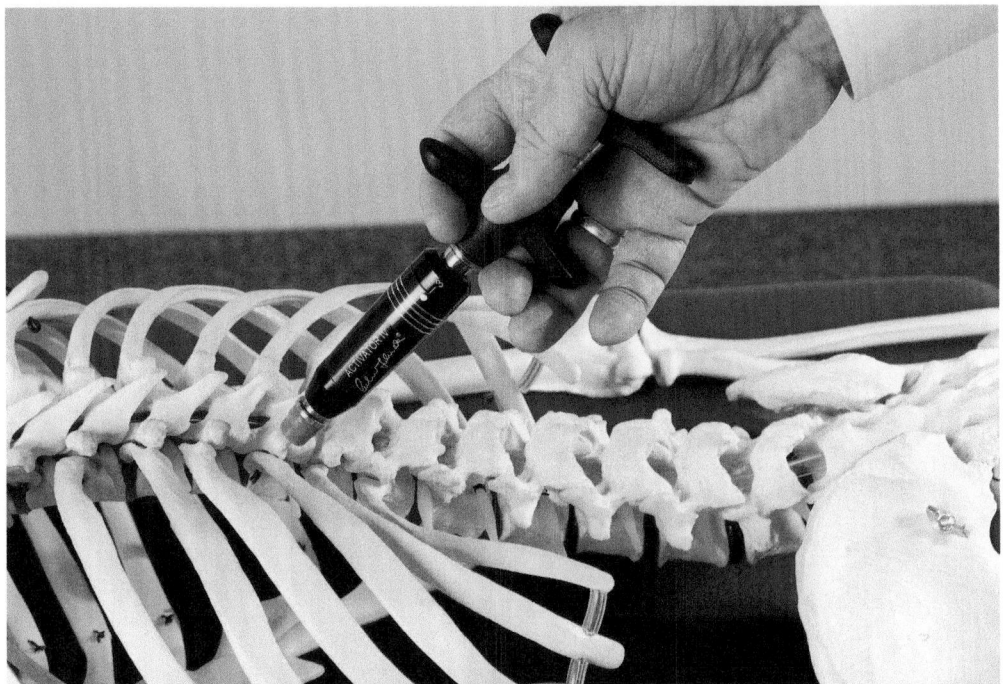

Figure 11-2   Adjustment for tenth thoracic. Line of Drive is anterior, superior, and slightly medial.

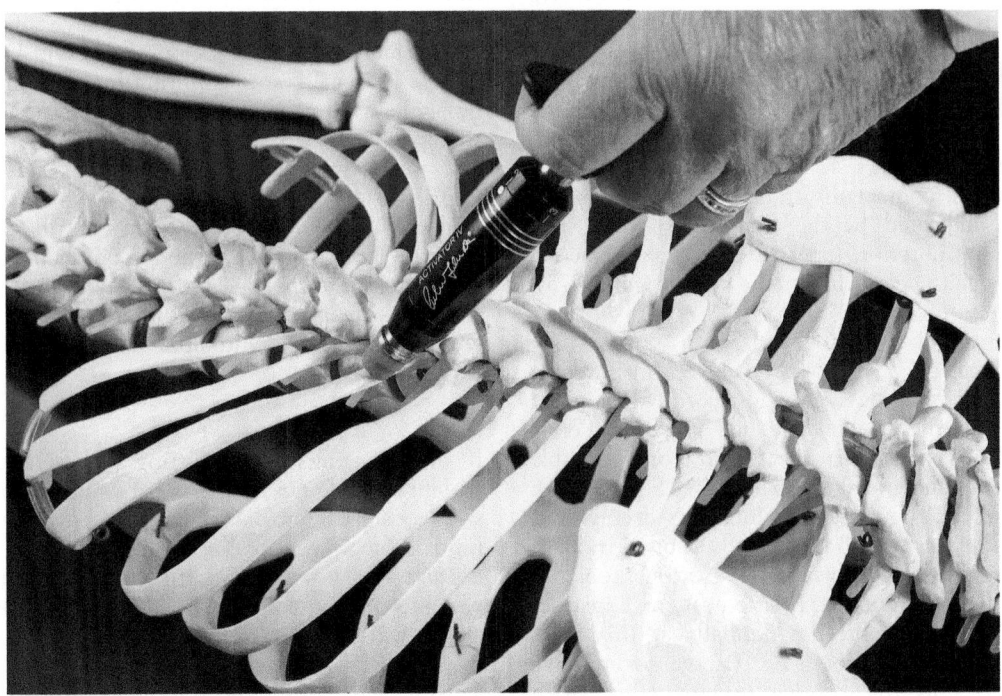

Figure 11-3   Adjustment for tenth rib. Line of Drive is lateral and inferior along longitudinal axis of rib.

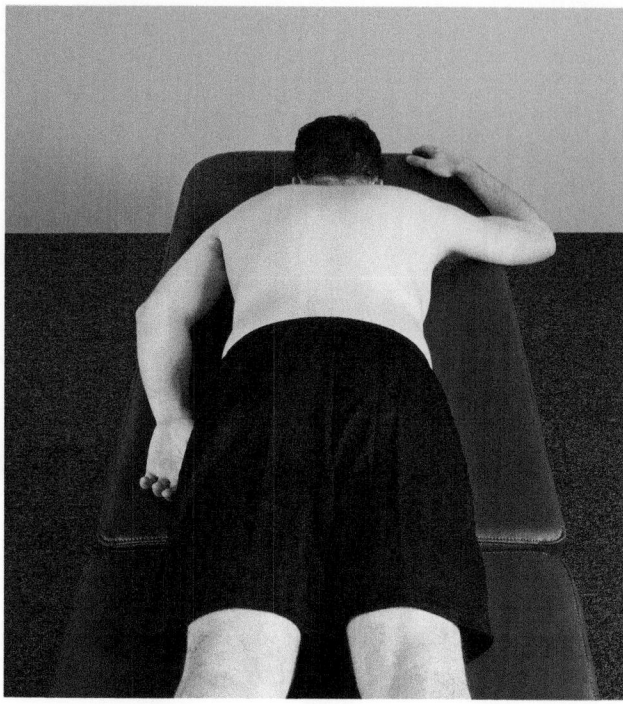

Figure 11-4 Isolation Test for eleventh thoracic.

If the PD leg lengthens in Position #2, eleventh thoracic motor unit involvement is on the side of Pelvic Deficiency. If the PD leg shortens in Position #2, eleventh thoracic motor unit involvement is on the side Opposite Pelvic Deficiency. Pressure Test to confirm by applying a firm but gentle anterior and superior pressure on the transverse process of the involved side.

Adjustment. To adjust the eleventh thoracic vertebra, contact the transverse process on the side indicated by the Short/Long Rule. The LOD is anterior, superior, and slightly medial through the plane line of the facet (Figure 11-5).

Eleventh Rib Involvement

Isolation Test. To test the eleventh rib, repeat the T11 Isolation Test by instructing the patient to raise the arm on the side Opposite Pelvic Deficiency and rest the forearm on the table superior and lateral to the head (see Figure 11-4). Next, ask the patient to inhale as deeply as is comfortable and to hold briefly. This is thought to stress the costovertebral junction. Look for PD leg reactivity in Position #1, and instruct the patient to breathe normally at this time. Proceed to Position #2. Observe for relative changes in the PD leg in comparison with Position #1. Follow the Short/Long Rule.

If the PD leg lengthens in Position #2, the test suggests eleventh rib involvement on the side of Pelvic Deficiency. If the PD leg shortens in Position #2, the test suggests eleventh rib involvement on the side Opposite Pelvic Deficiency. Pressure Test to confirm rib involvement by applying firm but gentle thumb pressure on the body of the rib. Direct the pressure laterally and inferiorly along the longitudinal axis of the rib.

Adjustment. To adjust the eleventh rib, contact the body of the rib about one-half inch lateral to the transverse process on the side of rib involvement. The LOD is lateral and inferior along the longitudinal axis of the rib (Figure 11-6).

Ninth Thoracic (T9)

If after testing and adjusting of T11, the patient's legs do not balance, or if symptoms persist, consider motor unit involvement of the ninth thoracic vertebra.

Isolation Test. After testing of T11, the patient's arm on the side Opposite Pelvic Deficiency will still be raised, with the forearm resting on the table superior and lateral to the head. To isolate the ninth thoracic vertebra, instruct the patient to lower the arm back down to the

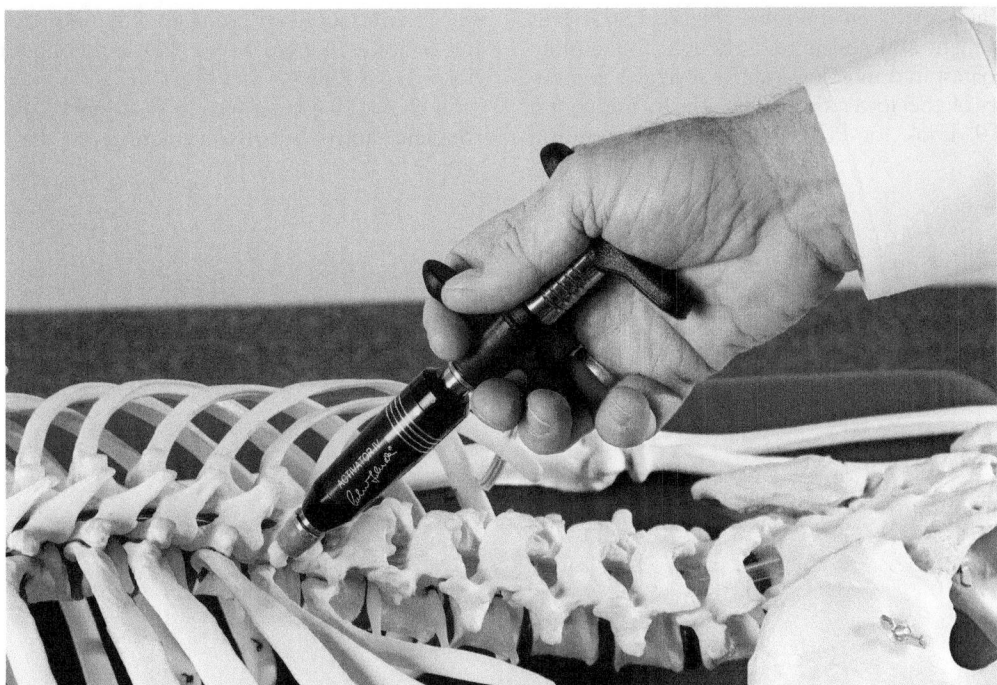

Figure 11-5 Adjustment for eleventh thoracic. Line of Drive is anterior, superior, and slightly medial.

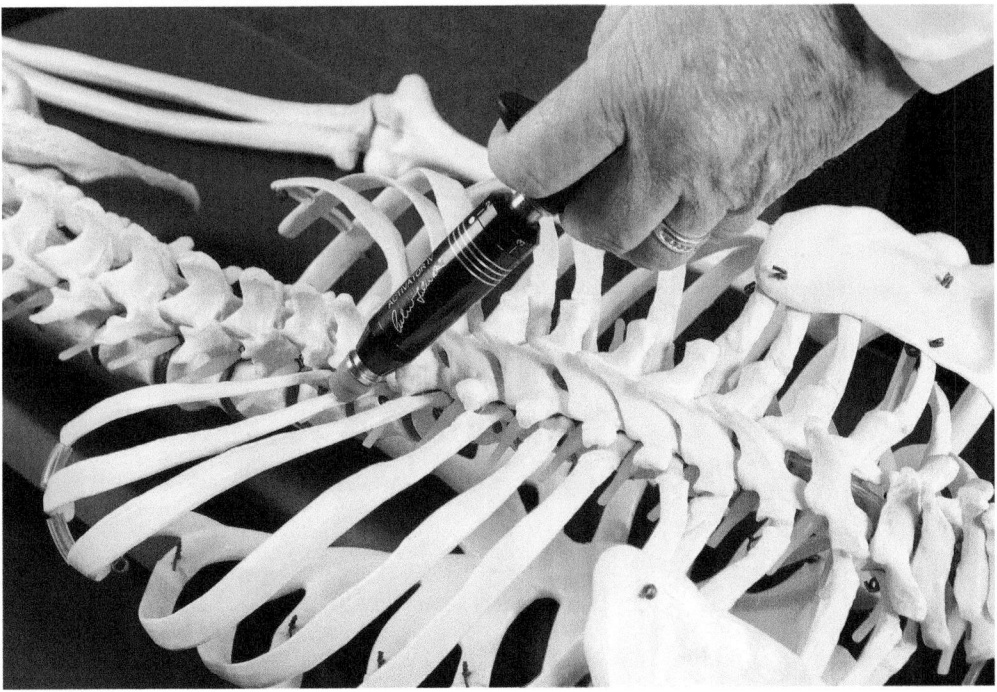

Figure 11-6 Adjustment for eleventh rib. Line of Drive is lateral and inferior along longitudinal axis of rib.

side and rest it on the table (Figure 11-7). This movement and position are thought to facilitate the paraspinal muscles and the articular components of the lower thoracic spine in the region of T9. Look for PD leg reactivity in Position #1. Then proceed to Position #2, while observing relative changes in the PD leg. Follow the Short/Long Rule.

If the PD leg lengthens in Position #2, ninth thoracic motor unit involvement is on the side

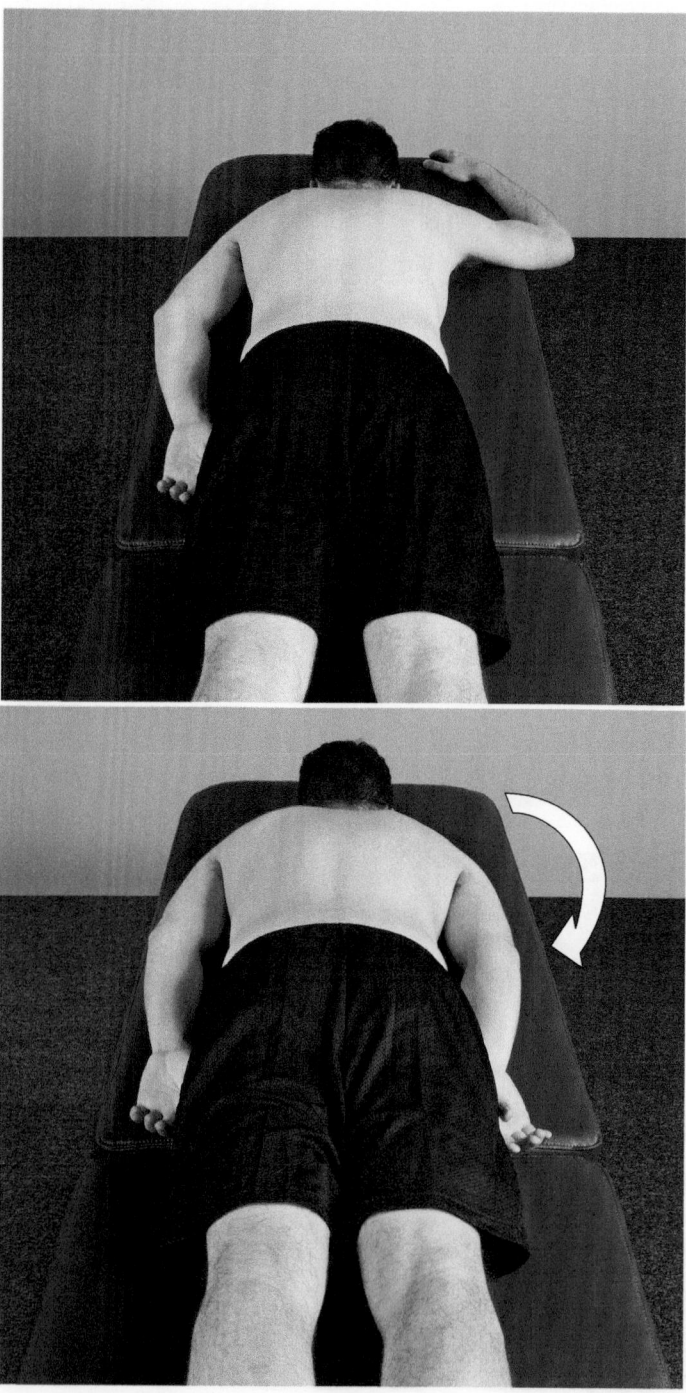

Figure 11-7   Isolation Test for ninth thoracic; patient returns arm to side after eleventh thoracic test.

of Pelvic Deficiency. If the PD leg shortens in Position #2, ninth thoracic motor unit involvement is on the side Opposite Pelvic Deficiency. Pressure Test to confirm by applying a firm but gentle anterior and superior pressure on the transverse process of the involved side.

Adjustment. To adjust a ninth thoracic vertebra, contact the transverse process on the side indicated by the Short/Long Rule. The LOD is anterior, superior, and slightly medial through the plane line of the facet (Figure 11-8).

After the ninth thoracic vertebra has been adjusted, adjust the ninth rib on the side opposite the vertebral adjustment.

Corresponding Ninth Rib Adjustment. The ninth rib is adjusted on the side opposite vertebral adjustment. To adjust the ninth rib, contact the body of the rib about one-half inch lateral to the transverse process on the side of rib involvement. The LOD is lateral along the longitudinal axis of the rib (Figure 11-9).

To ensure an effective adjustment and to minimize discomfort for the patient, use the thumb of the free hand to take a lateral and inferior tissue pull over the contact point on the rib. Use the thumb to stabilize the tip of the instrument on the body of the rib during the adjustment.

Seventh Thoracic (T7)

If both T8 and T6 were involved, consider involvement of the seventh thoracic vertebra as well. The combination of costovertebral articulations and the hypertonicity of paraspinal muscles is likely to involve T7 in the same direction as T8 or T6; however, counterinvolvement is possible. Therefore the seventh thoracic vertebra should be examined independently through its specific Isolation Test.

Isolation Test. After testing and adjustment of T8, both arms will be raised, with the forearms resting on the table superior and lateral to the head. To isolate the seventh thoracic vertebra, ask the patient to lower the arms back down to the sides and rest them on the table. Next, instruct the patient to raise both shoulders posterior away from the table, and then relax (Figure 11-10). This movement and position are thought to facilitate the paraspinal muscles and the neuroarticular components of the lower thoracic spine in the region of T7. Look for PD leg reactivity in Position #1. Then proceed to Position #2, while observing relative changes in the PD leg. Follow the Short/Long Rule.

If the PD leg lengthens in Position #2, seventh thoracic motor unit involvement is on the side of Pelvic Deficiency. If the PD leg

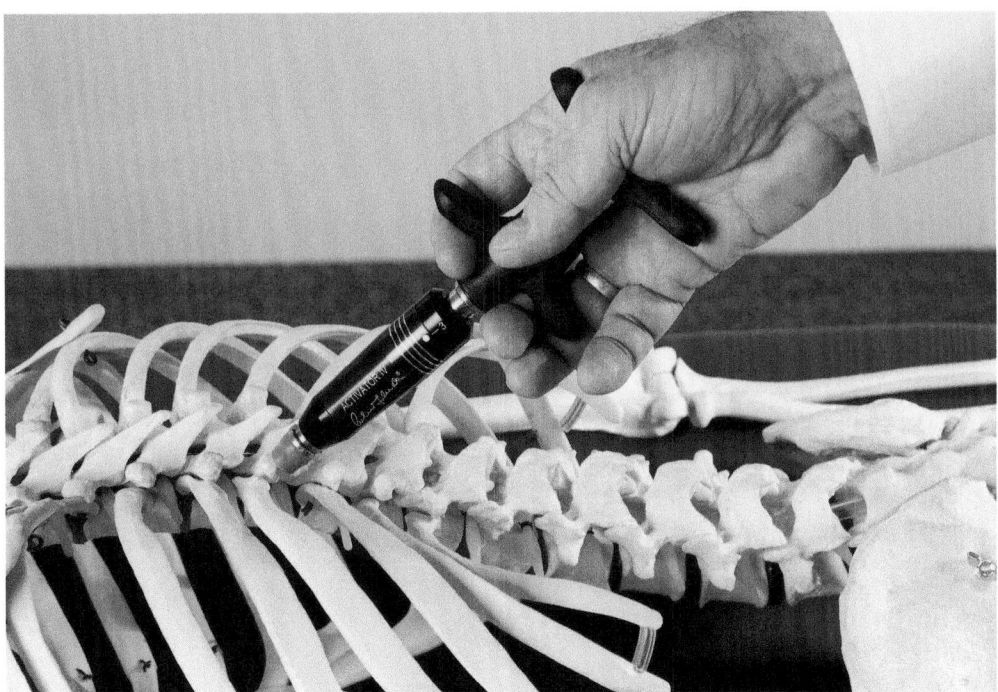

Figure 11-8 Adjustment for ninth thoracic. Line of Drive is anterior, superior, and slightly medial.

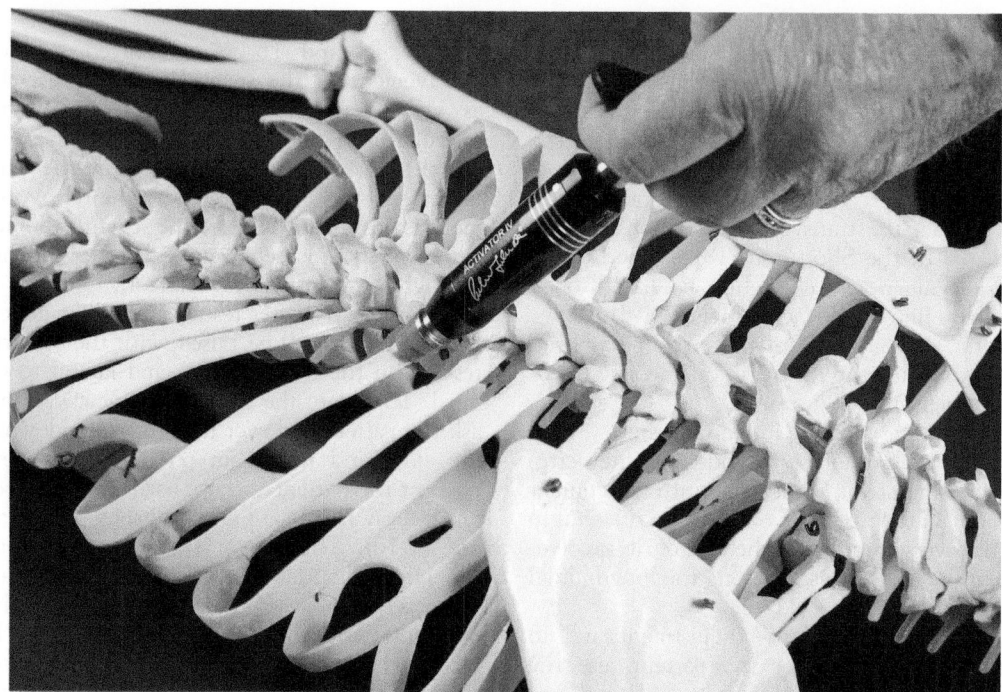

Figure 11-9 Adjustment for ninth rib. Line of Drive is lateral and inferior along longitudinal axis of rib.

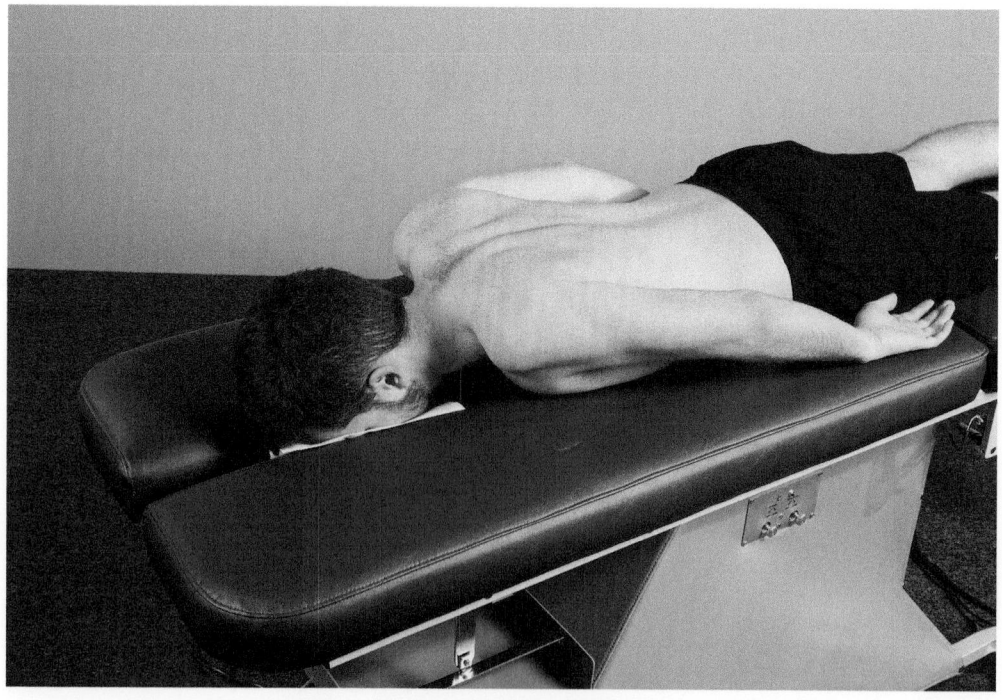

Figure 11-10 Isolation Test for seventh thoracic.

shortens in Position #2, seventh thoracic motor unit involvement is on the side Opposite Pelvic Deficiency. Pressure Test to confirm by applying a firm but gentle anterior and superior pressure on the transverse process of the involved side.

Adjustment. To adjust a seventh thoracic vertebra, contact the transverse process on the side indicated by the Short/Long Rule. The LOD is anterior, superior, and slightly medial through the plane line of the facet (Figure 11-11).

After the seventh thoracic vertebra has been adjusted, adjust the seventh rib on the side opposite the vertebral adjustment.

Corresponding Seventh Rib Adjustment. The seventh rib is adjusted on the side opposite the vertebral adjustment. To adjust the seventh rib, contact the body of the rib about one-half inch lateral to the transverse process on the side of rib involvement. The LOD is lateral and inferior along the longitudinal axis of the rib (Figure 11-12).

To ensure an effective adjustment and to minimize discomfort for the patient, use the thumb of the free hand to take a lateral and inferior tissue pull over the contact point on the rib. Use the thumb to stabilize the tip of the instrument on the body of the rib during the adjustment.

Fifth Thoracic (T5)

If testing indicates involvement of both T6 and T4, consider involvement of the fifth thoracic vertebra as well.

Isolation Test. After testing and adjustment of the sixth thoracic vertebra, instruct the patient to keep the face turned to the side of Pelvic Deficiency. To isolate the fifth thoracic vertebra, instruct the patient to raise the arm on the side Opposite Pelvic Deficiency and rest it on the table superior and lateral to the head (Figure 11-13). This movement and position are thought to facilitate the paraspinal muscles and the neuroarticular components of the upper thoracic spine in the region of T5. Look for PD leg reactivity in Position #1. Then proceed to Position #2, while observing relative changes in the PD leg. Follow the Short/Long Rule.

If the PD leg lengthens in Position #2, fifth thoracic motor unit involvement is on the side of Pelvic Deficiency. If the PD leg shortens in Position #2, fifth thoracic motor unit involvement is on the side Opposite Pelvic Deficiency. Pressure Test to confirm by applying a firm but gentle anterior and superior pressure through the plane line of the facet on the transverse process of the involved side.

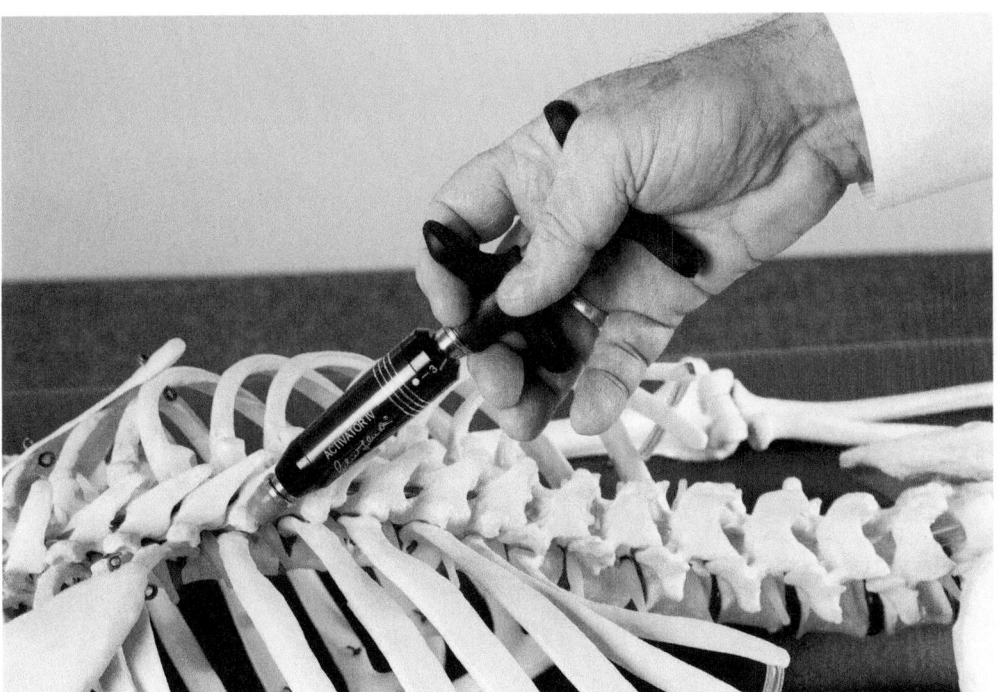

Figure 11-11 Adjustment for seventh thoracic. Line of Drive is anterior, superior, and slightly medial.

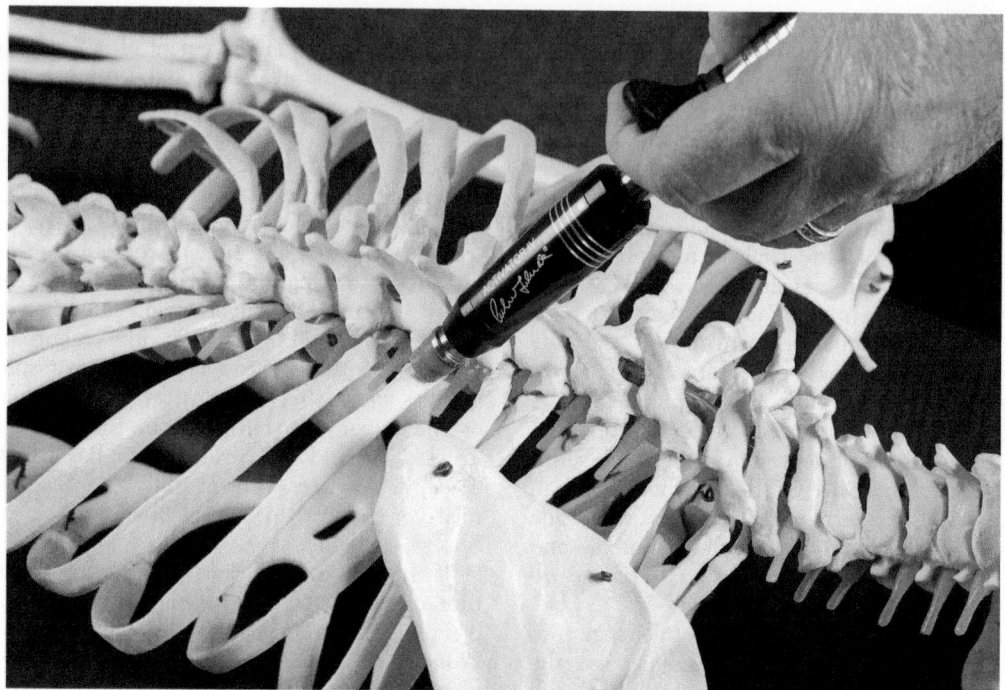

Figure 11-12   Adjustment for seventh rib. Line of Drive is lateral and inferior along longitudinal axis of rib.

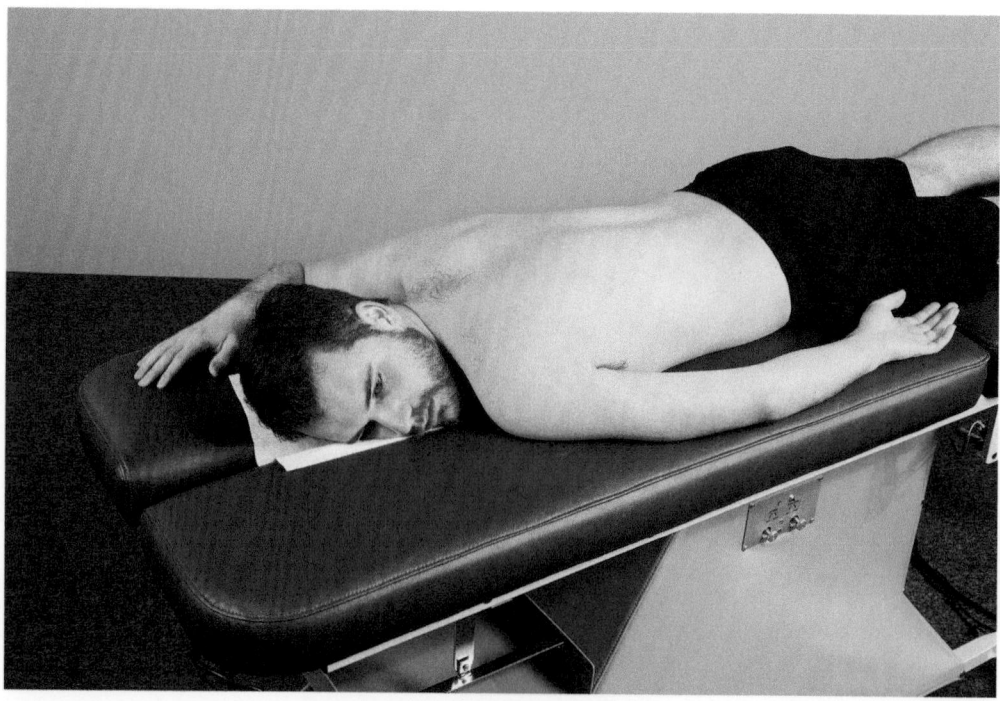

Figure 11-13   Isolation Test for fifth thoracic.

Adjustment.   To adjust a fifth thoracic verte-bra, contact the transverse process on the side indicated by the Short/Long Rule. The LOD is anterior, superior, and slightly medial through the plane line of the facets (Figure 11-14).

After the fifth thoracic vertebra has been adjusted, adjust the fifth rib on the side opposite the vertebral adjustment.

Corresponding Fifth Rib Adjustment.   The fifth rib is adjusted on the side opposite verte-bral adjustment. To adjust the fifth rib, contact the body of the rib about one-half inch lateral to the transverse process on the side of rib involve-ment. The LOD is lateral and inferior along the longitudinal axis of the rib (Figure 11-15).

To ensure an effective adjustment and to minimize discomfort for the patient, use the thumb of the free hand to take a lateral and inferior tissue pull over the contact point on the rib. Use the thumb to stabilize the tip of the instrument on the body of the rib during the adjustment.

Third Thoracic (T3)

When a patient presents with persistent upper thoracic spinal pain and recurrent T4 neuroarticular dysfunctions, consider involve-ment of the third thoracic vertebra.

Isolation Test.   After testing and adjustment of T4, the patient's face will be turned to the side of Pelvic Deficiency, and the arms will be down at the sides resting on the table. To isolate the third thoracic vertebra, instruct the patient to keep the head turned to the PD side, and to raise the arm on the side of Pelvic Deficiency and rest the forearm on the table superior and lateral to the head (Figure 11-16). This move-ment and position are thought to facilitate the paraspinal muscles and the neuroarticular com-ponents of the upper thoracic spine in the region of T3. Look for PD leg reactivity in Posi-tion #1. Then proceed to Position #2, while observing relative changes in the PD leg. Follow the Short/Long Rule.

If the PD leg lengthens in Position #2, third thoracic motor unit involvement is on the side of Pelvic Deficiency. If the PD leg shortens in Position #2, third thoracic motor unit involve-ment is on the side Opposite Pelvic Deficiency. Pressure Test to confirm by applying a firm but gentle anterior and superior pressure through the plane line of the facet on the transverse pro-cess of the involved side.

Adjustment.   To adjust a third thoracic verte-bra, contact the transverse process on the side indicated by the Short/Long Rule. The LOD is

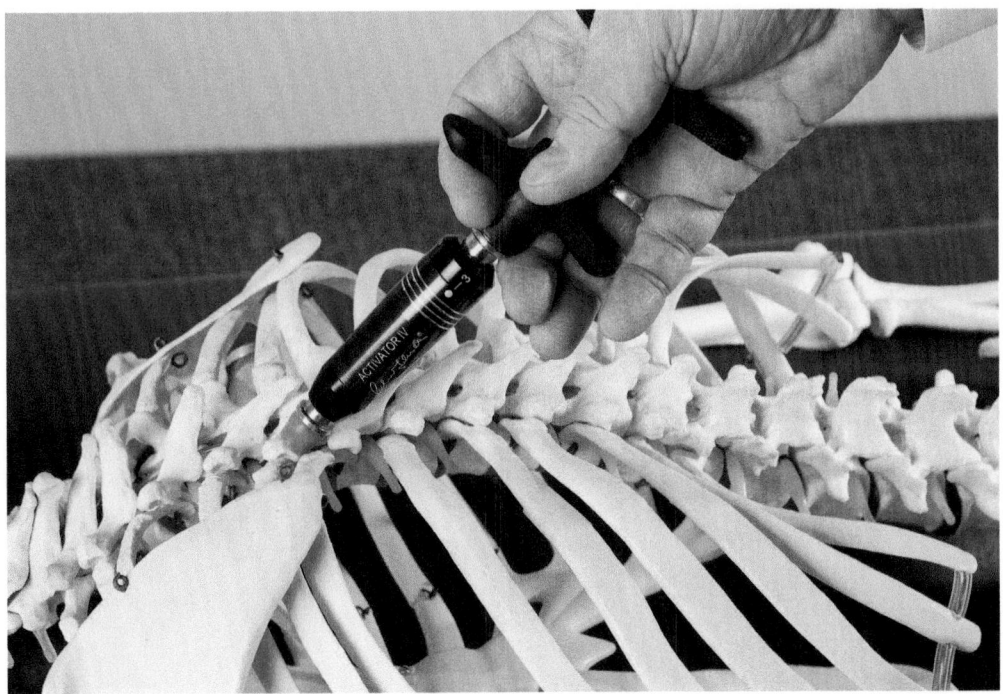

Figure 11-14   Adjustment for fifth thoracic. Line of Drive is anterior, superior, and slightly medial.

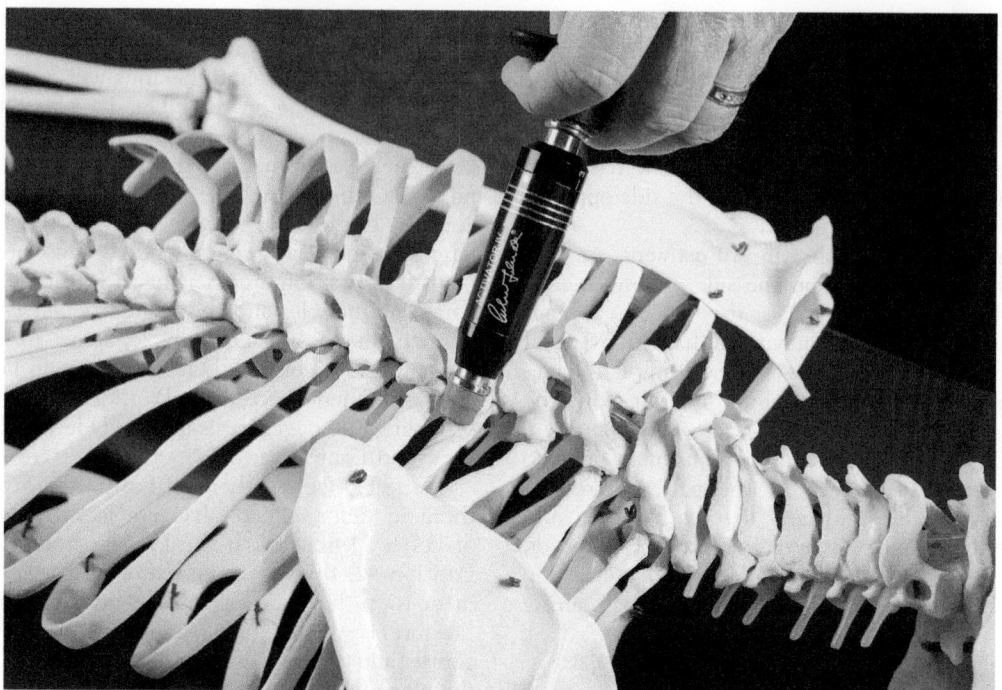

Figure 11-15   Adjustment for fifth rib. Line of Drive is lateral and inferior along longitudinal axis of rib.

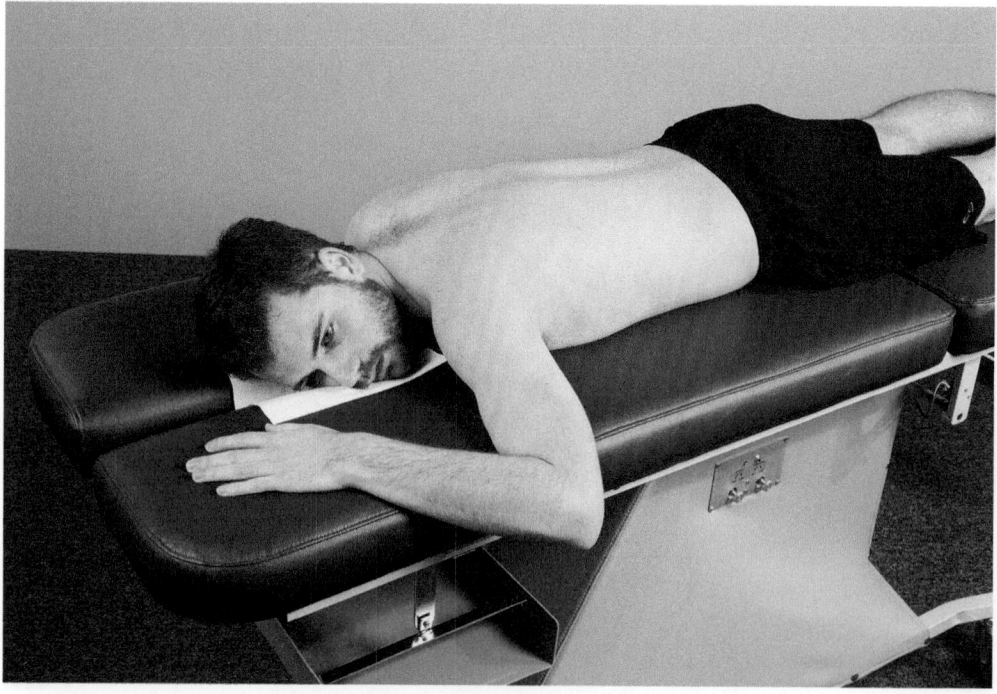

Figure 11-16   Isolation Test for third thoracic.

anterior, superior, and slightly medial through the plane line of the facet (Figure 11-17).

After the third thoracic vertebra has been adjusted, adjust the third rib on the side opposite the vertebral adjustment.

Corresponding Third Rib Adjustment. The third rib is adjusted on the side opposite vertebral adjustment. To adjust the third rib, contact the body of the rib about one-half inch lateral to the transverse process on the side of the rib involvement. The LOD is lateral and inferior along the longitudinal axis of the rib (Figure 11-18).

To ensure an effective adjustment and to minimize discomfort for the patient, use the thumb of the free hand to take a lateral and inferior tissue pull over the contact point on the rib. Use the thumb to stabilize the tip of the instrument on the body of the rib during the adjustment.

Second Thoracic (T2)

If testing and adjusting of T3 as indicated does not balance the legs, or if examination findings so indicate, test the second thoracic vertebra for neuroarticular dysfunction.

Isolation Test. After testing of T3, the patient's head will be turned to the PD side, and the arm on the side of Pelvic Deficiency will be raised, with the forearm resting on the table superior and lateral to the head. To isolate the second thoracic vertebra, ask the patient to keep the head turned to the side of Pelvic Deficiency. Then instruct the patient to bring the arm back down to the side and rest it on the table (Figure 11-19). This movement and position are thought to facilitate the paraspinal muscles and the neuroarticular components of the upper thoracic spine in the region of T2. Look for PD leg reactivity in Position #1. Then proceed to Position #2, while observing relative changes in the PD leg. Follow the Short/Long Rule.

If the PD leg lengthens in Position #2, second thoracic motor unit involvement is on the side of Pelvic Deficiency. If the PD leg shortens in Position #2, second thoracic motor unit involvement is on the side Opposite Pelvic Deficiency. Pressure Test to confirm by applying a firm but gentle anterior and superior pressure on the transverse process of the involved side.

Adjustment. To adjust a second thoracic vertebra, contact the transverse process on the side indicated by the Short/Long Rule. The LOD is anterior, superior, and slightly medial through the plane line of the facets (Figure 11-20).

After the second thoracic vertebra has been adjusted, adjust the second rib on the side opposite the vertebral adjustment.

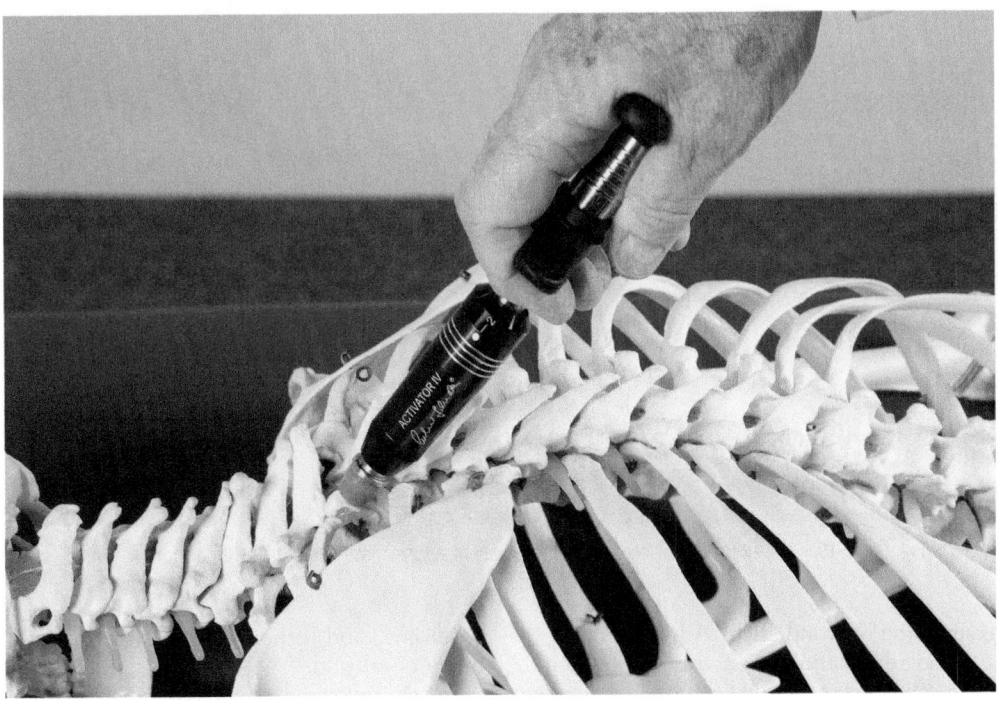

Figure 11-17 Adjustment for third thoracic. Line of Drive is anterior, superior, and slightly medial.

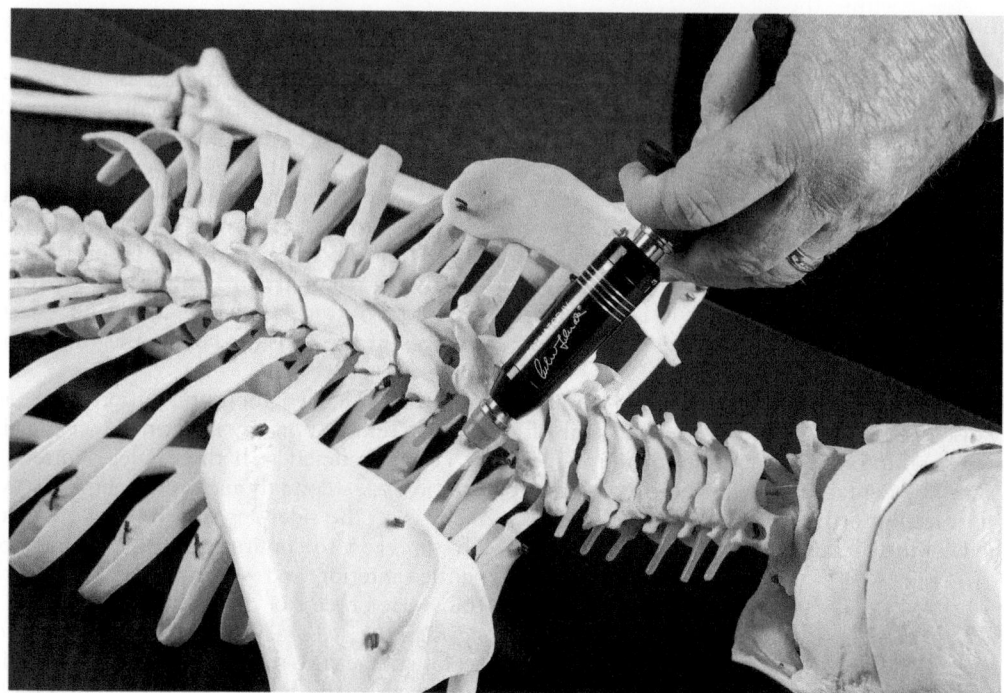

Figure 11-18 Adjustment for third rib. Line of Drive is lateral and inferior along longitudinal axis of rib.

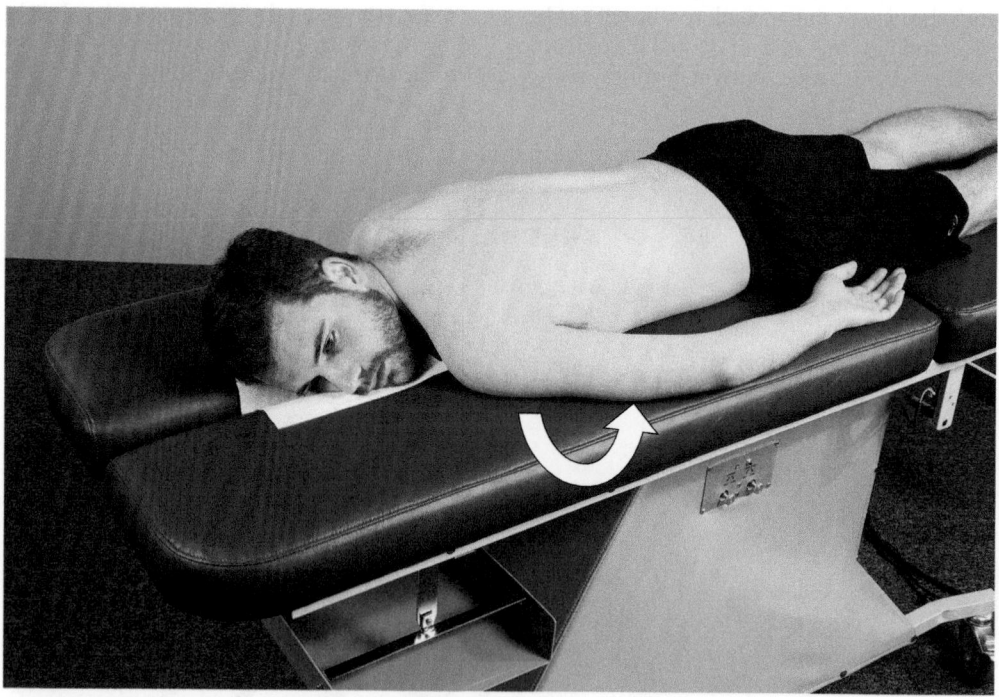

Figure 11-19 Isolation Test for second thoracic; patient returns arm to side after third thoracic test.

Corresponding Second Rib Adjustment.
The second rib is adjusted on the side opposite vertebral adjustment. Second rib neuroarticular dysfunction may also occur with frozen shoulder syndrome and other restrictions to shoulder range of motion.[22]

To adjust second rib neuroarticular dysfunction, contact the body of the rib about one-half inch

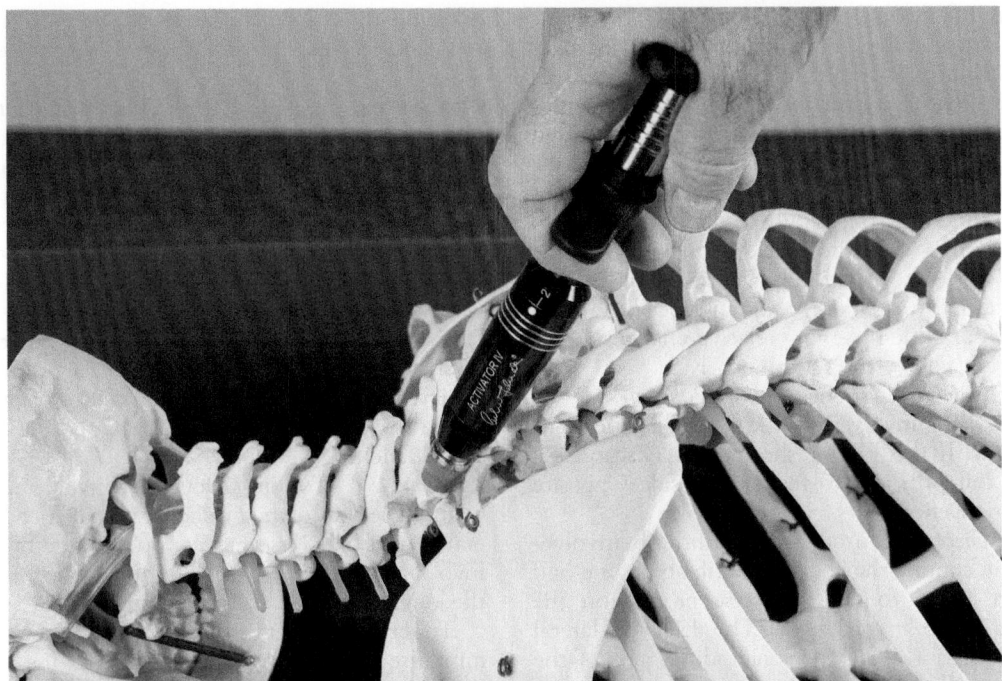

Figure 11-20 Adjustment for second thoracic. Line of Drive is anterior, superior, and slightly medial.

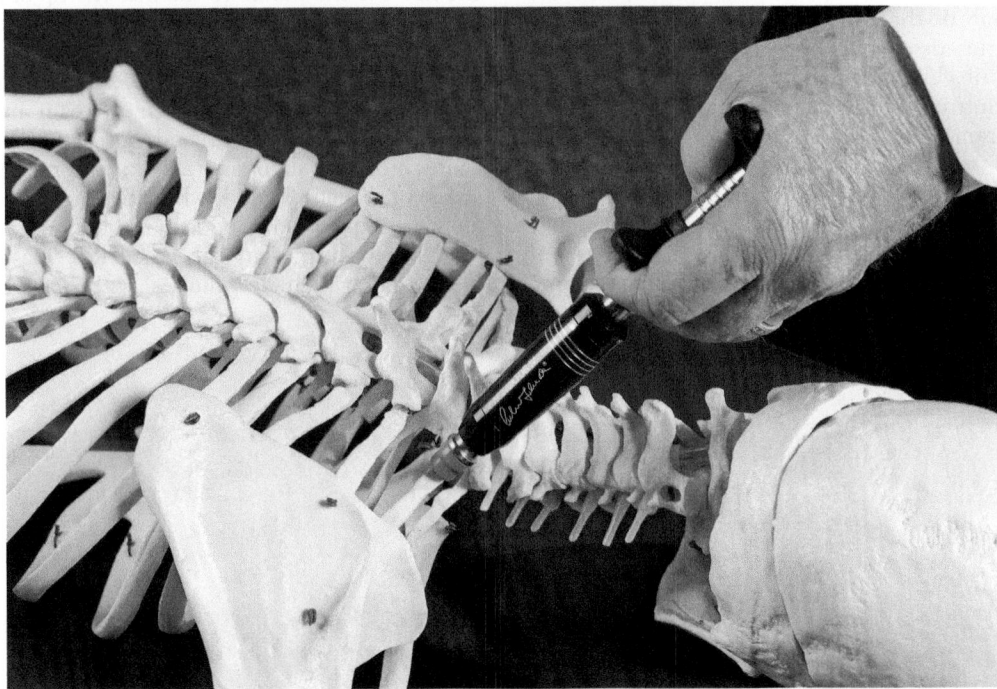

Figure 11-21 Adjustment for second rib. Line of Drive is lateral and inferior along longitudinal axis of rib.

lateral to the transverse process on the side of rib involvement. The LOD is lateral and inferior along the longitudinal axis of the rib (Figure 11-21).

To ensure an effective adjustment and to minimize discomfort for the patient, use the thumb of the free hand to take a lateral and inferior tissue pull over the contact point on the rib. Use the thumb to stabilize the tip of the instrument on the body of the rib during the adjustment.

Third Rib Involvement

If third thoracic vertebral motor unit involvement testing was not reactive, and the patient reports neck, upper back, and shoulder problems, test and correct for third rib involvement alone.

Isolation Test. To isolate the third rib, instruct the patient to bilaterally abduct the arms to 90 degrees with the palms facing up, holding this position (Figure 11-22). Look for PD leg reactivity in Position #1. Then proceed to Position #2, while observing relative changes in the PD leg. Follow the Short/Long Rule.

If the PD leg lengthens in Position #2, the third rib is involved on the side of Pelvic Deficiency. If the PD leg shortens in Position #2, the third rib is involved on the side Opposite Pelvic Deficiency.

Adjustment. To adjust for third rib involvement, contact the body of the rib about one-half inch lateral to the transverse process on the side of rib involvement. The LOD is lateral and inferior along the longitudinal axis of the rib (see Figure 11-18).

To ensure an effective adjustment and to minimize discomfort for the patient, use the thumb of the free hand to take a lateral and inferior tissue pull over the contact point on the rib. Use the thumb to stabilize the tip of the instrument on the body of the rib during the adjustment.

Fourth Rib Involvement

If fourth thoracic vertebral neuroarticular dysfunction during the Basic Scan did not reveal involvement, but the patient complains of upper and mid thoracic pain and shoulder problems, test and correct for fourth rib involvement alone.

Isolation Test. To isolate the fourth rib alone, instruct the patient to bilaterally abduct the arms to 90 degrees with the palms up and then return the hands to the table in neutral position (Figure 11-23). Look for PD leg reactivity in Position #1. Then proceed to Position #2, while observing relative changes in the PD leg. Follow the Short/Long Rule.

If the PD leg lengthens in Position #2, the fourth rib is involved on the side of Pelvic Deficiency. If the PD leg shortens in Position #2, the fourth rib is involved on the side Opposite Pelvic Deficiency.

Adjustment. To adjust a fourth rib involvement, contact the body of the rib about one-half inch lateral to the transverse process on the side of rib involvement. The LOD is lateral and inferior along the longitudinal axis of the rib (Figure 11-24).

To ensure an effective adjustment and to minimize discomfort for the patient, use the thumb of the free hand to take a lateral and inferior tissue pull over the contact point on the rib. Use the thumb to stabilize the tip of the instrument on the body of the rib during the adjustment.

Additional Rib Involvement Isolation Tests. When a patient experiences localized rib pain upon inhalation or exhalation and has suffered an acute bronchopulmonary attack, chronic episodes of coughing and wheezing, noncardiac chest pain, pain radiating into the breast, a previous open heart surgical procedure, mastectomy, motor vehicle injuries with seat belt

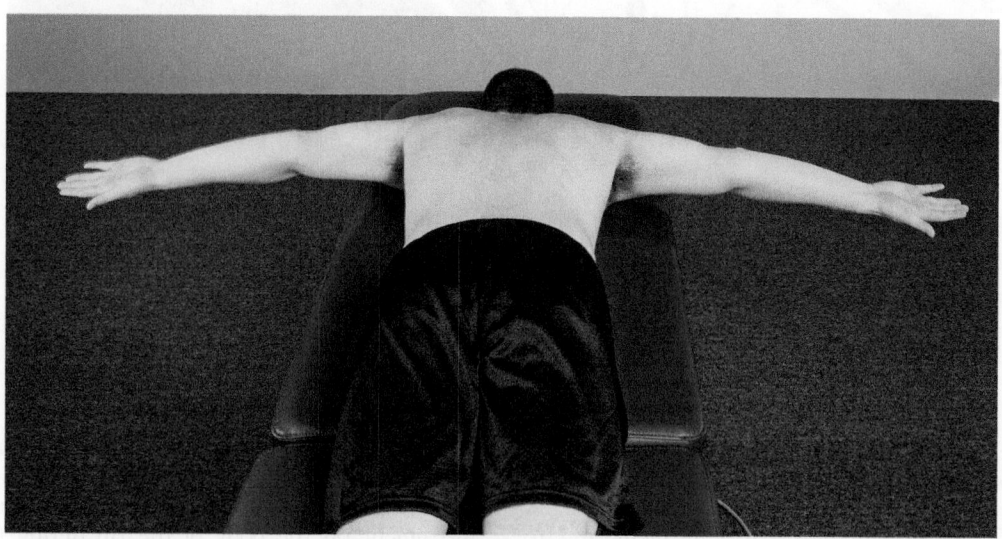

Figure 11-22 Isolation Test for third rib.

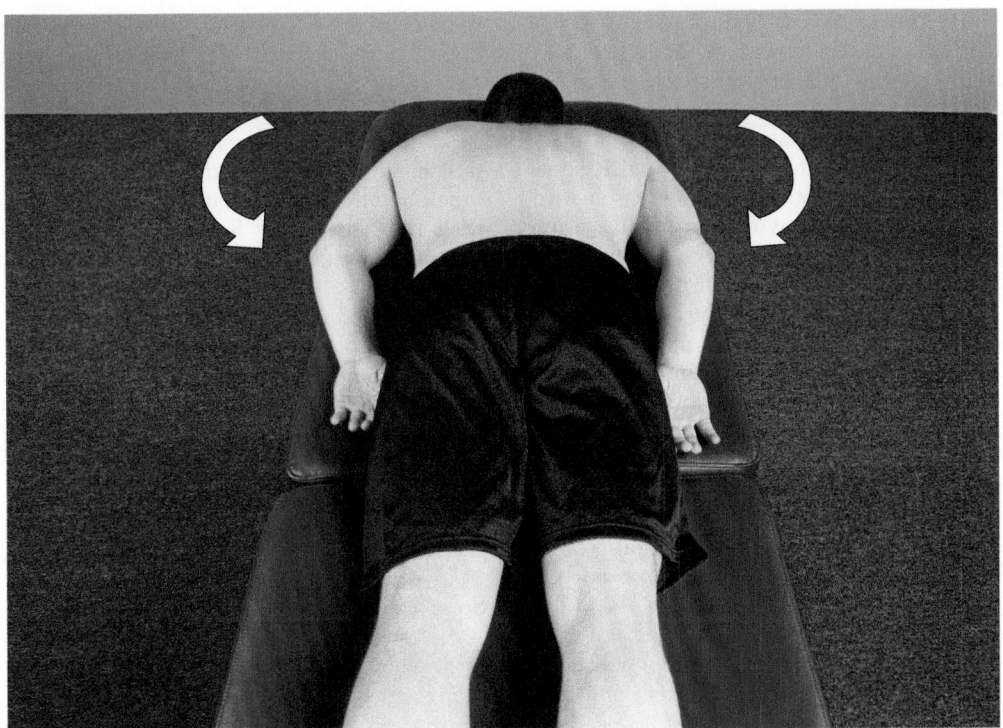

Figure 11-23 Isolation Test for fourth rib; patient returns arms to side after third rib test.

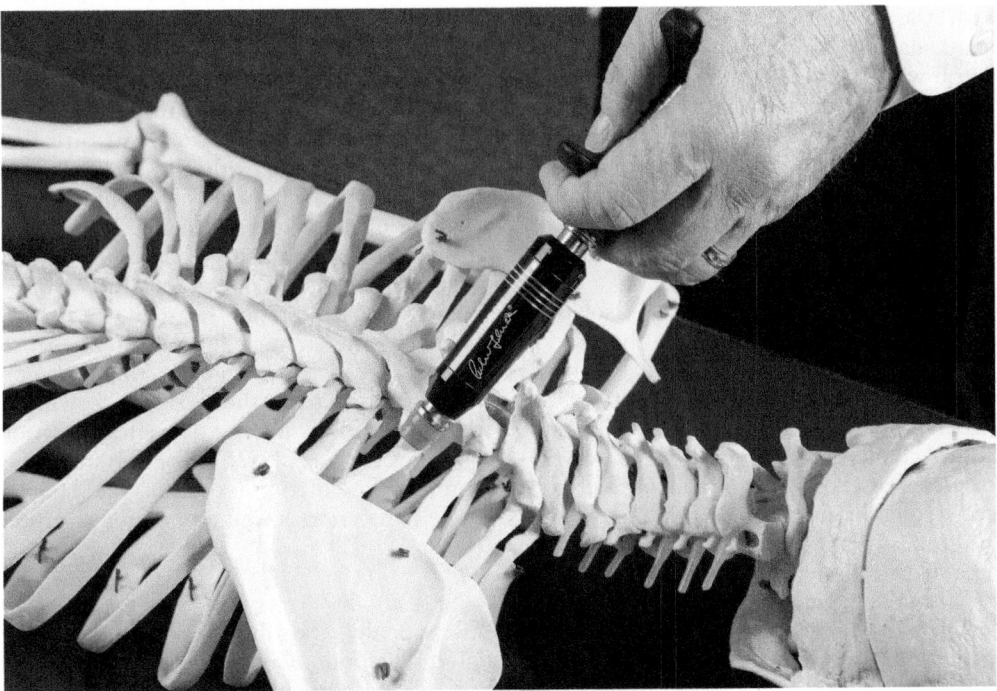

Figure 11-24 Adjustment for fourth rib. Line of Drive is lateral and inferior along longitudinal axis of rib.

utilization and/or air bag deployment, gastrointestinal reflux, and repetitive activities that strain the costal articulations, consider more specific testing for rib involvement. Examples of repetitive activity that is out of the ordinary could occur in winter climates with snow shoveling and at the start of spring season with repetitive athletic endeavors that involve using the driving range for golf and the batting cages for baseball and softball. Confirm adjustments and LODs by Pressure Testing. Adjustments are used with the lowest instrument setting. Before adjustments are made, the integrity of the osseous structure should be intact. Rib fractures are not readily identified through plain radiographs. History of trauma and pathological fractures should be kept in mind. Rib fractures that occur within close proximity to the spine should be considered highly suspicious, especially in children. In all, 98% of posterior rib fractures that occur within 2 cm of the spine are the result of child abuse.[12]

Costovertebral (Posterior) Rib Isolation Test. Isolate the vertebral segment with the use of its Isolation Test, and adjust accordingly if indicated. With the Isolation Test still active, ask the patient to inhale briefly to the fullest comfortable breath. Look for PD leg reactivity in Position #1, and instruct the patient to breathe normally at this time. Then proceed to Position #2, while observing relative changes in the PD leg. Follow the Short/Long Rule.

With the patient in the prone position, neuroarticular stress occurs at the articulation of the rib with the vertebral junction or at the posterior aspect of the rib cage.

Adjustment. Contact the body of the rib about one-half inch lateral to the transverse process on the side of rib involvement as indicated by the Short/Long Rule. The LOD is lateral and interior along the longitudinal axis of the rib involved.

Costosternal (Anterior) Rib Isolation Test. Isolate the vertebra with the use of its Isolation Test, and adjust accordingly if indicated. With the Isolation Test still active, ask the patient to inhale briefly and then exhale to the fullest comfortable excursion. Look for PD leg reactivity in Position #1, and instruct the patient to breathe normally at this time. Then proceed to Position #2, while observing relative changes in the PD leg. Follow the Short/Long Rule. With the patient in the prone position and in full exhalation, neurobiomechanical stress occurs at the articular junction of the rib with the sternum.

Adjustment. Contact the body of the rib about one-half inch lateral to the sternum on the side of rib involvement as indicated by the Short/Long Rule. The LOD is posterior and lateral along the longitudinal axis of the rib involved. In this illustration, the Isolation Test for the third thoracic vertebra is performed (see Figure 11-16), and the patient is asked to inhale and then exhale completely. In accordance with the Short/Long Rule, relative shortening was noted in Position #2 (Figure 11-25).

Superior/Inferior Rib Involvement

After the Isolation Test for the involved vertebral segment and the Inhalation/Exhalation Tests have been completed, along with any adjustments that were indicated, use Position #3 to determine whether a superior or inferior misalignment is present. Follow these steps to combine and localize the involvement.

Step One: Perform the Isolation Test for the involved vertebral segment.

Step Two: Ask the patient to inhale to the fullest comfortable level for costovertebral articulation.

Step Three: Look for PD leg reactivity in Position #1, and instruct the patient to breathe normally at this time. Then proceed to Position #2, while observing relative changes in the PD leg. Follow the Short/Long Rule.

Step Four: Use Position #3 to determine superiority or inferiority. Lengthening of the PD leg in Position #3 would indicate superior involvement of the isolated rib. Shortening of the PD leg in Position #3 would indicate an inferior rib.

Repeat Step One, then change Step Two and ask the patient to exhale to the fullest comfortable excursion for costosternal articulation isolation. Continue with the remaining steps to identify the side of involvement, as well as superior or inferior involvement.

Adjustment. Contact the body of the involved rib one-half inch lateral to the transverse process for a posterior rib and one-half inch lateral to the sternum for an anterior rib (see Figure 11-25). For a superior rib, contact the superior aspect of the body; you will note that the LOD is inferior as well as anterior or posterior (Figure 11-26). For an inferior rib, contact the inferior aspect of the body; the LOD is superior as well as anterior or posterior (Figure 11-27).

Lateral Rib Involvement

Occasionally, the rib head will subluxate in a lateral direction. Consider this procedure when the legs do not level after adjustment of a thoracic vertebra and the corresponding rib, and persistent complaints describe rib symptoms.

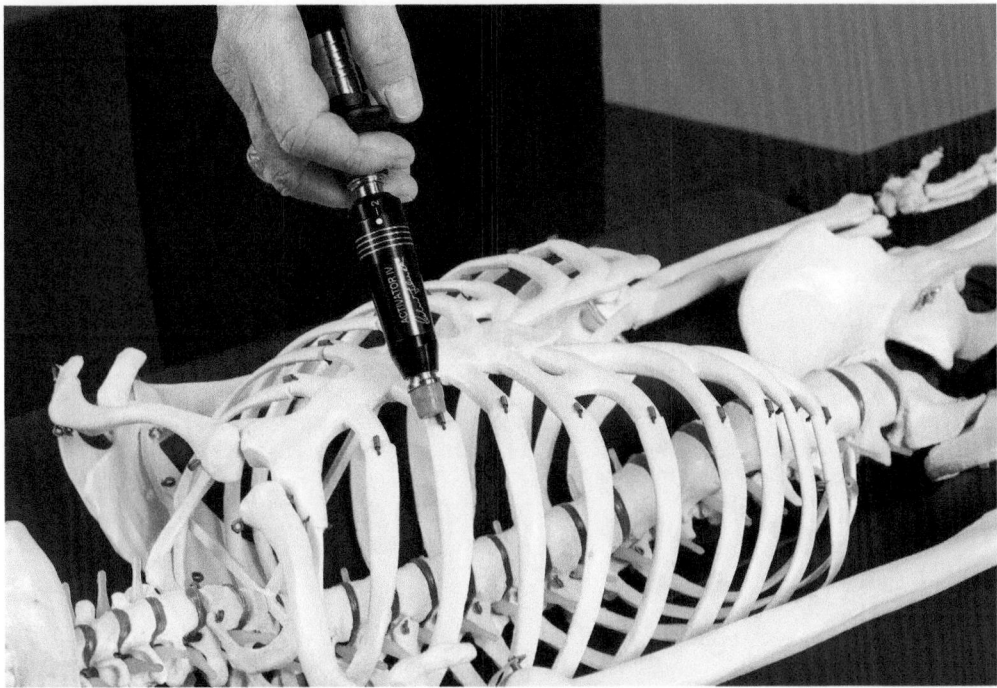

Figure 11-25   Adjustment for costosternal (anterior) rib. Line of Drive is posterior and lateral along longitudinal axis of rib.

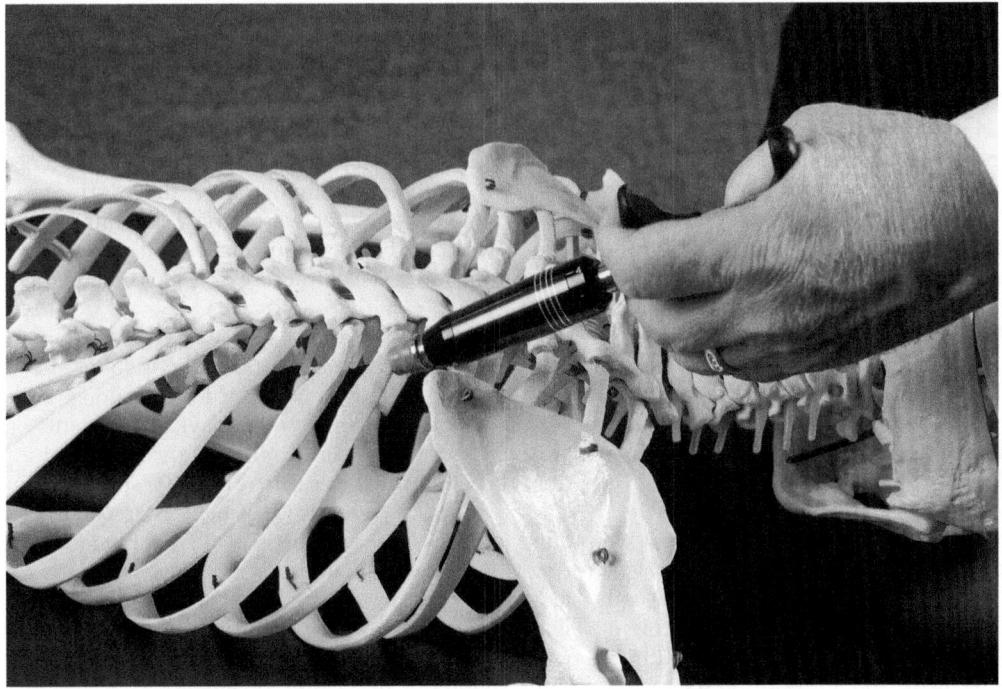

Figure 11-26   Adjustment for superior rib. Line of Drive is inferior and anterior.

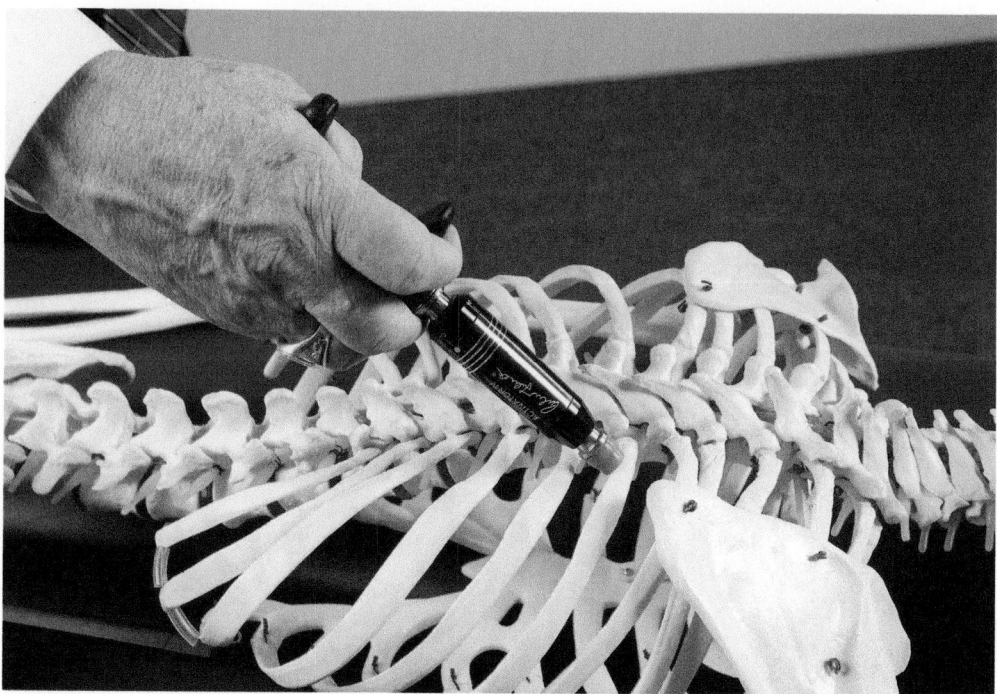

Figure 11-27 Adjustment for inferior rib. Line of Drive is superior and anterior.

Complete the following tests and adjust accordingly as they occur:
- The vertebral segment is isolated to reveal the level of involvement.
- Inhalation/Exhalation Testing is used to determine costovertebral and costosternal involvement.
- Position #2 determines the side of involvement through use of the Short/Long Rule.
- Position #3 determines superiority or inferiority of the structure.
- Position #4 can be used to determine laterality of the structure.

Adjustment. Contact the lateral aspect of the angle of the rib for costovertebral involvement and the body of the rib one-half inch lateral to the sternum for costosternal involvement. The LOD is medial and slightly superior according to the angle of the body of the rib. Stress Test and Pressure Test to confirm the contact point and LOD (see Figure 11-10 for the Isolation Test; Figure 11-28).

SIDE NOTE: The patient may report symptoms along the lateral aspects of the rib cage. Asking the patient to point to the area usually leads the doctor to the level of involvement. Then use Stress Tests to identify the direction of involvement and Pressure Tests to determine

the LOD for the adjustment. Involvement most frequently occurs in a superior (Figure 11-29) direction on the lateral aspect of the rib cage (Figure 11-30 illustrates inferior involvement). Patient history usually involves direct pressure to the actual area of complaint, for example, leaning over the arm rest of a car seat to reach for an object, or falling with the arm against the side of the rib cage. Other involvements have been reported in women who have recently undergone mammography diagnostic testing, lumpectomy, or mastectomy. Examination performed before adjustment would seek to rule out any type of fracture or osseous incongruence.

Anterior First Rib Involvement

Patient complaints typically involve the area along the supraclavicular fossa or along the inferior margin of the clavicle. Patients may describe pressure similar to the feeling of a golf ball in the lower throat near the sternoclavicular junction. This involvement is frequently associated with an anterior-inferior humerus and/or inferior-medial coracoid involvement. Also, clavicular injury of any type, shoulder dislocation, rotator cuff syndrome, and thoracic outlet syndrome should be viewed as indicators for anterior first rib involvement.

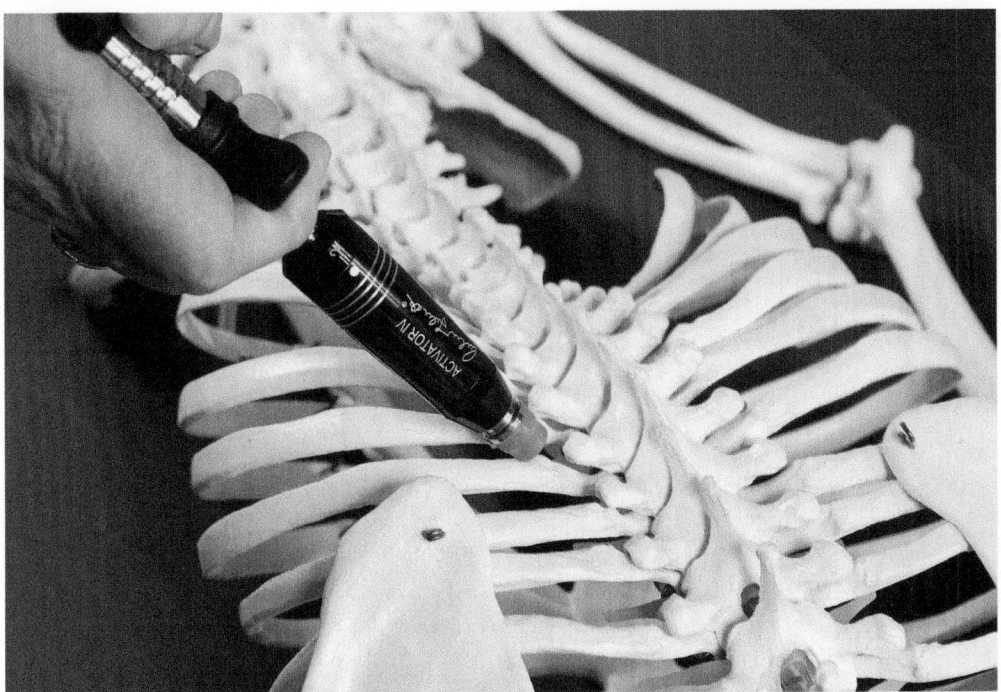

Figure 11-28   Adjustment for lateral rib. Line of Drive is medial and slightly superior.

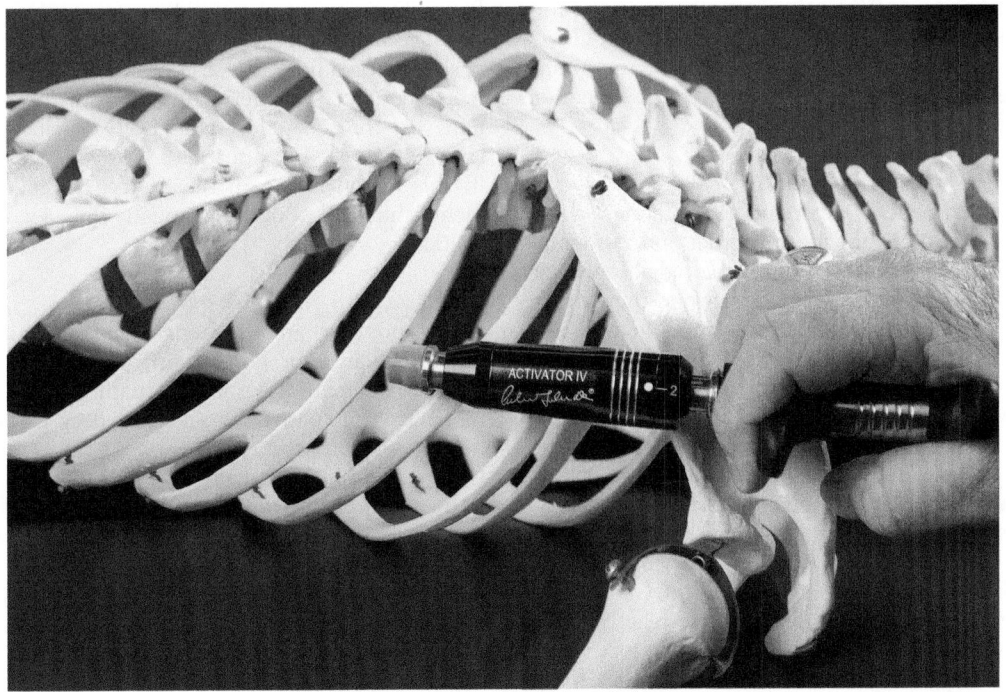

Figure 11-29   Adjustment for superior rib on lateral aspect of the rib cage. Line of Drive is inferior.

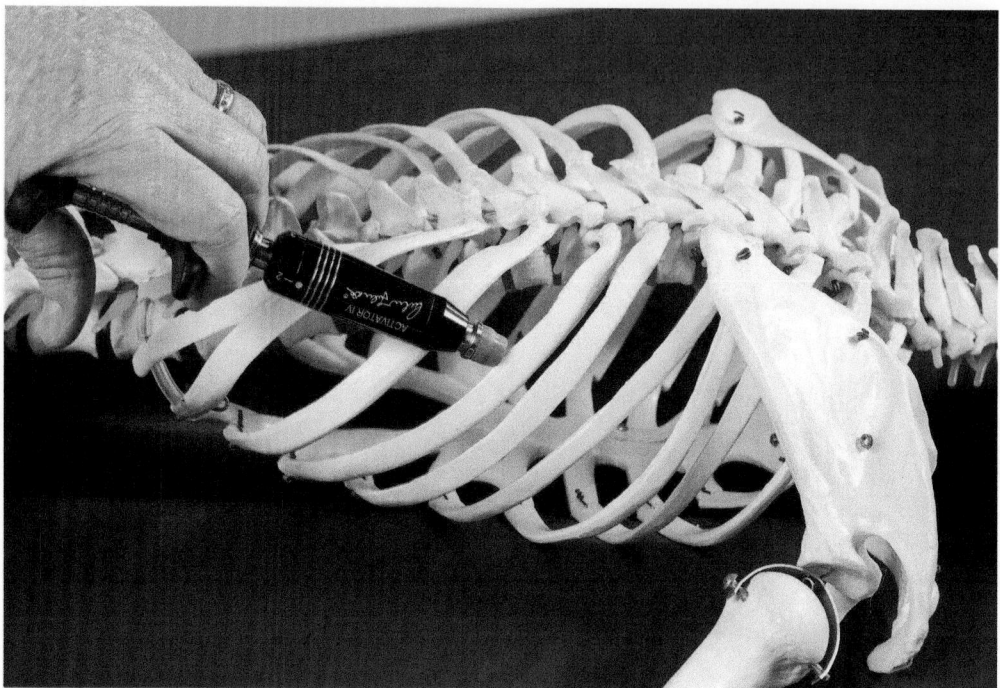

Figure 11-30   Adjustment for inferior rib on lateral aspect of the rib cage. Line of Drive is superior.

To assess involvement, instruct the patient to press the involved shoulder directly into the table. Look for PD leg reactivity in Position #1 (Figure 11-31).

Adjustment.   With the patient in a supine position, contact just below the involved clavicle about 2 inches lateral to the manubrium. The LOD is posterior and slightly superior (Figure 11-32).

Scalenus Anticus Involvement

When a patient experiences noncardiac chest pain, pain along the medial border of the scapula, or pain that is referred down the radial aspect of the arm, forearm, and hand, or when the patient experiences tingling and numbness in the arm and exhibits positive Adson's test findings, consider testing for scalene involvement. Consider as well the hallmark symptom of tingling in *all* of the fingertips, especially at night, as an indicator for the scalene test, especially after a cervical acceleration/deceleration trauma.

Isolation Test.   To isolate the scalenus anticus, ask the patient to make a fist with both hands and hold while shrugging both shoulders (Figure 11-33). Look for PD leg reactivity in Position #1. Then proceed to Position #2, while observing relative changes in the PD leg. Follow the Short/Long Rule.

If the PD leg lengthens in Position #2, the scalenus anticus on the side of Pelvic Deficiency is involved. If the PD leg shortens in Position #2, the scalenus anticus on the side Opposite Pelvic Deficiency is involved.

Adjustment.   Place the patient in the supine position. To adjust the scalene anticus attachment, contact the inferior insertion of the scalene at the clavicle. The LOD is inferior (Figure 11-34). Because of the delicate tissues in this region and pain sensitivity, the adjustment should be made through the doctor's thumb.

Superior Manubrium of the Sternum

Indications for involvement include patient reports of anterior chest pain, particularly in the sternal area, and shoulder pain. Isolate by instructing the patient to take in a deep breath, hold, and lift the head up off the table (Figure 11-35). Reactivity of the PD leg in Position #1 indicates involvement. Be sure to instruct the patient to breathe normally after the Isolation Test.

Adjustment.   With the patient in the supine position, instruct the patient to turn the head to the side to reach the contact point of the sternal notch. The LOD is inferior (Figures 11-36 and 11-37).

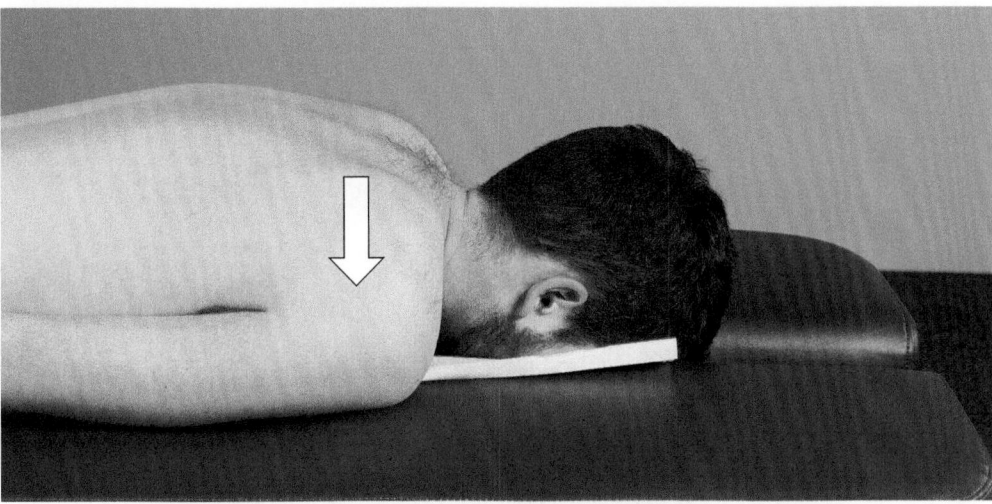

Figure 11-31 Isolation Test for anterior first rib; patient pushes involved shoulder into table.

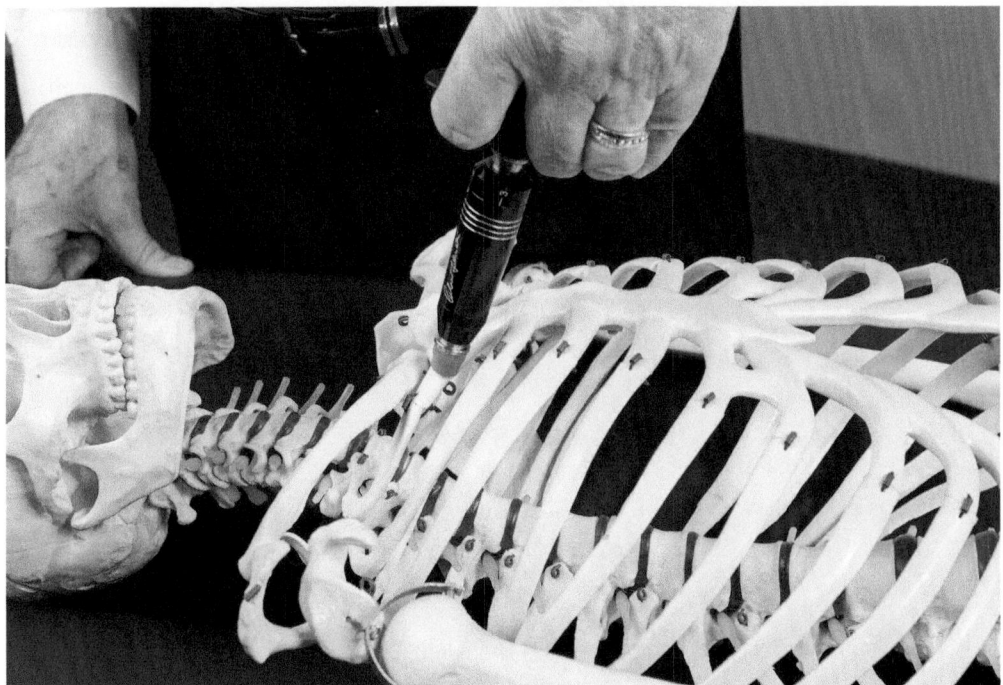

Figure 11-32 Adjustment for anterior first rib. Line of Drive is posterior and slightly superior.

Hiatal Hernia Symptoms

Patients present with symptoms of a "hiatal hernia" or gastrointestinal esophageal reflux disease (GERD). Symptoms are classic in occurrence at night when the patient has consumed a large meal within a couple hours before going to bed. While the patient is lying supine, gastric contents regurgitate, and symptoms of heartburn, upper stomach discomfort, dyspepsia, hiccups, noncardiac chest pain, and radiating pain to the mid and upper thoracic spine can occur. Stress Test by gently pushing superior in the epigastric region near the xiphoid process (Figure 11-38), and look for

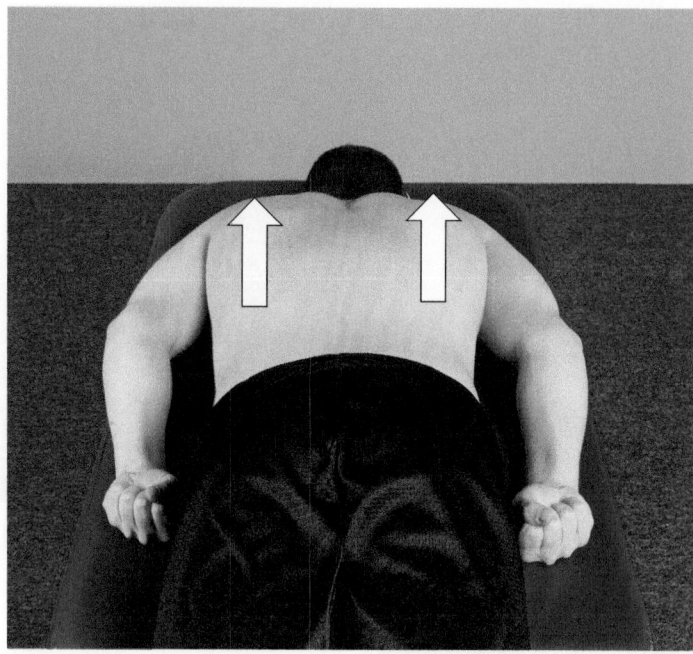

Figure 11-33   Isolation Test for scalenus anticus; patient makes fists with both hands and shrugs both shoulders.

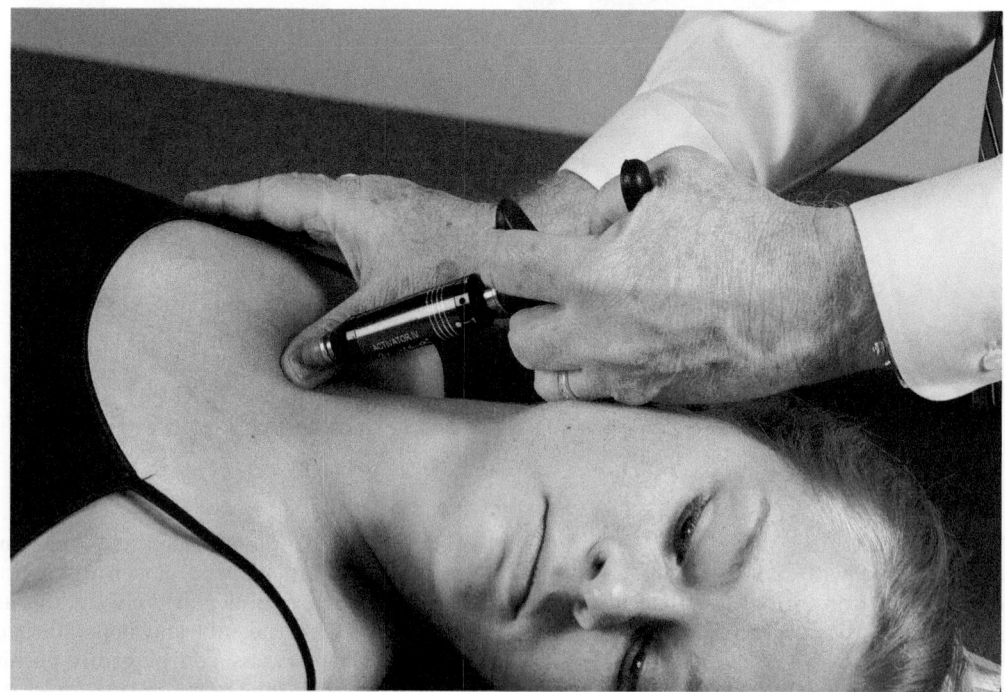

Figure 11-34   Adjustment for scalenus anticus. Line of Drive is inferior.

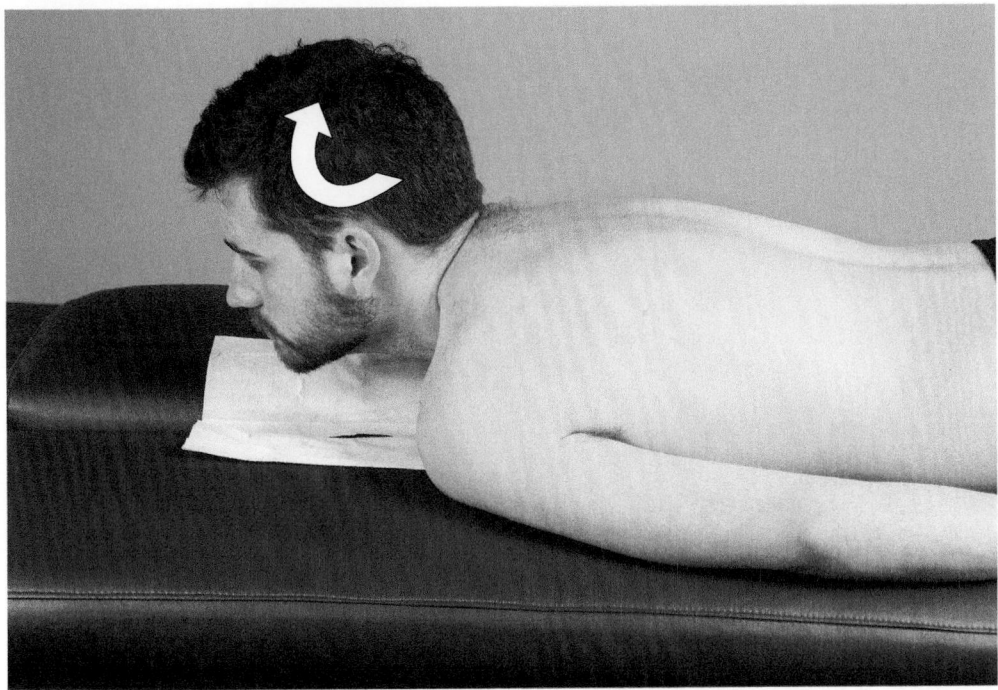

Figure 11-35 Isolation Test for superior manubrium; patient inhales and holds, then lifts head off table.

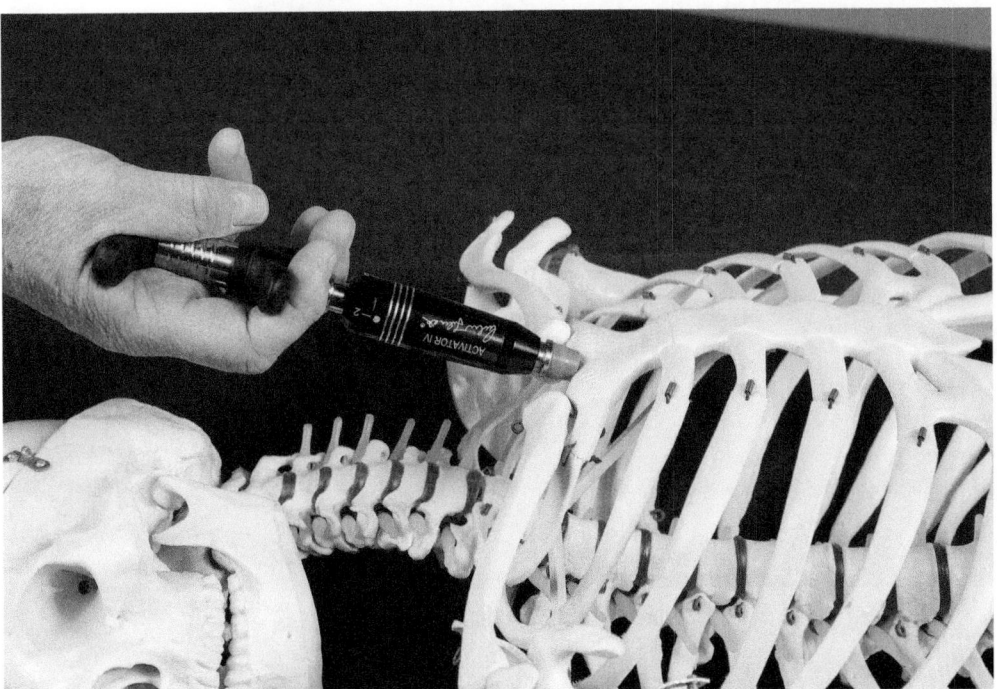

Figure 11-36 Adjustment for superior manubrium. Line of Drive is inferior.

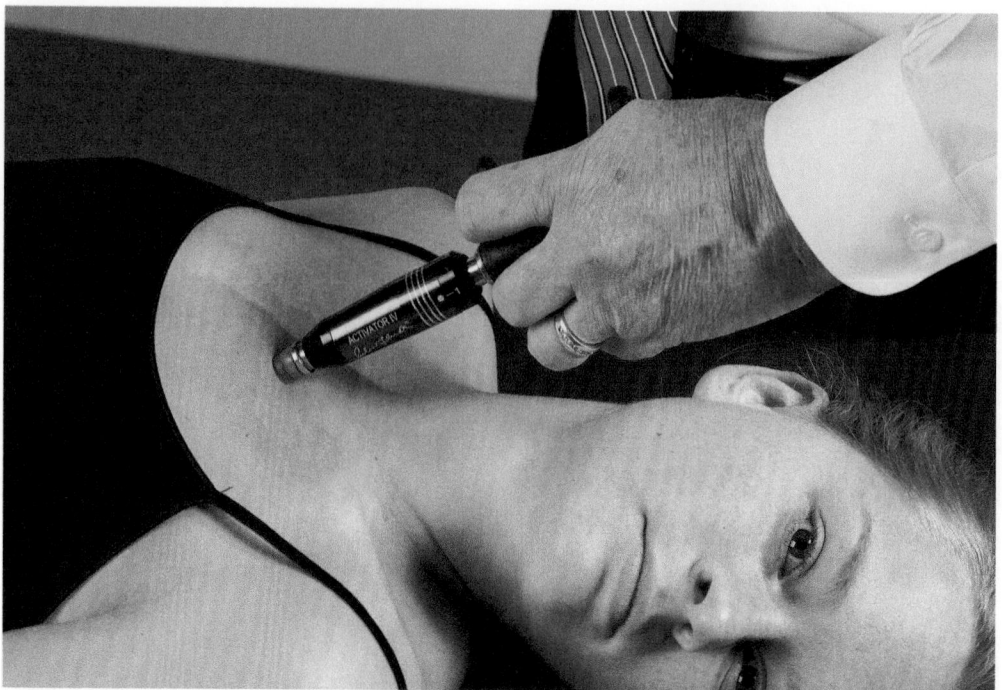

Figure 11-37   Adjustment for superior manubrium. Line of Drive is inferior.

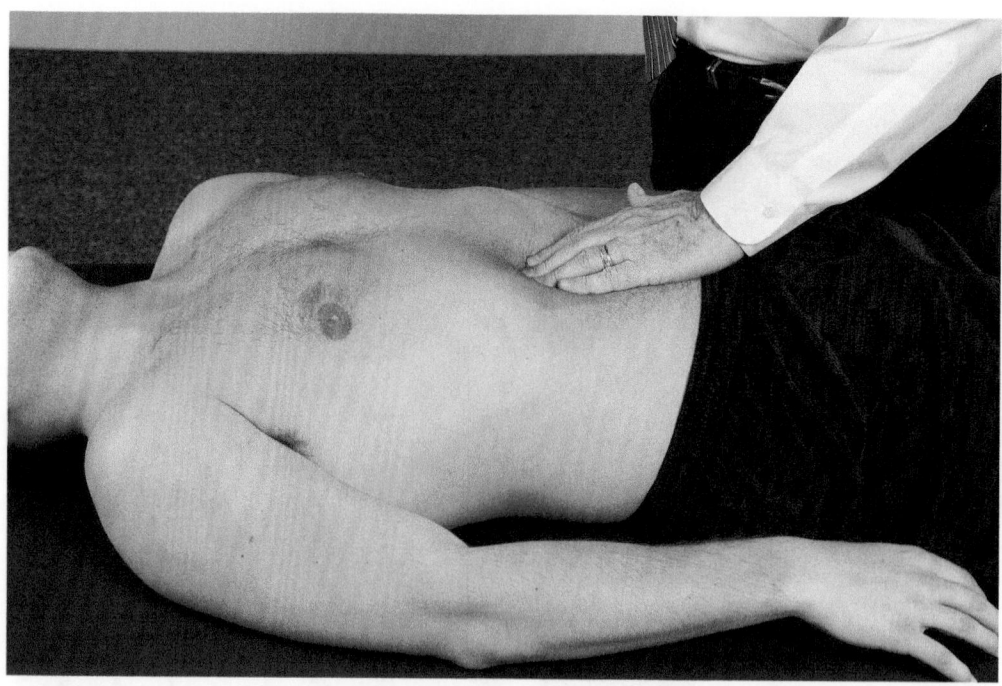

Figure 11-38   Stress Test for hiatal hernia.

reactivity of the PD leg in Position #1; if the patient is lying supine, perform a supine leg check. Adjustment is made to the left side of the abdomen.

Adjustment.   Three steps and contact points are used:

- Step One: 1 inch inferior to the xiphoid process (Figure 11-39)
- Step Two: 1 inch inferior and 2 inches lateral to the first contact point (Figure 11-40)
- Step Three: 1 inch inferior and 2 inches lateral to the second contact point (Figure 11-41)
   The LOD is inferior and lateral.

SIDE NOTE: A clinical tip to help with symptoms of hiatal hernia or GERD is to instruct the patient to sleep at night while lying on the left side. This position can usually replace elevation of the head of the bed and can give the patient significant relief of symptoms during sleep. The other primary consideration is that the patient should finish eating the evening meal at least four hours before retiring; preferably, portion size should be small.

Xiphoid Involvement

This test should be considered for patients who have previously undergone thoracic surgery, are experiencing flank-type pain (costal), have a dull lower thoracic area of pain that cannot be cleared by the usual means, or are exhibiting upper gastric symptoms similar to hiatal hernia symptoms. Stress Test to determine the direction of involvement of the xiphoid with the patient supine, while using a supine Leg Length Analysis. Involvement most commonly occurs in an inferior direction (Figure 11-42).

Adjustment.   Correct by adjusting through the doctor's thumb at the lowest instrument setting in the direction opposite to the Stress Test. After trauma and thoracic surgery, the xiphoid can be involved in any direction (Figure 11-43).

   Mechanical force, manually assisted chiropractic adjusting is summarized in Table 11-1. Boxes 11-1 through 11-3 present summaries of related research for the thoracic spine and related structures.

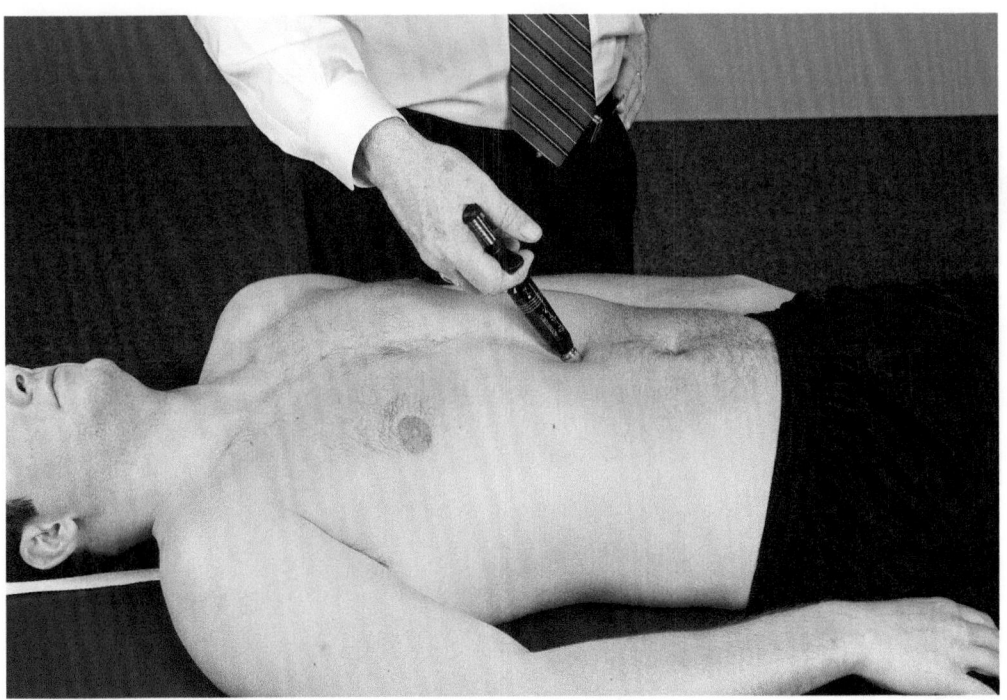

Figure 11-39   Adjustment for hiatal hernia, Step One. Line of Drive is inferior and lateral.

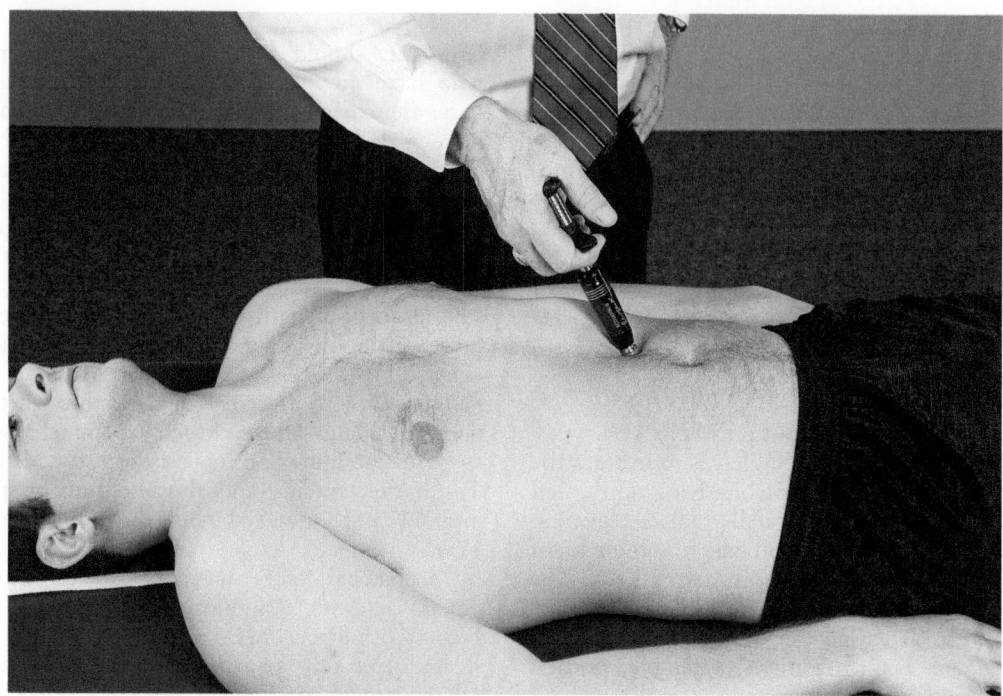

Figure 11-40   Adjustment for hiatal hernia, Step Two. Line of Drive is inferior and lateral.

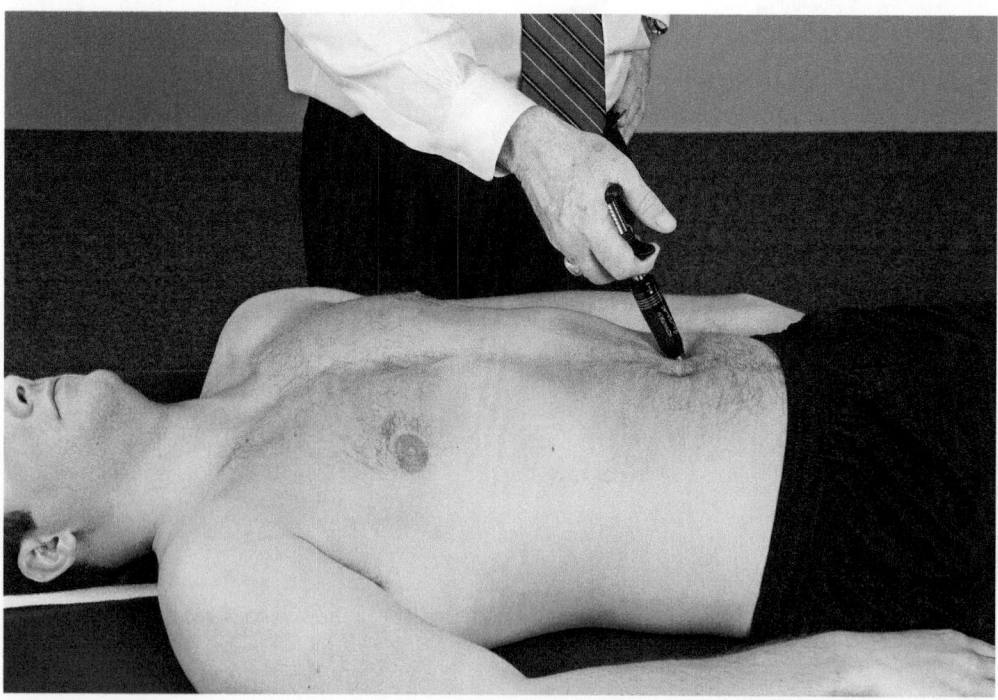

Figure 11-41   Adjustment for hiatal hernia, Step Three. Line of Drive is inferior and lateral.

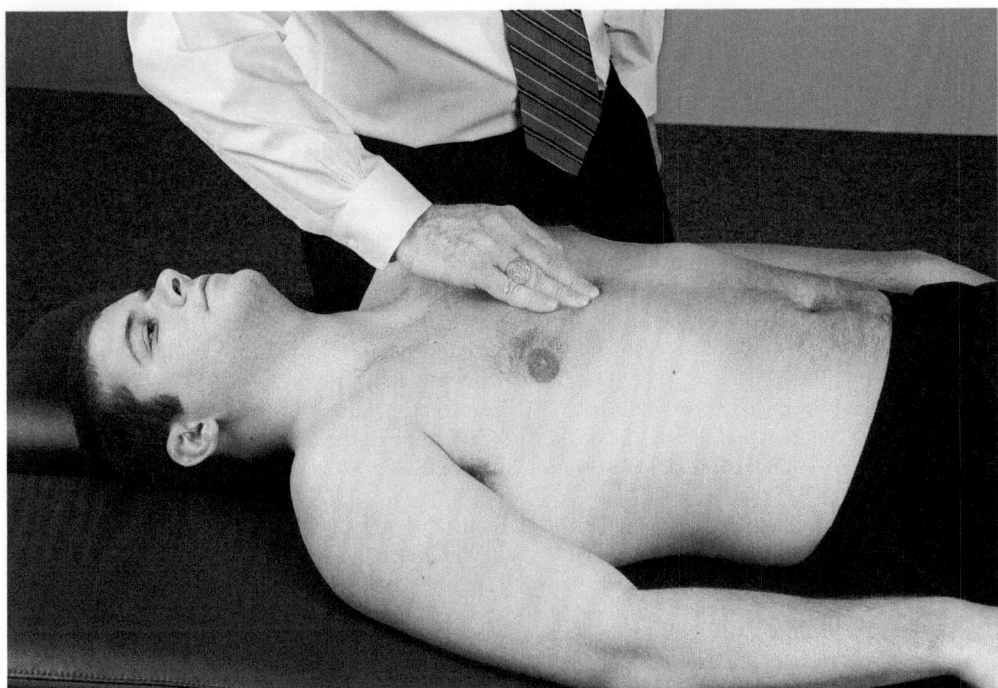

Figure 11-42   Stress Test for inferior xiphoid.

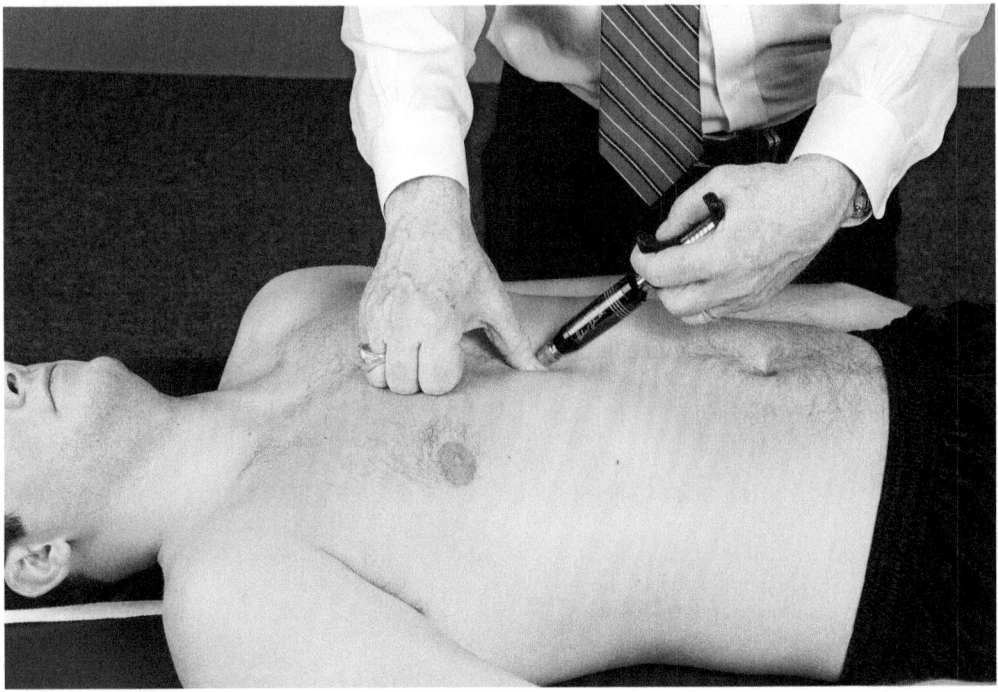

Figure 11-43   Adjustment for inferior xiphoid. Line of Drive is superior.

Table 11-1 Summary Table–Additional Tests and Adjustments for the Thoracic Vertebrae, Ribs, and Anterior Thorax

Articular Dysfunction	Test	ADJUSTMENT	
		Segmental Contact Point	Line of Drive
Tenth Thoracic (T10)	Instruct the patient to lower arm from the T12 test on the side of PD back along the side of the body	*Step One*: Transverse process according to the Short/Long Rule	Anterior, superior, and slightly medial
		Step Two: Proceed to contralateral corresponding rib	Lateral and inferior along longitudinal axis of rib
Eleventh Thoracic (T11)	Instruct the patient to raise arm on OPD side and rest forearm on table superior and lateral to head	Transverse process according to the Short/ Long Rule	Anterior, superior, and slightly medial
Eleventh Rib Involvement	Repeat T11 Isolation Test and have patient inhale	Body of rib one-half inch lateral to transverse process according to the Short/Long Rule	Lateral and inferior along longitudinal axis of rib
Ninth Thoracic (T9)	Instruct the patient to lower arm from T11 test on OPD side back along side of body	*Step One*: Transverse process according to the Short/Long Rule	Anterior, superior, and slightly medial
		Step Two: Proceed to contralateral corresponding rib	Lateral and inferior along longitudinal axis of rib
Seventh Thoracic (T7)	Instruct the patient to lower both arms from T8 test back along side of body, raise both shoulders posterior, then relax	*Step One*: Transverse process according to the Short/Long Rule	Anterior, superior, and slightly medial
		Step Two: Proceed to contralateral corresponding rib	Lateral and inferior along longitudinal axis of rib
Fifth Thoracic (T5)	Instruct the patient to keep face turned to PD side, raise the OPD forearm, and rest it on table superior and lateral to the head	*Step One*: Transverse process according to the Short/Long Rule	Anterior, superior, and slightly medial
		Step Two: Proceed to contralateral corresponding rib	Lateral and inferior along longitudinal axis of rib
Third Thoracic (T3)	Instruct patient to keep face turned to PD side, raise forearm on side of PD, and rest on table superior and lateral to head	*Step One*: Transverse process according to the Short/Long Rule	Anterior, superior, and slightly medial
		Step Two: Proceed to contralateral corresponding rib	Lateral and inferior along longitudinal axis of rib
Fourth Rib Involvement	Instruct the patient to bilaterally abduct the arms to 90 degrees, with the palms facing up, then to return arms to table	Body of rib one-half inch lateral to transverse process on side according to the Short/ Long Rule	Lateral and inferior along longitudinal axis of rib
Third Rib Involvement	Instruct the patient to bilaterally abduct the arms to 90 degrees with the palms facing up, and to hold	Body of rib one-half inch lateral to transverse process on side according to the Short/ Long Rule	Lateral and inferior along longitudinal axis of rib

		ADJUSTMENT	
Articular Dysfunction	Test	Segmental Contact Point	Line of Drive
Second Thoracic (T2)	Instruct patient to keep face turned to PD side and to lower arm from T3 test on side of PD back along side of body	*Step One:* Transverse process according to the Short/Long Rule *Step Two:* Proceed to contralateral corresponding rib	Anterior, superior, and slightly medial Lateral and inferior along longitudinal axis of rib
Costovertebral Rib (posterior)	Isolate the involved vertebral segment, and adjust accordingly. Patient to inhale deeply and hold briefly.	Contact point is one-half inch lateral to the transverse process	Lateral and inferior along longitudinal axis of rib
Costosternal Rib (anterior)	Isolate the involved vertebral segment, adjust accordingly. Patient inhales and then exhales to a deep level of excursion.	Contact point is one-half inch lateral to the sternal junction	Posterior and lateral along longitudinal axis of rib
Superior Rib Costovertebral	Isolate the involved vertebral segment. Inhale. Position #2 determines side per Short/Long Rule, Position #3 reveals relative lengthening.	One-half inch lateral to the transverse process on the superior aspect of the body of the rib	Inferior and anterior
Superior Rib Costosternal	Isolate the involved vertebral segment. Exhale. Position #2 determines side per Short/Long Rule, Position #3 reveals relative lengthening.	One-half inch lateral to the sternum on the superior aspect of the body of the rib	Inferior and posterior
Inferior Rib Costovertebral	Isolate the involved vertebral segment. Inhale. Position #2 determines side per Short/Long Rule, Position #3 reveals relative shortening.	One-half inch lateral to the transverse process on the inferior aspect of the body of the rib	Superior and anterior
Inferior Rib Costosternal	Isolate the involved vertebral segment. Exhale. Position #2 determines side per Short/Long Rule, Position #3 reveals relative shortening.	One-half inch lateral to the sternum on the inferior aspect of the body of the rib	Superior and posterior
Lateral Rib Costovertebral	Isolate the involved vertebral segment. Inhale. Position #2 determines side from Short/Long Rule, long leg in Position #4 reveals side of laterality.	Lateral aspect of the angle of the rib	Medial and slightly superior

Continued

		ADJUSTMENT	
Articular Dysfunction	Test	Segmental Contact Point	Line of Drive
Lateral Rib Costosternal	Isolate the involved vertebral segment. Exhale. Position #2 determines side per Short/Long Rule, long leg in Position #4 reveals side of laterality.	One-half inch lateral to the sternal junction of the rib	Medial and slightly superior
Anterior First Rib	Patient instructed to push the involved shoulder into the table	Patient supine, just below the clavicle, 2 inches lateral to the manubrium	Posterior and slightly superior
Scalenus Anticus	Make a fist with both hands, shrug both shoulders. Position #1, Position #2 for side per Short/Long Rule.	Patient supine, doctor's digit on insertion of scalenus anticus muscle on tendon	Inferior
Xiphoid	Patient supine, Stress Test, usually inferior, supine leg analysis	Through the doctor's thumb on the xiphoid	Opposite direction of Stress Test
Superior Manubrium of Sternum	Inhale deeply and hold. Lift head up.	Patient supine with head turned, contact sternal notch	Inferior
Hiatal Hernia Symptoms	Gently push superior in the epigastic region near the xiphoid process; check Position #1	On left abdomen: (1) 1 inch inferior to xiphoid process	Inferior and lateral
		(2) 1 inch inferior and 2 inches lateral to the first contact point	Inferior and lateral
		(3) 1 inch inferior and 2 inches lateral to the second contact point	Inferior and lateral

Table 11-1 **Summary Table–Additional Tests and Adjustments for the Thoracic Vertebrae, Ribs, and Anterior Thorax–cont'd**

OPD, Opposite Pelvic Deficiency; *PD*, Pelvic Deficiency.

RELATED RESEARCH

Box 11-1

Reference: Yates RG, Lamping DL, Abram NL, Wright C. Effects of chiropractic treatment on blood pressure and anxiety: a randomized controlled trial. J Manipulative Physiol Ther. 1988;11(6):484-8.

ABSTRACT

This study examined the effects of chiropractic adjustments of the thoracic spine (T1-T5) on blood pressure and state anxiety in 21 patients with elevated blood pressure. Subjects were randomly assigned to one of three treatment conditions: active treatment, placebo treatment, or no treatment control. Adjustments were performed with a mechanical chiropractic adjusting device (Activator Adjusting Instrument). Dependent measures obtained before and after treatment included systolic and diastolic blood pressure and state anxiety. Results indicated that systolic and diastolic blood pressure decreased significantly in the active treatment condition, whereas no significant changes occurred in the placebo and control conditions. The state of anxiety significantly decreased under active and control conditions. Results provide support for the hypothesis that blood pressure is reduced after chiropractic treatment. Further study is needed to examine the long-term effects of chiropractic treatment on blood pressure.

Box 11-2

Reference: Polkinghorn BS, Colloca CJ. Chiropractic management of chronic chest pain using mechanical force, manually assisted short-lever adjusting procedures. J Manipulative Physiol Ther. 2003;26(2):108-15.

ABSTRACT

OBJECTIVE

To discuss a case involving a patient with chronic chest pain, dyspnea, and anxiety. Although resistant to previous treatment regimens, the condition responded favorably to chiropractic manipulation of the costosternal articulations.

CLINICAL FEATURES

A 49-year-old man had chronic chest pain, dyspnea, and anxiety for longer than 4 months. The severity of the condition gradually progressed to the point of precluding the patient's active employment and most physical activity. Previous efforts to treat the condition had met with failure.

INTERVENTION AND OUTCOME

The patient received mechanical force, manually assisted short-lever chiropractic adjustment of the thoracic spine and, in particular, the costosternal articulations. Adjustments were made by means of an Activator Adjusting Instrument-II. The patient responded favorably to the intervention, obtaining prompt relief from his symptoms. Sustained chiropractic care rendered over a 14-week period resulted in complete resolution of the patient's previously chronic condition, with recovery maintained at 9-month follow-up.

CONCLUSIONS

Some types of chest pain may have their origin in a subluxation complex involving the costosternal articulation. Although the possibility of myocardial involvement must be considered with all patients whose symptoms include chest pain, musculoskeletal involvement, including costosternal subluxation complex, may be the underlying cause of the symptoms in some patients. When this is the case, chiropractic adjustment may provide an effective mode of treatment. Further study in an academic research venue is merited to investigate the role that conservative chiropractic care can play for patients with chest pain.

Box 11-3

OTHER THORACIC SPINE–RELATED REPORTS
- Nathan M, Keller TS. Measurement and analysis of the in vivo posteroanterior impulse response of the human thoracolumbar spine: a feasibility study. J Manipulative Physiol Ther. 1994;17 (7):431-41.
- Lehneman NM, Keller TS. The dynamic response of the human spine to low amplitude high velocity posteroanterior thrusts. Proceedings of the 1994 International Conference on Spinal Manipulation; 1994 June 10-11; Palm Springs, CA. p. 87.
- Fuhr AW, Smith DB. Accuracy of piezoelectric accelerometers measuring displacement of a spinal adjusting instrument. J Manipulative Physiol Ther. 1986;9(1):15-21.

REFERENCES

1. Armstrong TJ. Mechanical stressors. In: Rosenstock L, and Cullen MR, editors. Textbook of clinical occupational and environmental medicine. Philadelphia: Saunders; 1994.
2. Hoppenfeld S. Examination of the physical spine and extremities. Norwalk (CT): Appleton-Century-Crofts; 1976.
3. Nepola JV. Examination of the shoulder. In: Clark CR, Bonfiglio M, editors. Orthopaedics: essentials of diagnosis and treatment. New York: Churchill Livingstone; 1994.
4. Cramer GD, Darby SA. Basic and clinical anatomy of the spine, spinal cord, and ANS. St. Louis: Mosby; 1995.
5. Spapen HD, Reynaert H, Debeuckelaere S, Segers O, Somers G. The straight back syndrome. Neth J Med. 1990;36(1-2):29-31.
6. Chandrasoma P, Taylor CR. Concise pathology. 2nd ed. Norwalk (CT): Appleton and Lange; 1995.
7. Bates B. A guide to physical examination and history taking. 4th ed. Philadelphia: JB Lippincott; 1987.
8. Nilsson N, Christiansen B. Prognostic factors in bronchial asthma in chiropractic practice. J Australian Chiro Assoc. 1988;18(3):85-7.
9. Marasaky CS, Weber M. Chiropractic management of chronic obstructive pulmonary disease. J Manipulative Physiol Ther. 1988;11(6):505-10.
10. Taylor GW. Thoracic and lumbar injuries. In: Lillegard WA, Rucker KS. Handbook of sports medicine: a symptom-oriented approach. Boston: Andover; 1993.
11. Johnson RJ, Renström P. Injuries in Alpine skiing. In: Renström P, editor. The encyclopedia of sports medicine, vol v: clinical practice of sports injury prevention and care. London: Blackwell; 1994.
12. Rowe LJ. International Pediatrics Conference, Maui, Hawaii, November 2005.
13. Yochum TR, Rowe LJ. Essentials of skeletal radiology, vol I and II. Baltimore: Williams & Wilkins; 1987.
14. Taber's cyclopedic medical dictionary. 20th ed. Philadelphia: FA Davis; 2005.
15. Ford DM, Bagnall KM, McFadden KD, Greenhill BJ, Raso VJ. Paraspinal muscle imbalance in adolescent idiopathic scoliosis. Spine. 1984; 9(4):373-6.
16. Dixson R. Scoliosis in the community. Br Med J. 1983;286:615-18.
17. McCaw ST, Bates BT. Biomechanical implications of mild leg length inequality. Br J Sports Med. 1991;25(1):10-13.
18. Friberg O. Clinical symptoms and biomechanics of lumbar spine and hip joint in leg length inequality. Spine. 1983;8(6):643-51.
19. Giles LGF, Taylor JR. Lumbar spine structural changes associated with leg length inequality. Spine. 1982;7(2):159-62.
20. Aspegren DD. Scoliosis. In: Cox JM, editor, Low back pain—mechanism, diagnosis and treatment. 5th ed. Baltimore: Williams & Wilkins; 1990. p. 309-38.
21. Magee DJ. In: Orthopedic physical assessment. Philadelphia: Saunders; 1987. p. 266-313.
22. Polkinghorn BS. Chiropractic treatment of frozen shoulder syndrome (adhesive capsulitis): using mechanical force manually assisted short lever adjusting procedures. J Manipulative Physiol Ther. 1995;18(2):105-15.

12

ADDITIONAL TESTS AND ADJUSTMENTS FOR THE CERVICAL SPINE

In the experience of clinicians who use the Activator Method (AM), patient reports of neck pain and stiffness arising from cervical neuroarticular dysfunction complexes can often be resolved by testing for and adjusting, as indicated in the Basic Scan Protocol. Sound clinical procedure, however, still calls for appropriate examination and testing before any form of care is initiated.

When a patient's cervical complaints continue and/or examination findings so indicate, perform Isolation and Stress Tests for the following additional cervical neuroarticular dysfunctions:

- Sixth Cervical (C6)
- Enhancement of Sixth (C6) Cervical
- Enhancement of Fifth (C5) Cervical
- Fifth Cervical (C5) Inferior
- Hidden Posterior C5
- Fourth Cervical (C4)
- Third Cervical (C3)
- Third Cervical (C3) Opposite Pelvic Deficiency Alternative Test
- Second Cervical (C2)
- Second Cervical (C2) Enhancement
- Second Cervical (C2) Lateral
- Second Cervical (C2) with Pelvic Deficiency (PD) Side Levator Scapulae Contracture
- Second and Fifth Cervical (C2-C5 combination)
- Lateral Occiput
- Cervical Disc with Radiculopathy

COMMON CERVICAL COMPLAINTS

Neck pain and stiffness are common complaints of chiropractic patients. Many but not all patients report additional or related symptoms of headache, discomfort in the shoulder, arm, and upper back, and interscapular discomfort that is directly or indirectly associated with problems of the cervical spine.[1,2] Cervical complaints may be of sudden traumatic onset or may be related to falls, athletic injuries, or motor vehicle crashes. Onset may be more gradual and insidious when related to postural defects, inadequate workstations, or repetitive strain injury. Recent literature has implicated the cervical zygapophyseal joints as a common source of idiopathic neck pain.[3-6]

In acceleration/deceleration injuries, the cervical zygapophyseal joints are the most commonly injured tissues in the neck. According to Bogduk,[7] most patients have normal neurological examination findings and normal x-rays, and in patients with posttraumatic neck pain, the zygapophyseal joints are more often implicated as producing pain than are the discs.

Trauma to the cervical spine and related structures during motor vehicle collisions is a frequent cause of a wide variety of head, neck, and upper extremity complaints.[8-10] The precise incidence of motor vehicle collisions that result in whiplash injury or cervical acceleration/deceleration trauma is difficult to determine because of variability in reporting, in onset of signs and symptoms, and in duration of symptoms. However, several sources have conservatively estimated that more than 1 million cases of cervical acceleration/deceleration (CAD) injury occur per year in the United States.[11,12]

As the underlying cause, whiplash may present with the most complex clinical picture in patients with cervical complaints. In addition to altered ranges of motion, cervical complaints associated with CAD may include one or more of the following symptoms of more or less acute onset: neck pain and stiffness, trapezius pain and contracture or spasm, headache, upper extremity paresthesias, thoracic spine and low back pain, vertigo, ocular disturbances, dysphagia, and hoarseness. The full extent of injury to the cervical spine and to related structures may take days or weeks to manifest fully.[13] Delayed signs and symptoms associated with CAD injury can also include thoracic outlet syndrome, carpal tunnel syndrome, temporomandibular joint dysfunction, postconcussion syndrome, and myofascial pain disorder.[11,14]

Head and neck injuries are also common with athletic activities, especially in body contact sports.[15,16] Collision impact to the head with the neck in flexion appears to be most injurious to the cervical spine and is associated with a risk of posterior disc rupture and sprain/strain syndrome to posterior ligamentous and musculotendinous structures.[17] Athletic endeavors in which falls are likely, such as rodeo and equestrian events, cycling, skiing, and gymnastics, may also present risks for cervical trauma.

When a cervical complaint can be related to a specific event, the exact circumstances of the injury can play a valuable role in patient assessment, diagnosis, and prognosis. After a motor vehicle crash, include as many specific details as possible about the collision in the patient record. Details should include exact time and location of the incident, direction or vector of the collision, use and type of seat belt, head restraint adjustment, position of the patient at time of impact, and at least estimates of the speed of impact. Because transient amnesia is a frequent manifestation of mild traumatic brain injury, it may also be valuable to include observations and recollections of witnesses to the injury.[18] Of course, a thorough history and specifics of the precipitating incident that resulted in cervical trauma and acute or delayed onset of symptoms are important not only from a clinical perspective but also from a medicolegal point of view.

When cervical complaints are of gradual onset or cannot be related to specific traumatic or stressful events, consider postural, occupational, or environmental factors that might contribute to cumulative microtrauma to the cervical spine and related structures. Occupational activities that require work to be performed above eye or head level, such as electrical work, pipefitting, painting, and dry walling, often require that the head and neck be held in forced extension for long periods of time.[15]

Cumulative strain and sprain injury to the cervical spine is associated with other trades as well. For those workers who use a computer as a significant part of their task assignment, placement of the keyboard and especially the monitor may cause adverse postural effects. A monitor placed to one side of the workstation, for example, causes the worker to turn the head and neck to that side during operation of the computer. Muscles on the side of head and neck rotation may become mildly hypertonic, while the corresponding muscles on the opposite side may tend to lose tone. Monitors may also be placed too high for the worker's normal field of vision, and the head and neck may have to be held in unnatural extension for much or all of a work shift.

Sustained flexion postures of the cervical spine further cause abnormal loading to spinal structures and tissues. Breig[19] demonstrated that flexion of the head tractioned the cervical cord, nerve roots, and hindbrain; this normally would be well tolerated. However, a flexed posture in the presence of space-occupying lesions such as disc protrusions and posterior osteophytes may create deformation of neural structures and subsequent development of symptoms. A forward head posture or anterior translation further places abnormal loads on tissues, predisposing them to deformation. Calliet[20] states that if the head weighs ten pounds, for every inch of anterior weight bearing of the head, a tenfold increase in muscle effort of the posterior cervical musculature is required to offset this load, leading to fibrous infiltration, pain, and reduced motion.[21] On the contrary, a cervical lordosis is implicated as a state of static equilibrium[20,22,23] while dynamic investigation is pending.

The effects of such postural adaptation to an ergonomically unsound workstation are, of course, cumulative and gradual. Early complaints of cervical pain and stiffness and examination findings of altered range of motion may be very subtle and may not be recognized until they become clinically significant. Unfortunately for the patient, by that time, signs and symptoms may be part of a larger and more complex clinical picture of significant disability or at least impairment of lifestyle. In addition to complaints of neck pain and stiffness, cumulative stress injury to the cervical spine may produce fatigue, headache, eyestrain, and myofascial pain disorder.

EXAMINATION PROCEDURES FOR THE CERVICAL SPINE

When a patient first presents with a cervical problem, be sure to take a thorough history and to perform an appropriate examination, including range-of-motion testing, orthopedic and neurological assessment, and instrumentation as indicated. Examination findings and clinical judgment may indicate the need for additional special tests and radiographic analysis or other diagnostic imaging. If a complaint appears to arise from a work-related injury, a motor vehicle crash, or any other situation in which personal injury claims may result, make a special point to carefully document patient statements, examination findings, treatment plans, and outcome measurements.

Overt signs of cervical injury or dysfunction may include antalgic posture, guarded motion, abnormal head tilt and rotation, or a compensatory "high shoulder." Reduced or asymmetrical range of motion of the cervical spine is likely to accompany paravertebral muscle spasm with acute injury or contracture with chronic complaints.[24] Evaluate the cervical spine in its six standard ranges of motion: flexion, extension, lateral flexion (lateral bending) to the right and left, and rotation to the right and left. Average range-of-motion values for the cervical spine are listed in Box 12-1.[25,26]

Evaluate both active and passive ranges of motion for the cervical spine with particular attention to pain-limited motion, bilateral symmetry, and fluid motion in all directions. During passive range-of-motion testing, note evidence of soft tissue swelling, inflammation, muscle spasm, or contracture, as well as palpable or audible joint crepitus.

In addition to range-of-motion testing, examination of the cervical spine includes neurological and orthopedic testing.[24] Neurological tests should include assessment of the cranial nerves in terms of motor, sensory, and autonomic functions. Reflex testing of the upper extremity provides further evaluation of the peripheral nervous system and cervical spinal nerves. Standard reflex testing involves the biceps brachii (C5 nerve root and musculocutaneous nerve), the brachioradialis (C6 nerve root and radial nerve), and the triceps (C7 nerve root and radial nerve). Muscle strength testing with resisted range of motion of the biceps brachii, brachioradialis, and triceps muscles also may be used to evaluate the functional integrity of the nerve roots and peripheral nerves of the upper extremity.

Several orthopedic tests may be used to assess the cervical spine. The Valsalva maneuver and Naffziger's test can be used to identify disc lesions and other space-occupying lesions of the cervical spine.[25] The Valsalva maneuver is performed by having the patient seated comfortably, with the arms slightly flexed at the elbows. The patient is instructed to take a deep breath and hold it. While holding the deep breath, the patient is asked to bear down to create greater intra-abdominal pressure. Reproduction of radicular pain is indicative of nerve root compression caused by a space-occupying mass in the spine.[27] This can result from nerve root entrapment at an intervertebral foramen or within the neural canal and may indicate a herniated intervertebral disc. A more ominous finding is bilateral radiating pain that suggests a posterior, midline disc lesion. With Naffziger's test, compression of the jugular veins while the supine patient coughs may produce unilateral or bilateral radiating pain suggestive of a cervical disc lesion.

Dysphagia may be an indication of prevertebral soft tissue swelling—a relatively common sequela to cervical acceleration/deceleration injury.[28-30] Osteophytic changes associated with osteoarthritis or degenerative disc disease of the cervical spine may also contribute to difficult or painful swallowing when bony spurs develop on the anterior aspects of cervical vertebral bodies. Ask the patient to swallow, and note pain or difficulty when he or she performs the motion. Obstructive dysphagia may occur when the patient tries to swallow solid foods like bread or meat, but liquids do not present problems. Be sure to rule out other possible causes of dysphagia, including infection or tumors of the esophagus or paraesophageal tissues.

The shoulder depression test evaluates muscles and ligamentous tissues, as well as cervical nerve root involvement.[24] Apply a downward force on the patient's shoulder while simultaneously flexing the head and neck to the opposite side. Local pain and restricted motion suggest hypertonicity of the superior trapezius. Radiating pain into the shoulder and upper extremity is more indicative of nerve root involvement with possible intervertebral foramen encroachment.

The cervical compression test is useful for identifying and isolating specific levels of nerve root involvement.[24,25] A downward axial compressive force is applied to the head of the seated patient. Radiating pain into the shoulder or upper extremity suggests nerve root compression at the intervertebral foramen. Pain or nerve root impingement tends to distribute along the dermatomal region of the involved nerve root. Unilateral foraminal compression with extension, lateral flexion, and rotation will be more likely to result in radiating pain in mild cases of nerve root encroachment.

Box 12-1 **Cervical Ranges of Motion**	
Flexion	55 to 75 degrees
Extension	45 to 65 degrees
Lateral flexion	45 to 55 degrees
Rotation	65 to 85 degrees

The average range-of-motion values listed here and elsewhere in *The Activator Method* are averages of values published in various sources and should not be interpreted as "normal for a given patient." Ranges of motion may be influenced by such factors as age, gender, weight, build, and general physical activity.

The cervical distraction test helps to differentiate nerve root compression or entrapment from musculotendinous or ligamentous involvement of the cervical spine.[24,25] A gentle but firm lifting force is applied to the head and neck by cupping the hands under the patient's chin and occiput. If pain increases with distraction, muscular or ligamentous injury may be present. If pain is relieved, nerve impingement at the intervertebral foramen is suggested.

ADDITIONAL TESTING AND ADJUSTMENTS FOR THE CERVICAL SPINE

Additional cervical involvement is suggested when the patient complains of point tenderness at specific vertebral levels, when leg lengths do not balance following testing and adjustment of the Basic Scan Protocol, or when examination findings so indicate.

Sixth Cervical (C6)
Consider a sixth cervical neuroarticular dysfunction when the lower cervical spine shows restricted range of motion or palpable crepitus or tenderness on passive range of motion.

Isolation Test. After isolation of C7, the head will be in the neutral, face-down position. To isolate the sixth cervical vertebra, ask the patient to shrug both shoulders toward the ears (Figure 12-1). This movement is thought to facilitate the spinal intrinsic muscles and the neuroarticular components of the lower cervical spine in the region of C6. Look for PD leg reactivity in Position #1. Then proceed to Position #2, while observing relative changes in the PD leg. Follow the Short/Long Rule. If the PD leg lengthens in Position #2, sixth cervical vertebra involvement is on the side of Pelvic Deficiency. If the PD leg shortens in Position #2, sixth cervical vertebra involvement is on the Opposite PD (OPD) side. Pressure Test to confirm by applying a gentle but firm anterior-to-superior pressure on the pedicle-lamina junction through the joint plane line of the facets on the side of involvement indicated by the Short/Long Rule.

Adjustment. To adjust a sixth cervical vertebra, contact the pedicle-lamina junction on the side of involvement. The Line of Drive (LOD) is anterior, superior, and slightly medial through the plane line of the facets (Figure 12-2).

Enhancement of the Sixth Cervical (C6)
When the patient has undergone treatment and has recurrent or persistent cervical complaints and symptoms involving a C6 neuroarticular dysfunction that does not react to the C6 test, consider using the following enhancement of

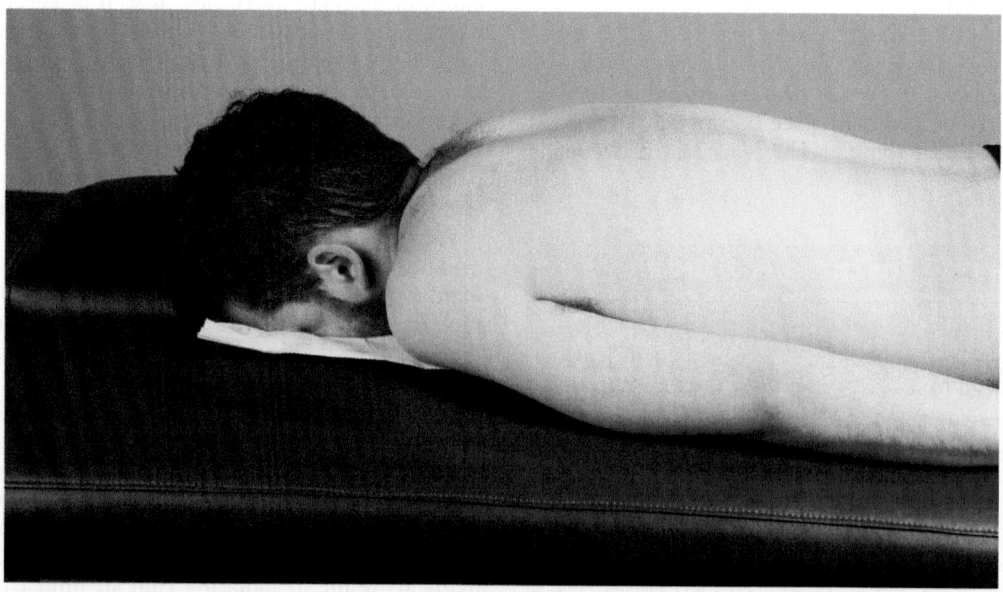

Figure 12-1 Isolation Test for sixth cervical. Patient shrugs the shoulder.

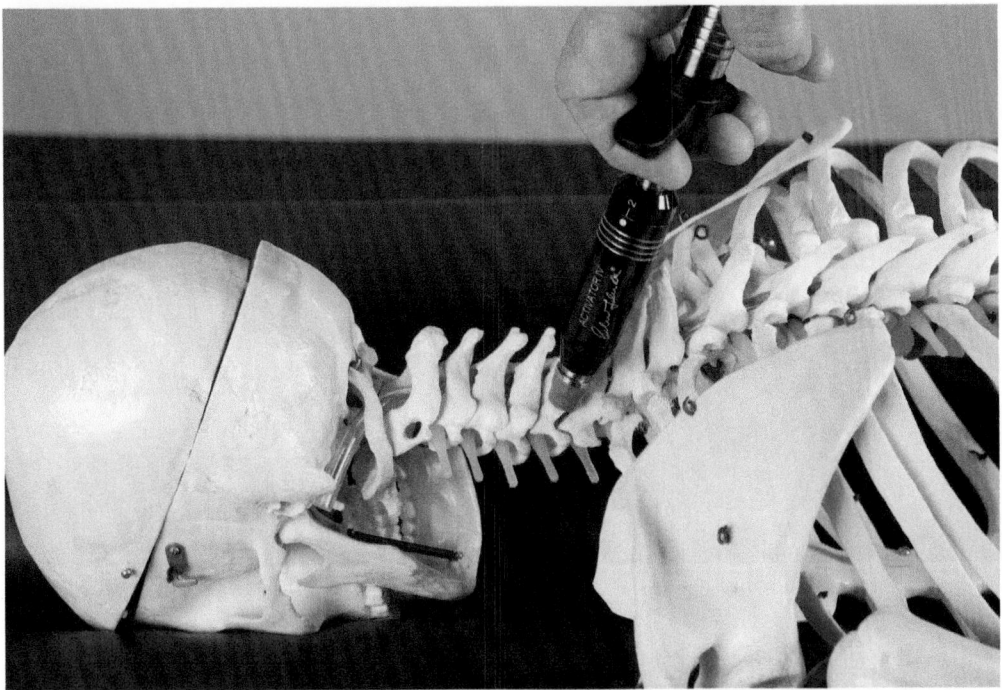

Figure 12-2 Adjustment for sixth cervical. Line of Drive is anterior, superior, and slightly medial.

the sixth cervical test as a more sensitive test for C6 neuroarticular dysfunction.

Isolation Test. After isolation of C7, the head will be in the neutral, face-down position. To isolate the sixth cervical vertebra, instruct the patient to return the head to the PD side. Ask the patient to shrug and hold both shoulders toward the ears as he or she returns the head to the neutral position (Figure 12-3). This movement is thought to facilitate the spinal intrinsic muscles and the neuroarticular components of the lower cervical spine in the region of C6. Look for PD leg reactivity in Position #1. Then proceed to Position #2, while observing relative changes in the PD leg. Follow the Short/Long Rule.

If the PD leg lengthens in Position #2, sixth cervical vertebra involvement is on the side of Pelvic Deficiency. If the PD leg shortens in Position #2, sixth cervical vertebra involvement is on the OPD side. Pressure Test to confirm by applying a gentle but firm anterior-to-superior pressure on the pedicle-lamina junction through the joint plane line of the facets on the side of involvement indicated by the Short/Long Rule.

Adjustment. To adjust a sixth cervical vertebra, contact the pedicle-lamina junction on the side of involvement. The LOD is anterior, superior, and slightly medial through the plane line of the facets. (see Figure 12-2).

Enhancement of Fifth (C5) Cervical

With recurrent or persistent cervical complaints at the fulcrum of flexion and extension and without evidence of C5 neuroarticular dysfunction during the traditional Basic Scan test, consider using the following test to enhance or exacerbate a C5 involvement.

Isolation Test. Instruct the patient to slide the chin up the table to produce cervical extension, then ask him or her to press the chin into the table (Figure 12-4). This movement is believed to exaggerate facilitation of the spinal intrinsic muscles and the neuroarticular components in the region of C5. Look for PD leg reactivity in Position #1. Then proceed to Position #2, while observing relative changes in the PD leg. Follow the Short/Long Rule.

If the PD leg lengthens in Position #2, fifth cervical vertebra involvement is on the side of Pelvic Deficiency. If the PD leg shortens in Position #1, fifth cervical vertebra involvement is on the OPD side. Pressure Test to confirm by applying a gentle but firm anterior-to-superior pressure on the pedicle-lamina junction through the plane line of the facets on the side of involvement indicated by the Short/Long Rule.

Adjustment. To adjust a fifth cervical vertebra, contact the pedicle-lamina junction on the side of involvement. The LOD is anterior, superior, and slightly medial through the plane line of the facets (Figure 12-5).

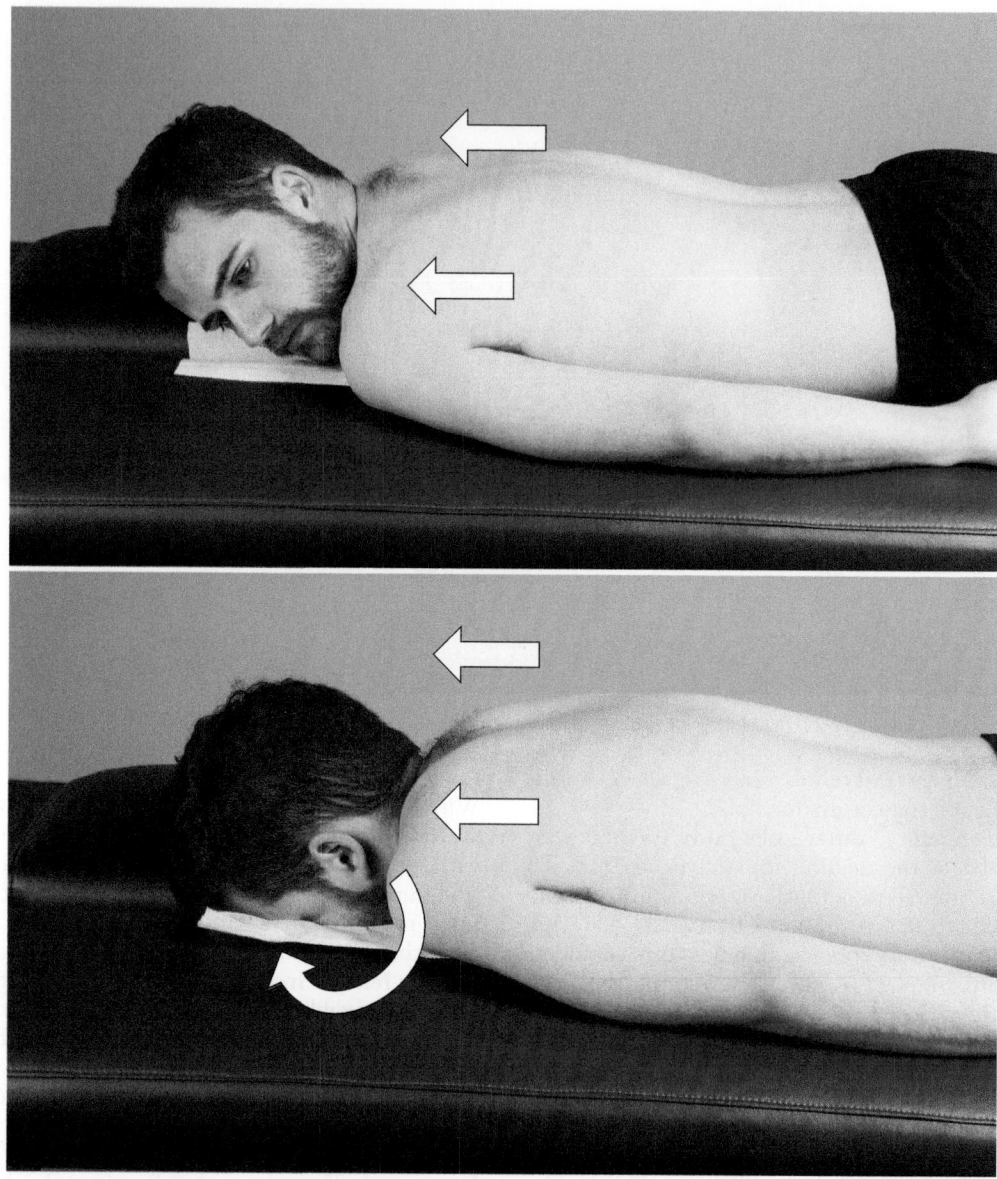

Figure 12-3 Isolation Test for enhancement of sixth cervical. Patient's face is toward Pelvic Deficiency side; patient shrugs shoulders and holds while returning to neutral posture.

Fifth Cervical (C5) Cervical Vertebra Inferior

After the AM Basic Scan Protocol for the fifth (C5) cervical vertebra has been completed and the patient continues to exhibit cervical kyphosis, or a loss of anterior curve is noted radiographically, consider this enhanced stress test for an inferior or hyperextension malposition of C5 when Position #3 was nonresponsive.

Isolation Test. After completion of all cervical testing procedures, instruct the patient to tuck the chin to his or her chest and then to press the forehead into the table and relax (Figure 12-6). This movement is thought to facilitate the spinal intrinsic muscles and the neuroarticular components of the lower cervical spine in the sagittal plane of C5. If the PD leg shortens in

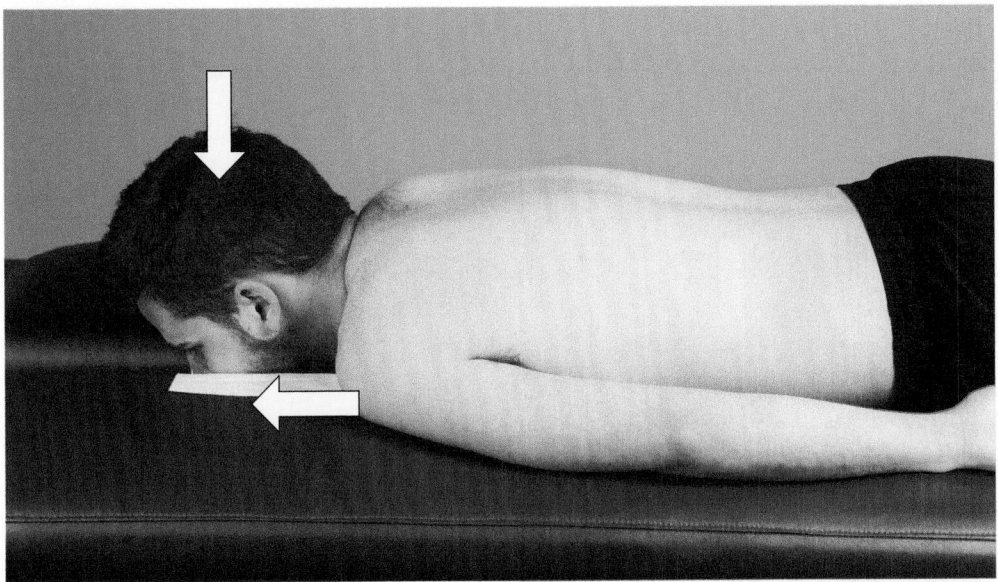

Figure 12-4   Isolation Test for enhancement of fifth cervical. Patient slides chin up in the face slot and then presses it into the table.

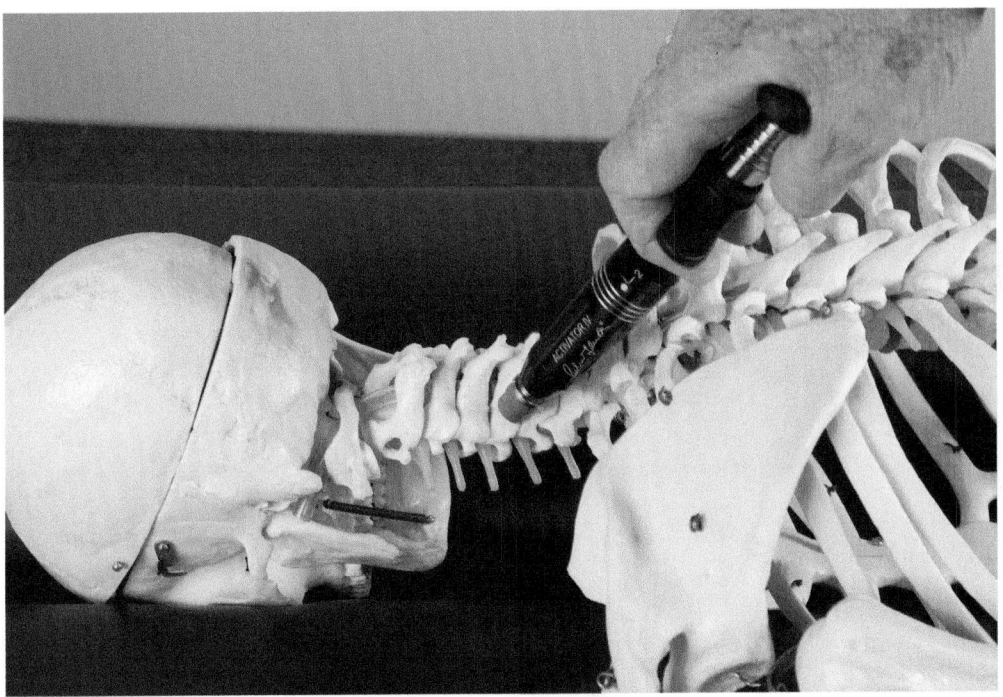

Figure 12-5   Adjustment for enhancement of fifth cervical. Line of Drive is anterior, superior, and slightly medial.

Position #1, the fifth cervical vertebra is considered to be in hyperextension, or the spinous process of the vertebra is inferior. Pressure Test to confirm by applying a gentle but firm superior pressure on the inferior aspect of the spinous process of the fifth cervical vertebra.

Adjustment.   Contact the inferior portion of the fifth (C5) cervical spinous process. The LOD is anterior and superior (Figure 12-7).

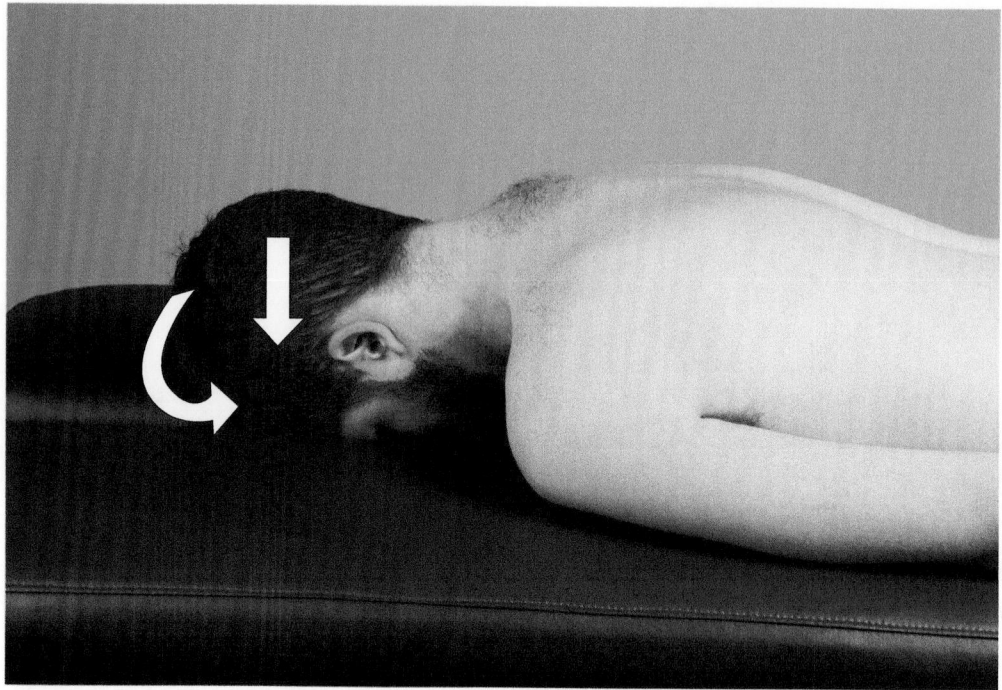

Figure 12-6   Isolation Test for fifth cervical inferior. Patient tucks the chin toward the chest and then presses the forehead into the table.

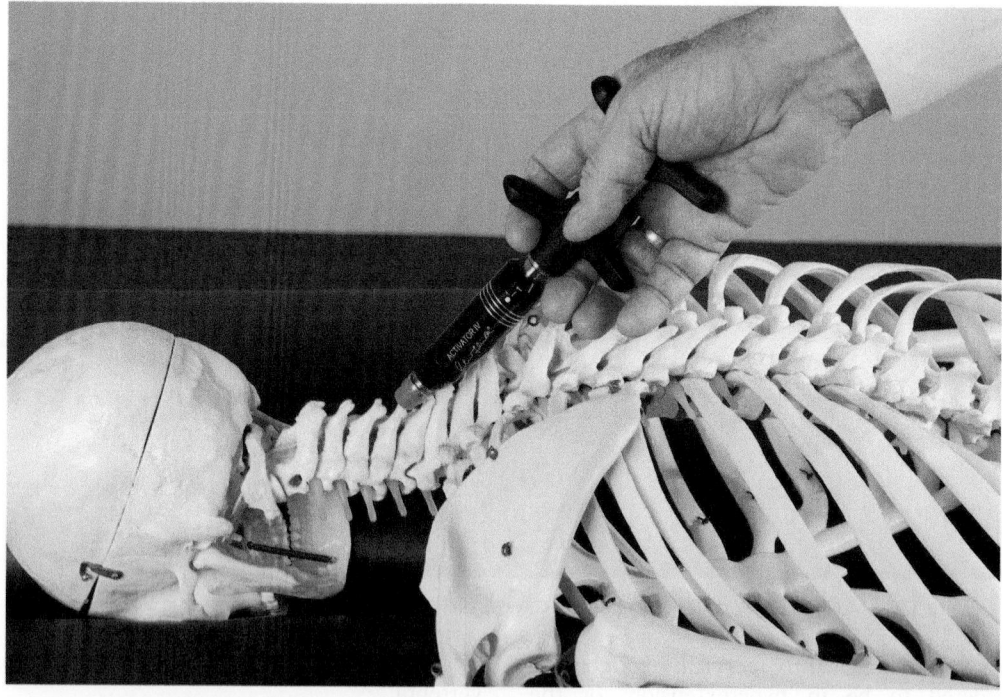

Figure 12-7   Adjustment for fifth cervical inferior. Line of Drive is anterior and superior.

Hidden Posterior Fifth (C5) Cervical Vertebra

After testing and adjusting of the sixth (C6) cervical vertebra and the fifth (C5) cervical vertebra tests, if the patient persists with complaints of neck pain, particularly after a motor vehicle collision, consider testing for a Hidden Posterior Fifth (C5) vertebra. This test will facilitate the involvement of a posterior neuroarticular dysfunction of the fifth (C5) cervical vertebra after a motor vehicle mechanism of injury, even when other tests of the fifth (C5) and sixth (C6) cervical vertebrae are not evident.

Isolation Test. After all C6 and C5 tests have been performed and the positive ones have been cleared, do the following:

1. Instruct the patient to shrug the shoulders toward the head.
2. Hold the shrug.
3. Then raise the head up slightly off of the table (Figure 12-8).

Look for PD leg reactivity in Position #1 for involvement.

Adjustment. Contact the posterior-inferior aspect of the C5 spinous process and Pressure Test to confirm. The LOD is anterior-superior with the instrument on the lowest setting (see Figure 12-7).

Fourth (C4) Cervical

With recurrent or persistent cervical neuroarticular dysfunction and especially with evidence of loss of the normal anterior (lordotic) cervical curve, consider involvement of the fourth cervical vertebra.

Isolation Test. After testing of C5, the head will be in the neutral, face-down position. Instruct the patient to raise the head, turn to the side of Pelvic Deficiency, and look superiorly, and then to return the head to the neutral, face-down position (Figure 12-9). This maneuver puts the head and neck into rotation on the side of Pelvic Deficiency and extension on the OPD side. This movement is believed to facilitate the spinal intrinsic muscles and the neuroarticular components in the mid cervical spine in the region of C4. Look for PD leg reactivity in Position #1. Then proceed to Position #2, while observing relative changes in the PD leg. Follow the Short/Long Rule.

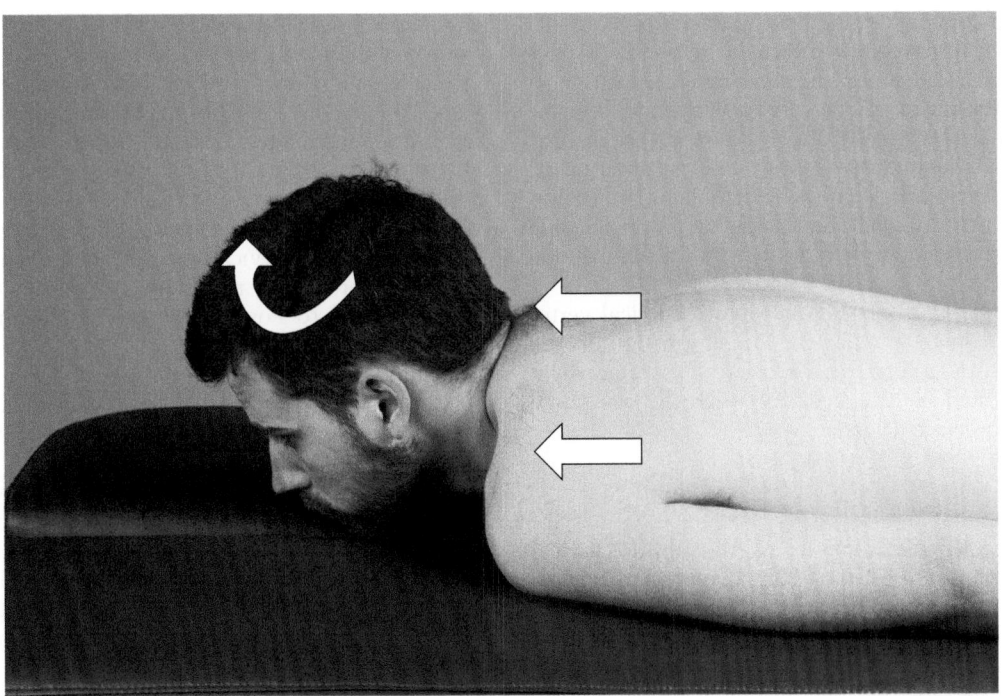

Figure 12-8 Isolation Test for fifth cervical hidden posterior. Patient shrugs the shoulders, holds the shrug, and then raises the head off the table.

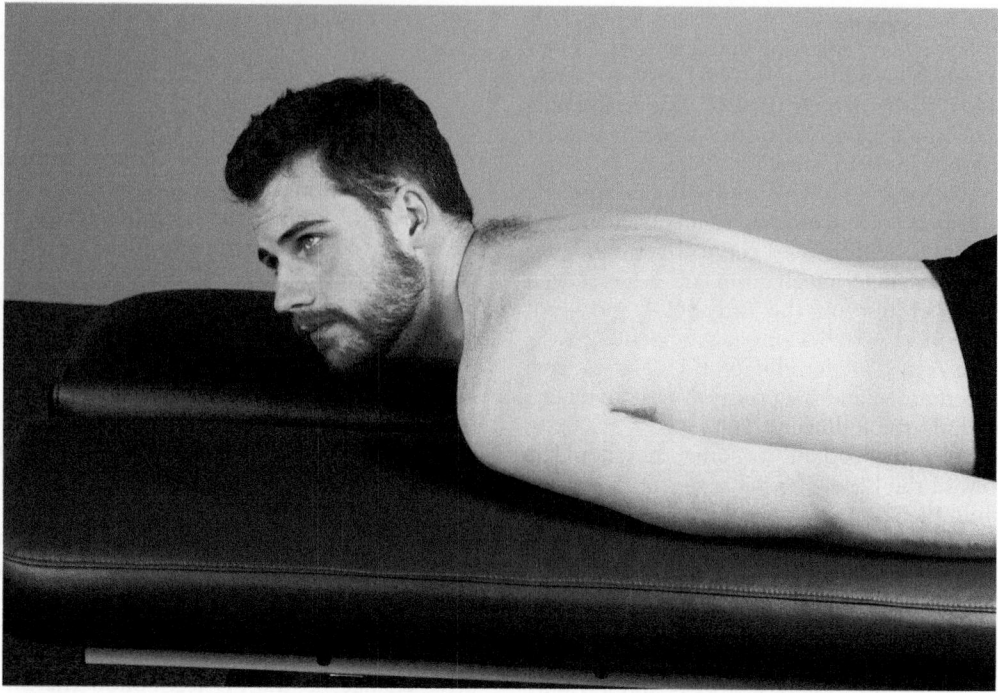

Figure 12-9 Isolation Test for fourth cervical. Patient turns the head toward the Pelvic Deficiency side and then tips the head superior.

If the PD leg lengthens in Position #2, fourth cervical vertebra involvement is on the side of Pelvic Deficiency. If the PD leg shortens in Position #2, fourth cervical vertebra involvement is on the OPD side. Pressure Test to confirm by applying a gentle but firm anterior-to-superior pressure on the pedicle-lamina junction through the plane line of the facets on the side of involvement as indicated by the Short/Long Rule.

Adjustment. To adjust a fourth cervical vertebra, contact the pedicle-lamina junction on the side of involvement. The LOD is anterior, superior, and slightly medial through the plane line of the facets (Figure 12-10).

Third (C3) Cervical

Consider involvement of the third cervical vertebra when the patient complains of tightness or discomfort while flexing the cervical spine.

Isolation Test. After testing of C4, the head will be in the neutral, face-down position. Instruct the patient to raise the head, turn to the side of Pelvic Deficiency, and look inferiorly toward the tip of the shoulder, and then to return the head to the neutral, face-down position (Figure 12-11). This maneuver puts the head and neck into rotation on the side of Pelvic Deficiency and into flexion on the OPD side. This movement is thought to facilitate the spinal intrinsic muscles and articular components in the mid cervical spine in the region of C3. Look for PD leg reactivity in Position #1. Then proceed to Position #2, while observing relative changes in the PD leg. Follow the Short/Long Rule.

If the PD leg lengthens in Position #2, third cervical vertebra involvement is on the side of Pelvic Deficiency. If the PD leg shortens in Position #2, third cervical vertebra involvement is on the OPD side. Pressure Test to confirm by applying a gentle but firm anterior-to-superior pressure on the pedicle-lamina junction through the joint plane line of the facets on the side of involvement indicated by the Short/Long Rule.

Adjustment. To adjust a third cervical vertebra, contact the pedicle-lamina junction on

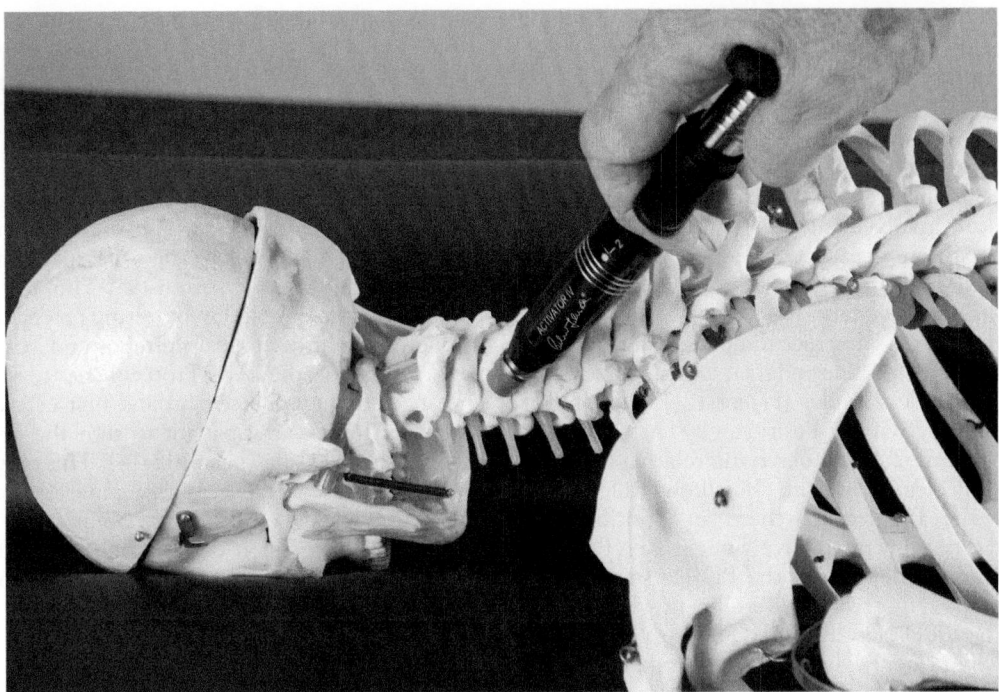

Figure 12-10 Adjustment for fourth cervical. Line of Drive is anterior, superior, and slightly medial.

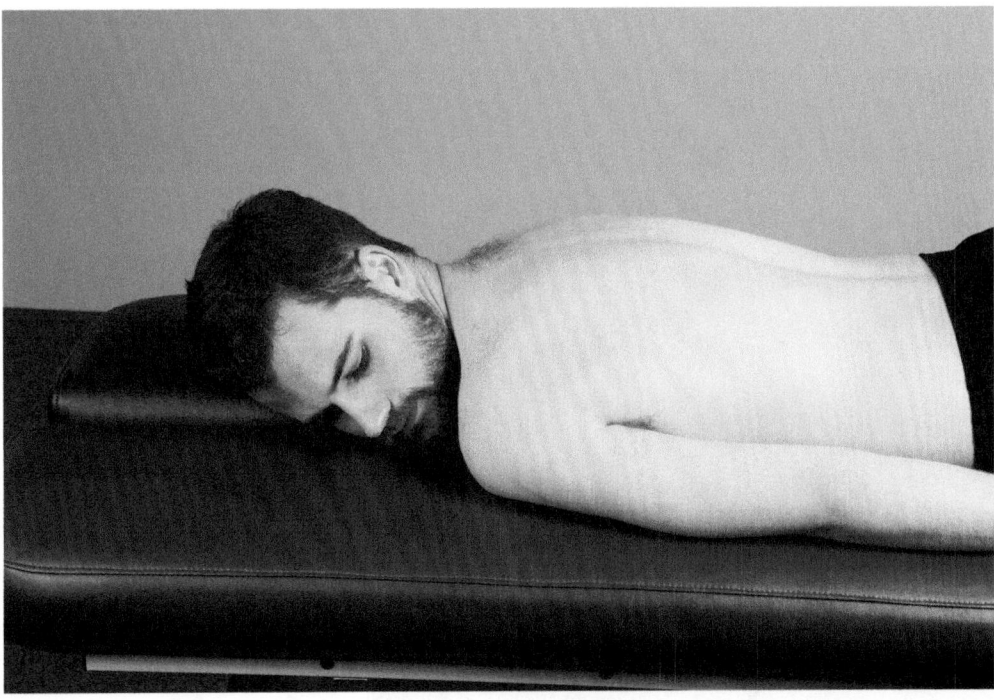

Figure 12-11 Isolation Test for third cervical. Patient turns the head toward the Pelvic Deficiency side and then tips the head inferiorly toward the shoulder.

the side of involvement. The LOD is anterior, superior, and slightly medial through the plane line of the facets (Figure 12-12).

Third (C3) Cervical Opposite Pelvic Deficiency

When routine testing fails to reveal a third (C3) cervical involvement, yet clinical signs and symptoms are apparent, especially on the OPD side, consider this alternative test for the third (C3) cervical vertebra.

Isolation Test. Instruct the patient to turn the head to the OPD side and then look down toward the same side shoulder (Figure 12-13). Look for PD leg reactivity in Position #1. Then proceed to Position #2, while observing relative changes in the PD leg. Follow the Short/Long Rule.

If the PD leg lengthens in Position #2, third cervical vertebra involvement is on the side of Pelvic Deficiency. If the PD leg shortens in Position #2, third cervical vertebra involvement is on the OPD side. Pressure Test to confirm by applying a gentle but firm anterior-to-superior pressure on the pedicle-lamina junction through the joint plane line of the facets on the side of involvement indicated by the Short/Long Rule.

Adjustment. Use the Short/Long Rule to determine the side for adjustment, and Pressure Test to confirm. The contact point is the pedicle-lamina junction of the third (C3) cervical vertebra. The LOD is anterior, superior, and slightly medial through the plane line of the facets (see Figure 12-12).

Second Cervical (C2) Vertebra

Patient complaints relative to the second cervical vertebra may include headaches, sinus problems, neck pain, cervicogenic vertigo, dizziness, eye, and nonpathological hypertension. This test is performed after completion of testing procedures through the third cervical vertebra and before performance of the AM Protocol Basic Scan chin-tuck test for the second and first cervical vertebrae. Instruct the patient to turn the head toward the OPD side (Figure 12-14). This movement is thought to facilitate the spinal intrinsic muscles and the neuroarticular components of the spine in the region of C2. Look for PD leg reactivity in Position #1. Then proceed to Position #2, while observing relative changes in the PD leg. Follow the Short/Long Rule.

Pressure Test to confirm by applying a gentle but firm anterior-to-superior pressure on the pedicle-lamina junction through the plane line of the facets on the side of the second cervical vertebra, as indicated by the Short/Long Rule.

Adjustment. Contact the second cervical vertebra on the pedicle-lamina junction at the

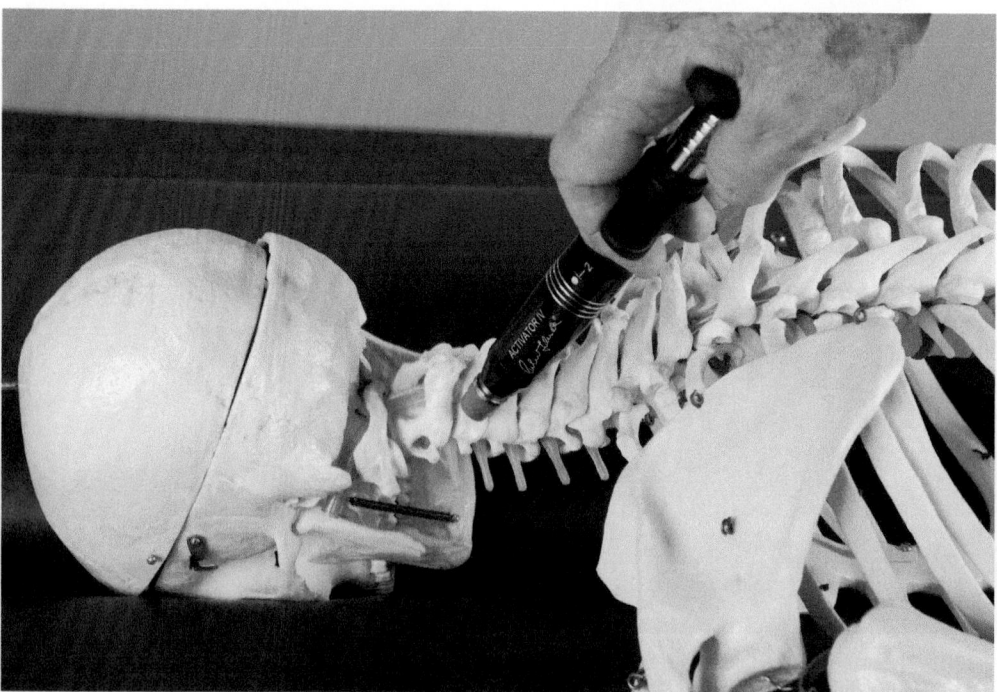

Figure 12-12 Adjustment for third cervical. Line of Drive is anterior, superior, and slightly medial.

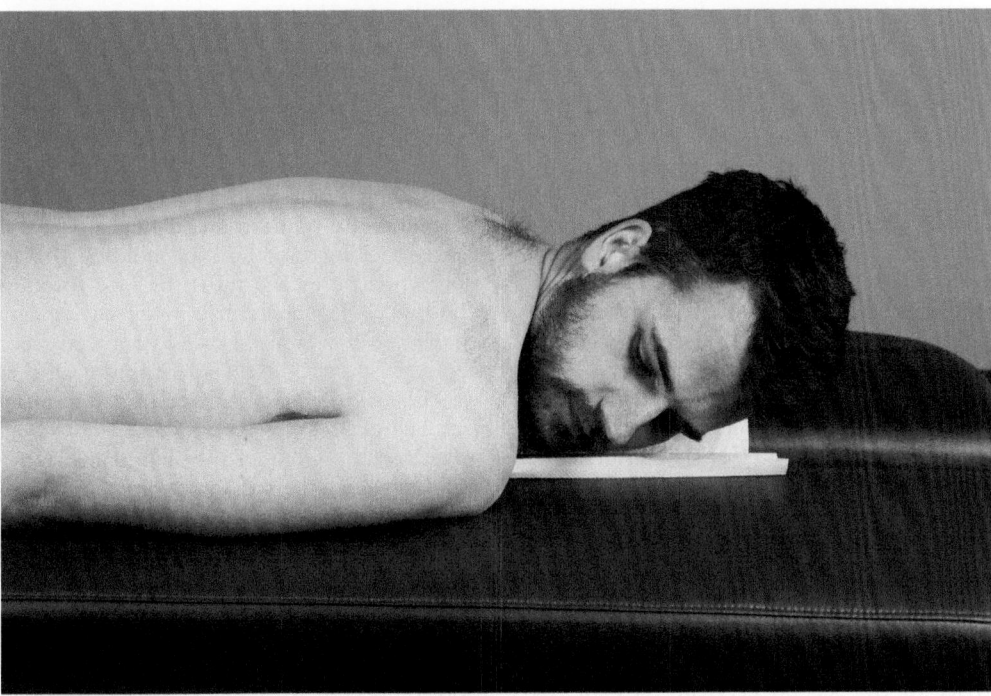

Figure 12-13 Isolation Test for Opposite Pelvic Deficiency third cervical. Patient turns the head toward the Opposite Pelvic Deficiency side and tips the head inferiorly toward the shoulder.

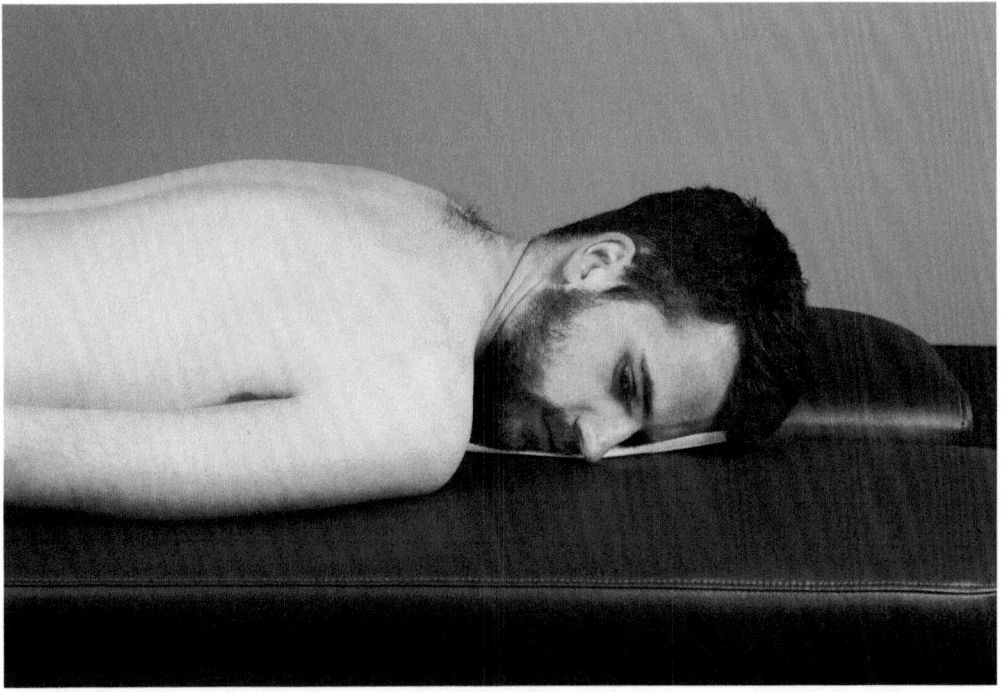

Figure 12-14 Isolation Test for second cervical. Patient turns head toward Opposite Pelvic Deficiency side.

side of the second cervical vertebra, as indicated by the Short/Long Rule. The LOD is anterior, superior, and slightly medial and is directed toward the tip of the nose (Figure 12-15).

If no change in relative leg length is noted in Position #1, the patient is instructed to return the head to the neutral position (Figure 12-16). Look for PD leg reactivity in Position #1. If present, this indicates involvement of the second cervical vertebra on the side of Pelvic Deficiency. Pressure Test to confirm involvement on the pedicle-lamina junction of the second cervical vertebra on the side of Pelvic Deficiency.

Adjustment. Contact the second cervical vertebra on the pedicle-lamina junction on the side of Pelvic Deficiency. The LOD is anterior, superior, and slightly medial and is directed toward the tip of the nose (Figure 12-17).

Second Cervical (C2) Enhancement
Any upper cervical complaints, especially limited neck rotation, or persistent complaints as listed in the previous C2 test that showed no reactivity to the second cervical vertebra test would indicate performance of this test. After the AM Basic Scan Protocol has been completed (through the occiput), instruct the patient to "gently" tuck the chin and hold it in this position while he or she turns the face toward the PD side. A relative leg length change in Position #1 would indicate second cervical vertebral involvement on the side of Pelvic Deficiency, or the side the patient is facing (see Figure 12-17). This movement is typically restricted (Figure 12-18). If no reaction occurred, instruct the patient to return the head to the neutral position and to repeat the test of gently tucking the chin and holding this position while he or she turns the face toward the OPD side (Figure 12-19). Relative leg length change in Position #1 would indicate second cervical vertebral involvement to the OPD side, which generally is noted as restricted movement (see Figure 12-15).

Adjustment. Contact the side of involvement on the pedicle-lamina junction of the second cervical vertebra. The LOD is anterior, superior, and slightly medial and is directed toward the tip of the nose.

Second and Fifth Cervical Combination (C2-C5)
The second and fifth cervical vertebra combination is conceptually similar to the superior-inferior sacrum neuroarticular dysfunction or the superior-inferior spinous concept for lumbar vertebrae. Evaluation by Isolation Testing of the C2-C5 combination requires a two-step testing procedure and Leg Length Analysis in Position #3.

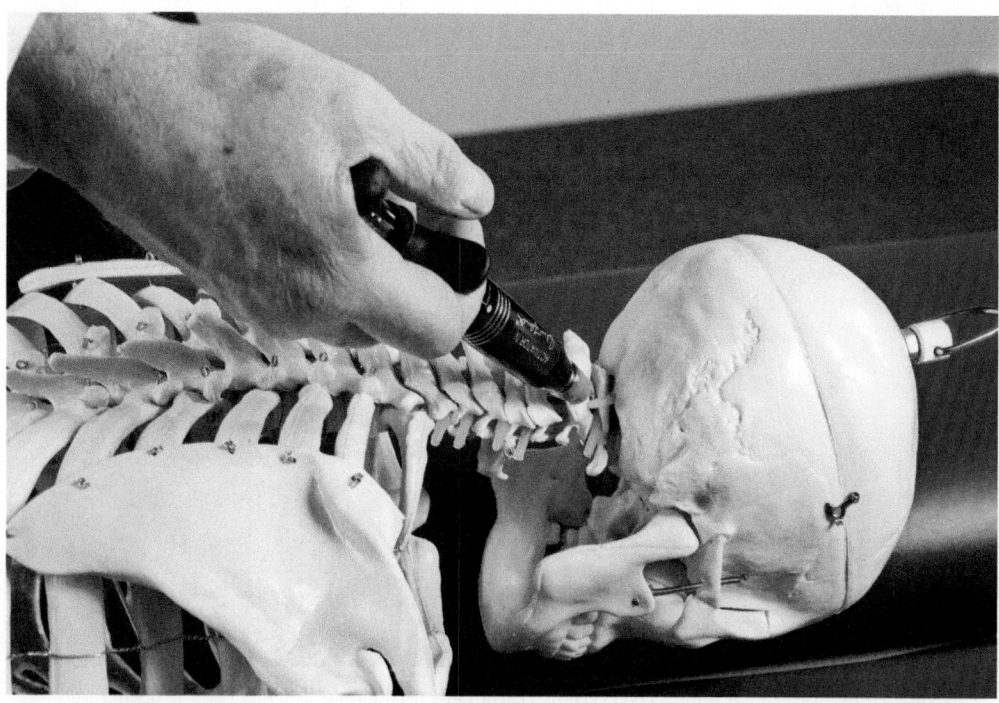

Figure 12-15 Adjustment for second cervical. Line of Drive is anterior, superior, and slightly medial.

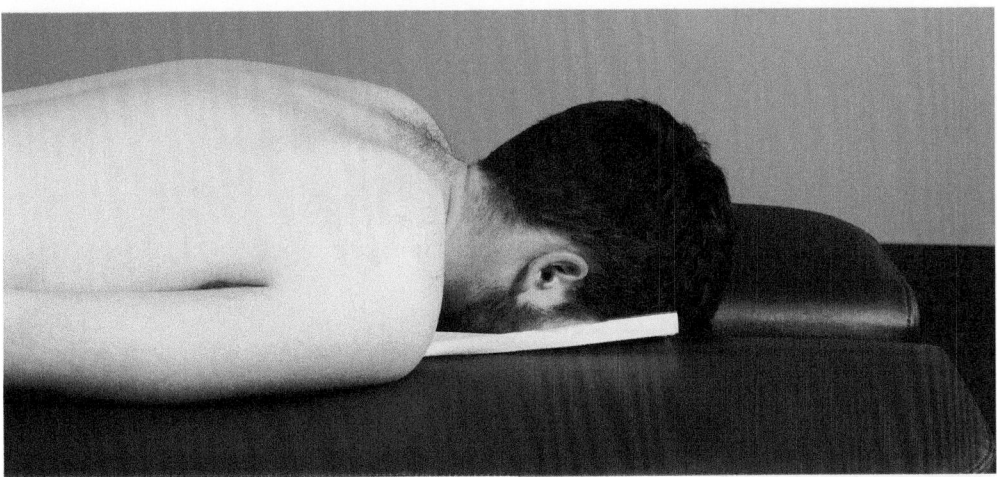

Figure 12-16 Isolation Test for second cervical Pelvic Deficiency (PD) side. The patient returns head to neutral from looking at the Opposite PD side for the second cervical.

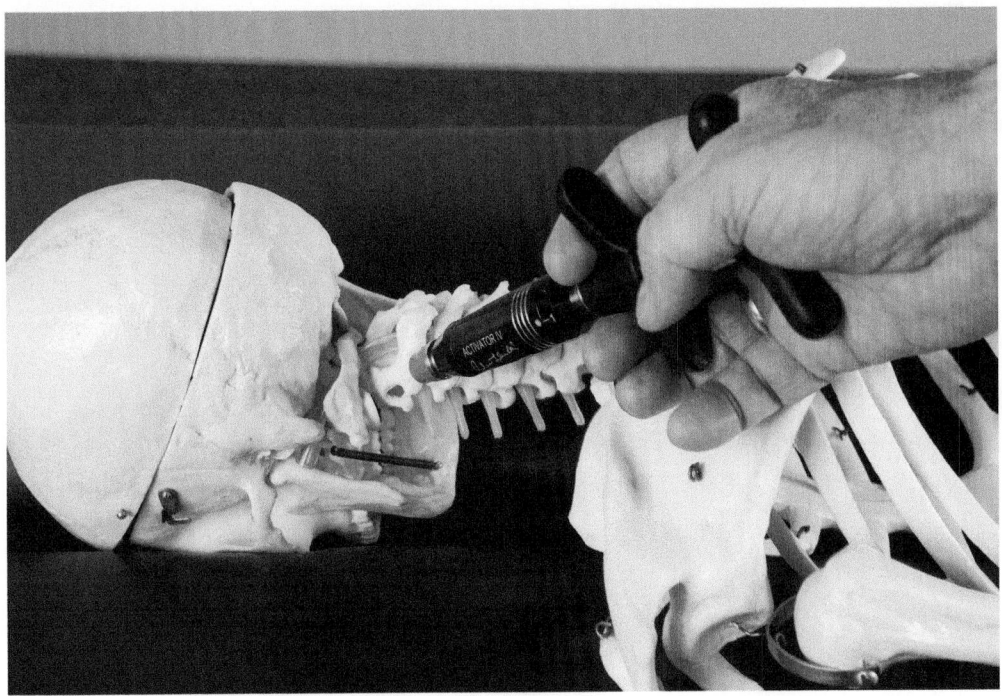

Figure 12-17 Adjustment for second cervical. Line of Drive is anterior, superior, and slightly medial.

Isolation Test for C2. The Isolation Test for the axis-atlas involves having the patient flex the cervical spine by tucking the chin to the chest. After adjustment of C1 or C2 has been performed according to the Basic Scan Protocol, instruct the patient to tuck the chin to the chest again to isolate the second cervical vertebra (Figure 12-20). This movement and position are thought to facilitate the spinal intrinsic muscles and the neuroarticular components of the

upper cervical spine at the level of C2. Look for PD leg reactivity in Position #1, and proceed to Position #3 by flexing the knees past 90 degrees to resistance, while observing for changes in relative leg length. If the PD leg lengthens in Position #3, the test indicates a superior spinous or flexion malposition of the second cervical vertebra (Figure 12-21). If the PD leg shortens in Position #3, the test indicates an inferior spinous or extension malposition of

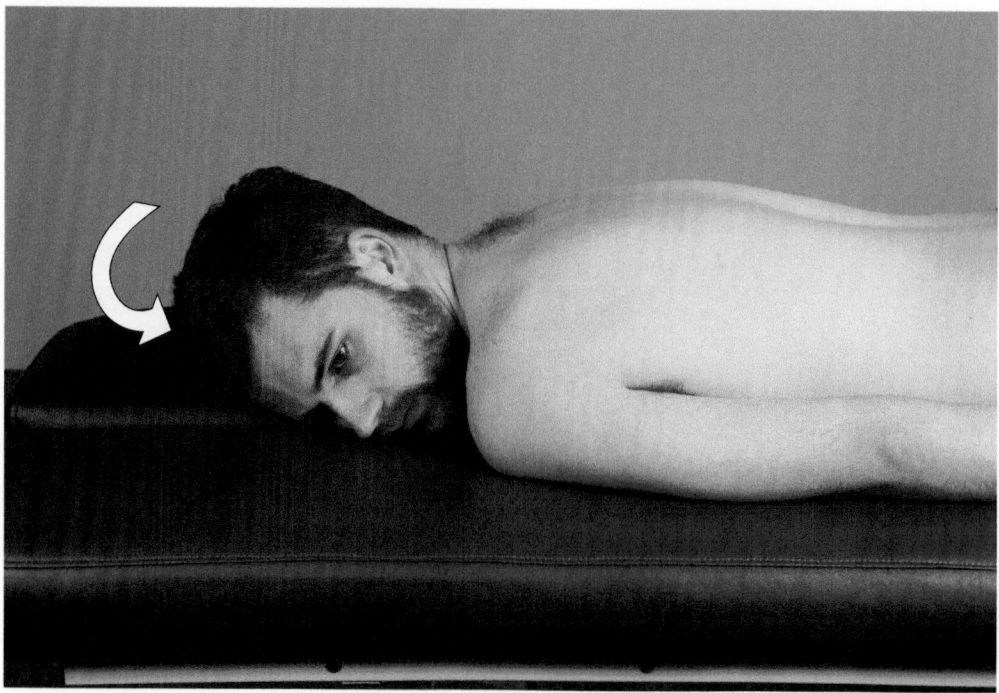

Figure 12-18   Isolation Test for second cervical enhancement. Patient tucks chin slightly to chest and holds while turning to the Pelvic Deficiency side.

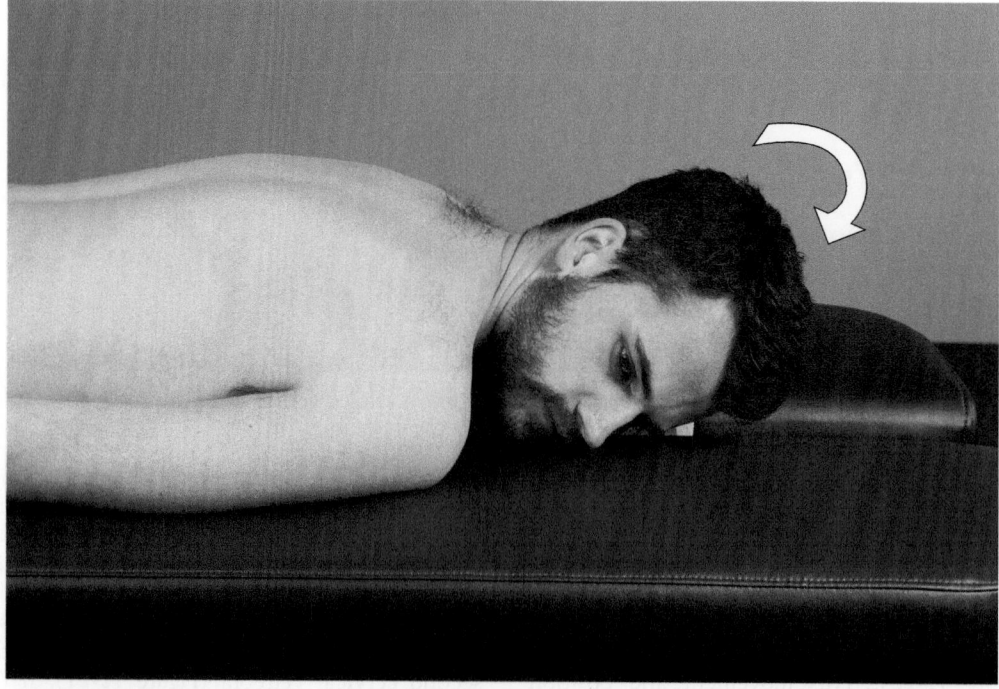

Figure 12-19   Isolation Test for second cervical enhancement. Patient tucks chin slightly to chest and holds while turning to the Opposite Pelvic Deficiency side.

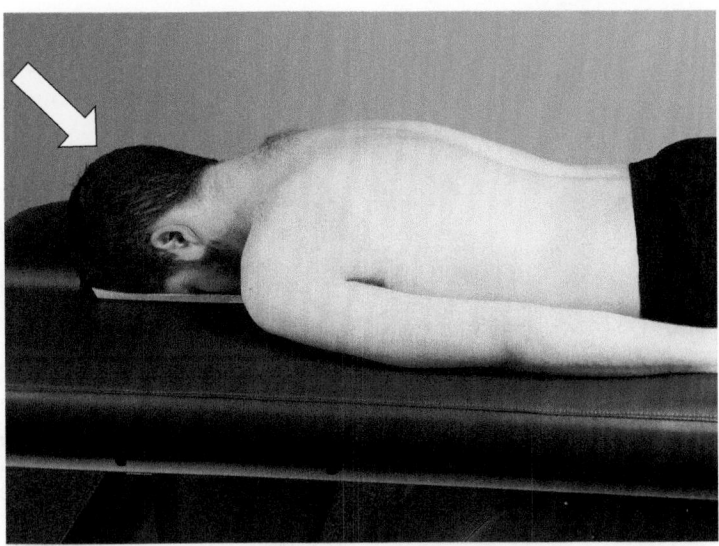

Figure 12-20   Isolation Test for superior or inferior spinous of the second cervical.

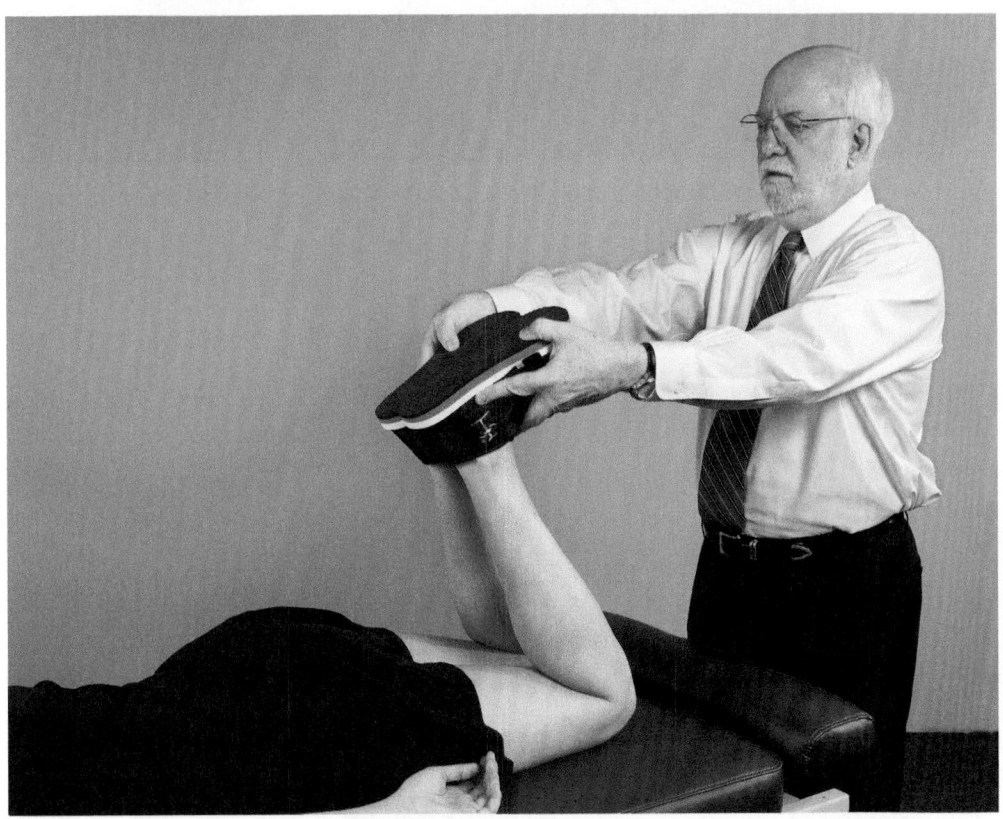

Figure 12-21   Position #3: Leg Length Analysis for superior spinous of the second cervical.

the second cervical vertebra (Figure 12-22). Pressure Test to confirm by applying gentle but firm inferior or superior pressure on the spinous process in the direction that is indicated by the response in Position #3.

Adjustment.   To adjust a superior second cervical vertebra, contact the superior aspect of the spinous process. The LOD is straight inferior (Figure 12-23). *Note:* In the second and fifth cervical combination, C2 is usually superior.

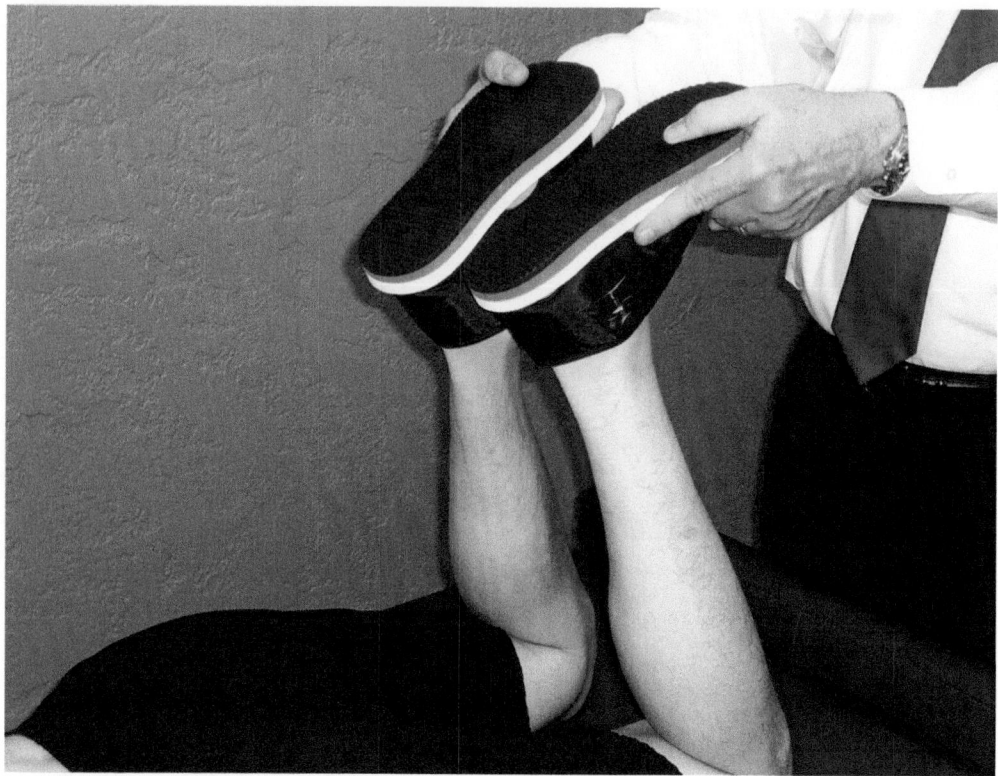

Figure 12-22 Position #3: Leg Length Analysis for inferior spinous of the second cervical.

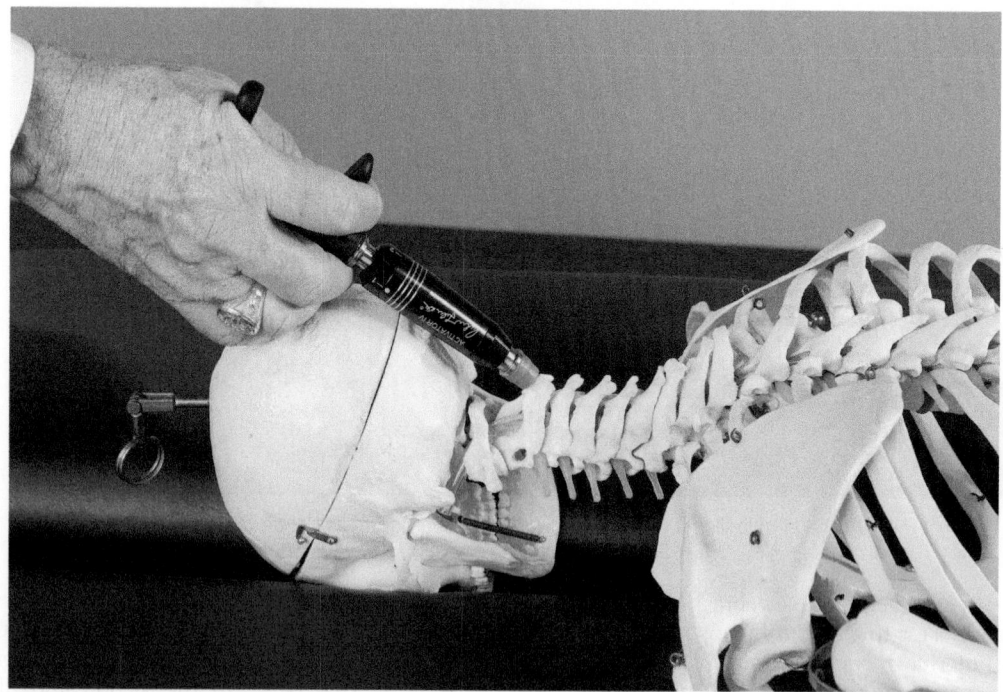

Figure 12-23 Adjustment for superior second cervical. Line of Drive is straight inferior.

To adjust an inferior second cervical vertebra, contact the inferior aspect of the spinous process. The LOD is straight superior (Figure 12-24).

Isolation Test for C5.   After Isolation Testing and adjustment as indicated for the superior or inferior spinous of C2, instruct the patient to flex the cervical spine one more time by tucking the chin to the chest (see Figure 12-20). Look for PD leg reactivity in Position #1, and proceed to Position #3 by flexing the knees past 90 degrees to resistance, while observing for changes in relative leg length. If the PD leg lengthens in Position #3, the test indicates superior spinous or flexion malposition of the fifth cervical vertebra (see Figure 12-21). If the PD leg shortens in Position #3, the test indicates inferior spinous or extension malposition of the fifth cervical vertebra (see Figure 12-22). Pressure Test to confirm by applying a gentle but firm inferior or superior pressure on the spinous process in the direction that is indicated by interpretation of Position #3.

Adjustment.   To adjust a superior fifth cervical vertebra, contact the superior aspect of the spinous process. The LOD is straight inferior (Figure 12-25).

To adjust an inferior fifth cervical, contact the inferior aspect of the spinous process. The LOD is straight superior (Figure 12-26).

SIDE NOTE: In the second and fifth cervical combinations, the C5 spinous is usually inferior.

Lateral Occiput (C0)

When a patient presents with headaches, upper cervical complaints or lateral head translation, or imbalanced tone of the sternocleidomastoid muscles or the upper trapezius, consider testing for and adjusting a lateral occiput. It may accompany a lateral atlas.

Isolation Test.   To isolate a lateral occiput, instruct the patient to turn the head to the PD side and to push the head into the table (Figure 12-27). If the PD leg shortens in Position #1, this indicates that the occiput has lateralized to the PD side. If there is no reaction, instruct the patient to turn the head to the OPD side and push the head into the table. If the PD leg shortens in Position #1, this indicates a lateral occiput on the OPD side.

Adjustment.   To adjust a lateral occiput, contact the lateral aspect of the occiput, making sure to be superior to the mastoid process on

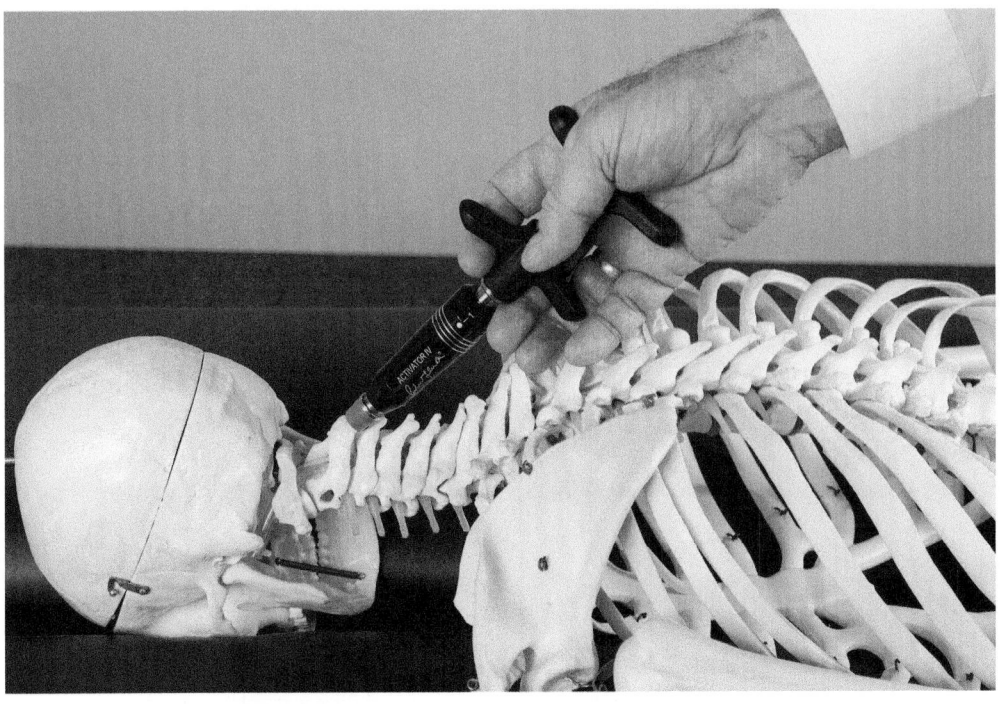

Figure 12-24   Adjustment for inferior second cervical. Line of Drive is straight superior.

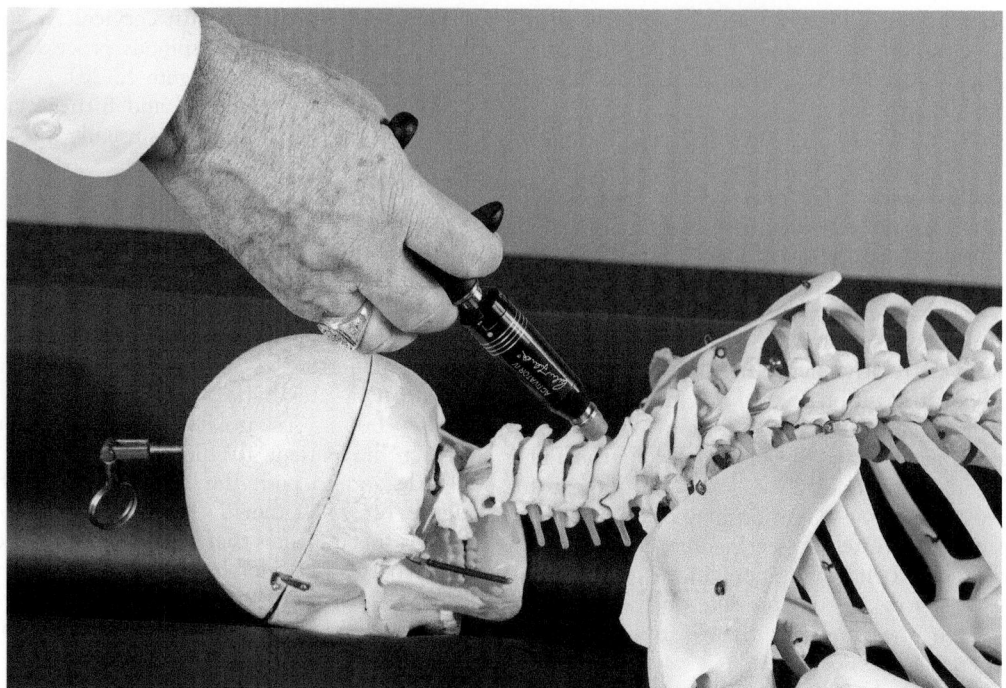

Figure 12-25 Adjustment for superior fifth cervical. Line of Drive is straight inferior.

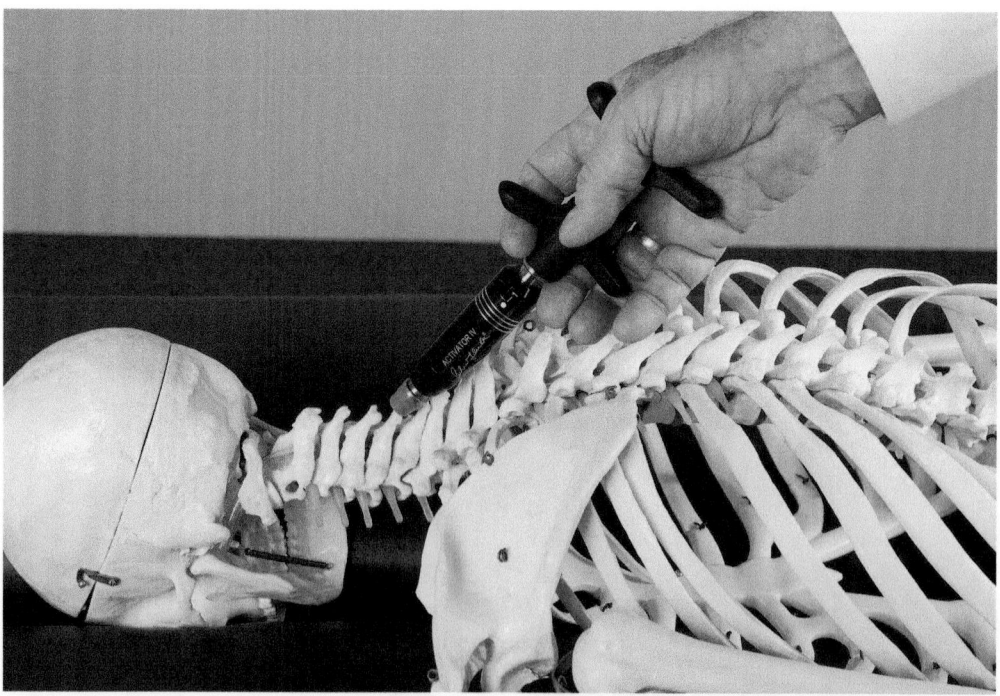

Figure 12-26 Adjustment for inferior fifth cervical. Line of Drive is straight superior.

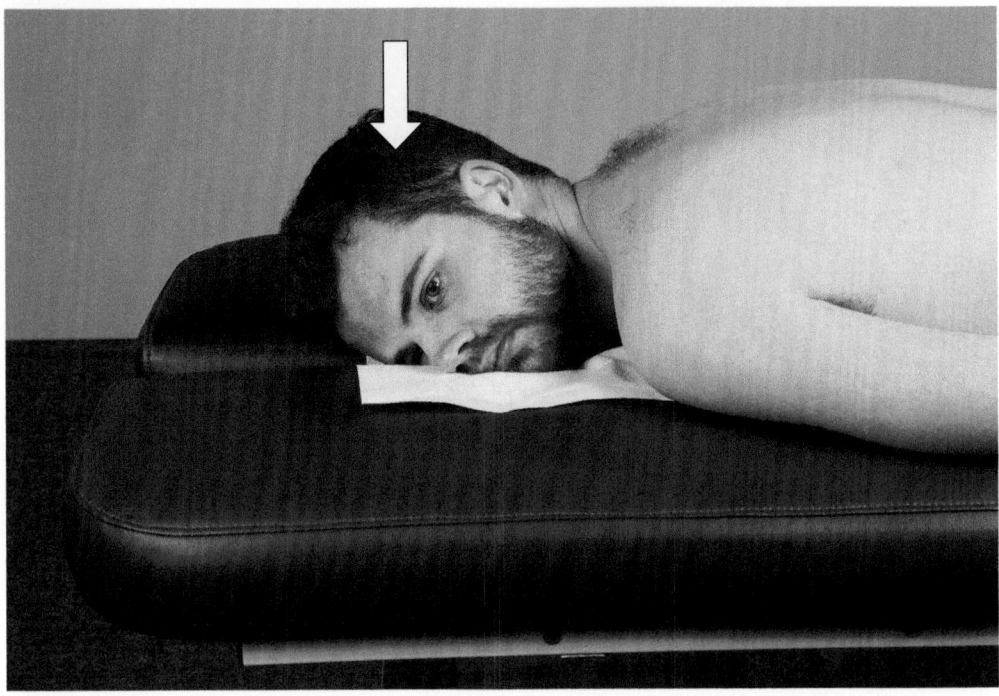

Figure 12-27 Isolation Test for lateral occiput. Patient turns head to Pelvic Deficiency side and pushes side of head into the table.

the involved side while stabilizing the tip of the instrument with your thumb or fingertip. The LOD is lateral to medial (Figure 12-28).

SIDE NOTE: After the posterior occiput test has been performed, Position #4 can be used to determine a lateral occiput neuroarticular dysfunction. After asking the patient to press the forehead into the table, perform the Position #4 test by raising the PD leg to resistance, evaluating for reactivity in Position #1 and using the Short/Long Rule to determine the side of global laterality.

Cervical Disc with Radiculopathy

A patient presents with symptoms relative to disc disease and has examination findings that correlate clinically. The patient may have a positive Bakody's sign, wherein the patient experiences relief of symptoms when he or she places the hand of the involved side on the head.

Isolation Test. After clearing the patient with the AM Protocol for all cervical involvement, instruct the patient to laterally flex the head so as to "close down" on the suspected disc

involved (Figure 12-29). For example, if the patient has signs of left-sided sixth (C6) cervical radiculopathy, ask the patient to laterally flex the head to the left. Look for PD leg reactivity in Position #1 as a positive sign of involvement.

Adjustment. Determine the level of involvement on the basis of clinical findings and previously adjusted levels. Pressure Test to confirm the level to be adjusted. Have the patient slightly laterally flex the head away from the side to be adjusted and contact the pedicle- lamina junction of the involved segment; the LOD is superior and medial (Figure 12-30). The second contact will be the pedicle-lamina junction of the vertebra below the one previously adjusted. With the patient maintaining slight lateral flexion of the cervical spine, the LOD is inferior and medial (Figure 12-31).

Mechanical force, manually assisted chiropractic adjusting (AM) is summarized in Table 12-1. Relevant published research for the cervical spine and related structures is presented in Boxes 12-2 through 12-8.

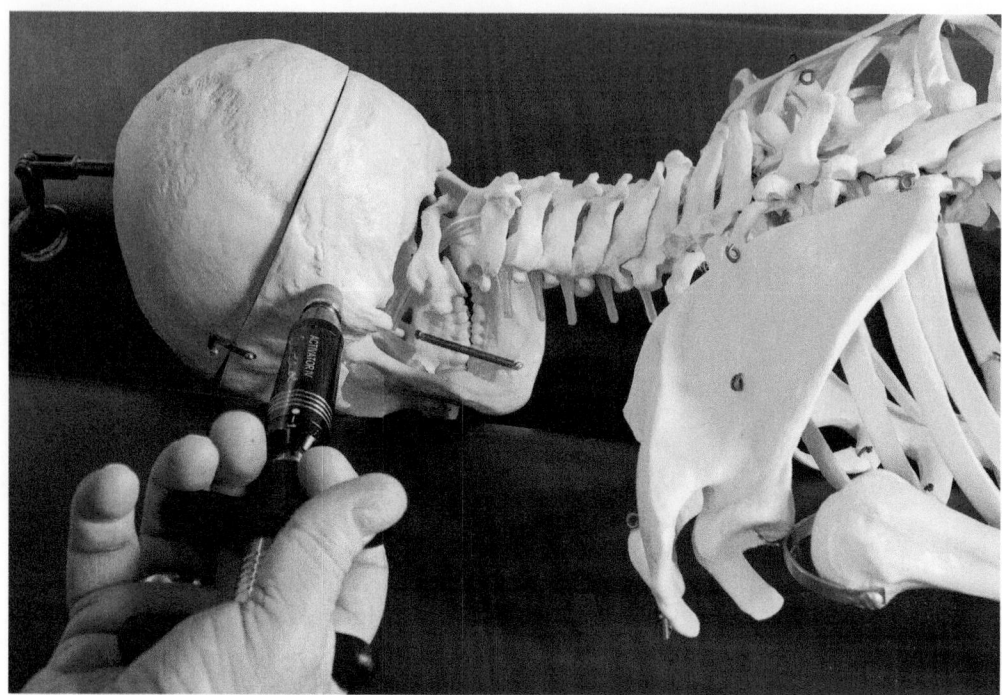

Figure 12-28   Adjustment for lateral occiput. Line of Drive is lateral to medial.

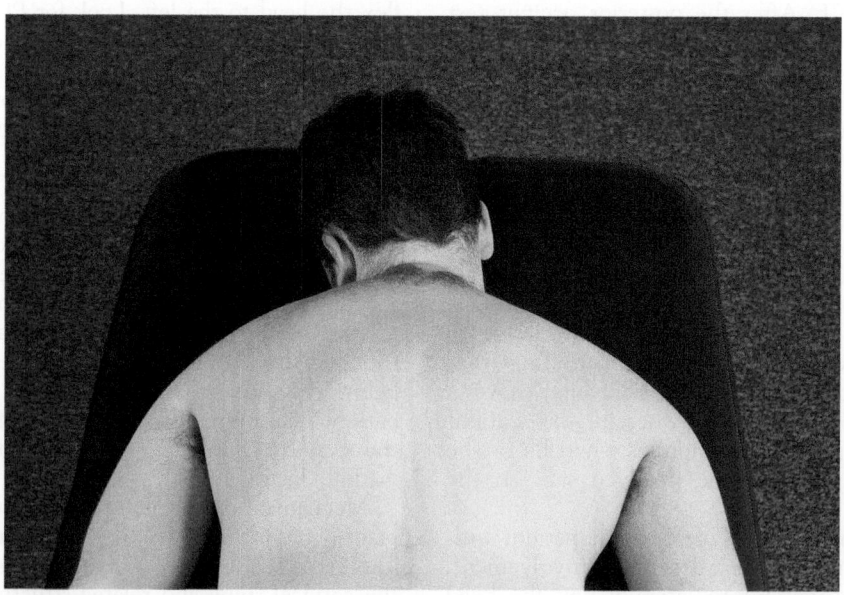

Figure 12-29   Test for cervical disc with radiculopathy. The patient laterally flexes the head to the involved side.

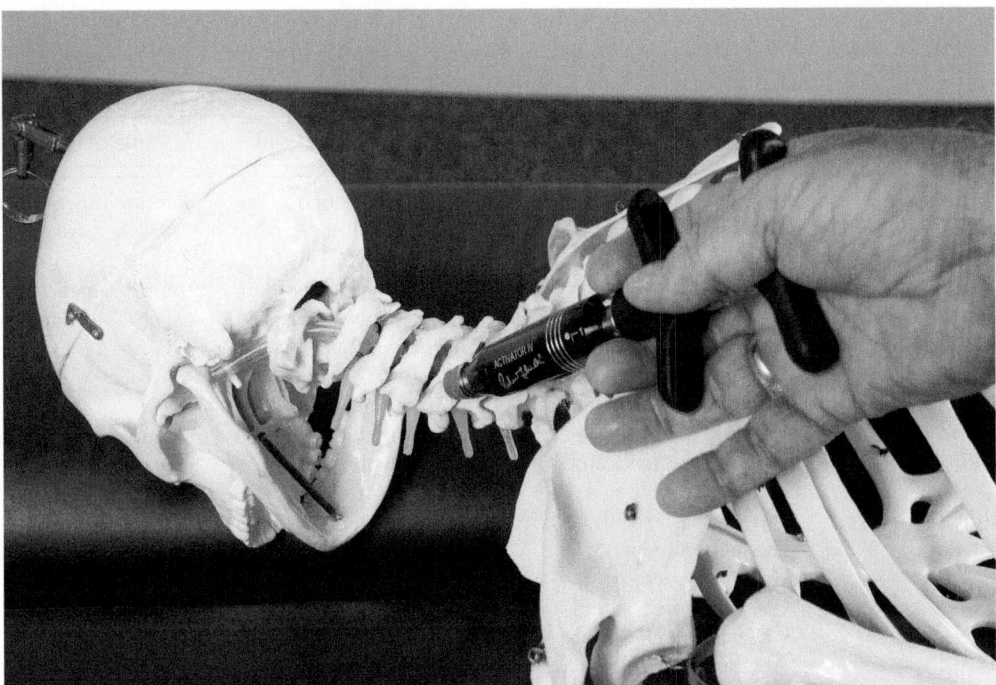

Figure 12-30   Adjustment for cervical disc with radiculopathy, Step One. The patient is laterally flexed away from side tested. Line of Drive is superior and medial.

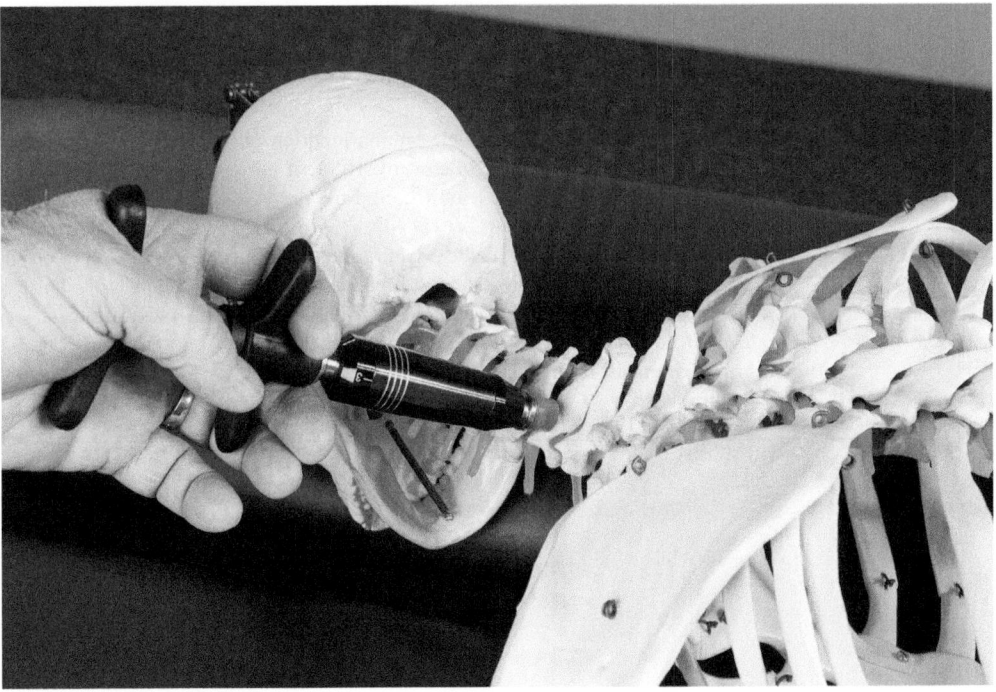

Figure 12-31   Adjustment for cervical disc with radiculopathy, Step Two. The patient is laterally flexed away from side tested. Line of Drive is inferior and medial.

Table 12-1 Summary Table of Tests and Adjustments for the Cervical Spine

Articular Dysfunction	Test	ADJUSTMENT	
		Segmental Contact Point	Line of Drive
Sixth Cervical (C6)	Instruct patient to shrug both shoulders toward the head	Pedicle-lamina junction on side of involvement per Short/Long Rule	Anterior, superior, and slightly medial
Enhancement of Sixth Cervical (C6)	Instruct patient to return the face to PD side, shrug both shoulders, and hold while returning the head to neutral	Pedicle-lamina junction on side of involvement per Short/Long Rule	Anterior-superior, and slightly medial
Enhancement of Fifth (C5) Cervical	Instruct patient to slide the chin up the table and push it into the table	Pedicle-lamina junction on side of involvement per Short/Long Rule	Anterior, superior, and slightly medial
Fifth (C5) Cervical Inferior	After testing C5 with normal procedures, instruct patient to tuck the chin to chest and press the forehead into the table and relax	Inferior portion of C5 spinous process	Anterior, superior
Hidden Posterior Fifth (C5) Cervical	Instruct patient to (1) shrug the shoulders, (2) hold the shrug, and (3) raise the head up slightly	Posterior-inferior aspect of C5 spinous process	Anterior-superior
Fourth Cervical (C4)	Instruct patient to raise head and turn toward side of PD and look superiorly	Pedicle-lamina junction on side of involvement per Short/Long Rule	Anterior, superior, and slightly medial
Third Cervical (C3)	Instruct patient to raise head and turn toward side of PD and look inferiorly	Pedicle-lamina junction on side of involvement per Short/Long Rule	Anterior, superior, and slightly medial
Third Cervical (C3) OPD Alternative Test	Instruct patient to raise the head and turn toward OPD side and look inferiorly	Pedicle-lamina junction on side of involvement per Short/Long Rule	Anterior, superior, and slightly medial
Second Cervical (C2)	*Step One*: Instruct patient to turn toward OPD side	Pedicle-lamina junction on side of involvement per Short/Long Rule	Anterior-superior, slightly medial to tip of nose
	Step Two: If no reaction, instruct patient to return to neutral	Pedicle-lamina junction on the PD side. Pressure Test to confirm.	Anterior-superior, slightly medial to tip of nose

		Adjustment	
Articular Dysfunction	**Test**	**Segmental Contact Point**	**Line of Drive**
Second Cervical (C2) Enhancement	*Step One:* Instruct patient to slightly tuck chin toward chest and hold while turning the head toward PD side	Pedicle-lamina junction on the PD side	Anterior-superior, slightly medial to tip of nose
	Step Two: If no reaction, instruct patient to slightly tuck chin toward chest and hold while turning the head toward OPD side	Pedicle-lamina junction on the OPD side	Anterior-superior, slightly medial to tip of nose
Cervical Disc with Radiculopathy	Instruct patient to laterally flex the head on the involved side. Before adjustment, patient is positioned so he or she is slightly laterally flexed away from the tested side.	*Step One:* Pedicle-lamina on tested side of involved segment	Superior and medial
		Step Two: Head still flexed laterally away, pedicle-lamina junction of the segment below	Inferior and medial
C2-C5 Combination: Second Cervical Vertebra (C2)	Instruct patient to flex neck by tucking chin toward chest. Check legs in Position #3.	Superior C2: Superior aspect of spinous process	Inferior
		Inferior C2: Inferior aspect of spinous process	Superior
Fifth Cervical Vertebra (C5) (Position #3)	Instruct patient to flex neck by tucking chin toward chest. Check legs in Position #3.	Superior C5: Superior aspect of spinous process	Inferior
		Inferior C5: Inferior aspect of spinous process	Superior
Lateral Occiput (C0)	Instruct patient to turn the head to the PD side and push it into the table. If PD shortens in Position #1, contact PD side. If no change, instruct patient to turn the head to the OPD side and push it into the table. If PD shortens in Position #1, contact the OPD side.	Lateral aspect of occiput, superior to mastoid process	Medial

Table 12-1 Summary Table of Tests and Adjustments for the Cervical Spine—cont'd

OPD, Opposite Pelvic Deficiency; *PD,* Pelvic Deficiency.

RELATED RESEARCH

Box 12-2

Reference: Youngquist MW, Fuhr AW, Osterbauer PJ. Interexaminer reliability of an Isolation Test for the presence of an upper cervical isolation subluxation. J Manipulative Physiol Ther. 1989; 12(2):93-7.

ABSTRACT

A reliability study was conducted to determine whether prone Leg Length Analysis in association with an Isolation Test maneuver was reproducible. A total of 72 subjects were evaluated by two examiners on separate occasions for the presence of C1 subluxation. Concordance was assessed by the kappa statistic, and interexaminer percentage of agreement was compared. Agreement beyond chance for the two groups was $\kappa = 0.52$ (p < .01 and 0.55, p < .001, respectively). Results indicate good reliability with this method of analysis for putative upper cervical subluxation in this patient population. Further investigation is necessary to correlate this method of analysis with empirical evidence of manipulable lesions or subluxations.

Box 12-3

Reference: De Witt JK, Osterbauer PJ, Stelmach GE, Fuhr AW. Optoelectric measurement of changes in leg length inequality resulting from Isolation Tests. J Manipulative Physiol Ther. 1994; 17(8):530-8.

ABSTRACT
OBJECTIVE

(a) Establish a precise, standardized method to assess prone leg alignment changes (functional "Leg Length Inequality") that have, until now, been reported clinically to occur as a result of putative chiropractic subluxation Isolation Tests (neck flexion [C1-C2] and extension [C5]); and (b) describe differences in leg alignment changes in a group of healthy subjects and patients with chronic spinal complaints.

DESIGN
Two groups, two Isolation Tests, descriptive, repeated measure analysis of variance

SETTING
Exercise and Sport Research Institute, Arizona State University

PARTICIPANTS
Eight healthy controls, eight patients with a history of chronic spinal complaints and observable leg alignment reactivity

INTERVENTIONS
Active cervical flexion/extension maneuvers

OUTCOME
Opto-electrical markers affixed to heels and occiput, as subjects lay prone

MARKER MEASURES
Locations sampled at 100 Hz for 10 seconds during (a) three no movement trials, (b) three cervical extension trials, and (c) three flexion trials. Data transformed approximately to local reference frame each subject's longitudinal axis before analysis.

RESULTS
Heel position movement occurred during trials and was highly individualistic. Patients exhibited more asymmetrical movements than did controls during the head-up trials. No differences existed between controls and patients for range of heel displacement or net displacement.

CONCLUSIONS
Results of this study allow the following to be concluded: (1) Small leg displacements (<1 mm) were recorded by the opto-electrical measurement system; (2) heel position changes during Isolation Tests were identifiable; (3) as a result of head-up maneuvers, patients exhibited more asymmetrical heel movement than controls ($t = 8.743$, p < .01); (4) heel range of motion was not different between the groups; and (5) net change in heel position was not different between the groups. Patients exhibited more asymmetrical heel motion during head-up Isolation Tests, suggesting that some phenomena may separate these two groups; this warrants future study.

Box 12-4

Reference: Osterbauer PJ, Derickson KL, Peles JD, DeBoer KF, Fuhr AW, Winters JM. Three-dimensional head kinematics and clinical outcome of patients with neck injury treated with spinal manipulative therapy: a pilot study. J Manipulative Physiol Ther. 1992;15(8):501-11.

ABSTRACT
OBJECTIVE
Finite helical axis parameters (FHAPs) of the cervical spine and clinical measures were obtained to evaluate neck function and the clinical effects of spinal manipulative therapy in patients with "whiplash"-type neck injury.

DESIGN
Descriptive case series, 1-year follow-up

SETTING
Three private chiropractic practices

SUBJECTS
Ten consecutive new patients with a history of neck injury; nine asymptomatic, volunteer controls

INTERVENTIONS
A 6-week regimen of short lever manually assisted adjustments with an Activator Instrument; while acute, four patients received interferential electrotherapy

OUTCOME
Cervical FHAP during normal movements, neck pain (visual analog scale)

ACTIVE MEASURES
Cervical range of motion and follow-up questionnaire

RESULTS
On the basis of data from six patients, the FHAPs appeared to mirror the clinical condition, being markedly deviant from patterns observed in the control group for one or more of the tracking tasks for all but one of the patients. Mean pain scores decreased from 44.1 to 10.5 (t = 4.93; p < .0001), and mean total range of motion increased from 234 to 297 degrees (t = 5.68; p < .0001). At 1 year, seven respondents noted stability of their symptoms at or near the level reported immediately after the 6-week treatment period.

CONCLUSIONS
On the basis of these preliminary data, (a) FHAPs may aid in diagnosing and monitoring treatment of neck dysfunction, (b) spinal manipulative therapy may be beneficial to some patients with neck injury, and future study is warranted as a means to promote recovery of patients with neck injuries.

Box 12-5

Reference: Wood TG, Colloca CJ, Matthews R. A pilot randomized clinical trial on the relative effect of instrumental (MFMA) versus manual (HVLA) thrust manipulation in the treatment of cervical spine dysfunction. J Manipulative Physiol Ther. 2001; 24(4):260-71.

ABSTRACT
OBJECTIVE
To determine the relative effect of instrument-delivered as compared with traditional manual-delivered thrust cervical manipulations in the treatment of cervical spine dysfunction

DESIGN
Prospective, randomized, comparative clinical trial

SETTING
Outpatient chiropractic clinic

SUBJECTS
Thirty patients diagnosed with neck pain and restricted cervical range of motion

INTERVENTIONS
Two randomized groups. One group received mechanical force, manually assisted (MFMA) manipulation delivered with the Activator Adjusting Instrument II. The other group received high-velocity, low-amplitude (HVLA) Diversified adjustments to the cervical spine.

Continued

Box 12-5—cont'd

OUTCOME MEASURES
Subjective (Pain Rating Scale, McGill Short-Form Pain Questionnaire, and Neck Disability Index) and objective goniometer cervical ranges of motion during treatment and at 1-month follow up

RESULTS
Both treatment methods had a positive effect on both clinical outcome measures with no significant difference noted between the two groups.

CONCLUSIONS
Results indicate that instrumental (MFMA) and manual (HVLA) manipulation have beneficial effects associated with reduced pain and disability and improved cervical range of motion. A large, randomized controlled clinical trial is necessary to verify these findings.

Box 12-6

Reference: Polkinghorn BS. Treatment of cervical disc protrusions via instrumental chiropractic adjustment. J Manipulative Physiol Ther. 1998; 21(2):114-21.

ABSTRACT
OBJECTIVE
To present a case of posttraumatic cervical syndrome involving multiple protrusions of cervical intervertebral discs, successfully treated with conservative instrumental chiropractic adjusting procedures

CLINICAL FEATURES
A 42-year-old woman suffered acute neck and arm pain after a motor vehicle accident. Radiological examination revealed complete reversal of cervical lordosis, and magnetic resonance imaging study revealed four separate disc protrusions.

INTERVENTION AND OUTCOME
After initially aggravating her symptoms by treating with manual manipulation of the cervical spine, the patient was treated with the Activator Adjusting Instrument. Treatment was well tolerated, and subsequently, the patient experienced complete resolution of her presenting symptoms.

CONCLUSION
Instrument-delivered adjustments may benefit those patients whose conditions were exacerbated by manual adjusting or in those cases in which manual manipulation is contraindicated. Further study is needed.

Box 12-7

Reference: Yurkiw D, Mior S. Comparison of two chiropractic techniques on pain and lateral flexion in neck pain patients: a pilot study. Chiropr Tech. 1996;8(4):155-62.

ABSTRACT
Musculoskeletal disorders affect 5% to 7% of the population in Canada. Neck pain is one of the more common musculoskeletal complaints. Spinal manipulative therapy attempts to reduce pain and increase range of motion. Treatments from any profession require valid evidence of efficacy. This study examines two popular treatments used by Canadian chiropractors: a mechanically assisted device commonly known as the Activator Adjusting Instrument and spinal manipulative therapy. Fourteen subjects were randomly assigned to two groups. Each subject was assigned by a blind examiner and then was given one of the two treatment interventions, which was provided by an experienced chiropractor. Outcome measures used included lateral flexion and a subjective pain rating scale. Results revealed that no statistically significant differences before and after the interventions. Further study is required with larger sample sizes before conclusions can be made regarding the efficacy of the selected interventions. However, the importance of the need for future comparative studies is discussed.

Box 12-8

Reference: Polkinghorn BS, Colloca CJ. Chiropractic treatment of postsurgical neck syndrome utilizing mechanical force, manually-assisted short lever spinal adjustments. J Manipulative Physiol Ther. 2001;24(9):589-95.

ABSTRACT
OBJECTIVE

To describe a case of postsurgical neck pain, after multiple spinal surgeries, that was successfully treated by chiropractic intervention with instrumental adjustment of the cervical spine

CLINICAL FEATURES

A 35-year-old woman had chronic neck pain for longer than 5 years after two separate surgeries of the cervical spine: a diskectomy at C3/4 and a fusion at C5/6. Surgeries were performed 6 months apart in an attempt to resolve persistent neck pain and spasm of the cervical musculature. Neither surgery was effective in relieving the patient's pain. Five years after the second surgery had been performed, a third surgery was recommended by the patient's physicians to alleviate the chronic pain. The patient sought chiropractic evaluation of her condition to avoid further surgical intervention.

INTERVENTION AND OUTCOME

The patient was treated with conservative instrumental chiropractic manipulation, consisting of mechanical force, manually assisted short-lever

spinal adjustments rendered with an Activator Adjusting Instrument (AAI)-II. She comfortably tolerated the treatment and responded favorably to this therapy. All chronic symptoms had resolved within 30 days of initiation of chiropractic instrumental adjustments made with an AAI. Even more interesting is the fact that longitudinal examination over the next 2 years showed that the patient experienced no residual effects or additional recurrences of her previous chronic problem after the initial course of chiropractic care.

CONCLUSION

Chiropractic treatment of postsurgical neck syndrome may be effective, in some cases, with use of mechanical force, manually assisted adjusting procedures performed with an AAI. The use of instrumental adjustment methods may provide chiropractic physicians with an effective alternative to manual manipulation in those cases in which the patient's surgical history or presenting symptoms make forceful manipulation of the spine, particularly performed at end range, inappropriate. This approach may be contemplated by physicians who are faced with managing this type of condition. Further study should be made in this regard, in an academic research setting, to determine the safest and most effective approaches for managing the treatment of postsurgical patients in a chiropractic setting.

REFERENCES

1. Spangfort E. Clinical aspects of neck-and-shoulder pain. Scand J Rehabil Med Suppl. 1995;32:43-6.
2. Vernon H, Steiman I, Hagino C. Cervicogenic dysfunction in muscle contraction headache and migraine: a descriptive study. J Manipulative Physiol Ther. 1992;15(7):418-29.
3. Bogduk N, Marsland A. The cervical zygapophysial joints as a source of neck pain. Spine. 1988;13(6):610-17.
4. Dwyer A, Aprill C, Bogduk N. Cervical zygapophyseal joint pain patterns. I: A study in normal volunteers. Spine. 1990;15(6):453-7.
5. Aprill C, Dwyer A, Bogduk N. Cervical zygapophyseal joint pain patterns. II: A clinical evaluation. Spine. 1990;15(6):458-61.
6. Aprill C, Bogduk N. The prevalence of cervical zygapophyseal joint pain. A first approximation. Spine. 1992;17(7):744-7.
7. Bogduk N, Aprill C. On the nature of neck pain, discography and cervical zygapophysial joint blocks. Pain. 1993;54(2):213-17.
8. Barnsley L, Lord S, Bogduk N. Clinical review: whiplash injury. Pain. 1994;58:283-307.
9. Barnsley L, Lord SM, Wallis BJ, Bogduk N. The prevalence of chronic cervical zygapophysial joint pain after whiplash. Spine. 1995;20(1):20-6.
10. Murphy DJ. Whiplash distortions, cervical zygapophysial joint injury, and chronic post traumatic neck pain. Am J Clin Chiro. 1995;5(2):31.
11. Spitzer WO, Skovron ML, Salmi LR, Cassidy JD, Duranceau J, Suissa S, et al. Scientific monograph of the Quebec Task Force on Whiplash-Associated Disorders: redefining "whiplash" and its management. Spine. 1995;20(8 Suppl):1S-73S.
12. Foreman SM, Croft AC. Whiplash injuries: the cervical acceleration deceleration syndrome. Baltimore: Williams & Wilkins; 1988.

13. Hodgson SP, Grundy M. Whiplash injuries: their long-term prognosis and its relationship to compensation. Neuro Orthop. 1989;7:88-91.

14. Braaf MM, Rosner S. Symptomatology and treatment of injuries of the neck. NY State J Med. 1955;55(2):237-42.

15. Garrick JG, Webb RD. Sports injuries: diagnosis and management. Philadelphia: Saunders; 1990.

16. Hagberg M. Neck and shoulder disorders. In: Rosenstock L, Cullen MR, editors. Textbook of clinical occupational and environmental medicine. Philadelphia: Saunders; 1994.

17. Vafidis JA. Injuries to the head and spine. In: McLatchie GR, Lennox CME, editors. The soft tissues: trauma and sports injuries. London: Butterworth-Heinemann; 1993.

18. Katz RT, DeLuca J. Sequelae of minor traumatic brain injury. Am Fam Physician. 1992;46(5):1491-8.

19. Breig A. Adverse mechanical tension in the central nervous system. New York: Wiley; 1978.

20. Calliet R. Neck and arm pain. Philadelphia: FA Davis; 1981.

21. Harrison DD, Jackson BL, Troyanovich S, Robertson GA, de George D, Barker WF. The efficacy of cervical extension-compression traction combined with diversified manipulation and drop table adjustments in the rehabilitation of cervical lordosis: a pilot study. J Manipulative Physiol Ther. 1994;17(7):454-64.

22. Clemente CD. Gray's anatomy. 30th American ed. Philadelphia: Lea & Febiger; 1985.

23. Cramer GD, Darby SA. Basic and clinical anatomy of the spine, spinal cord, and ANS. St. Louis: Mosby; 1995.

24. Jirout J. Effect of variations in mobility in the frontal plane at the occiput-atlas level on the dynamics of the atlas-axis segment during side bending of the head and neck. J Manual Med. 1992;6:182-4.

25. Cipriano JJ. Photographic manual of regional orthopaedic tests. Baltimore: Williams & Wilkins; 1985.

26. Hoppenfeld S. Physical examination of the spine and extremities. Norwalk (CT): Appleton-Century-Crofts; 1976.

27. Evans RC. Illustrated orthopedic physical assessment. 2nd ed. Philadelphia: Saunders; 1992. p. 149-51.

28. Pollock RA, Apple DF, Purvis JM, Murray HH. Esophageal and hypopharyngeal injuries in patients with cervical spine trauma. Ann Otolaryngol. 1981;90:323-7.

29. Reddin A, Mirvis SE, Diaconis JN. Rupture of the cervical esophagus and trachea associated with cervical spine fracture. J Trauma. 1987;27(5):564-76.

30. McLauchlan CAJ, Pidsley R, Vandenberk PJM. Minor trauma—major problem: neck injuries, retropharyngeal hematoma, and emergency airway management. Arch Emerg Med. 1991;8(2):135-9.

13

THE TEMPOROMANDIBULAR JOINT AND RELATED TESTS AND ADJUSTMENTS

James DeVocht and Wally Schaeffer

The temporomandibular joint (TMJ) itself, as shown in Figure 13-1, is fairly complex as far as joints in the human body go. It is also unique in that left and right synovial joints are separate, and yet they are connected by the essentially rigid mandible. Therefore the biomechanical functioning of one is inherently influenced by that of the other. It is functionally complex in that movement of the mandible relative to the temporal bone consists of both rotation and translation. In addition, the anatomy of the TMJ is relatively sophisticated inasmuch as a disk, or meniscus, is present between the articulating surfaces, and associated soft tissue structures have functions and implications that are not yet fully understood. Despite the considerable translation and rotation of the mandible relative to the temporal bone, the articular disk is able to maintain its position between the two in the normal TMJ. The articular disk itself has a complex anatomy in terms of the nature of its biconcave shape and variable composition, along with its posterior attachment, the bilaminar zone. As a true synovial joint, the entire TMJ is enclosed within the articular capsule and is bathed in synovial fluid.

Not only is the anatomy of the TMJ complex, but virtually all of the components are quite variable, even among the normal population—with no discernible abnormalities of function. Considerable variation is noted in the geometric shape of the articular eminence, the anterior slope of the mandible, and the shape of the mandibular condyle, articular disk, articular capsule, and discal attachments. The composition and points of attachment of the bilaminar zone are very inconsistent among normal individuals. Considerable variation also is noted in the manner of insertion of the muscles of mastication. All of this variation adds to the difficulty involved in understanding the mechanisms of biomechanical functioning of the normal TMJ.

NORMAL FUNCTION

The sequence of events for the opening of the normal TMJ is depicted in Figure 13-2. In the relaxed position with the mouth closed, the condyle of the mandible is nestled down in the mandibular fossa (sometimes referred to as the glenoid fossa) of the temporal bone (see Figure 13-2, A). When the mouth is opened, the condyle first rotates somewhat within the fossa, on the articular disk, and then begins to translate anteriorly as it continues to rotate (see Figure 13-2, B). As the mandible translates anteriorly, the disk moves along with it, always separating the articular surface of the mandibular condyle from the articular surface of the temporal bone (see Figure 13-2, C). In normal maximal mouth opening, the condyle translates to just beyond the high point of the articular eminence, which forms the anterior side of the mandibular fossa (see Figure 13-2, D). The mandible essentially retraces that pattern in reverse when the mouth is closed. Considerable stresses are applied to the disk during normal mastication, resulting in repeated deformation of the disk during the course of a normal cycle.[1] The topology of the disk is conducive to its being carried along mechanically during normal mandibular motion. It is thought that the coordinated contraction of muscles might be an essential part of keeping the disk in proper position throughout normal movement, although it is possible that the geometry and proximity of the involved structures may be sufficient to accomplish this under normal conditions without active muscular control.

DYSFUNCTION

Virtually any sort of abnormal condition that pertains to the TMJ is included within the general term *temporomandibular disorder* (TMD). Many different types of aberrations related to the TMJ itself are observed to occur, although

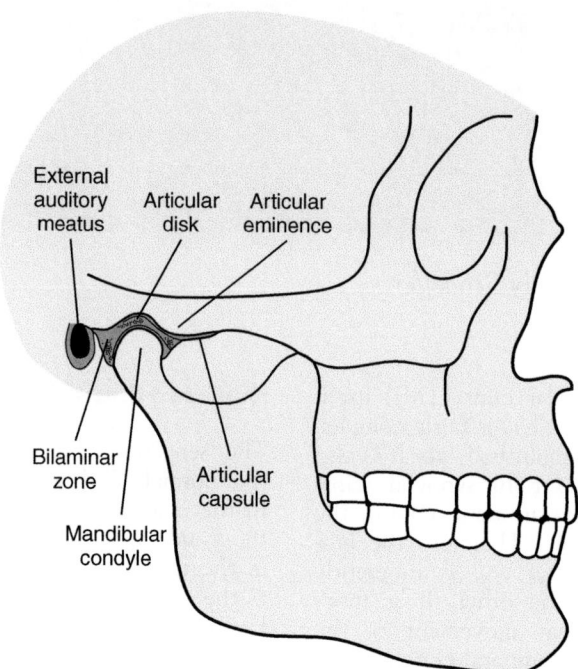

Figure 13-1 Anatomy of the temporomandibular joint. *(Copyright © 2006 by Data Trace Publishing Company, originally published in DC Tracts, 2006, Volume 18, Number 4, pages 4 and 5 and reproduced here with permission.)*

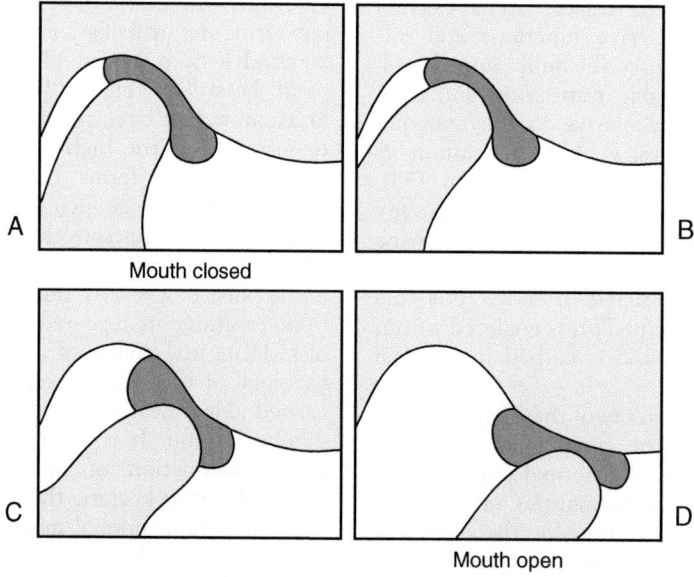

Figure 13-2 Sequence of *normal* opening of the temporomandibular joint. **A,** Mouth is closed, and the condyle is in the mandibular fossa (glenoid fossa). **B,** Beginning mouth opening condyle rotates on the articular disk. **C,** Continued mouth opening; the mandibular condyle moves anteriorly with the disk separating it from the articular surface of the temporal bone. **D,** Maximal mouth opening; the condyle translates just beyond the high point of the articular eminence, which forms the anterior side of the mandibular fossa. *(Copyright © 2006 by Data Trace Publishing Company, originally published in DC Tracts, 2006, Volume 18, Number 4, pages 4 and 5 and reproduced here with permission.)*

little is known of their origin. It has been noted universally that women are several times more likely to suffer from TMD than men, but the reason for this imbalance remains unknown. Poor posture of the head has been purported to cause muscle imbalance that may make one more susceptible to developing some forms of TMD.[2] It has also been noted that TMD sometimes appears to be associated with trauma, especially whiplash-type trauma.[3] If trauma is involved, magnetic resonance imaging (MRI) has become the current standard technique for demonstrating that a disk injury has occurred.[4] However, no detectable difference has been noted in symptoms for those cases of TMD that appear to be related to trauma.[5] In spite of years of work by numerous parties, we still do not know much about the causes of TMD at the individual level.[6] Whatever the uncertain causes of TMD may be, there is no doubt that it is a significant issue; some 10 million TMD sufferers have been identified in the United States, most of whom are young adults, female, and between 20 and 40 years of age.[7]

Not only is the cause of TMD basically unknown, but the full extent of ramifications of TMD remains unknown as well. It has been shown that induced malocclusion in rats leads to scoliotic curves in the spine that return to normal when proper occlusion is restored.[8] Such experiments cannot be conducted with humans, but TMD is frequently observed to occur in conjunction with other pathological conditions such as bad posture or headaches. Causal relationships have not yet been determined but it seems likely that connections with at least some such conditions will be discovered.

Inasmuch as TMD can be presented in any of a wide variety of different forms, the Research Diagnostic Criteria for Temporomandibular Disorders (RDC/TMD)[9] was developed some time ago through a combination of questionnaires and an extensive clinical examination that would serve as a method of classifying specific cases into fairly well-defined categories. It seems to be the best method currently available for doing so and is used frequently in the research community in an effort to document just what types of TMD are being included in various studies. Unfortunately, the method is time consuming, and proper use requires considerable training. Furthermore, it does not always reveal abnormalities that are apparent on MRI.[10] Consequently, it is seldom if ever used in clinical practice. In common clinical practice, TMD remains a highly nonspecific term.

The most general classification that is usually made regarding TMD is articular versus myofascial. That is, the problem is associated with the structures of the TMJ itself, or it results from some sort of aberrant activity of the musculature that affects the TMJ in some way.

Within the articular division of TMJ, perhaps the most common general type is biomechanical derangement of the articular disk, which can occur in two different main ways. In one

category of patients, the disk slips out of its normal position (between the condyle of the mandible and the articular surface of the temporal bone) for one part of the opening and closing cycle, but then it slips back into place for another part of that cycle. This is called disk displacement with reduction (DDwR). It usually involves anterior displacement of the disk and generally is accompanied by a clicking sound. Typically, this type of derangement is not associated with much if any pain or other symptoms. Therefore, even though it is fairly common, DDwR often is not a serious concern. Individuals with this type of TMD (and others around them) may well note the clicking sound in their jaw, but most often they do not seek treatment if this is the only perceptible abnormality.

In the other general category of disk derangement, displacement of the disk never reduces to the normal position. This category is consequently known as disk displacement without reduction (DDw/oR). The acute stages of DDw/oR often are quite painful and may be accompanied by a reduction of maximum mouth opening. After a period of some months, the pain associated with DDw/oR often decreases, but chronic cases of this situation often continue on to be quite problematic as a result of the level of pain or restriction of mouth opening.

When the articular disk dislocates, it usually does so anteriorly, although it can go laterally as well and even posteriorly (rarely). Not all dislocations involve large displacements, and many produce no symptoms at all. In a study involving 40 symptom-free healthy subjects, MRI showed that 9 of 80 TMJs displayed some degree of disk displacement at occlusion.[11]

Myofascial types of TMD are much more difficult to describe or categorize. Typically, pain is associated with the musculature around the joint, but often, it is not well localized to a specific spot. The most common distinction among individuals with these forms of TMD involves whether myofascial pain is accompanied by a limitation in mouth opening. Often times, no clear distinction can be made between articular and myofascial types; many individuals will show characteristics of both.

CURRENT STATUS OF TREATMENT MODES FOR TEMPOROMANDIBULAR DISORDERS

Over the years a large number of treatment protocols for TMD have been developed and used by a wide range of health care providers. The first major, multidisciplinary conference dedicated to TMD was conducted by the National

Institutes of Health in 1996.[7] It was concluded in that conference there were no data to support the superiority of any treatment. That finding was reiterated in 2001 in a major study by the Lewin Group, Inc.[12] It appears that up to 75% of TMD cases may resolve spontaneously, and little evidence is currently available to confirm that any form of treatment will increase that rate very much.[13] Many of the cases that go on to become chronic do not cause major issues in the lives of patients, but rather they learn to live with the disorder, and such individuals often get along well. On the other hand, some cases do become very problematic over time and can result in almost constant suffering and misery over many years. Anecdotal evidence suggests that treatment provided by the Activator Method (AM) Protocol may well be effective in at least some such cases of TMD.[14,15]

ACTIVATOR METHOD PROTOCOL FOR TREATMENT OF TEMPOROMANDIBULAR DISORDERS

The protocols and procedures described herein seek to establish normal, or as near normal as possible, biomechanics of the TMJ in order to restore jaw function that is as normal as possible. This, in turn, relieves many of the symptoms that are associated with, and a result of, aberrant jaw mechanics. This research-based protocol for the treatment of patients with TMJ disorders has been in development for over 15 years.

This approach is about joint function (e.g., a bilaterally hinged joint that is designed to operate smoothly and evenly on both sides). It is about subsequent joint dysfunction/derangement with the adverse effects of uneven force load distribution throughout the joint complex. These adverse effects may involve accessory structures such as muscles, tendons, ligaments, and secondarily involved joint complexes (e.g., the cervical spine, in which there may be some shared or associated anatomy and therefore function). A review of anatomy recalls the proximity of the head, neck, and jaw structures in an anatomically functional context.

This approach involves the neurological control of the TMJ and is targeted at restoring neurobiomechanical function that is as near normal as possible. It is not about dental or bite work, although there may be dentition/occlusal consequences. Therefore it may be of benefit to maintain a referral relationship with a compatible dentist for concurrent care. This understanding, as well as communication of this information to patients, is essential for developing supportive relationships with dental and other health care professionals.

Case History

The case history specific to TMJ/TMD issues would again include the view of the head, neck, and jaw as a motor unit and would be taken accordingly. Therefore the usual and appropriate protocols would be used for the head and neck in addition to the TMJ protocols.

TMJ disorders are seldom the primary or chief complaint; patients more often present with neck pain, headaches, facial neuralgias, or whiplash trauma. Specific TMJ issues include questions regarding trauma, abuse, dental work, pain in the TMJs and face, joint crepitus (which also would include bruxism [grinding]), intraoral bite plates or appliances, auditory changes and tinnitus, multiple ear infections, headaches, facial palsies, jaw locking open or closed, surgery, decreased mouth opening, difficulty chewing, biting of the lips, tongue, or cheeks, and motor vehicle collisions. This is by no means an exhaustive list, but it should serve to direct your thoughts and attention not only to specific issues but to a more global approach as well.

Some items particular to the above include early childhood traumas that are often forgotten; these usually include such accidents as falling from playground equipment and striking the chin, or a bicycle fall with jaw impact on the handlebars. These are often revealed by faint scars underneath the chin.

Physical abuse is frequent and often is not revealed during a case history, particularly with females, as occurrences may include family members and friends. Strong emotional reactions may occur if abuse is revealed, and if not, memories may be too painful to be shared.

Extensive dental work, including surgeries and other procedures with prolonged jaw extension, is often involved with TMJ dysfunction. A mouth opening measurement (MOM) of less than 30 mm is often thought to be pathognomonic for TMJ disorders.

A strong relationship has been noted between the TMJ and ear function. Thus questions of ear fullness and pressure, auditory changes, and tinnitus are appropriate. Proper jaw function facilitates the movement of debris, including bacteria, through the Eustachian tube to the esophagus, where it is resorbed and/or eliminated. Bacteria are always present. An infection results when the bacterial population becomes so numerous and virulent that it overwhelms the body's immune response. This may result from stasis caused by compromised jaw function. Jaw movement also assists in equalizing pressure on both sides of the eardrum.

Croft et al.[3] have described and documented the effects of motor vehicle collisions, particularly whiplash types, on the TMJ for many years; these events should be considered in treatment of jaw pain and dysfunction.

A thorough case history would include the interrelationship of the head, neck, and jaw to establish an anatomically functional context in all cases. Several questionnaires would be important in this approach: TMJ Patient Information, Jaw Symptom Questionnaire, Neck Pain Disability Index, and TMJ Pain Visual Analog Scale (VAS). These instruments provide thorough baseline information for a complete history and assessment in TMJ/TMD cases. These instruments may be obtained through Activator Methods International.

Examination

The examination should provide a clear indication of the presence and nature of TMJ dysfunction for both the clinician and the patient. It should be noted that dysfunction may be present in the absence of symptoms.

Examination Step One: Visual Inspection The first step in the examination process is a visual inspection for physical distortions. These distortions may be seen as unilateral cheek fullness, disproportionate muscle definition, uneven approximation of the teeth, and lower jaw imbalance with mouth function during conversation. Common visible areas of imbalance are the approximation of the central incisors and the areas just inferior to the lateral portion of the zygomatic arches.

The facial area should be inspected for any evidence of scars indicating surgery or trauma, particularly underneath the chin and the throat area. This would also apply to the head and neck regions. A visual inspection should be made of the dentition for evidence of extensive dental repair.

Examination Step Two: Mouth Opening Measurement The second step would be to take a MOM, obtained with a metric ruler in millimeters. The patient is asked to open the mouth as wide as possible without pain. The measurement is then taken with the ruler from the bottom of the patient's right maxillary (upper) central incisor (#8) to the top of the patient's right mandibular (lower) central incisor (#25). This measurement is then recorded in the patient's records for later reference as a baseline. Again, some dental institutions assess clinical significance with a MOM of less than 30 mm (Figure 13-3).

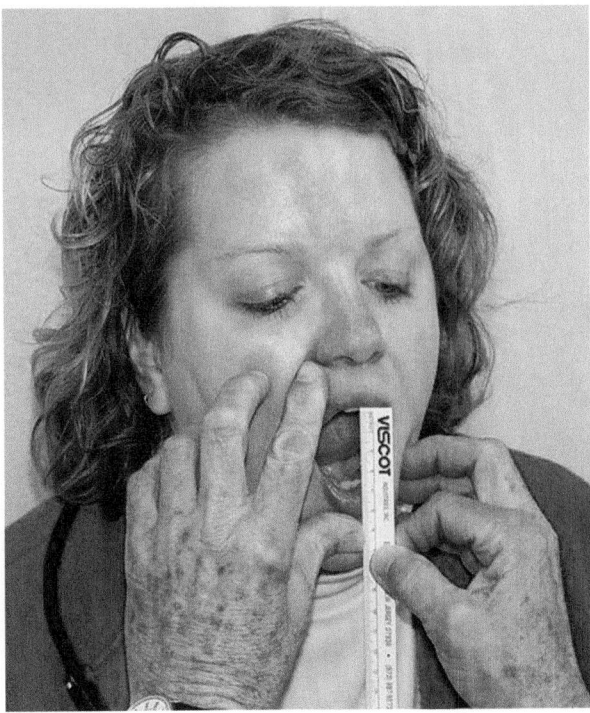

Figure 13-3 Mouth opening measurement.

Examination Step Three: Visual Observation of Motion The clinician will observe the jaw function for evidence of aberrant motion, as well as the patient for signs of pain and crepitus (look, listen, and feel). Aberrant movement usually includes lateral translation and ratchet closure (i.e., first one side approximating, then the other).

The doctor places the index fingers bilaterally on the condyles of the ramus just inferior to the zygomatic arches. The patient is asked to open the mouth wide, then close slowly as mild pressure is applied. Emphasize a slow closing movement to exaggerate any aberrant motion that may be present. Instruct the patient to "open your mouth and then close *slowly* while I apply mild pressure to the sides of your jaw. . . . Tell me what you notice" (Figure 13-4). The doctor visually observes as the patient opens and closes for any deviation throughout the movement and palpates for any open or closing clicks, crepitus, or locking.

Examination Step Four: Physical Examination The fourth step is to assess jaw function through three physical examination procedures that will exaggerate the extent of the jaw's dysfunction, providing palpatory, visual, and/or auditory evidence of the dysfunction.

Mild to moderate pressure is provided evenly, bilaterally, and simultaneously by the clinician at three points on the mandible. The patient should be advised that this process may be tender and may provoke pain. The clinician will observe jaw motion for evidence of aberrant movement, as well as the patient for signs of pain and crepitus. Aberrant movement usually includes lateral translation and ratchet closure (i.e., first one side approximating, then the other).

This step involves the doctor creating passive movement into the TMJ by applying pressure at two different mandibular contact points, and palpating at a third contact point during active movement of the jaw. These should be performed in the following order:

1. The doctor places the index fingers bilaterally on the condyles of the ramus just inferior to the zygomatic arches. Instruct the patient to open the mouth slightly so the teeth are clearly separated. Let the patient know, "I am going to apply some pressure to the sides of your jaw. Open your mouth so the teeth are clearly separated, and relax your muscles so I can apply pressure and move the jaw slightly. Tell me what you notice and whether you feel any pain. This may be tender."

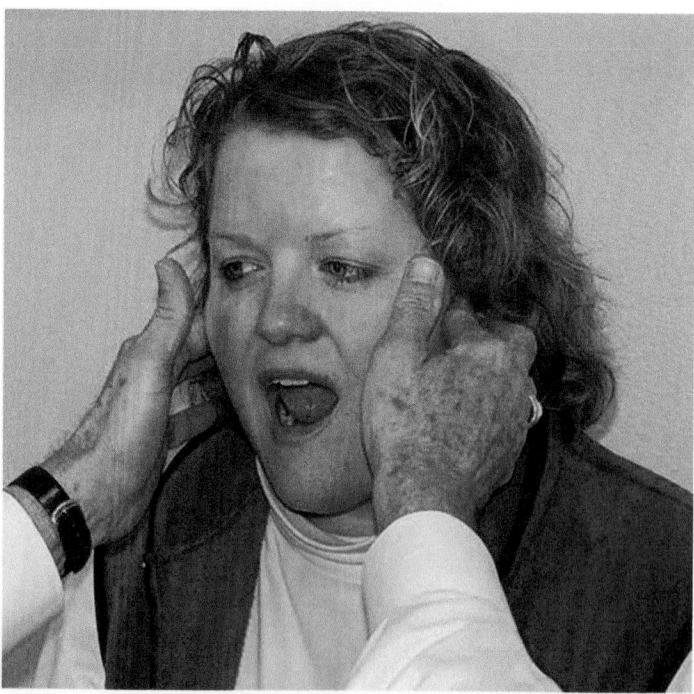

Figure 13-4 Observing and palpating for aberrant movement and crepitus throughout opening and closing movements.

The doctor applies gentle pressure in a lateral-to-medial direction (Figure 13-5).

2. The doctor places the thumbs on the lateral aspects of the frontal bone, and the second or third fingers are placed on the posterior aspect of the angle of the mandible. Pressure is applied in a posterior-to-anterior direction to assess passive joint motion and evaluate for any crepitus, catching, locking, or pain. The patient is instructed, "Open your mouth so the teeth are clearly separated and relax your muscles so I can apply pressure and move the jaw slightly. Tell me what you notice and if you feel any pain. This may be tender" (Figure 13-6).

3. Instruct the patient, "I will place my little fingers in your ears to assess the back of your jaw joints while you open your mouth. This is usually the most tender test." The doctor then places the little fingers bilaterally posterior to the condyles inside the ear canal. Pressure is applied lightly but firmly to the posterior aspect of the condyle. The patient is then instructed, "Open your mouth, then close *slowly*. . . . Tell me what you notice" (Figure 13-7).

This last test may be very sensitive and may elicit a sharp pain response that usually recedes quickly. It is not unusual to abort the test before complete jaw closure is achieved, but the clinician most likely will have obtained the necessary clinical information at this point.

Although this completes the physical examination process, additional information will be obtained with the application of the appropriate AM Isolation Tests and the Short/Long Rule in order to obtain specific correction points on the side of involvement.

Treatment

Five Isolation Tests are done in the order given: three primary (anterior extension, superior, and lateral) and two secondary (posterior and anterior). AM Protocol uses the Short/Long Rule in the assessment of most of the tests to identify the side of involvement for the adjustment procedure. This differentiates TMJ testing from other extremity testing where only Position #1 is used. Always go to Position #2 if results are inconclusive or if there is any uncertainty, especially if symptoms are present but a lack of reactivity in leg length is noted in Position #1.

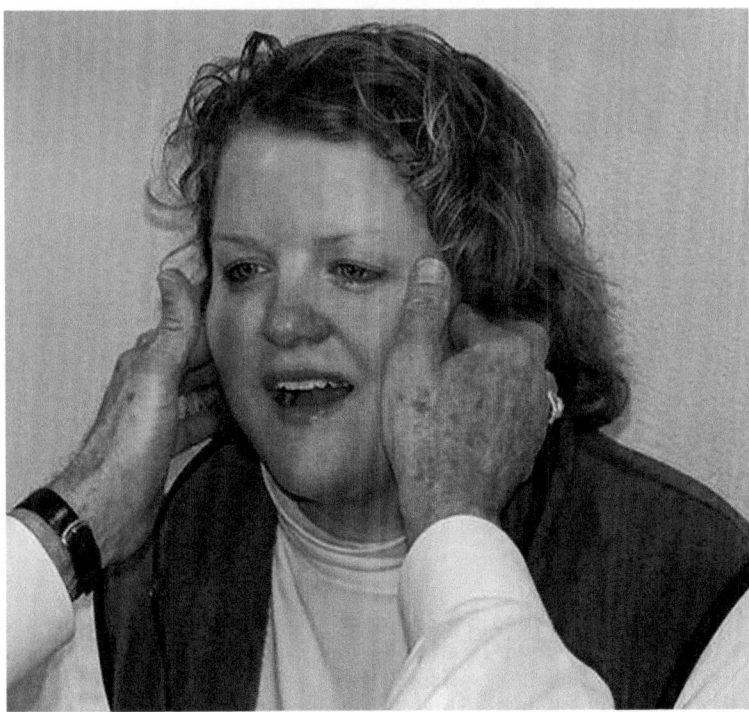

Figure 13-5 Passive movement applied in a lateral-to-medial direction.

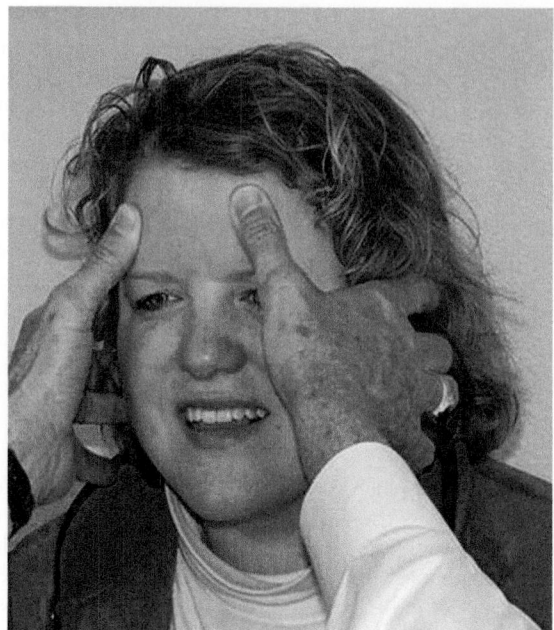

Figure 13-6   Passive movement applied in a posterior-to-anterior direction.

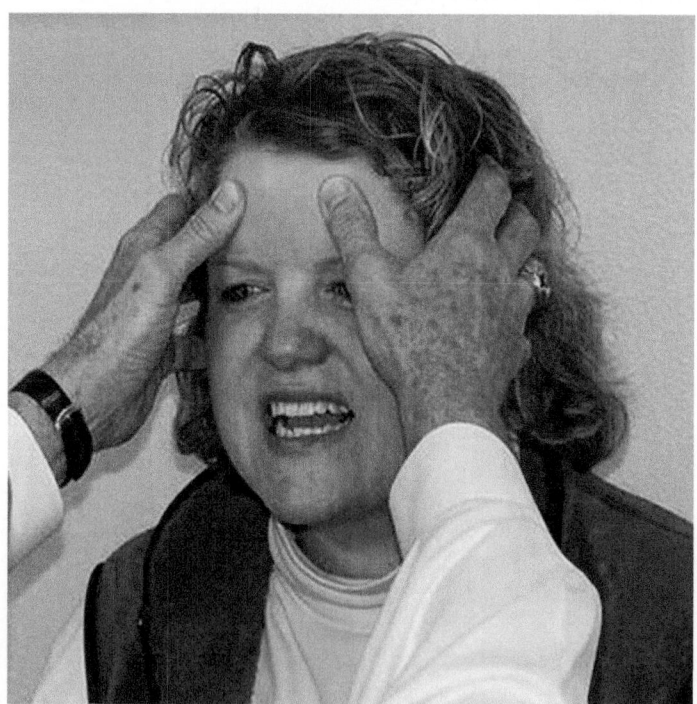

Figure 13-7   The doctor places the little fingers into the ear canal and palpates the posterior aspect of the condyles as the patient opens.

After performing the Isolation Test, look for Pelvic Deficiency (PD) leg reactivity in Position #1. Then proceed to Position #2, while observing relative changes in the PD leg. Follow the Short/Long Rule to identify the side of correction.

When adjusting with the Activator Instrument, use the lowest setting and always deliver the adjustment through the finger or thumb. Adjustments are performed near enough to the joint to affect the related mechanoreceptors, proprioceptors, and nociceptors. Adjustments should avoid contact over or near the joint that could directly affect the joint capsule and its discal attachments. Special care must be taken to AVOID contact with any teeth.

ALL palpatory contacts should be performed gently as the area involved may be tender.

Anterior Extension Test

- With the patient in the prone position, instruct the patient to "open your mouth wide" (Figure 13-8). (*Note:* The patient's head is turned for visualization of the illustration.) Look for PD leg reactivity in Position #1. Then proceed to Position #2, while observing relative changes in the PD leg. Follow the Short/Long Rule to determine the side of correction.
- Palpate gently with your thumb for the contact point at the anterior and inferior aspect of the neck of the coronoid process on the side determined by the Short/Long Rule (Figure 13-9, A and B).
- Ask the patient to open and then slowly close the mouth.
- As the mouth slowly closes, make your correction as you feel the head of the condyle begin to "seat," or rock back into the mandibular fossa; the mouth should still be open at the moment of correction.
- A coronoid contact is taken in order to influence "seating" at the condylar articulation.

- It may be helpful to ask the patient to open and close slowly several times first so you can correctly assess this "seating" motion for the instant of correction.
- The Line of Drive (LOD) is anterior to posterior and inferior to superior without any medial or lateral angle (Figure 13-10). The Activator Instrument should be directed toward the external auditory meatus (EAM).
- Correction is to be made at the lowest instrument setting and over the finger or thumb.
- Special caution must be taken to avoid contact with any teeth.

Superior Test

- Instruct the patient to "bite down" (Figure 13-11). (*Note:* The patient's head is turned for visualization of the illustration.) Look for PD leg reactivity in Position #1. Then proceed to Position #2, while observing relative changes in the PD leg. Follow the Short/Long Rule to determine the side of correction.
- Palpate gently for the contact point on the body of the ramus of the mandible inferior to the zygomatic arch and the mandibular incisure on the side determined from the Short/Long Rule (Figure 13-12, A and B).
- The LOD is superior to inferior down the ramus with as little angle as possible (Figure 13-13).
- Correction is to be made at the lowest instrument setting and over the finger or thumb.

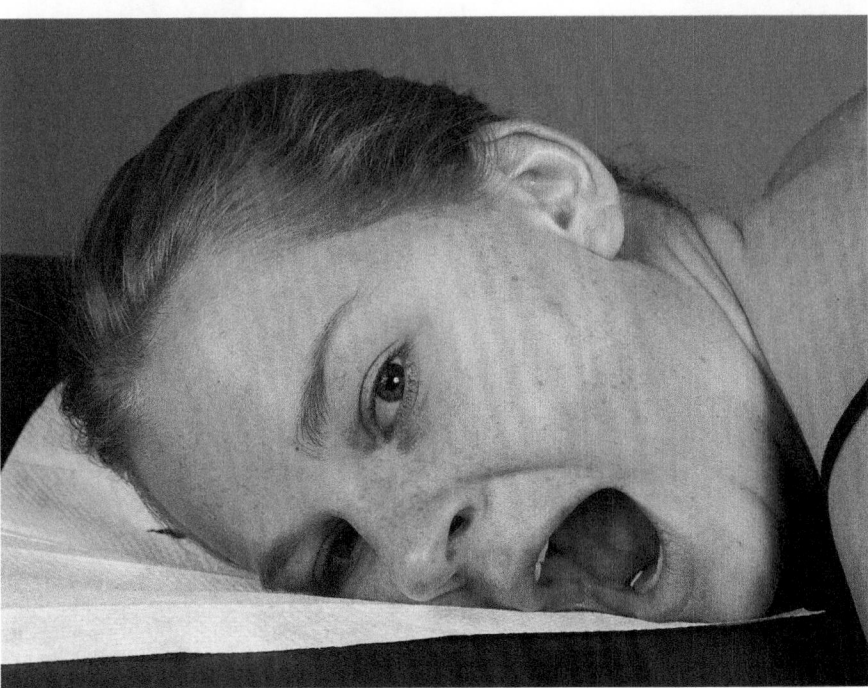

Figure 13-8   Isolation Test for anterior extension of the temporomandibular joint; open mouth. All tests are to be performed in a neutral prone position with the face down.

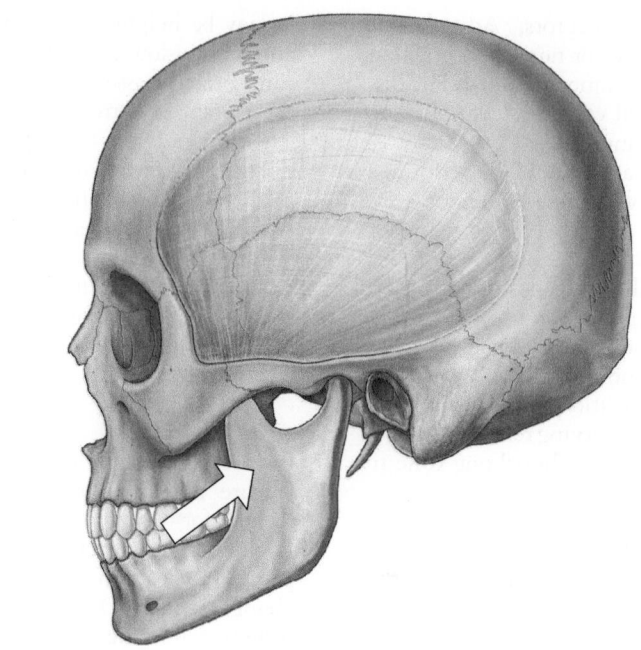

A

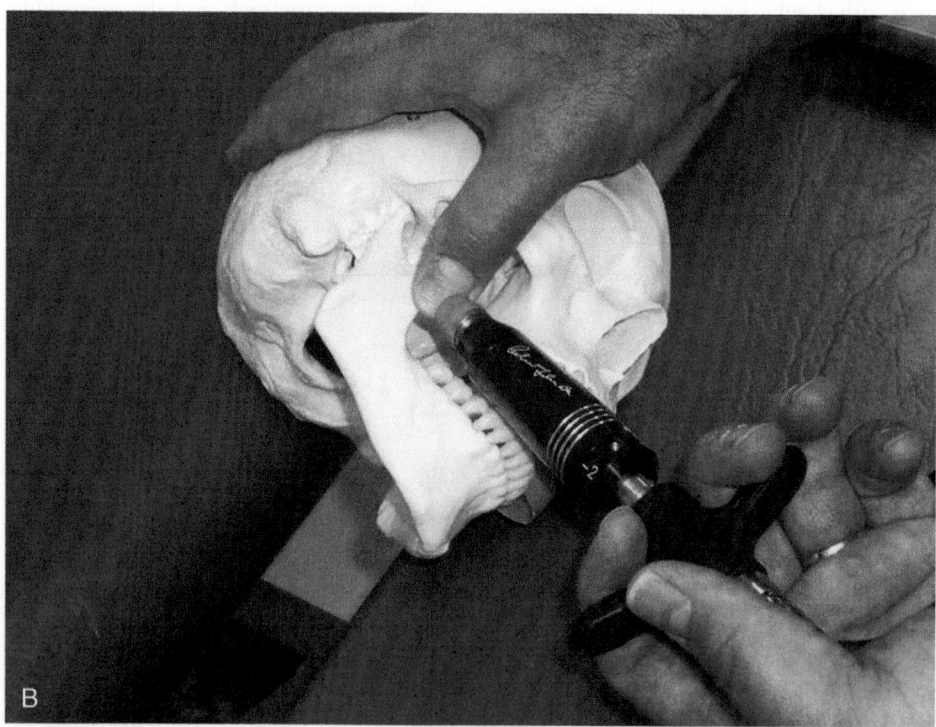

B

Figure 13-9 **A,** Anatomical Line of Drive (LOD) for anterior extension temporomandibular joint (TMJ). **B,** Contact point and LOD for anterior extension TMJ. *(**A**, Modified from Drake RL, Vogl W, Mitchell AWM. Gray's anatomy for students. Edinburgh: Churchill Livingstone; 2005.)*

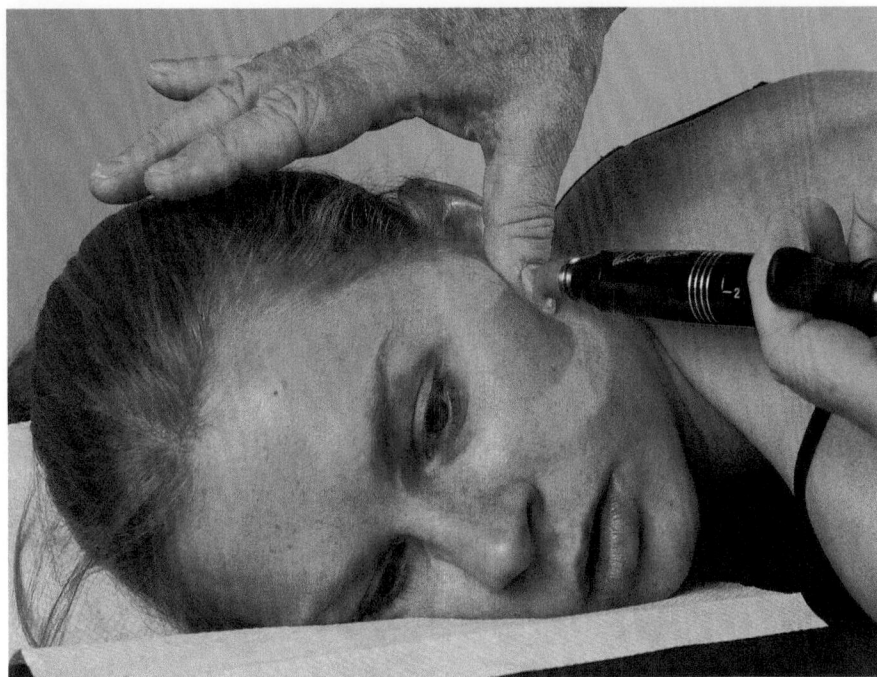

Figure 13-10 Adjustment for anterior extension temporomandibular joint. Line of Drive is anterior to posterior and inferior to superior.

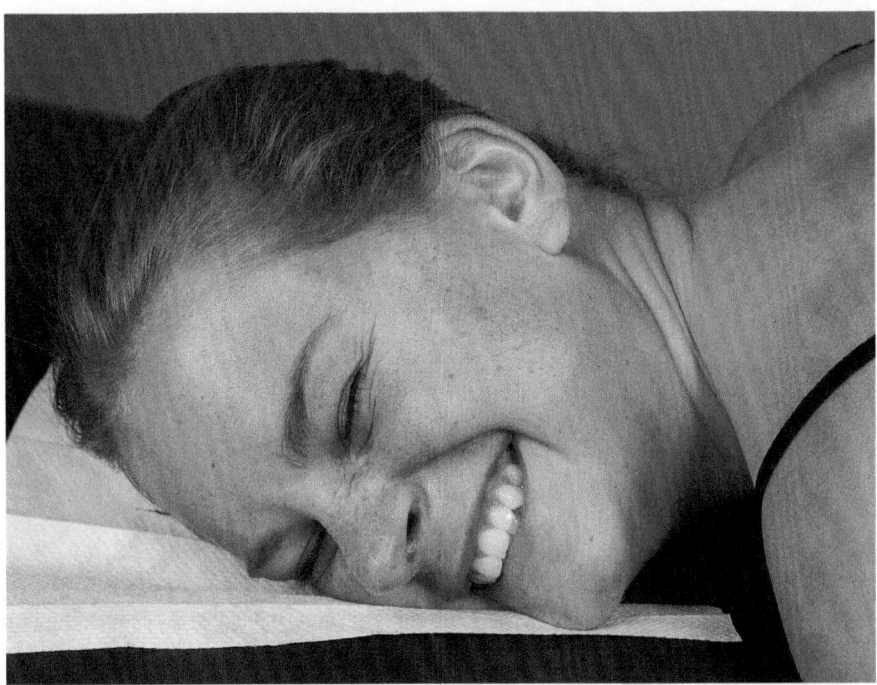

Figure 13-11 Isolation Test for superior temporomandibular joint; the patient is asked to bite down. All tests are to be performed in a neutral prone position with the face down.

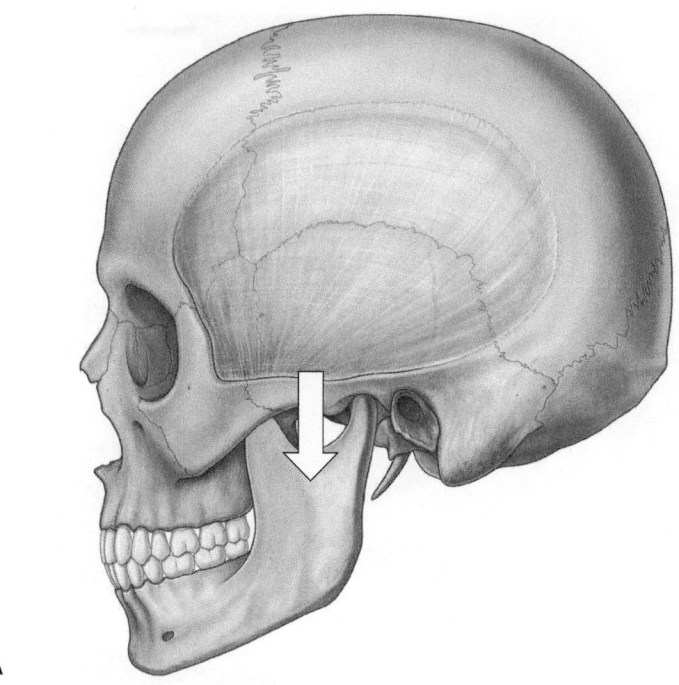

A

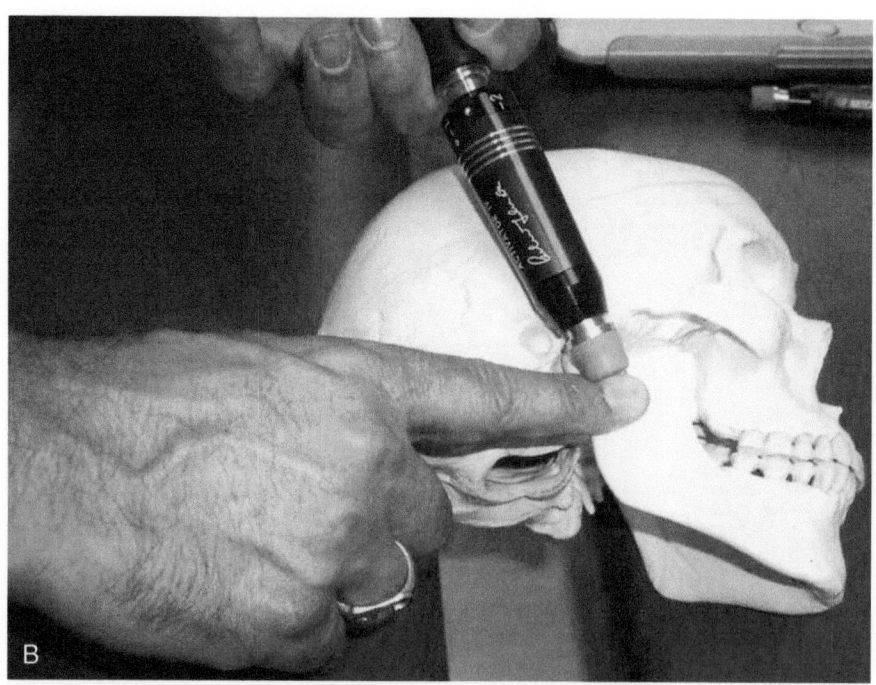

B

Figure 13-12   A, Anatomical Line of Drive (LOD) for superior temporomandibular joint (TMJ). **B,** Contact point and LOD for superior TMJ. (*A, Modified from Drake RL, Vogl W, Mitchell AWM. Gray's anatomy for students. Edinburgh: Churchill Livingstone; 2005.*)

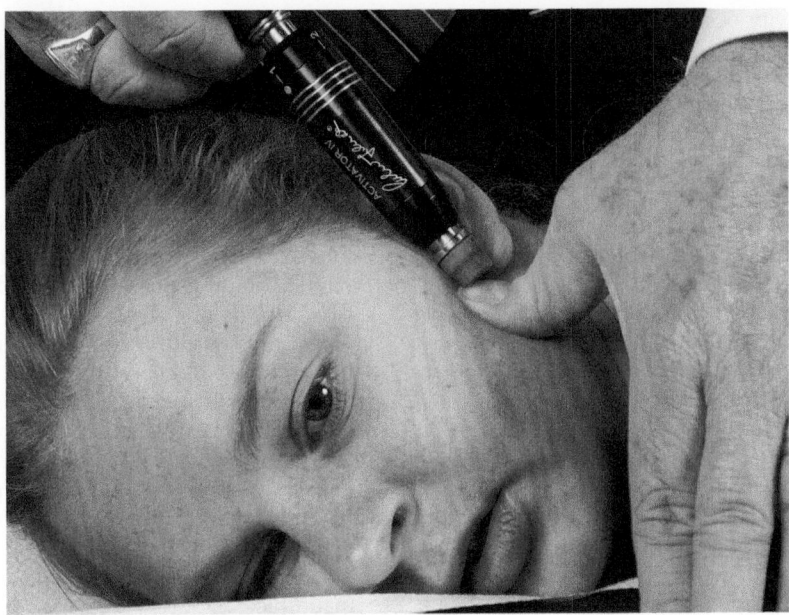

Figure 13-13   Adjustment for superior temporomandibular joint. Line of Drive is inferior through the ramus.

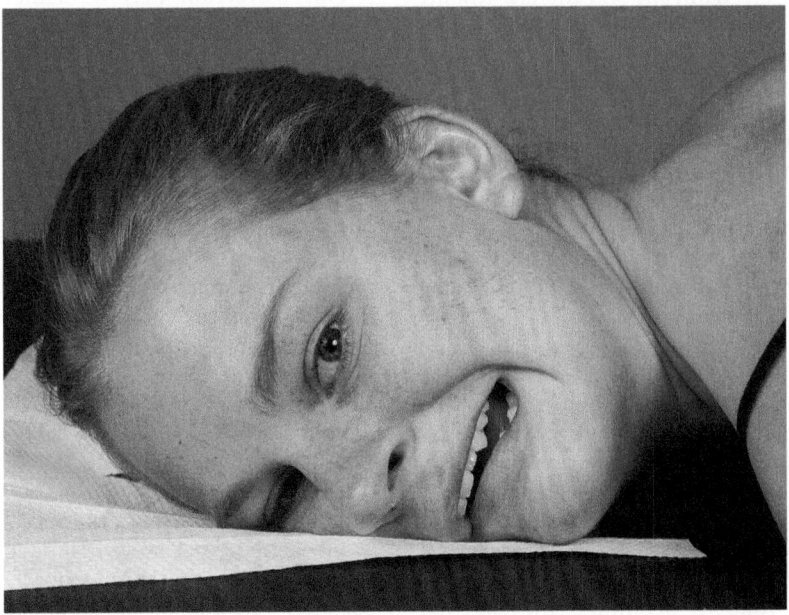

Figure 13-14   Isolation Test for lateral temporomandibular joint. Step One: Move jaw sideways toward the Pelvic Deficiency side. All tests are to be performed in a neutral prone position with the face down.

Lateral Test

- Instruct the patient to "slide or push your jaw sideways to the right/left" (PD side first) (Figure 13-14). (*Note:* The patient's head is turned for visualization of the illustration.) Look for PD leg reactivity in Position #1.

If reactivity occurs after this test, proceed to Pressure Testing to confirm the adjustment on the side of Pelvic Deficiency. Position #2 is not used with the lateral test. *Note:* This is the only TMJ test that does not use Position #2.

- If no reactivity occurred, instruct the patient to slide the jaw to the Opposite PD (OPD) side, and observe for reactivity in Position #1. Pressure Test to confirm the adjustment on the side Opposite Pelvic Deficiency.
- Palpate gently for the contact point on the ramus halfway between the condyle and the angle of the mandible on the side determined from the Pressure Test (Figure 13-15, A and B).
- The LOD is straight lateral to medial (Figure 13-16).
- Correction is to be made at the lowest instrument setting and over the finger or thumb.

CLINICAL NOTE: In some complicated cases, reactivity may not occur as expected. For example, the patient slides the jaw to the PD side, and there is reactivity. But, upon Pressure Testing on the PD side before the adjustment, there is no balancing in Position #1. Protocol would then call for Pressure Testing on the OPD side. If this creates balance, the adjustment would be performed on the OPD side, even though the patient biomechanically slid the jaw toward the PD side. Keep in mind that the TMJ is a complicated, two-sided structure. Leg length reactivity may be more responsive to a stretch type of stimulus on the OPD side than to the actual movement of the mandibular swing motion (biomechanically) to the PD side. This is an Isolation Test that accesses kinetic chains that are individualized; it may not always follow the more traditional chiropractic biomechanical view of the bone as subluxated in a particular direction.

Posterior Test

- Instruct the patient to "put the tip of your tongue on the *back* of the roof of your mouth" (Figure 13-17). (*Note:* The patient's head is turned for visualization of the illustration.) Look for PD leg reactivity in Position #1. Then proceed to Position #2, while observing relative changes in the PD leg. Follow the Short/Long Rule to determine the side for correction.
- This maneuver is performed to provide jaw retraction, the opposite of the next test.
- Palpate gently for the contact point at the posterior edge of the ramus where it meets the angle of the mandible on the side determined from the Short/Long Rule (Figure 13-18, A and B).
- The LOD is posterior to anterior (Figure 13-19).

- Special caution must be taken as this is usually a very tender contact point; it is best to advise the patient appropriately.
- Correction is to be made at the lowest instrument setting and over the finger or thumb.

Anterior Test

- Instruct the patient to "push your *jaw* straight forward" or "jut your jaw forward into the table" (not the head) (Figure 13-20). (*Note:* The patient's head is turned for visualization of the illustration.) Look for PD leg reactivity in Position #1. Then proceed to Position #2, while observing relative changes in the PD leg. Follow the Short/Long Rule to determine the side for correction.
- Palpate gently for the contact point at the mental tubercle on the side of correction as indicated by the Short/Long Rule (Figure 13-21, A and B)—not in the center of the mandible.
- The LOD is inferior to superior and anterior to posterior. The Activator Instrument should be directed toward the EAM (Figure 13-22).
- This correction may be achieved with the patient's head turned toward the side, or the patient may have to be repositioned supine.
- Correction is to be made at the lowest instrument setting and over the finger or thumb.

Clinical Notes

Patients typically expect the involvement to be on the same side as their symptoms, which may well be the case. However, as in many instances, referral or compensatory mechanisms may dictate the opposite side for treatment. It is helpful to address this with the patient at the time of treatment.

Shoulder or scapular involvement often attends the TMD. A recent case study provides examples of this and other clinical issues discussed in this chapter.[15]

Differential diagnoses that may be applicable would include, but are not limited to, mastoiditis, tooth abscess or infection, osteomyelitis, occipital neuralgia, stylomandibular sprain/strain (Ernest syndrome) and temporal tendonitis. TMJ adjusting may alleviate functional pain, but an underlying pathology may be present, thus confusing the clinical picture.

Outcome measures that would be particularly helpful would include a repeat of the instruments previously mentioned (MOM, VAS, various questionnaires) in addition to the TMJ Patient Outcome Questionnaire.

Text continued on p. 352

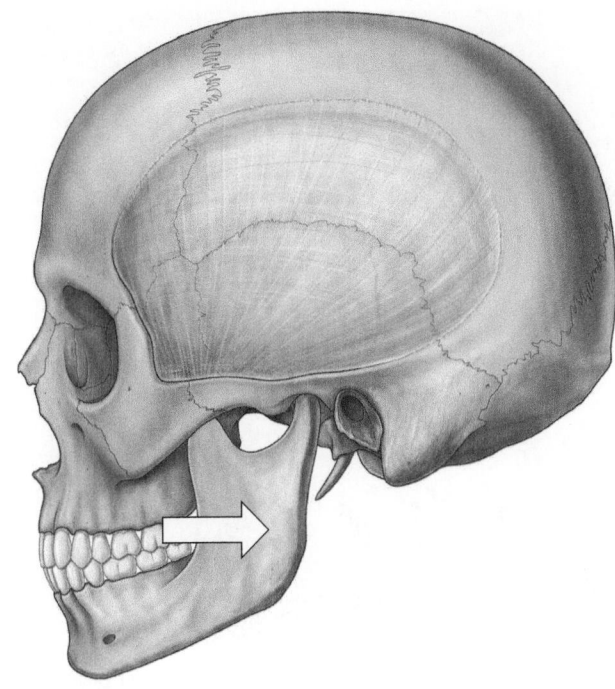

A

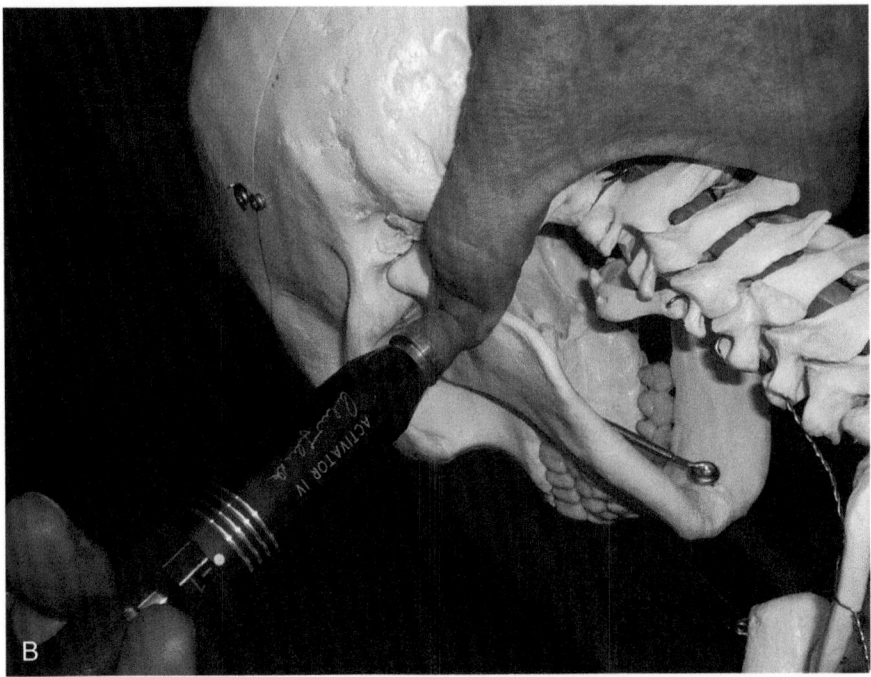

B

Figure 13-15 **A,** Anatomical Line of Drive (LOD) for lateral temporomandibular joint (TMJ). Refer to **B** for further clarity. **B,** Contact point and LOD for lateral TMJ. (*A, Modified from Drake RL, Vogl W, Mitchell AWM. Gray's anatomy for students. Edinburgh: Churchill Livingstone; 2005.*)

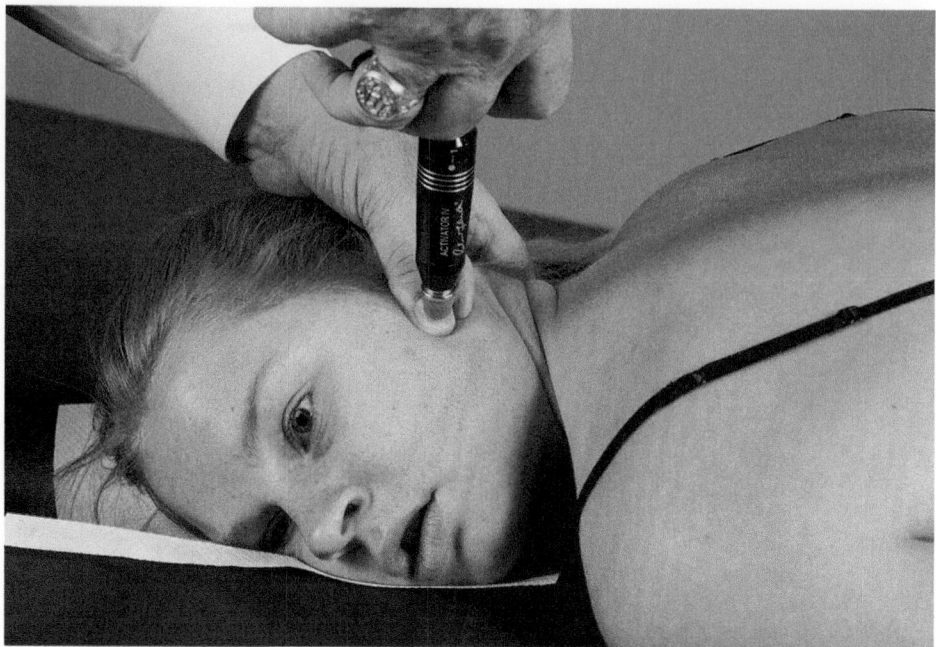

Figure 13-16 Adjustment for lateral temporomandibular joint. Line of Drive is lateral to medial.

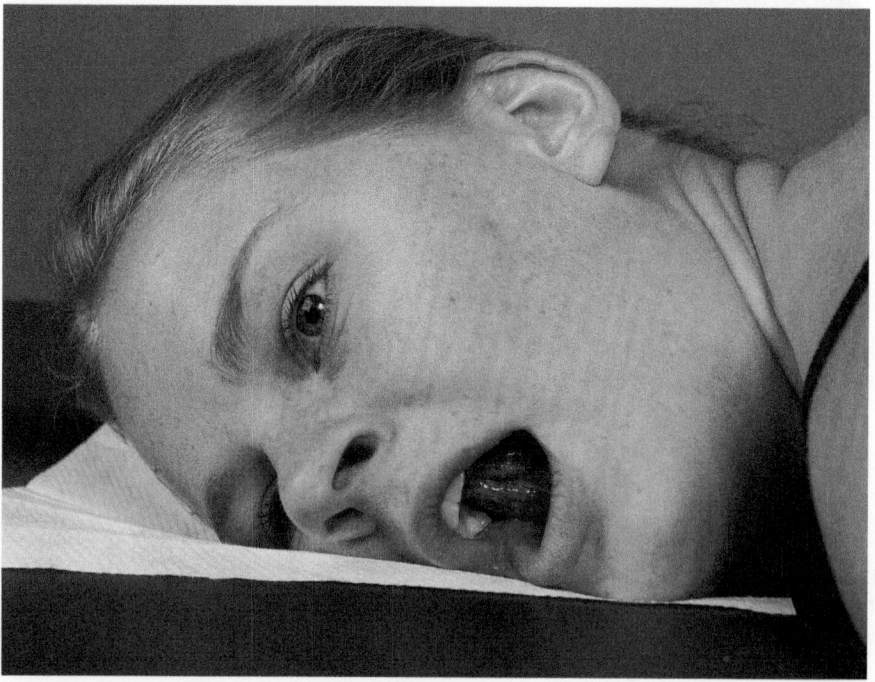

Figure 13-17 Isolation Test for posterior temporomandibular joint. Put the tip of the tongue on the roof of the mouth. All tests are to be performed in a neutral prone position with the face down.

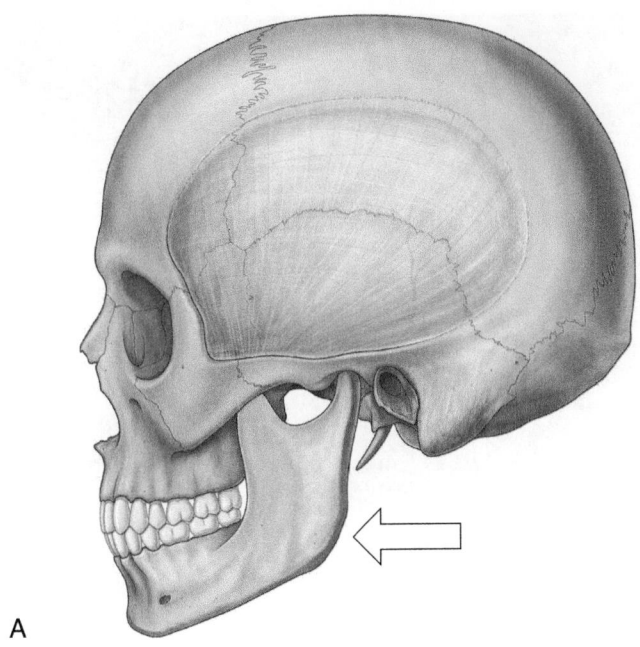

A

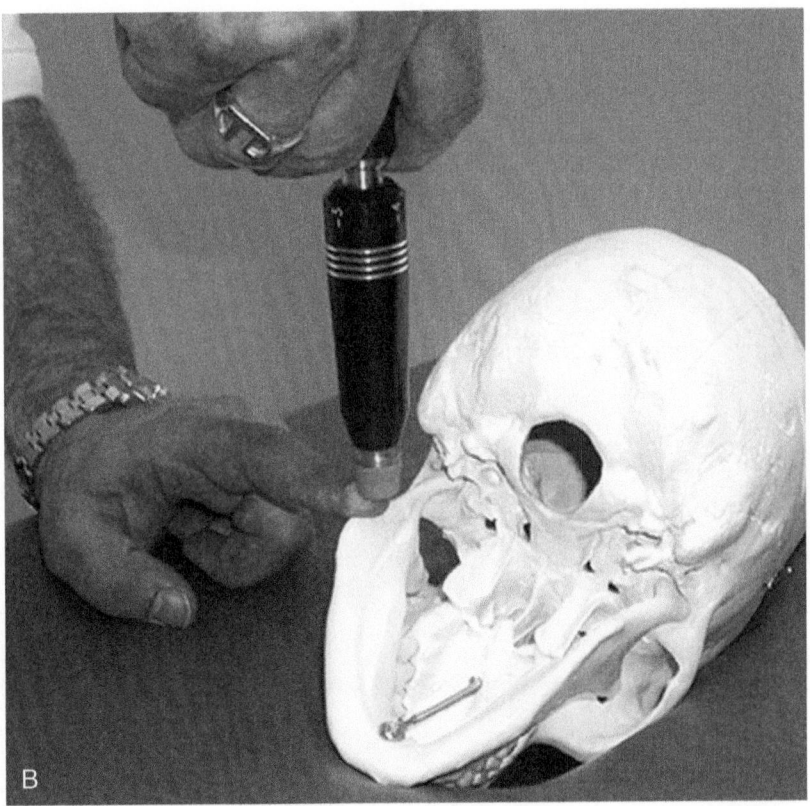

B

Figure 13-18 **A,** Anatomical Line of Drive (LOD) for posterior temporomandibular joint (TMJ). **B,** Contact point and LOD for posterior TMJ. *(A, Modified from Drake RL, Vogl W, Mitchell AWM. Gray's anatomy for students. Edinburgh: Churchill Livingstone; 2005.)*

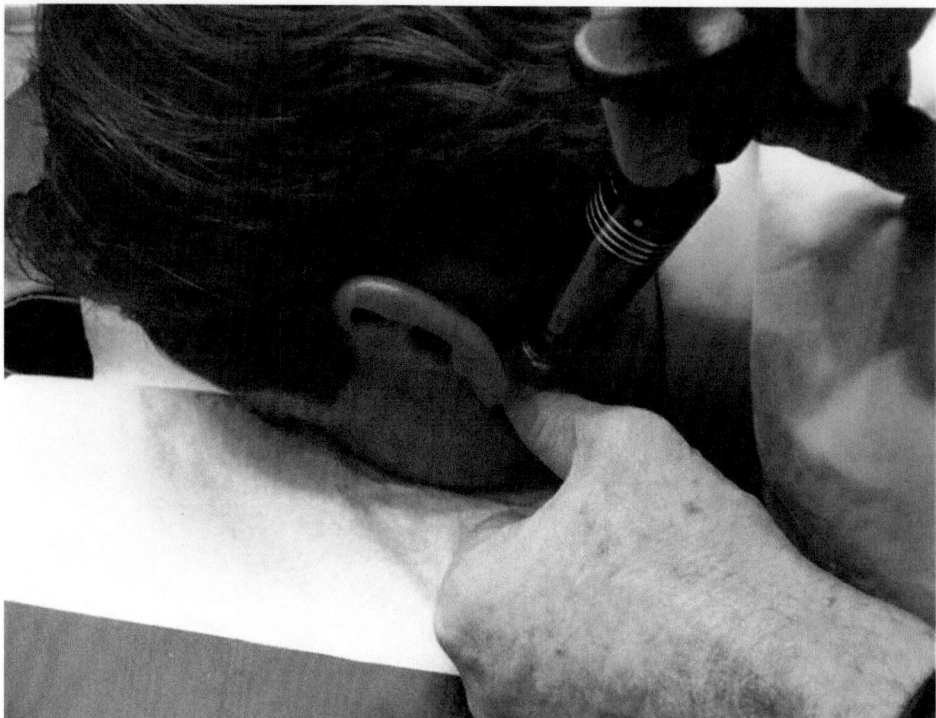

Figure 13-19   Adjustment for posterior temporomandibular joint. Line of Drive is posterior to anterior.

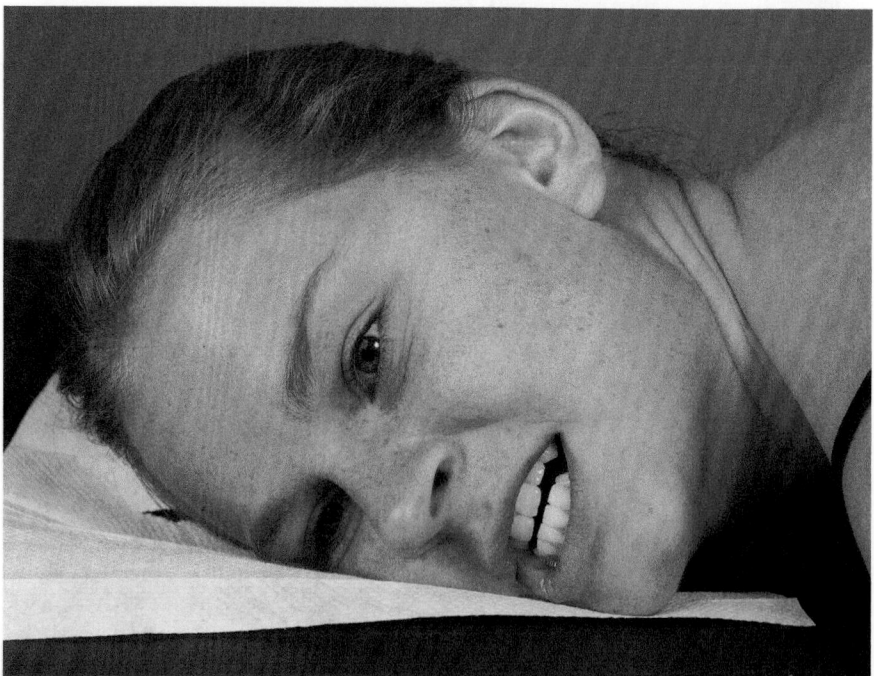

Figure 13-20   Isolation Test for anterior temporomandibular joint. The patient pushes or juts the jaw straight forward. All tests are to be performed in a neutral prone position with the face down.

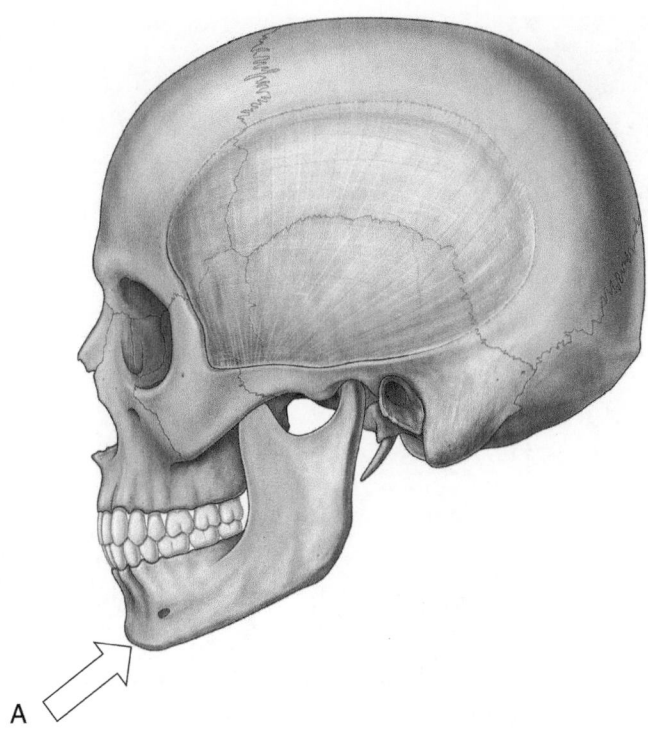

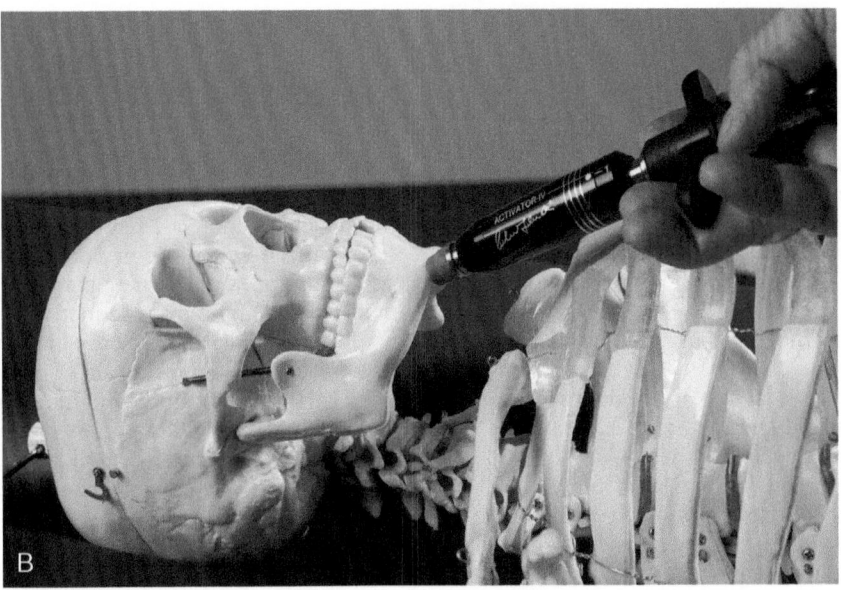

Figure 13-21 **A,** Anatomical Line of Drive (LOD) for anterior temporomandibular joint (TMJ). **B,** Contact point and LOD for anterior TMJ. *(A, Modified from Drake RL, Vogl W, Mitchell AWM. Gray's anatomy for students. Edinburgh: Churchill Livingstone; 2005.)*

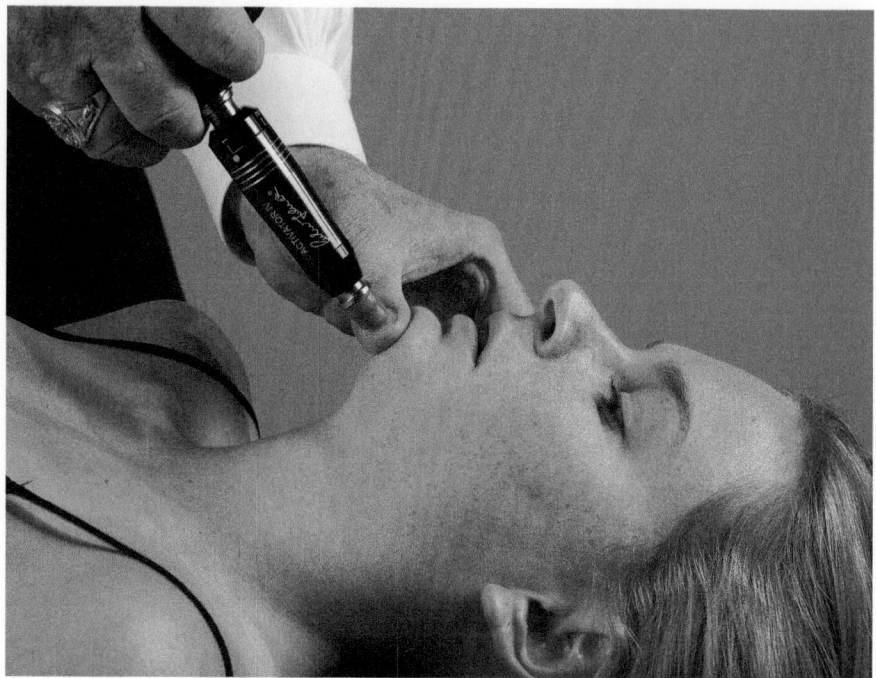

Figure 13-22   Adjustment for anterior temporomandibular joint. Line of Drive is inferior to superior and anterior to posterior.

Clinical Pearls

- Examine and treat the head, neck, and jaw as a motor unit.
- Referral or compensatory mechanisms may indicate adjusting on the opposite side of the pain.
- Allow for hidden abuse trauma in the case history.
- It is about reducing or eliminating unequal load distribution on the TMJs, and the adverse consequences thereof.
- It involves the restoration of functional balance and symmetry, as much as possible, of two joints connected by a single bone.

SUMMARY

We are performing joint adjustment/stabilization relative to the TMJs to balance neuroarticular function as best as possible. This is about joint function (i.e., bilaterally hinged joints that are designed to operate smoothly and evenly on both sides). It is about subsequent joint dysfunction/derangement with the adverse effects of uneven force load distribution throughout the joint complex(es). This also includes accessory structures such as muscles, tendons, ligaments, and secondarily involved joint complexes (e.g., the cervical spine), where there may be some shared or associated anatomy and function.

Restoring balance removes or minimizes the adverse affects of unequal load distribution on the TMJs, in effect improving function, motion, and the reduction/elimination of pain. This is joint work, not bite/occlusal work, although there may be occlusal consequences. This is a joint complex for which symmetry, balance, and neuronal control are the issues, similar to any other joint complex that we address, whether spinal or otherwise.

Our desire is for whole structure balance and symmetry; the more integrated our approach, the more stable the structure, and ultimately the function. Thus the global view of the head, neck, and jaw as a motor unit. Normal function is without restriction or pain, and it is as balanced and symmetrical as possible.

See the summary for testing and adjusting of the TMJ in Table 13-1.

Table 13-1 Summary Table of Tests and Adjustments for the Temporomandibular Joint

Articular Dysfunction	Test	ADJUSTMENT	
		Contact Point	Line of Drive
Anterior Extension	Instruct the patient to "open your mouth wide"	Anterior and inferior aspect of the neck of the coronoid process as indicated by the Short/Long Rule	Anterior to posterior and inferior to superior without any medial or lateral angle, with the instrument directed toward the EAM
Superior	Instruct the patient to "bite down"	Body of the ramus of the mandible inferior to the zygomatic arch as indicated by the Short/Long Rule	Superior to inferior through the plane of the ramus
Lateral	Instruct the patient to "slide or push your jaw sideways" toward the PD side. If no reactivity, instruct the patient to slide the jaw to the Opposite PD side.	The ramus, halfway between the angle of the mandible and the condyle on the side indicated by Pressure Testing	Lateral to medial
Posterior	Instruct the patient to "put the tip of your tongue on the back of the roof of your mouth"	Posterior edge of the ramus where it meets the angle of the mandible as indicated by the Short/Long Rule	Posterior to anterior
Anterior	Instruct the patient to "push/jut your *jaw* straight forward"	Mental tubercle on the side of correction as indicated by the Short/Long Rule	Inferior to superior and anterior to posterior with the instrument directed toward the EAM

EAM, External auditory meatus; PD, Pelvic Deficiency.

RELATED RESEARCH

Boxes 13-1 and 13-2 provide related research on the AM of TMJ disorders.

Box 13-1

Reference: DeVocht JW, Long CR, Zeitler DL, Schaeffer W. Chiropractic treatment of temporomandibular disorders using the Activator Adjusting Instrument: a prospective case series. J Manipulative Physiol Ther. 2003;26(7):421-5.

ABSTRACT
OBJECTIVE
To determine whether there was a basis for the treatment of temporomandibular disease (TMD) using the chiropractic protocol developed by Activator Methods, International

SETTING
Private, solo practice of an Activator Advanced Proficiency Rated chiropractor with 15 years' experience

DESIGN
Prospective case series

PARTICIPANTS
Nine adult volunteers with articular TMD recruited from the practice of the treating clinician

MAIN OUTCOME MEASURES
Change from baseline to follow-up of Visual Analog Scale (VAS) for temporomandibular joint (TMJ) pain and maximum active mouth opening without pain

INTERVENTIONS
Full spine and TMJ adjusting in accordance with the advanced protocol of Activator Methods, International. Participants were typically seen

Continued

Box 13-1—cont'd

three times per week for 2 weeks and according to ndividual progress thereafter for 6 additional weeks.

RESULTS
Eight participants completed outcome assessments. The median VAS decrease was 45 mm (range, 21-71 mm); all experienced improvement. The median increase in mouth opening was 9 mm (range, 1-15 mm); all showed improvement.

CONCLUSION
Results of this prospective case series indicated that the TMD symptoms of these participants improved after a course of treatment that used the Activator Methods, International Protocol. Consequently, further investigation into this type of chiropractic treatment for patients with the articular type of TMD is warranted.

Box 13-2

Reference: DeVocht JW, Schaeffer W, Lawrence DJ. Chiropractic treatment of temporomandibular disorders using the Activator Adjusting Instrument and protocol. Alternative Therapies. 2005; 11(6):70-3.

ABSTRACT
OBJECTIVE
To describe the chiropractic management of a 30-year-old woman with temporomandibular joint (TMJ) pain and to discuss the general origin and management of TMJ conditions

CLINICAL FEATURES
The patient suffered from daily unremitting jaw pain for 7 years; this pain was the apparent sequela of a series of eight root canals performed on the same tooth. Pain radiated from her TMJ into her shoulder and was accompanied by headache, tinnitus, impaired hearing, and a feeling of congestion in her right ear. Symptoms were not reduced by medication or other dental treatments.

OUTCOME AND INTERVENTION
The patient underwent a series of chiropractic treatments with the instrument and protocol of Activator Methods, International. During the first 5 months, her Visual Analog Scale rating of jaw pain decreased from 60 (on a scale of 1 to 100) to 9, her ability to eat solid foods increased, her headache intensity and frequency diminished, and her maximum mouth opening without pain measurement increased from 22 to 28 mm. Overall, 20 months of chiropractic treatment along with 2 concurrent months of massage therapy yielded slow but continual progress that finally resulted in total resolution of all symptoms except some fullness in the right cheek.

CONCLUSION
Use of the Activator Method Protocol of chiropractic treatment was beneficial for this patient and merits further study in similar cases.

ACKNOWLEDGMENT

The graphics for Figures 13-1 and 13-2 were generated by Glen Williamson of the Palmer Center for Chiropractic Research. They are copyrighted © 2006 by Data Trace Publishing Company, originally published in *DC Tracts*, 2006, Volume 18, Number 4, pages 4 and 5, and are reproduced here with permission.

REFERENCES

1. Sindelar BJ, Herring SW. Soft tissue mechanics of the temporomandibular joint. Cells Tissues Organs. 2005;180(1):36-43.
2. Evcik D, Aksoy O. Relationship between head posture and temporomandibular dysfunction syndrome. J Musculoskel Pain. 2004;12(2):19-24.
3. Curl DD. Whiplash and temporomandibular joint injury: principles of detection and management. In: Foreman S, Croft A, editors.

Whiplash injuries: the cervical acceleration/deceleration syndrome. 3rd ed. Philadelphia: Lippincott Williams & Wilkins; 2007. p. 452-98.

4. Tomas X, Pomes J, Berenguer J, Quinto L, Nicolau C, Mercader JM, et al. MR imaging of temporomandibular joint dysfunction: a pictorial review. Radiographics. 2006;26(3):765-81.

5. Steed PA, Wexler GB. Temporomandibular disorders—traumatic etiology vs. nontraumatic etiology: a clinical and methodological inquiry into symptomatology and treatment outcomes. Cranio. 2001;19(3):188-94.

6. Greene CS. The etiology of temporomandibular disorders: implications for treatment. J Orofac Pain. 2001;15(2):93-105.

7. National Institutes of Health (NIH). NIH technology assessment statement: management of temporomandibular disorders. Bethesda (MD): NIH; 1996. p. 1-31.

8. D'Attilio M, Filippi MR, Femminella B, Festa F, Tecco S. The influence of an experimentally-induced malocclusion on vertebral alignment in rats: a controlled pilot study. Cranio. 2005;23(2):119-29.

9. Dworkin SF, LeResche L. Research diagnostic criteria for temporomandibular disorders: review, criteria, examinations and specifications, critique. J.Craniomandib Disord. 1992;6(4):301-55.

10. Schmitter M, Kress B, Rammelsberg P. Temporomandibular joint pathosis in patients with myofascial pain: a comparative analysis of magnetic resonance imaging and a clinical examination based on a specific set of criteria. Oral Surg Oral Med Oral Pathol Oral Radiol Endod. 2004;97(3):318-24.

11. Haiter-Neto F, Hollender L, Barclay P, Maravilla KR. Disk position and the bilaminar zone of the temporomandibular joint in asymptomatic young individuals by magnetic resonance imaging. Oral Surg Oral Med Oral Pathol Oral Radiol Endod. 2002;94(3):372-8.

12. Agency for Healthcare Research and Quality (AHRQ). Study of the per-patient cost and efficacy of treatment for temporomandibular joint disorders (AHRQ Publication No. 290-96-0009). Washington (DC): The Lewin Group; 2001. p. 1-72.

13. ECRI. Temporomandibular articular disorders: selected treatments. Plymouth Meeting (PA): Health Technology Assessment Information Service (ECRI); 2001.

14. DeVocht JW, Long CR, Zeitler DL, Schaeffer W. Chiropractic treatment of temporomandibular disorders using the Activator Adjusting Instrument: a prospective case series. J Manipulative Physiol Ther. 2003;26(7):421-5.

15. DeVocht JW, Schaeffer W, Lawrence DJ. Chiropractic treatment of temporomandibular disorders using the Activator Adjusting Instrument and protocol. Altern Ther Health Med. 2005;11(6):70-3.

14

ADDITIONAL TESTS AND ADJUSTMENTS FOR THE KNEE AND RELATED STRUCTURES

Evaluation of the knee and related structures is indicated when a patient complains of pain within the joint or periarticular soft tissue, swelling with or without pain, joint instability, or joint stiffness. The knee is a complex joint, and its fluid motion is essential for normal gait, posture, and balance.

A thorough assessment of the knee and its related structures should be performed when a patient suffers from any of the following conditions:

- Reduction or alteration of knee range of motion
- Chondromalacia of the patella
- Osgood-Schlatter syndrome
- Shin splints
- Overpronation of the ankle
- Patellar effusion or bursitis of the knee
- Posterior thigh/knee pain
- Referred pain to the ankle or foot

Complaints of knee pain or discomfort include intermittent clicking or locking of the joint and pain exacerbated by long periods of standing. Because of its role in weight bearing, gait, and mobility, the knee is subject to the degenerative changes characteristic of osteoarthritis.[1,2]

KNEE RANGES OF MOTION

The knee is a complex bicondylar joint. The freely movable articulation between the femur and the tibia is anatomically classified as a ginglymus, or hinge joint, although its movements are more complex in that they involve both rotation and sliding movements.[3] An important feature of the knee is its cartilaginous meniscus, with biconcave discs located between the femoral condyles and the tibial plateau. A torn meniscus can produce fragments of cartilage, often referred to as "joint mice," that can migrate around the interior of the joint capsule and restrict range of motion or produce pain.[4]

The patella glides in the trochlear groove on the anterior aspect of the distal femur between the femoral condyles as the knee is extended and flexed. Erosion or other damage to the articular cartilage on the posterior surface of the patella or on the articular surfaces of the trochlear groove can impair the normally smooth gliding motion of the patella during flexion and extension. As a result, a patellar misalignment syndrome may develop.[5,6]

Four major ligaments maintain the anatomical integrity of the knee joint: the medial and lateral collateral ligaments and the anterior and posterior cruciate ligaments.[3] Ligamentous laxity, especially of the cruciate and medial collateral ligaments, can make the knee unstable and vulnerable to both recurrent injury and degenerative changes.[6] Instability of the joint typically leads to gait irregularities that affect the toe-off, swing-through, and heel-strike phases of gait. Be especially alert for "stiff-legged" or arching motion during the swing-through phase of gait. After toe-off, the knee normally flexes and then extends just before heel-strike. In a normal walking gait, knee flexion enables the foot to clear the ground during swing-through. The patient with an unstable knee, regardless of whether it is painful, often adapts to the instability by habitually keeping the knee in extension between toe-off and heel-strike.[7,8]

Stiffness or swelling that limits range of motion of the knee can contribute to gait irregularity. The primary motions of the knee are flexion and extension in the sagittal plane. In addition, the bicondylar structure of the joint allows limited external and internal rotation of the tibia. Average range of motion values for the knee are listed in Box 14-1.[7,9,10]

Active range of motion of the knee can be assessed in part by observing gait. In addition, active extension, internal rotation, and external rotation ranges of motion can be evaluated while the patient sits on the edge of the adjusting or examining table with the legs hanging over the side. Ask the patient to fully extend

Box 14-1	**Knee Ranges of Motion**
Flexion/Extension	135 degrees*
Internal Rotation	10 degrees
External Rotation	10 degrees

The range-of-motion values listed here and elsewhere in *The Activator Method* are averages of values published in various sources and should not be interpreted as "normal" for a given patient. Ranges of motion may be influenced by factors such as age, gender, weight, build, and general physical activity.[15,17,18]

*Average flexion of the knee from a straight, neutral position is 135 degrees. Normal extension from the neutral position is 0 degrees, although there may be a few degrees of hyperextension as part of joint end play.

each leg at the knee. Then ask the patient to demonstrate active internal and external rotation by rotating the feet medially and laterally. Examine active flexion of the knee by positioning the patient prone on the table. Then ask the patient to bring each knee into full flexion. Inspect active ranges of motion, while observing for smooth, fluid movements and bilateral symmetry. Examine the knee for passive range of motion in all four directions. Be alert for crepitus, pain, limited motion, and restricted joint end play.

When a patient shows evidence of reduced or altered range of motion of the knee, perform Stress Tests and adjustments as necessary for the following misalignments:

- External rotation of the proximal tibia
- Internal rotation of the proximal tibia
- Anterior proximal head of the tibia
- Posterior proximal head of the tibia

ORTHOPEDIC TESTING OF THE KNEE

The primary flexors of the knee are the hamstrings in the posterior thigh; the extensors are the quadriceps group of muscles on the anterior thigh.[3] Muscle strength can be assessed by resisted range of motion testing performed manually.[11] Another effective way of testing muscle strength, however, is to ask the patient to squat down from a standing position and then to slowly stand up again using the muscles of the legs. Look for symmetry and coordinated movement as the patient squats and stands back up. Weakness in the quadriceps may be evident if the patient has difficulty returning to an upright position.

Stretching or tears in the medial collateral ligament are relatively common in athletes involved in body contact sports.[12] A blow to the lateral aspect of the knee tends to open the medial joint compartment by applying a valgus force to the medial knee tissues. Apley's distraction test can be used to identify collateral ligament involvement after a knee injury.[4] To perform the distraction test, place the patient prone. Passively flex the knee to 90 degrees by firmly grasping the lower leg near the ankle with one hand. Rotate the tibia laterally (externally) and pull up on the lower leg while using the other hand to keep the thigh from lifting off the table. An alternate method of performing the test is for the examiner to place one knee or shin on the posterior aspect of the patient's thigh and to use both hands to laterally rotate and lift the lower leg. Medial knee pain with the distraction maneuver suggests injury to the medial collateral ligament.

To assess the integrity of the medial collateral ligament, perform a valgus stress maneuver.[4,7] Have the patient sit on the side of the table. Passively lift the leg into extension and hold the lower leg firmly with one hand. Use the palm of the other hand to apply lateral-to-medial stress to the knee. Opening of the joint space on the medial aspect of the knee indicates laxity or tearing of the medial collateral ligament.

Although it is damaged far less frequently than the medial collateral ligament, the lateral collateral ligament of the knee can be tested in similar fashion. To perform Apley's distraction test, place the patient prone and flex the knee to 90 degrees. Rotate the tibia medially (internally) and pull up on the leg while applying resistance to the posterior thigh. Lateral knee pain during this maneuver indicates lateral collateral ligament involvement. To check the integrity of the ligament, use a varus stress maneuver.[4,7] With the patient seated on the side of the table, passively extend the knee and hold the leg firmly with one hand while using the palm of the other hand to apply medial-to-lateral stress to the knee. Look for opening of the joint space on the lateral aspect of the knee.

The intracapsular cruciate ligaments stabilize the knee joint by restricting glide of the tibia relative to the femur in an anterior and posterior direction.[3] Evaluate the integrity of the cruciate ligaments with anterior and posterior drawer maneuvers.[12] To perform the drawer maneuvers, position the patient supine on the table with the knees flexed and the feet flat on the table. Sit on the feet, trapping them between the posterior thigh and the table to prevent them from sliding during performance of the maneuver.

To perform the anterior drawer maneuver, grasp the proximal tibia firmly with both hands and attempt to pull it anteriorly relative to the femur. More than a few millimeters of anterior movement suggests laxity or a possible tear of the anterior cruciate ligament. To perform the posterior drawer maneuver, keep the patient in the same position. Grasp the proximal tibia firmly with both hands and attempt to push it posteriorly relative to the femur. Again, movement of more than a few millimeters of posterior motion suggests laxity or a possible tear of the posterior cruciate ligament.

It should be noted there is considerable variation among writers regarding the patient's leg position during performance of the anterior and posterior drawer sign for assessment of the anterior and posterior cruciate ligaments of the knee. Both Hoppenfeld and Mazion instruct the examiner to sit on the patient's feet during performance of the drawer tests, but Hoppenfeld recommends the test be performed with the patient's knees flexed to 90 degrees; Mazion suggests that they should be flexed to 45 degrees.[7,13] Kulund[14] recommends that the anterior drawer test should be performed with the knees flexed to 25 degrees at one point in his text, and to only 15 degrees at another point. (The posterior drawer maneuver described by Kulund is still performed with the knees flexed to 90 degrees.) The reason for reducing flexion of the knees during the anterior drawer test, Kulund contends, is to limit hamstring restriction and the restraints to joint motion provided by the menisci.[14] Kulund further recommends that, instead of stabilizing the patient's feet by sitting on them, the examiner should stabilize the knee by pushing superiorly on the thigh while pulling anteriorly and inferiorly on the lower leg.[14]

Diagnostic Imaging

Joint integrity, especially of the meniscus, can be evaluated through magnetic resonance imaging (MRI). Its use and the improved quality of images can be beneficial in determining the need for orthopedic referral and surgical intervention. The number one orthopedic procedure that is performed is meniscectomy. Within weeks of a partial meniscectomy, acceleration of the degenerative process occurs in the knee joint. Standard orthopedic procedure dictates surgical removal of a documented torn meniscus. MRI is the preferred diagnostic evaluation tool; however, MRI cannot differentiate between an active meniscal tear and healing via fibrovascular scar tissue, that is, a stable tear. A definitive meniscus tear can be evaluated only by visual inspection as in arthroscopic invasion or possibly by gadolinium injection imaging.[15,16] Each patient should be assessed through review of the results of examination, range of motion, orthopedic tests, and symptoms; MRI findings alone should not be relied on to determine the difference between an active meniscal tear and a stable tear.[16]

COMMON CONDITIONS

Because the knee, the largest joint in the body, is a major weight-bearing articulation, acute and chronic injuries have a substantial impact on patient mobility and comfort. A 1980 study reported that injuries to the knee and ankle accounted for 25% of all athletic injuries.[17] Problems with the knee can manifest through a wide variety of symptoms.

Although a high proportion of knee injuries result from frank trauma, overuse injuries and biomechanical dysfunction account for a significant proportion of knee problems as well. Leg Length Inequality (LLI) causes unequal stresses and strains to the supporting knee joints and has been implicated in numerous lower extremity pain and stress syndromes such as patellar tendonitis, patellofemoral pain syndrome, and iliotibial band syndrome with lateral knee pain.[18,19] Klein[1] examined the relationship between gait alteration and LLI and found a mechanism for increased potential for knee injury. On the side of LLI, the ankle was found to be commonly pronated as the foot was planted, which forces the foot outward. Consequently, the knee is forced into valgus, causing an excessive tibial torsion and creating undue stress on the medial knee ligaments, thereby increasing the potential for knee injury.[20,21]

A growing body of evidence suggests that conservative management and injury prevention strategies for even serious injuries to the knee yield the most effective clinical outcomes.[12,22,23] Many of the following conditions may be related to neuroarticular dysfunction of the knee that can be adjusted with the use of low force and the highly specific Activator Adjusting Instrument.

Chondromalacia of the Patella

Anterior knee pain due to patellofemoral dysfunction or chondromalacia patella may be the most troublesome, ubiquitous overuse syndrome in athletics.[24] When a patient suffers from knee pain that is exacerbated by climbing stairs or standing up from a sitting or squatting position, consider misalignment of the patella in the trochlear groove. Inspect the patellae for bilateral positional symmetry and fluid motion during extension and flexion.

The patella rides up and down the trochlear groove of the femur as the knee extends and flexes. Tension in the patellar tendon locks the patella into the groove when the knee is flexed, and in this position, only the bony anterior surface is palpable. When the knee is fully extended with the quadriceps muscles relaxed, however, the patella is normally quite mobile and can be pushed laterally, medially, inferiorly, and superiorly.[24]

Also, when the knee is in an extended, neutral position, portions of the cartilage-covered posterior surface of the patella are palpable from both medial and lateral aspects. Examination findings of roughness on the borders of the patellar cartilage may be early indications of osteoarthritis, or they may indicate *chondromalacia patella* (literally, a degenerative softening of the articular cartilage), which can impair the smooth motion of the patella in the trochlear groove.[3,24-26]

Further examination of the patella may include the patellar grind test. With the patient supine and the knee in a relaxed, extended position, press down on the superior border of the patella. Apply light resistance to the patella as the patient contracts the quadriceps muscle of the anterior thigh. Note any crepitus as the patella slides proximally in the trochlear groove, and be alert to patient complaints of pain during the maneuver. Pain or grinding associated with the motion of the patella suggests chondromalacia or other cartilage defects of the articulation.[14] Patellofemoral instability and resultant anterior knee pain have been associated with external tibial rotation.[27]

When patellar motion is not smooth, or when pain accompanies the motion, perform Stress Tests and adjustments as necessary for the following involvements:
- Inferior patella
- Lateral patella
- External rotation of the tibia
- Superior patella
- Quadriceps

Detailed instructions for performing Stress Tests and adjustments where indicated for these neuroarticular dysfunctions are given later in this chapter.

Osgood-Schlatter Syndrome

Tenderness and swelling at the insertion of the patellar tendon on the tibia is an indication of osteochondrosis of the tibial tubercle, or Osgood-Schlatter syndrome. The condition is frequently referred to as Osgood-Schlatter *disease*, although that descriptor may be a little extreme. Nevertheless, Osgood-Schlatter syndrome is a relatively common cause of knee complaints, especially in active adolescents and young adults.[5-7,14]

Because the epiphyseal growth plate in youngsters is not fully ossified, tension in the patellar tendon can irritate and provoke a local inflammatory response in the region of the tibial tubercle. The inflammatory response is variously described as an apophysitis, a tibial epiphysitis, or a patellar ligament (tendon) avulsion. Osgood-Schlatter syndrome is exacerbated by strenuous physical activity with forceful extension of the knee by the quadriceps group of muscles. Activities such as competitive running, tennis, snow and water skiing, skateboarding, basketball, and cycling all can contribute to development of osteochondrosis of the tibial tubercle.[6,28]

Occasionally, it may be advisable to tape and limit knee mobility during an acute exacerbation of Osgood-Schlatter syndrome. A simple infrapatellar or knee strap with a velcro closure is suggested as one method of limiting the symptoms of Osgood-Schlatter syndrome, although the benefit of such an intervention may be more psychological than physical.[6,14] Most often, however, the condition is self-limiting if the activities that provoke it are restricted. That, of course, is the biggest challenge in managing most cases of Osgood-Schlatter syndrome, because healthy children are rarely willing to stay inactive.

On rare occasions, the patellar tendon can be avulsed from its tibial insertion. The tendon will be flaccid and very painful on palpation, and the patella may be drawn asymmetrically up the trochlear groove. Other complications of recurring or unresolved Osgood-Schlatter syndrome may include genu recurvatum (reverse curvature or hyperextension malposition of the knee), malposition of the patella, and chondromalacia patella.[6]

Pain at the insertion of the patellar tendon on the tibia can result from increased tension on the tendon with a torqued tibia or with hypertonicity of the quadriceps muscle group. Pain from increased tension in the tendon is exacerbated when the leg is extended against resistance, as when climbing stairs or standing up from a sitting or squatting position.

For a patient who presents with a history of Osgood-Schlatter syndrome, perform Stress Tests and adjustments as necessary for at least the following involvements:
- Anterior proximal head of the tibia
- External rotation of the proximal head of the tibia

- Lateral patella
- Superior patella
- Inferior patella

Detailed instructions for performing Stress Tests and adjustments when indicated for these neuroarticular dysfunctions are given later in this chapter.

Shin Splints

Shin splints are painful contractures and spasms of leg muscles that occur frequently in runners and joggers, especially when they do not warm up before engaging in strenuous activity. Errors in training, muscle dysfunction or disease, improper biomechanics of running, and inadequate shock absorption capacity of running shoes can contribute to the development of shin splints.[14,29] The phenomenon of shin splints or runner's legs is familiar to those who run frequently and to the weekend athlete who participates only intermittently in running or related sports.

Pain on resisted dorsiflexion and inversion of the foot suggests strain injury to the tibialis anterior muscle whose belly makes up most of the soft tissue mass of the anterior tibial compartment. This muscle appears to be the most frequently involved in typical "anterior exertional compartment syndrome."[5] The compartment is bound medially by the shaft of the tibia and posteriorly by the fibula. Neuroarticular dysfunction of the fibula may increase tension in the anterior compartment muscles by stressing the interosseous ligament. Participation in contact sports like rugby, football, and hockey may predispose a patient to traumatic misalignment of the fibula. Other mechanisms in the development of shin splints include stress microfracture of the tibia, periostitis of the tibia, and ischemic or traumatic myositis of the soft tissues of the compartments that are symptomatic.[5]

The pain of shin splints, especially of the anterior leg compartment, is a relatively common complaint in physically active patients. Fortunately, the condition is generally self-limiting, and interventions such as change of foot wear, choice of running surface, and proper training can be productive in preventing runner's legs. Rest, elevation, and application of ice to the leg are generally recognized as appropriate and effective interventions with acute shin splints.[14] Be alert, however, to indications of the more serious anterior compartment syndrome. When leg pain is not relieved by normal conservative interventions and preventive strategies, consider injury to the microvasculature of the leg from overuse injury, trauma or thrombotic events.[24] Ischemic injury, muscle necrosis, fibrotic repair, and denervation or nerve entrapment can have devastating consequences for the patient with anterior compartment syndrome. If the condition develops into the full manifestations of Volkmann's ischemic contracture, the patient may experience chronic leg pain on exertion, paresthesias, and paralysis with foot drop on the side of involvement from ischemic atrophy of the tibialis anterior muscle.[5,14] When a patient presents with anterior leg pain or shin splints, perform Stress Tests and adjustments as necessary for the following neuroarticular dysfunctions:
- Lateral fibula
- Posterior-superior proximal head of the fibula
- Posterior distal fibula

Detailed instructions for performing Stress Tests and adjustments where indicated for these neuroarticular dysfunctions are provided later in this chapter.

Overpronation of the Ankle

With any knee complaint, it is very important to assess the biomechanics of the foot and ankle. Observation of wear patterns on the soles of the patient's shoes and weight-bearing evaluation of the ankles for excessive pronation should be performed. Almost all knee problems develop from poor biomechanics and overuse, and many of these injuries are associated with foot pronation.[30] Excessive and chronic pronation of the ankle tends to result in medial overstress of the Achilles tendon that causes an inflammatory process and thus, Achilles tendonitis (see Chapter 15). Because internal tibial torsion results from ankle overpronation, the iliotibial band is overstretched, causing friction at its insertion on the medial tibial plateau, leading to knee pain and misalignment and imbalance through the hips and pelvis. The vast majority of acute anterior cruciate ligament (ACL) tears actually occur without any contact or direct trauma to the athlete's knee,[31] and the highest risk factor for ACL rupture is directly correlated with the amount of ankle pronation of the athlete.[32] According to Liebenson, "the most common biomechanical problem in the lower extremity is excessive pronation."[33]

When a patient presents with knee pain or neuroarticular dysfunction due to overpronation of the ankle, perform Stress Tests and adjustments as necessary for the following neuroarticular dysfunctions:
- Internal rotation of the proximal tibia
- Anterior proximal tibia
- Medial calcaneus (see Chapter 15)

- Medial navicular (see Chapter 15)
- Inferior first metatarsal and inferior medial first cuneiform (see Chapter 15)

Detailed instructions for performing Stress Tests and adjustments where indicated for the knee are provided later in this chapter.

Patellar Effusions and Bursitis of the Knee

Soft tissue swelling in and around the knee joint is a common manifestation of acute and chronic injury to the joint. Edematous fluid in the anterior portion of the joint deep to the patellar tendon makes it difficult or painful for the patient to extend the knee fully. Similarly, retropatellar effusion, or fluid accumulation in the articulation between the patella and the trochlear groove of the femur, also will restrict extension of the knee.[34]

The patient with a joint effusion of the knee will demonstrate an antalgic gait in which normal heel-strike is prevented by restricted knee extension. Instead of contacting the ground with the heel first, the patient tends to land on the ball of the foot, with the knee flexed and the foot and ankle in slight plantar flexion. In addition to exhibiting a "hopping" limp, the patient will shift standing weight to the good leg while holding the knee in flexion.

The patellar ballottement or patellar tap test can be used to identify a major effusion in the retropatellar region.[4] With the patient supine and the knee relaxed in extension, gently press the patella in an anterior-to-posterior direction into the trochlear groove of the femur. The presence of significant edematous fluid in the joint space will cause the patella to rebound rapidly.

Several bursae around the knee joint can become inflamed and cause pain and limited range of motion. The prepatellar bursa is situated between the bony anterior surface of the patella and the thin layer of skin and fascia overlying the bone. Blunt trauma to the kneecap from falls or blows in body contact sports appears to be a common cause of prepatellar bursitis in athletes.[14] Such trauma can produce dramatic swelling in the bursa, and the patella will feel spongy on palpation.

Prepatellar bursitis, also known as "housemaid's knee," can result from acute trauma to the knee. Often, however, the effusion can result from cumulative microtrauma as part of an occupational activity. The superficial and deep infrapatellar bursae can become irritated and swollen by prolonged kneeling, especially on rough surfaces. Carpet layers and roofers, for example, are especially vulnerable to developing infrapatellar effusion because so much of their work must be performed in a kneeling or squatting position.[35] When the bursae on the anterior aspect of the knee are inflamed, any movement toward full extension or flexion puts pressure on the swollen tissues and elicits an immediate pain response. A patient with bursitis of the knee tends to lock the knee into about 20 degrees of flexion and consequently adopts a stiff-legged antalgic gait. The pes anserine bursa is located just medial to the tibial tubercle, deep to the tendons of insertion of the sartorius, gracilis, and semitendinosus muscles. External rotation of the tibia exacerbates the pain of pes anserine bursitis, and the patient may adopt a toe-in gait and stance.

When a patient suffers from pain on extension or flexion of the knee and indications of subpatellar effusion or bursitis of the knee are noted, perform Stress Tests and adjustments as necessary for the following neuroarticular dysfunctions:
- Posterior proximal head of the tibia
- Externally rotated tibia
- Lateral patella
- Internally rotated tibia
- Inferior patella

Detailed instructions for performing Stress Tests and adjustments where indicated for these neuroarticular dysfunctions are given later in this chapter.

Posterior Thigh/Knee Pain

When the patient presents with pain behind the knee or into the posterior thigh, muscular hypertonicity or weakness may be involved. Both the hamstrings and the gastrocnemius cross the knee joint; therefore any imbalance in this functional unit may cause articular dysfunction, pressure, or pain in the knee. The biceps femoris in particular harbors trigger points that refer pain to the posterior knee and thigh. Active trigger points in both heads of the gastrocnemius muscle refer to the posterior knee.[36]

When a patient suffers from pain in the posterior thigh or knee, perform Stress Tests and adjustments as necessary for a posterior proximal tibia. It is most important to note that the hamstrings and gastrocnemius muscles should be assessed for neuroarticular dysfunction (see later in this chapter).

Pain Referred to the Ankle or Foot

The common peroneal nerve winds around the proximal fibula on its course down the lateral leg to the foot. Entrapment of the common peroneal nerve due to neuroarticular dysfunction of the fibula can refer pain to the lateral ankle and the dorsum of the foot. The common peroneal nerve is the lateral branch of the sciatic nerve; its terminal branches innervate the dorsiflexors and evertors of the foot and ankle. The deep peroneal nerve carries motor neurons from cord levels L4 and L5 to the anterior tibial muscle in the anterior tibial compartment. It is therefore the principal nerve that controls dorsiflexion of the foot. The superficial peroneal nerve, whose motor neurons are derived primarily from cord level S1, innervates the peroneus longus and brevis muscles, which are evertors of the foot. In addition to referred pain along the common peroneal nerve, entrapment of the nerve can produce foot drop.[37]

When a patient presents with referred pain to the foot and ankle or shows evidence of weakness in the dorsiflexors and evertors of the foot, perform Stress Tests and adjustments as necessary for the following neuroarticular dysfunctions:

• Posterior-superior proximal head of the fibula
• Lateral fibula
• Externally rotated proximal tibia
• Lateral patella

Detailed instructions for performing Stress Tests and adjustments where indicated for these neuroarticular dysfunctions are given later in this chapter.

CONCURRENT CONDITIONS OF THE KNEE

As a major weight-bearing articulation, the knee is subject to many stresses. The femur and the tibia are the longest bones in the body, and their lever action at the knee involves very large biomechanical stresses during normal mobility. Compressive forces at the knee are also enormous. One study suggests that "a 59-kg (130-lb) person puts about 390 pounds of force on his tibial plateau with each walking step."[14] Consequently, altered anatomical relationships of the bones that make up the knee joint would likely contribute to rapid degenerative changes.

Osteoarthritis, with its characteristic bone lipping and spurring, limits knee joint range of motion, affecting gait, posture, and general mobility.[38] Gaits adapted to pain-limited range of motion or altered biomechanics of the joint can contribute to neuroarticular dysfunction of the knee itself, and can predispose the patient to articular dysfunction of the ankle and hip joints as ways of compensating for abnormal posture and weight bearing. Careful monitoring of the patient with degenerative joint disease of the knee and appropriate adjustments of the knee and appropriate adjustments of

neuroarticular dysfunction can help to maintain as much mobility as possible and may even slow the progression of osteoarthritis.

Inflammatory arthritides, including rheumatoid arthritis, systemic lupus erythematosus, and Sjögren's syndrome, all involve intermittent and unpredictable exacerbations and remissions.[39] During an acute exacerbation of these chronic inflammatory conditions, intracapsular synovitis and periarticular soft tissue swelling may create enough pressure to produce malpositions of the joint.

Adjunctive and conservative therapy may be beneficial. Recent advancements offer additional conservative treatment options; one of these is the injection of Synvisc (Hylan G-F 20; Genzyme, Ridgefield, N.J.), Hyalagen, or Supartz (Seikagaku Corporation, Tokyo, Japan). These materials are converted from the combs of chickens into an injectable form that is not readily absorbed or broken down. Typically, Synvisc is injected into the knee joint through a series of three injections, and Hyalagen a series of five injections. Research has demonstrated very minimal adverse effects. However, those who have known allergies to chickens and eggs should undergo more intensive screening. These products are considered drugs and were approved for knee injection by the U.S. Food and Drug Administration in 1996. Recently, approval for use has been granted for treatment of the ankle. Injections are typically performed by an orthopedic specialist. The substance acts to enhance the natural lubrication qualities of the joint, considerably reducing pain levels. This allows the patient to develop strength, be more active, and, as a result, lose weight if needed.

The strength of the musculature around the knee joint is critically important. In particular, quadriceps weakness has been shown to be a primary risk factor for knee pain, disability, and the progression of joint damage in people with osteoarthritis of the knee.[40] Quadriceps weakness also is strongly associated with knee pain and disability, even when other factors are taken into account.[41] The major shock-absorbing mechanism of the knee is not the cartilage, but the muscle. It has been found in the 50 to 59 age group that the average strength of knee extensors will be reduced by approximately 50%, and this strength drops even more dramatically in the 60 to 69 and 70 to 79 age groups.[42] When strength training of the knee extensors was performed among a group of patients with osteoarthritic knee, pain was reduced by 43% and physical function was increased by 44%.[43]

TESTING AND ADJUSTING THE KNEE AND RELATED STRUCTURES

When patient complaints or examination findings indicate involvement of the knee and related structures, the following Stress Tests and adjustments will be performed as necessary. For the knee joint, check for the following neuroarticular dysfunctions:

- External rotation of the proximal tibia
- Internal rotation of the proximal tibia
- Anterior proximal head of the tibia
- Posterior proximal head of the tibia
- Genu valgus
- Genu varus
- Medial knee joint
- Lateral knee joint
- Medial distal femur

Also, check for these neuroarticular dysfunctions of the patella:

- Inferior patella
- Lateral patella
- Superior patella

Because both signs and symptoms of knee involvement and referred pain to the foot and ankle can arise from neuroarticular dysfunction of the fibula, check for the following:

- Posterior-superior proximal head of the fibula
- Lateral fibula

Tests for these neuroarticular dysfunctions are known as *Stress Tests*, that is, movements or maneuvers performed by the practitioner intended to stress the structure into *the direction of neuroarticular dysfunction*. For the adjustment, the Line of Drive (LOD) is in the direction *opposite* to the direction of neuroarticular dysfunction.

Finally, because of the importance of the surrounding soft tissues in knee stability, check the following muscles:

- Hamstrings
- Quadriceps
- Gastrocnemius/Soleus

External Rotation of the Proximal Tibia

External rotation of the proximal tibia should be considered when a patient presents with inferior medial knee pain over the pes anserine bursa, chondromalacia patella or "runner's knee," or unilateral toe-out foot flare on the side of involvement. In addition, be alert to an increased Q angle with valgus deformity or neuroarticular dysfunction of the knee. The Q angle is the acute angle formed at the intersection of a line drawn from the middle of the patella to the tibial tubercle and a line drawn from the anterior-superior iliac spine to the middle of the patella. Controversy is found in the literature regarding the Q angle and its relationship to chondromalacia patella. A Q angle greater than 15 to 20 degrees can indicate neuroarticular dysfunction of the patella and can predispose the patient to chondromalacia patella.[6,29] Research indicates that muscle imbalance is a contributing factor. Chondromalacia patella, now known as patellofemoral dysfunction, traditionally has been thought to be due to inhibition or weakness of the vastus medialis muscles, thus allowing the patella to track out of the femoral groove.[23] Vastus medialis inhibition is now discredited; in electromyography studies, no differences in vastus medialis and vastus lateralis activity was observed during stair climbing in controls and patients with patellofemoral dysfunction.[44] Now, patellofemoral instability and resultant anterior knee pain have been found to be associated with external tibial rotation.[34]

Both toe-out foot flare and valgus deformity may be visible on inspection of patient gait. Even if foot flare is not readily visible during gait inspection, the foot on the side of knee involvement typically shows greater toe-out flare when the patient is on the adjusting table in Position #1. The patella may appear to have asymmetrically shifted laterally because external torquing of the tibia increases tension in the patellar tendon, drawing it toward the lateral aspect of the trochlear groove.

Stress Test. To Stress Test an externally rotated proximal tibia, take a firm grasp with one hand over the posterior aspect of the leg at the level of the belly of the gastrocnemius muscle. Rotate the proximal tibia externally relative to the femur (Figure 14-1). Look for reactivity of the Pelvic Deficient (PD) leg in Position #1.

Adjustment. To adjust an externally rotated proximal tibial involvement, contact the anterior tibia just lateral to the anterior tibial tubercle. The LOD is lateral to medial (Figure 14-2).

When a patient suffers from concurrent complaints of hip pain and tightness of the hamstring or quadriceps muscles, external rotation of the tibia could externally rotate the distal end of the femur. Similarly, swelling and stiffness of the knee may be caused by rotation of the tibia on the femur. To avoid an incorrect interpretation of the Stress Test for the externally rotated proximal tibia, stabilize the femur by placing one hand over the thigh just above the knee, and perform the Stress Test with the other hand.

To ensure an effective adjustment of an externally rotated proximal tibia, slide the fingers of the stabilization hand between the proximal tibia and the table. Position the index and middle fingers over the tibial tubercle and spread the fingers

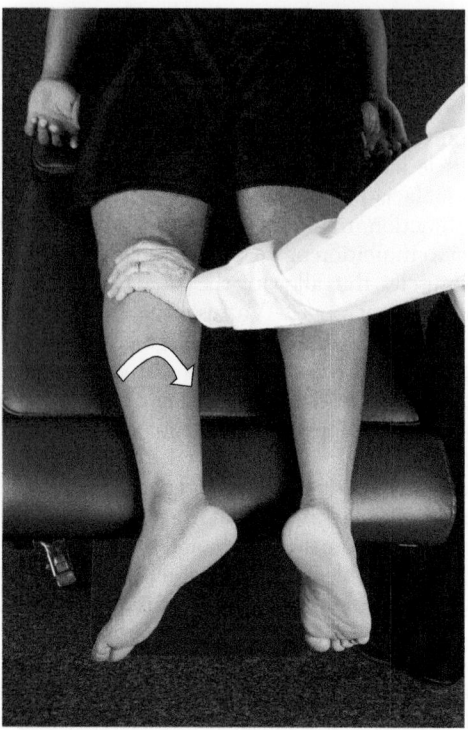

Figure 14-1 Stress Test for external rotation of the proximal tibia.

apart enough to accommodate the tip of the instrument. Use this "split-finger" position to stabilize the instrument during the adjustment.

Clinical Observations

External rotation of the proximal tibia is a relatively common occurrence that is associated with several sports activities. Sudden, forceful torquing forces can be applied to the tibia when an athlete pivots the body medially while keeping the foot planted firmly on the floor or ground. Activities like tennis, basketball, soccer, and football present risk of torquing the tibia when players make sudden, strenuous pivoting moves.

External rotation of the proximal tibia shifts the tibial tubercle away from the midline of the leg, thus increasing the Q angle. The patellar tendon is therefore pulled away from the midline and the patella is shifted laterally in the trochlear groove.[6,29]

Increased friction between the articular surface of the patella and the trochlear groove may then contribute to irritation and roughening of the articular cartilage characteristic of chondromalacia patella.

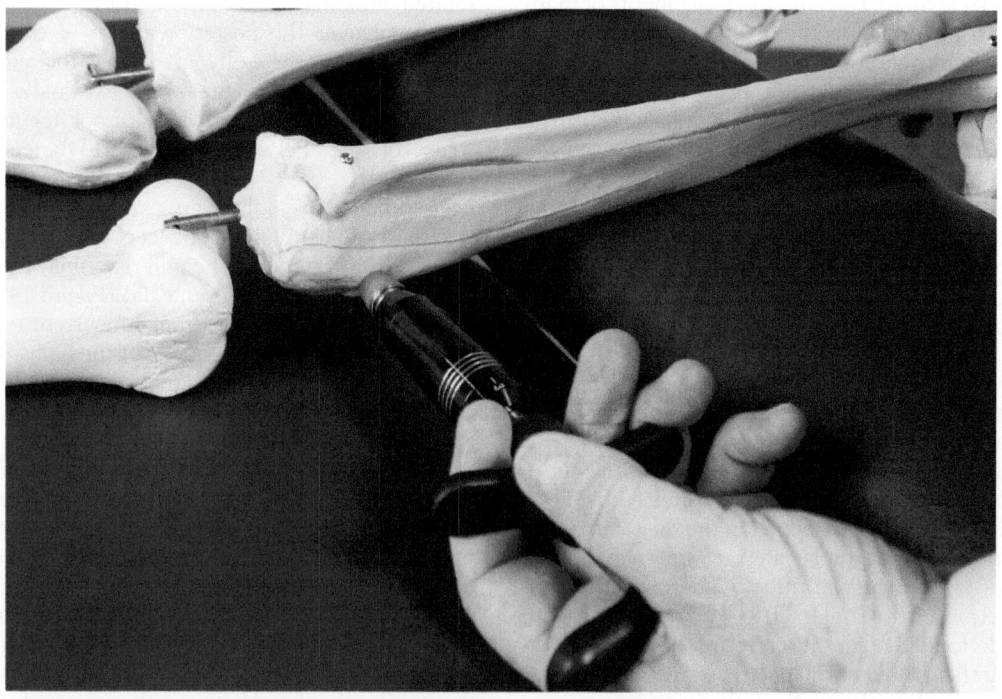

Figure 14-2 Adjustment for external rotation of the proximal tibia. Line of Drive is lateral to medial.

Internal Rotation of the Proximal Tibia

When a patient suffers from medial knee pain or pain referred to the calf muscles, restricted rotational range of motion, or swelling over the medial compartment of the knee joint, consider internal rotation of the proximal tibia.

Inspect the knee for a decreased Q angle with valgus deformity of the knee and toe-in foot flare. True toe-in foot flare or pigeon-toe is not likely to be observed, but the patient may demonstrate less than normal toe-out foot flare during gait or resting stance. Also, when the patient is in Position #1 on the adjusting table, the foot on the side of knee involvement may show less toe-out flare than the other foot.

Stress Test.   To Stress Test an internally rotated proximal tibia, take a firm grasp with one hand over the posterior aspect of the tibia at the level of the belly of the gastrocnemius. Rotate the proximal tibia internally relative to the femur (Figure 14-3). Look for reactivity of the PD leg in Position #1.

Adjustment.   To adjust an internally rotated proximal tibia, contact the anterior tibia just medial to the tibial tubercle. The LOD is straight medial to lateral (Figure 14-4).

To avoid incorrect interpretation of the Stress Test for medial rotation of the proximal tibia, stabilize the femur by placing one hand over the thigh, and perform the Stress Test with the other hand.

To ensure effective adjustment of an internally rotated proximal tibia, slide the fingers of the stabilization hand between the proximal tibia and the table. Position the index and middle fingers over the tibial tubercle, and spread the fingers apart enough to accommodate the tip of the instrument. Use the "split-finger" position to stabilize the instrument during the adjustment.

> ### Clinical Observations
> The mechanism of injury that produces an internally rotated proximal tibia is often traumatic strain or stretch to the tendons that define the medial border of the popliteal fossa. These are the tendons of the sartorius, gracilis, and semitendinosus muscles.
>
> Hyperextension injuries to the knee, blows to the anterolateral aspect of the shin, or sudden pivoting movements with the foot planted firmly on the ground can induce a torquing motion in the proximal tibia with internal rotation at the knee. Many athletic activities, including court games like tennis and basketball, as well as contact sports like soccer and rugby, can result in torquing injuries to the tibia, thereby producing internal or external rotation.[22,29]
>
> Consider the possibility of internal rotation of the proximal tibia when a patient presents with a recent history of inversion ankle sprain. The direction of injury can affect the knee as it is translated and even amplified by the long lever action of the tibia.

Anterior Proximal Tibia

When a patient presents with internal knee pain or restricted extension range of motion with loss of joint end play, consider an anterior proximal head of the tibia. Also, a history of trauma to the knee, such as a blow to the calf region, may subluxate the proximal tibia anteriorly.

Osgood-Schlatter syndrome, infrapatellar bursitis, or soft tissue swelling below the knee may cause the anterior portion of the proximal tibia to be tender to the touch. The rapid speed and specificity of the Activator Instrument help to minimize discomfort for the patient, but a direct thrust close to an inflamed tibial tubercle can hurt. An effective adjustment still can be made by using the split-finger stabilization described in the previous paragraph and positioning the instrument more inferior or distal and, if needed, laterally and away from sensitive tissue.

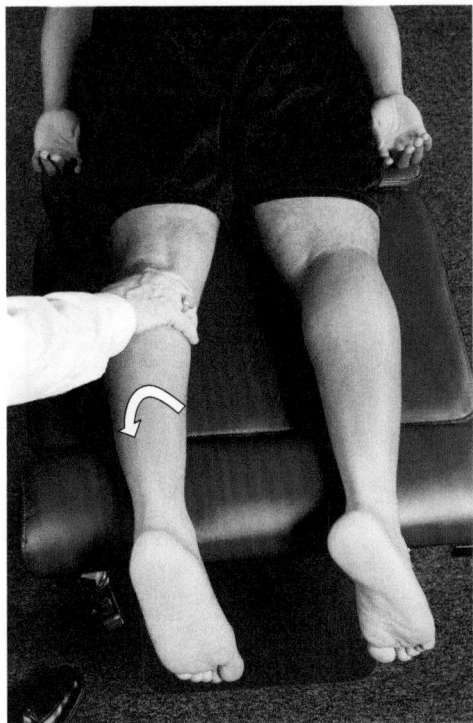

Figure 14-3   Stress Test for internal rotation of the proximal tibia.

Stress Test.   To Stress Test an anterior proximal tibia, take a broad contact with one hand over the posterior surface of the tibia at the level of the belly of the gastrocnemius. Push the tibia straight anterior relative to the femur

(Figure 14-5). Look for reactivity of the PD leg in Position #1.

Adjustment.   To adjust an anterior proximal tibia, flex the knee to 90 degrees. Position the tip of the instrument on the anterior tibia about

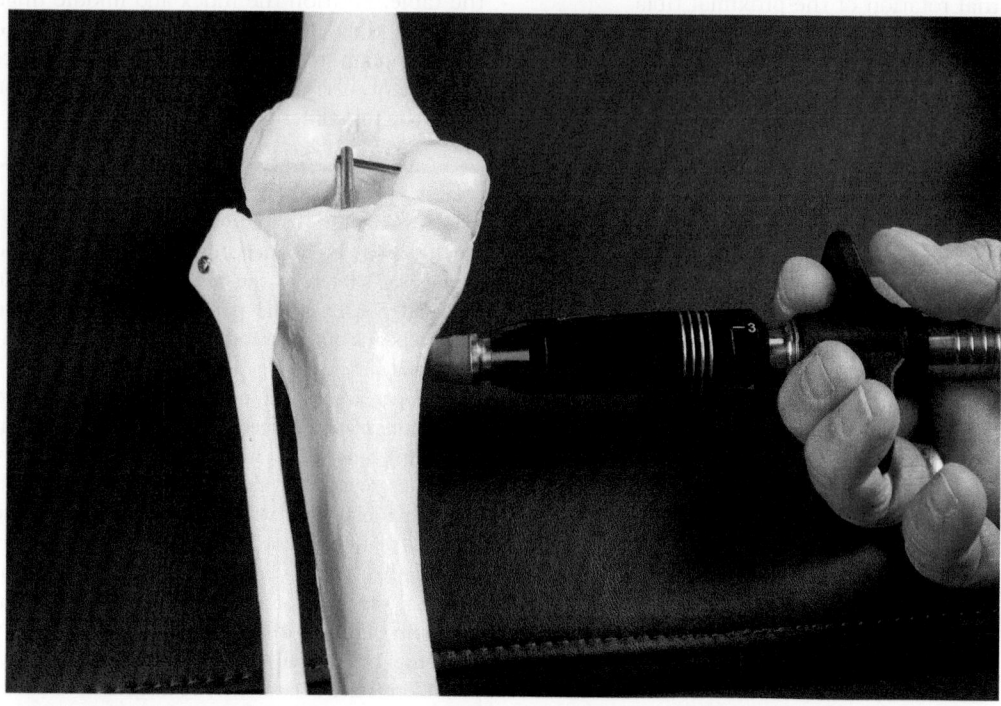

Figure 14-4 Adjustment for internal rotation of the proximal tibia. Line of Drive is medial to lateral.

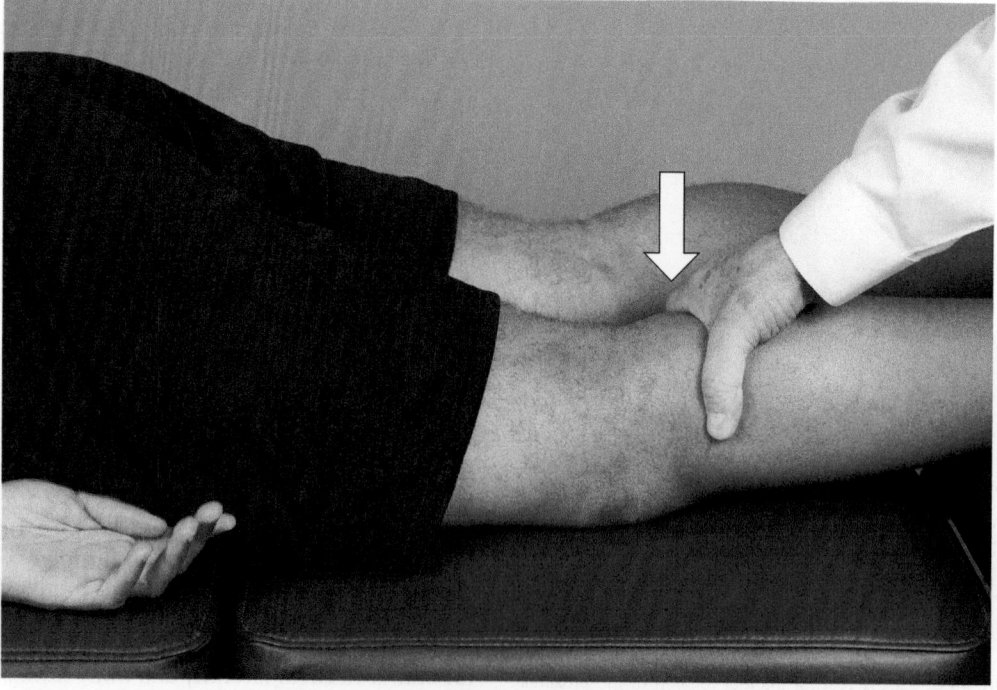

Figure 14-5 Stress Test for anterior proximal tibia.

½ inch distal to the tibial tubercle. The LOD is straight headward or superior (anatomically straight posterior) (Figure 14-6).

If the knee is especially stiff or painful, ensure a correct Stress Test for an anterior proximal tibia by sliding one hand between the anterior thigh just above the knee and the table. Use the other hand to push the tibia anteriorly relative to the femur.

Be sure to avoid the tibial tubercle with the tip of the instrument, especially if it is inflamed or swollen. In most patients, the contact point for the instrument is relatively easy to maintain. In some patients with particularly sharp shins, however, it may be advisable to reach around the leg when it is flexed to 90 degrees at the knee.

Clinical Observations

An anterior proximal tibia may present with pain in the region of the tibial tubercle. Increased tension in the patellar tendon from anterior displacement of the tibia may cause irritation at the tendon's insertion. Be sure to differentiate the pain finding from active Osgood-Schlatter syndrome. Also rule out injury to the anterior cruciate ligament by performing the anterior drawer maneuver.

Continued

Tightness in the patellar tendon can restrict the proximal glide of the patella in the trochlear groove during knee extension. Consequently, reduced joint end play at the limit of knee extension can compromise the shock-absorbing function of the knee during normal gait.[24]

Runners and joggers who run on hard surfaces without adequate footwear are prone to developing an anterior malposition of the proximal tibia. If the knee complaint appears to be related to running or other athletic or occupational activity, make a point of inspecting the patient's shoes.

Posterior Proximal Tibia

When a patient presents with capsular swelling of the knee, posterior knee pain, and a history of recent hyperextension injury, consider posterior proximal tibia. The knee is likely to demonstrate restricted range of motion on flexion, and the hamstring muscles tend to be hypertonic.

Stress Test. To Stress Test a posterior proximal tibia, slide the fingers of one hand between the table and the anterior tibia just below the knee at the level of the tibial tubercle. Lift the tibia straight posterior relative to the femur (Figure 14-7). It is not necessary to lift the leg up high off the table. Just break contact with the table surface while applying a hyperextension

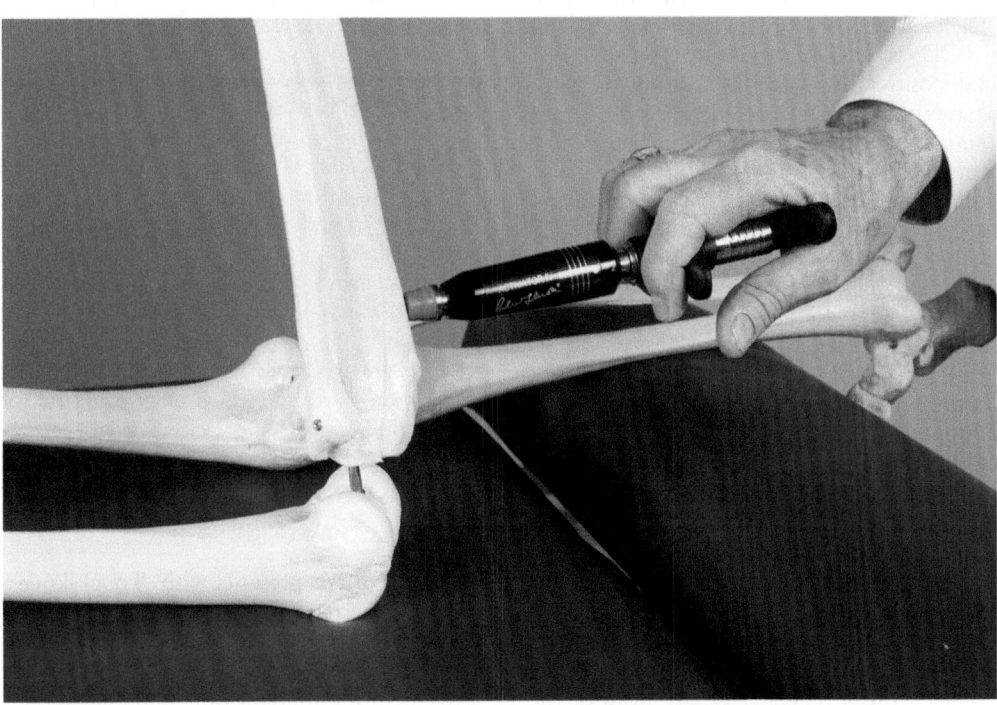

Figure 14-6 Adjustment for anterior proximal tibia. Line of Drive is superior (anatomically posterior).

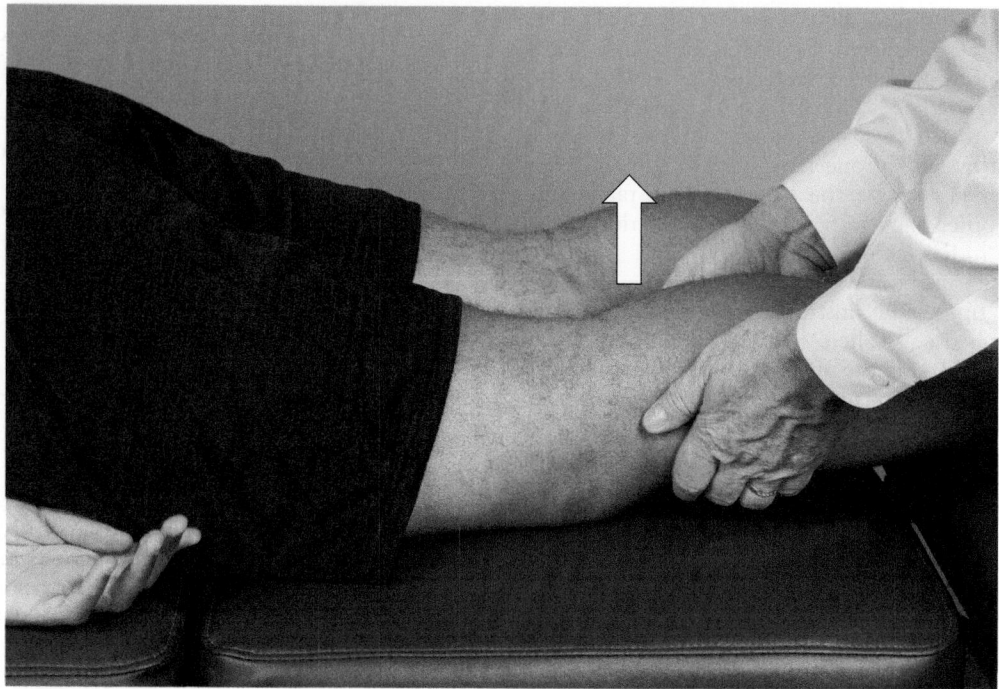

Figure 14-7 Stress Test for posterior proximal tibia.

stress to the knee. Look for reactivity of the PD leg in Position #1.

Adjustment. To adjust a posterior proximal tibia, use two contact points. First, position the tip of the instrument at the tibial insertion of the semimembranosus on the medial tibial condyle. The LOD is straight anterior (Figure 14-8). Second, position the tip of the instrument at the tibial insertion of the lateral head of the biceps femoris on the lateral tibial condyle. The LOD is straight anterior (Figure 14-9).

If the knee is particularly stiff or painful, or if there is obvious soft tissue swelling, perform the Stress Test by placing the palm of one hand over the posterior thigh just above the knee. Use the other hand to lift the lower leg or hyperextend the knee.

To locate the first contact point for adjustment, follow the tendons that make up the medial border of the popliteal fossa. These are the tendons of the semimembranosus and semitendinosus muscles. Their insertion point on the posterior aspect of the medial tibial condyle is the contact point for the first of two corrective thrusts.

To locate the second contact point, follow the tendon that makes up the lateral border of the popliteal fossa. This is mainly the tendon of the biceps femoris, which inserts on the lateral tibial condyle. Palpate for the head of the fibula, and place the tip of the instrument about

½ inch medial to the proximal tibiofibular joint on the lateral tibial condyle.

When performing this adjustment, be particularly attentive to any varicosities that may be present; alter your contact point if necessary to avoid them.

Clinical Observations

Persistent hamstring contractures and spasms may be an indication of a posterior proximal tibia. The patient may demonstrate Beery's sign, in which standing with the knees and hips in extension exacerbates hamstring pain, while sitting relieves the discomfort. Pain also may increase when a patient stands up from a sitting or squatting position.

Be sure to rule out intermittent claudication of the lower extremity, which often manifests with hamstring or calf pain exacerbated by exercise and relieved by rest.

Genu Valgus (Shear Test)

When a patient presents with "knock-knees" or medial knee pain, or when a valgus Stress Test is negative for instability of the medial collateral ligament yet pain is reported upon testing, assessment for a lateral tibia and a medial femur is indicated.

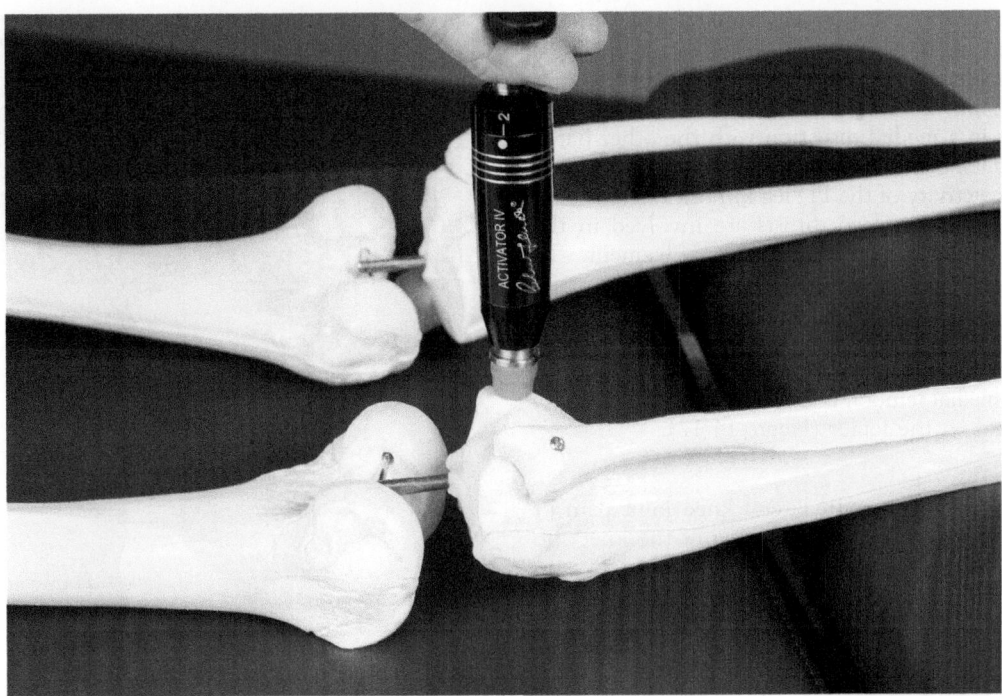

Figure 14-8   Adjustment for posterior proximal tibia. Step One: Contact the medial condyle. Line of Drive is anterior.

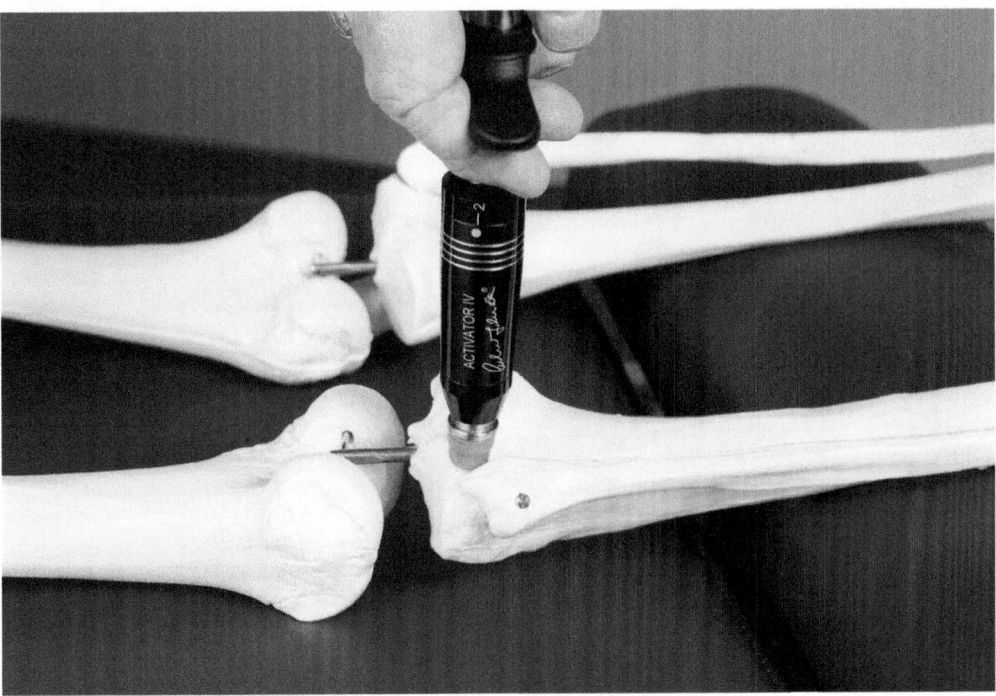

Figure 14-9   Adjustment for posterior proximal tibia. Step Two: Contact the lateral condyle. Line of Drive is anterior.

Stress Test. To stress the knee in a valgus direction, simultaneously push into the medial tibial condyle on the involved side in a lateral direction with one hand, and into the lateral femoral condyle in a medial direction with the other hand, producing a shear effect (Figure 14-10). Look for reactivity of the PD leg in Position #1.

Adjustment. Two thrusts are involved in the correction for genu valgus involvement. To adjust for lateral tibial involvement, contact the lateral aspect of the tibial condyle. The LOD is directly medial (Figure 14-11). To adjust for involvement of the medial femur, contact the medial femoral condyle. The LOD is directly lateral on the femur (Figure 14-12).

Genu Varus (Shear Test)

For the patient with lateral knee joint pain or who upon varus Stress Testing of the knee, no instability is noted yet the patient reports pain upon testing, assess for a medial tibia and a lateral femur.

Stress Test. To stress the knee in a varus direction, push into the lateral tibial condyle on the involved side in a medial direction with one hand, and simultaneously push into the medial femoral condyle in a lateral direction, thus creating a shear effect (Figure 14-13). Look for reactivity of the PD leg in Position #1.

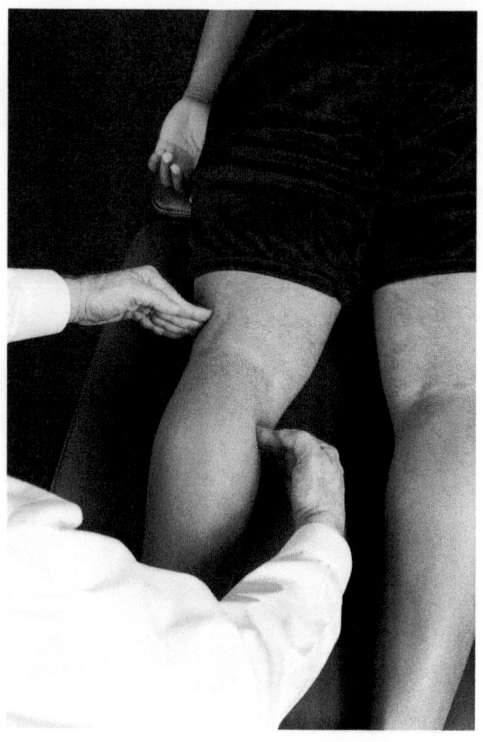

Figure 14-10 Stress Test for genu valgus knee (shear); doctor pushes laterally on the medial tibial condyle and medially on the lateral femoral condyle.

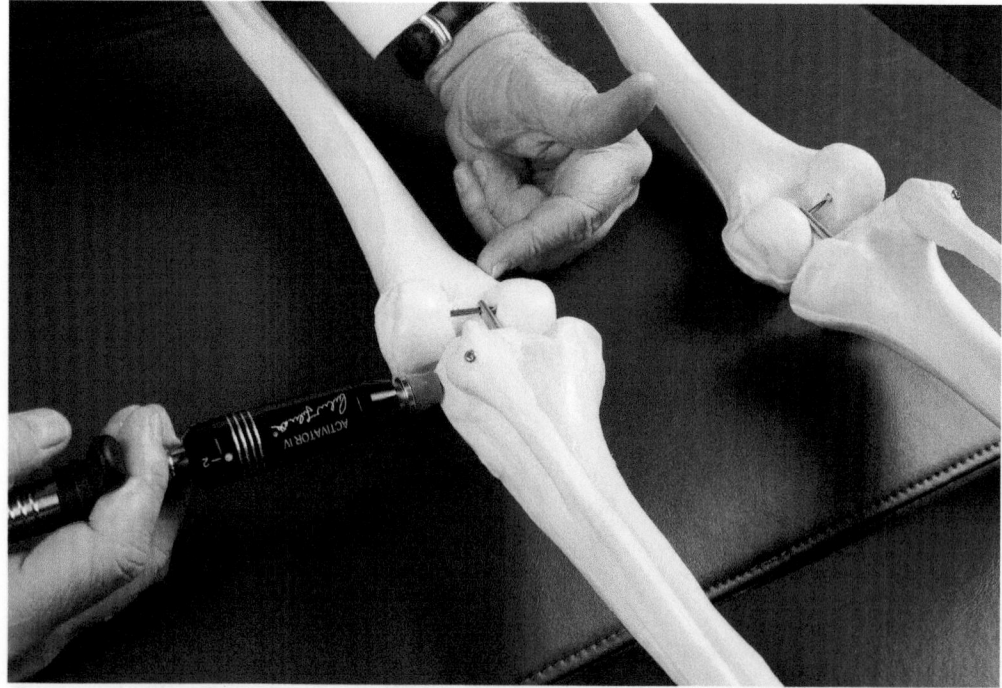

Figure 14-11 Adjustment for genu valgus knee: Step One: Contact the lateral aspect of the tibial condyle. Line of Drive is medial.

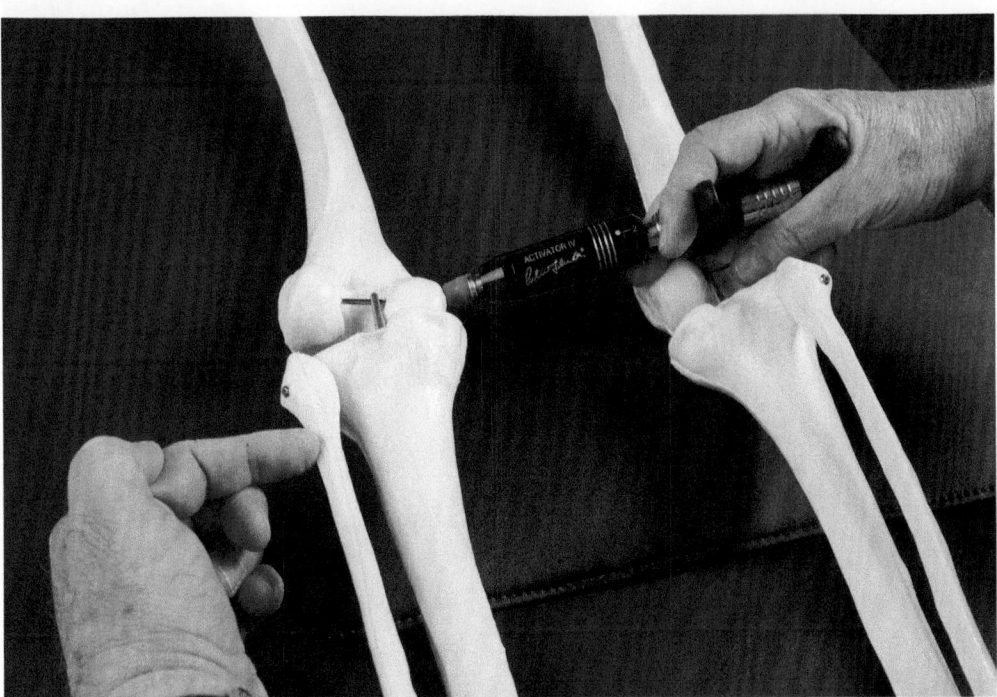

Figure 14-12 Adjustment for genu valgus knee. Step Two: Contact the medial aspect of the femoral condyle. Line of Drive is lateral.

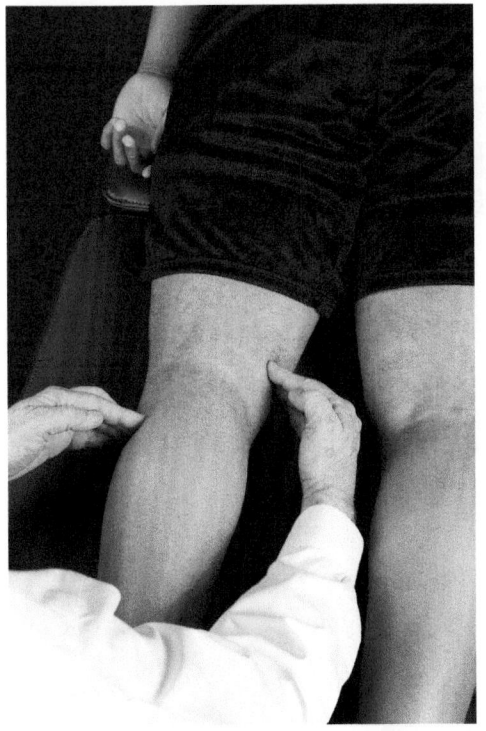

Figure 14-13 Stress Test for genu varus knee (shear): The doctor pushes medially on the lateral tibial condyle and laterally on the medial femoral condyle.

Adjustment. Two thrusts are involved in correction of genu varus involvement. To adjust for medial tibia involvement, contact the medial tibial condyle. The LOD is directly lateral (Figure 14-14). To adjust for lateral femoral involvement, contact the lateral femur condyle. The LOD is directly medial (Figure 14-15).

Medial Knee Joint Involvement

For persistent medial knee joint pain without response to standard protocol knee tests, further assessment of the medial knee joint for neuroarticular dysfunction is indicated. Upon examination, Apley's compression testing for a medial meniscal tear would be negative.

Stress Test. To assess for neuroarticular dysfunction of the medial knee, Stress Test the involved side by flexing the knee to 90 degrees, and while compressing the tibia, externally rotate the tibia to end range (Figure 14-16). Look for reactivity in Position #1.

Adjustment. To adjust the medial knee joint, contact the medial collateral ligament in the joint space. To accurately locate the medial collateral ligament, flex the knee to palpate inside the medial knee joint. The LOD is directly lateral (Figure 14-17).

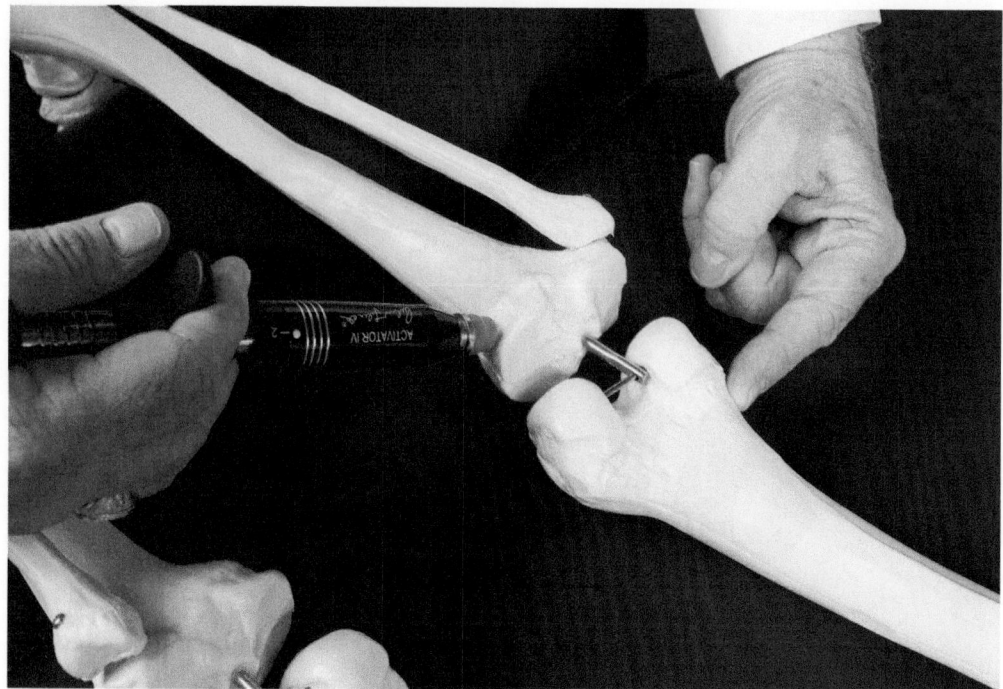

Figure 14-14   Adjustment for genu varus knee. Step One: Contact the medial tibial condyle. Line of Drive is lateral.

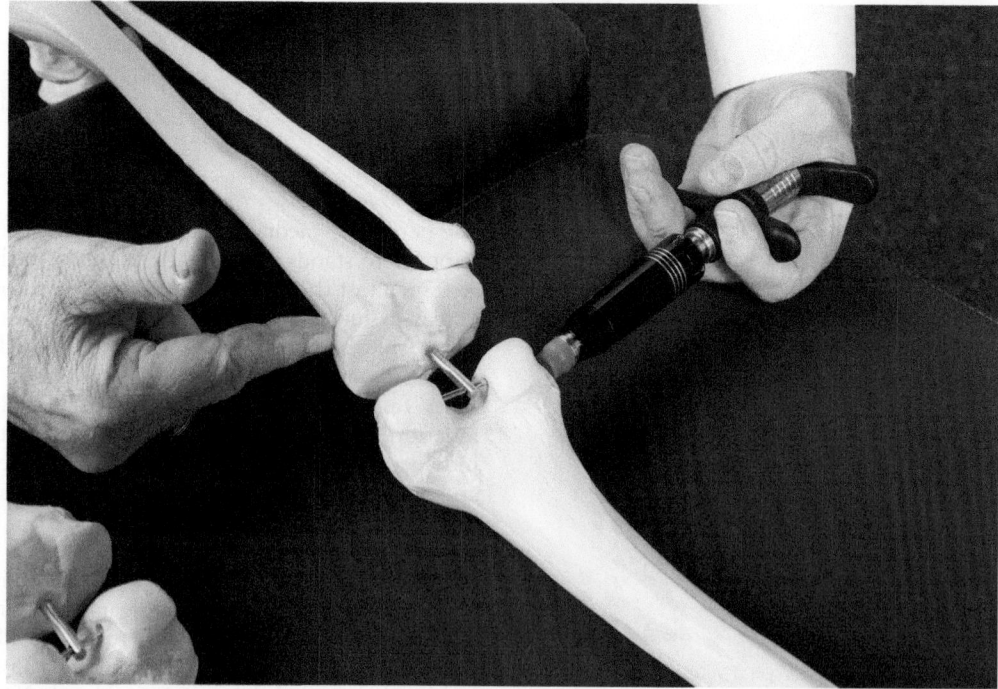

Figure 14-15   Adjustment for genu varus knee. Step Two: Contact the lateral femoral condyle. Line of Drive is medial.

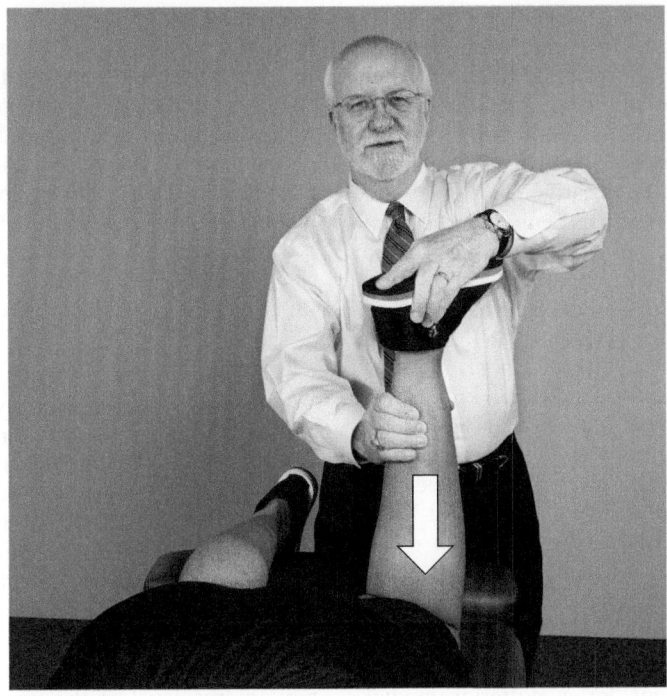

Figure 14-16 Stress Test for medial knee involvement: Doctor flexes knee to 90 degrees, compresses the tibia while externally rotating the tibia.

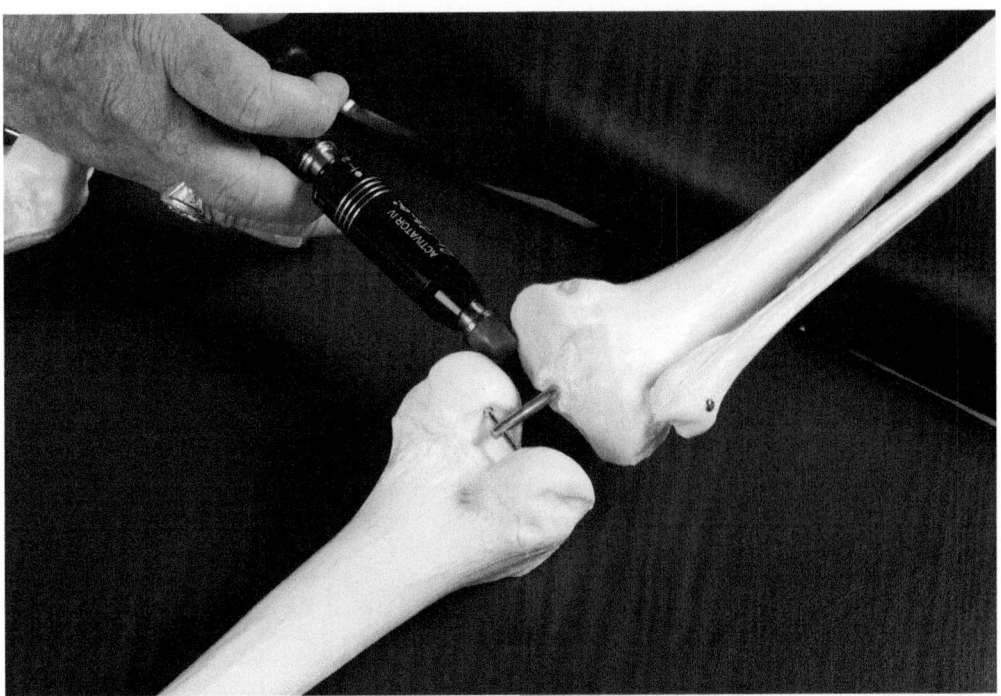

Figure 14-17 Adjustment for medial knee. Line of Drive is lateral.

Lateral Knee Joint Involvement

For persistent lateral knee joint pain without response to standard protocol knee tests, further assessment of the lateral knee joint for neuroarticular dysfunction is indicated. Upon examination, Apley's compression testing for a lateral meniscal tear would be negative.

Stress Test. To assess for neuroarticular dysfunction of the lateral knee, Stress Test the involved knee by flexing it to 90 degrees, and while compressing the tibia, internally rotate the tibia to end range (Figure 14-18). Look for reactivity of the PD leg in Position #1.

Adjustment. To adjust for lateral knee joint involvement, contact the lateral collateral ligament in the joint space. Accurately locate the ligament by flexing the patient's knee first and palpating into the lateral knee joint. The LOD is directly medial (Figure 14-19).

Posterior Medial Distal Femur/Internal Rotation

When a patient presents with knee stiffness or genu valgus (knock-knees), with or without pain or trauma, assessment for a posterior medial distal femur is indicated.

Stress Test. To Stress Test for posterior involvement of the medial distal femur, attempt to internally rotate the distal femur by rolling the distal femur in a lateral-to-medial direction while stabilizing the tibia and performing internal rotation of the femur (Figure 14-20). Look for reactivity of the PD leg in Position #1.

Adjustment. To adjust for involvement of the posterior medial distal femur, contact the posterior aspect of the medial femoral condyle. The LOD is directly anterior (Figure 14-21).

Involvement of the Inferior Patella

When a patient suffers from anterior knee pain or shows pain and limited extension of the knee, consider an inferior neuroarticular dysfunction of the patella. The patient also may demonstrate a positive patellar ballottement test, if subpatellar effusion is associated with the complaint. Inspect each patella for bilateral positional symmetry.

Stress Test. To Stress Test for involvement of the inferior patella, slide the fingers of one hand between the anterior thigh and the table at the level of the superior border of the patella. Gently push the patella inferiorly

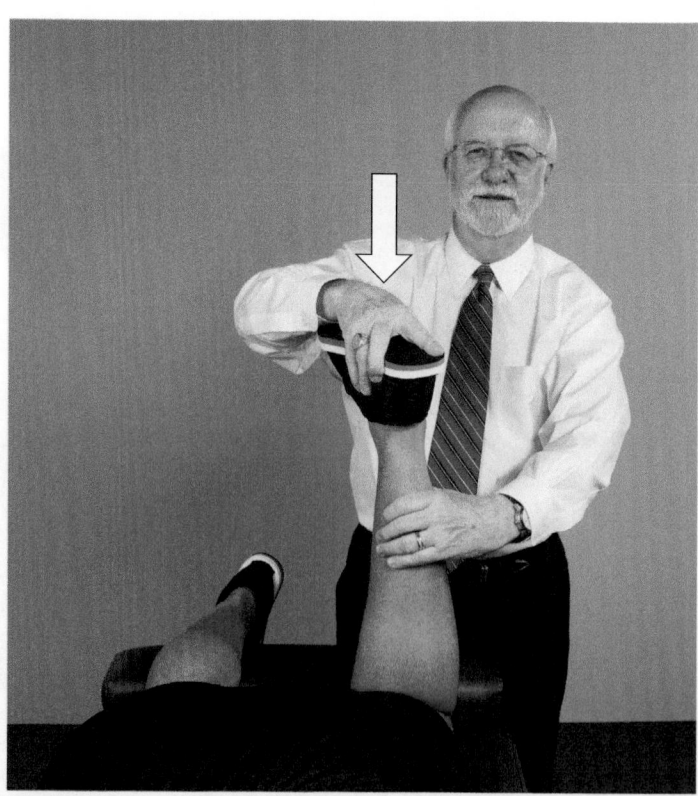

Figure 14-18 Stress Test for lateral knee involvement: Doctor flexes knee to 90 degrees, compresses the tibia while internally rotating the tibia.

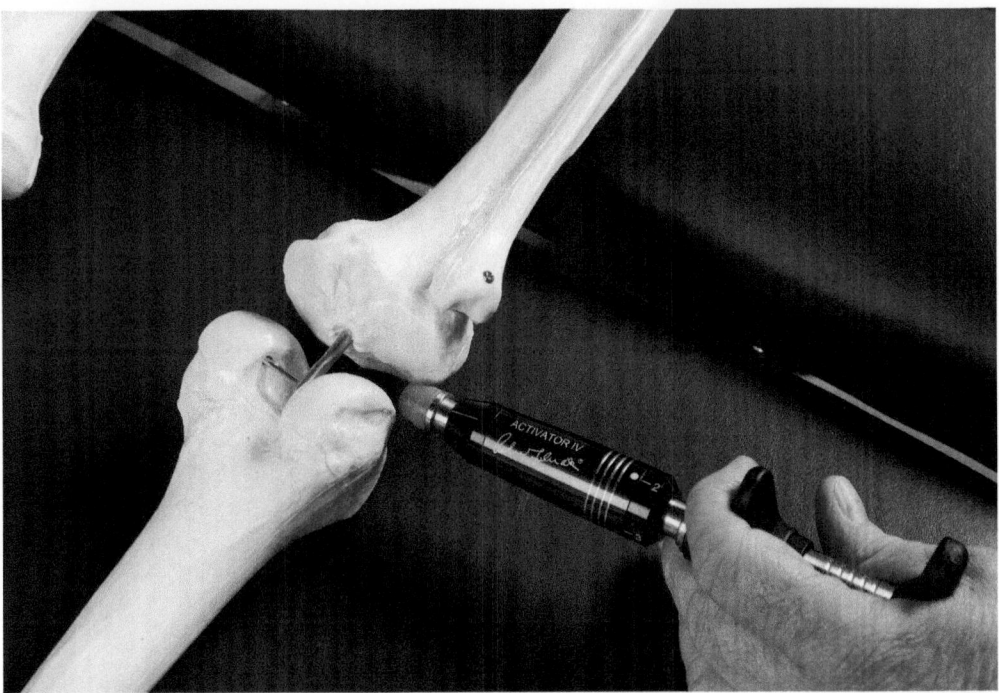

Figure 14-19 Adjustment for lateral knee. Line of Drive is medial.

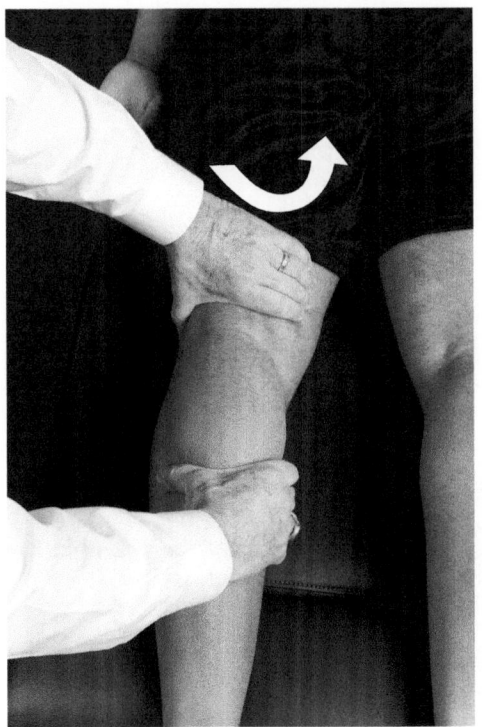

Figure 14-20 Stress Test for posterior medial distal femur (internal rotation).

(Figure 14-22). Look for reactivity of the PD leg in Position #1.

Adjustment. To adjust for inferior patellar involvement, flex the knee to 90 degrees. Contact the inferior aspect of the patella. The LOD is straight superior (proximal) (Figure 14-23). If the knee is unable to be flexed, perform the adjustment with the patient in the supine position.

If infrapatellar soft tissue swelling is noted, the patient may feel some discomfort during the Stress Test for the inferior patella, and range of motion of the knee may be restricted in flexion. Contact with the instrument during adjustment of the inferior patella may add to the discomfort of subpatellar swelling. Be sure to avoid direct contact over an inflamed bursa as well. To ensure a specific adjustment and to minimize patient discomfort, it may be advisable to place the thumb or a finger of the stabilization hand over the anterior aspect of the patella. Use the finger to prevent the tip of the instrument from slipping during placement and adjustment.

SIDE NOTE: SUPERIOR PATELLA If the patient continues to report pain above or behind the kneecap, consider testing for a superior

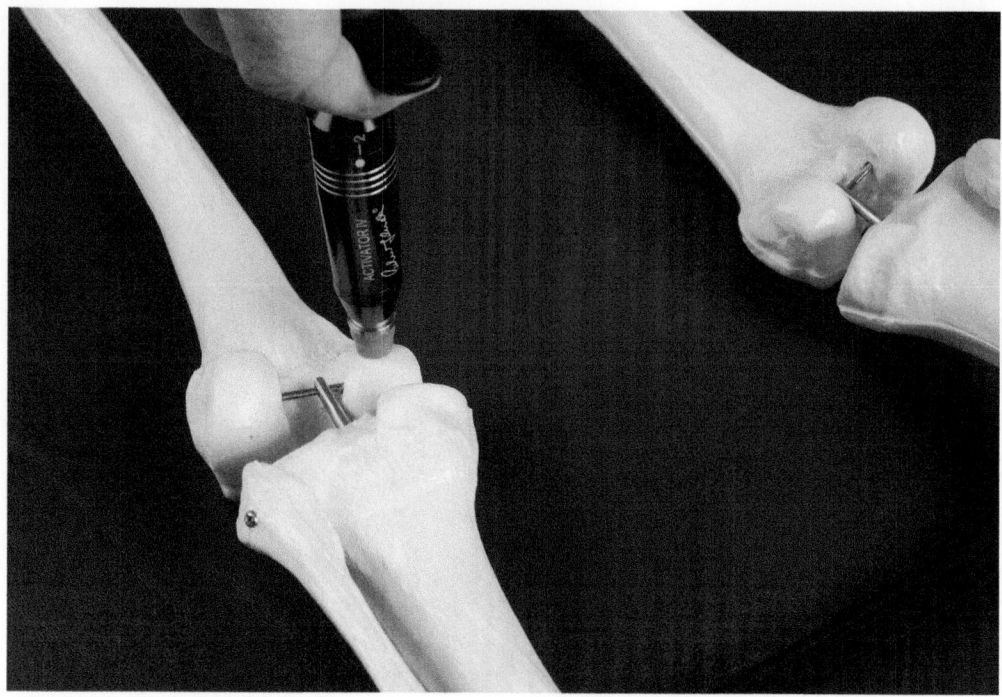

Figure 14-21 Adjustment for posterior medial distal femur. Line of Drive is anterior.

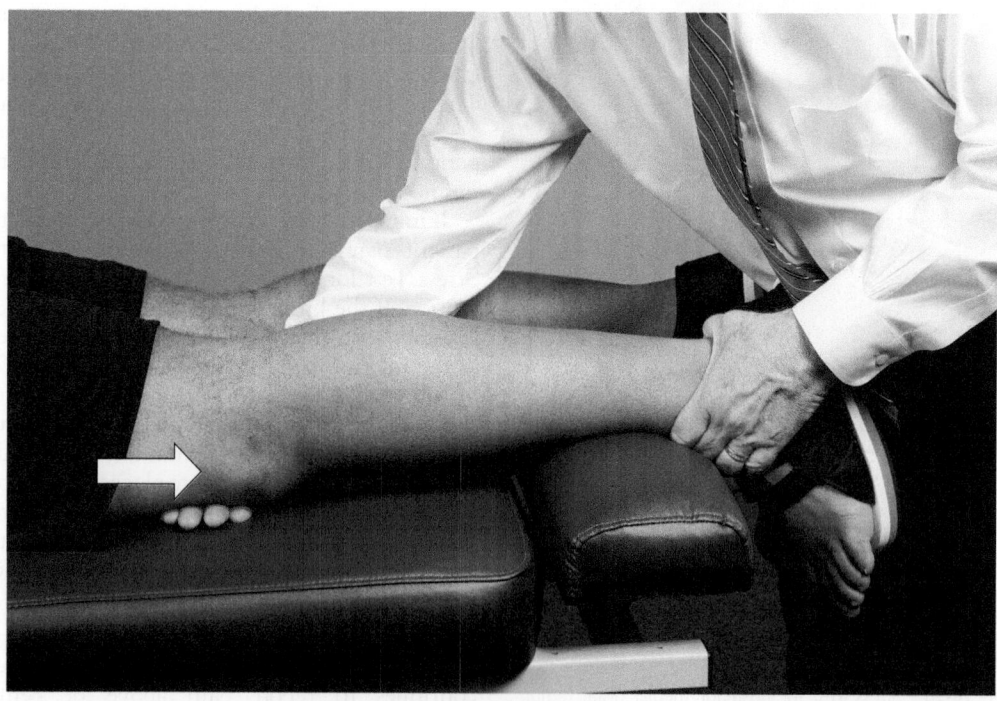

Figure 14-22 Stress Test for inferior patella.

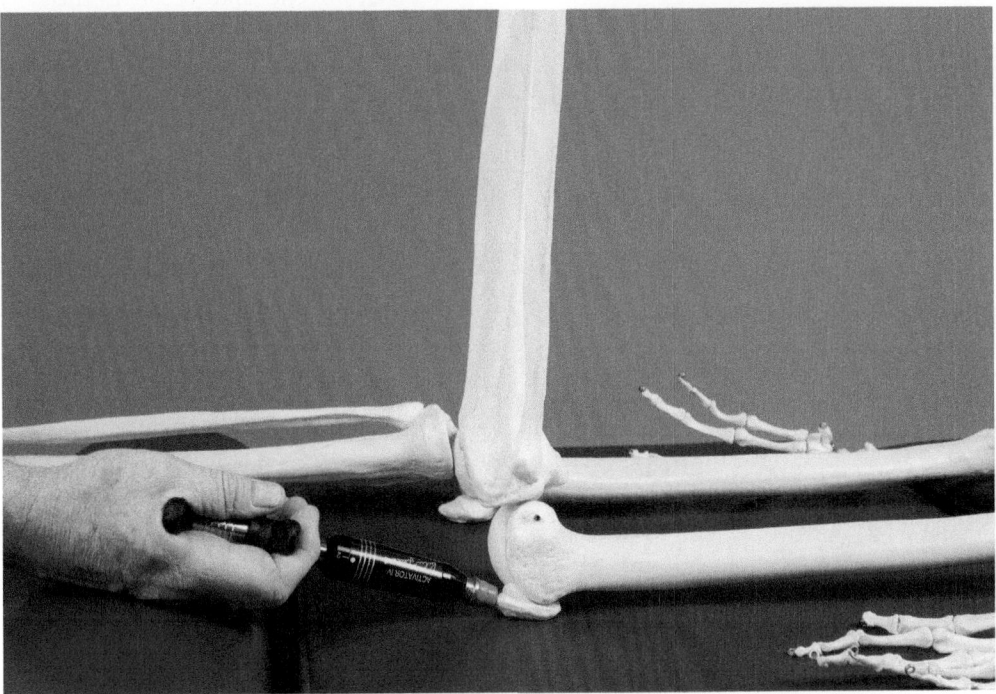

Figure 14-23   Adjustment for inferior patella. Line of Drive is straight superior (proximal).

patella. Stress Test by contacting the inferior border of the patella with the doctor's hand and pushing slightly in a headward, or superior, direction (Figure 14-24). Look for PD leg reactivity in Position #1 for involvement. For the adjustment, position the patient supine and contact the superior aspect of the patella. The LOD is inferior (Figure 14-25). Stabilize the contact of the instrument if needed with the thumb or a finger.

Clinical Observations

An inferior patella often is associated with subpatellar effusion, in which edematous fluid accumulates between the patella and the trochlear groove of the femur. Fluid pressure prevents the normal proximal glide of the patella during knee extension. As a result, the patient's gait may be irregular and antalgic.[35]

An inferior patella can manifest with pain and limited flexion range of motion, especially at its extreme. Pain or difficulty bending the knee in a squatting position or even a sitting position suggests limited travel of the patella in the trochlear groove.

Involvement of the Lateral Patella

When a patient experiences pain at or just medial to the tibial tubercle, consider lateral neuroarticular dysfunction of the patella. Also consider lateral patellar involvement in conjunction with an externally rotated proximal tibia, or when crepitus occurs with patellar movement during knee flexion and extension ranges of motion.

Stress Test.   To Stress Test a lateral patella, slide the fingers of one hand between the knee and the table. With the fingertips, gently push the patella laterally in the trochlear groove (Figure 14-26). Look for reactivity of the PD leg in Position #1.

Adjustment.   To adjust for lateral patellar involvement, position the tip of the instrument on the lateral border of the patella. The LOD is straight lateral to medial (Figure 14-27).

To ensure a correct LOD and to minimize discomfort for the patient, slide the fingers of the stabilization hand between the patella and the table, cupping the patella with the index and middle fingers. Spread the fingers enough to accommodate the tip of the instrument. Use the split-finger position to stabilize the instrument during the adjustment.

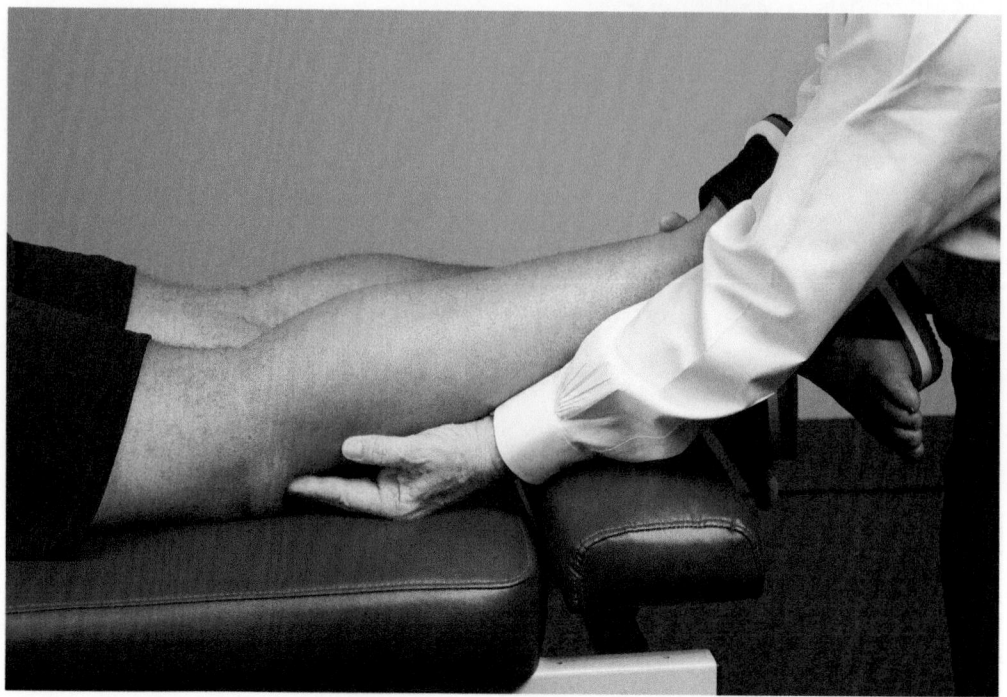

Figure 14-24 Stress Test for superior patella.

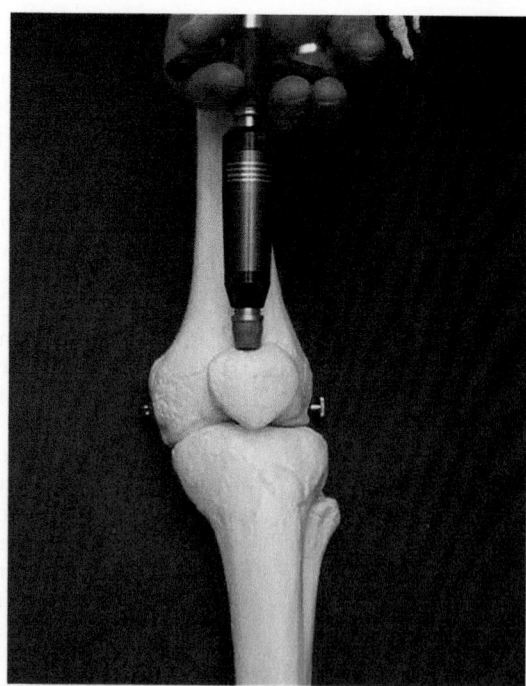

Figure 14-25 Adjustment for superior patella. Line of Drive is straight inferior (distal).

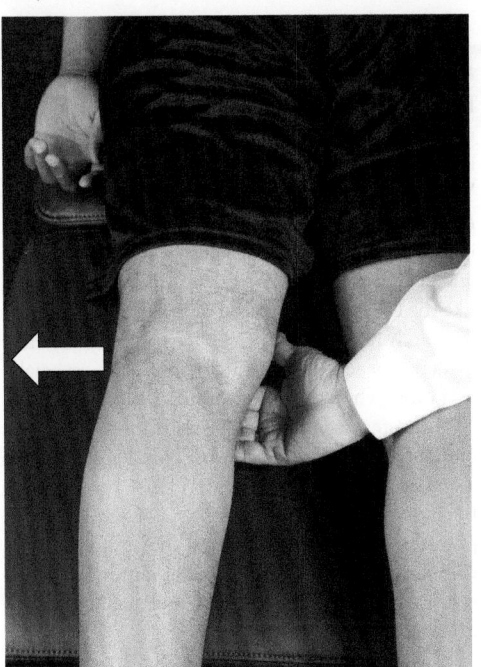

Figure 14-26 Stress Test for lateral patella. With the fingertips, gently push the patella laterally in the trochlear groove.

Clinical Observations

Lateral malposition of the patella can contribute to early degeneration of the patellar cartilage (chondromalacia patella) or to cartilaginous destruction of the trochlear groove on the femur. Because progression of this type of degenerative arthritis is rapid and progressive, early recognition and appropriate intervention are important.[29]

The patella may be shifted laterally by external torquing of the tibia, so that stresses are applied to the patella via the patellar tendon. The "screw home mechanisms" of the tibia on knee extension increase tension in the patellar tendon as the tibial tubercle rotates externally (laterally).[6] Therefore always perform the Stress Test and adjustment as necessary for external rotation of the proximal tibia.

Lateral Fibula

When a patient presents with shin pain or anterior compartment shin splints, consider a lateral malposition of the fibula.

Radiating pain by way of the common peroneal nerve from the knee to the foot and ankle

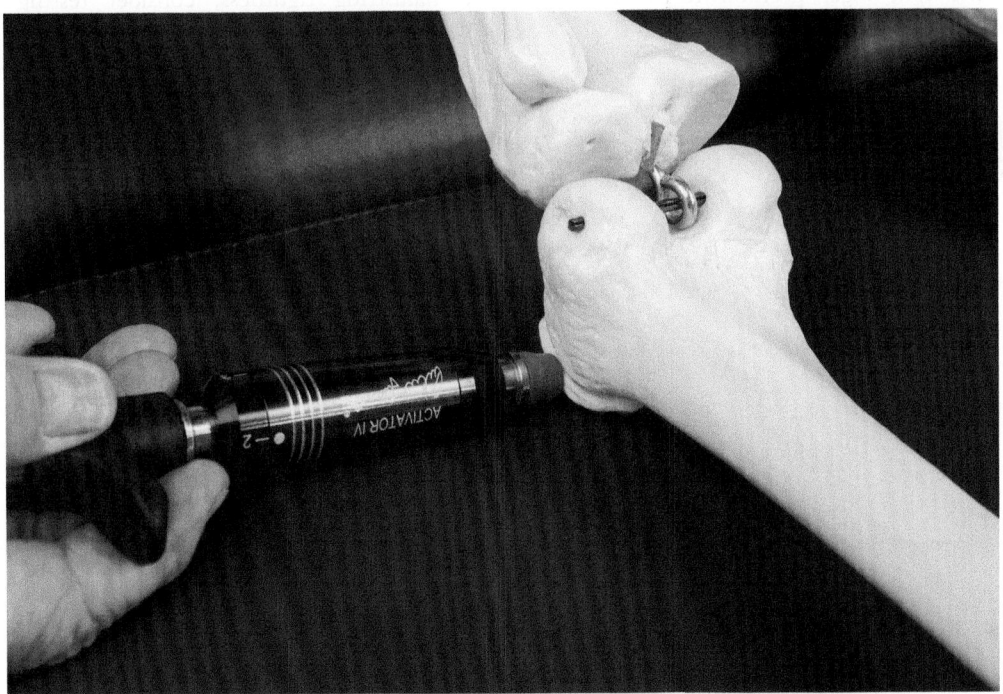

Figure 14-27 Adjustment for lateral patella. Line of Drive is medial to lateral.

can also indicate a lateral fibula. When a patient describes radiating pain from the knee, perform Stress Tests as necessary not only for the lateral fibula but also for the posterior-superior proximal fibula and the posterior distal fibula, as described in Chapter 15.

Stress Test.   To Stress Test for a lateral fibula, grasp the lateral aspect of the lower leg, at the proximal third point of the fibula. Using a tissue pull, gently distract laterally away from the tibia (Figure 14-28). Look for reactivity of the PD leg in Position #1.

Adjustment.   To adjust for involvement of a lateral fibula, contact the lateral aspect of the fibula at the proximal third level. The LOD is medial and slightly anterior (Figure 14-29).

With posterior lateral fibular involvement, soft tissue in the anterior tibial compartment is likely to be quite tender to deep palpation. During the Stress Test, try to keep broad contact over these tissues to avoid triggering muscle spasms or unnecessary discomfort for the patient.

Positioning the instrument is generally quite easy. To ensure specific contact on the shaft of the fibula, position the index and middle fingers of the stabilization hand anterior and posterior to the shaft. Spread the fingers enough to accommodate the tip of the instrument, and use the split-finger position to stabilize the instrument during the adjustment.

Clinical Observations

Because the common peroneal nerve follows the fibula down to the ankle and the dorsum of the foot, misalignment of the fibula may involve the nerve. When a patient presents with pain that is apparently radiating from the knee to the foot and ankle, be sure to rule out more proximal nerve root entrapment and sciatic neuralgia by performing standard tests like the Lasegue (straight leg raise) test, the Braggard test, and the Valsalva maneuver. Also look for any evidence of sensory deficit or motor loss, especially foot drop, when the peroneal nerve is involved.[5,29]

A posterior lateral malposition of the fibula is one of the risks attendant with contact sports such as soccer, rugby, football, and hockey. Blows to the anterior and lateral portion of the shin can put strain on the muscles of the anterior tibial compartment, like the tibialis anterior. As a result, painful shin splints, exacerbated by running, are likely to develop.

Hamstrings

For those patients who experience pain behind the knee, myofascial pain of the hamstrings, or decreased hip flexion (90 degrees is normal range of flexion during straight leg raise) due to hamstring tightness, consider testing for neuroarticular dysfunction of the hamstrings.

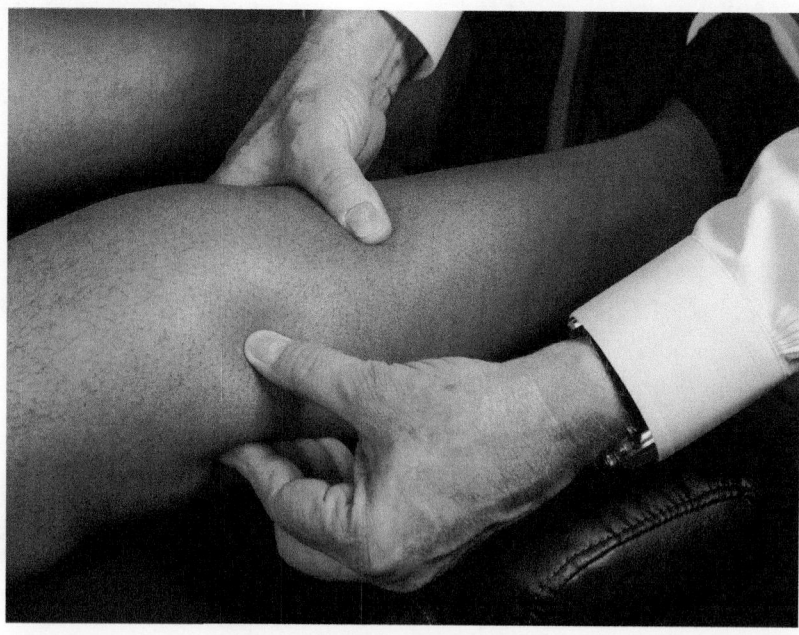

Figure 14-28   Stress Test for lateral fibula.

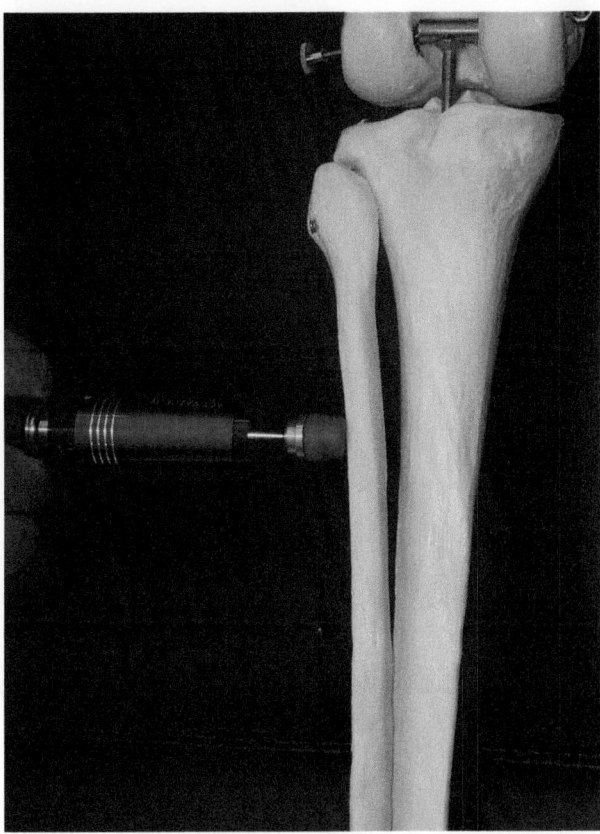

Figure 14-29 Adjustment for lateral fibula. Line of Drive is medial and slightly anterior.

Isolation Test. To isolate the hamstrings, use an active resistive manual muscle test. Instruct the patient to flex the knee on the involved side while the doctor contacts the posterior distal tibia with the palm of the hand to apply resistance to the knee flexion (Figure 14-30). Look for reactivity of the PD leg in Position #1.

Adjustment. To adjust for hamstring involvement, use two thrusts. First, contact the myotendon junction of the medial hamstrings. The LOD is directed posterior to anterior (Figure 14-31). The second contact is at the myotendon junction of the lateral hamstrings. The LOD is also directed posterior to anterior (Figure 14-32). Be aware of any varicosities or Baker's cysts in this area, and avoid adjustive contact with them by altering the contact point as needed.

Quadriceps Involvement

When a patient presents with a patellofemoral tracking problem, chondromalacia of the patella, external rotation of the tibia, or myofascial pain of the quadriceps muscles, consider testing for dysfunction of the quadriceps.

Isolation Test. To isolate for quadriceps involvement, use an active resistive manual muscle test. With the patient's knee in less than 90 degrees of flexion, instruct the patient to straighten the leg while the doctor contacts the anterior distal tibia and applies resistance to knee extension (Figure 14-33). Look for reactivity of the PD leg in Position #1.

Adjustment. Place the patient in a supine position. The contact point for quadriceps involvement is the vastus medialis myotendon junction, just medial and slightly superior to the patella. The LOD is anterior to posterior (Figure 14-34).

Gastrocnemius Involvement

When a patient presents with hypertonicity of the calf muscles, myofascial pain of the gastrocnemius muscle, chronic Achilles tendonitis, or a superior calcaneus, consider testing for neuroarticular dysfunction of the gastrocnemius muscle.

Isolation Test. To isolate the gastrocnemius, use an active resistive manual muscle test. With the patient's knee in less than 90 degrees of flexion, instruct the patient to plantarflex the foot while the doctor contacts the plantar surface of the foot, applying resistance to plantar flexion (Figure 14-35). Look for reactivity of the PD leg in Position #1.

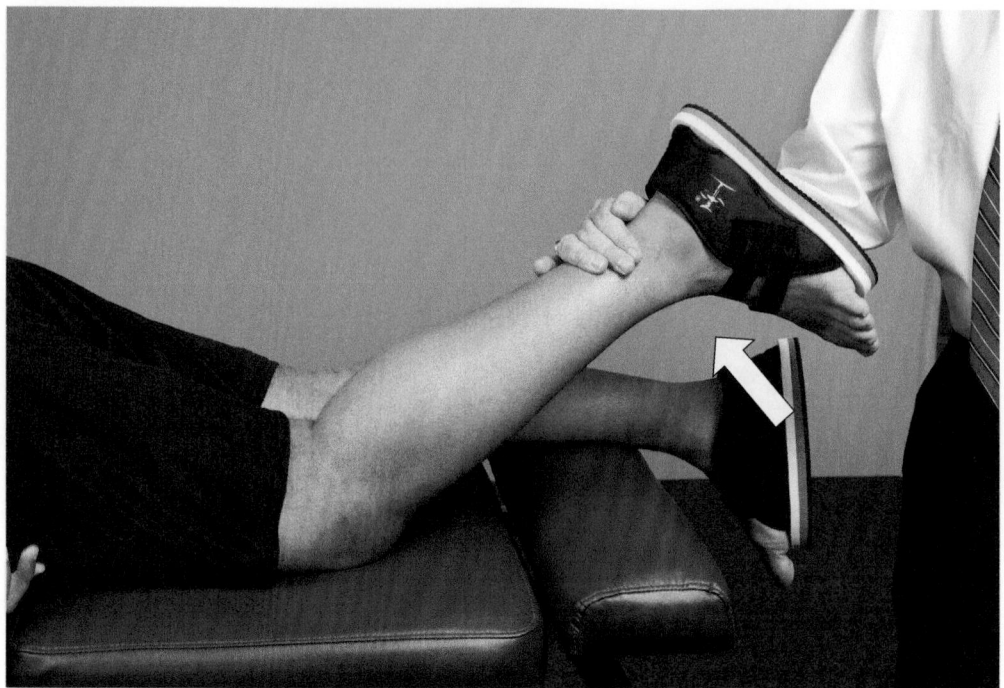

Figure 14-30 Active resistive muscle test for hamstrings.

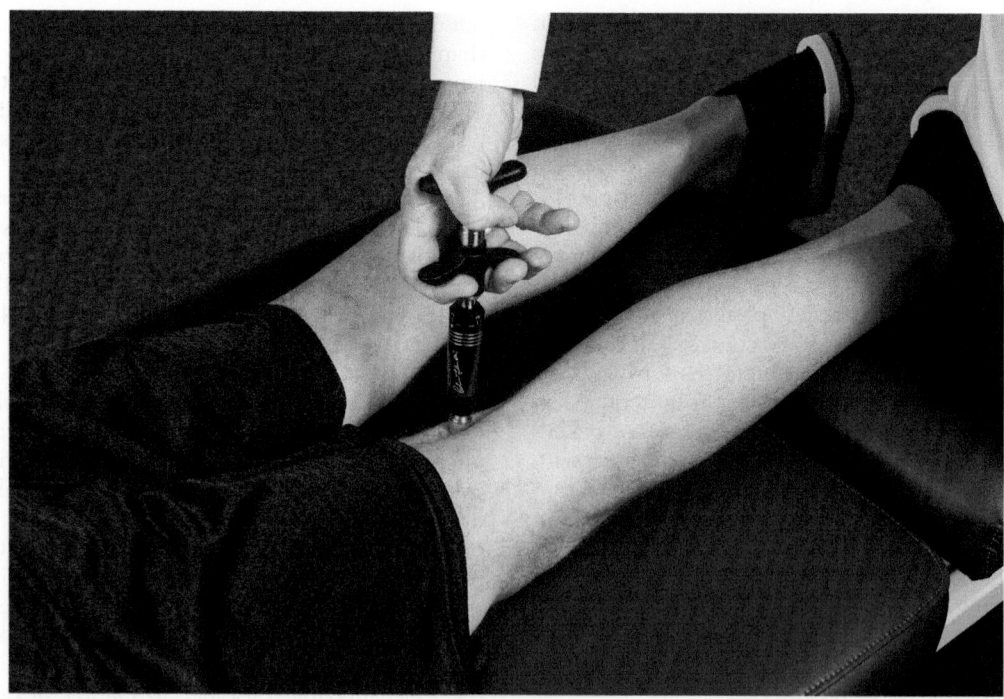

Figure 14-31 Adjustment for hamstrings. Step One: Contact the myotendon junction of the medial hamstrings. Line of Drive is posterior to anterior.

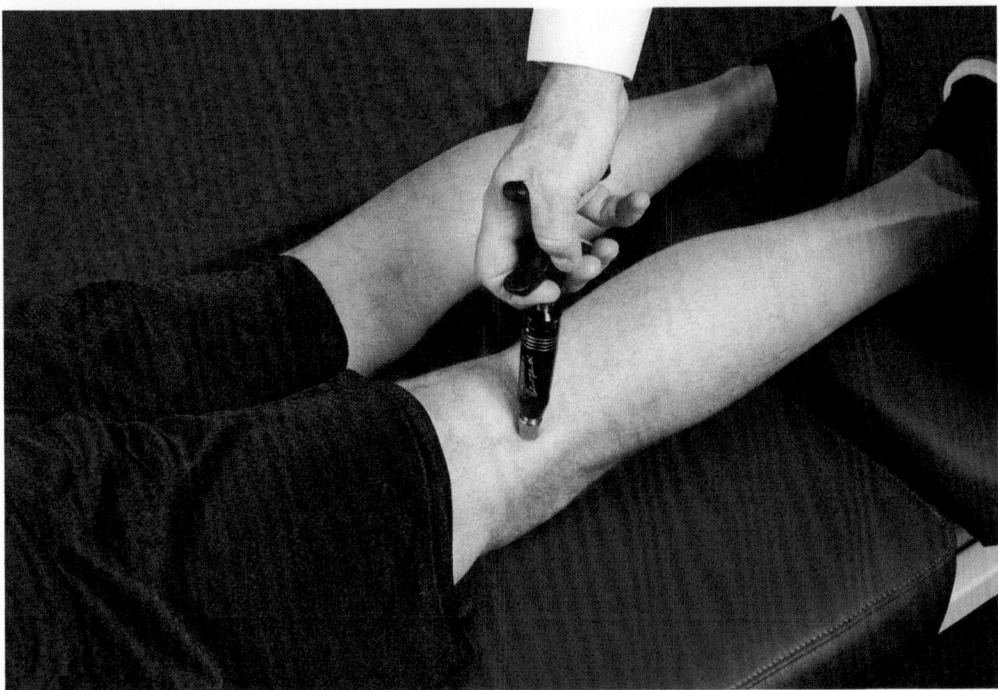

Figure 14-32   Adjustment for hamstrings. Step Two: Contact the myotendon junction of the lateral hamstrings. Line of Drive is posterior to anterior.

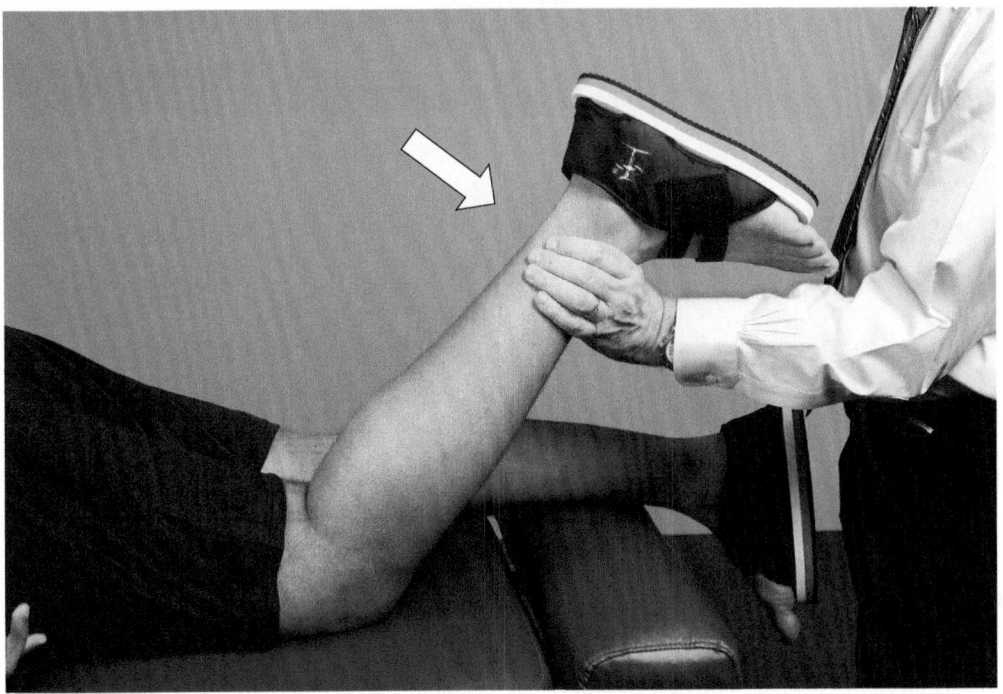

Figure 14-33   Active resistive muscle test for quadriceps.

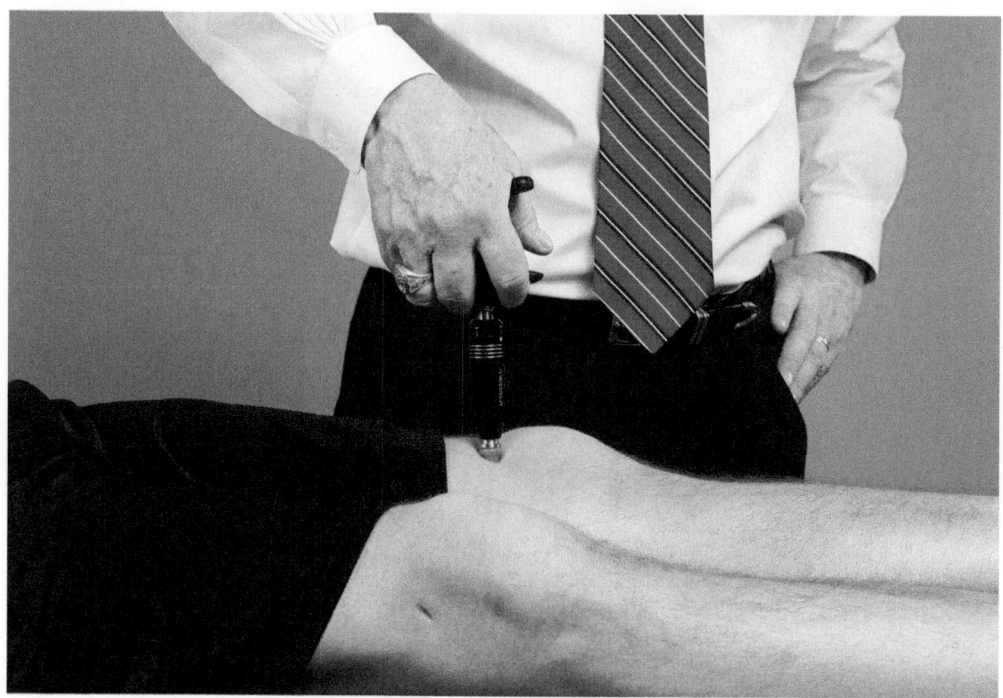

Figure 14-34 Adjustment for quadriceps. Line of Drive is anterior to posterior.

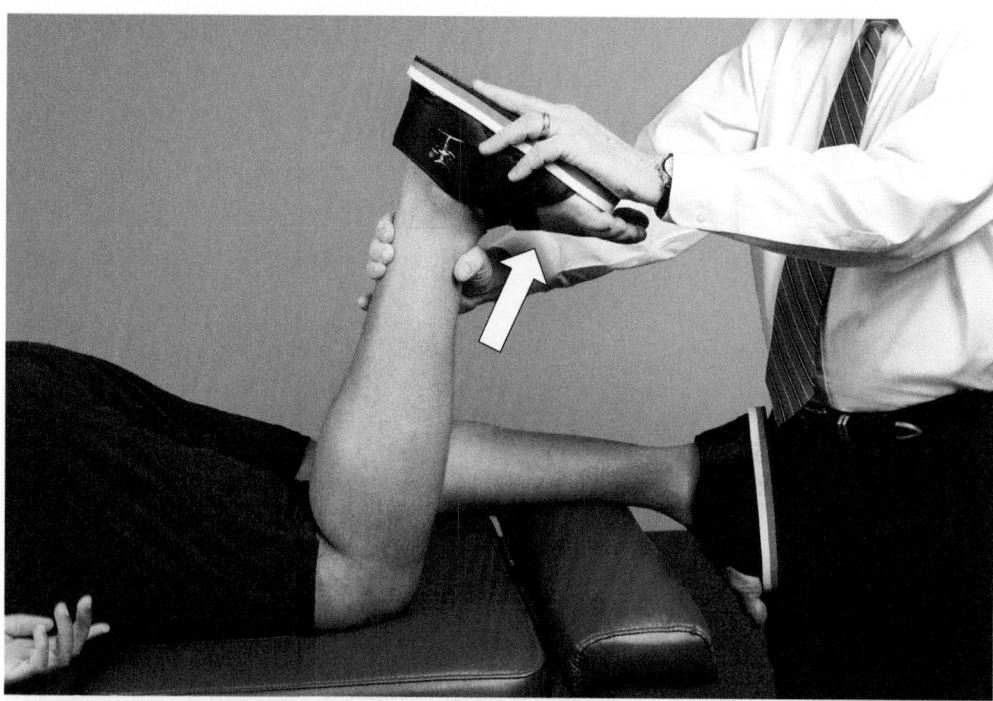

Figure 14-35 Active resistive muscle test for gastrocnemius.

Adjustment. To adjust for gastrocnemius involvement, use two thrusts. First, contact the medial head of the gastrocnemius ½ inch inferior to the medial tibial condyle. The LOD is anterior and slightly superior (Figure 14-36). The second contact is on the lateral head of the gastrocnemius ½ inch inferior to the lateral tibial condyle. The LOD is also anterior and slightly superior (Figure 14-37). When performing this adjustment, be particularly attentive to any varicosities

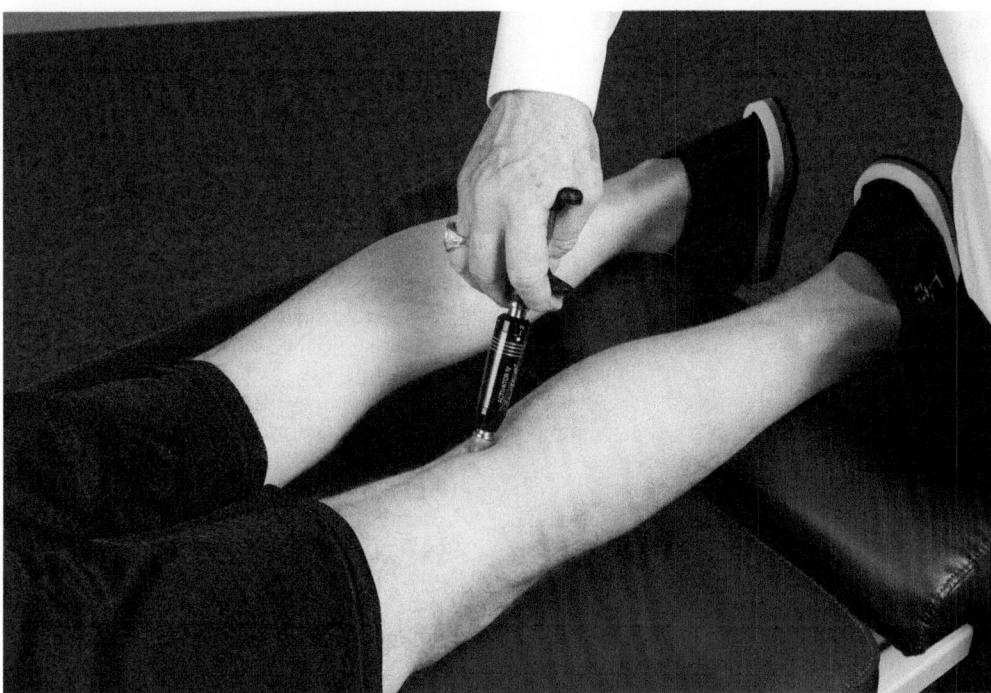

Figure 14-36 Adjustment for gastrocnemius. Step One: Contact the medial head of the gastrocnemius ½ inch inferior to the medial tibia condyle. Line of Drive is anterior and slightly superior.

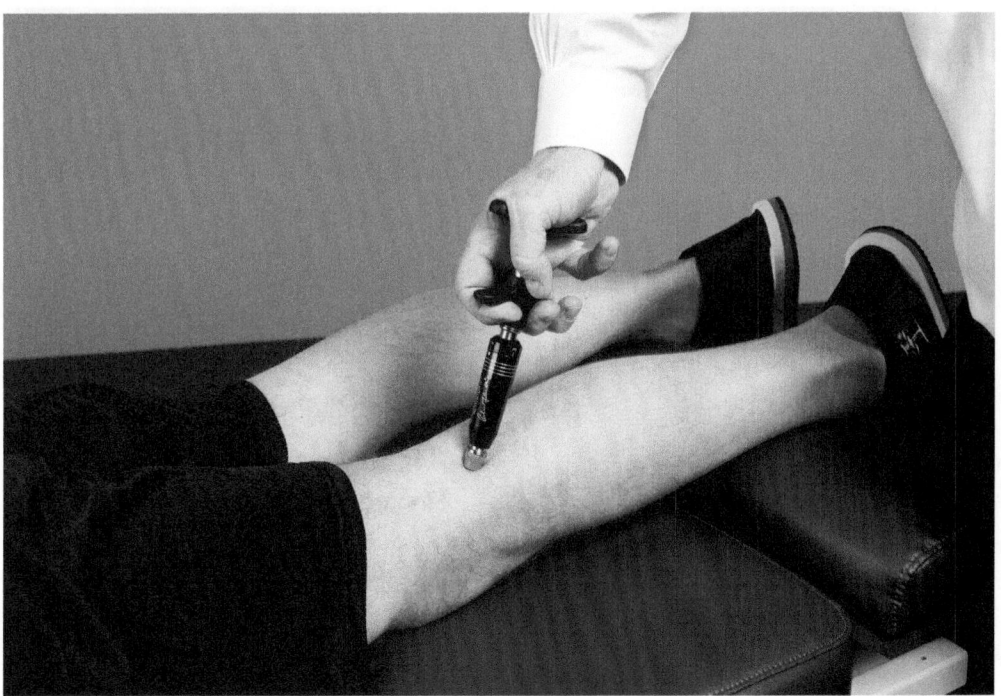

Figure 14-37 Adjustment for gastrocnemius. Step Two: Contact the lateral head of the gastrocnemius ½ inch inferior to the lateral tibia condyle. Line of Drive is anterior and slightly superior.

that may be present, and alter your contact point if necessary to avoid them.

Compressed/Impinged Femoral-Tibial Joint Involvement

When the patient has persistent knee pain and an inability to extend the knee completely, and a torn meniscus with locking of the joint is suspected, consider using this test after completing the tests described previously.

Isolation Test. There are two steps and options that may occur:

- **Medial Impingement:** The doctor grasps the involved posterior lateral distal end of the tibia with one hand, and the other hand is placed on the posterior medial distal end of the femur. A lateral-to-medial stress of the knee is performed by the doctor while moving the tibia toward the midline (Figure 14-38). (This is similar to testing for stability of the lateral collateral ligaments.) This movement compresses the medial knee joint. Look for reactivity of the PD leg in Position #1 for involvement.

- **Lateral Impingement:** The doctor grasps the involved posterior medial distal end of the tibia with one hand, and the other hand is

placed on the posterior lateral distal end of the femur. A medial-to-lateral stress is placed on the lateral knee joint by moving the tibia away from the midline (Figure 14-39). (This is similar to testing for stability of the medial collateral ligaments.) This movement compresses the lateral knee joint. Look for reactivity of the PD leg in Position #1.

Adjustment

- **Medial Impingement Involvement:** The first contact point is on the medial condyle of the femur. The LOD is superior and slightly lateral (Figure 14-40). The second contact point is on the medial aspect of the proximal tibia. The LOD is inferior and slightly lateral (Figure 14-41).

- **Lateral Impingement Involvement:** The first contact point is on the lateral condyle of the femur. The LOD is superior and slightly medial (Figure 14-42). The second contact point is on the lateral aspect of the proximal tibia. The LOD is inferior and slightly medial (Figure 14-43).

Mechanical force, manually assisted chiropractic adjusting (Activator Method) for the knee is summarized in Table 14-1.

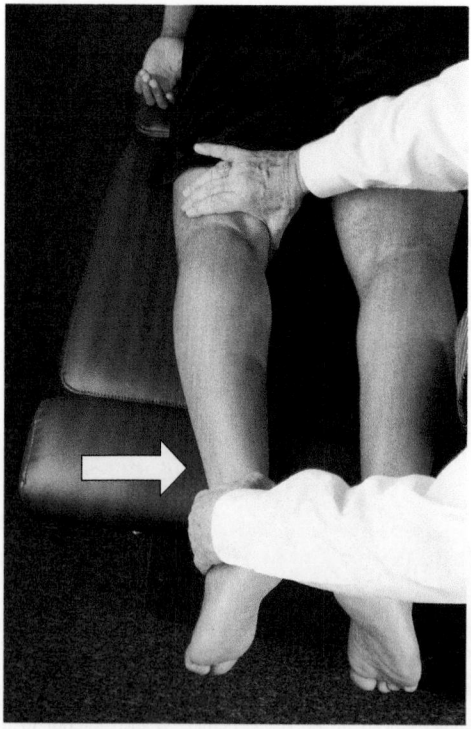

Figure 14-38 Stress Test for medial femoral/tibial impingement.

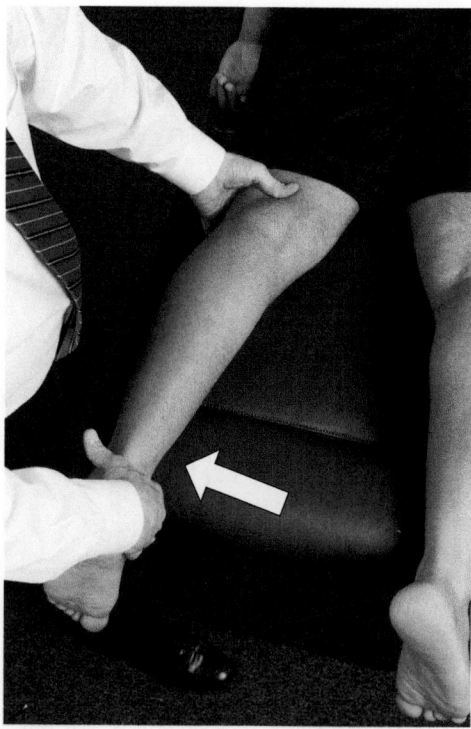

Figure 14-39 Stress Test for lateral femoral/tibial impingement.

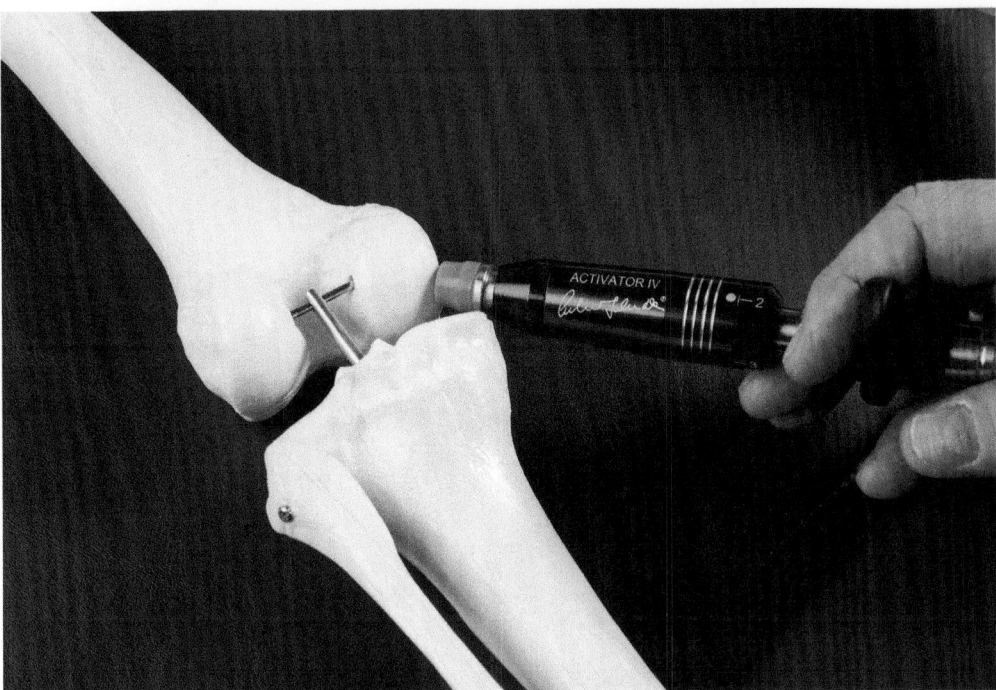

Figure 14-40 Adjustment for medial femoral/tibial impingement. Step One: Contact the medial femoral condyle. Line of Drive is superior and slightly lateral.

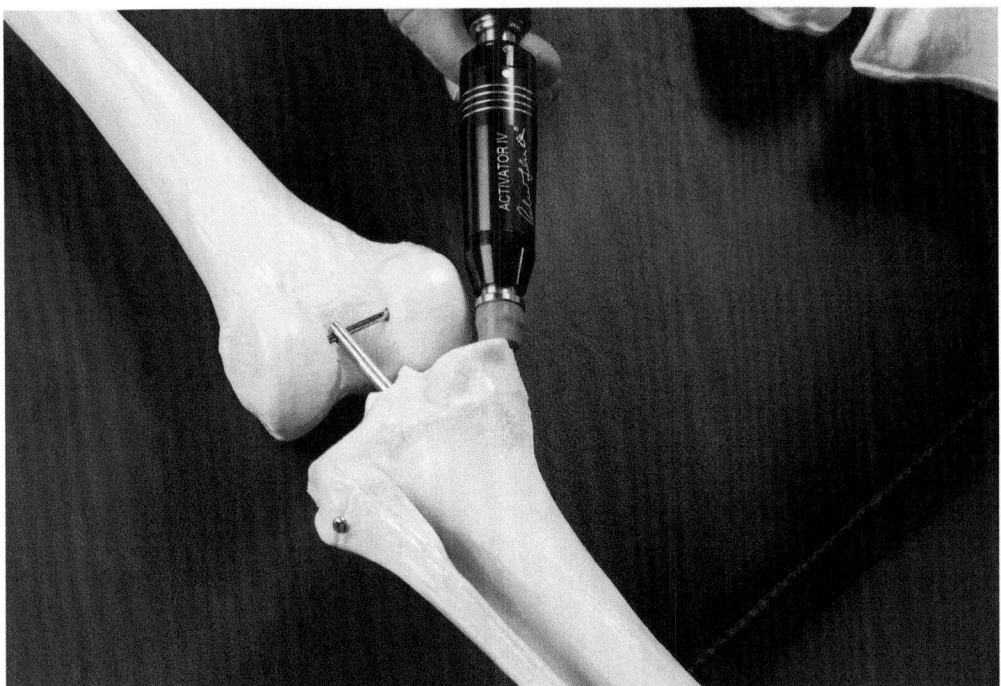

Figure 14-41 Adjustment for medial femoral/tibial impingement. Step Two: Contact the medial aspect of the proximal tibia. Line of Drive is inferior and slightly lateral.

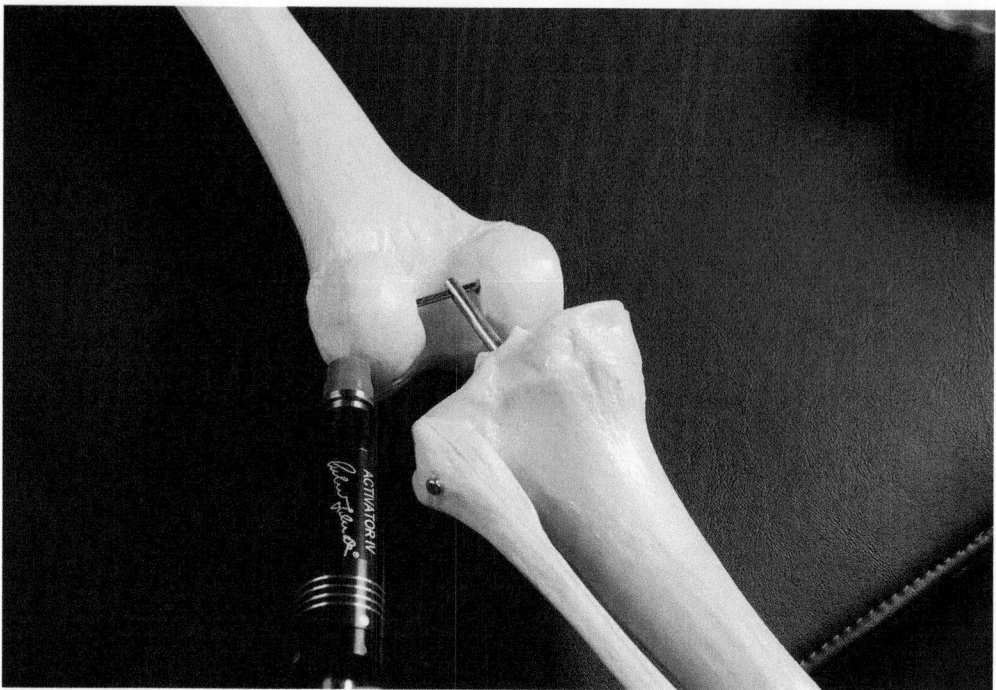

Figure 14-42 Adjustment for lateral femoral/tibial impingement. Step One: Contact the lateral femoral condyle. Line of Drive is superior and slightly medial.

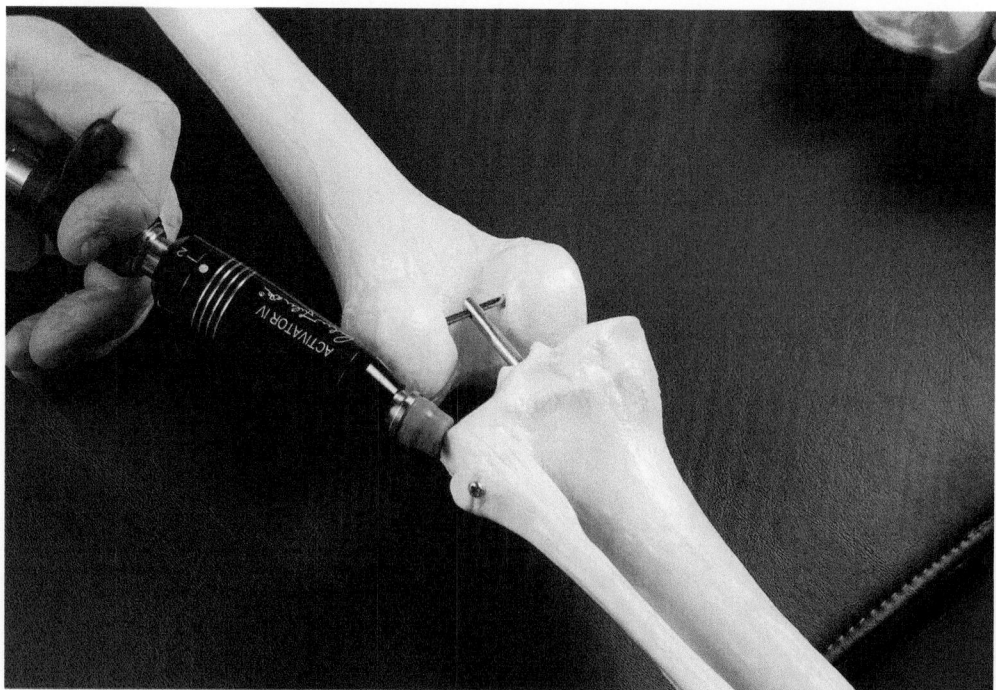

Figure 14-43 Adjustment for lateral femoral/tibial impingement. Step Two: Contact the lateral aspect of the proximal tibia. Line of Drive is inferior and slightly medial.

Table 14-1 Summary Table: Tests and Adjustments for the Knee and Related Structures

Articular Dysfunction	Test	ADJUSTMENT Segmental Contact Point	ADJUSTMENT Line of Drive
External Rotation of Proximal Tibia	Rotate proximal tibia laterally	Lateral tibial tubercle	Lateral to medial
Internal Rotation of Proximal Tibia	Rotate proximal tibia medially	Medial tibial tubercle	Medial to lateral
Anterior Proximal Tibia	Push proximal tibia anteriorly	Flex knee to 90 degrees and contact ½ inch below tibia tubercle	Posterior
Posterior Proximal Tibia	Lift proximal tibia posteriorly	*Step One:* Posterior medial condyle	Anterior
		Step Two: Posterior lateral condyle	Anterior
Genu Valgus	Push medial tibial condyle laterally and lateral femoral condyle medially	*Step One:* Lateral tibial condyle	Medial
		Step Two: Medial femoral condyle	Lateral
Genu Varus	Push lateral tibial condyle medially and medial femoral condyle laterally	*Step One:* Medial tibial condyle	Lateral
		Step Two: Lateral tibial condyle	Medial
Medial Knee Joint	Flex the knee to 90 degrees; compress and externally rotate the tibia	Medial collateral ligament in joint space	Lateral
Lateral Knee Joint	Flex the knee to 90 degrees; compress and internally rotate the tibia	Lateral collateral ligament in joint space	Medial
Medial (internal rotation) of the Distal Femur	Stabilize the tibia and roll the distal femur in a lateral-to-medial direction	Posterior medial femoral condyle	Anterior
Inferior Patella	Push patella inferiorly	Flex knee to 90 degrees inferior border of patella	Superior
Lateral Patella	Push patella laterally	Lateral border of patella	Medial
Lateral Fibula	Grasp lateral proximal third of fibula and pull laterally	Lateral fibula at proximal third of shaft	Medial and slightly anterior
Hamstrings	Doctor's hand on posterior distal tibia, resisting knee flexion	*Step One:* Myotendon junction of the medial hamstrings	Posterior to anterior
		Step Two: Myotendon junction of the lateral hamstrings	Posterior to anterior
Quadriceps Femoris	Doctor's hand on anterior distal tibia, resisting knee extension	Vastus medialis, myotendon junction	Anterior to posterior
Gastrocnemius	Patient's knee in less than 90 degrees of flexion; doctor's hand on plantar surface of foot; instruct the patient to plantarflex against resistance	*Step One:* Medial head of the gastrocnemius ½ inch inferior to the medial tibial condyle	Anterior and slightly superior
		Step Two: Lateral head of the gastrocnemius ½ inch inferior to the lateral tibial condyle	Anterior and slightly superior

Continued

Table 14-1 Summary Table: Tests and Adjustments for the Knee and Related Structures–cont'd

Articular Dysfunction	Test	Adjustment — Segmental Contact Point	Adjustment — Line of Drive
Compressed/ Impinged Femoral-Tibial Joint	*Medial Impingement:* Doctor grasps the involved posterior lateral distal tibia with one hand, and the other hand on the posterior medial distal femur. Doctor moves tibia toward midline, a lateral-to-medial stress.	*Step One:* Medial condyle of the femur *Step Two:* Medial aspect of the proximal tibia	Superior and slightly lateral Inferior and slightly lateral
	Lateral Impingement: Doctor grasps the involved posterior medial distal tibia with one hand, and the other hand on the posterior lateral distal femur. Move the tibia away from midline, a medial-to-lateral stress.	*Step One:* Lateral condyle of the femur *Step Two:* Lateral aspect of the proximal tibia	Superior and slightly medial Inferior and slightly medial

RELATED RESEARCH

Box 14-2 provides related research on the chiropractic treatment of the knee.

Box 14-2

Reference: Polkinghorn BS. Conservative treatment of torn medial meniscus via mechanical force, manually assisted short lever chiropractic adjusting procedures. J Manipulative Physiol Ther. 1994;17(7):474-84.

ABSTRACT
OBJECTIVE

To present the first reported case of successful chiropractic intervention in treatment of a torn medial meniscus of the knee; the meniscal tear was documented by magnetic resonance imaging (MRI).

CLINICAL FEATURES

A 54-year-old woman who reported right knee pain of several months' duration with accompanying marked functional impairment was given the diagnosis of a tear in the posterior horn of the ipsilateral medial meniscus, verified by MRI studies of the same. Independent consultation with three medical specialists resulted in the unanimous decision that surgical intervention for the purpose of meniscectomy provided the only therapeutic approach indicated for the problem. However, the patient was reticent to undergo said surgical procedure and chose, instead, to use chiropractic care and conservative management in an effort to resolve her condition without having to resort to surgery.

INTERVENTION AND OUTCOME

The patient received chiropractic treatment to the knee via mechanical force, manually assisted short lever chiropractic adjusting procedures performed with an Activator Adjusting Instrument. Auxiliary treatment included the use of homeopathic therapy as an adjunct to chiropractic care. Said treatment resulted in complete resolution of the patient's disability; the patient recovered full function of the knee joint and achieved asymptomatic status without having to submit to surgical intervention and its possible adverse sequelae.

CONCLUSIONS

Conservative management of meniscal tears via chiropractic treatment may provide a therapeutically effective and financial cost–containing alternative to routine meniscectomy in certain cases involving torn medial menisci of the knee.

REFERENCES

1. Klein KK. Development asymmetries of the weight bearing skeleton and its implications in knee stress and knee injury. Athlet Train. 1978;13:78-80.
2. Dixon AS, Campbell-Smith S. Long leg arthropathy. Ann Rheum Dis. 1969;28(4):359-64.
3. Clemente CD. Gray's anatomy. 30th American ed. Philadelphia: Lea & Febiger; 1985.
4. Magee DJ. The knee. In: Orthopedic physical assessment. Philadelphia: Saunders; 1987. p. 266-313.
5. Pecina MM, Bojanic I. Overuse injuries of the musculoskeletal system. Boca Rat (FL): CRC Press; 1993.
6. Marzo JM, Wickiewicz TL. Overuse knee injuries. In: Renström P, editor. The encyclopedia of sports medicine, Vol V: Clinical practice of sports injury prevention and care. London: Blackwell; 1994.
7. Hoppenfeld S. Physical examination of the spine and extremities. Norwalk (CT): Appleton-Century-Crofts; 1976.
8. Whittle MW. Gait analysis. In: McLatchie GR, Lennox CME. The soft tissues: trauma and sports injuries. London: Butterworth-Heinemann; 1993.
9. Bovee M. The essentials of orthopedic & neurological testing. Davenport (IA): Bovee/Palmer College of Chiropractic; 1977.
10. Cipriano JJ. Photographic manual of regional orthopaedic tests. Baltimore: Williams & Wilkins; 1985.
11. Peters LM. Manual muscle testing: a visual guide. Atlanta: Susan Hunter Publishing; 1986.
12. Moore KW, Frank CB. Traumatic knee injuries. In: Renström P, editor. The encyclopedia of sports medicine, Vol V: Clinical practice of sports injury prevention and care. London: Blackwell; 1994.
13. Mazion JM. Illustrated manual of neurological reflexes/signs/tests and orthopedic signs/tests/maneuvers for office procedures. Arizona City: Mazion; 1980.
14. Kulund DN. The injured athlete. 2nd ed. Philadelphia: Lippincott; 1988.
15. Deutsch AL, Mink JH, Fox JM, Arnoczky SP, Rothman BJ, Stoller DW, et al. Peripheral meniscal tears: MR findings after conservative treatment and arthroscopic repair. Radiology. 1990;176(2):485-8.
16. Polkinghorn BS. Conservative treatment of torn medial meniscus via mechanical force, manually assisted short lever chiropractic adjusting procedures. J Manipulative Physiol Ther. 1994;17(7): 474-84.
17. Pritchett JW. High cost of high school football injuries. Am J Sports Med. 1980;8(3):197-9.
18. Baylis WJ, Rzonca EC. Functional and structural limb length discrepancies: evaluation and treatment. Clin Podiatr Med Surg. 1988;5(3):509-20.
19. Subotnick DI. Limb length discrepancies of the lower extremity. J Orthop Sports Phys Ther. 1981;3:11-15.
20. Danbert RJ. Clinical assessment and treatment of leg length inequalities. J Manipulative Physiol Ther. 1988;11(4):290-5.
21. Lawrence DJ. Chiropractic concepts of the short leg: a critical review. J Manipulative Physiol Ther. 1985;8(3):157-61.
22. Henning CE, Griffis ND, Vequist SW, Yearout KM, Decker KA. Sport-specific knee injuries. In: Renström P, editor. The encyclopedia of sports medicine, Vol V: Clinical practice of sports injury prevention and care. London: Blackwell; 1994.
23. Henry JH. Conservative treatment of patellofemoral subluxation. Clin Sports Med 1989;8(2): 261-78.
24. Ireland ML. Patellofemoral disorders in runners and cyclists. Ann Sports Med. 1987;3:77-85.
25. Hughston JC. Patellar subluxation. A recent history. Clin Sports Med. 1989;8(2):153-62.
26. Hughston JC, Deese M. Medial subluxation of the patella as a complication of lateral retinacular release. Am J Sports Med. 1988;16(4):383-388.
27. Turner M. The association between tibial torsion and knee joint pathology. Clin Orthop Relat Res. 1994;(302):47-51.
28. Key J, Johnson D, Jarvis G, Ponsonby D. Knee and thigh injuries. In: Subotnick SI, editor. Sports medicine of the lower extremity. London: Churchill Livingstone; 1989.
29. Garrick JG, Webb RD. Sports injuries: diagnosis and management. Philadelphia: Saunders; 1990.
30. Christensen K. Preventing leg injuries. Dynamic Chiropractic, May 7, 2001.
31. McNair PJ, Marshall RN, Matheson JA. Important features associated with acute anterior cruciate ligament injury. N Z Med J. 1990;103(901): 571-9.
32. Loudon JK, Jenkins W, Loudon KL. The relationship between static posture and ACL injury in female athletes. J Orthop Sports Phys Ther. 1996;24(2):91-7.
33. Liebenson C. Rehabilitation of lower extremity disorders. Dynamic Chiropractic, January 1, 1997.
34. Roland GC, Beagley MJ, Cawley PW. Conservative treatment of inflamed knee bursitis. Phys Sports Med. 1992;20:60-77.
35. Castorina JS, Deyo RA. Back and lower extremity disorders. In: Rosenstock L, Cullen MR, editors. Textbook of clinical occupational and environmental medicine. Philadelphia: Saunders; 1994.
36. Travell J, Simons J. Myofascial pain and dysfunction, Vol 1, 2. Baltimore: Williams & Wilkins; 1998.
37. Orava S. Lower leg injuries. In: Renström P, editor. The encyclopedia of sports medicine, Vol V: Clinical practice of sports injury prevention and care. London: Blackwell; 1994.

38. Yochum TR, Rowe LJ. Essentials of skeletal radiology, Vol, I, II. Baltimore: Williams & Wilkins; 1987.

39. Katz JN, Brissot R, Liang MH. Systemic rheumatologic disorders. In: Rosenstock L, Cullen MR, editors. Textbook of clinical occupational and environmental medicine. Philadelphia: Saunders; 1994.

40. Slemenda C, Brandt KD, Heilman DK, Mazzuca S, Braunstein EM, Katz BP, et al. Quadriceps weakness and osteoarthritis of the knee. Ann Intern Med. 1997;127(2):97-104.

41. O'Reilly SC, Jones A, Muir KR, Doherty M. Quadriceps weakness in knee osteoarthritis: the effect on pain and disability. Ann Rheum Dis. 1998;57(10):588-94.

42. Lewis C, McAndrew J. Examining further treatment for osteoarthritis. Advance for Physical Therapists, June 24, 2002.

43. Baker KR, Nelson ME, Felson DT, Layne JE, Sarno R, Roubenoff R. The efficacy of home based progressive strength training in older adults with knee osteoarthritis: a randomized controlled trial. J Rheumatol. 2001;28(7): 1655-65.

44. Sheehy P, Burdett RG, Irrgang JJ, Van Swearingen J. An electromyographic study of vastus medialis oblique and vastus lateralis activity while ascending and descending steps. J Orthop Sports Phys Ther. 1998;27(6):423-9.

15

ADDITIONAL TESTS AND ADJUSTMENTS FOR THE FOOT AND ANKLE

E valuation of the foot and ankle is indicated when a patient complains of pain, weakness, or stiffness in the region, or biomechanical aberrancy is observed. A thorough screening of the foot, ankle, and related structures should be performed when a patient presents with any of the following:

• Reduction or alteration of ankle range of motion
• Plantar fasciitis and plantar soft tissue or toe pain
• Inversion sprain of the ankle
• Achilles tendonitis, posterior "shin splints," or calf muscle pain
• Biomechanical disorders of the foot and ankle

Frequent sites of pain are at the medial aspect of the plantar surface of the foot at the "instep," at the insertion of the Achilles tendon to the calcaneus, and at the region of the talofibular ligament just anterior and inferior to the lateral malleolus. Toe, heel, shin, and calf pain are common manifestations of biomechanical disorders of the foot and ankle.[1]

SPECIAL CONSIDERATIONS

Always inspect the shoes of a patient with foot and ankle complaints. Look for abnormal wear patterns, especially excessive unilateral heel wear. Normal heel-strike occurs at the posterior lateral aspect of the shoe heel, and shoes typically first show wear at that site.[2] If the heel on one side shows significantly greater wear at the posterior lateral aspect than the other, chronic inversion neuroarticular dysfunction of the ankle joint is the likely cause.

Also, inspect the leather uppers of the shoes. Bulging and distortion of the leather on the medial side of the foot toward the great toe indicate poorly fitting shoes that can cause corns, bunions, and displacement of the metatarsal bones, or may be an indication that such conditions already exist. Also note the wear pattern on the sole of the shoe. Excessive unilateral wear under the first metatarsophalangeal joint indicates overpronation, the most common biomechanical problem of the ambulatory patient.

If a patient experiences plantar foot pain, inspect the arch supports. Athletic and work shoes without adequate support for the medial longitudinal arch of the foot can contribute to plantar fasciitis and inferior neuroarticular dysfunction of the metatarsals, resulting in neuroarticular dysfunction of the tarsal-metatarsal joints.[2]

Patients who wear high-heeled shoes or Western boots frequently develop contractures of the gastrocnemius and soleus muscles of the calf. Calcaneal pain, especially at the insertion of the Achilles tendon, may occur when the patient walks in slippers, flat shoes, stockings, or bare feet. Calf muscle contracture should be considered when Activator Method Leg Length Analyses are conducted. It may be difficult to remove plantar flexion without distorting the leg test analysis. Thus the feet should be dorsiflexed just to the point of resistance in Position #1 and Position #2, if possible. If patient anatomy limits the correct position, perform Leg Length Analysis by avoiding any undue resistance of the patient.

COMMON COMPLAINTS

According to Magee,[3] at least 80% of people today have foot problems that can often be corrected by proper assessment and conservative treatment. Lesions of the ankle and foot can alter the mechanics of gait and, as a result, can affect the stress on joints of the lower limb, which may consequently lead to further neuroarticular dysfunction and pathology in these joints. The cause of most complaints in the lower extremity is traumatic injury; however, Leg Length Inequality (LLI) is also associated with various lower extremity pain and stress syndromes.

Individuals with LLI may pronate the foot on the side of the longer limb in an attempt to provide functional shortening of the longer leg.[4,5] Ankle plantar flexion with foot supination has been noted on the short leg side, also as a functional adaptation to LLI.[6-8]

Acute and chronic injury to articulations of the foot and ankle can result in a wide variety of problems. Many of the conditions discussed in the following sections are directly or indirectly related to neuroarticular dysfunction of structures in the lower extremity.

Reduction or Alteration of Ankle Range of Motion

The talocrural joint (ankle joint) is principally uniaxial and is classified as a ginglymoarthrodial, or hinge joint, located between the talus, the medial malleolus of the tibia, and the lateral malleolus of the fibula.[3,9] The superior articular surface of the talus articulates mainly with the distal portion of the tibia, at the medial malleolus. The strong distal tibiofibular joint forms a bridge or mortise over the superior talus, and the distal fibula forms the lateral malleolus. The deltoid ligament provides medial ankle support, and the anterior and posterior talofibular ligaments and the calcaneofibular ligaments collectively provide lateral ankle stability.

Ligamentous laxity, especially of the anterior talofibular ligament, can make the foot and ankle unstable and subject to recurrent inversion sprain.[10] The patient with a history of repeated ankle sprains is especially vulnerable to developing ligamentous laxity in the talocrural joint. The most common motion components of ankle sprain are inversion and plantar flexion of the foot. The anterior talofibular ligament therefore is subject to stretching, and the talus may be involved anteriorly and laterally. If left unaddressed, ligamentous laxity will almost invariably lead to chronic ankle pain or degenerative joint disease of the ankle and will have an impact on gait, mobility, and general body balance and posture.[10,11]

Stiffness or limited range of motion of the ankle joint can contribute to gait asymmetry or limp.[12] The normal motions of the ankle include plantar flexion, dorsiflexion, inversion (supination), and eversion (pronation). Average range of motion values for the ankle are listed in Box 15-1.[13-15]

Active plantar flexion and muscle strength of the gastrocnemius-soleus complex (calf muscles) can be assessed by having the patient walk a few paces on the balls of the feet. Active dorsiflexion and strength of the foot extensor muscles, especially of the tibialis anterior and the extensor hallucis longus, can be evaluated by having

Box 15-1	**Ankle Ranges of Motion**
Plantar flexion	50 degrees
Dorsiflexion	20 degrees
Inversion	5 degrees
Eversion	5 degrees

The range-of-motion values listed here and elsewhere in *The Activator Method* are averages of values published in various sources and should not be interpreted as "normal" for a given patient. Ranges of motion may be influenced by factors such as age, gender, weight, build, and general physical activity.[13-15]

the patient walk a few paces on the heels. The four motions of the ankle should be evaluated by passive range of motion testing, with comparison of left and right ankle and foot global ranges of motion. Be sure to note pain-limited range of motion, as well as tenderness to palpation. Be alert for crepitus and tenderness in and around the ankle joint on palpation.

Plantar Fasciitis

Strain and sprain injuries to the ligaments, muscles, and fascia of the plantar aspect of the foot can cause plantar fasciitis, an inflammatory reaction, in these soft tissues at or near the attachments to the calcaneus.[16] Plantar fasciitis typically results from repetitive microtrauma due to faulty mechanics (overpronation), muscular imbalance or fatigue, and training errors. This microtrauma leads to inflammation and tearing of the tissue at the attachment on the anterior tubercle of the calcaneus.[17] Fibrotic change in the tissues may result in a palpably firm mass near the region of the calcaneal tuberosity on the plantar surface of the calcaneus. Radiographical examination will rule out calcification of soft tissue and the formation of a true heel spur on the calcaneus.

The plantar tarsal ligaments, especially the long plantar ligament, provide important support to the plantar arches.[18] The long plantar ligament runs along the inferior aspect of the calcaneus from its tuberosity and inserts on the bases of the second through fifth metatarsals proximal to the toes. This strong ligament has bands of fibers that run to the cuboid, navicular, and cuneiform bones; it therefore plays a major role in maintaining the integrity of the transverse and longitudinal arches of the foot. The arches function as shock absorbers in diminishing the impact of each heel and foot-strike during walking or running.

Major muscles of the plantar aspect of the foot, originating on the calcaneus and inserting distally at the phalanges, are mainly flexors, adductors, and abductors of the toes.[9] The abductor of the great toe helps form the fleshy portion of the medial border of the sole of the foot. The short flexor muscles of the toes and the quadrate muscle of the sole make up most of the soft tissue mass of the plantar aspect of the foot. (The bellies of the long flexor muscles of the toes are located in the calf, but their tendons run through the plantar aspect of the foot.) Overlying the plantar musculature is the plantar aponeurosis, a sheet of strong fibrous tissue that runs from the calcaneal tuberosity to the phalanges. The plantar aponeurosis and the plantar muscle group also provide support for the medial longitudinal arch of the foot. The integrity of the plantar fascia plays a significant role in maintenance and stability of the medial longitudinal arch.[19]

The plantar soft tissue is subject to chronic or repetitive strain/sprain injury from long periods of standing, walking, or running, especially in shoes or boots without adequate arch support.[18] Patients who work in environments that require them to be on their feet for most of the day also may be particularly vulnerable to development of plantar fasciitis if they are not careful about their footwear. Occupations that require operation of a foot pedal, such as machinists, assemblers, tailors and seamstresses, and long distance drivers, can also produce stress in the plantar soft tissues by stretching the ligaments and muscles. Usually, the onset of plantar fasciitis is gradual and insidious. Signs and symptoms include plantar pain and swelling of the feet by the end of the workday. Pain may be diffused and may be distributed throughout the plantar soft tissue, or it may be focal, especially at the bottom of the heel near the calcaneal tuberosity, where even ordinary heel-strike during walking can exacerbate it.

The plantar soft tissues are subject to acute strain/sprain injury. Jumping from a high platform, such as a loading dock, the back of a truck, or scaffolding, can deliver enormous stresses to the plantar arches and the tissues that support them. Sudden, forceful plantar flexion of the foot in athletic activities such as sprinting, basketball, tennis, and even baseball can strain the plantar muscles and produce foot pain. Dancers, especially ballet performers dancing *en pointe*, are at risk of developing plantar fasciitis because of the extreme, forceful plantar flexion required by the position.[20] Signs and symptoms may include swelling and pain,

especially at the metatarsophalangeal joints. Point tenderness and edema may occur along the instep of the foot as well. Clinically, classic symptoms of plantar fasciitis are described as a sharp pain at the inferior calcaneal attachment of the plantar fascia. Patient symptoms include a distinct, "glasslike" pain that occurs after prolonged sitting, upon arising from sleep, or after a period of rest without support under the arch. As the condition develops, the patient will draw up the arch and walk on the outside of the foot to avoid pain on weight bearing.

Whether plantar fasciitis is of sudden or gradual onset, be sure to assess the patient for the following neuroarticular dysfunctions:
- Medial calcaneus
- Lateral calcaneus
- Superior calcaneus
- Posterior calcaneus
- Medial navicular
- Cuboid
- Anterior lateral talus
- Inferior first metatarsal and inferior medial first cuneiform
- Inferior metatarsal heads

Detailed instructions for performing Stress Tests and adjustments where indicated for these neuroarticular dysfunctions are provided later in this chapter. See the research related to plantar fasciitis in Box 15-2.

Metatarsalgia

When the patient reports pain at the ball of the foot, palpation of the metatarsophalangeal joints may reveal tenderness and inflammation, most often in the second and third joints. Metatarsalgia is aggravated by squatting down with toes extended (heels off the floor). An example would be in an elementary school teacher who repetitively squats to speak to children at eye level. Metatarsalgia also can be associated with foot pronation.[21] When a patient presents with metatarsalgia, assess the foot for the following neuroarticular dysfunctions:
- Inferior metatarsal heads
- Distal first metatarsal and superior proximal first phalanx

Detailed instructions for performing Stress Tests and adjustments where indicated for these involvements are given later in this chapter.

Retrocalcaneal Bursitis

Several bursae and synovial sheaths near the heel, when inflamed, can produce retrocalcaneal bursitis. A subcutaneous bursa on the posterior aspect of the calcaneus, for example, can become painful and swollen after a blow to the heel. Bursitis at this location is particularly painful at heel-strike during gait, and the patient may adopt an antalgic, flat-footed gait when the bursitis is active. Poorly fitted tight shoes will exacerbate bursitis at the posterior aspect of the heel.

The most common site of retrocalcaneal bursitis is the bursa between the calcaneus and the Achilles tendon; this condition is known as Haglund's syndrome.[22] Passive dorsiflexion of the ankle produces sharp, localized pain deep to the Achilles tendon near its insertion on the calcaneus. Point tenderness on deep palpation over the insertion of the Achilles tendon with the foot held in passive plantar flexion also helps to confirm bursitis at this site. The patient will adopt a flat-footed antalgic gait on heel-strike and will demonstrate a vaulting gait to avoid plantar flexion against resistance at the toe-off component of a normal gait cycle.

The tendons of the long flexor muscles of the toes pass posterior to the medial malleolus, through synovial sheaths located close to the bursa of the Achilles tendon. These sheaths are located deep to the flexor retinaculum, which itself runs from the medial malleolus to the medial aspect of the calcaneus. Passive dorsiflexion of the great toe and of other toes can produce pain over the medial and posterior regions of the calcaneus. Point tenderness on deep palpation and palpable swelling over the medial aspect of the calcaneus or just below the medial malleolus may signify inflammation of these synovial sheaths.[23]

When a patient presents with retrocalcaneal bursitis, assess the foot and ankle for the following neuroarticular dysfunctions:

- Medial calcaneus
- Superior calcaneus
- Inferior first metatarsal and inferior medial cuneiform
- Inferior metatarsal heads

Detailed instructions for performing Stress Tests and adjustments where indicated for these neuroarticular dysfunctions are given later in this chapter.

Inversion Ankle Sprains

The main components of a sprain injury to the talocrural ankle joint are inversion and plantar flexion.[3,9] As a result of inversion ankle sprains, the talus is forced anteriorly and laterally relative to the bridge formed by the distal fibula and tibia, and the navicular tends to be displaced anteriorly and superiorly.

A patient with a sprained ankle, with pain and swelling over the dorsolateral aspect of the foot, has point tenderness localized to the region of the *sinus tarsi*—that region of the talus just anterior and inferior to the lateral malleolus. During injury, the anterior portion of the talofibular ligament is stretched and may be torn. Passive inversion and plantar flexion of the foot and ankle produce pain near the anterior talofibular ligament.

In severe plantar flexion and inversion injury, avulsion fracture of the distal fibula is possible. Radiographical examination of the ankle may be necessary for differentiation. To assess the ankle for torn anterior or posterior talofibular ligaments, use the anterior-posterior drawer sign.[16] To perform the anterior ankle drawer test, stabilize the leg by taking a firm hold with one hand over the shin at the level of the distal tibiofibular joint. Grasp the calcaneus by cupping the heel in the other hand, and try to pull or draw the foot anteriorly. Anterior movement of more than 1 or 2 millimeters, accompanied by pain, suggests laxity and a possible tear of the anterior talofibular ligament. To perform the posterior ankle drawer sign, stabilize the leg by taking a firm hold with one hand over the calf at the level of the Achilles tendon. Grasp the calcaneus by cupping the plantar surface in the other hand, and try to push the tarsal bones as a unit posteriorly. Posterior movement of more than 1 or 2 millimeters, with pain, indicates laxity and a possible tear of the posterior talofibular ligament.

A patient with a history of "weak ankles" who is subject to recurrent sprains may have laxity of the talofibular ligaments (both anterior and posterior portions).[11] The joint itself may be hypermobile, and the patient will tend to show significant inversion on the side of involvement. When the patient is on the adjusting table with the legs in Position #1, abnormal inversion of greater than 10 to 15 degrees is readily visible. Another indicator of ligamentous laxity and ankle instability is the observation of greater inversion on the side of the Pelvic Deficiency. During initial patient placement, the Pelvic Deficient (PD) or reactive leg most often is on the side that shows greater inversion of the foot and ankle. Excessive unilateral heel wear on the side of ligamentous laxity can be an important indication of an ankle injury. If excessive shoe wear or greater than normal inversion of the foot is observed, ask the patient about past ankle injuries or a tendency to sprain the ankle frequently and easily.

When a patient experiences an inversion ankle sprain, weak, easily turned ankles, or excessive inversion of the ankles and feet, perform

Stress Tests and adjustments as indicated for the following neuroarticular dysfunctions:

- Anterior lateral talus
- Anterior-superior navicular
- Anterior distal tibia
- Medial calcaneus
- Superior calcaneus
- Posterior distal fibula

Detailed instructions for performing Stress Tests and adjustments where indicated for these neuroarticular dysfunctions are given later in this chapter.

Achilles Tendonitis

Strain injury with inflammation of the Achilles tendon is a common problem among dancers, runners, and other athletes.[20] Symptoms may occur at the insertion of the tendon on the posterior aspect of the calcaneus, or, more proximally, at the musculotendinous junction of the gastrocnemius-soleus complex. Most often, this is described as diffuse pain in or about the Achilles tendon that is aggravated by activity.

In more severe cases of a chronic inflammatory process, swelling, crepitus, and a palpable tender nodule are noted in the tendon.[24] Calf muscle hypertonicity, contracture, or sharply painful spasm may accompany Achilles tendonitis.[25]

Resisted dorsiflexion of the foot and ankle reproduces localized pain in the Achilles tendon. Pressure applied to the tendon while the foot is held firmly in a neutral or slightly dorsiflexed position also confirms Achilles tendonitis. The Achilles (S1) reflex is typically present, but it may be slightly exaggerated if calf muscles are hypertonic. On the other hand, the reflex may be apparently diminished if the peritendineum and surrounding tissues are boggy and edematous.

The pain of Achilles tendonitis is exacerbated when the patient climbs stairs or walks uphill because the forced dorsiflexion of the foot and ankle stretches the tendon. The patient may develop a limp or other antalgic gait to avoid pain, especially during the "toe-off" portion of the gait cycle.

A patient who frequently wears high heels or Western boots and changes abruptly to flat shoes, running shoes, or slippers can experience calf muscle pain similar to Achilles tendonitis after walking or running even a short distance. Runners, dancers, skaters, and skiers can experience moderate to severe calf muscle strain injury and Achilles tendonitis if they fail to warm up by passively stretching the calf muscles before beginning strenuous activity.[26-28]

When a patient experiences Achilles tendonitis or calf muscle pain, assess the patient for the following neuroarticular dysfunctions:

- Superior calcaneus
- Medial calcaneus

Detailed instructions for performing Stress Tests and adjustments where indicated for these neuroarticular dysfunctions are given later in this chapter.

CONCURRENT CONDITIONS

Several disorders can contribute to foot problems and altered biomechanics of the ankle. The source of foot pain may actually be referred from the knee, hip, or lumbosacral level of the spine. Syndromes, especially sciatic neuralgia, should be ruled out with appropriate orthopedic and neurological assessment. Nerve entrapment can produce sensory deficit (hypoesthesia), altered or painful sensation (dysesthesia), and atrophy of lower extremity muscles.[29] The most common motor deficit affects the evertors and dorsiflexors of the ankle, leading to foot drop.

Patients with diabetes mellitus are especially at risk of developing foot and lower extremity problems.[30] Good patient education for the diabetic patient emphasizes meticulous care of the feet, including daily visual inspection for blisters, sores, and signs of poor circulation. In advanced diabetes mellitus, significant loss of vascular supply and sensory and proprioceptive innervation to the lower extremity can occur. Diabetic arthropathy, a painless degeneration of articular soft tissue and bone, can lead to changes in the structural and functional integrity of the foot, knee, and hip.

Atherosclerotic plaquing in the arterial circulation, with occlusion of the blood supply to tissues, underlies two of the top three causes of death in the North American population: heart disease and stroke.[31] In addition to the coronary and cerebral blood vessels, other branch points in the circulatory system are vulnerable to atherosclerosis. Intermittent claudication results when the common iliac arteries are occluded. Ischemic injury to active muscles, whose physiological demand for oxygen becomes greater than the supply, causes pain that can mimic sciatica, arthritis, or sprain/strain injuries. Diminished pulse pressures at the popliteal artery and dorsum of the foot can indicate vascular occlusion from intermittent claudication.[16]

TESTING AND ADJUSTING THE FOOT, ANKLE, AND RELATED STRUCTURES

When patient complaints or examination findings indicate involvement of the foot, ankle, or related structures, the following tests and adjustments should be performed as needed. For the ankle articulation, check for the following neuroarticular dysfunctions:

- Medial calcaneus
- Lateral calcaneus
- Superior calcaneus
- Inferior calcaneus
- Posterior calcaneus
- Anterior-superior navicular
- Cuboid
- Medial navicular
- Anterior lateral talus
- Anterior distal tibia
- Posterior distal fibula
- Posterior-superior proximal fibula

For the foot proper, check for these neuroarticular dysfunctions:

- Inferior first metatarsal and inferior medial cuneiform
- Inferior metatarsal heads
- Superior distal first metatarsal and superior proximal first phalanx
- Hallux valgus or first metatarsophalangeal joint (great toe)

Involvement of the fibula can occur proximally or distally, and can affect the role of the biomechanical and structural integrity of the ankle; therefore consider these neuroarticular dysfunctions:

- Posterior distal end of the fibula
- Posterior-superior proximal end of the fibula

Keep in mind the tests for neuroarticular dysfunction of these structures are *Stress Tests*, that is, patient movements or maneuvers performed by the practitioner are intended to stress the structure involved into the direction of neuroarticular dysfunction. For the adjustment or correction, therefore, the Line of Drive (LOD) is opposite the direction of the Stress Test.

Medial Calcaneus

Medial involvement of the calcaneus should be considered when a patient experiences posterior plantar arch pain, Achilles tendonitis, plantar fasciitis, retrocalcaneal bursitis, or a history of inversion ankle sprain. In addition, consider a medial calcaneus in a patient who shows excessive unilateral heel wear or a gait abnormality consistent with chronic ankle inversion.

Stress Test. To Stress Test for a medial calcaneus, apply a lateral-to-medial force at the lateral border of the affected calcaneus. The standard method for performing this Stress Test is to tap the lateral calcaneus using a percussive tap in the medial direction on the lateral surface of the calcaneus (Figure 15-1). Look for PD leg reactivity in Position #1.

Adjustment. To adjust for medial calcaneal involvement, contact the inferior medial border

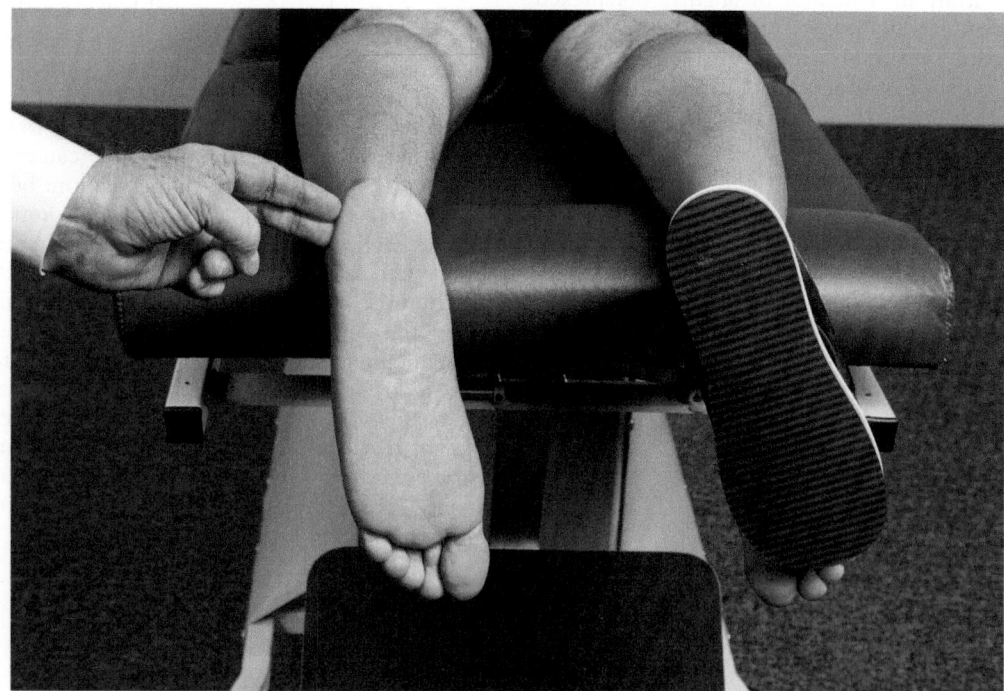

Figure 15-1 Stress Test for medial calcaneus.

of the calcaneus. The LOD is straight medial to lateral (Figure 15-2).

To maintain consistency of the leg test analysis for a medial calcaneus, perform the Stress Test by leaving the patient's shoes on. However, to ensure correct contact, LOD, and delivery of an effective thrust, remove the shoe on the affected side before adjusting the calcaneus.

> ## Clinical Observations
>
> Frequent inversion sprains of the ankle, excessive unilateral inversion of the foot, and plantar foot pain are consistent with a medial calcaneus. Assess the patient for improperly fitted or excessively worn shoes. Also, be alert to the patient's need for, or use of improperly fitted, orthotics.
>
> When a medial calcaneus does not respond to adjusting procedures, or if the adjustment does not hold, consider taping the foot for support until adjustments do hold.[35]

Lateral Calcaneus

Lateral involvement of the calcaneus should be considered when a patient experiences plantar fasciitis or an eversion ankle injury. The patient may present with heel pain at the fascial insertion at the anteromedial aspect of the calcaneus or along the longitudinal medial arch of the foot. In addition, consider a lateral calcaneus in a patient who shows excessive unilateral heel wear medially, a gait abnormality consistent with chronic ankle eversion, medial bowing of the Achilles tendon, or pes planus.

Stress Test. To Stress Test for lateral calcaneal involvement, apply a medial-to-lateral force at the medial border of the affected calcaneus. The standard method for performing this Stress Test is to tap the medial calcaneus using a percussive tap in the lateral direction on the medial surface of the calcaneus. Look for PD leg reactivity in Position #1 (Figure 15-3).

Adjustment. To adjust for lateral calcaneal involvement, contact the inferior lateral border of the calcaneus. The LOD is straight lateral to medial (Figure 15-4).

To maintain consistency of the leg test analysis for a lateral calcaneus, perform the Stress Test by leaving the patient's shoes on. However, to ensure correct contact, LOD, and delivery of an effective thrust, remove the shoe on the affected side before adjusting the calcaneus.

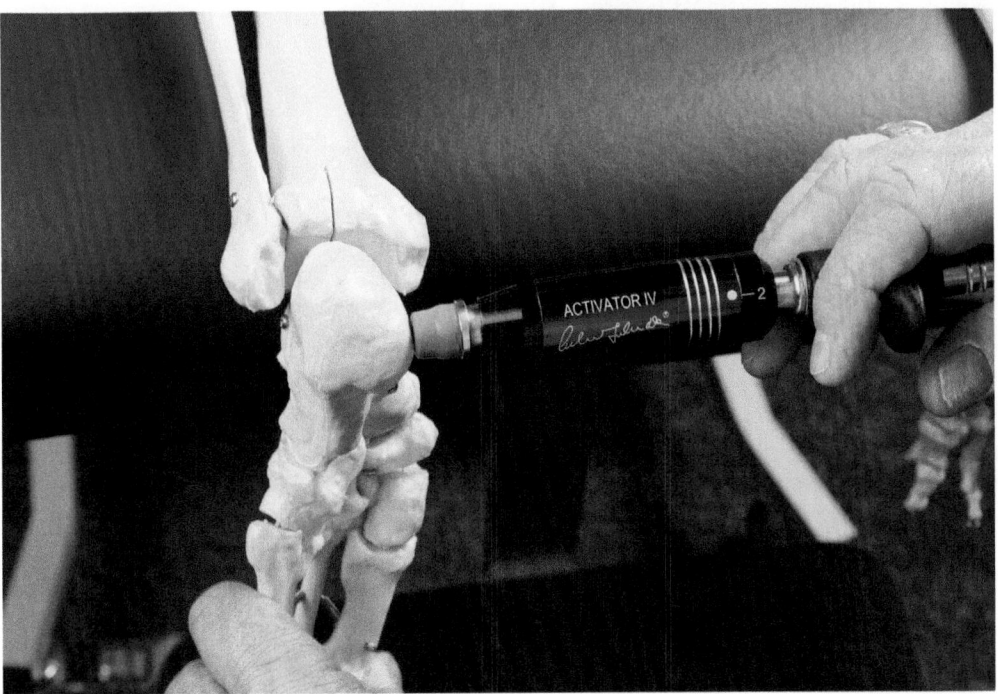

Figure 15-2 Adjustment for medial calcaneus. Line of Drive is straight medial to lateral.

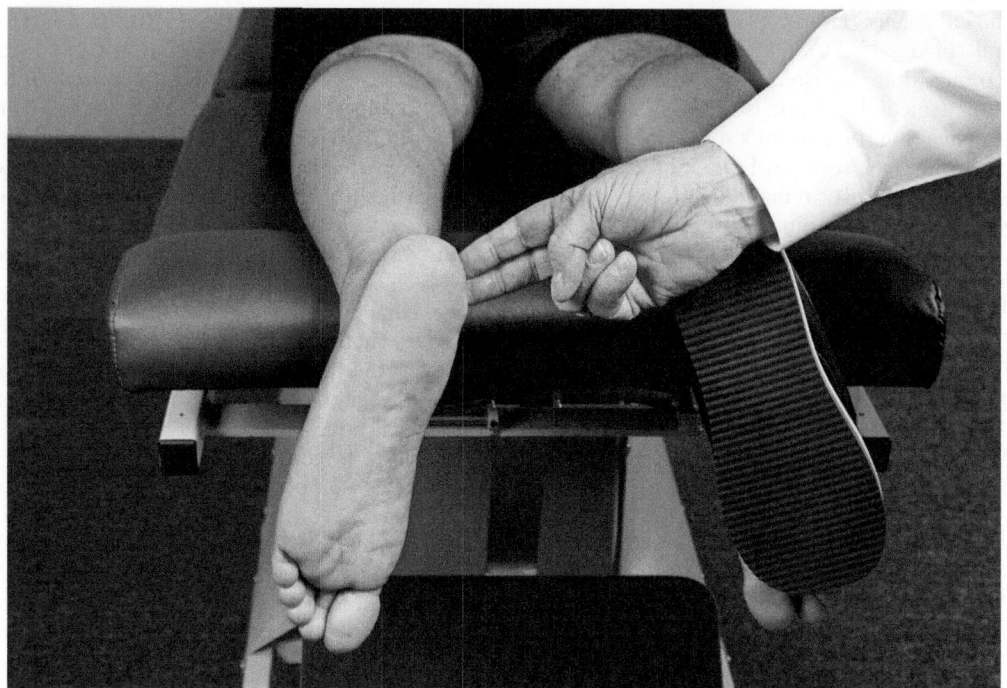

Figure 15-3 Stress Test for lateral calcaneus.

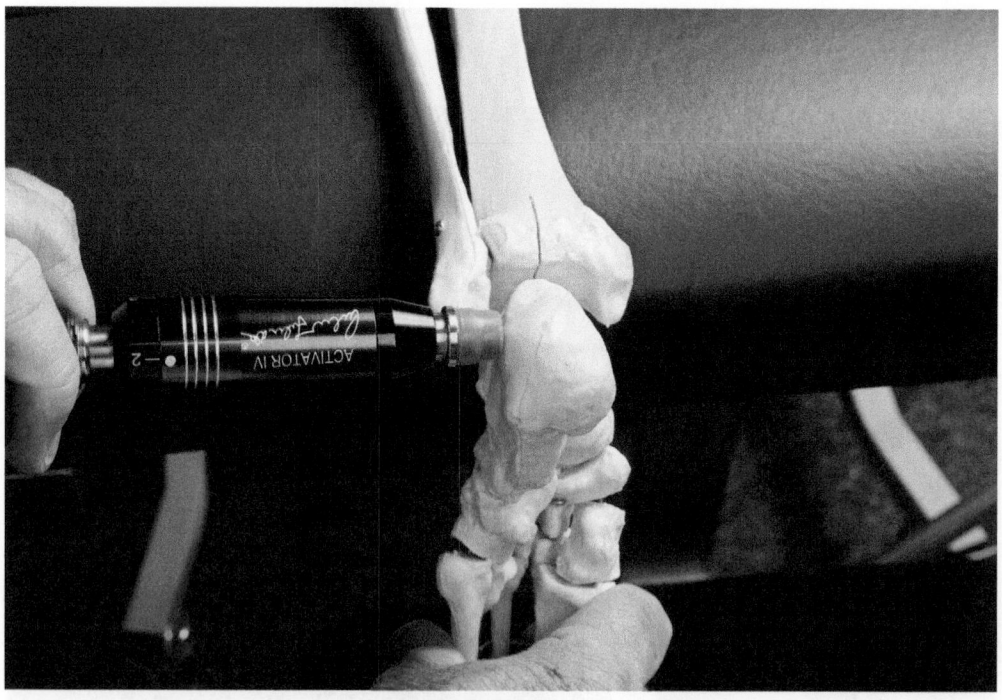

Figure 15-4 Adjustment for lateral calcaneus. Line of Drive is straight lateral to medial.

Clinical Observations

Traumatic injury to the heel or ankle can result in superior involvement of the calcaneus. Trauma may occur suddenly, caused for example by jumping from a height or stepping into a hole.[11] Onset also may be gradual, brought on by repeated impact of the heel on a hard surface.[10] Joggers whose shoes do not provide adequate impact protection to the foot are at risk of developing superior involvement of the calcaneus.

If correct adjusting procedures do not clear a superior calcaneus, or if adjustments will not hold, it may be advisable to tape or brace the foot and ankle until they stabilize. When a superior calcaneus is associated with Achilles tendonitis or contracture or spasm of the calf muscles, consider additional soft tissue therapy and therapeutic exercise for the patient.

Because superior and medial calcaneus neuroarticular dysfunctions are frequently due to plantar flexion and inversion ankle sprain, the patient who is vulnerable to recurrent sprain should be advised on appropriate supportive footwear. A high-top shoe or boot that can be laced firmly can help prevent further injury and can facilitate recovery from chronic neuroarticular dysfunction of the foot and ankle.

Superior Calcaneus

Acute or chronic ankle sprain is an indication of a possible superior calcaneus due to the typical plantar flexion component of the injury. Superior involvement of the calcaneus should be considered in Achilles tendonitis, calf muscle pain, and retrocalcaneal bursitis. The superior calcaneus involves rotation of the calcaneus around its transverse axis so that the heel portion is displaced superiorly (toward the calf) and the plantar surface is displaced inferiorly.

Stress Test. To Stress Test for superior calcaneal involvement, passively plantarflex the affected ankle to force the heel superior (Figure 15-5). To ensure that the calcaneus is actually stressed in the appropriate direction, firmly grasp the foot by cupping the fingers over the superior and lateral aspect of the foot; place the ball of the thumb of the same hand at or near the heel. Move the foot into plantar flexion, and use the thumb to maintain headward (superior) pressure on the posterior portion of the calcaneus. Look for PD leg reactivity in Position #1.

Adjustment. To adjust for superior calcaneal involvement, contact the posterior-superior border of the calcaneus as close to the insertion of the Achilles tendon as possible. The LOD is straight superior to inferior (Figure 15-6).

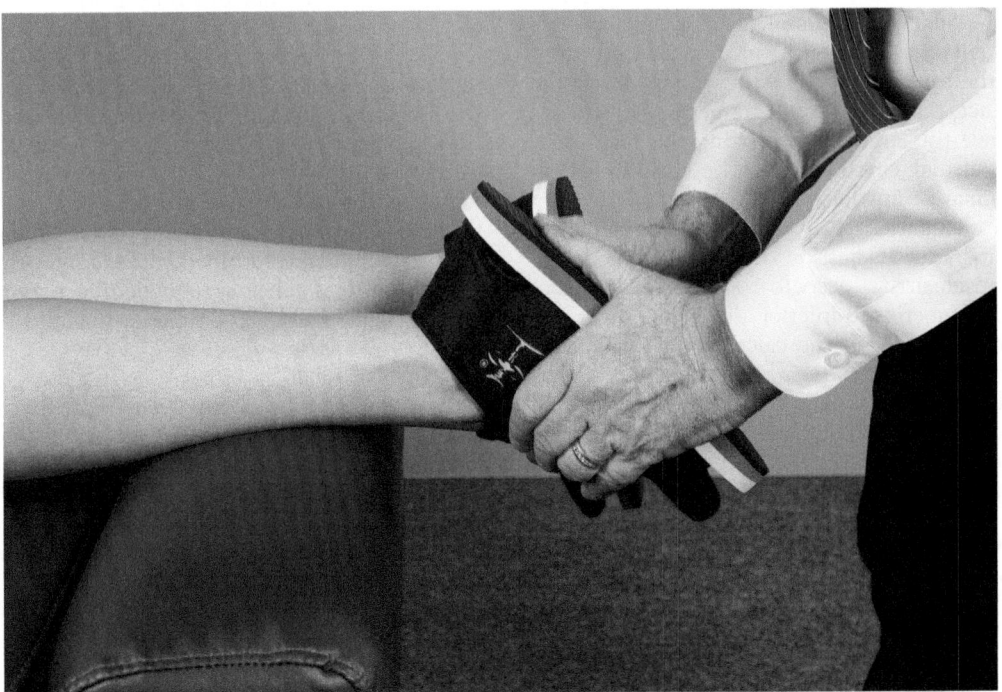

Figure 15-5 Stress Test for superior calcaneus.

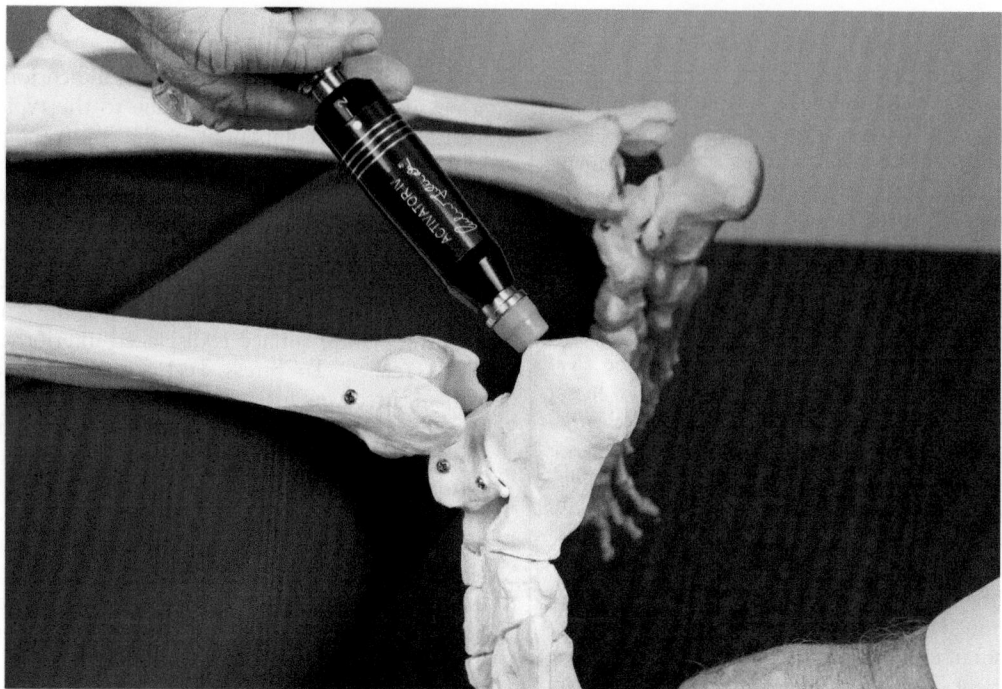

Figure 15-6 Adjustment for superior calcaneus. Line of Drive is straight superior to inferior.

In most cases, positioning the instrument and adjusting the superior calcaneus are straightforward. To ensure accurate positioning of the instrument and an effective adjustment, remove the patient's shoe before adjusting. Depending on the build of the patient, it may be advisable to stabilize the tip of the instrument by positioning the thumb of your free hand just below the contact point of the instrument. Be sure to remove the shoe before starting the procedure. The medial calcaneus and the superior calcaneus may be involved simultaneously.

If the patient has an active retrocalcaneal bursitis, avoid adjusting over the inflamed site. If the bursitis is deep to the Achilles tendon, take a superior-to-inferior tissue pull over the posterior aspect of the calcaneus with two fingers of the stabilization hand, hold the fingers slightly apart, and adjust by applying the tip of the instrument between the fingers. Use a split-finger position to stabilize the tip of the instrument during the adjustment.

Inferior Calcaneus

A patient report of pain across the medial aspect of the top of the foot is an indicator of inferior involvement of the calcaneus. Patient activity involving prolonged utilization of a ladder is also an indicator. Other symptoms and complaints include arch pain on the bottom of the heel,

especially in weight bearing, plantar fasciitis, and Morton's neuroma. Also consider any condition that alters the patient's gait and involves compensating weight-bearing postures.

Stress Test. The doctor firmly grasps the calcaneus and dorsiflexes the foot to resistance (Figure 15-7). If unable to perform this step, remove the patient's footwear and grasp around the calcaneus, stressing it in an inferior direction. Look for PD leg reactivity in Position #1.

Adjustment. The calcaneus is adjusted with the footwear removed. Palpate the inferior aspect of the calcaneus; vary the contact point if exquisite pain and a radiographically confirmed osteophyte are present. It is judicious to avoid direct contact with the spur. The LOD is superior (Figure 15-8).

Posterior Calcaneus

Indications of posterior involvement of the calcaneus include general heel or foot pain, but it is commonly associated with plantar fasciitis. Posterior involvement of the calcaneus may induce a longitudinal stretch of the plantar fascia, leading to irritation and resultant inflammation in the plantar tissues.

Stress Test. To Stress Test a posterior calcaneus, grasp the affected calcaneus between your thumb and fingertips and pull in a posterior direction (Figure 15-9) while stabilizing around the talus with your free hand. The patient's

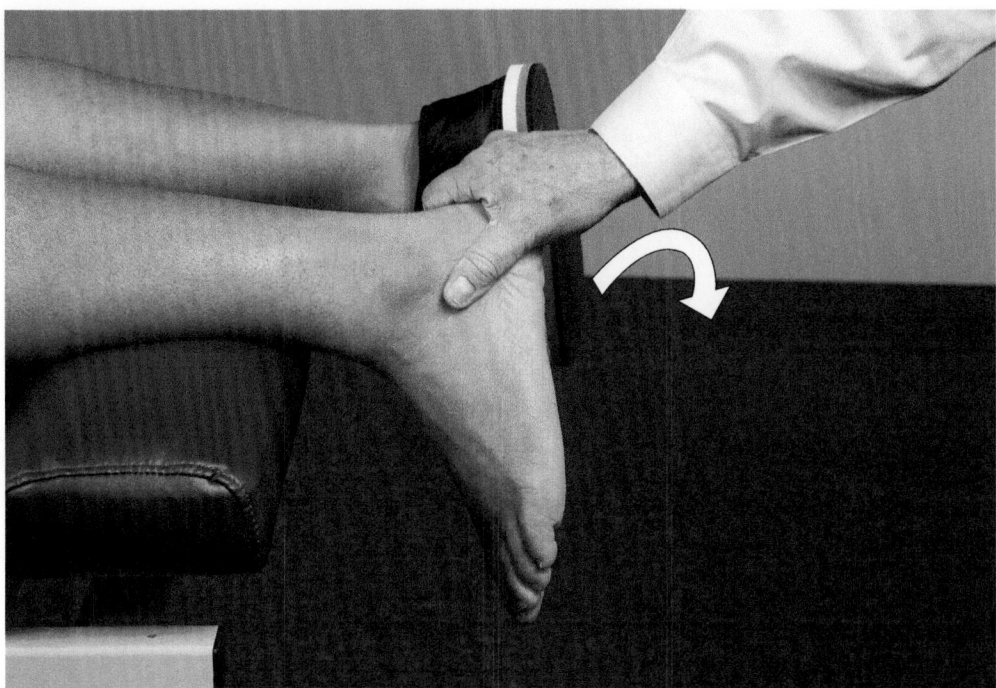

Figure 15-7 Stress Test for inferior calcaneus.

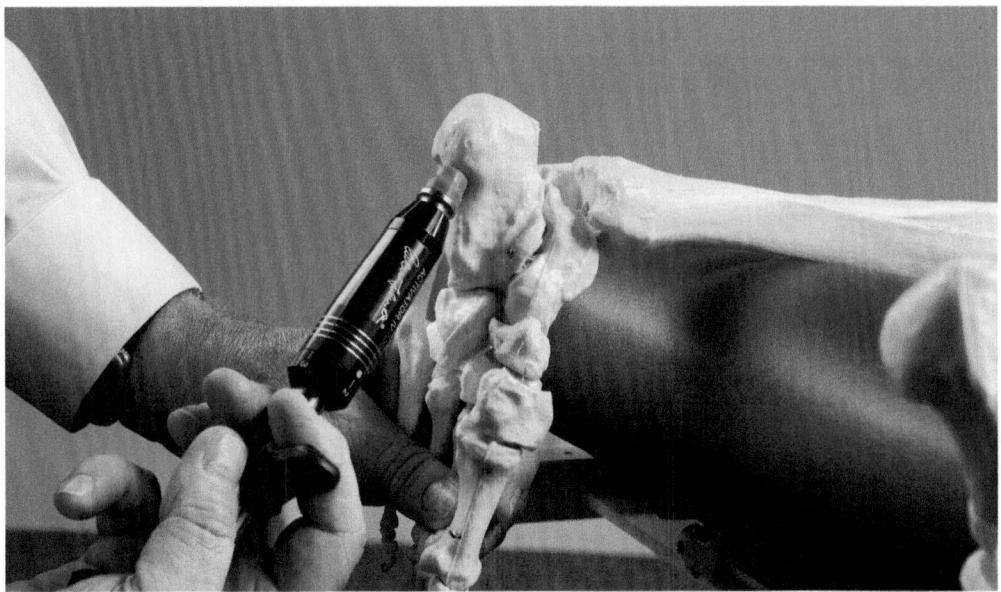

Figure 15-8 Adjustment for inferior calcaneus. Line of Drive is superior.

shoe must be removed for accurate perform-ance of this test. Look for PD leg reactivity in Position #1.

Adjustment. To adjust for posterior calcaneal involvement, contact the calcaneus distal to the insertion of the Achilles tendon, and stabilize the tip of the instrument with your free hand. The LOD is directly anterior (Figure 15-10).

Anterior-Superior Navicular
Anterior and superior displacement of the navicular commonly occurs as part of a plantar

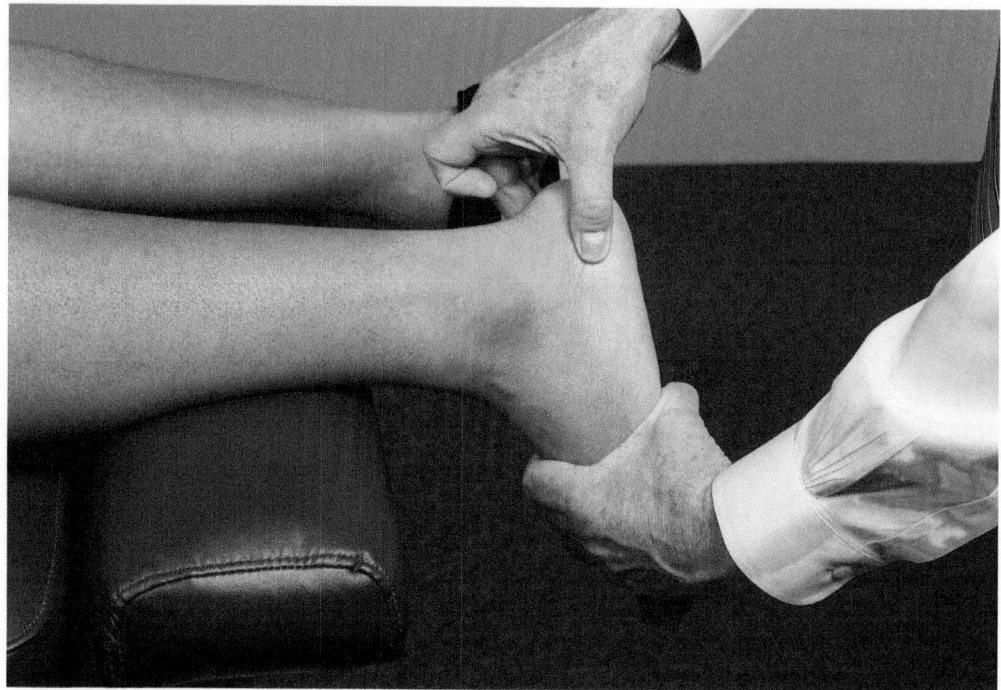

Figure 15-9 Stress Test for posterior calcaneus.

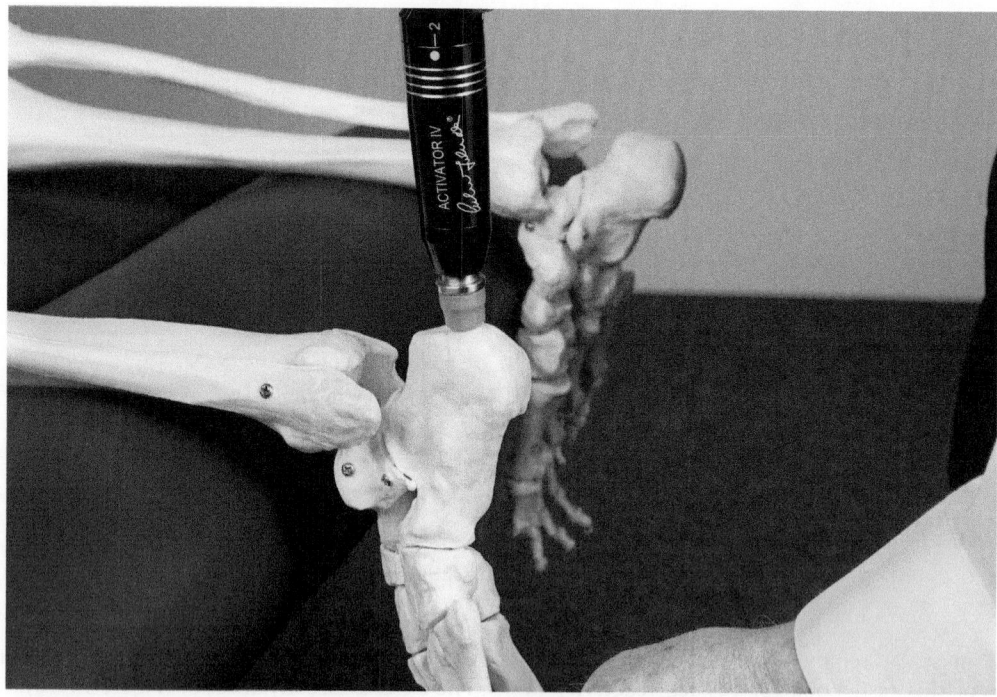

Figure 15-10 Adjustment for posterior calcaneus. Line of Drive is anterior.

flexion and inversion sprain of the ankle. Localized pain over the top of the foot at or near the talonavicular joint is an indication of navicular involvement, and the patient may walk with an antalgic gait that favors toe-off on the side of involvement.

Stress Test. To Stress Test an anterior-superior involvement navicular, take a firm tissue pull in an anterior-superior direction over the bony prominence of the navicular of the affected foot (Figure 15-11). If the patient is wearing low-cut loafers or shoes, it should be relatively easy to grasp the skin over the navicular between the thumb and forefinger to perform the Stress Test. Look for PD leg reactivity in Position #1.

Adjustment. To adjust for an anterior-superior navicular, contact the superior aspect of the navicular by positioning the tip of the instrument about 1 inch anterior to the joint between the talus and the tibia. The LOD is posterior and inferior toward the patient's heel (Figure 15-12).

To ensure a correct contact, LOD, and delivery of an effective thrust, remove the patient's shoe when adjusting an anterior-superior navicular. Adjust the navicular with the patient's leg flexed at the knee. This enables positioning

of the instrument without flexing or extending of the wrist and helps to avoid repetitive strain injury to the wrist.

Clinical Observations

Pain related to an anterior-superior neuroarticular dysfunction of the navicular may be exacerbated by Stress Tests for the medial and superior calcaneus. Because most Stress Tests are not painful, work with patients by having them tell you of any discomfort they experience during Activator Methods Stress Tests.

Pain over the navicular can result from poorly fitted shoes or shoes that are laced too tightly. Be sure to inspect the fit of shoes over the dorsal surface of the foot.

Medial Navicular

Indications for assessment of medial involvement of the navicular would be pain across the dorsum of the foot, edema over the dorsal-medial aspect of the foot, and observable deformity of the medial navicular.

Stress Test. To stress for medial navicular involvement, grasp the affected foot around the metatarsals and stabilize with one hand,

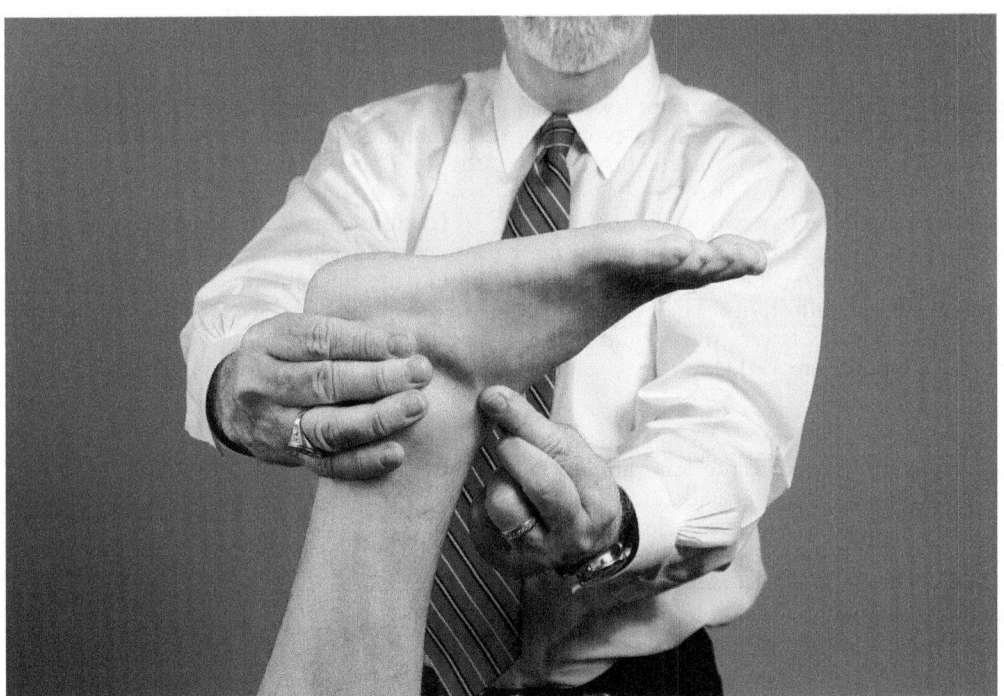

Figure 15-11 Stress Test for anterior-superior navicular.

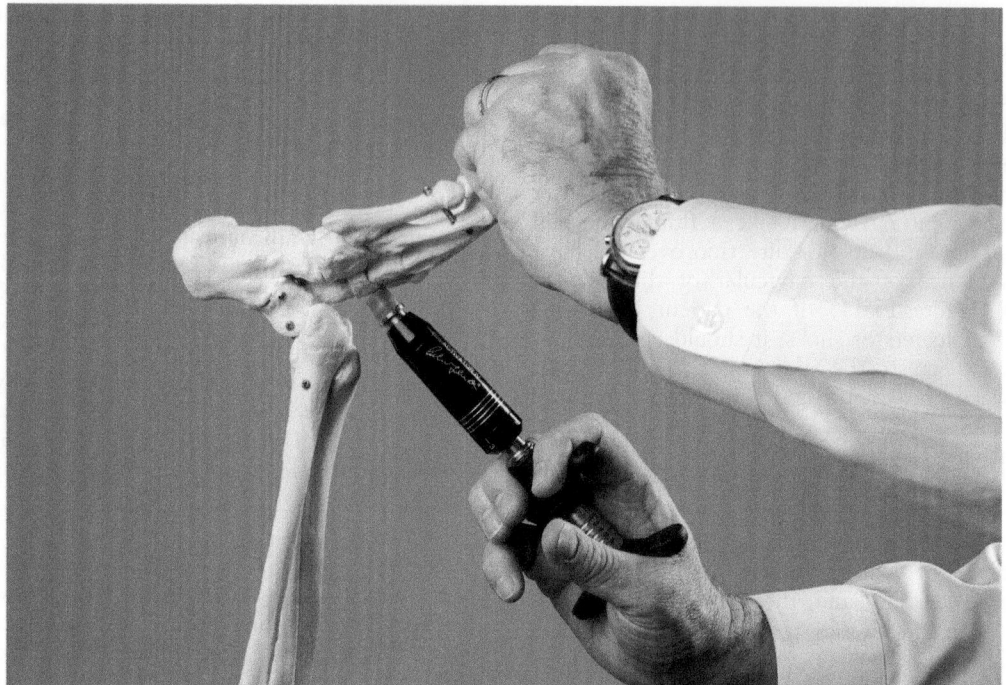

Figure 15-12 Adjustment for anterior-superior navicular. Line of Drive is posterior and inferior toward patient's heel.

while applying pressure by rolling in a lateral-to-medial direction across the navicular with the fingertips of the second and third digits of the other hand (Figure 15-13). Look for PD leg reactivity in Position #1.

Adjustment.   Find the medial tuberosity of the navicular by palpating from distal to proximal along the first metatarsal and over the first cuneiform to the superficial medial tuberosity of the navicular. Stabilize the foot with one hand while grasping around the metatarsals, and position the tip of the instrument on the medial plantar surface of the navicular tuberosity. The LOD is anatomically superior (i.e. toward the dorsum of the foot) and lateral (Figure 15-14).

Anterior Lateral Talus

The plantar flexion and inversion components of a typical ankle sprain force the talus anteriorly and laterally relative to its articulation with the tibia. Pain and swelling over the dorsal lateral aspect of the ankle in the region of the *sinus tarsi* are commonly noted. The sinus tarsi is the fossa or depression normally palpable just anterior and inferior to the lateral malleolus.

Stress Test.   To Stress Test for involvement of an anterior lateral talus, passively plantarflex the affected foot while inverting the ankle (Figure 15-15). Look for PD leg reactivity in Position #1.

Adjustment.   Contact the neck of the talus by positioning the tip of the instrument within the sinus tarsi. The LOD is posterior and medial toward the Achilles tendon (Figure 15-16).

To ensure an effective contact with the talus, it may be advisable to remove the patient's shoe during the adjustment, because lace-up shoes, athletic shoes, and boots make it difficult to obtain a good contact or LOD. When a patient describes ankle and foot problems, it is best to use a pair of surgical boots, or Activator modified shoes (Figure 15-17) to facilitate Leg Length Analysis and adjustment of the lower extremity.

Adjust for anterior lateral talus involvement by flexing the patient's leg to 90 degrees at the knee. This will ensure an accurate contact and LOD and will avoid unnecessary wrist flexion or extension during the adjustment.

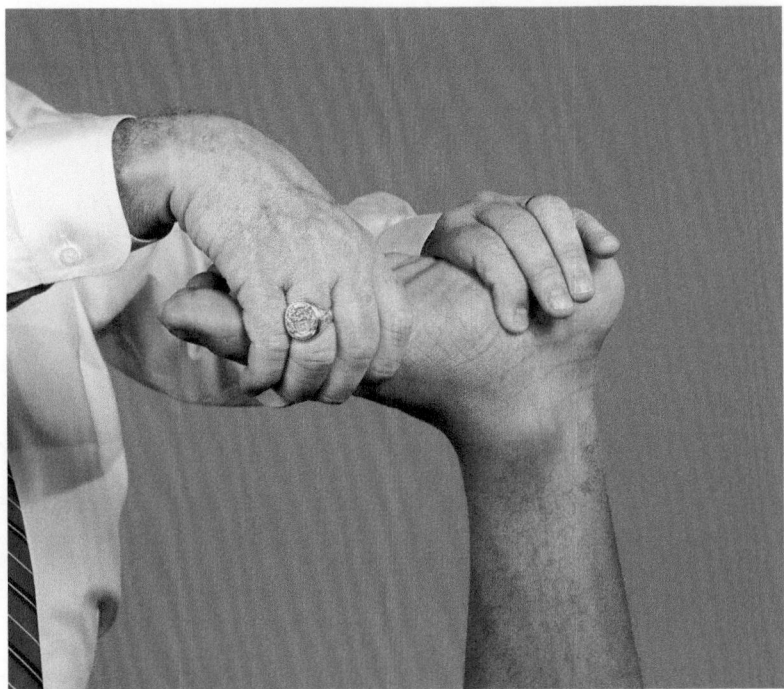

Figure 15-13 Stress Test for medial navicular.

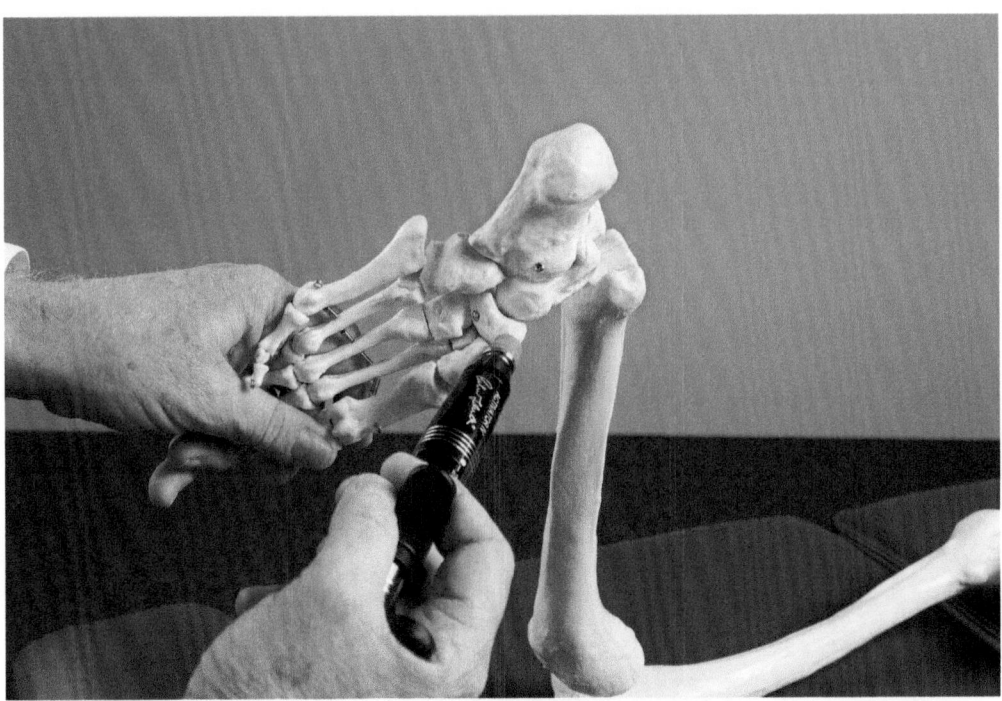

Figure 15-14 Adjustment for medial navicular. Line of Drive is anatomically superior (i.e., toward the dorsum of the foot) and lateral.

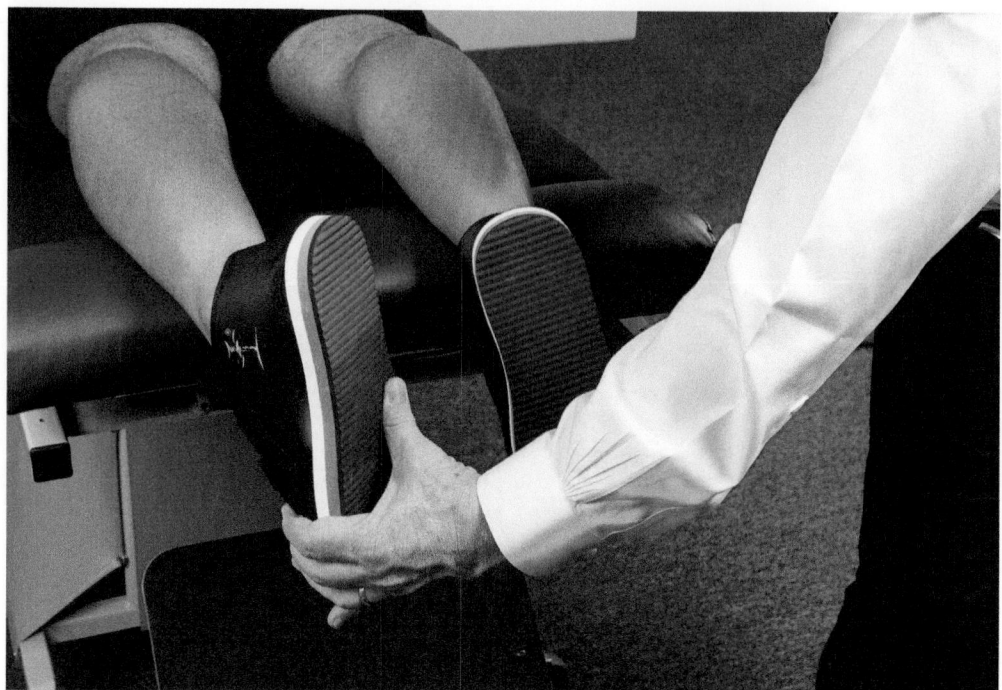

Figure 15-15 Stress Test for anterior lateral talus.

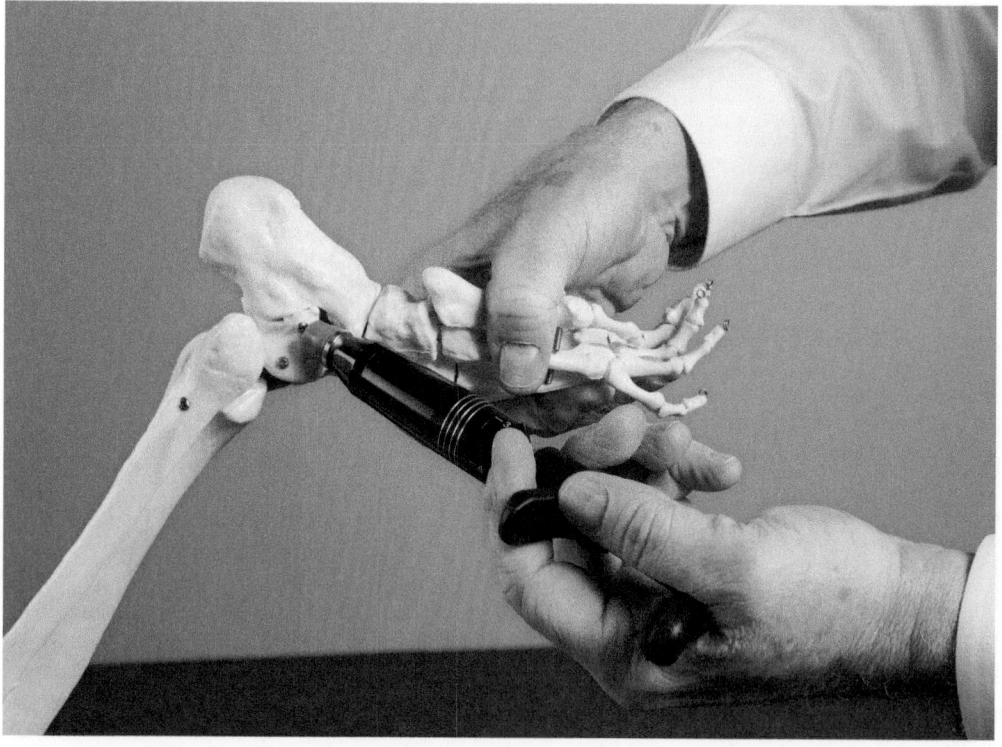

Figure 15-16 Adjustment for anterior lateral talus. Line of Drive is posterior and medial toward the Achilles tendon.

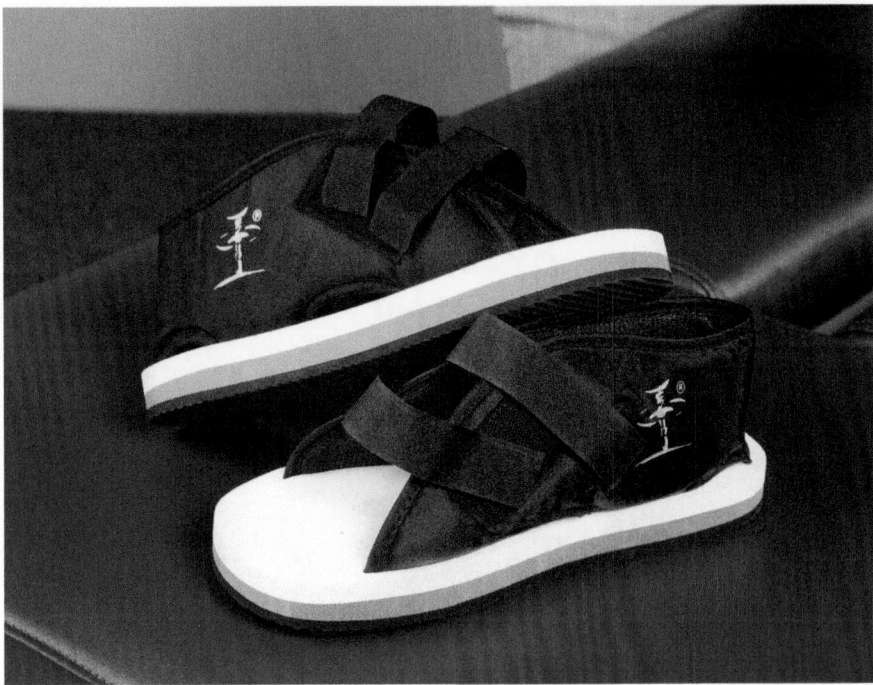

Figure 15-17   Activator adjusting shoes.

Clinical Observations

With moderate to severe sprain, significant swelling and possible hematoma may occur in the region of the sinus tarsi. The region will be very tender to touch. In an uncomplicated sprain, however, adjustment with the rapid low-force thrust of the Activator Instrument minimizes patient discomfort. The healing process after an ankle sprain may be enhanced if the bones of the talocrural joint are restored to their normal anatomical relationship.

With severe ankle sprain injuries, be sure to assess the ligaments using drawer sign maneuvers. When pain and swelling or hemorrhage is particularly pronounced after an acute injury of the ankle, application of ice or a cold pack before and after adjustment of the talus can be an effective intervention. Also, taping the foot and ankle into a neutral or slightly dorsiflexed position will facilitate repair of periarticular soft tissues.[11]

Anterior Distal Tibia

Although an anterior distal tibia may be found in patients with knee problems, whether ankle pain is associated or not, it also should be considered in those patients with a history of toe walking or wearing high heels. Evaluation of the gastrocnemius muscle would reveal hypertonicity and tenderness upon palpation. The patient will typically present with limited and possibly painful ankle dorsiflexion after ankle sprain/strain. Superior involvement of the calcaneus would also be assessed in this case.

Stress Test.   To stress for involvement of an anterior distal tibia, flex the knee on the affected side to 90 degrees, dorsiflex at the ankle, and stabilize the tarsals with one hand. Gently grasp the distal tibia and pull it anterior (Figure 15-18). Look for PD leg reactivity in Position #1.

Adjustment.   To adjust for anterior distal tibial involvement, flex the knee to 90 degrees, dorsiflex the ankle, and stabilize the tarsals with one hand. Contact the anterior distal tibia securely with the instrument. The LOD is posterior or headward in this position with the knee flexed (Figure 15-19).

Inferior First Metatarsal and Inferior Medial First Cuneiform

Pain at the instep or medial aspect of the plantar surface of the foot is a possible indication of involvement of the first metatarsal and first cuneiform articulation. Pain is exacerbated with walking, and the toe-off portion of gait may be

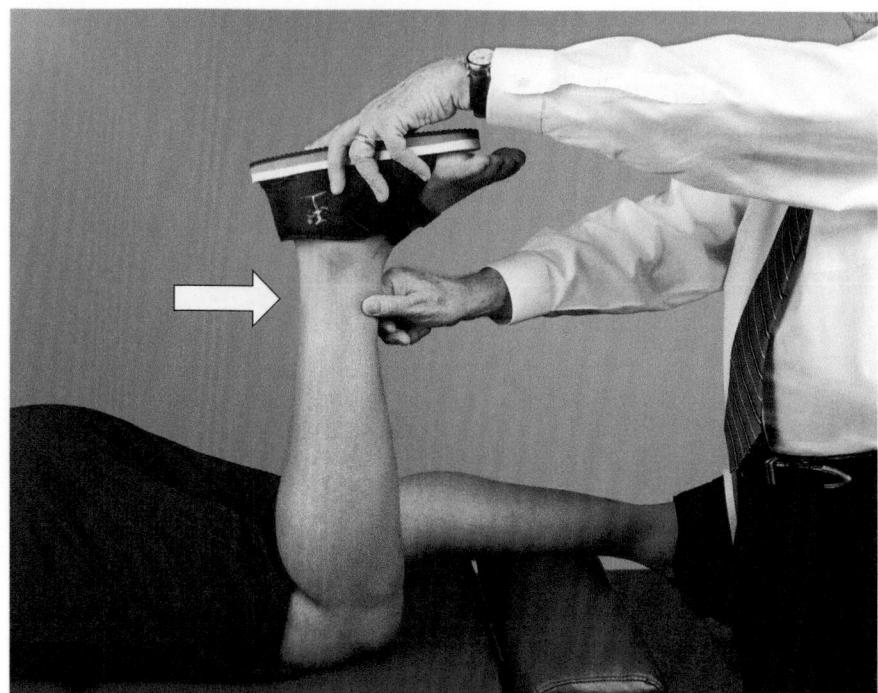

Figure 15-18   Stress Test for anterior distal tibia.

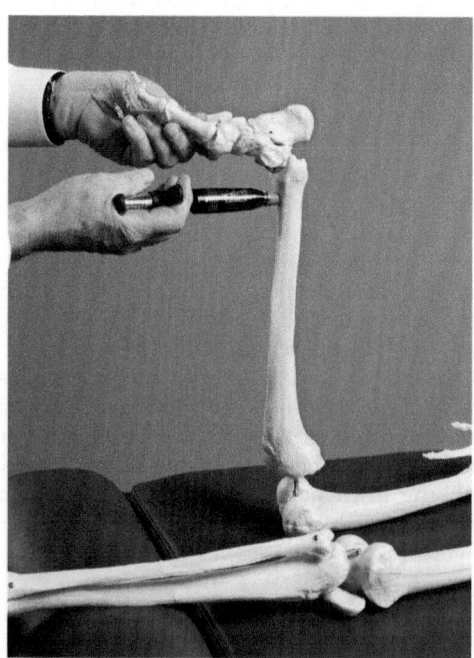

Figure 15-19   Adjustment for anterior distal tibia. Line of Drive is posterior.

affected, resulting in a limp.[13] This pain may be distributed throughout the sole of the foot, with symptoms similar to plantar fasciitis.

To locate the first metatarsal and the medial cuneiform, palpate the first metatarsophalangeal joint at the ball of the foot. Slide the fingers posteriorly along the shaft of the metatarsal until you feel the bone widen at the base. The medial cuneiform is located immediately posterior to the base of the first metatarsal.

Stress Test.   To Stress Test for involvement of the first metatarsal and first cuneiform, grasp the affected foot firmly and plantarflex while simultaneously everting the ankle (Figure 15-20). An alternate method of Stress Testing the articulation is to flatten the arch of the involved foot by pressing one hand down over the dorsum of the foot while supporting the plantar aspect with the other hand. Look for PD leg reactivity in Position #1.

Adjustment.   To adjust for inferior first metatarsal and inferior medial first cuneiform involvement, two contact points will be used. The first contact point is the plantar aspect of the base of the first metatarsal. The LOD is straight superior along the plane of the joint (Figure 15-21). The

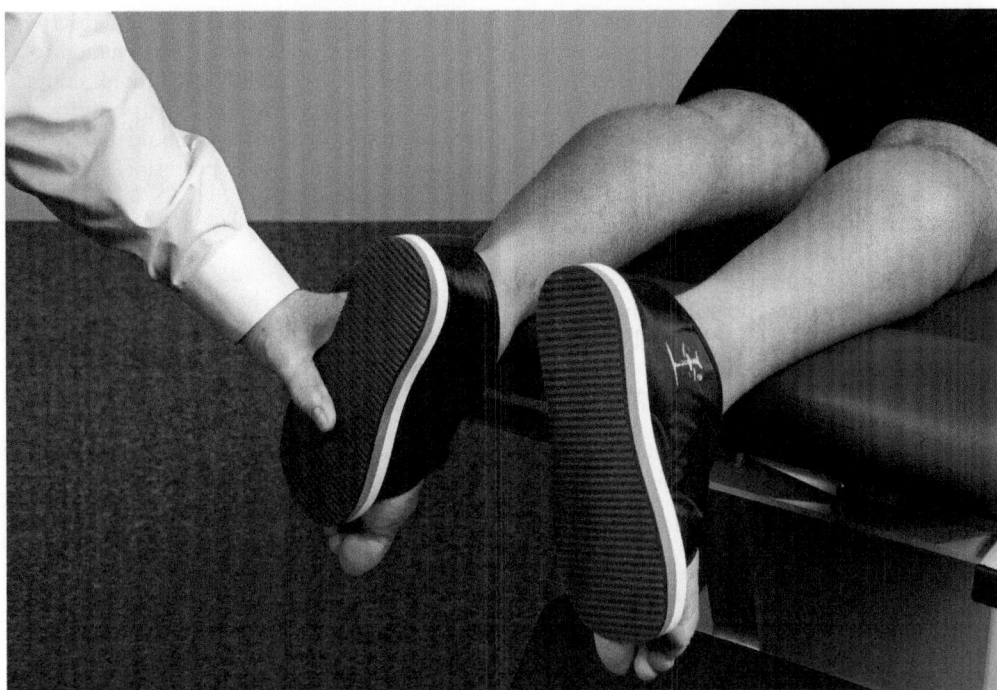

Figure 15-20 Stress Test for inferior first metatarsal and inferior medial first cuneiform; plantarflex the foot while simultaneously everting the ankle.

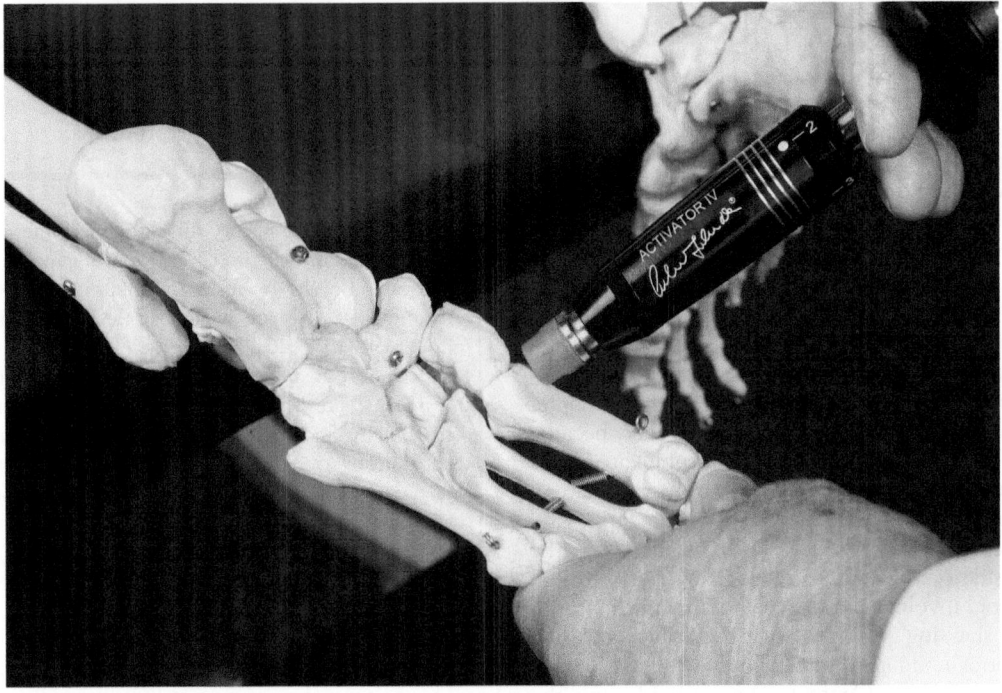

Figure 15-21 Adjustment for inferior first metatarsal. Line of Drive is straight superior.

second contact is on the medial surface of the first cuneiform, located in the fleshy part of the instep of the plantar arch. The LOD is superior and lateral (Figure 15-22).

To adjust for the inferior first metatarsal and the inferior medial first cuneiform, it will be necessary to remove the patient's shoe on the side of involvement. In some cases, it may even be necessary to remove the patient's shoe before performing the Stress Test. For the sake of efficiency, use Activator shoes, fracture boots, or other modified shoes for problems in the ankle and foot.

Clinical Observations

An inferior first metatarsal and inferior medial first cuneiform involvement can indicate a number of latent or developing biomechanical problems of the foot and associated structures.[36] Loss of resilience in the medial longitudinal arch is a serious concern for runners and other athletes, as well as for people who spend most of their workday on their feet—nurses, letter carriers, retail sales associates, construction workers, and chiropractors, to name a few. With recurrent inferior involvement of the first metatarsal and first cuneiform, make a point of examining the arch support of the patient's footwear. It may be advisable to fit the patient with orthotics and to make recommendations about footwear for work or other activities that exacerbate the condition.[37]

Unadjusted, the inferior first metatarsal can predispose the patient to developing corns and bunions. Furthermore, because this neuroarticular dysfunction of the metatarsals takes the foot into overpronation, compensatory stresses may occur in the knee and hip, and chondromalacia patellae or trochanteric bursitis may develop.

Cuboid

The cuboid is part of the adjustment for involvement of the lateral knee, as described in Chapter 7, in the Basic Protocol scan. However, because the cuboid is the most commonly subluxated bone in the foot, it can occur separately from lateral knee involvement. As the patient adapts gait, especially with plantar fasciitis, walking on the outside of the foot to avoid pain can result in cuboid involvement. The cuboid in the anatomical standing position usually exhibits anterior, inferior, and lateral involvement.[32,33]

Stress Test. Contact the cuboid on the anterior-superior aspect as the patient is lying in the prone position, and apply pressure anatomically in an inferior, lateral, and slightly anterior direction (Figure 15-23). Look for reactivity of the PD leg in Position #1 for involvement.

Adjustment. To adjust the cuboid, contact its inferior and lateral aspect, just posterior to the articulation between the cuboid and the fifth metatarsal. The LOD is posterior, superior, and medial (Figure 15-24).

Inferior Metatarsal Heads

Toe pain and pain in the ball of the foot, especially when exacerbated by the toe-off portion of gait, may be an indication of inferior involvement of the metatarsal heads, involving the metatarsophalangeal joints in toe flexion and extension.

Stress Test. To Stress Test for inferior metatarsal head involvement, extend the metatarsophalangeal joints by stabilizing the metatarsal heads and dorsiflexing the proximal phalanges (Figure 15-25). Look for PD leg reactivity in Position #1.

Adjustment. To adjust for inferior metatarsal head involvement, contact the inferior (plantar) aspects of the heads just proximal to the metatarsophalangeal joints. The LOD is straight superior (Figure 15-26). Adjust each metatarsal head or palpate each metatarsal head, and adjust only those described as tender by the patient. The most effective way to Stress Test and adjust for inferior metatarsal heads is to remove the patient's shoe first. Again, this is a good reason to use Activator shoes, surgical boots, or other modified footwear, especially when the patient presents with foot and ankle problems.

Clinical Observations

In addition to pain in the ball of the foot, inferior metatarsal heads may promote the development of calluses and corns at pressure points in the shoe. An antalgic or irregular gait may develop as the patient tries to avoid a painful toe-off component.

Be sure to inspect the patient's shoes or boots for pressure sites that force the metatarsals inferiorly. Bulging and worn spots on the leather uppers can indicate stress points on the foot. Shoes that are too tight across the dorsum of the foot also can apply inferior stress to the metatarsals.

Distal First Metatarsal and Superior Proximal First Phalanx

For those patients with great toe pain or a history or observable hiker's toe, assessment of the first metatarsophalangeal joint is indicated. Neuroarticular dysfunction may include distal first metatarsal and superior proximal involvement of the

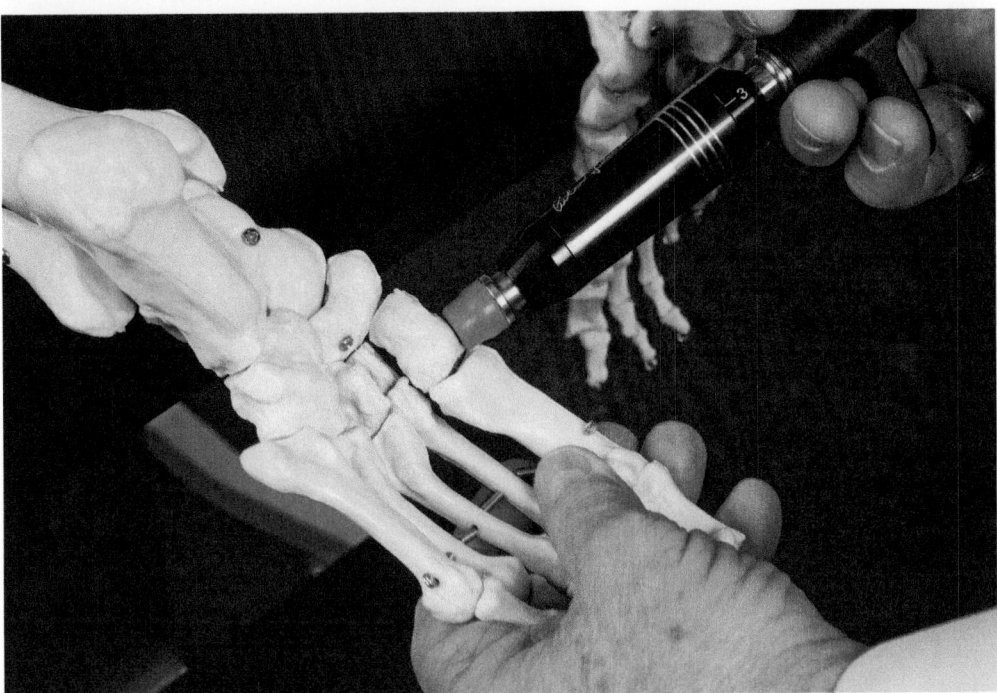

Figure 15-22   Adjustment for inferior medial cuneiform. Line of Drive is superior and lateral.

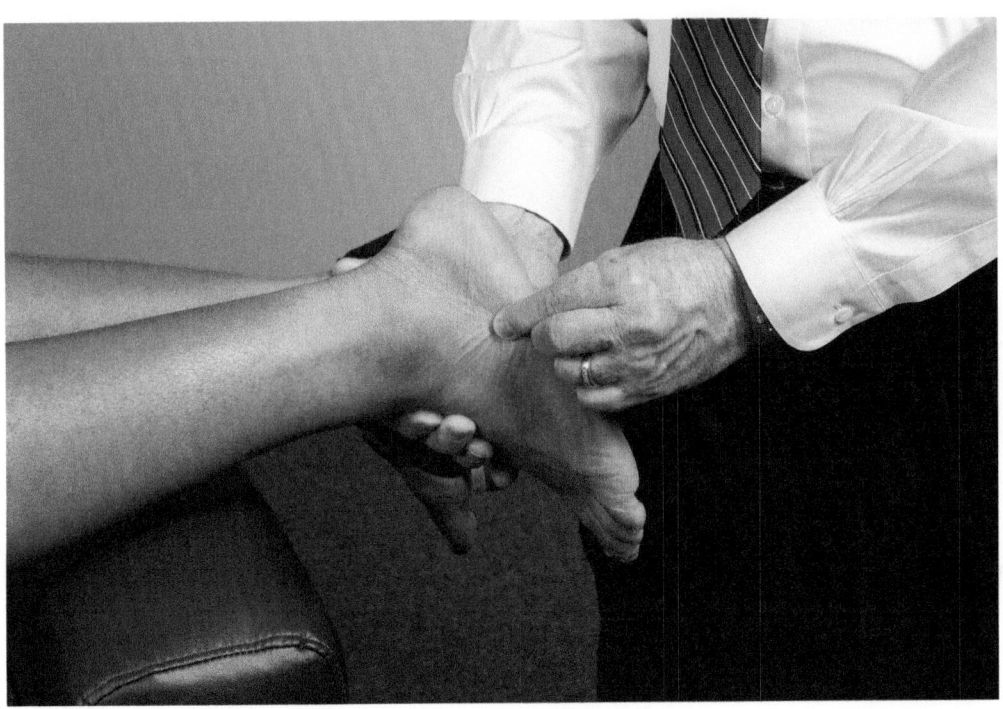

Figure 15-23   Stress Test for cuboid.

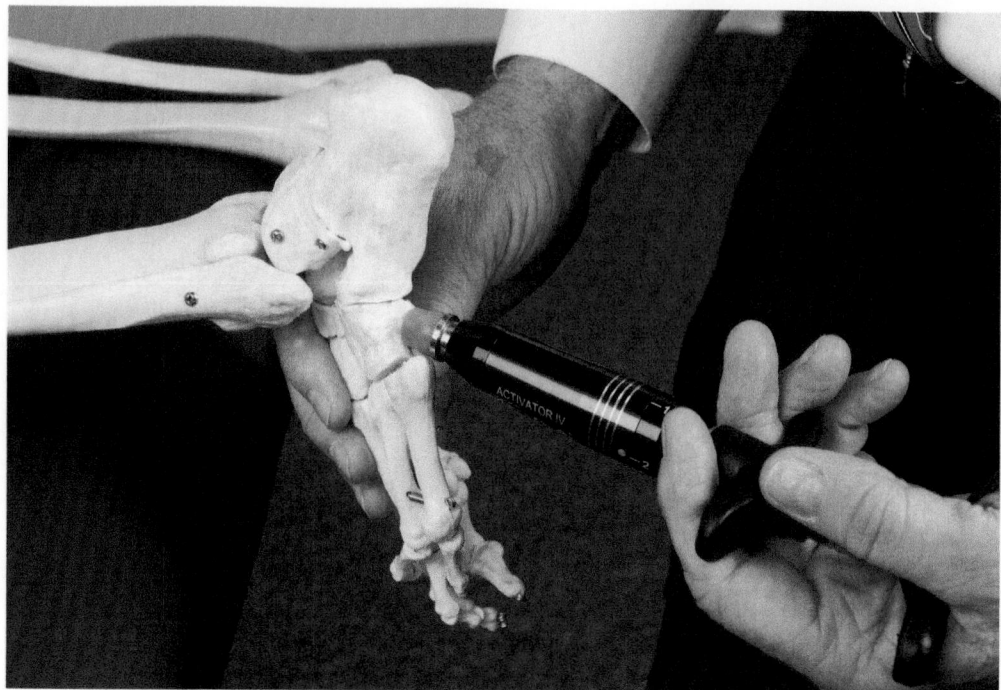

Figure 15-24   Adjustment for cuboid. Line of Drive is posterior, superior, and medial.

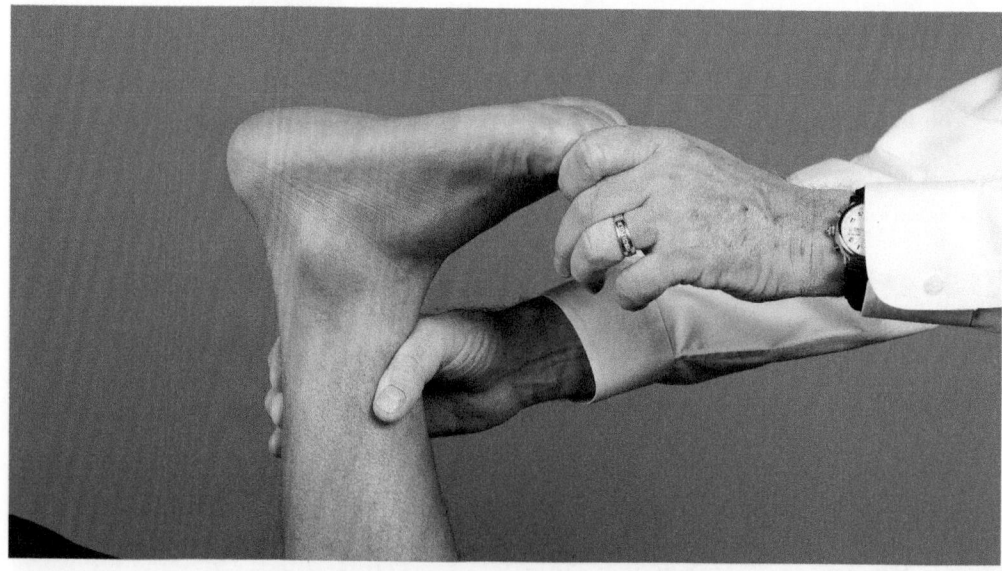

Figure 15-25   Stress Test for inferior metatarsal heads.

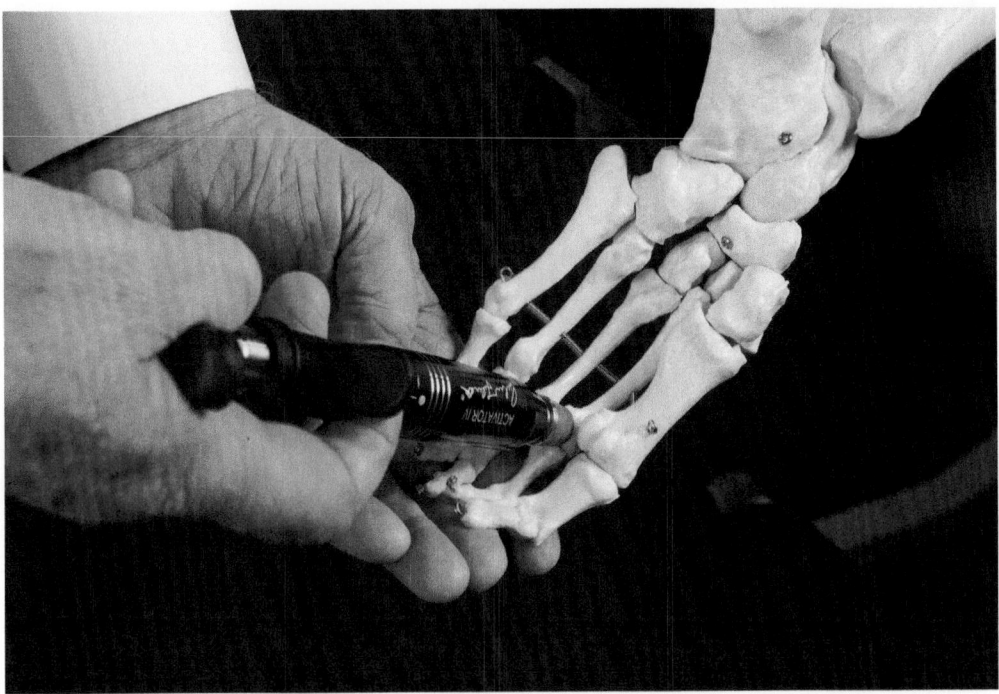

Figure 15-26 Adjustment for inferior metatarsal heads. Line of Drive is straight superior.

first phalanx due to axial compression of the great toe upon impact with the hiking boot during descent from a higher elevation.

Stress Test. To Stress Test for distal first metatarsal and superior proximal first phalangeal involvement, stabilize the plantar aspect of the first metatarsal with the thumb pad, and plantarflex the affected great toe at the metatarsophalangeal joint by flexing the first phalanx (Figure 15-27). Look for PD leg reactivity in Position #1.

Adjustment. To adjust for distal first metatarsal and superior proximal first phalangeal involvement, contact the dorsal surface of the first metatarsophalangeal joint while tractioning on the first proximal phalanx. Placing the knee into flexion will assist in contacting the dorsal surface of the joint. The LOD is anatomically inferior (Figure 15-28).

Hallux Valgus or First Metatarsophalangeal Joint (Great Toe)

General great toe pain, hallux valgus, degenerative joint disease, and bunions are common conditions in which first metatarsophalangeal joint involvement may be observed. A valgus deformity is commonly seen in patients with rheumatoid arthritis or severe osteoarthritis. Advanced joint destruction combined with dislocation of this joint in severe cases is known as Lanois deformity [34] and is diagnosed on radiography.

Stress Test. To induce valgus stress to the first metatarsophalangeal joint, push the proximal phalanx of the affected great toe in a lateral direction while stabilizing the first metatarsal head with the other hand (Figure 15-29). Look for PD leg reactivity in Position #1.

Adjustment. To adjust for valgus involvement of the first metatarsophalangeal joint, contact the medial aspect of the first metatarsophalangeal joint as you traction the proximal phalanx distally with your free hand. The LOD is directly lateral (Figure 15-30).

Posterior Distal Fibula

In ankle sprain injuries, articular dysfunction of the distal tibiofibular joint commonly results from involvement of the posterior lateral malleolus. As a result, tension on the anterior portion of the lateral collateral ligament is increased and instability can impair or delay recovery of the injured ankle joint. The patient may exhibit unilateral toe-out foot flare on the side of involvement.

Stress Test. To Stress Test for posterior distal fibular involvement, apply anterior-to-posterior

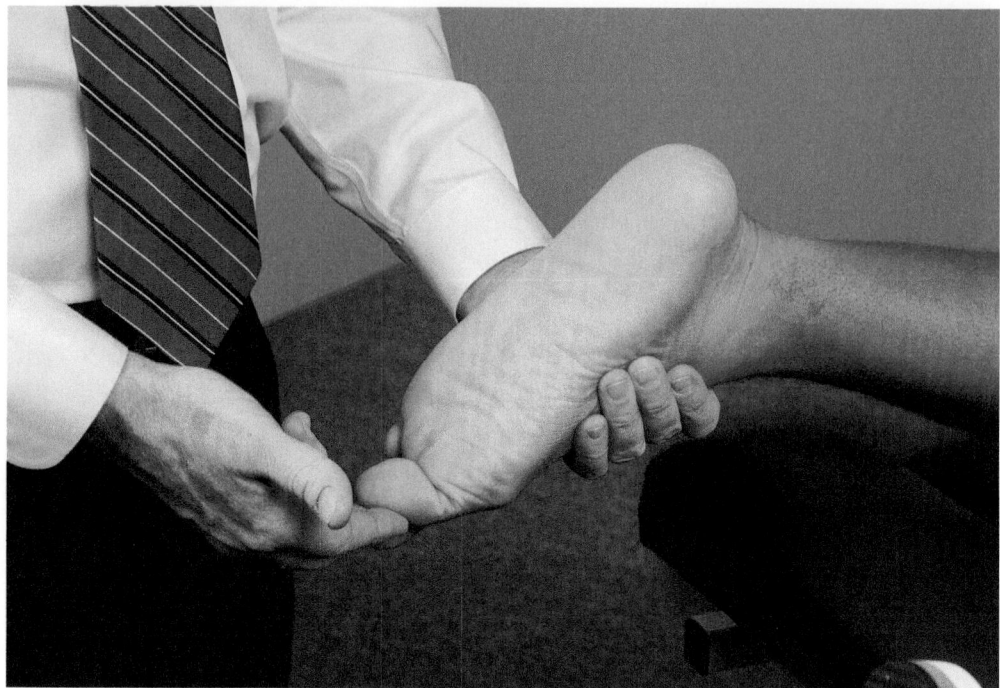

Figure 15-27   Stress Test for distal first metatarsal and superior proximal first phalanx.

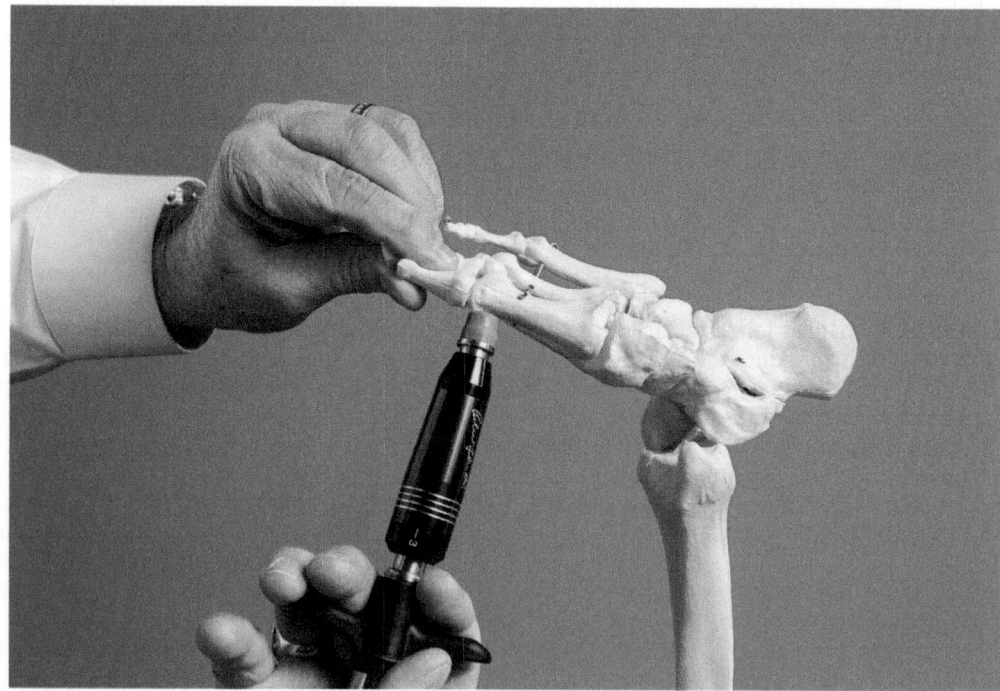

Figure 15-28   Adjustment for distal first metatarsal and superior proximal first phalanx. Line of Drive is anatomically inferior.

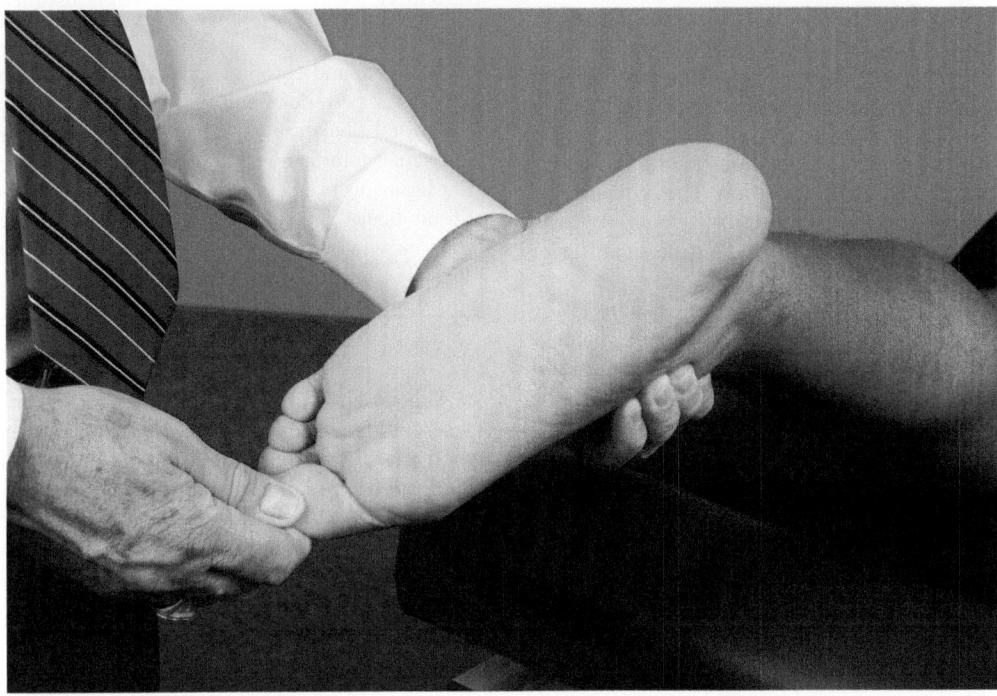

Figure 15-29 Stress Test for hallux valgus or first metatarsophalangeal joint (great toe).

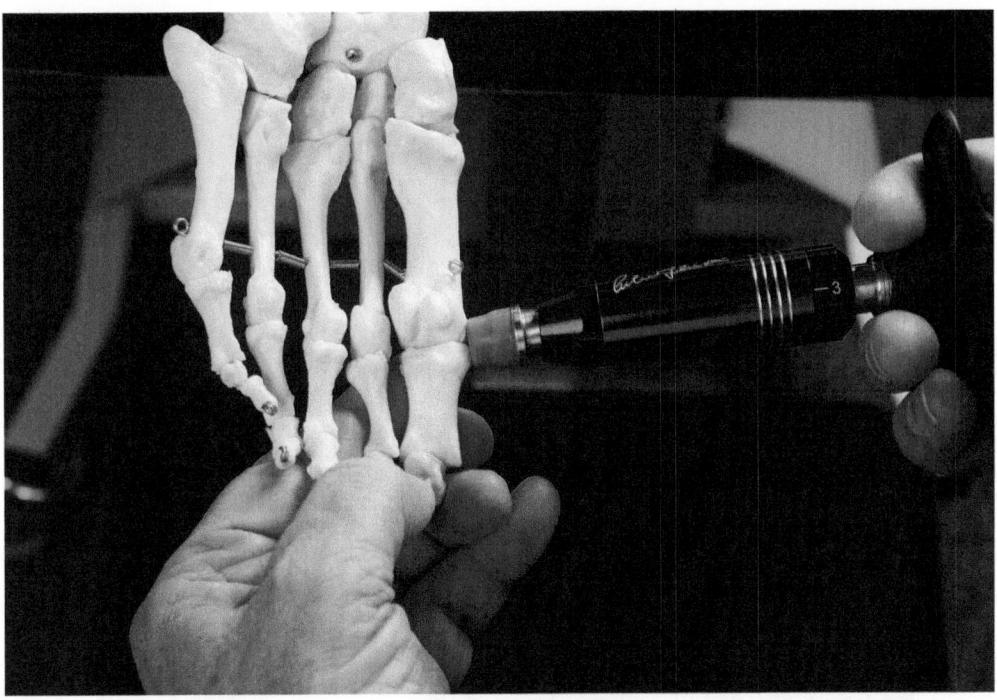

Figure 15-30 Adjustment for hallux valgus or first metatarsophalangeal joint (great toe); traction the proximal phalanx distally. Line of Drive is directly lateral.

pressure on the affected ankle at the lateral malleolus. Hook one or two fingers on the anterior aspect of the lateral malleolus, and pull the bony prominence straight posterior (Figure 15-31). Look for PD leg reactivity in Position #1.

Adjustment. To adjust for posterior distal fibular involvement, position the tip of the instrument on the posterior aspect of the lateral malleolus. The LOD is straight anterior (Figure 15-32).

In most ankle inversion sprains, soft tissue swelling and pain are concentrated in the region of the sinus tarsi, anterior to the lateral malleolus. There is, however, likely to be some point tenderness at the posterior aspect. To minimize discomfort for the patient, take a gentle tissue pull by sliding the ball of the thumb of the stabilization hand anterior from the Achilles tendon until it contacts the lateral malleolus. Use the thumb to stabilize the tip of the instrument when delivering the adjustment.

> **Clinical Observations**
> With acute and chronic ankle sprains, be sure to check for posterior neuroarticular dysfunction of the distal fibula. Severe inversion stresses to the talocrural joint can result in tears to the talofibular ligaments or fracture, including avulsion of the distal fibula. Use anterior and posterior drawer sign maneuvers to assess the ligaments. Radiographical examination will rule out fracture.

Posterior-Superior Proximal Fibula
Although the proximal tibiofibular joint is closest to the knee, it can become involved when the distal fibula is misaligned in an ankle injury. A complaint of pain along the lateral border of the fibula suggests posterior-superior involvement of the proximal fibula. A posterior-superior proximal fibula can be the source of referred pain to the ankle and foot region.

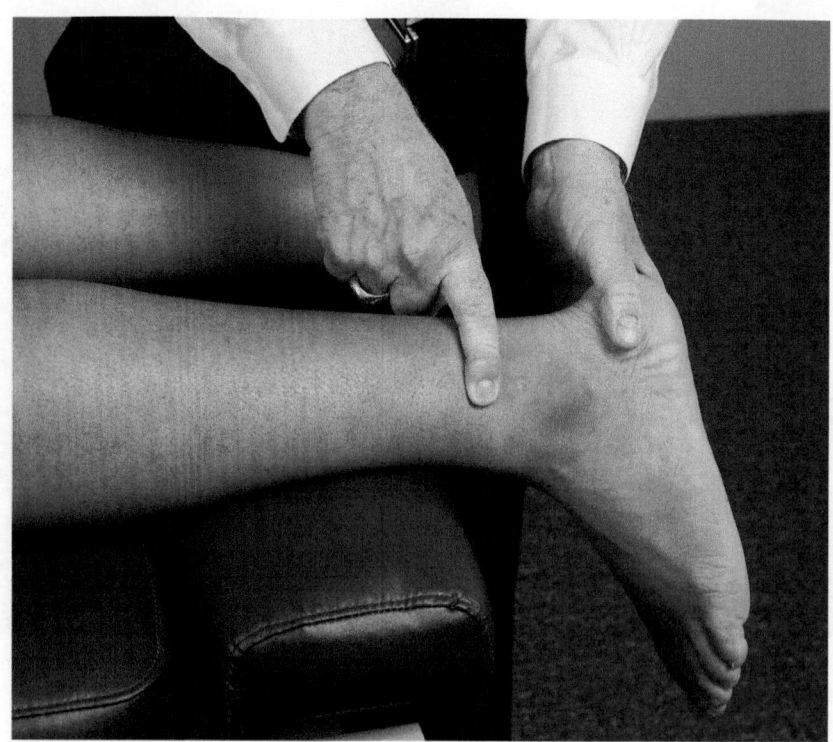

Figure 15-31 Stress Test for posterior distal fibula.

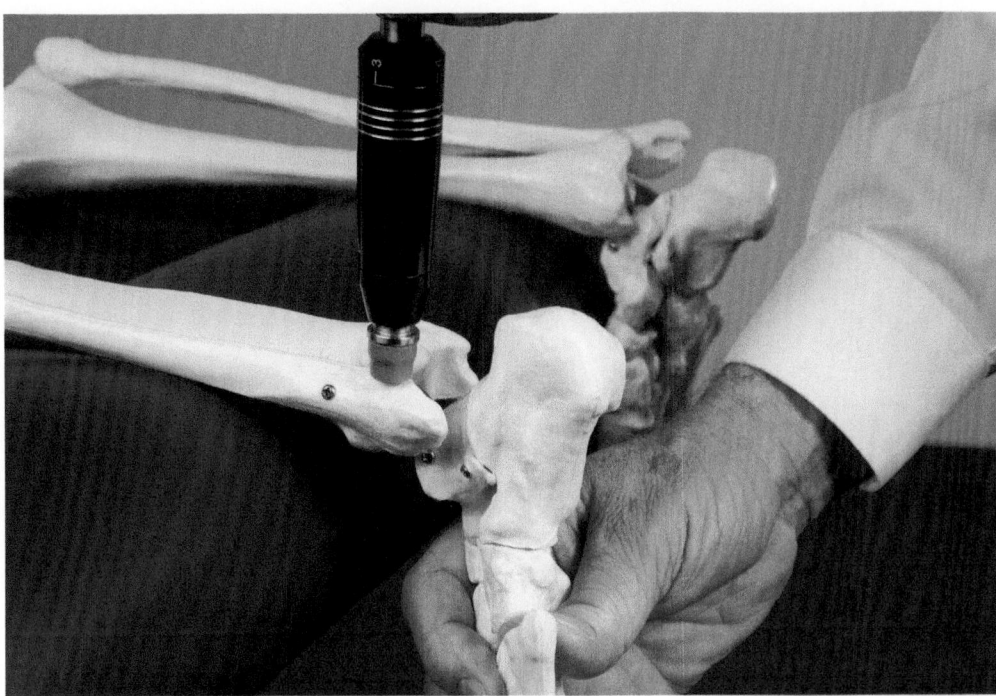

Figure 15-32 Adjustment for posterior distal fibula. Line of Drive is straight anterior.

Stress Test. To Stress Test for posterior-superior proximal fibular involvement, push or draw the fibular head on the affected side in the direction of neuroarticular dysfunction. Stabilize the medial leg with one hand, and use the thumb or index finger of the other hand to take a firm tissue pull over the proximal fibula in a posterior and superior direction (Figure 15-33). Look for PD leg reactivity in Position #1.

Adjustment. To adjust for posterior-superior proximal fibular involvement, contact the posterior aspect of the proximal fibular head. The LOD is anterior and inferior at an angle of about 45 degrees to the long axis of the fibula (Figure 15-34).

Because the proximal tibiofibular joint is 1 to 1½ inches below the knee joint, it is useful to flex and extend the knee to locate the lateral aspect of the tibial plateau. Then palpate inferiorly to find the bony prominence of the fibula.

To ensure an effective adjustment, take a tissue pull with the thumb or index finger of the stabilization hand over the proximal head of the fibula. Use the thumb to stabilize the tip of the instrument during the adjustment.

> **Clinical Observations**
> Involvement of the proximal head of the fibula can occur with injuries to the ankle and the knee. Posterior displacement can occur with ankle sprain injuries that primarily involve the distal portion of the fibula but also affect the proximal end of the bone as compensation. Twisting injuries to the knee, especially those that involve torque to the proximal tibia, can also involve the proximal tibiofibular articulation. When the joint is subluxated, normal fluid motion of the knee can be affected, and tissue swelling may produce referred pain to the ankle and dorsum of the foot via the superficial peroneal nerve.

Mechanical force, manually assisted chiropractic adjusting (Activator Method) and related investigation of lower extremities are summarized in Table 15-1.

RELATED RESEARCH

Box 15-2 presents related research to the Activator Method treatment of the foot and ankle.

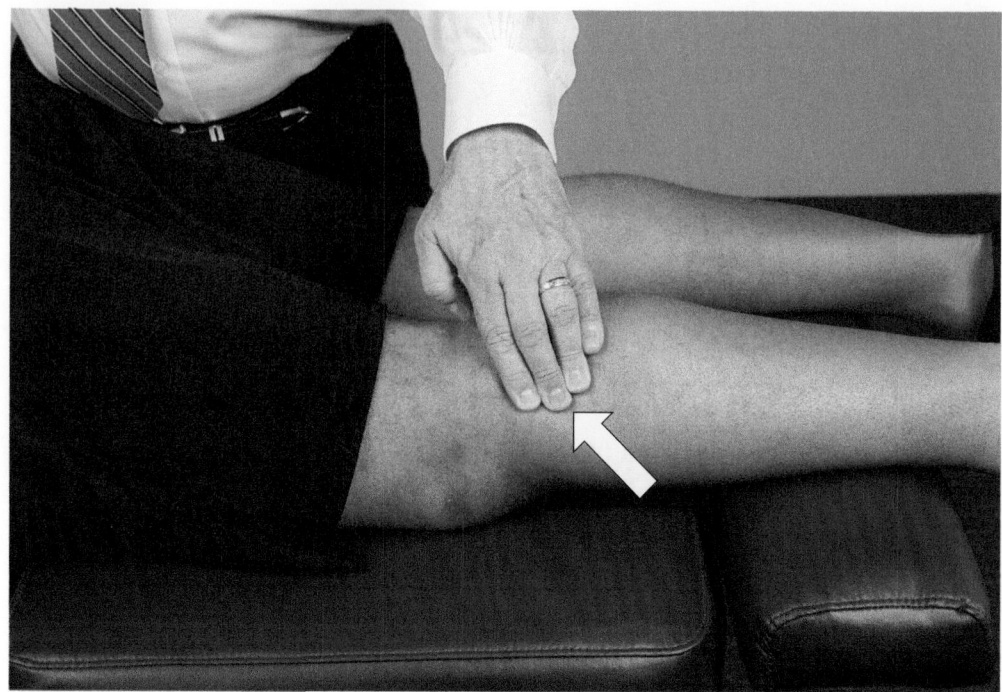

Figure 15-33   Stress Test for posterior-superior proximal fibula.

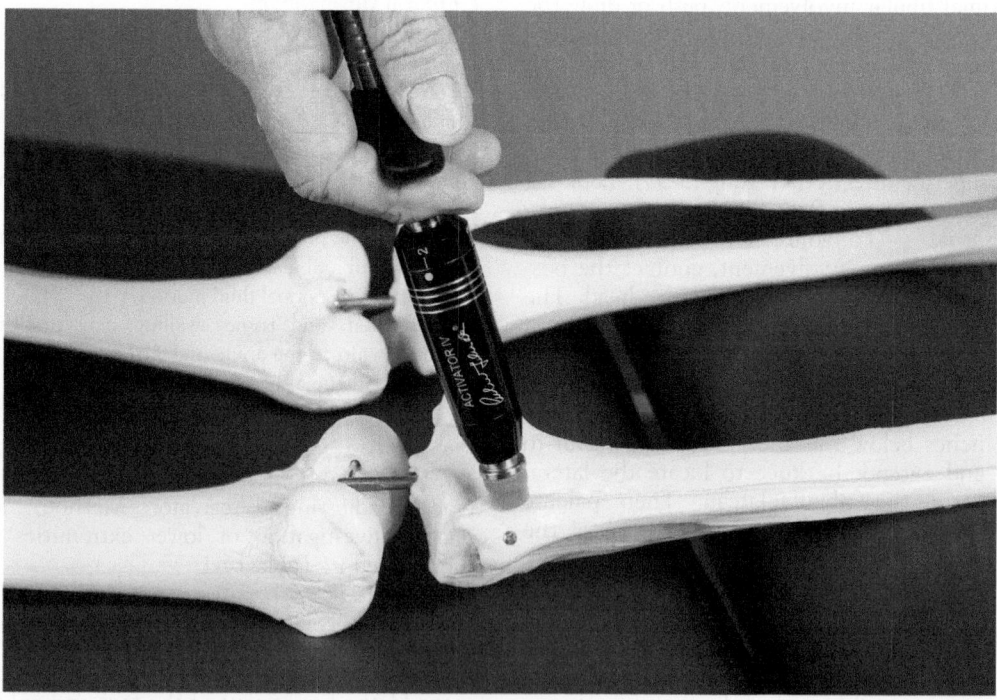

Figure 15-34   Stress Test for posterior-superior proximal fibula. Line of Drive is anterior and inferior at an angle of about 45 degrees to the long axis of the fibula.

Table 15-1 **Summary Table of Tests and Adjustments for the Foot, Ankle, and Related Structures**

Articular Dysfunction	Test	ADJUSTMENT	
		Segmental Contact Point	Line of Drive
Medial Calcaneus	Tap lateral border in a lateral-to-medial direction	Medial aspect of calcaneus	Medial to lateral
Lateral Calcaneus	Tap medial border in a medial-to-lateral direction	Lateral inferior calcaneus	Lateral to medial
Superior Calcaneus	Plantarflex the foot and ankle	Posterior aspect of calcaneus at insertion of Achilles tendon	Inferior
Inferior Calcaneus	Grasp calcaneus and dorsiflex to resistance	Inferior aspect of calcaneus	Superior
Posterior Calcaneus	Pull calcaneus posterior	Calcaneus distal to insertion of the Achilles tendon	Anterior
Anterior-Superior Navicular	Pull the tissue over the navicular in an anterior and superior direction	Superior aspect of navicular	Posterior and inferior
Medial Navicular	Roll lateral to medial across navicular	Medial tuberosity of the navicular	Superior and lateral
Anterior Lateral Talus	Plantarflex and invert the foot and ankle	Neck of talus in sinus tarsi	Posterior and medial
Anterior Distal Tibia	Pull the distal tibia anterior	Anterior distal tibia	Posterior
First Metatarsal and First Cuneiform	Plantarflex and evert the foot and ankle	*Step One:* Inferior or plantar aspect of first metatarsal head	Superior
		Step Two: Medial surface of first cuneiform	Superior and lateral
Inferior Metatarsal Heads	Push metatarsal heads inferior or extend toes against resistance	Inferior aspect of metatarsal heads	Superior
Distal First Metatarsal and Superior Proximal First Phalanx	Plantarflex at first metatarsophalangeal joint	Superior aspect of the first metatarsal joint	Inferior
Hallux valgus	Push distal first phalanx lateral	Medial first metatarso-phalangeal joint	Lateral
Posterior Distal Fibula	Pull lateral malleolus straight posterior	Posterior aspect of lateral malleolus	Anterior
Posterior-Superior Proximal Fibula	Push or take a tissue pull over the proximal, anterior-lateral fibula, posteriorly and superior	Posterior aspect of proximal fibular head	Anterior and inferior at about 45 degrees to long axis of fibular head
Cuboid	Pull the superior-anterior cuboid inferior and lateral	Inferior and lateral aspect, posterior to fifth metatarsal joint	Posterior, superior, and medial

Box 15-2

Reference: Polkinghorn BS. Posterior calcaneal subluxation: an important consideration in chiropractic treatment of plantar fasciitis (heel spur syndrome). Chiropractic Sports Med. 1995;9:44-51.

ABSTRACT

The objective of this article is to describe several cases (n = 3) in which patients with plantar fasciitis, associated with heel spurs, were successfully treated via chiropractic adjustments, emphasizing the correction of posterior calcaneal subluxation.

This particular group of patients presented with heel pain that ranged from 2 months to over 4 years in duration. Radiological confirmation of heel spur was evident in each case. Previously unsuccessful treatment regimens included oral antiinflammatory agents, steroid injections, orthotics, and sustained physical therapy. Two of the patients had been deemed candidates for surgical removal of the spurs but had declined to pursue this option, electing instead to use chiropractic care and conservative management in an effort to resolve the condition.

All patients were treated with short-lever mechanical force, manually assisted chiropractic adjusting procedures, with special emphasis on the foot, ankle, and calcaneus. Although the specific nature of the relevant subluxations varied among patients, a common denominator with this particular patient population group was the occurrence of a posterior subluxation of the calcaneus. All adjustments were delivered via the use of an Activator Adjusting Instrument and were comfortably tolerated by each patient. Said treatment resulted in complete resolution of all symptoms in this studied group of patients, and no recurrence was demonstrated over a protracted follow-up period.

Conservative management of heel spur syndrome may be effectively implemented through the use of specific chiropractic adjusting procedures in selected patients who present with this particular problem. Attention to the possibility of posterior subluxation of the calcaneus should be emphasized during the chiropractic examination process. Although other pedal subluxations may be involved as well, the posterior calcaneus is often a common denominator in the subluxation complex associated with this condition. The use of a mechanical force, manually assisted short-lever adjusting technique, such as with an Activator Adjusting Instrument, can provide effective delivery of chiropractic treatment. Further study of larger patient populations should be conducted to more thoroughly investigate this treatment on a wider scale.

REFERENCES

1. Orava S. Lower leg injuries. In: Renström P, editor. The encyclopedia of sports medicine, Vol V: Clinical practice of sports injury prevention and care. London: Blackwell; 1994.
2. Cook SD, Brinker MR, Poche M. Running shoes: their relation to running injuries. Sports Med. 1990;10(1):1-8.
3. Magee DJ. Lower leg, ankle, and foot. In: Orthopedic physical assessment. Philadelphia: Saunders; 1987. p. 314.
4. Langer S. Structural leg shortage: a case report. J Am Podiatry Assoc. 1976;66(1):38-40.
5. McCaw ST, Bates BT. Biomechanical implications of mild leg length inequality. Br J Sports Med. 1991;25(1):10-13.
6. Beal MC. The short leg problem. J Am Osteopath Assoc. 1977;76(10):745-51.
7. Bailey HW. Theoretical significance of postural imbalance, especially the "short leg." J Am Osteopath Assoc. 1978;77(6):452-5.
8. Beekman S, Louis H, Rosich JM, Coppola N. A preliminary study on asymmetrical forces at the foot to ground interphase. J Am Podiatr Med Assoc. 1985;75(7):349-54.
9. Clemente CD. Gray's anatomy. 30th American ed. Philadelphia: Lea & Febiger; 1985.
10. Karlsson J, Faxén E. Chronic ankle injuries. In: Renström P, editor. The encyclopedia of sports medicine, Vol V: Clinical practice of sports injury prevention and care. London: Blackwell; 1994.
11. Grana WA. Acute ankle injuries. In: Renström P, editor. The encyclopedia of sports medicine, Vol V: Clinical practice of sports injury prevention and care. London: Blackwell; 1994.
12. Whittle MW. Gait analysis. In: McLatchie GR, Lennox CME. The soft tissues: trauma and sports injuries. London: Butterworth-Heinemann; 1993.
13. Bovee M. The essentials of orthopedic & neurological testing. Davenport (IA): Bovee/Palmer College of Chiropractic; 1977.
14. Cipriano JJ. Photographic manual of regional orthopaedic tests. Baltimore: Williams & Wilkins; 1985.
15. Hoppenfeld S. Physical examination of the spine and extremities. Norwalk (CT): Appleton-Century-Crofts; 1976.
16. Kwong PK, Kay D, Voner RT, White MW. Plantar fasciitis—mechanics and pathomechanics of treatment. Clin Sports Med. 1988;7(1):119-26.

17. Kosmahl E, Kosmahl H. Painful plantar heel, plantar fascitis, and calcaneal spur: etiology and treatment. J Orthop Sports Phys Ther. 1987;9(1):17-24.
18. Warren BL. Anatomical factors associated with predicting plantar fasciitis in long-distance runners. Med Sci Sports Exerc. 1984;16(1):60-3.
19. Huang CK, Kitaoka HB, An KN, Chao EYS. Biomechanical evaluation of longitudinal arch stability. Foot Ankle. 1993;14(6):353-7.
20. Pecina MM, Bojanic I. Overuse injuries of the musculoskeletal system. Boca Raton (FL): CRC Press; 1993.
21. Hartley A. Practical joint assessment: a sports medicine manual. St. Louis: Mosby; 1991.
22. Rossi F, La Cava F, Amato F, Pincelli G. The haglund syndrome (H.s.): clinical and radiological features and sports medicine aspects. J Sports Med Phys Fitness. 1987;27(2):258-65.
23. Kelikian H, Kelikian S. Disorders of the ankle. Philadelphia: Saunders; 1985.
24. Travell J, Simons D. Myofascial pain and dysfunction: the trigger point manual. Baltimore: Williams & Wilkins; 1992.
25. Bottomley MB. Risks and injuries in athletics and running. In: McLatchie GR, Lennox CME, editors. The soft tissues: trauma and sports injuries. London: Butterworth-Heinemann; 1993.
26. Taunton JE, McKenzie DC, Clement DB. The role of biomechanics in the epidemiology of injuries. Sports Med. 1988;6(2):107-20.
27. Safran MR, Seaber AV, Garrett WE. Warm-up and muscular injury prevention. An update. Sports Med. 1989;8(4):239-49.
28. Williford HN, East JB, Smith FH, Burry LA. Evaluation of warm-up for improvement in flexibility. Am J Sports Med. 1986;14(4):316-19.
29. Styf J. Diagnosis of exercise-induced pain in the anterior aspect of the lower leg. Am J Sports Med. 1988;16(2):165-9.
30. Bates B. A guide to physical examination and history taking. 4th ed. Philadelphia: J.B. Lippincott; 1987.
31. McGinnis JM, Foege WH. Actual causes of death in the United States. JAMA. 1993;270(18):2207-12.
32. Schafer RC. Clinical biomechanics: musculoskeletal actions and reactions. Baltimore: Williams & Wilkins; 1983. p. 596.
33. Marshall P, Hamilton WG. Cuboid subluxation in ballet dancers. Am J Sports Med. 1992;20(2):169-75.
34. Yockum T, Rowe L. Essentials of skeletal radiology. Baltimore: Williams & Wilkins; 1987.
35. Buschbacher RM. Ankle sprain evaluation and bracing. In: Buschbacher RM, Braddom RL, editors. Sports medicine and rehabilitation: a sport-specific approach. Philadelphia: Hanley & Belfus; and St. Louis: Mosby. 1994.
36. Polkinghorn BS. Posterior calcaneal subluxation: an important consideration in chiropractic treatment of plantar fasciitis (heel spur syndrome). Chiropractic Sports Med. 1995;9:44-51.
37. McKenzie DC, Clement DB, Taunton JE. Running shoes, orthotics, and injuries. Sports Med. 1985;2(5):334-47.

ADDITIONAL TESTS AND ADJUSTMENTS FOR THE SHOULDER AND RELATED STRUCTURES

Evaluation of the shoulder and related structures is indicated when a patient suffers from any of the following complaints:

- Reduction or alteration of shoulder range of motion
- Frozen shoulder syndrome
- Sprain and strain injuries
- Rotator cuff weakness
- Subacromial bursitis
- Myofascial pain disorder of the shoulder

Shoulder pain may be referred via cervical spinal nerves and their branches.[1,2] If cervical neuroarticular dysfunction underlies shoulder complaints, spinal adjusting with the Activator Method (AM) Basic Scan Protocol for cervical motion units often alleviates symptoms.

Shoulder pain can be the product of visceral or organic disease.[3] The typical referral pattern of angina pectoris, for example, is to the neck, jaw, left arm, and shoulder region. Be alert to factors in a patient's history or chief complaint that might signal underlying or contributory disease. Use sound clinical judgment when shoulder complaints appear to be of suspicious origin.

Many shoulder problems directly involve the shoulder articulations and related structures, and careful attention to patient history and chief complaint will facilitate evaluation of acute and chronic problems in the shoulder and upper extremity. Common sites of pain are deep within the tissues surrounding the glenohumeral joint, in the bursae and synovial sheaths of adjacent soft tissue, and in the region of the scapula. Onset of shoulder symptoms may be sudden and related to falls. Sudden overloads that forcefully move the shoulder into extreme extension, abduction, or external rotation can injure soft tissue and cause instability of the shoulder joint complex. Impact trauma from contact sports, motor vehicle collisions, or industrial injuries also can displace the osseous elements of the shoulder, with resultant subluxation or dislocation. Frequently, shoulder problems are of insidious onset and may be related to occupational overuse or misuse, degenerative changes within the joint, or complications of concurrent disease.[4]

COMMON PROBLEMS

The shoulder is the most mobile complex of joints in the body, with an even greater versatility in some ways than the fingers and wrists. The shoulder consists of four joints and articulations. The major and most mobile of these is the glenohumeral joint.

The clavicle participates in two joints. At its proximal end, the clavicle articulates with the manubrium of the sternum. The soft tissues overlying the clavicle, including the skin, subcutaneous fat, fascia, and platysma muscle, are quite thin. The sternoclavicular (SC) joints are easily palpated just lateral to the suprasternal notch. At its distal end, the clavicle articulates with the acromion process of the scapula. The acromioclavicular (AC) joint is subcutaneous and is palpable where the bony prominence of the distal clavicle protrudes superiorly about 1 inch from the most lateral bony portion of the shoulder. Finally, the scapula articulates with the thoracic wall by way of its muscular connections to the second through seventh ribs.

The glenohumeral joint, like the hip, is a freely movable ball-and-socket joint or *enarthrodial diarthrosis*.[5] The glenoid fossa or socket portion of the glenohumeral joint, however, is not nearly as deep as the acetabulum of the hip. Consequently, a healthy glenohumeral joint and shoulder have much greater ranges of motion in all directions than the hip.

On the other hand, strength and stability of the glenohumeral joint are provided by soft tissues rather than by reciprocating osseous tissues and cartilage that provide stability and weight-bearing properties to the hip. Soft tissues that support the glenohumeral joint include the capsular ligament and other accessory ligaments.

It is mainly the muscles of the rotator cuff—the supraspinatus, infraspinatus, teres minor, and subscapularis (the SITS muscles)—that preserve the anatomical and functional integrity of the glenohumeral joint. Soft tissue injury therefore tends to have a fairly dramatic impact on the stability and mobility of the shoulder.

Many of the following complaints can be acute or chronic and can be related to dysfunction of the bony articulations of the soft tissues of the shoulder. An accurate assessment and adjustment of these misalignments and neuroarticular dysfunctions can relieve pain and help to restore strength and mobility.

Reduction or Alteration of Shoulder Range of Motion

Impaired mobility of the shoulder affects everything a patient does with the upper extremity. Not only are work and recreational activities restricted, but even personal activities such as dressing can be impaired. Altered range of motion of the shoulder, especially when pain limits mobility, can produce compensatory aberrant motion that can create postural defects or put excess strain on other joints of the upper extremity.[6]

Because the glenohumeral joint is a ball-and-socket joint, the shoulder is capable of the same seven major motions as the hip. These include flexion, extension, abduction, adduction, internal (medial) rotation, external (lateral) rotation, and circumduction. Average values for shoulder ranges of motion are listed in Box 16-1.[7-9]

Scapular motion must be considered in conjunction with glenohumeral motion or as a component of overall shoulder mobility. During abduction of the humerus, the first 20 degrees of motion occurs exclusively at the glenohumeral articulation. However, beyond 20 degrees of abduction, one third of the mobility occurs with scapular movement away from the midline, and two thirds of the mobility occurs at the glenohumeral joint.[9] Therefore, while observing active or passive abduction and adduction of the shoulder, be sure to assess scapular motion as well. Look for the inferior angle of the scapula to swing laterally as the arm is abducted, and medially as the arm is adducted.

Three other scapular movements occur with shoulder movement. Scapular elevation occurs as part of the "shoulder shrug" maneuver, along with contraction of the trapezius and levator scapular muscles. The rhomboids pull the scapulae toward the midline during retraction of the shoulders. Look for the medial border of the

Box 16-1	**Shoulder Ranges of Motion**
Flexion	180 degrees
Extension	45 degrees
Abduction	180 degrees
Adduction	45 degrees
Internal (medial) rotation	55 degrees in neutral position
	80 degrees with arm at 90 degrees abduction
External (lateral) rotation	45 degrees in neutral position
	90 degrees with arm at 90 degrees abduction
Horizontal abduction	50 degrees with arm at 90 degrees abduction
Horizontal adduction	120 degrees with arm at 90 degrees abduction

The range-of-motion values listed here and elsewhere in *The Activator Method* are averages of values published in various sources and should not be interpreted as "normal" for a given patient. Ranges of motion may be influenced by factors such as age, gender, weight, build, and general physical activity.

scapula to move toward the spinous processes of the thoracic vertebrae as the shoulders are pulled back. During protraction of the scapula, the serratus anticus muscle draws the scapula away from the midline and around the rib cage as the arm is flexed and is moved anteriorly in a reaching gesture.

Evaluate active ranges of motion for bilateral symmetry and fluid, coordinated motion of the shoulder. Many shoulder motions can be assessed by observing the patient taking off or putting on a jacket. The clinician who uses the AM has an opportunity to observe active shoulder ranges of motion during thoracic spine and shoulder Isolation Tests.

Ask the patient to demonstrate active flexion, extension, and circumduction of the shoulder by following you as you demonstrate these conventional motions. Then use Apley's "scratch" test to evaluate adduction, abduction, internal rotation, and external rotation.[10] First, ask the patient to reach across the chest and place the fingers on the opposite shoulder at or near the acromion process of the scapula. To accomplish this maneuver, the patient must be able to adduct the shoulder and demonstrate internal rotation at the glenohumeral joint. When the patient has the hand on the opposite shoulder, the upper arm and elbow should be able to rest against the chest. If the patient cannot bring the arm and elbow down against the chest, or if lowering the arm causes pain, suspect dislocation of or degenerative changes in the joint.

Next, ask the patient to reach behind the back and touch the inferior aspect of the scapula on the opposite side. To perform this action, the patient must adduct and internally rotate the humerus at the glenohumeral joint, but reaching behind the back requires several more degrees of internal rotation.

Finally, ask the patient to reach behind the head and touch the superior aspect of the scapula on the opposite side. To perform this third maneuver, the patient must be able to abduct the shoulder and perform external rotation at the glenohumeral joint. For a patient with frozen shoulder syndrome or restricted external rotation range of motion, the last part of the Apley's scratch test will be the hardest to perform. The arm generally can be actively abducted to about 90 degrees at the shoulder, even when there is muscle and soft tissue injury or degenerative changes. However, to abduct the humerus past 110 to 120 degrees at the glenohumeral joint, the patient must be able to externally rotate the head of the humerus, so that the surgical neck does not butt up against the acromion process of the scapula and stop further abduction at the glenohumeral joint.

Internal and external rotation of the humerus can be evaluated further, independently of adduction or abduction, by having the patient hold the arm against the lateral chest wall with the elbow flexed to 90 degrees. As the patient swings the forearm medially across the body, the humerus rotates internally at the glenohumeral joint. As the patient swings the forearm laterally away from the midline of the body, the humerus rotates externally at the glenohumeral joint.

Assess the shoulder by performing passive range of motion tests when a patient presents with shoulder complaints or when active range of motion appears altered or restricted. Always compare left and right motions, and be alert to pain limitation, crepitus, and changes in joint end play.

Frozen Shoulder Syndrome

Acute or chronic injury to the glenohumeral joint can lead to frozen shoulder syndrome. In this condition, the inflamed joint capsule becomes infiltrated with a proteinaceous exudate, and the interior of the joint becomes fixed. Frozen shoulder syndrome is a form of adhesive capsulitis in which the articular surface of the

head of the humerus binds to the articular surface of the shallow glenoid fossa. Any movement of the humerus, especially abduction or rotation, is likely to elicit pain deep in the shoulder joint.[11]

With frozen shoulder syndrome, the patient typically avoids activities that require abduction of the shoulder or develops compensatory movements that can stress other tissues. Activities like reaching for items from a high shelf or any other task in which the arms must be raised above shoulder level become problematic. Even more mundane activities like putting on or removing a sweater or T-shirt can be severely limited with frozen shoulder syndrome.

Compensatory and antalgic maneuvers related to frozen shoulder syndrome can create additional problems for the patient. During abduction of the humerus beyond 20 degrees from the neutral position, only two thirds of the motion occurs at the glenohumeral joint. The remaining one third occurs as the inferior angle of the scapula moves laterally and superiorly along the scapulothoracic articulation. Any reduction of this 2:1 ratio of abduction can be an early indicator of frozen shoulder syndrome.

When abduction of the humerus is compared bilaterally, be sure to compare movement of the inferior angles of both scapulae. The scapulae tend to travel more laterally and superiorly on the side of the restricted glenohumeral joint and tend to become fixated laterally. As a result, the rhomboids tend to become hypertonic and develop painful trigger points along the medial border of the scapula. The patient may describe "pain between the shoulder blades," a typical symptom associated with thoracic vertebral and costovertebral neuroarticular dysfunction. In this case, however, the discomfort occurs in reaction to frozen shoulder syndrome.

Another compensation associated with frozen shoulder syndrome is the "high shoulder" on the side of involvement. When abduction of the glenohumeral joint becomes limited by pain, the patient may compensate by hiking the shoulder assembly up to get an extra few inches of reach.[12] If job or home activities require frequent reaching for items on high shelves, the shoulder hiking adaptation develops gradually and inevitably. As part of the adaptive phenomenon, the superior trapezius and levator scapulae muscles become hypertonic, develop painful trigger points, and may even limit cervical range of motion. The patient may now demonstrate a positive shoulder depressor test, typical of the trapezius involvement associated with cervical subluxation complex. Once again, however, the signs and symptoms occur in reaction to frozen shoulder syndrome (the high shoulder adaptation is analogous to the "hip hiking" gait observed in patients with fusion or restricted mobility of a lower extremity joint).

The clavicle serves to stabilize the scapula anteriorly during abduction, extension, and external rotation of the shoulder.[9] Compensatory shoulder hiking adaptation to a frozen shoulder as described earlier is likely to involve the clavicular articulations. The distal clavicle at the AC joint is relatively stable with a frozen shoulder, but the proximal clavicle can be drawn superiorly and medially at its articulation with the manubrium of the sternum. The SC joint may become tender to palpation, and the clavicle on the side of involvement may become more visibly prominent.

When a patient experiences frozen shoulder syndrome, perform Stress Tests and adjustments as necessary for the following involvements:

- Lateral and medial scapula
- Superior scapula
- Superior proximal head of the clavicle
- Anterior-inferior humerus
- External rotation of the humerus
- Internal rotation of the humerus
- Posterior humeral head
- Medial (global) scapula
- Subscapularis

Sprain, Strain, and Dislocation Injuries to the Shoulder

The shoulder is the most frequently sprained, strained, and dislocated joint in the body. Its vulnerability is due in part to the shallowness of the glenoid fossa. Although the glenohumeral joint is anatomically classified as a ball-and-socket joint, the socket portion of the glenoid fossa surrounds only a small part of the ball of the humeral head. Andrews describes the relationship between the humerus and the glenoid fossa as "analogous to a golf ball on a tee."[13] The frequency of shoulder injuries is due in part to the exposed location of the joint complex on the body. It is an easy target in contact sports, and it is vulnerable to trauma in falls and motor vehicle accidents.

Acute sprain and strain injuries can occur with falls and direct traction and torquing stresses to the shoulder and upper extremity. Chronic shoulder sprain and strain syndrome has a more insidious onset and can be related to postural defects and overuse and misuse of the shoulder. Repetitive and cumulative stress injuries to the shoulder often are related to occupational activities and may result from ergonomically unsound workstations or equipment.

Acute shoulder complex injury can occur in several ways. A natural and involuntary reflex during a fall is for the arm to snap out in the direction of the fall to protect the head, neck, and torso. Properly trained athletes and martial arts participants are taught to use these reflexes both to break the fall and to minimize trauma to the upper extremity. However, for most people, slipping on ice, tripping on a loose carpet, or misjudging a stair tread can have serious and long-term consequences. Falling injuries are estimated to affect as many as 30% of elderly individuals, in whom gait and balance often are restricted or impaired.[14]

In a fall, the force of impact on the outstretched arm can displace the head of the humerus in the glenoid fossa, causing subluxation, dislocation, or neuroarticular dysfunction. The shallow labrum surrounds less than half of the humeral head. The same anatomical features that give universal motion to the glenohumeral joint provide little protection against forceful displacement of the humerus in the joint.

Of course, soft tissues also are stressed through the impact of a fall on the outstretched arm. The capsular ligament may be stretched or distorted, and ligaments, especially the inferior glenohumeral ligaments, can be stretched or torn. When passive range of motion with abduction or rotation of the humerus produces pain, suspect a sprain or a ligamentous injury. Muscles and tendons of the rotator cuff also may be injured in a fall. Pain on resisted range of motion suggests a strain injury to the tissues of the rotator cuff. The labrum can be susceptible to tearing, especially when the impact force is directed at the glenohumeral joint. In motor vehicle collisions, the combined force directed posteriorly from the hand on the steering wheel through the forearm and humerus, and the ramping effect forces against the shoulder restraint, can cause labrum tears. Onset of this symptom is frequently delayed. When the patient has difficulty performing shoulder abduction within the first third of motion and externally rotates to make this movement more comfortable, consider a labrum tear. Persistent clicking, catching, and locking may be signs of a labrum tear during shoulder movement; the clinician should consider additional diagnostic testing or referral to an orthopedic specialist for further evaluation if sufficient improvement is not obtained.

The direction of a fall, the position of the outstretched arm, and the angle of impact all can determine the direction of misalignment of the humerus at the glenohumeral joint. For example, a forward fall in which one or both arms flex anteriorly to break the fall tends to misalign the head of the humerus posteriorly. When a patient has a shoulder problem related to a fall, get a complete description of the accident or circumstances of the injury. This can guide the examination of the shoulder and which combination of Isolation and Stress Tests to perform.

Sudden forceful torquing and traction stresses applied to the shoulder also can produce sprain and strain injuries.[15] Participants in body contact sports like football, rugby, and wrestling often get painful reminders of the vulnerability of the shoulder. Motions in overhand and underhand throwing and in racquet sports can induce destabilizing stresses to the osseous and soft tissue integrity of the shoulder.[13]

Workers in many occupational groups are at risk for sprain and strain injuries to the shoulder. Farmers, truckers, and warehouse workers often must perform awkward lifting tasks or make adjustments to bulky, heavy equipment. Agricultural workers who tend livestock know how large animals can tug on a tether or bridle.

Both direction and magnitude of torquing and tractioning stresses can determine the direction and severity of misalignment, dislocation, and soft tissue involvement of the shoulder. Although displacement of the humeral head potentially can occur in any direction, the greatest injury is likely to occur when the arm is forced into abduction, external rotation, or extension. The most common direction for glenohumeral dislocation is anterior; clinically, it appears that anterior, medial, and inferior dislocations occur 95% of the time. The other 5% of dislocations occur posteriorly or inferiorly, or involve global instability. Global instability allows dislocation or subluxation in all planes as the result of overstretching and ligamentous laxity of the shoulder complex.[16] Once again, when a patient presents with shoulder pain after a twisting or pulling injury occurs to the shoulder, get as complete a description of the event as possible to guide the examination and the AM Isolation and Stress Test analyses.

Often, patients who present with mild to moderate shoulder sprain and strain with resultant or concurrent misalignment respond to effective conservative care.[11] Care includes appropriate adjusting procedures and rehabilitative therapy and exercise when indicated. When signs and symptoms are severe, or when complaints are related to on-the-job injuries, it makes good clinical sense to conduct a thorough regional examination of the shoulder. Findings of the examination provide the baseline data essential for outcomes measurement. The examination should include at least active and passive ranges of motion, muscle testing, and orthopedic assessment. Frank dislocation and fracture can be ruled out by radiographic examination, and x-rays should be taken when there is marked visible deformity of the shoulder, or when motion and static palpatory findings suggest pronounced displacement of the humeral head.[17]

When a patient has a history of recurrent shoulder sprains and strains or signs and symptoms that suggest repetitive motion sprain and strain injury, perform Isolation Tests and adjustments as necessary for the following involvements:
- Anterior-inferior humerus
- External rotation of the humerus
- Internal rotation of the humerus
- Posterior humeral head

Rotator Cuff Involvement

Acute or chronic injury to the rotator cuff muscles can contribute to the inherent instability of the glenohumeral joint. The wide, flat tendons of the rotator cuff are subject to degenerative changes caused by vascular compression during work against high resistance.[18] For example, in *swimmer's shoulder,* the tendon of the supraspinatus is compressed by forceful adduction of the arm against water resistance during the downstroke portion of many swimming maneuvers.[19] Similar injuries are likely to occur with some body building activities and gymnastics.

Repeated forceful adduction of the shoulder occurs with several occupational tasks. Many equipment operators operate levers or crank handles that require considerable force. Automotive and heavy equipment mechanics and tire repair workers are required to perform forceful shoulder adduction as part of their work activities. Epidemiological studies comparing a cohort of welders and platers and another cohort of automotive workers with control groups of office workers found at least an elevenfold increase in cumulative trauma injury to the rotator cuff and the bicipital tendon.[4]

Assess the rotator cuff by active shoulder range of motion and muscle testing. The supraspinatus muscle appears to be the most frequently injured member of the rotator cuff group. Several tests and maneuvers have been developed to test it for injury.[8,10] An injured supraspinatus typically produces pain at between 60 and 120 degrees of active abduction in the "painful arc" portion of the motion. The supraspinatus also performs most of the first 30 degrees of abduction of the humerus. (It works as a synergist to the deltoid for abduction greater than 30 degrees.) Therefore pain over the superior aspect of the humerus or weakness on resisted abduction between 0 and 30 degrees suggests supraspinatus involvement. Codman's test of the supraspinatus can isolate a weakened or damaged muscle. In this test, also known as the "drop arm" test, the patient is asked to lower the arm slowly to the side from a starting position of 90 degrees of abduction. Inability to perform this maneuver, so that the arm drops rapidly and without control, suggests supraspinatus weakness and possible tear. An alternate method of performing the test is to have the patient hold the arm in horizontal (90 degrees) abduction. If the arm drops suddenly, or if the patient is unable to resist when gentle downward pressure is applied, supraspinatus involvement is confirmed.

When a patient experiences rotator cuff and other shoulder muscle weakness, perform Isolation and Stress Tests and adjustments where indicated for the following involvements:

- Anterior-inferior humerus
- Posterior humeral head
- External rotation of the humerus
- Internal rotation of the humerus
- Superior distal clavicle
- Inferior medial coracoid
- T2-T3 facet
- Supraspinatus

Subacromial Bursitis

Pain at or just deep to the acromion process that is exacerbated by resisted abduction or rotation of the humerus suggests subacromial bursitis.[20] Inflammation of a strained rotator cuff provokes swelling in and around the bursae of the shoulder, and resultant friction between swollen tissues produces pain during motion.

Subacromial bursitis may occur as a consequence of acute injury to the rotator cuff, but it is more likely to result from chronic or repetitive strain injury. Wrestling, football, and throwing activities, for example, may contribute to subacromial bursitis in youngsters.[20] Workers in many occupational groups also are at risk of developing subacromial bursitis, especially when their jobs require overhead work. Painting, drywalling, wallpapering, electrical work, and carpentry are only a few examples of such occupations.

Upon clinical presentation, subacromial bursitis frequently is described as an impingement syndrome.[13,15,19] The principal finding is pain on abduction, as the greater tuberosity of the humerus rises and closes the gap between the humerus and the acromion process. If soft tissue is inflamed and swollen, it is pinched between the humerus and the acromion, and this produces the sharp localized pain of subacromial bursitis.[21] Pain tends to be maximal during the painful arc of abduction.

During abduction past 90 degrees, the head of the humerus must rotate externally to enable the greater tuberosity to clear the acromion. When bursae and other soft tissues are inflamed, however, attempts to rotate the humerus externally stress affected tendons and produce more pain by increasing friction in the already swollen tissues.

Because so many everyday activities, not to mention occupational and athletic activities, involve at least some shoulder abduction, the individual with subacromial bursitis is likely to develop an adaptive compensatory posture and antalgic maneuvers to avoid shoulder pain. As was noted with the frozen shoulder syndrome, a high shoulder may develop when a patient adapts to subacromial bursitis. Rather than abducting the arm when reaching for items on a high shelf, the patient may increase reach by flexing the arm anteriorly and hiking the shoulder to get a few extra inches of lift at the shoulder. As a result, the trapezius and levator scapulae muscles may become hypertonic and produce a superior scapula. Compensatory and antalgic maneuvers may add to shoulder instability and perpetuate pain, placing awkward and unintended loads on other muscles.

Multiple factors contribute to subacromial bursitis; these eventually can result in osteoarthritis or degenerative joint disease of the shoulder. Unresolved acute rotator cuff injury with ongoing inflammation can predispose the patient to bursitis. Unresolved inflammation also may lead to precipitation of calcium phosphate in the tendons and bellies of affected muscles. Calcific densities can develop in the ligaments, bursae, and tendon sheaths, resulting in severe loss of shoulder mobility.[15]

Application of eccentric loading to the soft tissues of the shoulder can contribute to instability of the glenohumeral joint. Overhand throwing and overhead work with the abducted shoulder in forced external rotation perpetuate instability as a form of repetitive strain injury. Loss of muscle tone and coordination with concurrent soft tissue degeneration leads ultimately to misalignment and impingement.[15]

When a patient describes signs and symptoms suggestive of subacromial bursitis, perform

Isolation Tests, Stress Tests, and adjustments where necessary for the following involvements of the shoulder:

- External rotation of the humerus
- Internal rotation of the humerus
- Anterior-inferior humerus
- Superior scapula
- Superior proximal head of the clavicle
- Inferior medial coracoid
- Superior distal clavicle
- Supraspinatus

Myofascial Pain of the Shoulder

In the syndromes variously described as fibromyalgia, fibrositis, and myofascial pain disorder, muscles become hypertonic and painful when stretched and develop trigger points or foci that are exquisitely tender to deep palpation. Several possible causes, including exercise, fatigue, and stress, have been implicated.[22] Fibromyalgia now is thought to arise from miscommunication between the nerve impulses of the central nervous system. The neurons, which supply the brain, become more excitable, exaggerating the pain sensation. This overamplification of pain is referred to as "central sensitization."[23] The development of trigger points in the bellies and at the musculotendinous junctions of hypertonic muscles is a familiar phenomenon to massage therapists, physical therapists, and other practitioners of manual therapeutics.[24,25] Bottomley points out that the shoulder region "contains several of the 14 or so trigger sites in the body [associated with] fibromyalgia or fibrositis."[26]

Myofascial pain may develop as a consequence of acute or chronic injury to shoulder soft tissue as described in previous sections. Several possible mechanisms have been proposed for the changes that occur in the shoulder muscles. Chronic, low-level irritation of muscles, for example, may result in gradual infiltration of the muscle bellies with collagenous matrix deposited by fibroblasts. If a mild, active inflammatory process is ongoing, the fibroblastic activity is essentially a misdirection of the body's defense cells as they attempt to repair damaged tissue. Collagen has great tensile strength but very little ability to relax or contract. Consequently, buildup of collagenous fibers in the contractile parts of muscle tissue can limit motion and cause pain when muscles are stretched or worked against resistance.

The clinical presentation of myofascial pain disorder is extremely variable; the syndrome itself is somewhat controversial.[27] Nevertheless, at least one study suggests that the condition may affect 1 in 20, or 5% of the American population.[28] More than 10 million Americans suffer from fibromyalgia; 90% of these are women between the ages of 25 and 45 years.[29] In addition to trigger points and muscle pain with movement, the patient may be sensitive to cold, changes in humidity, and a variety of emotional and workplace stresses. Patients may report fatigue and an inability to "get a good night's sleep." Symptoms may be relieved by massage and the application of heat.[15]

Chronic compensation for shoulder instability and altered mobility of the glenohumeral joint may contribute to myofascial pain disorder. Malposition of the humeral head also may result in facilitation of the rotator cuff muscles and associated muscles of the shoulder, with the development of hypertonicity and trigger point sensitivity. Shoulder range of motion may be limited by pain, but there may not be ready evidence of biomechanical disturbance of the joint structures. Passive ranges of motion of the shoulder are likely to be greater than active ranges of motion, but the patient may demonstrate apprehension when passive ranges of motion are performed.

When a patient presents with the clinical picture of myofascial pain disorder, conduct a thorough history. An occupational history may be especially valid for a patient with such complaints. Because the syndrome has an insidious onset, and because structural and functional changes are challenging to assess, it is important to identify physical and environmental stressors that may contribute to the patient's concerns.

One factor that deserves special attention is the patient's workstation, especially if the job involves use of a computer. Most occupations use computer technology and require that part of a workday be devoted to data entry, record searches, or inventory management. Although the new technology often has increased the speed of the job and has enhanced productivity, it has created problems in the workforce, too.

Often PCs or computer terminals are unceremoniously placed on a worker's desk or bench with a minimum of instruction in their usage and virtually no attention paid to the ergonomics of their placement. Too often, keyboards are placed on the surface of a desk at standard height rather than on a lower typing height table or under-the-desk tray. As a result, the worker may have to adapt posture to work at an awkward height. The ideal position for typing or keyboarding is a relaxed but erect posture with the forearms parallel to the floor, the elbows flexed at 90 degrees, and the wrists in a neutral position, neither flexed nor extended.

When a keyboard is too high, the worker may be able to type for a limited time with the elbows flexed more tightly and the wrists in flexion, but fatigue quickly takes its toll. To adapt, the worker may retract and raise the shoulders, shifting the burden to the muscles of the shoulder and the upper back. When this adaptation is repeated day after day, even for a few hours of a shift, hypertonicity may develop in the shoulder and other upper extremity muscles.

Be sure to question the patient about previous treatments. Because fibromyalgia is so nonspecific, many patients are treated as if their complaints were hysterical, and muscle relaxants and antidepressants may be prescribed.[27,28] During examination of the patient, note the presence and location of trigger points. Be observant for antalgic movements and compensatory postures such as a high shoulder, head tilt, or shoulders thrown back as if at rigid attention.

For the patient whose clinical presentation suggests myofascial pain disorder, perform Isolation Tests, Stress Tests, and adjustments where necessary for the following neuroarticular dysfunctions:
- Lateral and medial scapula
- Superior scapula
- Second rib
- External rotation of the humerus
- Internal rotation of the humerus
- Anterior-inferior humerus

CONCURRENT CONDITIONS

Keep in mind that the shoulder is a target of referred pain for a number of visceral disorders.[9] The cardiogenic pain of angina, for example, is described as substernal compressive pain that typically radiates to the neck, jaw, and left arm, including the shoulder.

Lung diseases may radiate to the shoulder or related structures.[3] Pleuritic pain, accompanied by pain-limited inspiration, can be localized to the subscapular region and may manifest with shoulder pain. With chronic obstructive pulmonary disease, fibrotic lung disease, and pneumoconioses such as silicosis or emphysema, biomechanical changes occur to the spine and rib articulations, as do soft tissue changes to the lung tissues. The patient often develops a "barrel chest" with an increase in the anteroposterior diameter of the thoracic cavity, so that costovertebral articulations may be stressed. Pain radiating along an intercostal nerve may give the impression of shoulder pain.

Cervicogenic pain referral also must be differentiated from a shoulder complaint.[30] Referred pain from the fifth cervical nerve, for example, may radiate out to the tip of the shoulder near the insertion of the superior portion of the trapezius muscle.[1,2] Care must be taken to differentiate referred pain from a cervical disc lesion or intervertebral entrapment syndrome from the impingement syndrome observed in subacromial bursitis, rotator cuff muscle injury, or degenerative changes to the glenohumeral joint.

TESTING AND ADJUSTING THE SHOULDER AND RELATED STRUCTURES

With involvement of the shoulder and related structures, the following Isolation Tests and adjustments of the glenohumeral joint should be performed:
- Anterior-inferior humerus
- External rotation of the humerus
- Internal rotation of the humerus
- Posterior humeral head

When clinical judgment and patient symptoms indicate involvement of structures other than the glenohumeral joint, the following Isolation and Stress Tests and adjustments also will be performed:
- Second rib
- Superior scapula
- Inferior scapula
- Superior proximal head of the clavicle
- Inferior medial coracoid
- T2-T3 facet syndrome
- T3-T4 facet syndrome

Bear in mind the Isolation Tests and Stress Tests for neuroarticular dysfunction and misalignments of these structures are performed by maneuvers that stress them *into the direction of misalignment, or neuroarticular dysfunction.* Adjustments therefore are applied in the opposite direction to the Stress Test. As with the lower extremity, the legs will be even in Position #1 before the Stress Test is performed. After the test, look for reactivity, typically shortening of the Pelvic Deficient (PD) leg in Position #1, to identify the presence of dysfunction. Note that except for Basic Scan Protocol scapular pattern isolations, all Isolation Tests for the shoulder are performed with the patient in the neutral (face-down) position.

Anterior-Inferior Humerus

Anterior-inferior involvement of the humeral head in the glenoid fossa should be considered when a patient reports pain in the anterior aspect of the shoulder. Anterior flexion of the shoulder and rotational motion may be limited by pain. It is also typically involved with bicipital tendonitis and in most cases of dislocation of the humerus, which is in the anterior-inferior direction.

Isolation Test.   To isolate an anterior-inferior humerus, ask the patient to pronate the forearm with the palm facing up. Then ask the patient to extend the arm at the shoulder by raising it toward the ceiling (Figure 16-1). Be sure to have the patient keep the elbow fully extended. Look for reactivity of the PD leg in Position #1 for involvement.

Adjustment.   To adjust an anterior-inferior humerus in the supine position, place the tip of the instrument on the intertubercular groove. The Line of Drive (LOD) is superior and posterior (Figure 16-2).

In most cases, the anterior-inferior humerus can be adjusted without turning the patient over. Reach under the shoulder and palpate for the contact point by locating the groove between the greater and lesser tubercles on the anterior aspect of the proximal humerus. Be careful when positioning the instrument if examination findings indicate irritation of the sheath of the long head of the bicipital tendon as it passes through the intertubercular groove. For the heavy patient and the patient with well-developed shoulder musculature, take an inferior-to-superior tissue pull over the proximal humerus with the index and middle fingers. Place the fingers on the two tubercles and wide enough apart to accommodate the tip of the instrument. Use the split-finger position to stabilize the instrument during the adjustment. Another aid to adjusting the anterior-inferior

humerus is to have the treating doctor stand close to the table and allow the patient to rest the forearm on the doctor's shoulder to act as a support while adjusting the anterior-inferior humerus. This takes the strain off the biceps tendon (Figure 16-3).

Clinical Observations

In the experience of most chiropractors, the most frequent direction of subluxation and dislocation of the shoulder is anterior and inferior.[15] Consequently, examination and Activator Method Isolation Test analysis of virtually all patients with shoulder complaints should, at the very least, include the anterior-inferior humerus.

When the shoulder is subluxated anteriorly and inferiorly, the supraspinatus muscle tendons may also be stretched, and an unadjusted anterior-inferior humerus may contribute to degenerative joint disease of the glenohumeral joint.

External Rotation of the Humerus

Restricted internal rotation of the humerus may indicate external involvement of the humerus (externally rotated head of the humerus). Difficulty performing part of Apley's maneuver, specifically, touching the shoulder opposite the side of involvement or reaching behind the back to touch the inferior angle of the opposite scapula, suggests restriction of internal rotation.

Isolation Test.   To test for an external humerus, begin with the palm facing up toward the ceiling

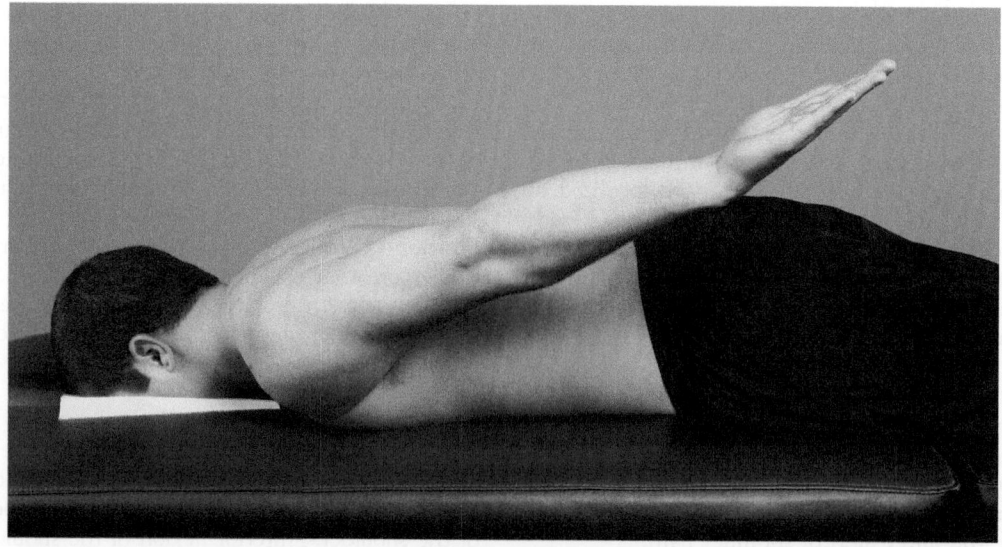

Figure 16-1   Isolation Test for anterior-inferior humerus; with palm facing up, extend the arm at the shoulder by raising it toward the ceiling.

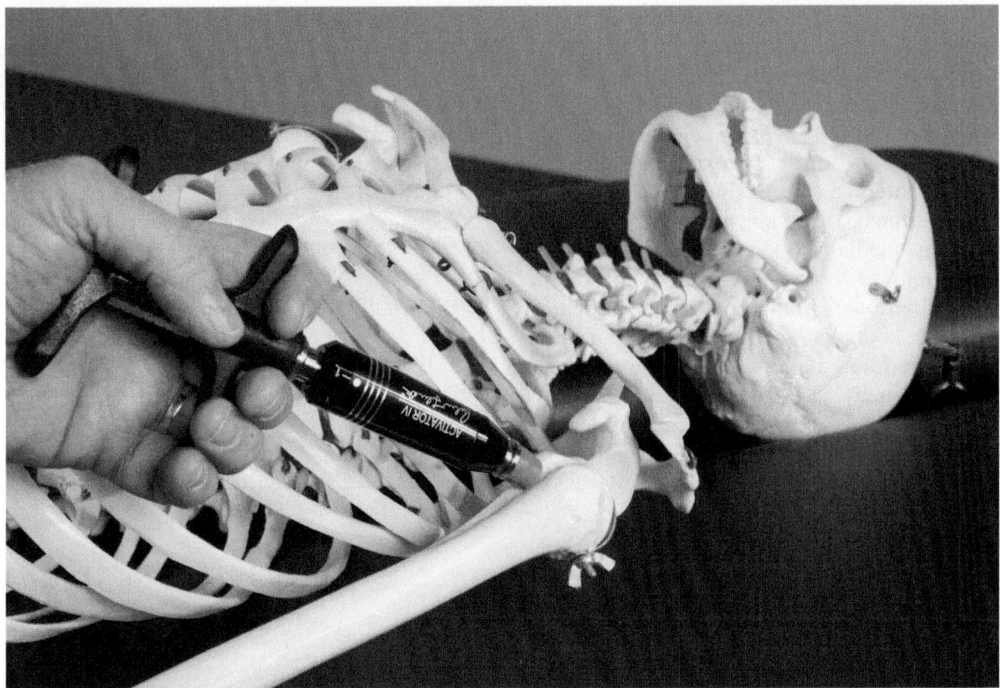

Figure 16-2   Adjustment for anterior-inferior humerus. Line of Drive is superior and posterior.

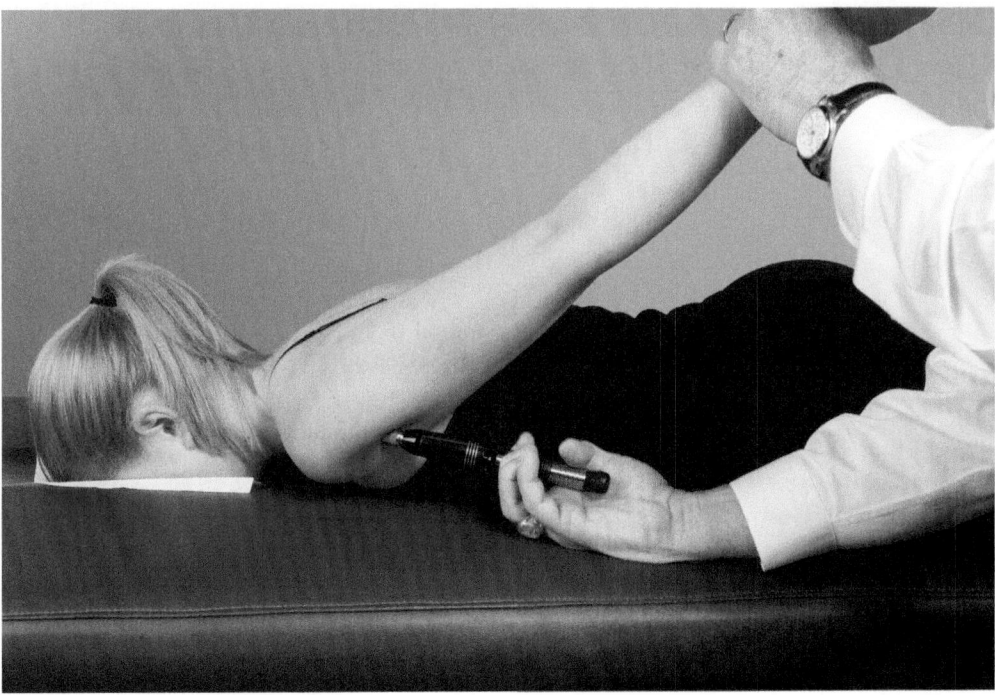

Figure 16-3   Alternate adjusting position for anterior-inferior humerus.

and the elbow locked in full extension. Instruct the patient to rotate the arm so that the palm ends up flat against the table (Figure 16-4). Look for reactivity of the PD leg in Position #1 for involvement.

Adjustment.   To adjust an external humerus, contact the lateral aspect of the greater tubercle. The LOD is medial and slightly anterior to drive the humerus medially (Figure 16-5).

If a patient has a concurrent elbow problem, or if examination of the elbow joints indicates ligamentous laxity or aberrant motion, it may be best to perform the external rotation of the shoulder manually. Take a firm grasp on the arm below the shoulder with one hand, and stabilize the elbow with the other. Using both hands, rotate the humerus externally.

To palpate for the greater tubercle, slide a finger from the lateral aspect of the humerus medially until the bony prominence is felt. Keep a finger on the greater tubercle to stabilize the instrument during the adjustment, to minimize discomfort for the patient and to ensure a firm contact with the humerus.

Clinical Observations

External rotation of the humerus is a common companion to the anterior-inferior subluxation of the humeral head. Contact sports, racquet sports, and falls to the side may force the humerus both anterior and inferior as well as into external rotation.

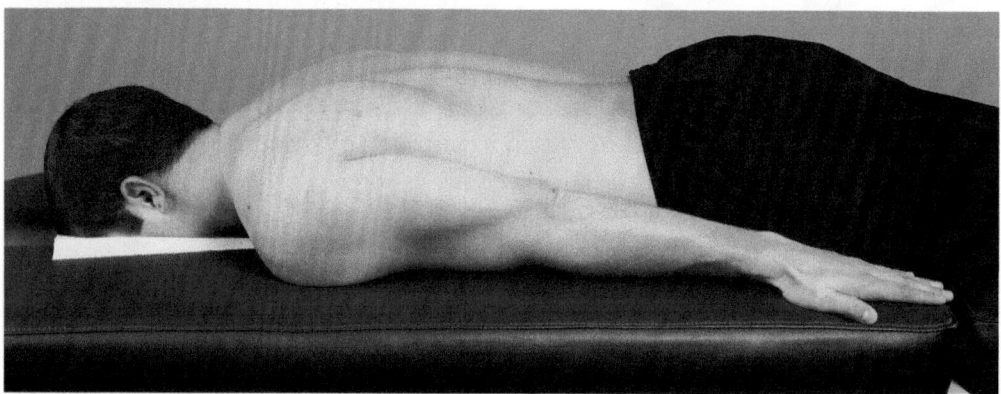

Figure 16-4   Isolation Test for external humerus; rotate the arm so that the palm ends up flat against the table.

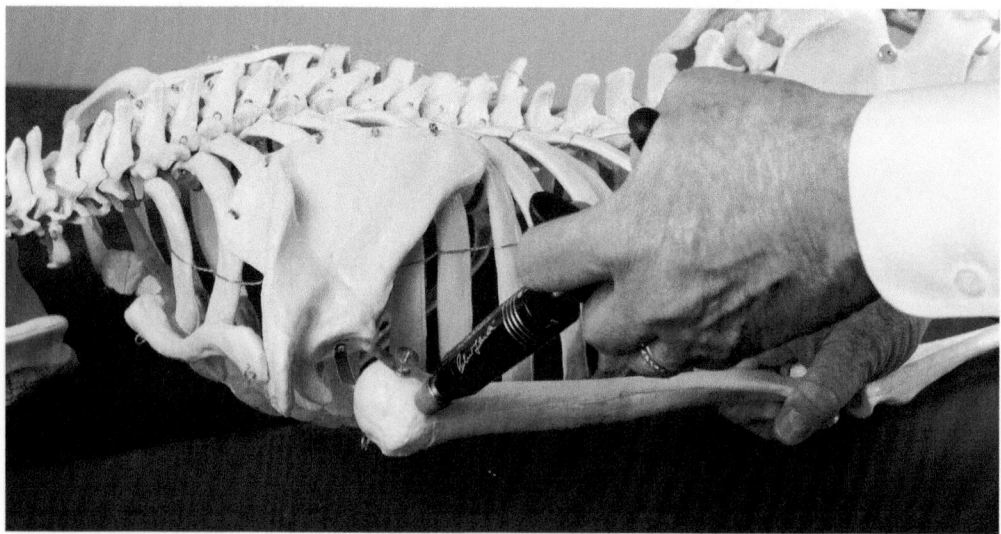

Figure 16-5   Adjustment for external humerus. Line of Drive is medial and slightly anterior.

Internal Rotation of the Humerus

Inability to externally rotate the shoulder may indicate internal involvement of the humeral head. Examination of active range of motion may show that the patient has difficulty abducting the arm past 90 degrees. The portion of Apley's test in which the patient is asked to touch the superior aspect of the scapula on the side opposite the shoulder involvement also may be difficult to perform.

Isolation Test. To test for an internal humerus, first turn the palm of the hand on the side tested toward the ceiling, with the elbow locked in full extension. Instruct the patient to continue turning the arm so that the pronated palm faces away from the midline of the body and the thumb will point upward or posterior (Figure 16-6). Look for reactivity of the PD leg in Position #1 for involvement.

Adjustment. To adjust an internal humerus, contact the posterior aspect of the head of the humerus. The LOD is directly medial to derotate the humeral head (Figure 16-7).

If the patient has a concurrent elbow problem, or if examination of the elbow joints indicates ligamentous laxity or aberrant motion, perform the Stress Test manually. Grasp the arm below the shoulder with one hand, and stabilize the elbow with the other. Using both hands, rotate the humerus internally.

To ensure good contact and an effective LOD, it may be advisable to take a tissue pull with the thumb of the stabilizing hand over the posterior aspect of the proximal humerus. Use the thumb to stabilize the tip of the instrument during the adjustment.

Posterior Humeral Head

Acute or chronic pain in the posterior portion of the deltoid that is exacerbated by abduction and extension of the arm suggests a posterior humeral head. A forward fall on an outstretched arm may force the head of the humerus posteriorly in the glenoid fossa.

Isolation Test. To test for a posterior humeral head, ask the patient to abduct the humerus to 90 degrees and let the forearm drop down beside the table (Figure 16-8). The weight of the forearm hanging over the edge of the table will push the proximal humerus posteriorly at the shoulder. Look for reactivity of the PD leg in Position #1 for involvement.

Adjustment. To adjust a posterior humeral head, reposition the arm on the table at the patient's side. Contact the posterior aspect of the proximal greater tubercle at the insertion point of the infraspinatus tendon (middle facet). The LOD is straight anterior (Figure 16-9).

The test for a posterior humerus works very effectively on a table designed for the AM, because for most patients the table is wide

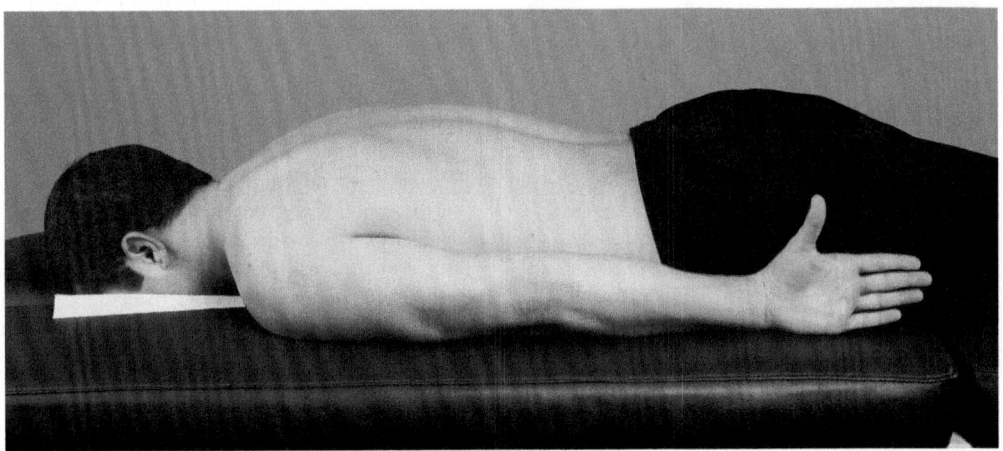

Figure 16-6 Isolation Test for internal humerus; turn the arm so the pronated palm faces away from the midline of the body.

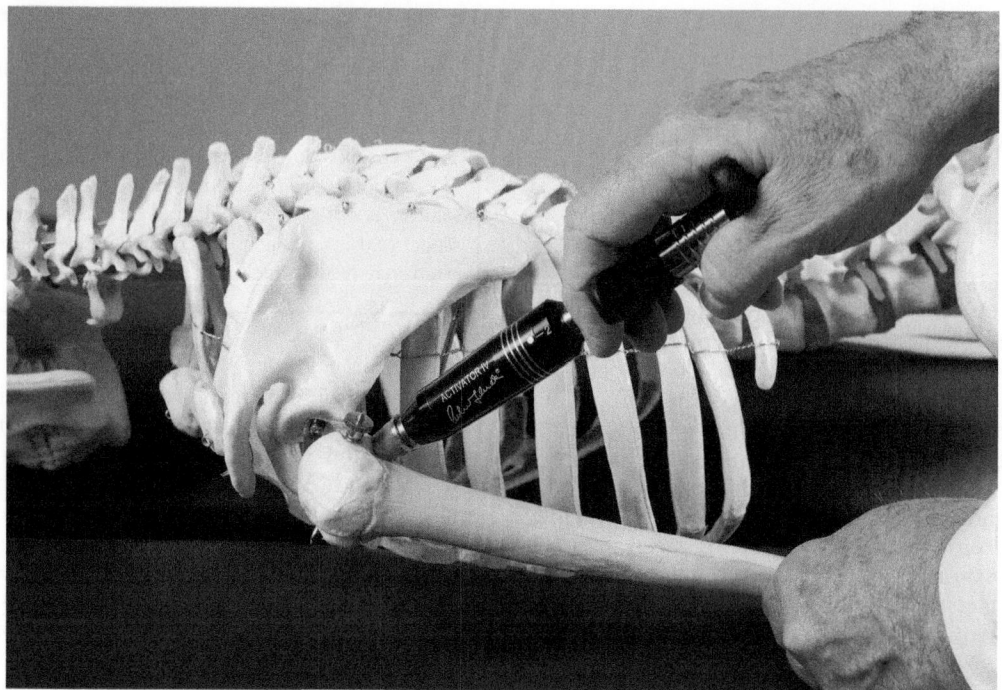

Figure 16-7   Adjustment for internal humerus. Line of Drive is directly medial.

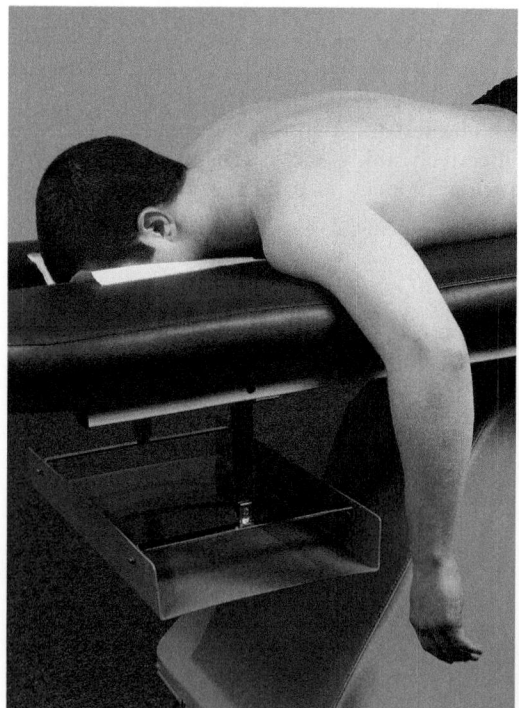

Figure 16-8   Isolation Test for posterior humerus; let the forearm drop down beside the table.

enough for just enough leverage to be applied to the humerus to stress the head posteriorly at the glenohumeral joint. For a child or a small patient, or when a full-sized AM table is not available, the Isolation Test for a posterior humerus may be performed manually. Grasp the humerus just distal to the shoulder with one hand, and swing it into 90 degrees of abduction. Support the humerus with that hand while gently pushing down (anatomically anterior) on the patient's elbow to stress the proximal humerus posteriorly.

Clinical Observations

The labrum or cartilaginous lip of the glenoid fossa is least developed at the posterior border. Furthermore, there is no significant glenohumeral ligamentous structure protecting the posterior aspect of the joint. As a result, posterior subluxation of the humerus increases the burden on the infraspinatus muscle of the rotator cuff. The strained muscle and tendon tend to be more painful on flexion, adduction, and internal rotation of the shoulder.

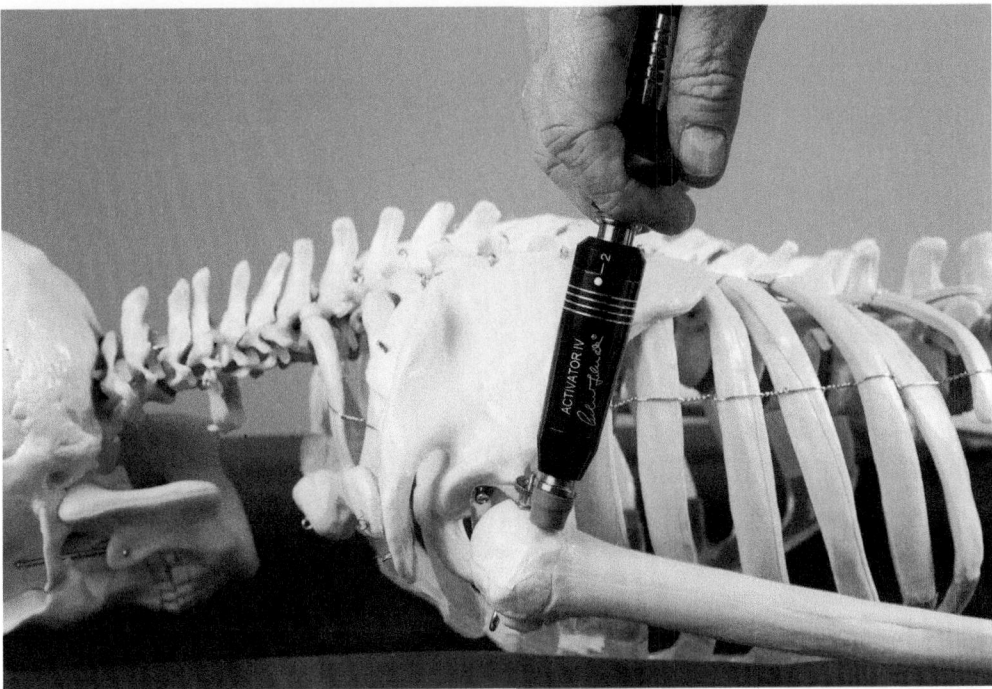

Figure 16-9   Adjustment for posterior humerus. Line of Drive is anterior.

Second Rib Involvement

For a patient with restricted glenohumeral joint range of motion such as frozen shoulder syndrome, or when scapular motion is limited during protraction or retraction of the shoulder, consider involvement of the second rib.

Isolation Test.   To test for the presence of second rib involvement, ask the patient to abduct the arm on the side of involvement to 90 degrees with the hand and the forearm pronated. (The patient's palm will be facing upward toward the ceiling [Figure 16-10].) Look for reactivity of the PD leg in Position #1 for involvement.

Adjustment.   To adjust a second rib, contact the nonarticular portion of the tubercle just lateral to the costotransverse joint. The LOD is lateral and slightly inferior along the longitudinal axis of the rib (Figure 16-11).

If the patient has the full clinical manifestations of frozen shoulder syndrome, abduction of the arm during the Isolation Test for a second rib fixation may be difficult or painful. In such a case, it is not essential for the patient to achieve the full 90 degrees of abduction. Simply ask the patient to abduct the arm with the hand pronated to the point of pain, but not beyond.

Clinical Observations

During shoulder abduction, two thirds of the motion occurs at the glenohumeral joint and the remaining one third is accomplished by the scapulothoracic articulation.[9] With frozen shoulder syndrome, hypertonicity of the rhomboids and weakness of the serratus anticus and subscapularis muscles may develop, with restricted travel of the scapula. Rhomboid muscle hypertonicity may indirectly involve the second rib by generating a muscle imbalance affecting the muscle's insertion on the thoracic vertebrae.

Second rib involvement may also be a consequence of scapulothoracic bursitis, in which tissues deep to the scapula become inflamed and swollen. The bursitis is associated with the "snapping scapula" condition associated with throwing sports.[13] Movement of the scapula creates painful friction between the inflamed tissues, and with chronic inflammation or recurrent injury, fibrotic repair can cause adhesions. Both the scapula and the second rib become hypomobile.

Superior Scapula

Frozen shoulder syndrome, antalgic "high shoulder," and hypertonicity over the upper trapezius

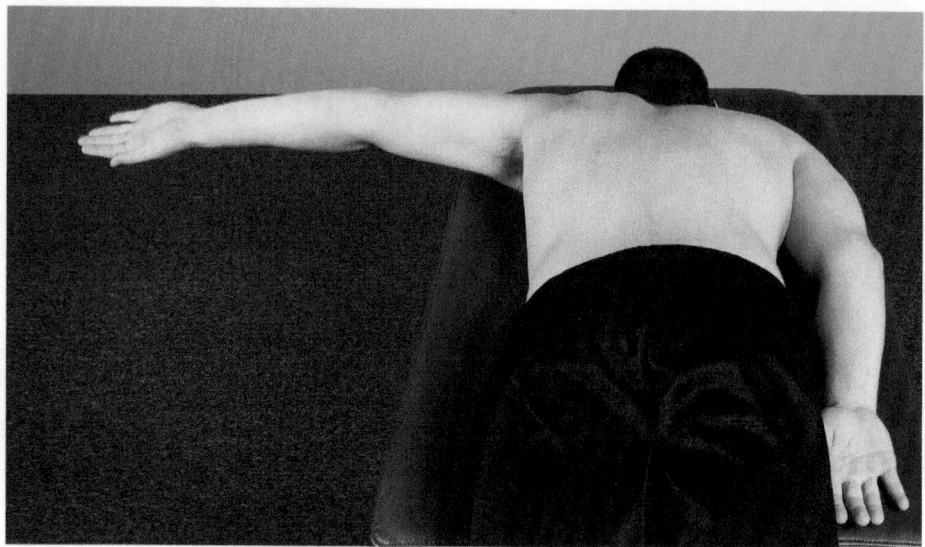

Figure 16-10   Isolation Test for second rib.

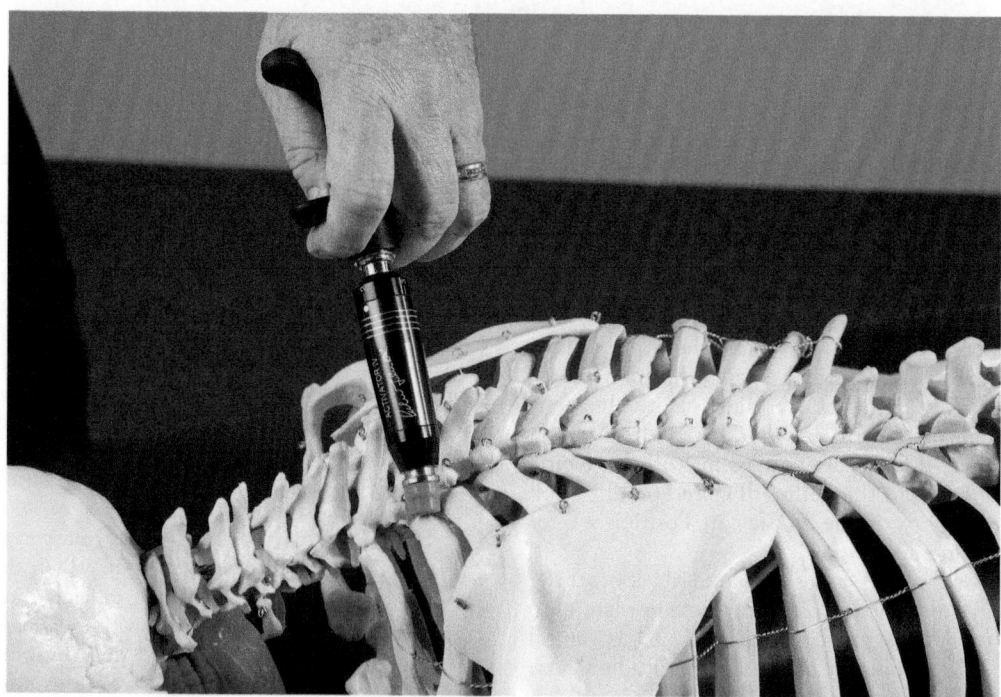

Figure 16-11   Adjustment for second rib. Line of Drive is lateral and slightly inferior along the longitudinal axis of the rib.

and levator scapulae muscles suggest superior malposition of the scapula. The levator scapula is often in spasm as a result of glenohumeral instability or AC dysfunction. Forward head posture, rounded shoulders, and thoracic kyphosis are commonly associated with superior scapular involvement resulting from long hours of computer use and prolonged sitting postures.

Isolation Test.   To test for a superior scapula, ask the patient to abduct the arm on the side of involvement, and place the palm of the hand over the lower cervicals of the neck

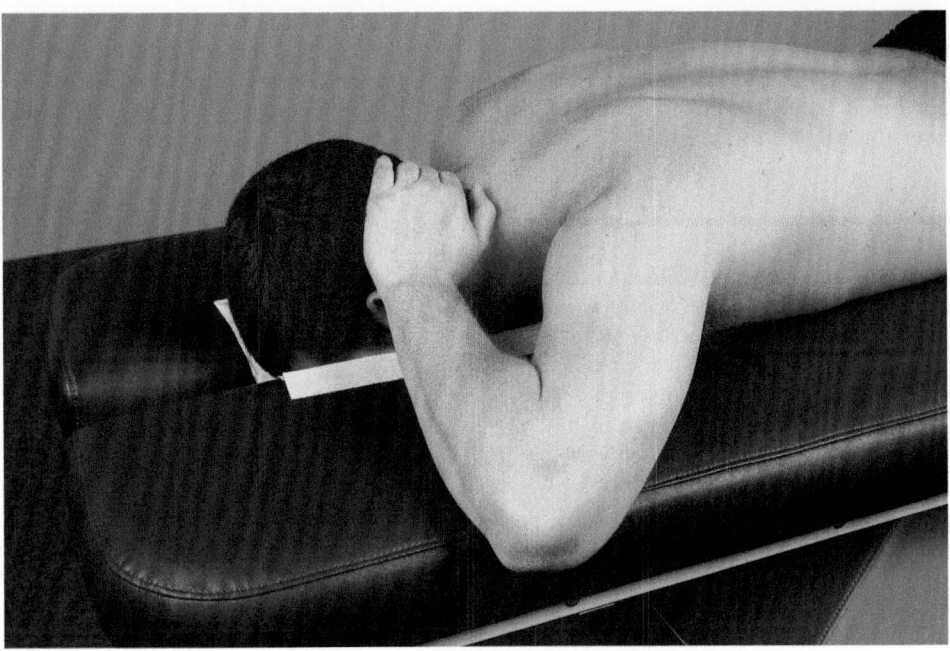

Figure 16-12 Isolation Test for superior scapula.

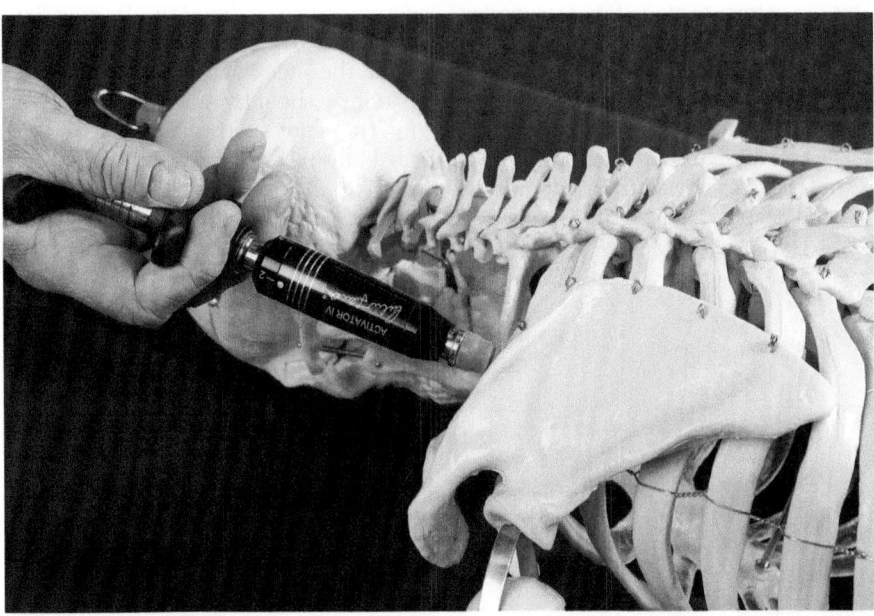

Figure 16-13 Adjustment for superior scapula. Line of Drive is straight inferior.

(Figure 16-12). Look for reactivity of the PD leg in Position #1 for involvement.

Adjustment. To adjust a superior scapula, contact the midpoint of the spine of the scapula on the superior aspect. The LOD is straight inferior (Figure 16-13).

For the patient with frozen shoulder syndrome or other severe restriction to shoulder abduction and external rotation, it may be difficult to perform the Isolation Test maneuver through active range of motion. Perform a Stress Test by abducting and externally rotating the humerus to patient tolerance, or until free movement of the shoulder no longer occurs. Then gently traction the scapula superiorly by taking a broad contact with the palm of the hand over the wing of the scapula.

Clinical Observations

A common cause of superior subluxation of the scapula is hypertonicity of the levator scapulae and superior portion of the trapezius muscle. The hypertonicity may be a result of antalgic compensation for a frozen shoulder, or it could be the result of cervical subluxation. Be sure to take a detailed case history and perform a full examination of the shoulder and cervical spine. Also test for medial or lateral scapula as part of the Activator Method Basic Scan Protocol.

Inferior Scapula

For cases in which a shoulder problem is recurrent or nonresponsive, or when a patient reports pain under the shoulder blade, check for an inferior scapula on the side of involvement.

Isolation Test. After testing for a superior scapula with the patient's hand on the back of the neck, instruct the patient to bring the arm back down to the side (Figure 16-14). Look for reactivity of the PD leg in Position #1 for involvement.

Adjustment. To adjust for an inferior scapula, contact the inferior aspect, at the midpoint of the spine of the scapula. The LOD is superior (Figure 16-15).

Superior Proximal Clavicle

Point tenderness at the SC joint or a compensatory high shoulder suggests superior involvement of the proximal clavicle at its articulation with the manubrium of the sternum. Consider a superior proximal clavicle also when a patient suffers from sternocleidomastoid and other cervical muscle hypertonicity as a result of whiplash injury, wry neck, or torticollis.

Isolation Test. To test a superior proximal clavicle, ask the patient to abduct the arm on the involved side and place the palm of the hand over the lower cervicals of the neck. Then have the patient push the elbow of the abducted arm into the table (Figure 16-16). Look for reactivity of the PD leg in Position #1 for involvement.

Adjustment. Before adjusting a superior proximal clavicle, raise the table and reposition the patient in the supine position. Contact the proximal end of the clavicle. The LOD is inferior and slightly lateral through the plane line of the SC joint (Figure 16-17).

When shoulder motion is severely restricted by pain or degenerative changes, it may be too difficult for the patient to perform the Isolation Test for the superior proximal clavicle with active range of motion. It may be advisable therefore to perform a Stress Test manually. Slide the index and middle fingers between the patient's shoulder and the table, and palpate for the shaft of the clavicle. Slide the fingers medially to a point as close to the sternum as possible. The fingers used to palpate are likely to encounter the bulge of the first rib before they get to the sternum. Hook the fingers on

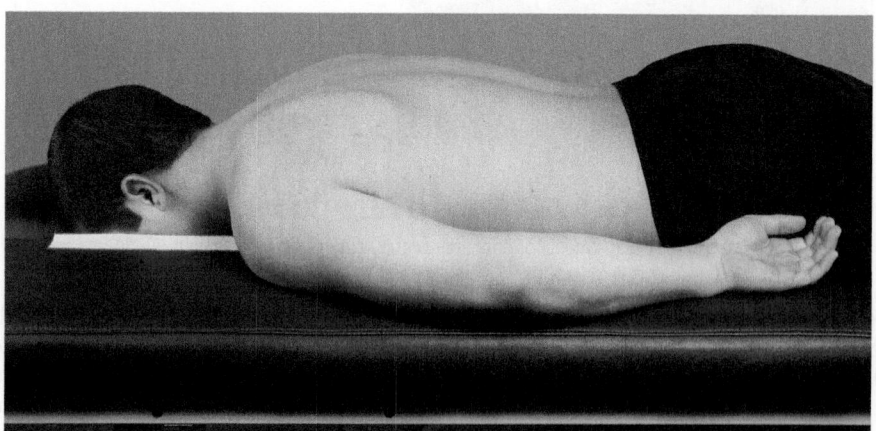

Figure 16-14   Isolation Test for inferior scapula; return arm to side after testing for superior scapula.

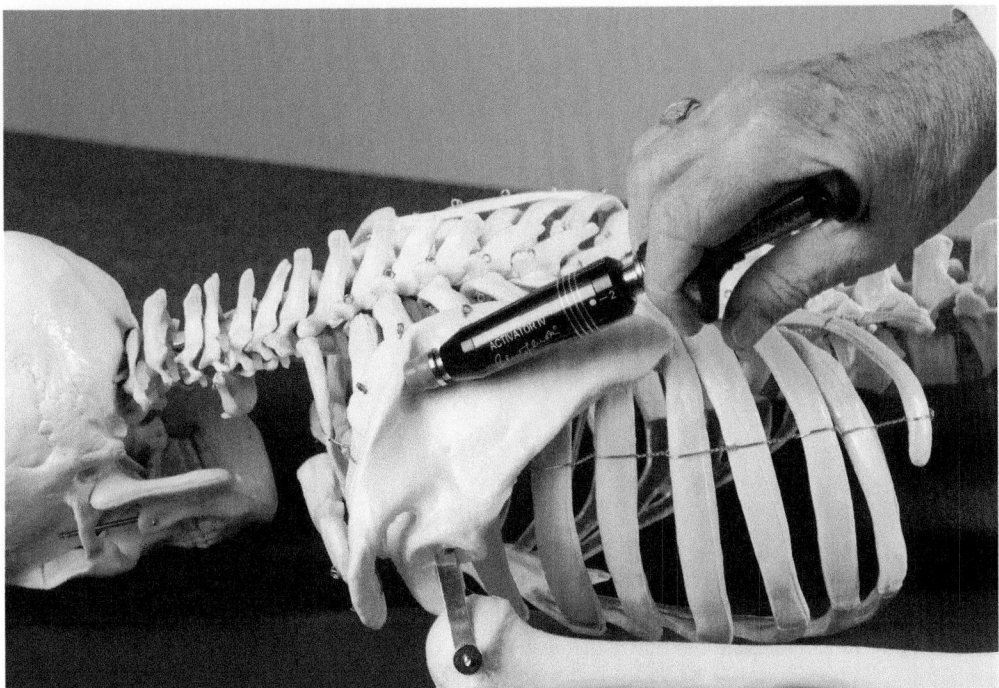

Figure 16-15   Adjustment for inferior scapula. Line of Drive is superior.

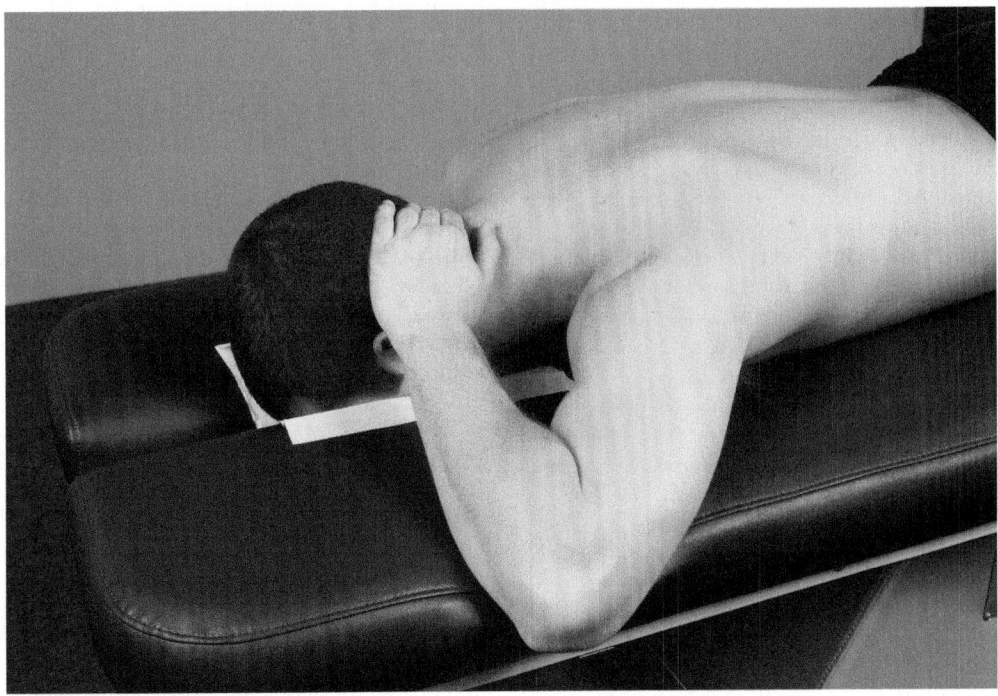

Figure 16-16   Isolation Test for superior proximal clavicle; with palm of the hand over the lower neck, push the elbow of the abducted arm into the table.

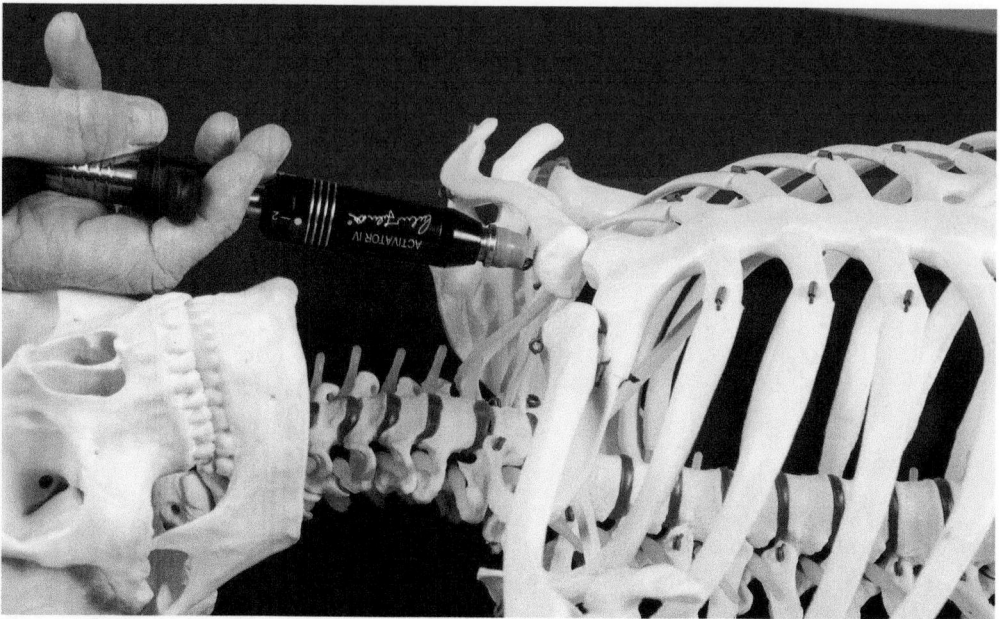

Figure 16-17 Adjustment for superior proximal clavicle. Line of Drive is inferior and slightly lateral.

the inferior border of the clavicle, and pull it gently but firmly in a superior and slightly medial direction. Look for reactivity of the PD leg in Position #1 for involvement.

To ensure optimal contact during adjustment, locate the SC joint by palpating just lateral to the episternal notch. To avoid discomfort to the patient, take a gentle tissue pull by drawing the thumb inferiorly over the proximal clavicle. Use the thumb to stabilize the tip of the instrument during the adjustment.

Before proceeding with additional Isolation and Stress Tests, raise the table and reposition the patient in the prone position.

Clinical Observations

The clavicle stabilizes the scapula anteriorly during most normal ranges of motion of the shoulder. Furthermore, the sternoclavicular (SC) joint is the only osseous articulation between the shoulder assembly and the axial skeleton. Consequently, aberrant motion, hypertonicity of soft tissues, and direct trauma to the shoulder can displace the proximal head of the clavicle.

A subluxated SC joint may be painful during hyperabduction of the shoulder, as when a patient works with the arms over the head or reaches for

Continued

---

an object on a high shelf. The joint may also show crepitus during external and internal rotation as well as during resisted horizontal abduction and adduction.

Inferior Medial Coracoid

When a patient is unable to abduct the arm above shoulder height (90 degrees of abduction) without biomechanical compensation, consider scapular involvement along with an inferior medial coracoid.

Stress Test.   To test an inferior medial coracoid, stroke the soft tissue over the coracoid process inferiorly and medially in the direction of the fibers of the pectoralis minor muscle (Figure 16-18). Look for reactivity of the PD leg in Position #1 for involvement.

Adjustment.   To adjust for an inferior medial coracoid, raise the table and place the patient in the supine position. Contact the inferior and medial aspect of the coracoid process. The LOD is superior and lateral at a 45-degree angle (Figure 16-19).

Locate the coracoid process by palpating the shaft of the clavicle about 2 inches medial to the AC joint. Slide the fingers inferiorly

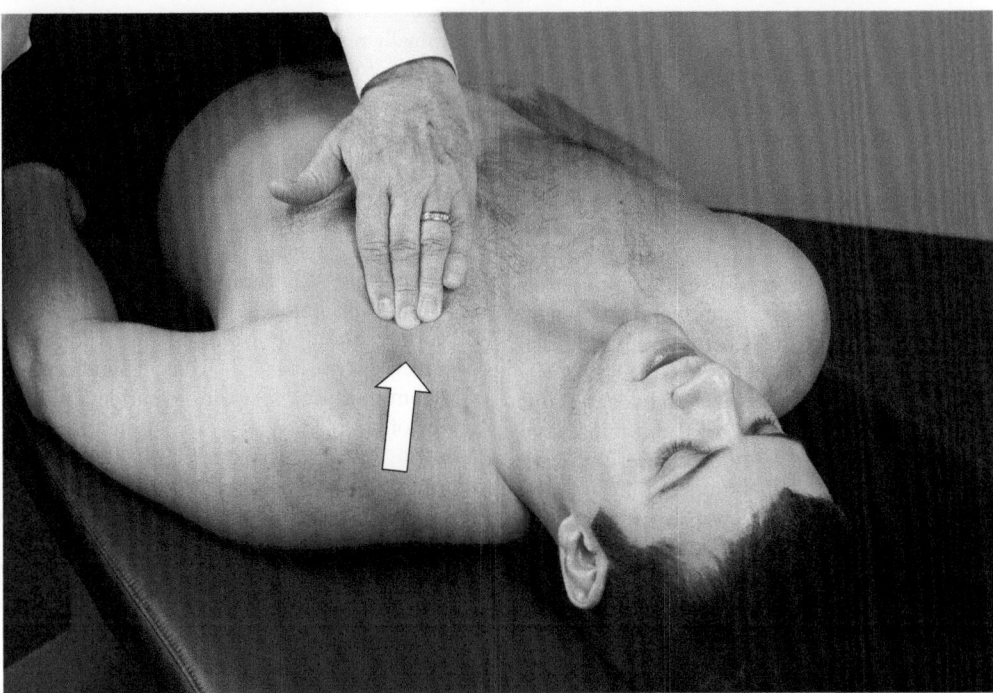

Figure 16-18 Stress Test for inferior medial coracoid; stroke the soft tissue over the coracoid process inferiorly and medially in the direction of the fibers of the pectoralis minor muscle.

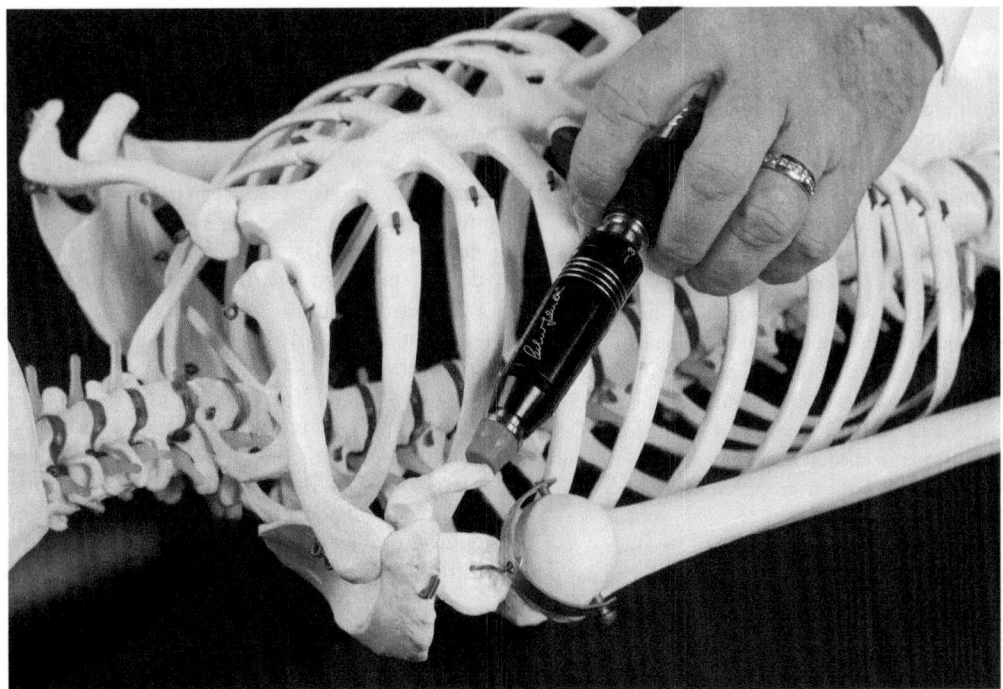

Figure 16-19 Adjustment for inferior medial coracoid. Line of Drive is superior and lateral at a 45-degree angle.

into the infraclavicular fossa, and locate the bony prominence of the coracoid process. An alternative method of identifying the bony prominence of the coracoid process is by placing the palm of one hand just medial to the anterior aspect of the AC joint, and the second hand on the posterior aspect of the acromion. When pressure is applied from a posterior-to-anterior medial direction, the coracoid process will be felt. Soft tissue over the coracoid is usually tender to deep palpation and is exquisitely tender when the patient also has subacromial bursitis. To ensure an effective contact and correct LOD, take a superior and lateral tissue pull over the coracoid process with the thumb of the stabilization hand. Use the thumb to stabilize the tip of the instrument during the adjustment.

For the patient with an acute shoulder injury, degenerative changes to the shoulder, or impingement syndrome, abduction, and external rotation, will be pain limited, and attempts to get the arm into position may be counterproductive. In such a case, have the patient move the shoulder into abduction to the point of tolerance, flex the elbow to 90 degrees, and rotate the forearm laterally to gain as much external rotation as possible.

Clinical Observations

Onset of scapular subluxation with inferior-medial malposition of the coracoid process may be acute or insidious. A fall on the back of the shoulder during a football game or wrestling match, for example, can force the scapula superiorly and traumatize the soft tissue of the scapulothoracic articulation. When a patient presents with restricted shoulder motion related to a fall, rule out fracture of the scapula with a radiographic examination.

Gradual onset of scapular malposition with a frozen shoulder or chronic inflammation of the scapulothoracic soft tissues can also present as an inferior-medial coracoid. Patients with the mixed clinical picture of fibromyalgia may demonstrate hypertonicity of shoulder and cervical musculature and trigger points in the region of the trapezius, levator scapulae, and rhomboid muscles. For such a patient, performance of the Stress Test for the inferior-medial coracoid may be uncomfortable when palpation pressure is applied to the coracoid process.

The long head of the biceps brachii passes through the intertubercular groove of the humerus and provides part of the soft tissue network that stabilizes the glenohumeral joint. If the tendon is stretched or if there is laxity in the fibers that

Continued

---

normally retain the tendon in the intertubercular groove of the humerus, the coracoid process may more easily subluxate inferiorly and medially. Evaluate the tendon of the long head of the biceps brachii by performing Yergason's test.

T2-T3 Facet Syndrome

If the patient still complains of pain in the T2-T3 area that radiates into the shoulder, after all upper thoracic Isolation Tests have been completed, consider T2-T3 facet syndrome. This is a common area for pain in patients with high levels of stress.

Isolation Test.   To test for T2-T3 facet syndrome, instruct the patient to anteriorly flex the arm off the table and rotate it 360 degrees in a freestyle swimming stroke, and place it back on the table alongside of the body (Figure 16-20). Look for reactivity of the PD leg in Position #1 for involvement.

Adjustment.   Adjustment for T2-T3 facet syndrome is made with two contacts and thrusts. First, contact the transverse process of T2 on the affected facet side. The LOD is superior and anterior (Figure 16-21). Next, contact the transverse process of T3. The LOD is inferior and anterior (Figure 16-22).

T3-T4 Facet Syndrome

If a patient continues to have pain from the upper thoracic region that radiates out into the shoulder, consider testing for T3-T4 facet syndrome.

Isolation Test.   To isolate the T3-T4 facets, instruct the patient to place the hand on the involved side on the back of the neck and raise the elbow off the table (Figure 16-23). Look for reactivity of the PD leg in Position #1 for involvement.

Adjustment.   To adjust for a T3-T4 facet syndrome, make two thrusts. First, contact the T3 transverse process. The LOD is anterior and superior (Figure 16-24). Next, contact the T4 transverse process. The LOD is anterior and inferior (Figure 16-25).

After adjustments have been made for the patient through a series of treatments for neuroarticular dysfunctions, and the patient has reached a subacute stage, consider the following neuromuscular involvements: supraspinatus, infraspinatus, subscapularis, and medial scapula.

Supraspinatus

For patients who exhibit difficulty when abducting the arm (especially during early range of abduction before the middle deltoid takes over

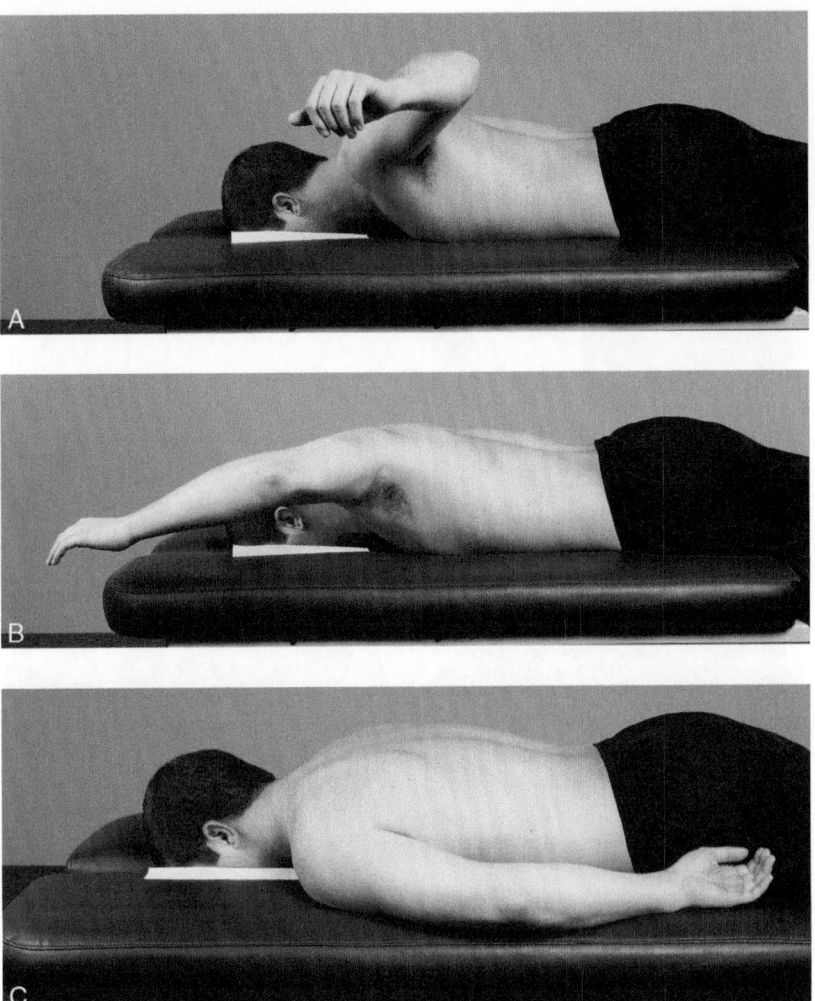

Figure 16-20 **A** through **C,** Isolation Test for T2-T3 facet syndrome; arm off the table, and rotate it 360 degrees in a freestyle swimming stroke.

the main component of abduction), and for those with pain due to tendonitis, signs of rotator cuff impingement, subacromial bursitis, shoulder instability, and trigger point pain referral into the mid-deltoid region and the lateral epicondyle of the humerus, consider testing for dysfunction of the supraspinatus muscle. Popping and clicking also may be palpated during glenohumeral range of motion when degeneration of the supraspinatus tendon occurs.

Isolation Test. The AM Isolation Test can be performed, after the patient has been cleared for any scapular patterns and all related shoulder biomechanical dysfunctions, by instructing the patient to reach behind the back in an attempt to touch the opposite scapula. Reactivity of the PD leg in Position #1 indicates involvement of

the supraspinatus tendon as it is stretched. The procedure of reaching behind the back toward the opposite scapula is part of Apley's scratch test and involves the motion that places the greatest stress on the supraspinatus tendon (Figure 16-26).

Adjustment. The adjustment involves three contact points and adjustments. First contact is the medial aspect of the supraspinatus muscle belly, and the LOD is inferior (Figure 16-27). The second contact is the lateral aspect of the supraspinatus muscle belly, and the LOD is inferior (Figure 16-28). The third contact is the musculotendinous junction of the supraspinatus on the proximal, lateral aspect of the humerus. The LOD is inferior and slightly medial (Figure 16-29).

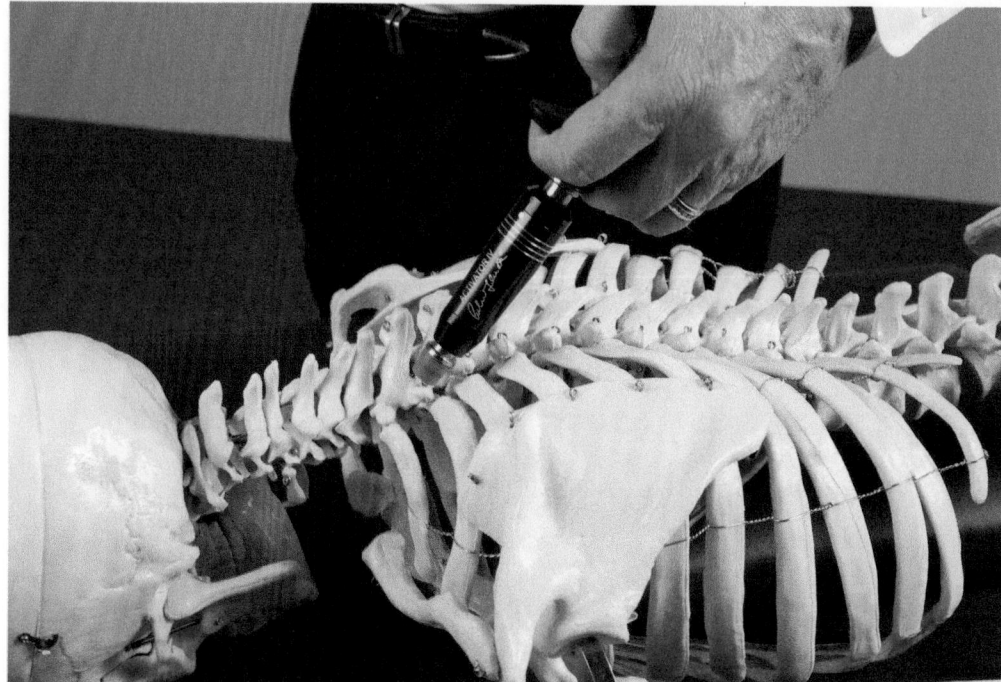

Figure 16-21   Adjustment for T2 facet. Contact the transverse process of T2. Line of Drive is superior and anterior.

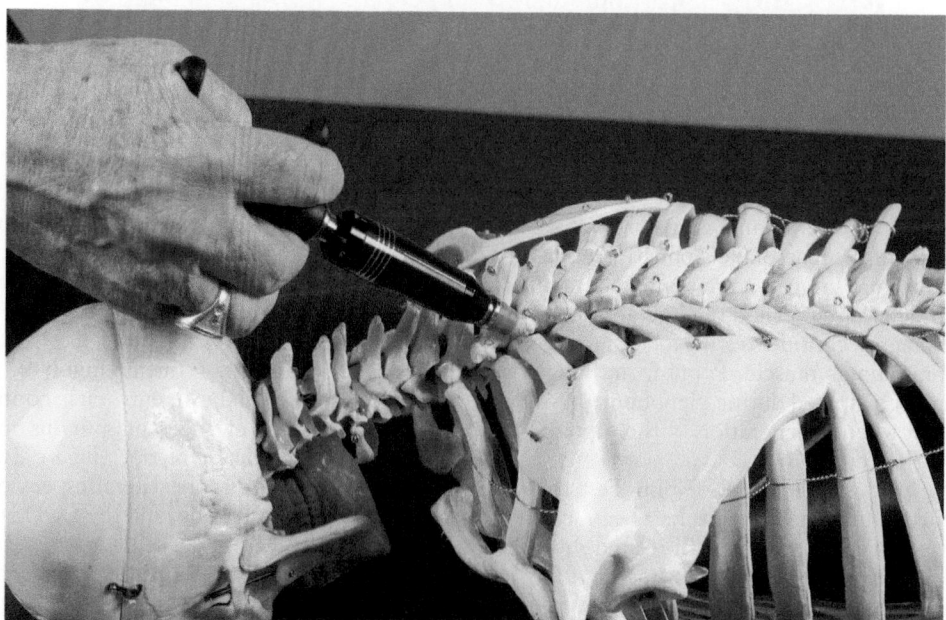

Figure 16-22   Adjustment for T3 facet. Contact the transverse process of T3. Line of Drive is inferior and anterior.

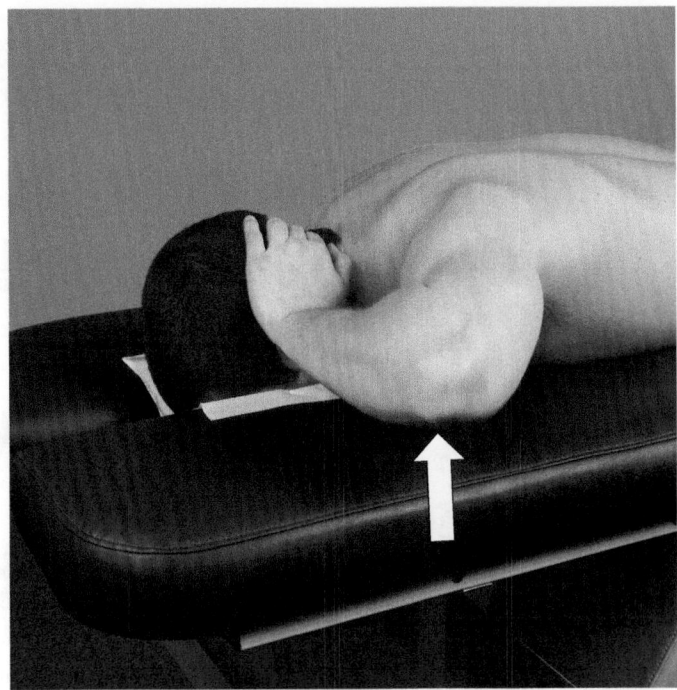

Figure 16-23 Isolation Test for T3-T4 facet syndrome; hand on the back of the neck and raise the elbow off the table.

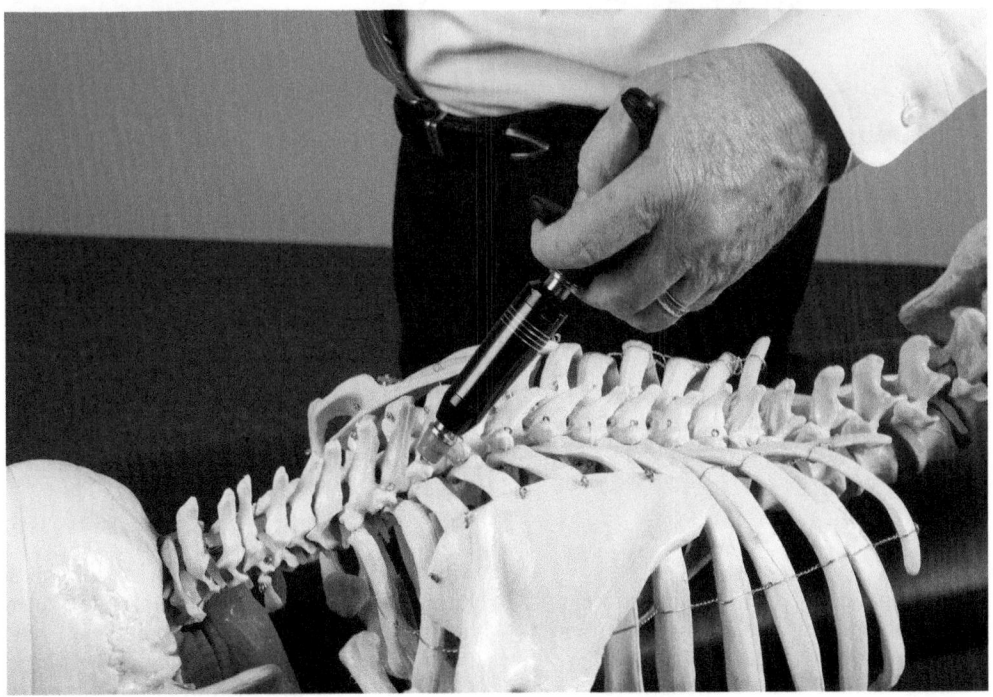

Figure 16-24 Adjustment for T3 facet. Contact the transverse process of T3. Line of Drive is superior and anterior.

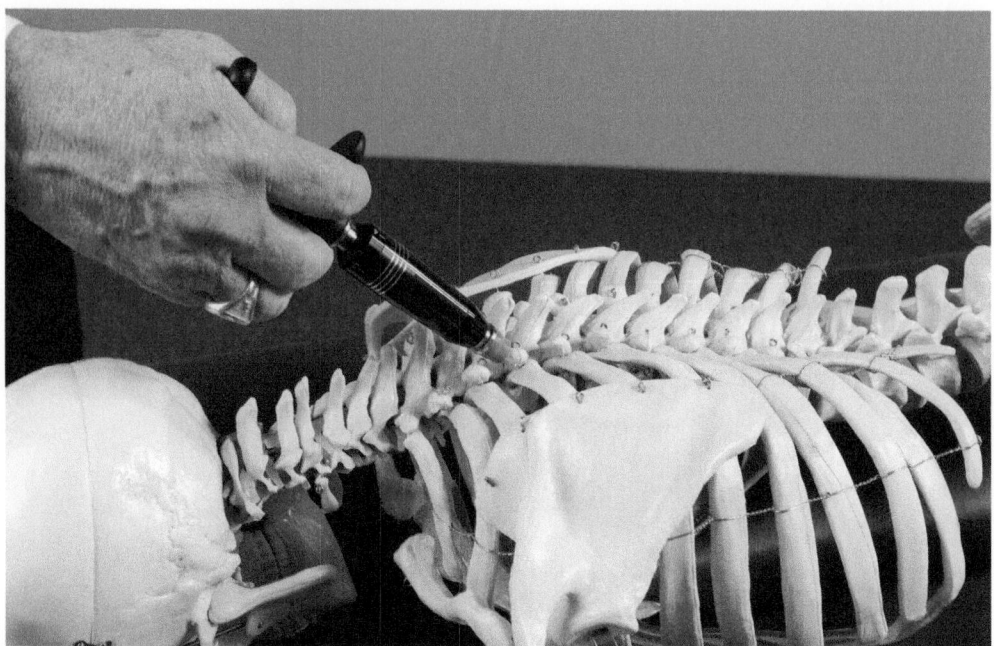

Figure 16-25 Adjustment for T4 facet. Contact the transverse process of T4. Line of Drive is inferior and anterior.

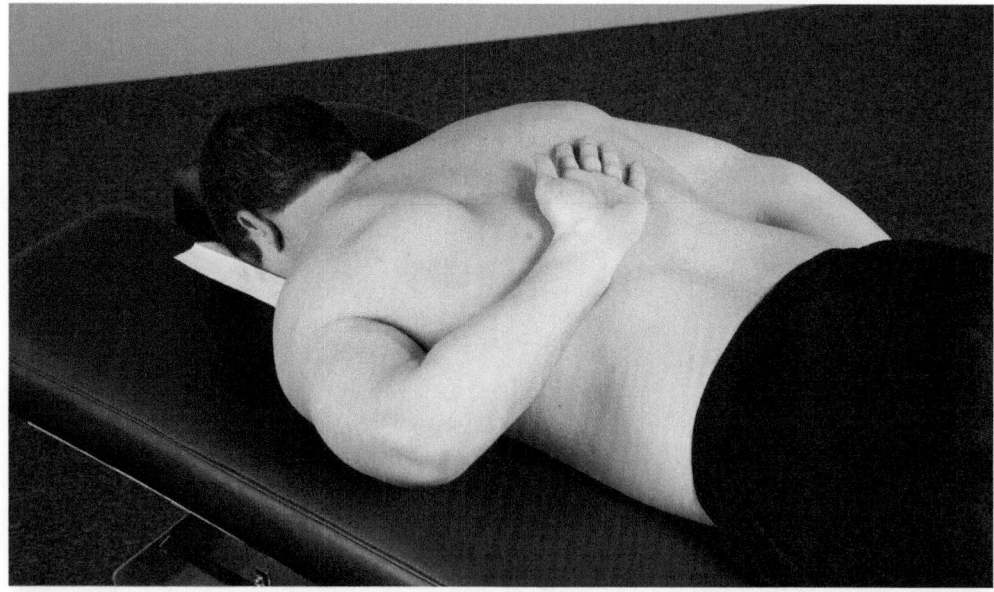

Figure 16-26 Isolation Test for supraspinatus; reach behind the back in an attempt to touch the opposite scapula.

Infraspinatus

In those patients who demonstrate (1) decreased range of motion in internal rotation of the humerus upon Apley's testing, (2) weakness during manual muscle strength testing of the external rotators of the humerus with or without pain at the insertion of infraspinatus into the middle facet of the greater tubercle upon testing, or (3) trigger point pain referral to the anterior deltoid and down the arm, consider testing for dysfunction of the infraspinatus muscle.

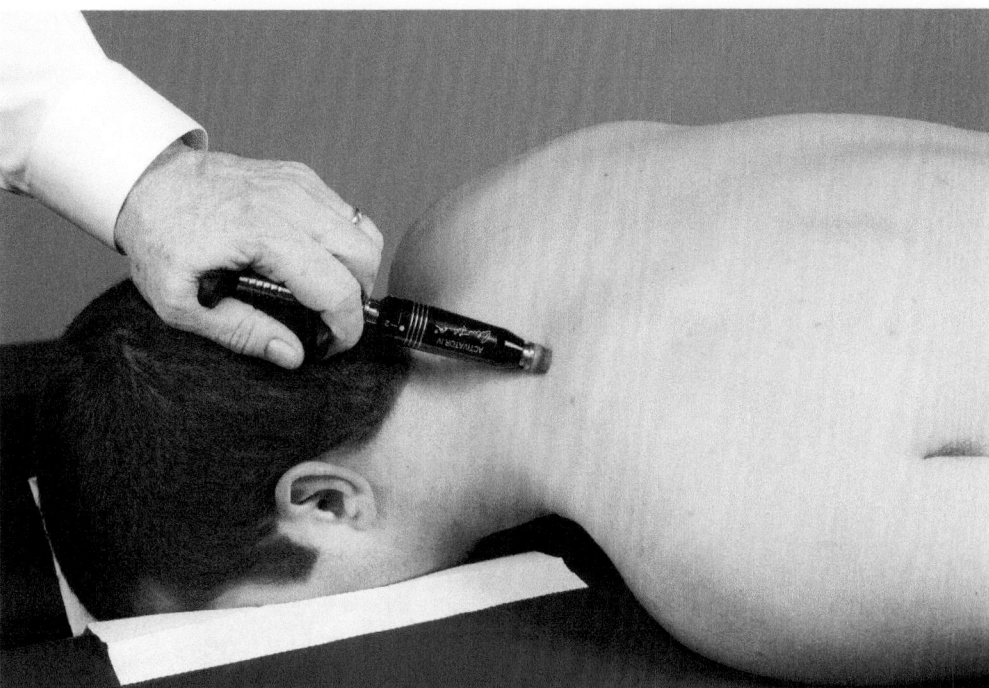

Figure 16-27 Adjustment for supraspinatus. First contact is the medial aspect of the supraspinatus muscle belly. Line of Drive is inferior.

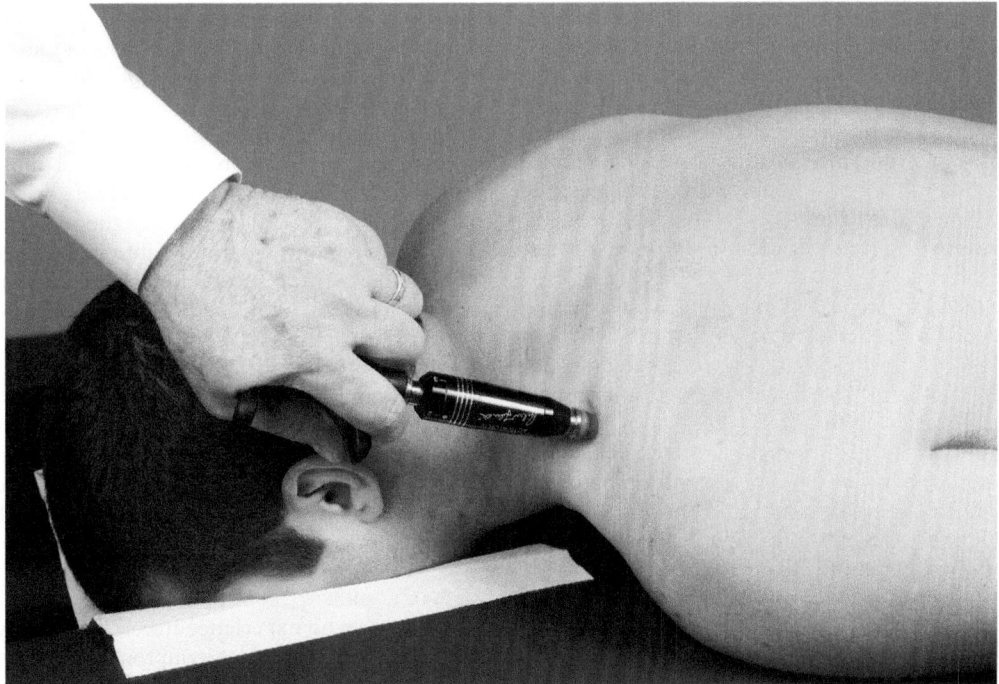

Figure 16-28 Adjustment for supraspinatus. Second contact is the lateral aspect of the supraspinatus muscle belly. Line of Drive is inferior.

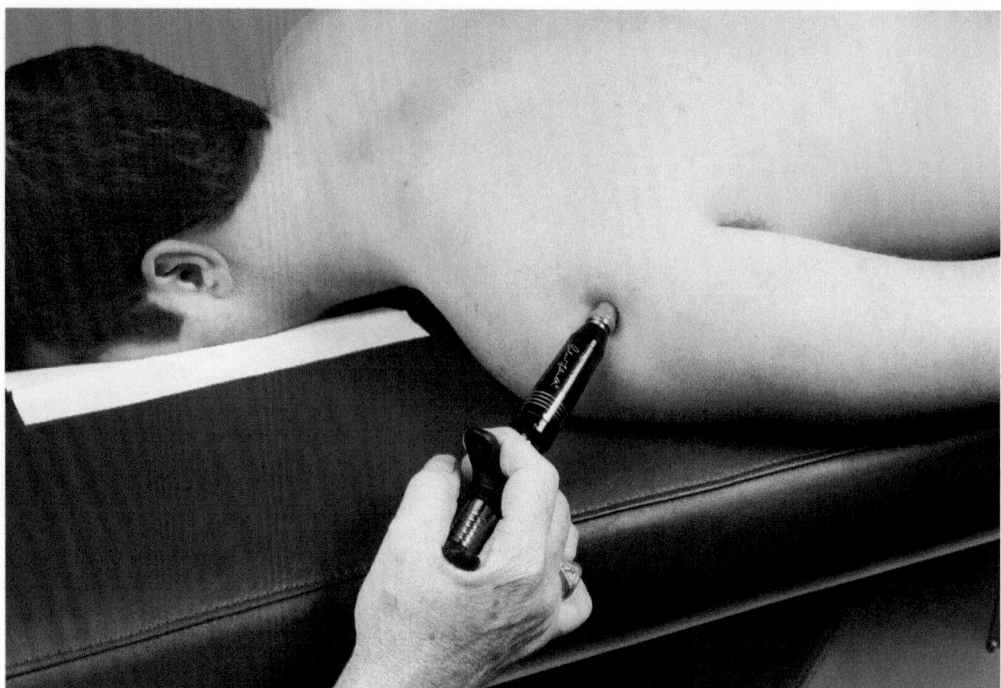

Figure 16-29   Adjustment for supraspinatus. Third contact is the musculotendinous junction of the supraspinatus on the proximal, lateral aspect of the humerus. Line of Drive is inferior and medial.

Isolation Test.   To isolate the infraspinatus muscle, use an active resistive manual muscle test. With the arm on the involved side dropped off the side of the table, instruct the patient to push the forearm headward (superior), against the doctor's resistance on the posterior forearm. The patient's elbow should exhibit 90 degrees of flexion during the test (Figure 16-30). Look for reactivity of the PD leg in Position #1 for involvement.

Adjustment.   To adjust the infraspinatus muscle, one thrust is required on each of the two contact points. The first contact occurs at the medial aspect of the muscle belly in the infraspinous fossa. The LOD is anterior, medial, and superior (Figure 16-31). The second contact occurs at the myotendon junction of the infraspinatus at the lateral aspect of the scapula and just inferior to the spine of the scapula. The LOD is anterior, medial, and superior (Figure 16-32).

Subscapularis

For those patients who present with restricted motion in external rotation, weakness or pain upon manual muscle strength testing of the internal rotators of the humerus, bursitis, shoulder instability or trigger point referred pain down the posterior aspect of the humerus and around the elbow, consider testing for dysfunction of the subscapularis muscle.

Isolation Test.   To isolate the subscapularis muscle, use an active resistive manual muscle test. With the arm on the involved side dropped off the side of the table, instruct the patient to push the forearm footward (inferior), against the doctor's resistance on the anterior forearm. The patient's elbow should be at 90 degrees of flexion during the test (Figure 16-33). Look for reactivity of the PD leg in Position #1 for involvement.

Adjustment.   To adjust the subscapularis muscle, drop the arm on the involved side off the table. Contact the subscapularis muscle under the lateral border of the scapula. The LOD is medial and superior (Figure 16-34).

Medial Scapula

For patients who experience frozen shoulder syndrome, chronic shoulder symptoms, and persistent pain along the medial border of the scapula, consider testing for medial scapular involvement. This is different from medial

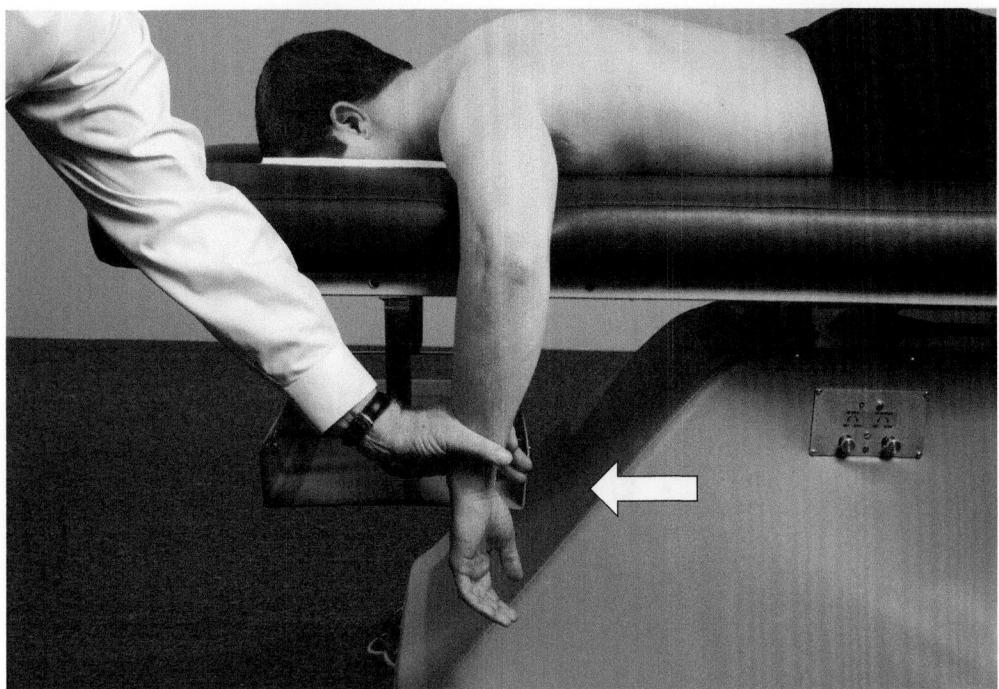

Figure 16-30 Isolation Test for infraspinatus. Push the forearm headward (superior) against the doctor's resistance on the posterior forearm; resist headward pressure.

scapular involvement as described in the AM Basic Scan Protocol; consider this a "global" medial scapula.

Instruct the patient to place the arm of the involved shoulder over the lumbars on the side of pain.

The doctor places the hand against the lateral aspect of the distal humerus (outside area) to provide resistance.

The patient then is instructed to push out against the resistance of the doctor's hand, constituting isometric shoulder abduction (Figure 16-35).

Look for reactivity of the PD leg in Position #1 for involvement.

Adjustment. The adjustment consists of a thrust on each of the three contact points:
- Superior aspect of the medial border of the scapula (Figure 16-36)
- Midpoint of the medial border of the scapula (Figure 16-37)
- Inferior aspect of the medial border of the scapula (Figure 16-38)

All LODs are lateral.

Mechanical force, manually assisted chiropractic adjusting (AM) of the shoulder is summarized in Table 16-1. Sequential testing for shoulder cases is summarized in Box 16-2.

ADDITIONAL TESTS AND ADJUSTMENTS FOR THE CLAVICLE

Evaluation of the clavicle is indicated when a patient presents with any of the following:
- Restricted or altered range of motion of the clavicle
- Pain at the AC joint
- Pain at the SC joint
- Persistent shoulder complaints
- Torticollis or wry neck
- History of trauma to the clavicle

The clavicle is an important structure in relation to the upper extremity; it provides the bony framework for the AC and SC joints. Because of its anatomical makeup, the shoulder greatly depends on its supporting soft tissues for stability and support.[15] Pain that arises from the clavicle or its associated soft tissues and articulations must be distinguished from referred pain syndromes. Clavicular symptoms may be related to cervical spine disorders due to referred pain syndromes or radiculopathies.[4,15] Overuse injuries, postural faults, and frank trauma all are involved in clavicular dysfunction and symptom-related causes. Careful history and examination will help to differentiate cervical spine involvement from clavicular problems.

Text continued on p. 456

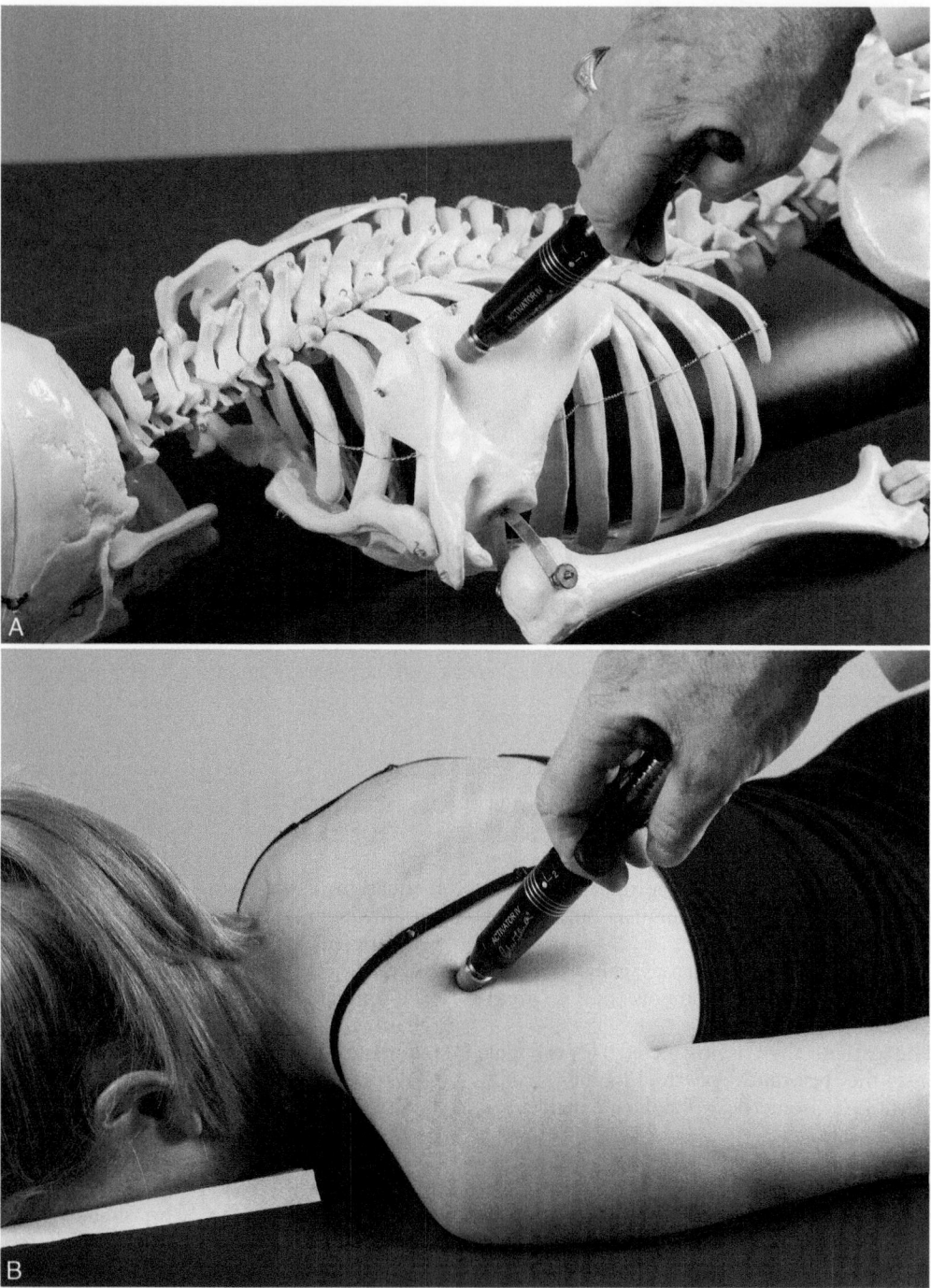

Figure 16-31 **A** and **B,** Adjustment for infraspinatus. First contact is at the medial aspect of the muscle belly in the infraspinous fossa. Line of Drive is anterior, medial, and superior.

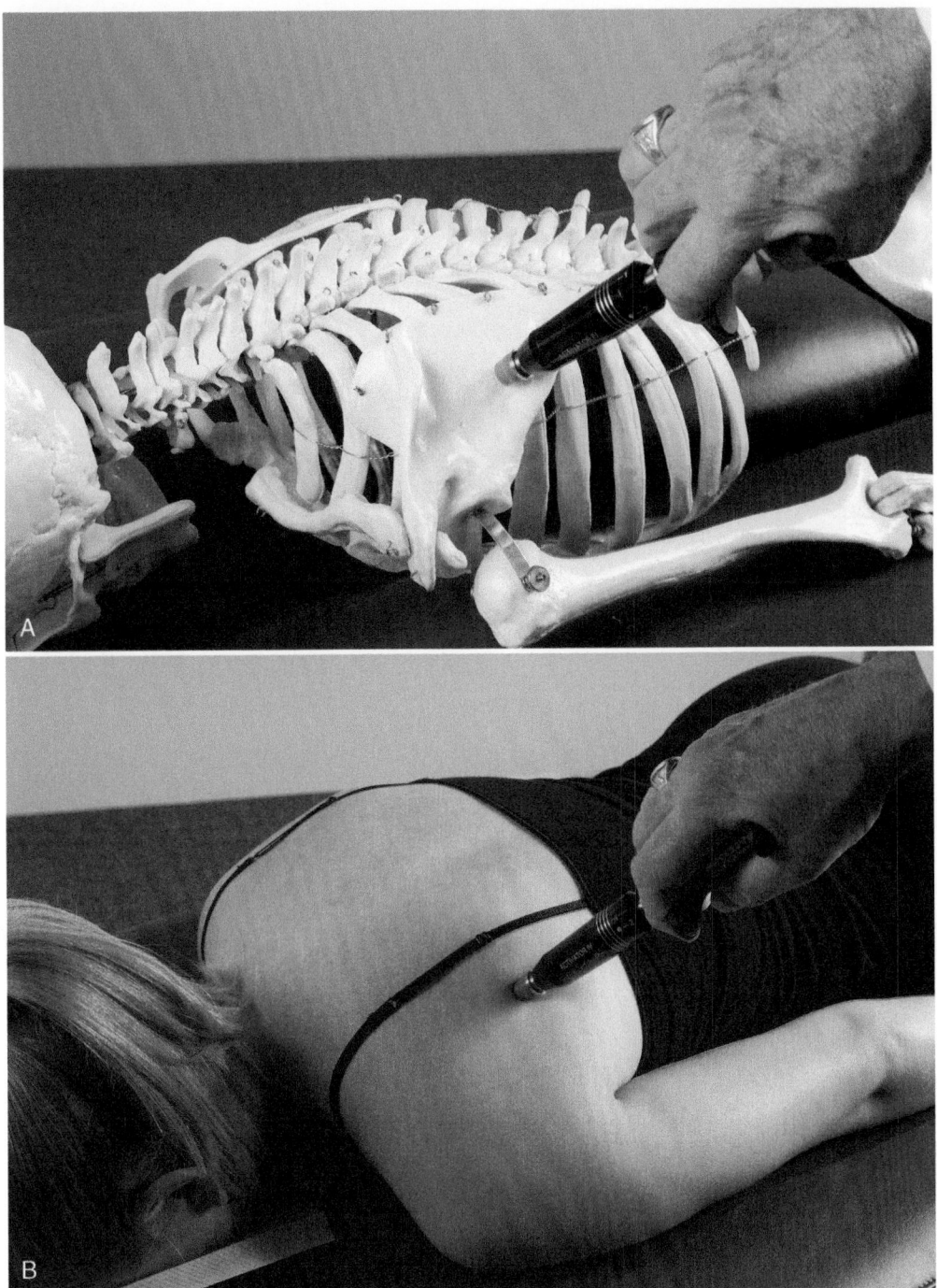

Figure 16-32 **A** and **B,** Adjustment for infraspinatus. Second contact is at the myotendon junction of the infraspinatus at the lateral aspect of the scapula and just inferior to the spine of the scapula. Line of Drive is anterior, medial, and superior.

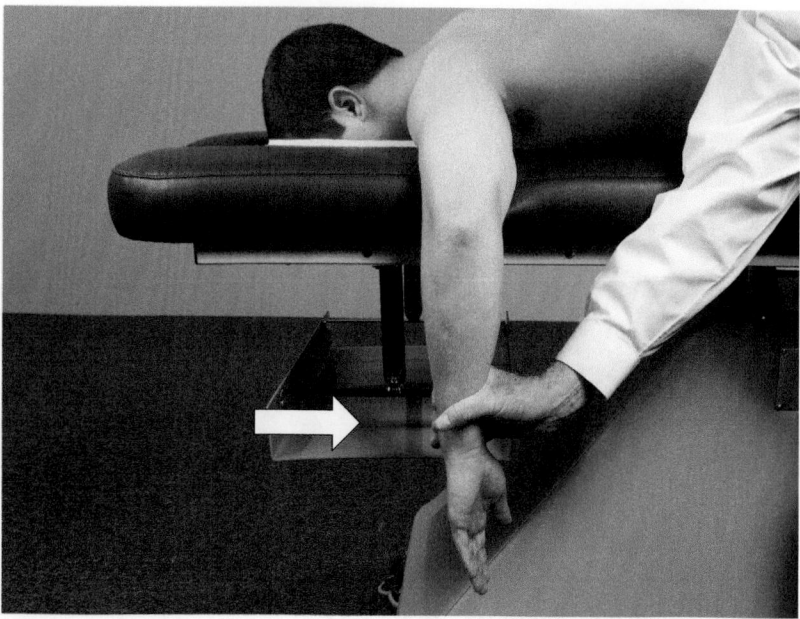

Figure 16-33   Isolation Test for subscapularis. Push the forearm footward (inferior) against the doctor's resistance on the anterior forearm.

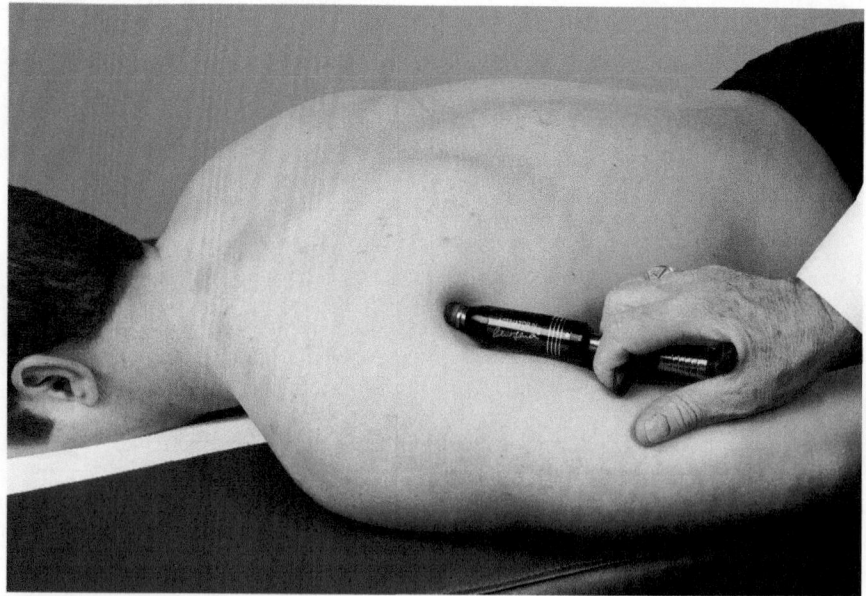

Figure 16-34   Adjustment for subscapularis. Contact the subscapularis muscle under the lateral border of the scapula. Line of Drive is medial and superior.

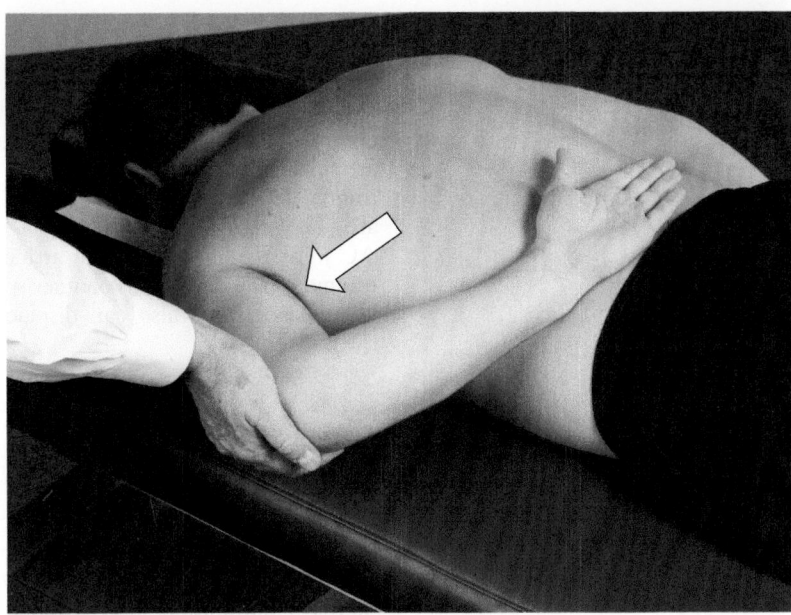

Figure 16-35 Isolation Test for medial scapula. Place arm over the lumbars; doctor places hand against the lateral aspect of the distal humerus, providing resistance for isometric shoulder abduction.

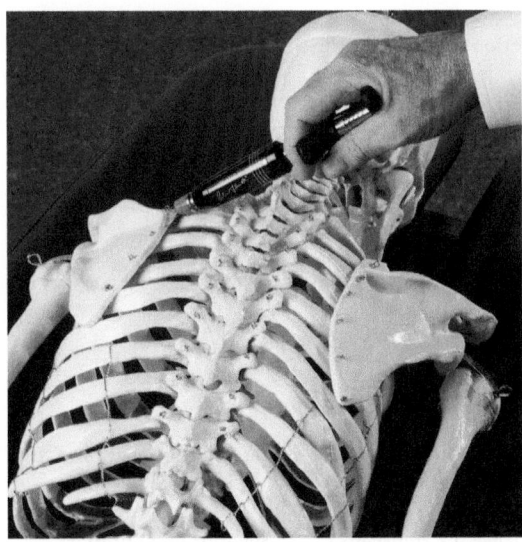

Figure 16-36 Adjustment for medial scapula. First contact is the superior aspect of the medial border of the scapula. Line of Drive is lateral.

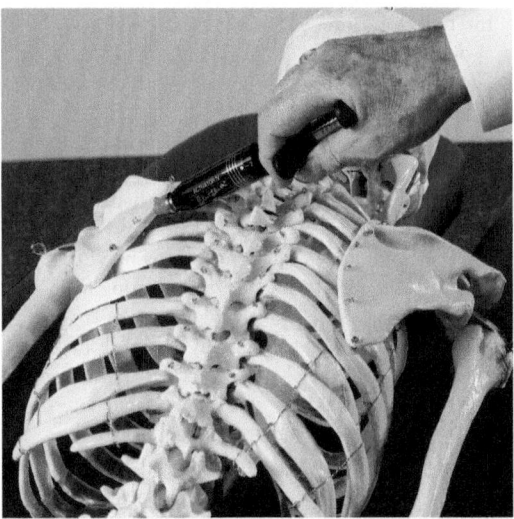

Figure 16-37 Adjustment for medial scapula. Second contact is the midpoint of the medial border of the scapula. Line of Drive is lateral.

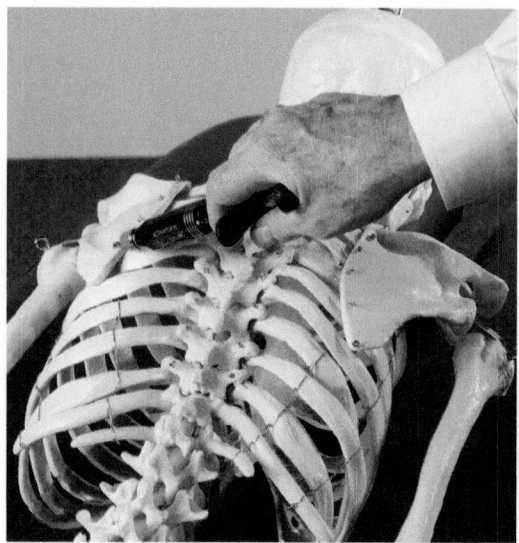

Figure 16-38 Adjustment for medial scapula. Third contact is the inferior aspect of the medial border of the scapula. Line of Drive is lateral.

COMMON PROBLEMS

Because of its anatomical makeup, the clavicle and associated articulations are commonly susceptible to injury.[9] Injury to the clavicle and its articulations may result from acute or repetitive trauma to the shoulder. A fall on an abducted arm may result in a sprain or a dysfunctional AC joint or coracoclavicular articulation. Blunt trauma to the clavicle in contact sports or motor vehicle accidents also can displace or fracture the clavicle.[17]

Restricted or Altered Range of Motion of the Clavicle

The shoulder girdle is a term that refers to the means by which the upper limb is appended to the trunk; it consists of the clavicles and scapulae.[5] For the shoulder to function with optimal proficiency in daily activities and in sports, a harmonious and synchronous balance must be achieved between muscular action and

Table 16-1   Summary Table for Tests and Adjustments of the Shoulder

Articular Dysfunction	Test	Adjustment	
		Segmental Contact Point	Line of Drive
Anterior-Inferior Humerus	Patient extends arm, palm up	Intertubercular groove	Superior and posterior
External Rotation of the Humerus	Patient turns palm down onto table	Lateral greater tubercle	Medial and slightly anterior
Internal Rotation of the Humerus	Patient turns palm away from midline	Posterior greater tubercle	Medial
Posterior Humeral Head	Patient drops arm off side of table	Posterior greater tubercle	Anterior
Second Rib Involvement	Patient abducts arm to 90 degrees, palm up	Lateral to costotransverse joint	Lateral and slightly inferior
Superior Scapula	Patient places hand on back of neck	Superior angle of scapula	Inferior
Inferior Scapula	Patient returns hand to side, after testing for a superior scapula	Inferior aspect, midpoint of spine of the scapula	Superior
Superior Proximal Clavicle	With hand on back of neck, patient pushes elbow into table	Patient supine. Superior proximal clavicle	Inferior and slightly lateral
Inferior Medial Coracoid	Soft tissue pull over the coracoid process inferiorly and medially	Inferior and medial aspect of coracoid process	Lateral and superior at 45 degrees
T2-T3 Facet Syndrome	Patient performs freestyle swimming stroke	*Step One*: T2 transverse process	Superior and anterior
		Step Two: T3 transverse process	Inferior and anterior

Table 16-1	**Summary Table for Tests and Adjustments of the Shoulder—cont'd**		
Articular Dysfunction	**Test**	**ADJUSTMENT**	
		Segmental Contact Point	**Line of Drive**
T3-T4 Facet Syndrome	Patient places hand on back of neck and lifts elbow off table	*Step One*: T3 transverse process	Superior and anterior
		Step Two: T4 transverse process	Inferior and anterior
Supraspinatus	Patient reaches behind the back toward the opposite scapula	*Step One*: Medial aspect of supraspinatus muscle belly	Inferior
		Step Two: Lateral aspect of the supraspinatus muscle belly	Inferior
		Step Three: Proximal lateral humerus on musculotendon junction of supraspinatus	Inferior, and slightly medial
Infraspinatus	Patient places arm over the edge of the table and pushes the hand and forearm headward against resistance of the doctor	*Step One*: Medial aspect of the infraspinatus fossa of the scapula	Medial and superior
		Step Two: Lateral aspect of the infraspinatus fossa of the scapula	Medial and superior
Subscapularis	Patient places arm over the edge of the table and pushes the hand and forearm footward against resistance of the doctor	Lateral aspect of the subscapularis under the scapula	Medial and slightly superior
Medial (Global) Scapula	Patient places arm over low back. Doctor places hand against the lateral distal humerus, and patient pushes out against resistance (isometric shoulder abduction).	*Step One*: Superior aspect of medial border of scapula	Lateral
		Step Two: Mid-aspect of medial border of scapula	Lateral
		Step Three: Inferior aspect of medial border of scapula	Lateral

coordinated joint movements.[13] The clavicle plays an important role in the intricate shoulder joint. The clavicle acts as a strut and moves in complex unison with the scapula, providing stability in the scapulothoracic component of shoulder movement.[15]

At its distal end, the clavicle participates in the AC joint and is palpable as the most lateral and superior bony prominence of the shoulder. At its proximal end, the clavicle articulates with the manubrium of the sternum, forming the SC joint. The proximal clavicle is palpable immediately lateral to the episternal notch. The AC and SC joints are freely movable saddle joints or *sellar diarthroses*. Strong fibrous ligaments reinforce these joints; each contains a fibrous meniscus.[5] The clavicle also has ligamentous attachments to the coracoid process of the scapula. The two-part coracoclavicular ligament is made up of coracoid and trapezoid portions. During elevation, depression, and longitudinal rotation of the clavicle, the coracoid functions as a stabilizing fulcrum to clavicular motion.

The fibrous nature of the proximal and distal clavicular joints, as well as their saddle shape, gives them multiaxial movement capability. Values for clavicular ranges of motion are not typically measured as part of the examination, but

---

Box 16-2   Sequential Testing Procedure of the Shoulder

1. External Rotation of the Humerus
2. Internal Rotation of the Humerus
3. Second Rib Involvement
4. Posterior Humeral Head
5. T2-T3 Facets
6. Superior Scapula
7. Superior Proximal Clavicle
8. T3-T4 Facets
9. Inferior Scapula
10. Acromioclavicular Joint Separation
11. Anterior-Inferior Humerus
12. Superior Distal Clavicle

13. Inferior Medial Corocoid
14. Anterior First Rib
15. Lateral Distal Humerus
   After stabilizing the above listed neurobiomechanical dysfunctions through a series of treatments, and after the patient's condition is subacute, add the following:
16. Supraspinatus
17. Medial (Global) Scapula
18. Subscapularis
19. Infraspinatus

---

when a patient describes a shoulder complaint, the clavicles and the clavicular joints should be evaluated. Inspect the clavicles for bilateral symmetry. Palpate for elevation of the distal clavicle when the patient shrugs the shoulders or abducts the arms past shoulder height. Note the depression of the distal clavicles when the patient adducts the arms.

During horizontal adduction and protraction of the shoulder, the clavicle should swing forward, pivoting at the SC joint. During horizontal abduction, the distal clavicle should swing back. If the clavicle is moving freely, shoulder flexion, extension, internal rotation, and external rotation should be accompanied by slight rotation of the clavicle along its longitudinal axis.[12] Be alert to any audible or palpable crepitus in the SC and AC joints during shoulder motion.

Pain at the Acromioclavicular Joint

A fall on the shoulder, blunt trauma to the acromion process, and carrying of heavy weights supported by the shoulder can cause varying degrees of separation of the AC joint. A grade I sprain injury produces some tearing of the AC ligaments. A grade II injury also produces tearing of the coracoclavicular ligaments.[15,17] Grade I and II injuries are amenable to conservative care.[15] AC separation is suggested by a "step-off" visual and palpatory finding at the AC joint. Normally, the distal clavicle rises slightly above the acromion at the joint. With separation of the joint, marked elevation of the distal clavicle occurs, as do point tenderness on palpation and passive motion of the joint.

Subacromial bursitis can cause point tenderness at the AC joint, especially during abduction and rotation of the glenohumeral joint.[15] To differentiate AC joint involvement from subacromial bursitis, perform the "coracoid push button" test. Apply digital pressure into the belly of the anterior portion of the deltoid, lateral to the coracoid process. Sharp pain on deep palpation suggests inflammation, with pain and swelling of the subacromial bursitis.

Degenerative changes of osteoarthritis may be a source of pain in the AC joint.[19] Osteophytes, as well as fibrotic and calcific changes to related soft tissues, can generate an impingement syndrome, as was noted previously.

Perform a thorough examination of the AC joints to compare palpatory findings and ranges of motion bilaterally. Radiographic examination with anterior-to-posterior views will help to rule out degenerative joint disease, fracture, and gross dislocation of the AC joint. More subtle separation injuries of the joint may be revealed by stress-weighted anteroposterior views, and the shoulders should be compared for bilateral asymmetry of the joints.

When a patient experiences AC joint pain, perform Isolation Tests, Stress Tests, and adjustments as necessary for the following clavicular misalignments and associated joint dysfunctions:
- Anterior distal clavicle
- Posterior distal clavicle
- Superior distal clavicle
- AC joint separation
- AC joint impingement

Pain at the Sternoclavicular Joint

Tractioning trauma, an anterior blow to the shoulder, or incorrect lifting of heavy objects may cause neuroarticular dysfunction and instability of the SC joint. Crepitus and pain in the joint on protraction and internal and external rotation of the shoulder suggest SC joint dysfunction.

In a traction injury to the shoulder, the clavicle may be pulled laterally. Direct trauma to the chest can displace it anteriorly or posteriorly at the SC joint. Anterior displacement is the most common direction of misalignment of the proximal clavicle.[17] Posterior malposition of the proximal clavicle can apply pressure to the trachea or neurovascular structures deep to the bone. The patient may describe a feeling of pressure in the throat with involvement of a proximal clavicle neuroarticular dysfunction.

Malposition of the proximal clavicle can produce palpable asymmetry of the SC joints and point tenderness on palpation and passive motion.

When a patient experiences SC joint involvement, perform Isolation Tests, Stress Tests, and adjustments as necessary for the following misalignments:
- Lateral clavicle
- Inferior proximal clavicle
- Superior proximal clavicle
- Anterior first rib
- Scalenus anticus

Persistent Shoulder Complaints

For the patient with persistent or recurrent shoulder complaints, or for shoulder misalignment that does not respond well to the adjustments described in the chapter on shoulder and related structures, consider clavicular instability at the AC and SC joints.[11] Because the clavicle provides stability for the scapula during shoulder ranges of motion, as well as during work against resistance, instability of the proximal or distal clavicular joint can affect the whole kinetic chain of the shoulder complex.

Persistent shoulder problems may result from unresolved acute injury to the shoulder complex. The severity of the initial injury and the extent to which articular and soft tissues are damaged will determine the rate of healing for an acute injury. Mild to moderate shoulder injury with neuroarticular dysfunction frequently resolves with conservative care. More severe injuries with tearing of soft tissue, especially of the poorly vascularized ligaments, require much more protracted healing and repair times, and during the healing period, the tissues are vulnerable to reinjury. Of course, factors such as general health, nutritional status, mobility, and age play significant roles in healing. Stability of the healing tissues is also a major factor. If the clavicle does not provide its normal stabilizing effect for the scapula and the rest of the shoulder assembly because of fixation or aberrant motion, the healing soft tissues will be subject to increased stresses that will delay healing or increase the risk of reinjury.

Persistent shoulder complaints may be an indication of overuse or repetitive motion injury to the shoulder with chronic dysfunction of the clavicular joints. Throwing sports, for example, can generate very high stresses in the rotator cuff and in the AC joint.[13] The cocking motion of an overhand throw takes the shoulder into extreme external rotation and abduction, approaching the limit of normal glenohumeral and AC joint ranges of motion. The effects of sudden loading and unloading of the AC ligaments are cumulative and can predispose the joint to instability, as many baseball pitchers can confirm.

Another form of repetitive injury to the clavicular joints occurs in weight lifters and body builders who perform presses, dips, and push-ups.[31] Instability of the AC joint can ultimately lead to calcific changes in the soft tissues, erosion of articular cartilage, and osteolytic changes in the clavicle and acromion.[19] These persistent injuries and changes are not unique to competitive weight lifters or body builders. Warehouse workers, truckers, auto body mechanics, and construction workers typically partake in frequent lifting as part of their jobs.[6] Moreover, the materials these workers lift are not well designed ergonomically, in contrast to weights found in a gymnasium or home workout equipment.

Yet another form of repetitive injury to the clavicular articulations is even subtler in its onset. Backpackers and students who carry heavy bookbags slung over the shoulder are at risk of developing clavicular malposition from constant pressure on the shoulder structures. Quality backpacks for hikers and climbers generally are well constructed, with padding and struts designed to distribute the weight evenly over the back and pelvis. However, overloading the pack or failing to distribute contents evenly can create load stresses on the shoulder and clavicle. The weight stress is compounded when the hiker walks over uneven ground, so that jostling of the pack constantly loads and unloads the clavicular joints. "Severe and prolonged disability" associated with back injury to the brachial plexus has been observed in major dysfunction of the radial and musculocutaneous nerves with occasional involvement of the median nerve.[32]

Most school backpacks have two straps and are meant to be worn over both shoulders. Some brands have wide, padded shoulder straps, which help to distribute the weight, but many lower priced packs have simple webbed straps with no padding. An informal survey of students shows that many adult students tend to carry bookbags slung over only one shoulder, which, of course, defeats any attempt by the manufacturer to achieve sound ergonomic design. A combination of carrying the bookbags the "cool way," over one shoulder, and overloading the bag with heavy textbooks, predisposes the student to shoulder problems of insidious onset.

When a patient suffers from recurrent or persistent shoulder misalignments, be sure to perform a full evaluation of clavicular motion and integrity of the clavicular joints. When onset of a shoulder complaint is sudden and is related to a specific event that causes injury, try to get as much specific information as possible about the injury. When onset is insidious, be sure to take a complete history, including not only the parameters of the shoulder complaint but also occupational and social histories. With the patient's help, analyze job and recreational pursuits for activities and specific movements that may cause or exacerbate the shoulder condition.

For the patient who suffers from persistent or recurrent shoulder complaints, or when the shoulder adjustments described in the previous section do not hold, perform Isolation Tests, Stress Tests, and adjustments as necessary for the following clavicular involvements:
- Anterior distal clavicle
- Posterior distal clavicle
- Lateral clavicle
- Superior clavicle
- AC joint separation
- AC joint impingement

Torticollis and Wry Neck
In its strictest sense, torticollis describes a lateral flexion deformity of the neck with axial rotation of the head so that the chin points away from the side of involvement. Torticollis occurs with spasm or contracture of the sternocleidomastoid muscle, which attaches to the medial aspect of the clavicle, as well as to the sternum and mastoid process. Torticollis may be congenital or may be acquired through infection or trauma such as cervical acceleration/deceleration injury (whiplash). Attempts to straighten the neck produce extreme pain for the patient. Hypertonicity and spasm in the sternocleidomastoid muscle may contribute to superior involvement of the proximal clavicle, and certainly restrict motion at the SC joint.

Wry neck, on the other hand, manifests with lateral flexion deformity of the neck and a high shoulder but does not include axial rotation of the head. The sternocleidomastoid muscle may be hypertonic in wry neck, but the principal muscular involvement is the superior portion of the trapezius. The trapezius originates on the spinous processes of the cervical and thoracic vertebrae and inserts on the base of the spine of the scapula, acromion process, and clavicle. A patient with wry neck will demonstrate a positive shoulder depressor test. Perform this test by pushing down on the shoulder while passively flexing the head and neck to the opposite side. Pain and restricted lateral flexion indicate hypertonicity, spasm, or contracture of the superior portion of the trapezius muscle on the side of involvement. If the patient has wry neck, the trapezius muscle usually can be tractioned if the maneuver is performed slowly and gently. Hypertonicity or spasm of the superior trapezius may draw the distal clavicle superiorly, compromising the AC joint and predisposing it to dysfunction.

When a patient suffers from torticollis or wry neck, perform Isolation Tests, Stress Tests, and adjustments as necessary for the following involvements of the clavicle:
- Superior distal clavicle
- Posterior distal clavicle
- Anterior distal clavicle
- Superior proximal clavicle

History of Trauma to the Clavicle
Football, hockey, rugby, and other contact sports tend to provide ample opportunity for direct trauma to the clavicle. For this reason, many of these sports require the use of standard equipment such as shoulder pads, which are designed to protect the clavicle. A direct blow to the clavicle can result in fracture or dislocation of the SC or AC joints.[12,17] A careful history, thorough examination, and radiographic examination help to rule out fractures and frank dislocations.

A forceful blow to the anterior clavicle may have serious consequences. If the clavicle is dislocated posteriorly at the SC joint, the risk of neurovascular compression is present. Recall that the subclavian vessels are located just deep to the clavicle. Compromise of the subclavian artery and the nerves of the brachial plexus through direct compression of a posteriorly displaced clavicle or by inflamed and swollen soft tissues can impair the blood supply and innervations to the upper extremity.[33] Be alert to indications of thoracic outlet syndrome associated with direct trauma to the clavicle.[34] When a patient presents with a history of direct trauma to the clavicle, perform the necessary tests and examinations to rule out neurovascular compromise. Question the patient about any loss of sensation or dysesthesias in the upper extremity. Check the hands and distal extremities for temperature. If the vascular supply is compromised, the hand on the side of involvement may feel cooler to the touch than the hand on the opposite side.

Perform Adson's test in three stages. First, palpate the radial pulse on the side of involvement while the patient extends and rotates the head and neck to the opposite side and holds the breath. Second, palpate the radial pulse on the side of involvement while tractioning the arm down to depress the clavicle at the shoulder. Third, palpate the radial pulse on the side of involvement while passively abducting and hyperextending the arm. All three maneuvers are meant to decrease the space between the clavicle and the first rib. Diminishment or cessation of the radial pulse or exacerbation of pain or paresthesia in the extremity may indicate neurovascular entrapment by a malpositioned clavicle or swollen subclavicular soft tissue.[8,10,35] Another indicator of possible neurovascular compromise secondary to clavicular trauma is Eden's costoclavicular test. To perform Eden's test, palpate the radial pulses bilaterally as the patient retracts and depresses the shoulders while taking and holding a deep breath. Diminishment of the radial pulse, pain, or paresthesia can indicate neurovascular entrapment between the clavicle and the rib cage on the side of involvement.

A third test of neurovascular compromise is the Wright hyperabduction test. To perform the Wright test, palpate the radial pulse on the side of involvement, with the arm in a neutral, relaxed position. Then raise the arm into 180 degrees of abduction. Diminishment or cessation of the pulse suggests vascular entrapment between the pectoralis major muscle and the rib cage just deep to the pectoralis insertion on the coracoid process.

When a patient suffers from direct trauma to the clavicle, rule out more serious injury by a thorough history and examination and by appropriate orthopedic and neurological assessment. Perform Isolation Tests, Stress Tests, and adjustments as necessary for the following involvements and associated joint dysfunctions:
- Posterior distal clavicle
- Superior distal clavicle
- Lateral clavicle

- Superior proximal clavicle
- Inferior proximal clavicle
- AC joint separation
- AC joint impingement
- Inferior medial coracoid

TESTING AND ADJUSTING THE CLAVICLE

When patient complaints or examination findings indicate involvement of the clavicle and its articulations, the following Isolation Tests, Stress Tests, and adjustments for the clavicle may be indicated:
- Anterior distal clavicle
- Posterior distal clavicle
- Lateral clavicle
- Superior distal clavicle
- AC joint separation
- AC joint impingement
- Inferior proximal clavicle
- Superior proximal clavicle

Anterior Distal Clavicle
Patient complaints of chronic shoulder pain, pain on shoulder flexion and external rotation, or a persistent dysfunctional scapular pattern suggest anterior involvement of the distal clavicle.
Stress Test. To Stress Test for anterior distal clavicle, use a finger to push on the posterior aspect of the clavicle as close as possible to the AC joint. Press the distal clavicle straight anterior (Figure 16-39). Look for reactivity of the PD leg in Position #1 for involvement.

Be sure to perform the Stress Test for the anterior distal clavicle by contacting the posterior aspect of the bone, taking care to be well lateral to the coracoid process. The coracoid functions as a fulcrum to support the clavicle during its motions. Therefore pressure on the clavicle medial to the coracoclavicular articulation would stress the SC joint instead of the AC joint. To ensure a correct contact for the Stress Test, place the thumb in the supraclavicular fossa and slide it laterally along the posterior aspect of the clavicle toward the AC joint. For a patient with well-developed trapezius muscles, it may be advisable to retract the muscle while performing the Stress Test.
Adjustment. To adjust an anterior distal clavicle, first raise the table and place the patient in the supine position. Contact the anterior border of the distal clavicle at the AC joint. The LOD is posterior and slightly superior through the plane line of the articulation (Figure 16-40).

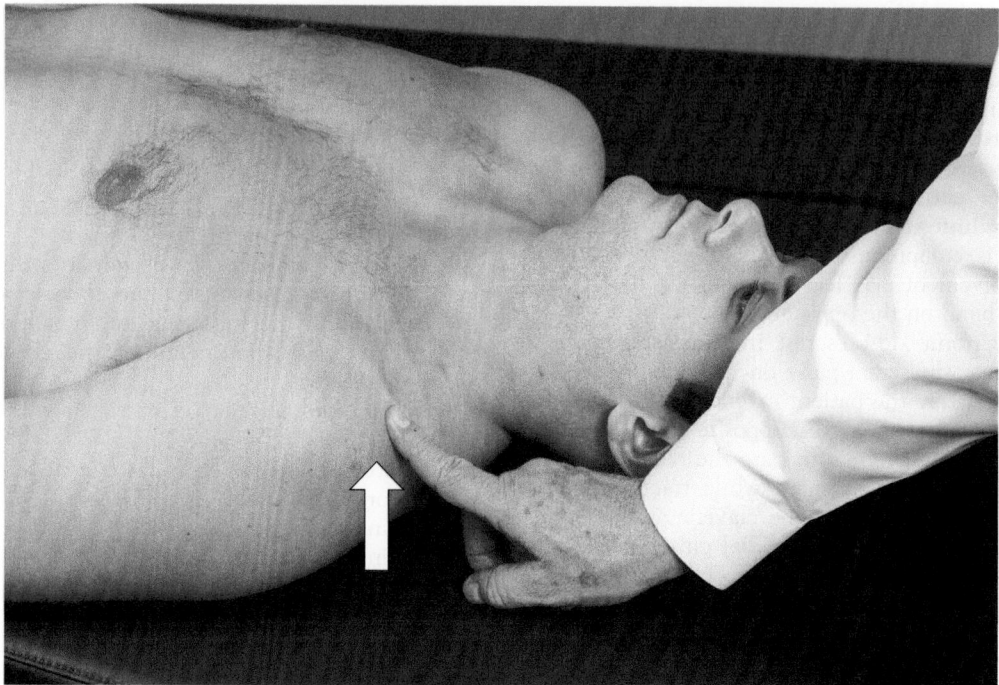

Figure 16-39   Stress Test for anterior distal clavicle.

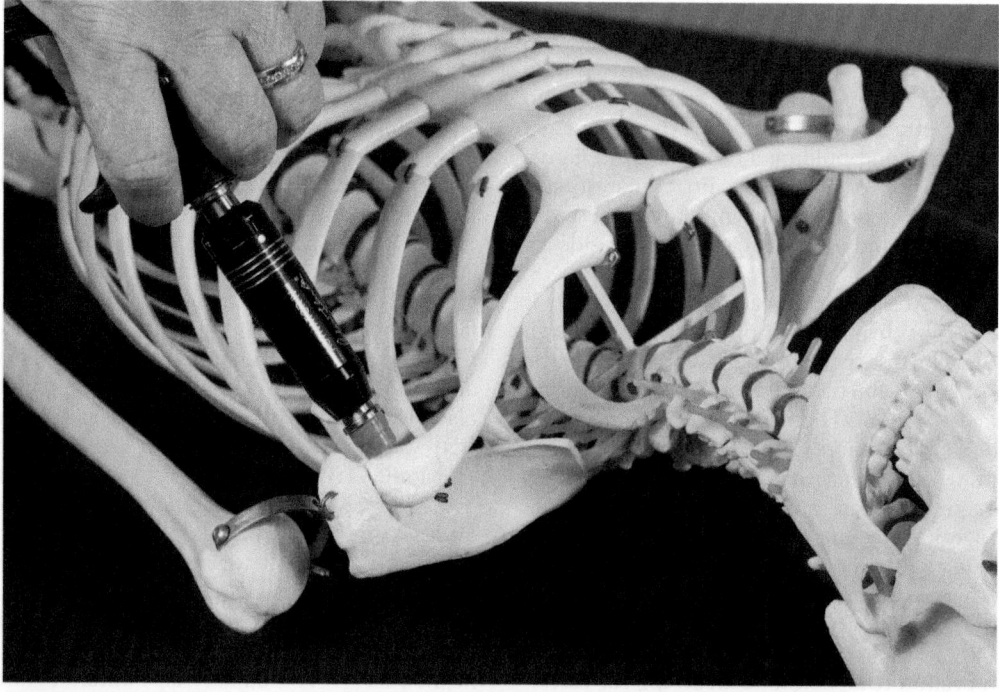

Figure 16-40   Adjustment for anterior distal clavicle. Line of Drive is posterior and slightly superior through the plane line of the articulation.

To locate the head of the distal clavicle, palpate medially over the flat surface of the acromion process until the slightly elevated and rounded prominence of the clavicle is encountered. To ensure an effective contact and adjustment, take an anterior-to-posterior tissue pull over the AC joint. Use the thumb of the stabilization hand to stabilize the tip of the instrument on the clavicle during the adjustment.

Clinical Observations

Anterior involvement of the distal clavicle can stress the fibrous ligaments of the acromioclavicular (AC) joint, as well as the insertion point of the trapezius on the acromion and clavicle. Point tenderness at the AC joint and pain on active and passive flexion and external rotation of the shoulder suggest an anterior distal clavicle.

Anterior involvement of the distal clavicle can destabilize the scapula, allowing it to ride up the scapulothoracic articulation. A persistent or recurrent superior scapula can therefore indicate an otherwise "silent" anterior distal clavicle.

Posterior Distal Clavicle

Pain at the AC joint during active or passive internal rotation and extension of the shoulder suggests posterior malposition of the distal clavicle.

Stress Test. To Stress Test for a posterior distal clavicle, contact the anterior border of the clavicle as close to the AC joint as possible. Pull the clavicle in a straight posterior direction (Figure 16-41). Look for reactivity of the PD leg in Position #1 for involvement.

Stress Test for posterior distal clavicle involvement by contacting the anterior border of the shaft of the bone lateral to the coracoid process, while keeping in mind that the coracoid functions as a fulcrum to support the clavicle during its motions. Therefore pressure on the clavicle medial to the coracoclavicular articulation would stress the SC joint instead of the AC joint.

Adjustment. To adjust for a posterior distal clavicle, contact the posterior aspect of the clavicle at the AC joint. The LOD is straight anterior (Figure 16-42).

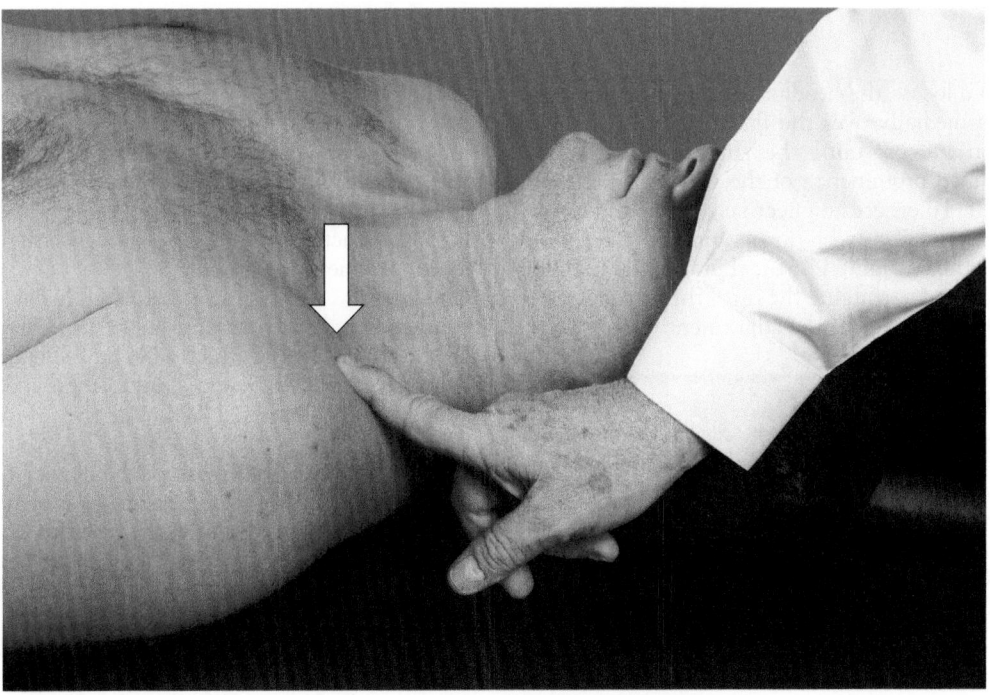

Figure 16-41 Stress Test for posterior distal clavicle.

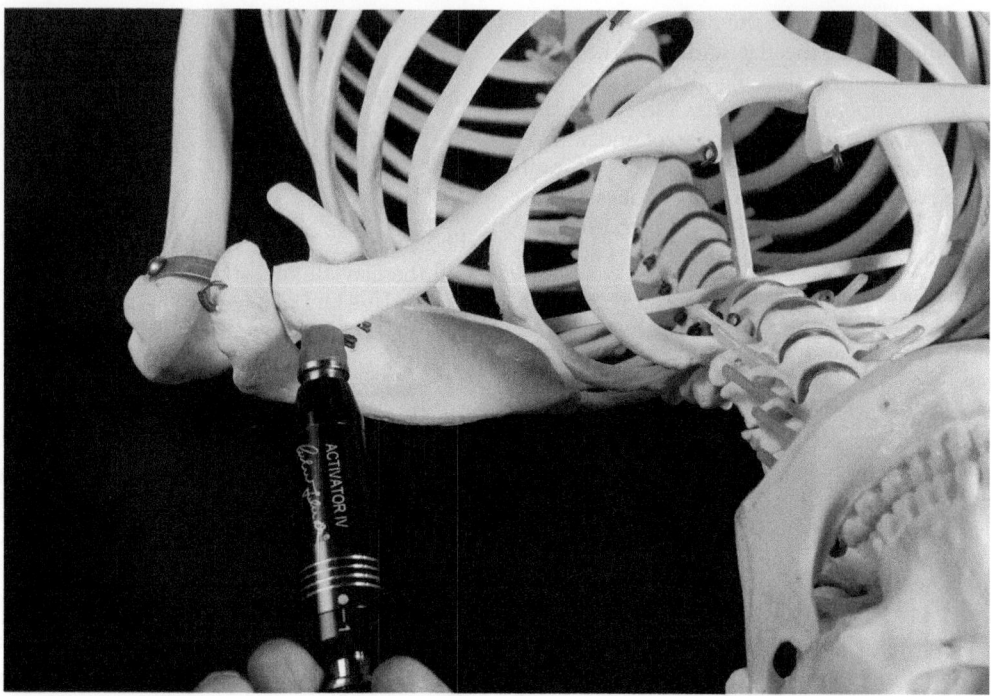

Figure 16-42   Adjustment for posterior distal clavicle. Line of Drive is straight anterior.

To locate the head of the distal clavicle, palpate medially over the flat surface of the acromion process until the slightly elevated and rounded prominence of the clavicle is encountered. To ensure an effective contact and adjustment, take a posterior-to-anterior tissue pull over the AC joint. Use the thumb of the stabilization hand to stabilize the tip of the instrument on the clavicle during the adjustment.

Clinical Observations

A direct frontal blow to the clavicle can misalign it posteriorly at the acromioclavicular joint. Posterior displacement may narrow the space between the clavicle and the chest wall with the risk of neurovascular compromise. Be alert to numbness, paresthesias, and other indicators of possible thoracic outlet syndrome in patients who test positive for a posterior distal clavicle.

Lateral Clavicle

Consider a lateral clavicle when a patient has a recurrent medial scapula, or when the AM Basic Scan Protocol fails to clear a medial scapula.

Stress Test.   To Stress Test for a lateral clavicle, position the shaft of the clavicle between the index and middle fingers, and gently traction the clavicle laterally or simply push the distal clavicle in a lateral direction (Figure 16-43). Look for reactivity of the PD leg in Position #1 for involvement.

Adjustment.   To adjust for a lateral clavicle, contact the distalmost portion of the clavicular head just where the bony prominence is palpable at the AC joint. The LOD is medial along the longitudinal axis of the clavicle (Figure 16-44).

With lateral involvement of the clavicle, the distal head tends to ride up the articular plane of the AC joint. Consequently, the rounded prominence of the distal clavicle may appear higher than normal. Compare the involved side with the asymptomatic side.

Lateral involvement of the clavicle also may be associated with hypertonicity of the trapezius, and the muscle may develop trigger points near its insertion on the distal clavicle and acromion. As a result, the joint and associated soft tissues are likely to be tender to touch and deep palpation. To minimize patient

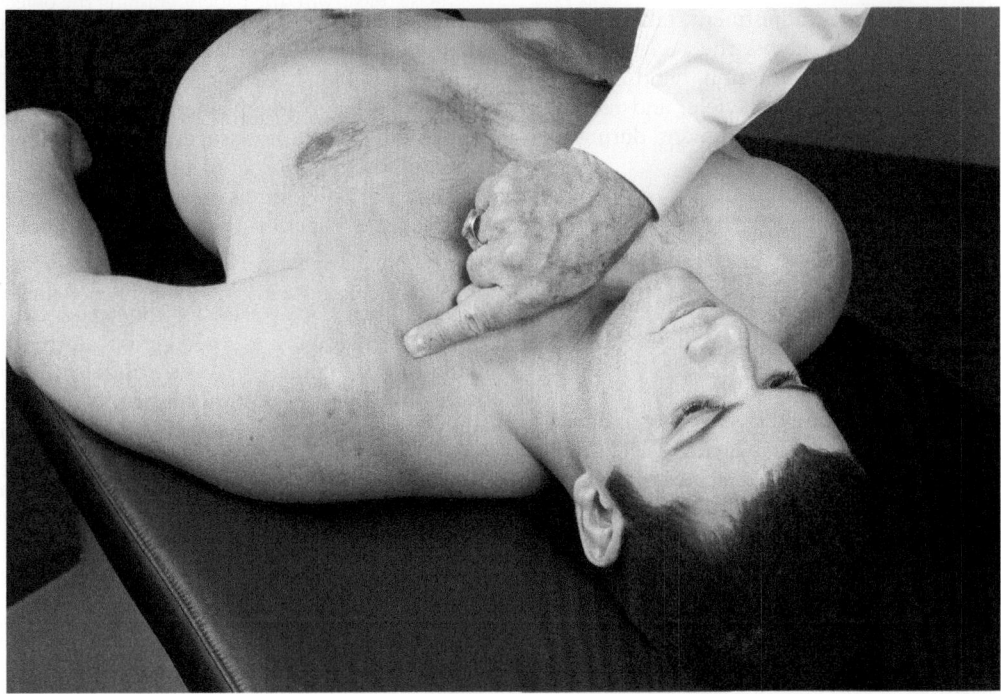

Figure 16-43 Stress Test for lateral distal clavicle.

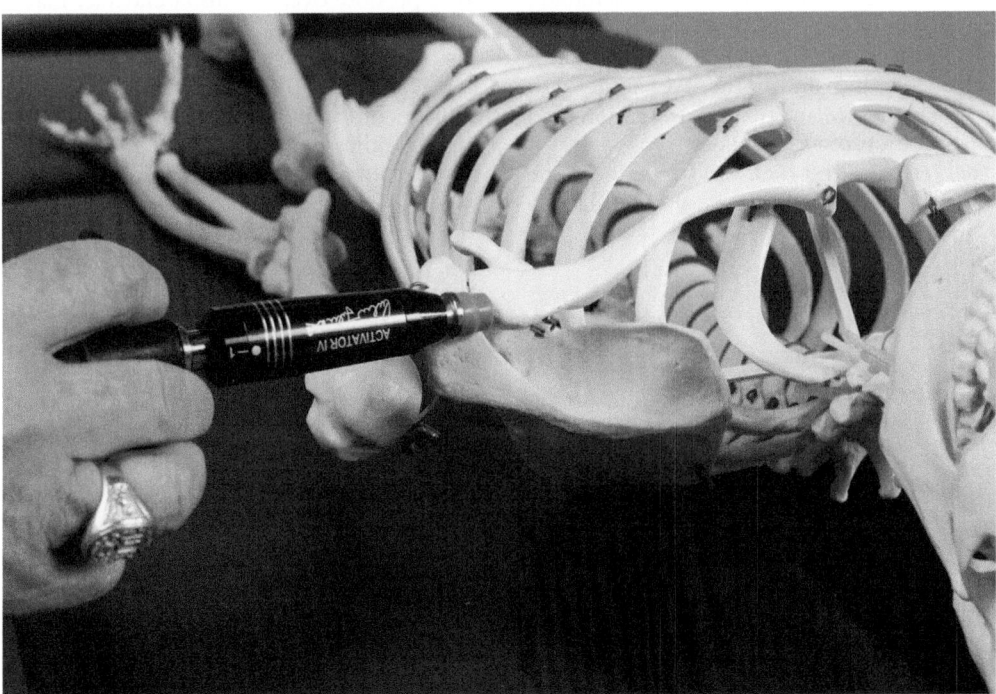

Figure 16-44 Adjustment for lateral distal clavicle. Line of Drive is medial along the longitudinal axis of the clavicle.

discomfort during the adjustment, take a lateral-to-medial tissue pull across the AC joint with the thumb of the stabilization hand. Position the thumb on the distal clavicle, and use it to stabilize the tip of the instrument during the adjustment.

Clinical Observations

Lateral malposition of the clavicle may occur with a blow to the lateral arm or from a fall on an out-stretched arm. A motor vehicle collision in which the driver or a passenger is thrown against the door could contribute to lateral malposition of the clavicle. In all these scenarios, the acromion is driven medially and under the distal clavicle. The "laterality" of the clavicle therefore is relative to the acromioclavicular (AC) joint, and the adjustment is meant to open and restore mobility to the joint.

The relationship of a lateral clavicle to medial scapular pattern arises from restriction of the superior and slightly medial rotation of the acromion during abduction of the scapula. Consequently, the patient with a lateral clavicle is likely to experience pain at the AC joint during attempts to abduct the arm at the shoulder.

Superior Distal Clavicle

A high shoulder or head tilt associated with a hypertonic trapezius or a visible "step-off" between the distal clavicle and the acromion process suggests superior involvement of the distal clavicle. Another indicator of a superior distal clavicle is pain in the AC joint with resisted adduction, and external rotation and internal rotation of the shoulder.

Isolation Test or Stress Test. To perform the Isolation Test for superior distal clavicle involvement, instruct the patient to shrug the involved shoulder upward, toward the ear (Figure 16-45). Look for PD leg reactivity in Position #1 for involvement. To Stress Test for involvement of a superior distal clavicle, contact the inferior border of the clavicle as close to the AC joint as possible. Draw the clavicle straight superior (Figure 16-46). Look for reactivity of the PD leg in Position #1 for involvement.

During the Stress Test for the superior distal clavicle, be sure to get a good grasp on the shaft lateral to the coracoid process. Slide the thumb laterally along the posterior aspect of the clavicle in the supraclavicular fossa while contacting the anterior aspect with the index finger. It may be helpful to retract the muscle while performing the Stress Test for a patient with well-developed trapezius musculature.

Adjustment. To adjust for a superior distal clavicle, position the tip of the instrument on the superior aspect of the distal head, just medial to the AC joint. The LOD is straight inferior (Figure 16-47).

The superior aspect of the distal clavicle is a relatively wide and flat bony prominence that provides a readily accessible contact point for the instrument. However, the joint and the soft tissues may be tender with a superior distal clavicle. To minimize discomfort for the patient, use the index and middle fingers to apply inferior-ward pressure over the distal clavicle. Place the fingers wide enough apart to accommodate the tip of the instrument, and use the split-finger position to stabilize the instrument during the adjustment. Stand at the head of the table during the adjustment to be in proper ergonomic form, maintaining neutral posture at the wrist while adjusting.

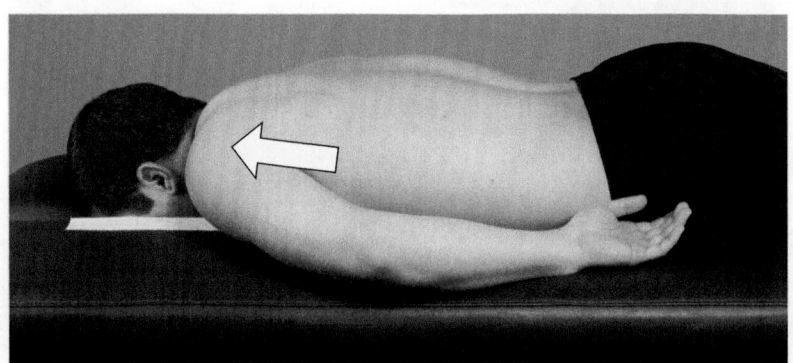

Figure 16-45 Isolation Test for superior distal clavicle; shrug shoulder.

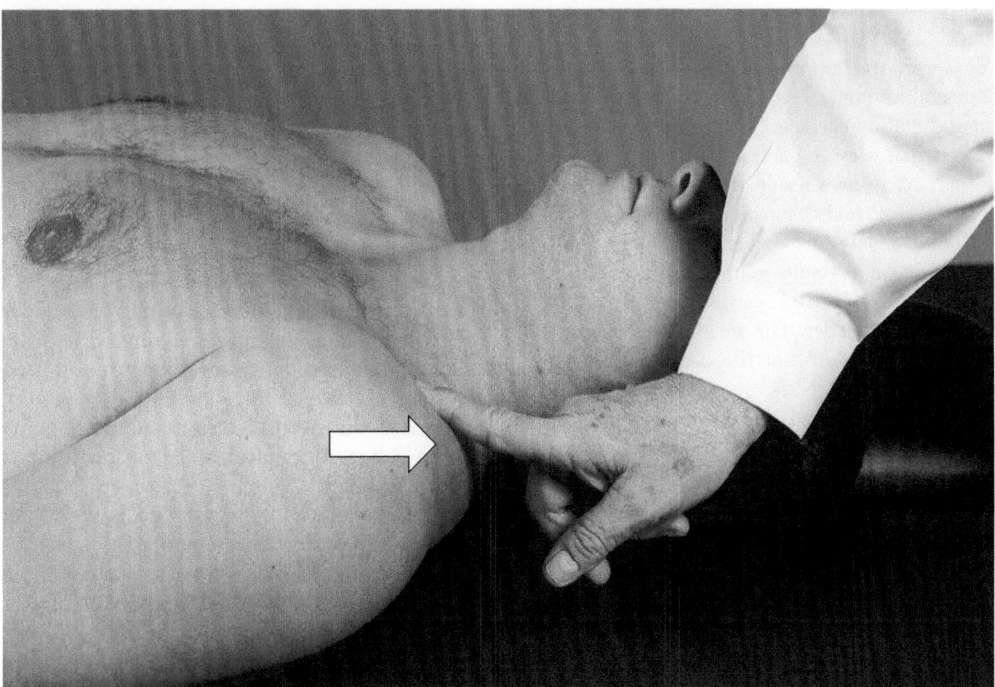

Figure 16-46   Stress Test for superior distal clavicle.

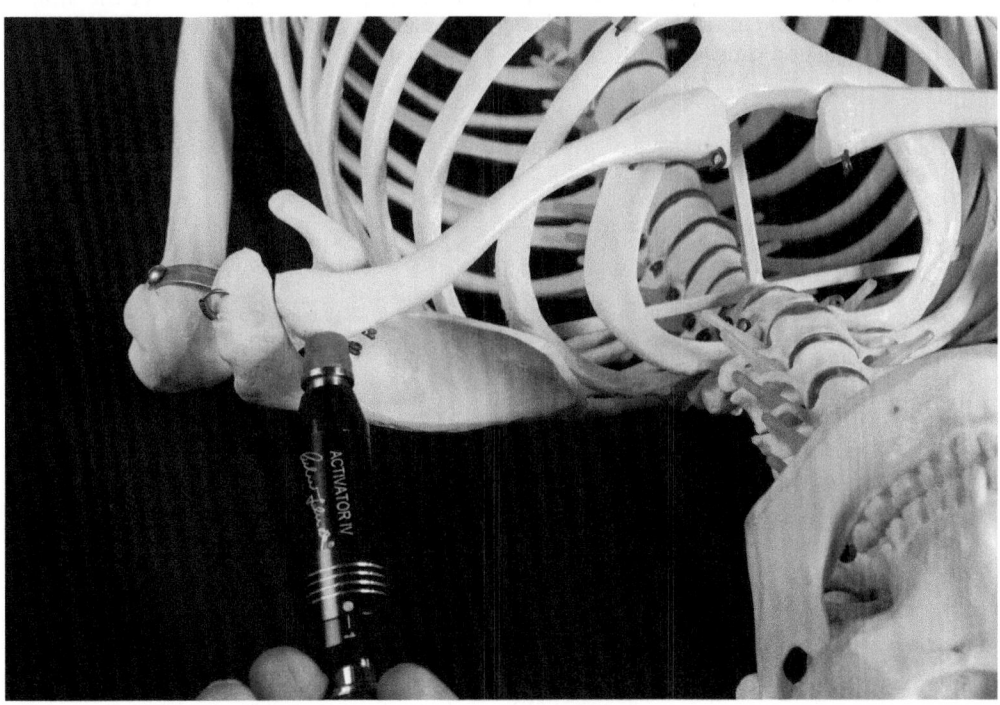

Figure 16-47   Adjustment for superior distal clavicle. Line of Drive is straight inferior.

Clinical Observations

A downward traction injury to the arm at the glenohumeral joint may precipitate superior malposition of the distal clavicle. Such injuries can occur in sports like wrestling and martial arts, but they also may occur as a result of heavy lifting done for recreational and occupational purposes.

More insidious development of a superior distal clavicle may result from hanging a heavy bookbag, purse, or baby carrier over the distal aspect of the shoulder. The weight and repetitive loading and unloading of the acromioclavicular (AC) joint may drop the acromion process and scapula down relative to the distal clavicle.

When a patient presents with significant visible or palpable step-off between the distal clavicle and the acromion process, be sure to evaluate the AC joint for separation.

Acromioclavicular Joint Separation

When a patient presents with a history of a fall on the point of the shoulder or direct trauma downward over the shoulder such that movement of the shoulder is severely restricted, suspect an AC joint separation.[13] Another indicator of an AC joint separation is a marked visible and palpable step-off between the distal clavicle and the acromion process. The patient is likely to hold the arm in a guarded position and may even support the injured arm with the opposite hand acting as a sling.

Isolation Test. To perform the Isolation Test for AC joint separation involvement, ask the patient to anchor the hand on the side of involvement firmly on the hip (ilium) so that the elbow is flexed at about 45 degrees and the shoulder is internally rotated. Then ask the patient to push the hand straight medially toward the body (Figure 16-48). Look for reactivity of the PD leg in Position #1 for involvement.

The Isolation Test for AC joint separation is based on the biomechanics of resisted adduction of the shoulder. Adduction swings the scapular ala medially and depresses the acromion process. Normally, the distal clavicle also would be depressed during adduction, but with laxity of the AC ligaments after a separation injury, the joint will open.

The Isolation Test is a relatively gentle maneuver; however, a separated AC joint can be very painful. Give the patient plenty of time to perform the test, because apprehension of pain can generate enough muscle tension to obscure test results.

If the Isolation Test maneuver for the AC joint separation is too difficult or painful for the patient to perform independently, the test can be performed with manual assistance. Hold the patient's arm in slight internal rotation at approximately 25 degrees of abduction. Apply resistance just proximal to the elbow while the patient tries to adduct the arm. Look for reactivity of the PD leg in Position #1 for involvement.

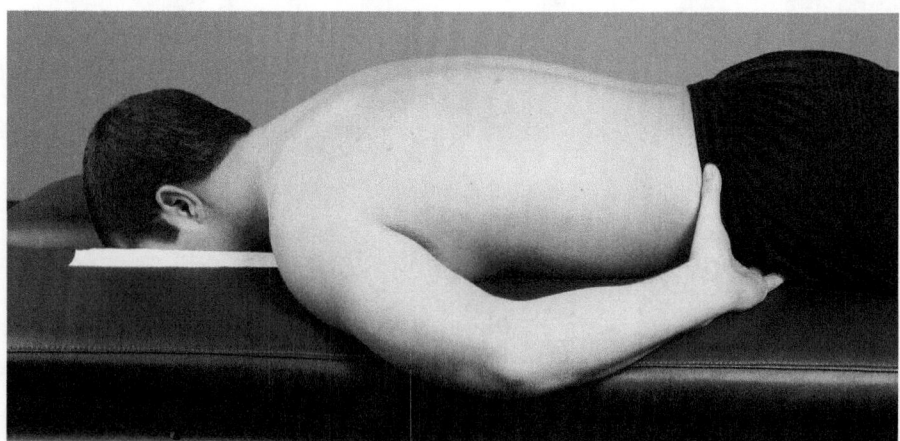

Figure 16-48 Isolation Test for acromioclavicular joint separation. Place hand firmly on the hip (ilium) so that the elbow is flexed at about 45 degrees and the shoulder is internally rotated, and push the hand straight medially toward the body.

Adjustment.   Adjustment for an AC joint separation is performed in two steps. First, contact the superior aspect of the distal clavicle with the tip of the instrument. Use the thumb of the stabilization hand to anchor the acromion process by applying firm lateral-to-medial pressure on the acromion. The LOD is lateral and slightly inferior to close the joint space (Figure 16-49). (*Note:* For photographic reasons, Figures 16-49 and 16-50 are shown on the right side. This Isolation Test was performed on the left, which is side specific, and the adjustment should be performed on the left side.) Second, contact the lateral aspect of the acromion process with the tip of the instrument. Use the thumb of the stabilization hand to anchor the distal clavicle by applying firm medial-to-lateral pressure on the head. The LOD is medial and slightly superior to close the joint space (Figure 16-50).

With AC joint separation, periarticular soft tissue and especially fibers of the trapezius at its insertion on the distal clavicle and acromion process are likely to be tender to touch and deep palpation. To minimize discomfort during Step One of the adjustment, take a medial-to-lateral tissue pull over the distal clavicle, position the tip of the instrument, and hold until the acromion process is anchored. During Step Two of the adjustment, take a lateral-to-medial tissue pull across the acromion process, position the tip of the instrument, and hold until the distal clavicle is anchored.

Clinical Observations

An acromioclavicular (AC) joint separation is a grade II sprain with partial displacement of the acromion process relative to the distal clavicle, with laxity of the AC ligaments and possible involvement of the coracoclavicular ligaments.[36,37] Until healing is complete, soft tissues are extremely vulnerable to reinjury. Although grade II sprains are amenable to conservative therapy,[15] it is important for the patient to avoid excessive use of the shoulder during the acute phase and during recovery. For the patient with an acute AC separation, use of a simple sling for at least a few days is recommended.[37]

Monitor the healing process carefully, adjust as necessary, and advise the patient on participating in or resuming activities that could delay repair or cause serious and degenerative injury to the AC joint.

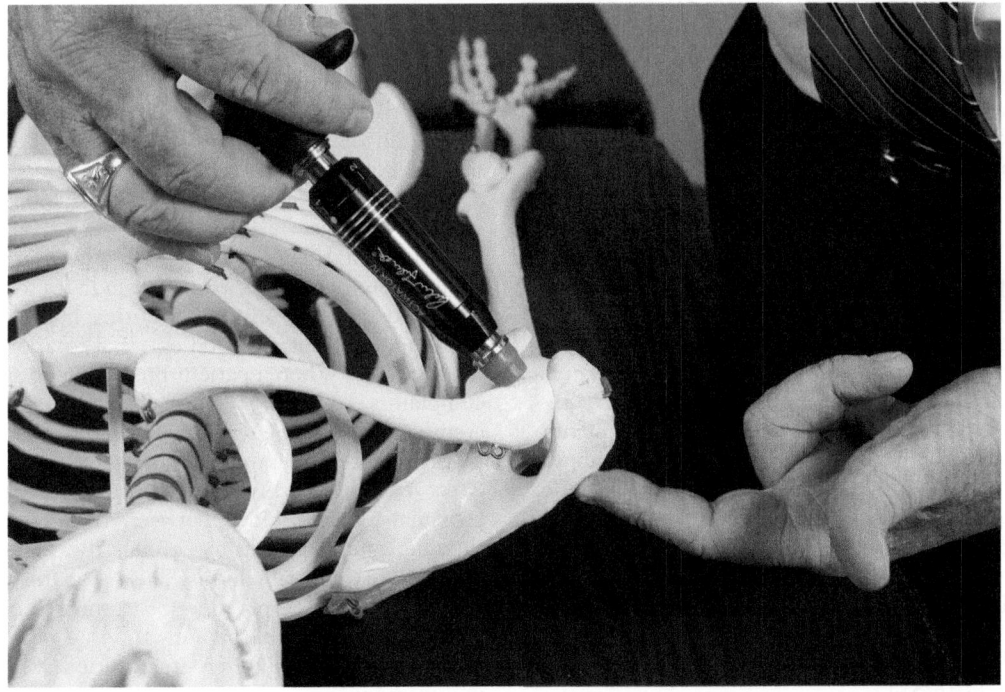

Figure 16-49   Adjustment for acromioclavicular joint separation. Step One: Contact superior aspect of the distal clavicle. Line of Drive is lateral and slightly inferior to close the joint space.

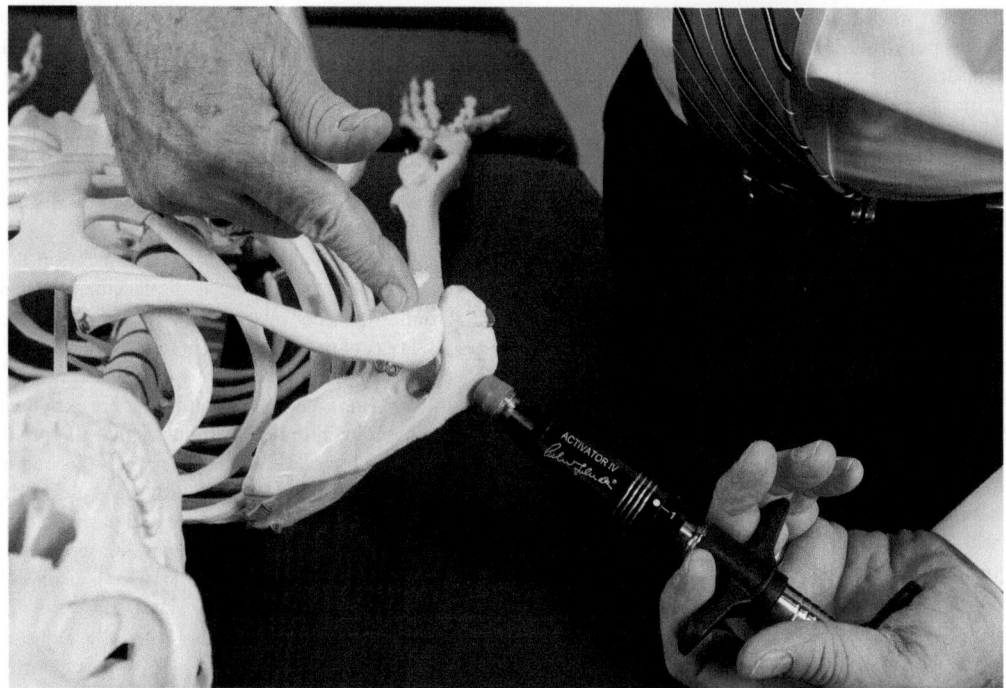

Figure 16-50 Adjustment for acromioclavicular joint separation. Step Two: Contact lateral aspect of the acromion process. Line of Drive is medial and slightly superior to close the joint space.

Acromioclavicular Joint Impingement

When a patient presents with frozen shoulder syndrome, limited shoulder range of motion, or arm pain or numbness and tingling, consider testing for AC joint impingement. Upon physical examination, internal rotation and adduction of the humerus (impingement sign) will be positive for pain, and tenderness of the AC joint will be evident.

Stress Test. To Stress Test for AC joint impingement, gently pinch the acromion and the lateral clavicle together (Figure 16-51). Look for reactivity of the PD leg in Position #1 for involvement.

Adjustment. Adjustment for AC joint impingement is performed in two steps. First, contact the posterior distal clavicle with the tip of the instrument. The LOD is anterior and medial (Figure 16-52). Second, contact the anterior and superior acromion process with the tip of the instrument. The LOD is posterior, lateral, and slightly inferior to open the joint space (Figure 16-53).

To minimize discomfort during Step One of the adjustment, take a lateral-to-medial tissue pull over the distal clavicle, position the tip of

the instrument, and stabilize it. During Step Two of the adjustment, take a medial-to-lateral tissue pull over the acromion, position the tip of the instrument, and stabilize it.

Inferior Proximal Clavicle

Instability of the proximal clavicle can cause localized sternal pain or pain that radiates to the back and shoulder, especially during horizontal abduction, and internal and external rotation of the shoulder. When a patient presents with such complaints, or when shoulder motion produces crepitus in the SC joint, consider inferior involvement of the proximal clavicle.

Stress Test. To Stress Test for an inferior proximal clavicle, reach between the patient's shoulder and the table to contact the superior border of the clavicle as close to the SC joint as possible. Apply superior-to-inferior pressure to the clavicle (Figure 16-54). Look for reactivity of the PD leg in Position #1 for involvement.

When Stress Testing for an inferior clavicle, be sure to contact the bone medial to the coracoid process. Recall that the coracoid functions

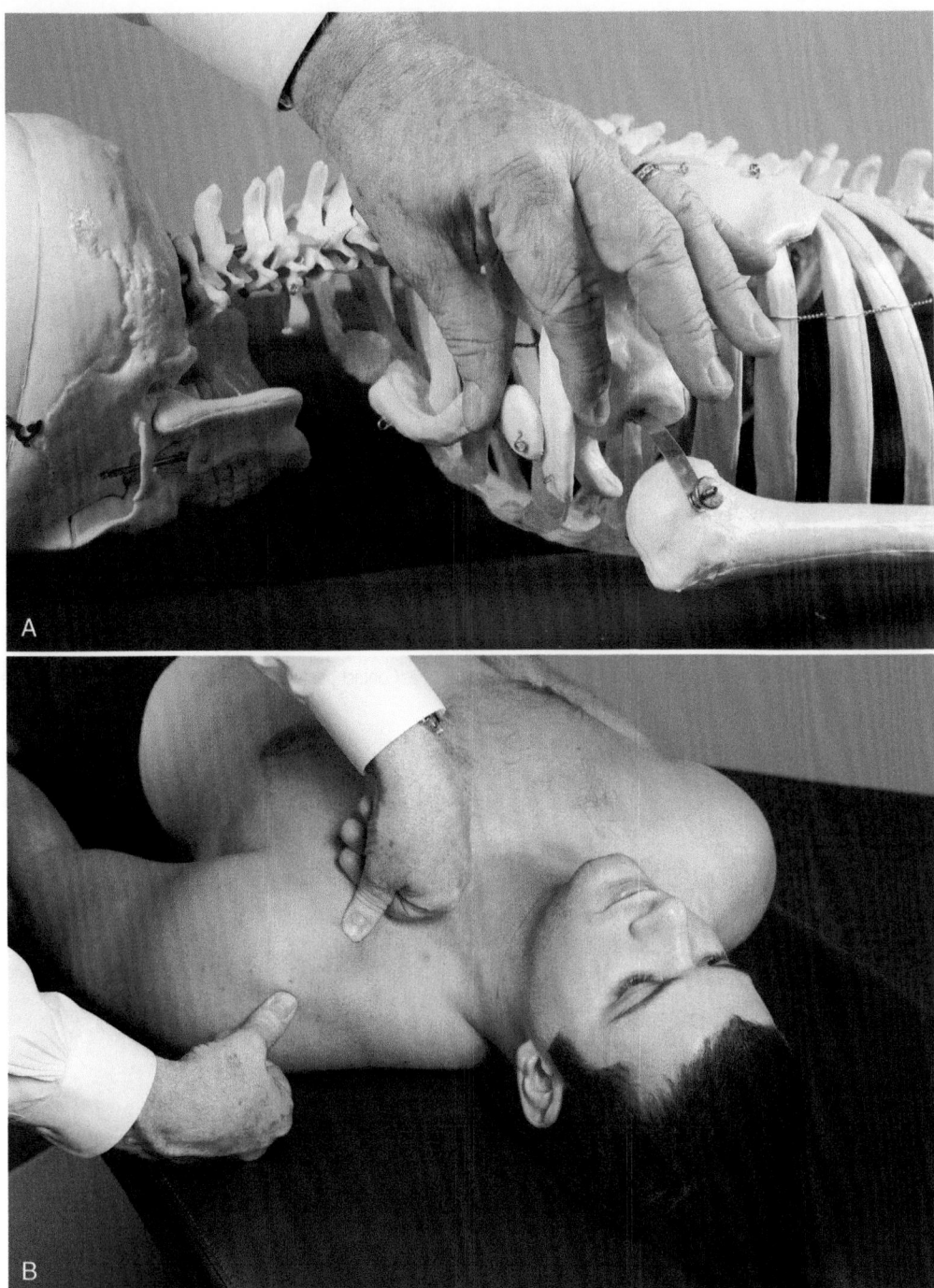

Figure 16-51 **A** and **B**, Stress Test for acromioclavicular impingement.

as a fulcrum to stabilize the clavicle during its motions. Applying pressure lateral to the coracoid would stress the AC joint instead of the SC joint. **Adjustment.**   To adjust an inferior proximal clavicle, first raise the table and place the patient in the supine position. Contact the inferior aspect of the proximal clavicle just inferior and lateral to the SC joint. The LOD is superior and slightly medial along the plane line of the SC joint (Figure 16-55).

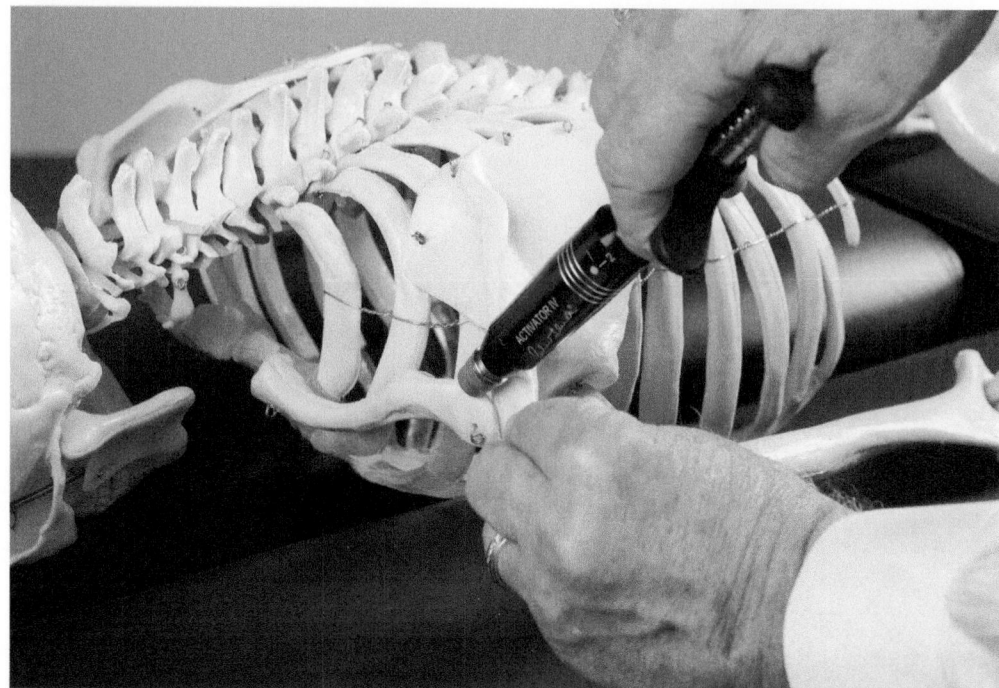

Figure 16-52   Adjustment for acromioclavicular impingement. Step One: Contact posterior distal clavicle. Line of Drive is anterior and medial.

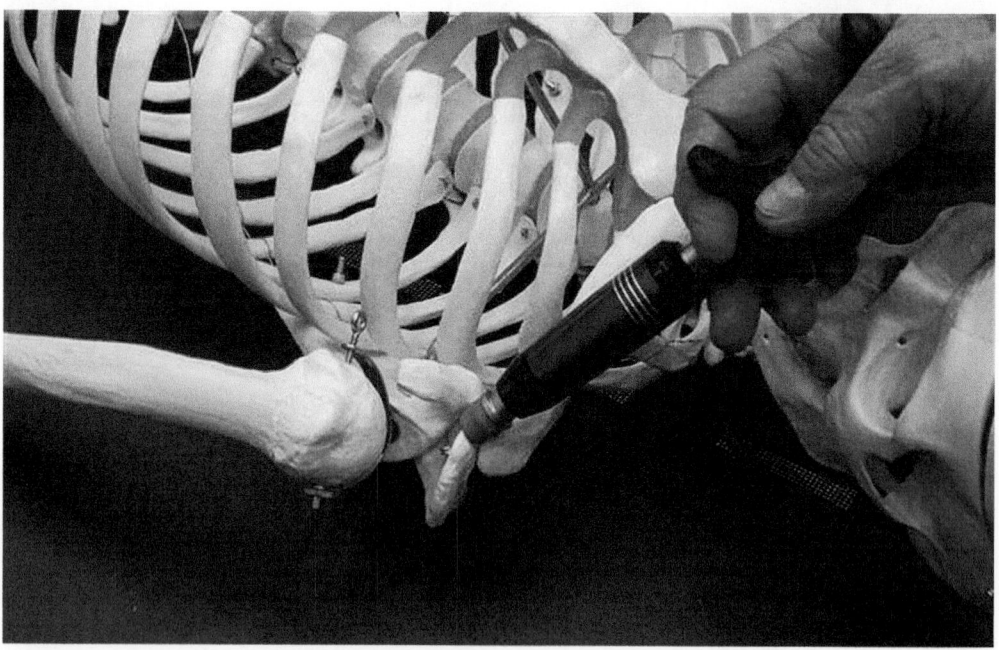

Figure 16-53   Adjustment for acromioclavicular impingement. Step Two: Contact anterior and superior acromion process. Line of Drive is posterior, lateral, and slightly inferior to open the joint space.

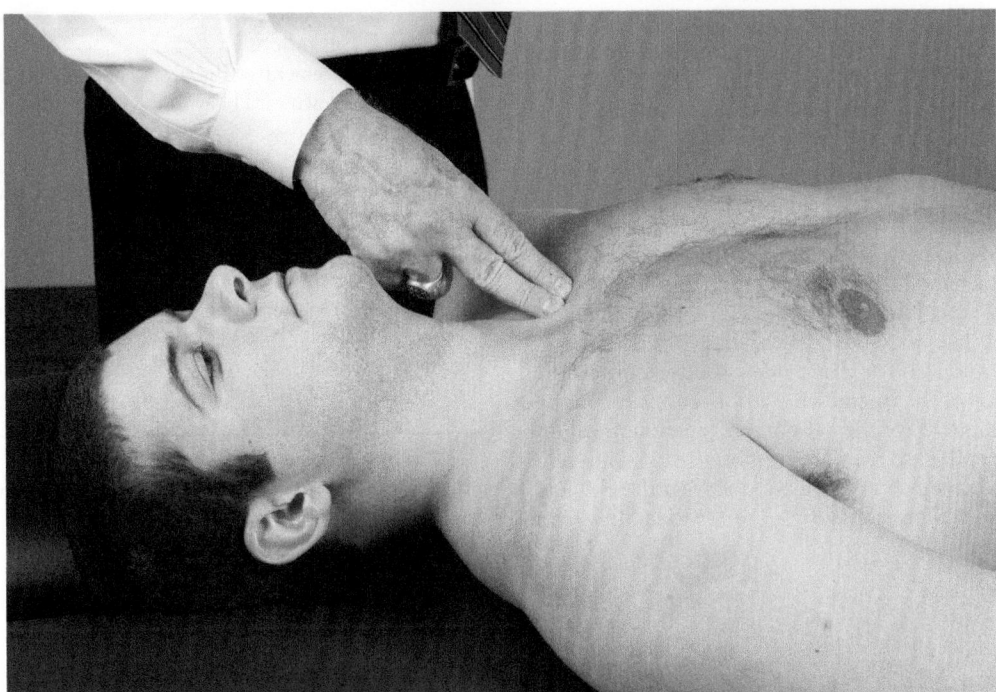

Figure 16-54 Stress Test for inferior proximal clavicle.

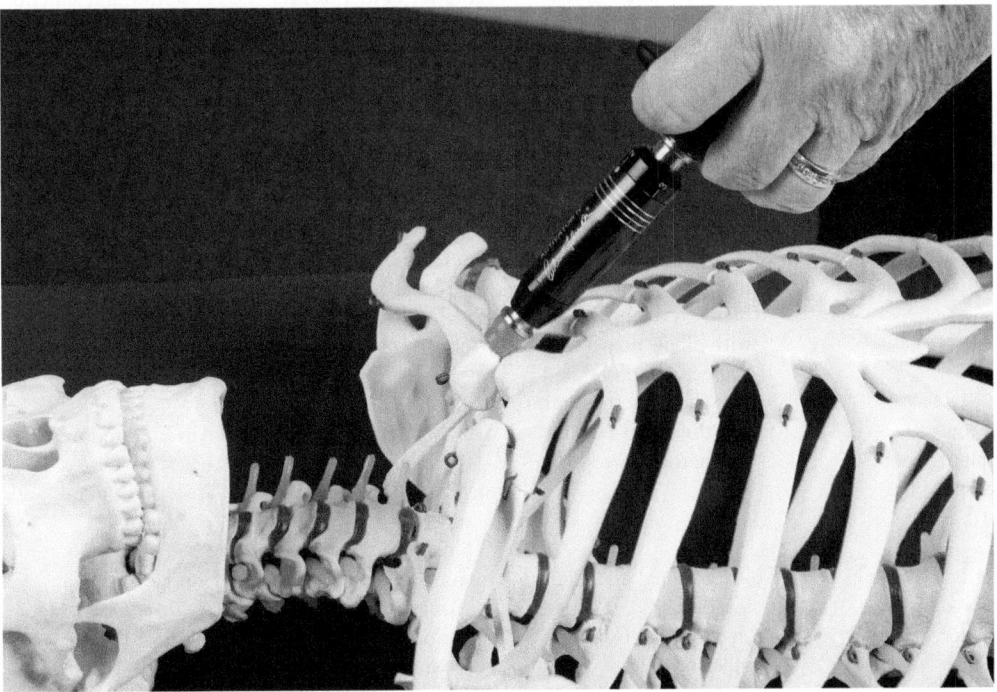

Figure 16-55 Adjustment for inferior proximal clavicle. Line of Drive is superior and slightly medial along the plane line of the sternoclavicular joint.

A dysfunctional SC joint can be tender to touch and to deep palpation. To minimize patient discomfort during the adjustment, take an inferior-to-superior tissue pull over the SC joint with the thumb of the stabilization hand. Use the thumb to stabilize the tip of the instrument during the adjustment.

If the proximal clavicle is displaced posteriorly, it may be difficult to attain an effective contact and LOD. It may help to have the patient place the forearm of the side of involvement across the abdomen. This will swing the scapula anteriorly and will provide a better contact for the tip of the instrument. Another option, if possible, is to have the patient reach across the abdomen and grasp the iliac crest on the opposite side. This maneuver not only will protract the clavicle, it also will pre-stress the SC joint to facilitate the adjustment.

Clinical Observations

Inferior displacement of the proximal clavicle can occur with a downward blow to the bone medial to the coracoid process. Contact sports like football and rugby provide likely conditions for such an injury. A traction injury to the shoulder during abduction or hyperabduction could contribute to an inferior malposition of the proximal clavicle as the shaft rocks over the fulcrum of the coracoid process.

Whenever a patient tests positive for an inferior proximal clavicle, be especially alert to neurovascular compression syndromes that may arise from narrowing of the costoclavicular space.

Mechanical force, manually assisted adjusting (AM) for the clavicle is summarized in Table 16-2.

Table 16-2 Summary Table for Tests and Adjustments of the Clavicle

Articular Dysfunction	Test	Segmental Contact Point	Line of Drive
Anterior Distal Clavicle	Stress Test distal clavicle anterior	Anterior border at AC joint	Posterior and superior
Posterior Distal Clavicle	Stress Test clavicle posterior	Posterior aspect at AC joint	Anterior
Lateral Clavicle	Traction clavicle laterally	Distal clavicle	Medial
Superior Distal Clavicle	Instruct patient to shrug involved shoulder or Stress Test by pulling clavicle superior	Distal clavicle	Inferior
AC Joint Separation	Instruct patient to place involved side palm of hand on the hip (ilium) with elbow flexed to 45 degrees and push hand into the body (medially)	Step One: Superior aspect of distal clavicle	Lateral
		Step Two: Lateral aspect of acromion process	Medial
AC Joint Impingement	Pinch the distal clavicle and acromion together	Step One: Posterior distal clavicle	Anterior and medial
		Step Two: Anterior and superior acromion process	Posterior, lateral, and inferior
Inferior Proximal Clavicle	Push proximal clavicle inferior	Inferior aspect of proximal clavicle	Superior
Superior Proximal Clavicle	Push proximal clavicle superior	Superior aspect of proximal clavicle	Inferior

AC, Acromioclavicular.

RELATED RESEARCH

Related published research for this chapter is summarized in Boxes 16-3 and 16-4.

Box 16-3

Reference: Polkinghorn BS. Chiropractic treatment of frozen shoulder syndrome (adhesive capsulitis) using mechanical force manually assisted short lever adjusting procedures. J Manipulative Physiol Ther. 1995;18(2):105-15.

ABSTRACT
OBJECTIVE

To describe treatment of frozen shoulder syndrome (adhesive capsulitis) via conservative chiropractic treatment to the shoulder joint, using specific contact, low-force instrumental adjusting procedures. A case report, providing an illustrative example of the same, is presented along with a review of the relevant literature.

CLINICAL FEATURES

A 53-year-old woman suffered severe shoulder pain of over 6 months' duration. The patient had been diagnosed as having adhesive capsulitis and had undergone a variety of treatment regimens without obtaining relief, including various nonsteroidal antiinflammatory drugs, analgesics, and physical therapy. At the time of examination, her condition had progressed to the point of near total immobility of the shoulder joint, accompanied by severe pain with resulting marked restriction in her normal activities of daily living.

INTERVENTION AND OUTCOME

The patient's shoulder was conservatively managed with chiropractic adjustments to the affected shoulder joint, as well as to the cervicothoracic spine. Treatment consisted of mechanical force, manually assisted short lever chiropractic adjustments, delivered with an Activator Adjusting Instrument. Successful resolution of the presenting symptomatology was achieved.

CONCLUSION

Chiropractic care may be able to provide an effective mode of therapeutic treatment for certain types of these difficult cases. Low-force instrument adjustments, in particular, may present certain benefits in these cases that the more forceful manipulations and/or mobilizations cannot. A larger-scale formal investigation of this type of therapeutic intervention for treatment of frozen shoulder may be warranted.

Box 16-4

Reference: Polkinghorn BS. Instrumental chiropractic treatment of frozen shoulder associated with mixed metastatic carcinoma. Chiropr Tech. 1995;7:98-102.

ABSTRACT
OBJECTIVE

Patients often present themselves for chiropractic treatment with conditions that may include contraindications for manipulative therapy.

CLINICAL FEATURES

This report describes successful chiropractic treatment, with an Activator Adjusting Instrument, of acute shoulder pain, involving a patient who presented with mixed metastatic carcinoma that affected the humerus, scapula, and clavicle. The successful outcome of the case demonstrates the possible value of instrumental chiropractic adjustment in treating neuromusculoskeletal cases where a forceful, high-velocity adjustment or manipulation would be contraindicated because of the underlying osseous disease involved. Further study into this possibility should be pursued to train those physicians who are called upon to treat these patients, and to better define risk management protocols for the chiropractic profession.

REFERENCES

1. Dwyer A, Aprill C, Bogduk N. Cervical zygapophyseal joint pain patterns. I: A study in normal volunteers. Spine. 1990;15(6):453-7.
2. Aprill C, Dwyer A, Bogduk N. Cervical zygapophyseal joint pain patterns. II: A clinical evaluation. Spine. 1990;15(6):458-61.
3. Bates B. A guide to physical examination and history taking 4th ed. Philadelphia: J.B. Lippincott; 1987.
4. Hagberg M. Neck and shoulder disorders. In: Rosenstock L, Cullen MR, editors. Textbook of clinical occupational and environmental medicine. Philadelphia: Saunders; 1994.
5. Clemente CD. Gray's anatomy 30th American ed. Philadelphia: Lea & Febiger; 1985.
6. Cherniack M. Upper extremity disorders. In: Rosenstock L, Cullen MR, editors. Textbook of clinical occupational and environmental medicine. Philadelphia: Saunders; 1994.
7. Bovee M. The essentials of orthopedic & neurological testing. Davenport (IA): Bovee/Palmer College of Chiropractic; 1977.
8. Cipriano JJ. Photographic manual of regional orthopaedic tests. Baltimore: Williams & Wilkins; 1985.
9. Magee DJ. The shoulder. In: Orthopedic physical assessment. Philadelphia: Saunders; 1987. p. 62-91.
10. Hoppenfeld S. Physical examination of the spine and extremities. Norwalk (CT): Appleton-Century-Crofts; 1976.
11. Polkinghorn BS. Chiropractic treatment of frozen shoulder syndrome (adhesive capsulitis) using mechanical force manually assisted short lever adjusting procedures. J Manipulative Physiol Ther. 1995;18(2):105-15.
12. Nepola JV. Examination of the shoulder. In: Clark CR, Bonfiglio M, editors. Orthopaedics: essentials of diagnosis and treatment. New York: Churchill Livingstone; 1994.
13. Andrews JR, Whiteside JA, Wilk KE. Rehabilitation of throwing and racquet sport injuries. In: Buschbacher RM, Braddom RL, editors. Sports medicine and rehabilitation: a sport-specific approach. Philadelphia: Hanley & Belfus; and St. Louis: Mosby; 1994.
14. Tinetti ME, Liu WL, Claus EB. Predictors and prognosis of inability to get up after falls among elderly persons. JAMA. 1993;269(1):65-70.
15. Chase J, Carnine K. Injuries to the upper limb. In: McLatchie GR, Lennox CME, Percy EC, Davies J. The soft tissues: trauma and sports injuries. London: Butterworth-Heinemann; 1993.
16. Evans RC. Illustrated orthopedic physical assessment. 2nd ed. St. Louis: Mosby; 1994. p. 206.
17. Krieg JC, Nepola JV. Fractures of the shoulder and humerus. In: Clark CR, Bonfiglio M, editors.

Orthopaedics: essentials of diagnosis and treatment. New York: Churchill Livingstone; 1994.
18. Rathbun JB, MacNab I. The microvascular pattern of the rotator cuff. J Bone Joint Surg Br. 1970;5(3):540-532.
19. Wei F. Swimming injuries: diagnosis, treatment. In: Buschbacher RM, Braddom RL, editors. Sports medicine and rehabilitation: a sport-specific approach. Philadelphia: Hanley & Belfus; and St. Louis: Mosby; 1994.
20. Bryant PR, Koch B. Pediatric sports issues. In: Buschbacher RM, Braddom RL, editors. Sports medicine and rehabilitation: a sport-specific approach. Philadelphia: Hanley & Belfus; and St. Louis: Mosby; 1994.
21. Neer CS, 2nd Impingement lesions. Clin Orthop Relat Res. 1983;173:70-7.
22. Cinque C. Fibromyalgia: is exercise the cause or the cure? Physician Sports Med. 1989;17:181-4.
23. Staud R, Smitherman ML. Peripheral and central sensitization in fibromyalgia: pathogenetic role. Curr Pain Headache Rep. 2002;6(4):259-66.
24. Travell JG, Simons DG. Myofascial pain and dysfunction: the trigger point manual. Baltimore: Williams & Wilkins; 1983.
25. Silverstolpe L. A pathological erector spinae reflex: a new sign of mechanical pelvis dysfunction. J Manual Med. 1989;4:28.
26. Bottomley MB. Risks and injuries in athletics and running. In: McLatchie GR, Lennox CME, editors. The soft tissues: trauma and sports injuries. London: Butterworth-Heinemann; 1993.
27. Pascarelli E, Quilter D. Repetitive strain injury: a computer user's guide. New York: Wiley; 1994.
28. Katz JN, Brissot R, Liang MH. Systemic rheumatologic disorders. In: Rosenstock L, Cullen MR, editors. Textbook of clinical occupational and environmental medicine. Philadelphia: Saunders; 1994.
29. Murphee RH. Nutrition Reviews. 1994;52(7):249.
30. Spangfort E. Clinical aspects of neck-and-shoulder pain. Scand J Rehab Med. 1995;32S:43-6.
31. Millard RS. Body-building and weight-lifting: special issues in rehabilitation. In: Buschbacher RM, Braddom RL, editors. Sports medicine and rehabilitation: a sport-specific approach. Philadelphia: Hanley & Belfus and St. Louis: Mosby; 1994.
32. Kulund DN. The injured athlete 2nd ed. Philadelphia: Lippincott; 1988.
33. Bracker MD, Ralph LP. The numb arm and hand. Am Fam Physician. 1995;51(1):103-16.
34. Szaraz ZT. The thoracic outlet syndrome: first rib subluxation syndrome. In: Gatterman MI, editor. Foundations of chiropractic: subluxation. St. Louis: Mosby; 1995. p. 359-77.

35. Mazion JM. Illustrated manual of neurological reflexes/signs/tests and orthopedic signs/tests/ maneuvers for office procedures. Arizona City: Mazion; 1980.

36. Paulos L, Kody M. Management of the acutely injured joint. In: McLatchie GR, Lennox CME, editors. The soft tissues: trauma and sports injuries. London: Butterworth-Heinemann; 1993.

37. Fukuda K, Craig EV, Kai-Nan A, Cofiel RH, Chao EY. Biomechanical study of the ligamentous system of the acromioclavicular joint. J Bone Joint Surg Am. 1986;68(3):434-41.

17 ADDITIONAL TESTS AND ADJUSTMENTS FOR THE ELBOW, WRIST, AND HAND

Attention to the elbow, wrist, and hand is indicated when a patient suffers from any of the following:

- Restricted or altered range of motion
- Point tenderness
- Lateral or medial epicondylitis
- Peripheral nerve entrapment syndrome
- Olecranon bursitis

Elbow, wrist, and hand problems may occur suddenly or may have a gradual onset. Problems that occur suddenly include sprains, strains, dislocations, and fractures. Such trauma often is associated with sports activities but also can result from work-related injuries, motor vehicle collisions, and falls.

The cumulative effects of microtrauma produce elbow, wrist, and hand problems of more insidious onset. Often, the development of signs and symptoms is slow and subtle, and both the patient and the clinician may miss early warning indications. Cumulative microtrauma, also known as repetitive strain injury (RSI) or repetitive motion injury (RMI), may be associated with sports activities such as racquet and throwing sports; however, RMI associated with occupational activity is a major cause of lost work time and productivity. The rapid increase in the number of jobs that require at least some computer work as part of employment tasks has led to an enormous increase in the number of cases of RSI.[1]

There is by no means universal agreement on the origin, mechanism, diagnosis, or treatment of RMI of the elbow, wrist, and hand. Ireland, for example, discusses the "epidemic" of occupational arm pain or RSI that occurred in Australia during the early 1980s.[2] This condition was attributed to rapid, repetitive motion typical of keyboarding and other occupational activities; the rising incidence coincided with technological changes in many occupations. Ireland therefore describes RSI as a "sociopolitical phenomenon" and concludes, "The self-generating term RSI is misleading, for there is no scientific evidence proving that repetitive work causes either tissue strain or injury."[2] Terrono and Millender, on the other hand, cite the role in "... acute or chronic [wrist] disorders of forceful pulling or grasping, as well as repetitive activities incurred in work and everyday activities."[3] Similarly, Simmons and Wyman report a significant increase in the incidence of work-related elbow injuries, "...when rapid and repetitive arm motion, particularly in the wrist and fingers, is involved."[4]

Elbow, wrist, and hand pain, numbness, and paresthesias may result from referred neurovascular problems that arise in the shoulder and upper thoracic and cervical regions. Brachial plexus involvement associated with soft tissue injury of the shoulder, for example, can affect sensory and motor functions of the ulnar, radial, and median nerves. Cervical spinal nerve root injury or entrapment can refer pain and other symptoms to the distal upper extremity. Neurovascular compromise in thoracic outlet syndrome must be ruled out when patients report elbow, wrist, and hand problems.

COMMON PROBLEMS

The upper extremity is used so frequently and requires such precision that even minor disturbances to function, range of motion, and sensation significantly influence work and personal activities. Many of the conditions described in the following sections may be related to neuroarticular dysfunction of the elbow, wrist, and hand, or to more proximal involvement of the shoulder, clavicle, and cervical vertebrae. When a patient experiences upper extremity problems, be sure to conduct a comprehensive history including occupational history, a thorough regional assessment including relevant orthopedic and neurological examinations, and appropriate radiological examinations where indicated.

Restricted or Altered Range of Motion

The elbow is a complex set of three synovial joints with coordinated interaction that enables the elbow to assume precise positions and provide the support necessary for fine motor activities of the hands and fingers.[5] The humeroulnar and humeroradial joints form the medial and lateral portions of the elbow joint proper. The two articulations constitute a freely movable hinge joint or *diarthrodial ginglymus*. As a hinge joint, the elbow is uniaxial and enables flexion and extension of the forearm. The proximal radioulnar joint is anatomically a *diarthrodial trochoid* or pivoting synovial joint. It consists of the head of the radius and the annular ligament—a loop of strong fibrous tissue that extends from the radial notch on the ulna to encircle the radial head. The osteoligamentous nature of the annular ligament gives it enough strength to maintain the anatomical proximity of the proximal ulna and the radial head while at the same time allowing the radius to turn freely during the actions of pronation and supination of the forearm and hand. Average range of motion values for the elbow are listed in Box 17-1.[6-8]

Because fluid-coordinated motion of the elbow is essential for so many upper extremity functions, any reduction or alteration of elbow range of motion can impair activity.

Two principal ligaments provide ligamentous stability of the elbow. The medial or ulnar collateral ligament runs from the medial epicondyle of the humerus to the proximal shaft of the ulna. It provides stability to the medial compartment of the elbow joint by resisting valgus stress or distortion. Supporting the patient's forearm while simultaneously trying to stress the elbow joint medially constitutes a valgus stress maneuver. Pain or excessive laxity in the medial aspect of the elbow joint suggests tearing or stretching of the medial collateral ligament.

The lateral or radial collateral ligament runs from the lateral epicondyle of the humerus to insert on the annular ligament, the proximal shaft of the radius, and the proximal ulna. It provides stability to the lateral compartment of the elbow joint by resisting varus bending or distortion. A varus stress maneuver is performed by supporting the patient's forearm while simultaneously trying to stress the elbow joint laterally. Pain or excessive laxity in the lateral aspect of the elbow joint suggests tearing or stretching of the lateral collateral ligament. In addition, the lateral collateral ligament functions to check elbow extension and maintain proximity of the annular ligament and humerus during pronation and supination of the forearm.

Examine the elbow for passive and active ranges of motion. Ask the patient to try to touch the shoulder of the arm that is being tested to demonstrate active flexion. A patient with developed biceps muscles may not be able to achieve the full 130 to 140 degrees of flexion because of muscle mass. Always compare left and right arms for symmetry and coordinated motion. Note any evidence of tremor, muscle weakness, or pain-limited motion during active flexion.

To assess passive range of motion of the elbow, cup the posterior aspect of the proximal forearm with one hand so that the fingers extend over the elbow. Grasping the forearm or wrist with the other hand, gently move the elbow into full flexion. Palpate for movement of the olecranon process of the ulna as it opens outward from the olecranon fossa on the posterior humerus. Palpate for the head of the radius as it swings anteriorly over the capitulum of the humerus. Note any pain, crepitus, or aberrant motion of the elbow during passive flexion.

Have the patient actively extend the arm at the elbow. On full extension, the arm typically forms an angle of 180 degrees at the elbow. Hypertonicity of flexor muscles from heavy lifting resulting in hypertrophy may restrict extension slightly as a normal physiological variant to range of motion. Many female patients and some males may be able to demonstrate hyperextension of the elbow up to 5 degrees. Again, this hyperextensibility is a normal variant if bilateral.

To examine passive extension of the elbow, begin by asking the patient to hold the arm relaxed with the elbow flexed to about 25 to 30 degrees. Cup the posterior aspect of the proximal forearm with one hand so that the fingers extend over the elbow. Place the thumb and

Box 17-1	**Elbow Ranges of Motion**
Flexion	130 to 140 degrees
Extension	0 to 5 degrees
Pronation	90 degrees
Supination	90 degrees

The range-of-motion values listed here and elsewhere in *The Activator Method* are averages of values published in various sources and should not be interpreted as "normal" for a given patient. Ranges of motion may be influenced by factors such as age, gender, weight, build, and general physical activity.

middle fingers on the lateral and medial epicondyles of the humerus, and position the index finger on the olecranon process of the ulna. Grasp the forearm or wrist with the other hand, and gently straighten the arm into full extension at the elbow. As the olecranon process closes into the olecranon fossa with extension, the three fingers of the stabilizing hand should line up such that the olecranon process is on a line between the two humeral epicondyles. The small gap between the posterior aspect of the head of the radius and the capitular process of the humerus should close with extension of the elbow. Note any pain, palpable or audible crepitus, or aberrant motion of the elbow during extension.

To assess active pronation and supination of the forearm, have the patient stand or sit with elbows flexed, forearms directed forward, and palms of the hands parallel and facing each other. First, ask the patient to demonstrate pronation by medially rotating the forearms and hands 90 degrees so that the palms are parallel to the floor. Next, ask the patient to return the hands to the neutral starting position. Finally, ask the patient to demonstrate supination by laterally rotating the forearms and hands 90 degrees so that the palms are parallel to the ceiling. Observe the motions of supination and pronation, and note any lack of symmetry from side to side and any restriction to the full 90 degrees of rotation in each direction.

When assessing passive supination and pronation, grasp the wrist or forearm firmly. Rotate the forearm into supination and pronation with one hand while palpating the radial head with the other hand. The head of the radius should roll smoothly within the annular ligament; this motion is readily palpable on the posterior lateral aspect of the forearm, about ½ inch distal to the lateral epicondyle of the humerus.

The radiocarpal joint or wrist is an *ellipsoidal diarthrosis* in which the distal radius articulates with the two carpal bones, the carpal scaphoid or navicular, and the lunate.[9] The ellipsoidal configuration of the wrist permits motion in two axes. Normal motions of the wrist include flexion, extension, radial deviation, and ulnar deviation. Average values for wrist range of motion are listed in Box 17-2.[6-8]

Restricted range of motion of the wrist due to pain, degenerative changes, and fibrotic and calcific infiltration caused by RMI can be severely debilitating to the patient.

Before evaluating passive and active range of motion of the wrist, inspect the patient's hands

Box 17-2	**Wrist Ranges of Motion**
Flexion	70 to 90 degrees
Extension	70 degrees
Radial deviation	20 degrees
Ulnar deviation	20 degrees

The range-of-motion values listed here and elsewhere in *The Activator Method* are averages of values published in various sources and should not be interpreted as "normal" for a given patient. Ranges of motion may be influenced by factors such as age, gender, weight, build, and general physical activity.

and wrists in a neutral, relaxed position. If a patient reports wrist or hand pain, especially from RSI, this part of the examination is crucial. Visualize the longitudinal axis of the hand and wrist by sighting a straight line along the third metacarpal, the lunate, and Lister's tubercle on the posterior aspect of the distal radius. Angulation of the axial line to the thumb side suggests radial deviation deformity, and angulation to the little finger side suggests ulnar deviation deformity of the wrist.

Ask the patient to demonstrate active flexion, extension, and radial and ulnar deviation of the wrist. Note pain-restricted movement in any of the four ranges of motion, and observe for symmetrical, fluid motion. Next, have the patient extend the wrists by placing the palms together in a "praying hands" position. Finally, ask the patient to flex the wrists by placing the backs of the hands together. Again, note symmetry of flexion and extension and any pain associated with the motions.

To assess passive range of motion of the wrist, support the forearm by grasping it firmly at the distal radioulnar joint. Hold the patient's hand and place a thumb over the radiocarpal joint. Gently bend the wrist into flexion. Note joint end play, and palpate for the lunate to protrude as the limit of flexion is attained. Then bend the wrist into extension. The lunate, if mobile, should slide anteriorly with extension. Next, reposition the thumb in the patient's anatomical snuff box. The carpal scaphoid or navicular forms the floor of the snuff box. Gently bend the wrist into ulnar deviation, and palpate for the scaphoid to slide out from under the radial styloid process. Finally, move the thumb to the opposite side of the hand, and palpate for the triquetrum bone, the most medial of the proximal carpal bones. As the hand is gently bent into radial deviation, palpate for the triquetrum bone to slide out from the styloid process of the distal ulna. Note any point tenderness, crepitus, or aberrant motion of the wrist on passive range of motion.

Medial and Lateral Epicondylitis

A relatively common painful condition of the medial compartment of the elbow is medial epicondylitis, also known as "golfer's elbow," "bowler's elbow," and "little leaguer's elbow." The cause of pain or discomfort could be a sprain injury of the medial collateral ligament or a strain injury affecting the tendons of the common flexor muscles of the forearm. Examination of the elbow may reveal point tenderness over the medial epicondyle or in the soft tissue just distal to the epicondyle. The patient may hold the elbow in a guarded and partially flexed position.[10]

If pain is a consequence of a sprain injury to the medial collateral ligament of the elbow, passive extension of the elbow and supination of the forearm will likely reproduce or exacerbate the pain by stretching the ligament. To perform a more definitive assessment of the medial collateral ligament, use a valgus stress maneuver. With the patient's elbow extended, support the forearm with one hand on the medial or ulnar side. Cup the elbow with the other hand such that the fingers extend over the medial epicondyle and the proximal ulna. Simultaneously apply gentle lateral-to-medial pressure at the elbow while applying medial-to-lateral pressure on the forearm. If tearing or laxity of the medial collateral ligament occurs, a palpable gap will open between the medial epicondyle and the proximal ulna. Because the maneuver is performed by passive range of motion testing, reproduction of pain at or immediately distal to the medial epicondyle indicates ligamentous injury.

Medial collateral ligament sprains of the elbow are frequently encountered in throwing sports. Windup and tension in the elbow just before the ball is released generate a strong valgus force on the humeroulnar joint. Repetitive throwing, especially when tissues have become fatigued, increases the risk of medial collateral ligament sprain. Other factors that can contribute to medial collateral ligament injury are awkward throwing mechanics and failure to perform warm-up stretching exercises before throwing.[11]

Medial epicondylitis may result from a strain injury. The common flexor muscles of the forearm, whose bellies make up most of the soft tissue mass of the medial forearm, originate on the medial epicondyle of the humerus and insert on the distal radius, the carpal bones and palmar fascia, the metacarpals, and the phalanges of the fingers. This muscle group includes the flexor carpi ulnaris, flexor carpi radialis, palmaris longus, pronator teres, and flexor digitorum superficialis. Repetitive motion, especially motion involving forceful flexion of the wrist, may lead to a periosteal inflammatory reaction or tendinitis at the medial epicondylar attachment of the flexor muscles.[4] Throwing activities, especially those requiring a forceful snap of the wrist into flexion, also can produce medial epicondylitis.[12,13]

To test for strain injury at the medial epicondyle, position the patient with the arm in slight flexion at the elbow. Cup the patient's elbow with one hand positioned so the fingers extend over the medial epicondyle. Use the other hand to resist motion while the patient attempts to flex the wrist and simultaneously pronate the forearm. Make sure the resisted motion increases tension in the muscles and tendons of the flexor group. Reproduction or exacerbation of pain on resisted motion indicates that the medial epicondylitis is a result of strain injury to the flexor and pronator muscles or their common tendinous attachment at the medial epicondyle.[11] Regardless of whether medial epicondylitis results from a sprain injury, a strain injury, or both, the risk of degenerative changes to osseous, cartilaginous, and other tissues is present. "Little leaguer's elbow," for example, can include not only injury to muscles and ligaments but also stress and avulsion fractures of the medial epicondyle.[12] In children and adolescents, in whom endochondral ossification is still under way, the inflammatory reaction at the symphysis of the medial epicondyle can be extremely painful and debilitating. In an acute condition or with acute exacerbation of chronic medial epicondylitis, rest, ice, and compression with an elastic wrap or elbow brace may be warranted.[14]

Complications of unresolved or recurrent medial epicondylitis may include fibrotic and calcific infiltration of the periarticular soft tissues, with the characteristic changes of osteoarthritis. In addition, the ulnar nerve may become entrapped as it courses posterior to the medial epicondyle. Be alert to loss of sensation in the little finger and ring finger and to motor deficits that cause weakness in the flexors of the wrist and fingers.

A novel method for assessing elbow pain from epicondylitis was developed and is known as Polk's test (see Box 17-4). There are two phases to the test, one for lateral epicondylitis (see Figure 17-47) and for medial epicondylitis (see Figure 17-48). Pain associated with lateral epicondylitis, commonly known as "tennis elbow," occurs more frequently than medial epicondylitis.[15] Similar to medial epicondylitis, lateral epicondylitis may be the clinical manifestation of a strain or sprain injury. However, epidemiological studies suggest that most cases involve musculotendinous tissue and therefore are classified as strain injuries.[13]

The lateral epicondyle is the proximal attachment of the common extensor muscles of the forearm, whose bellies make up most of the soft tissue mass of the lateral forearm. The extensor muscle group inserts on the radius, posterior carpal bones, metacarpals, and phalanges of the fingers. A partial list of the extensor muscles that originate on the lateral epicondyle includes brachioradialis, supinator, extensor carpi radialis longus and brevis, extensor carpi ulnaris, and extensor digitorum. In addition, the anconeus, a synergist of the triceps in elbow extension, originates on the lateral epicondyle of the humerus.

To assess lateral epicondylitis of musculotendinous origin, test resisted extension and supination of the wrist and forearm. Cup the patient's elbow with one hand positioned so that the thumb contacts the lateral epicondyle. Hold the patient's forearm in moderate flexion and pronation. Grasp the patient's hand by taking a firm grip of the posterior carpals. Ask the patient to attempt to extend the wrist while simultaneously attempting to extend the elbow and supinate the forearm. Be sure to palpate for increased tension in the extensor muscles and their common tendinous attachment at the lateral epicondyle. Reproduction or exacerbation of pain on resisted extension and supination suggests a strain injury and is indicative of lateral epicondylitis of musculotendinous origin.

Lateral epicondylitis from strain injuries to the common extensor muscle group of the forearm and its tendinous attachment may be of acute onset and associated with a specific activity or injury. The condition also may be of insidious onset yet still be classified as a strain injury. With gradual onset, soft tissues exhibit the effects of cumulative microtrauma frequently associated with repetitive motions involving forceful or resisted extension and supination of the wrist and forearm.

The mechanism of injury in acute onset of lateral epicondylitis appears to be sudden forceful overload of the wrist extensors and the forearm extensors and supinators. The classic case of tennis elbow, for example, is related to the biomechanics of the backhand stroke.[13] In a backhand serve or volley, several events occur simultaneously that place a powerful longitudinal stretching force into the muscles and tendons of the wrist and forearm extensors. In anticipation of the backhand shot, the player's

finger flexion increases on the grip, simply to hold onto and maintain control of the racquet. At the same time, wrist extensors exert tension at the carpal and metacarpal insertions, to keep the wrist and racquet in line with the longitudinal axis of the arm. Last but not least, the player tends to lock the elbow in partial or full extension with the triceps and its synergist, the anconeus, which originates on the lateral epicondyle.

When the backhanded racquet strikes the ball, the force of the impact is amplified through the already contracted extensor muscles. Amplification of force is a function of the simple physics of torque and angular momentum. A force applied to a lever is multiplied by a factor proportionate to the length of the moment arm. In a tennis backhand stroke, the moment arm consists of the length of the forearm *plus* the length of the racquet. Slow motion cinematography of a tennis racquet striking a ball indicates the force of impact on the racquet itself. The force is enough to bend the handle and bow the strings. Clearly, the stretching forces applied to the extensor muscles of the forearm and wrists are enormous. When the stretching forces exceed the tolerances of soft tissues, injury can occur. One study suggests that as many as 50% of all tennis players are affected at some point during their playing career.[16] On the other hand, another study suggests that athletes with reports of humeral epicondylitis account for "... only five percent of the cases in clinical [orthopedic] practice."[14]

Lateral epicondylitis of insidious onset appears to have essentially the same biomechanical origins as the acute case, that is, forceful or resisted extension and supination of the wrist and forearm. Many occupations require activities that can contribute to the gradual development and chronic recurrence of lateral epicondylitis. In fact, occupational injury may explain the observation that less than 5% of patients who seek care for tennis elbow are actually tennis players.[15]

Workers in manual trades, such as electricians, carpenters, and pipe fitters, as well as construction and assembly line workers, typically must perform repetitive tasks that predispose them to strain injuries of the wrist extensors. Use of manual tools such as screwdrivers and wrenches requires forceful extension and supination of the wrist and forearm. Although many manual tools have been redesigned with ergonomically improved hand grips, driving a conventionally threaded screw, bolt, or nut still requires significant work by the extensor and supinator muscles of the wrist and forearm. When the task is repeated hundreds or thousands of times, chronic strain injury is almost inevitable.[17]

Building and mechanical trades are not the only occupations with a high incidence of lateral elbow strain injury. Data entry during computer operation, now a job requirement of a vast number of occupations, increases the risk of lateral epicondylitis, as well as other upper extremity conditions. Repetitive motion strain to wrist extensors is most likely to occur when the keyboard is too high for the operator. Desks and tabletops of conventional height, as well as customer service counters, are common yet poor locations for keyboards. By eliminating keystrokes, the use of a mouse often speeds up computer activity and reduces the number of motions required. However, use of a mouse on too high a surface or for extended periods can cause chronic injury to the muscles and tendons of the wrist and forearm. Other factors such as chair height and support, reach and skill of the operator, and frequency and duration of the task can contribute to the development of repetitive motion or strain injury associated with computer operation and keyboarding.

At an ergonomically sound workstation, a computer operator should be able to sit in a relaxed but erect and alert position. The operator's chair should provide firm support, especially to the lumbar spine. The keyboard must be positioned so that the operator can reach it comfortably with the elbows at the sides and flexed at 90 degrees with the forearms parallel to the floor. In addition, work on the keyboard optimally should be performed with the wrist in a neutral position. Keyboarding should not require the wrists to be held in extension or flexion during work. Furthermore, the operator should not have to bend the wrists into radial or ulnar deviation to achieve the "home position" for typing, or to reach the keys used in most keyboard operations.

When a keyboard is positioned too high for the operator, several problems may result. To reach and work on a keyboard that is too high, the operator must extend the wrists or abduct the shoulders. Normally, neither motion is especially stressful or difficult, but when an operator must hold the position for hours, fatigue, muscle contracture, and joint hypomobility may develop. A typical scenario begins with the operator's wrists held in extension to reach the improperly placed keyboard. Because the wrists are extended, the operator may have to exert more forceful finger flexion than normal to strike the keys.

As the muscles of the hands and the wrist extensors fatigue and become uncomfortable or painful, the operator may compensate by raising the arms into enough shoulder abduction to bring the forearms parallel to the floor. Another compensatory maneuver that the operator may make is to elevate the shoulders and arch the back into extension to get enough lift to relieve the discomfort of the extended wrists. Compensatory shoulder abduction or elevation may give the operator temporary relief from the discomfort felt in the wrists and hands, but these compensations also have their price. Sooner or later, the supraspinatus muscles fatigue and are unable to sustain shoulder abduction. The trapezius and levator scapulae muscles, as well as the paraspinal muscles of the back, will fatigue. The computer user then goes back to keyboarding with the wrists extended. Of course, lateral epicondylitis from chronic strain of the wrist extensor muscles is only one part of the vicious cycle of RMI that is associated with ergonomically unsound computer operation.

Although most cases of lateral epicondylitis present as manifestations of acute or chronic musculotendinous strain injury, the condition also can result from sprain injury to the lateral or radial collateral ligament.[5,10,18] Sudden forceful extension or hyperextension of the elbow may cause stretching or even tearing of the lateral collateral ligament. Body contact sports such as wrestling, martial arts, football, and rugby present many opportunities for hyperextension injury of the elbow. Sudden, forceful torquing motions of the wrist and forearm into pronation (such as those that might be delivered by power tools such as an electric drill, post hole or ice auger, or pneumatic wrenches) can put operators of such equipment at risk for lateral collateral ligament strain.

If pain is a consequence of a sprain injury to the lateral collateral ligament of the elbow, passive extension of the elbow and pronation of the forearm will likely reproduce or exacerbate the pain by stretching the ligament. To perform a definitive assessment of the lateral collateral ligament, use a varus stress maneuver. With the patient's elbow extended, support the forearm with one hand on the lateral or radial side. Cup the elbow with the other hand such that the fingers extend over the lateral epicondyle and the proximal radius. Simultaneously apply gentle medial-to-lateral pressure at the elbow while applying lateral-to-medial pressure on the forearm. If tearing or laxity of the lateral collateral ligament occurs, a palpable gap will open between the lateral epicondyle and the proximal radius. Because the maneuver is performed by passive range of motion testing, reproduction of pain at or immediately distal to the lateral epicondyle also indicates ligamentous injury.

When a patient experiences the signs and symptoms of medial or lateral epicondylitis, perform a thorough assessment of the elbow, to rule out fracture, dislocation, or nerve entrapment. The primary Isolation Test and adjustment for lateral elbow involvement would include the posterior-superior radius and an anterior lunate. When medial elbow involvement is present, the primary Isolation Test and adjustment are for an inferior medial ulna and posterior carpals.

Peripheral Nerve Entrapment Syndromes

Radiating pain, paresthesias, and muscle weakness are classic signs of peripheral nerve entrapment syndrome. The most common examples of nerve entrapment in the distal upper extremity involve the ulnar and median nerves. The ulnar nerve is vulnerable to impingement by soft tissue swelling as it passes posterior to the medial epicondyle. The median nerve is subject to distal entrapment by degenerative or adaptive changes that cause narrowing of the carpal tunnel and proximal entrapment between the ulnar and humeral heads of the pronator teres muscle.[19]

Sprain and strain injuries associated with medial epicondylitis may result in soft tissue swelling that could encroach on the ulnar nerve. Repetitive throwing motions, especially when muscles are fatigued or when poor throwing technique is used, make an athlete vulnerable to ulnar neuritis and neuralgia.[19] The primary site of ulnar nerve entrapment is the ulnar sulcus. a groove on the posterior aspect of the medial epicondyle of the humerus. The nerve is sometimes palpable (and tender) in the sulcus just medial to the olecranon process of the ulna. Palpation of the nerve and soft tissues around it is best performed with the elbow held in moderate flexion at about 45 to 60 degrees less than full extension.

Pain in the ulnar nerve may be obscured by the discomfort of medial epicondylitis. One indication of ulnar nerve entrapment is radiation of pain along the medial aspect of the forearm. A key feature is numbness or altered sensation in the ring and little fingers of the hand on the side of involvement. True weakness and atrophy of the flexor muscles of the fourth and fifth fingers are difficult to detect and, in fact, may not manifest with ulnar nerve entrapment syndrome. One way to test for entrapment of the ulnar nerve is to perform the Tinel or

"tap" test.[20] Palpate for the sulcus, and use the fingers to deliver a sharp, percussive tap to the site. A positive Tinel's sign is reproduction or exacerbation of sharp, electric-like, neuralgic pain, indicative of ulnar nerve entrapment. The ulnar nerve also can be entrapped as it travels through the canal of Guyon in the wrist. The canal of Guyon is formed by the hook of the hamate. Patient complaints are distal to the wrist and are primarily paresthesia types of symptoms. Symptoms are elicited along the medial aspect of the fourth finger, the fifth finger, and the medial aspect of the palm of the hand. Palpation reveals distinct tenderness at the hamate. Repetitive pressure on the palm of the hand, for example, with the use of a stapler and pressing down with the palm of the hand, can result in irritation, hamate involvement, narrowing of the canal of Guyon and entrapment.

Median nerve entrapment is the principal feature of carpal tunnel syndrome. Compression of the median nerve may result from thickening and distortion of soft tissues investing the carpal tunnel, from repetitive strain or sprain injury to the wrist, or from direct compression during use of vibrating hand tools. Along with tenosynovitis, it is one of two diagnoses most frequently ascribed to repetitive workplace injury.[5] Cardinal signs of carpal tunnel syndrome are numbness or tingling and pain and muscle weakness in the thumb, index finger, and middle and lateral aspects of the ring finger. Atrophic changes may include flattening of the thenar eminence of the palm of the hand, coldness in the distal extremity, and gradual, progressive deterioration of peripheral vasculature. In advanced cases, blackening of the nail beds and fingertips can indicate that mummification or dry gangrene is occurring from chronic atrophic and ischemic compression of the median nerve and associated structures.

Two tests that suggest median nerve entrapment and carpal tunnel syndrome can be performed quickly and conveniently. The first is Phalen's test. Instruct the patient to place the backs of the hands together and to hold the wrists in sustained flexion for a period of 1 minute. Reduction in sensation and reproduction or exacerbation of the signs and symptoms of median nerve entrapment strongly suggest active carpal tunnel syndrome. The second test is another Tinel or "tap" test, as noted earlier. Electrodiagnostic studies may be essential for differential diagnosis in some cases.[5]

Although median nerve entrapment can occur at the carpal tunnel, it is important to rule out entrapment proximally between the ulnar and humeral attachments of the pronator teres muscle, commonly known as pronator syndrome. It may be possible to differentiate carpal tunnel syndrome with pronator syndrome if there is an absence of diffuse forearm symptoms, palpable tenderness at the attachment sites of the pronator teres on the proximal ulna and distal medial humerus, and normal muscle strength in the forearm pronators and wrist flexors upon manual resistive strength testing. Ultimately, neurodiagnostic studies are essential for differentiating the location of median nerve entrapment.

Radial Nerve Entrapment

At the proximal area of the forearm, the radial nerve can become entrapped within the radial tunnel. This occurs most commonly in individuals who have highly developed forearm muscles; in a small percentage of cases, it is associated with lateral epicondylitis. Anatomically, the radial nerve pierces the aponeurosis of the radius and ulna, in the area of the supinator muscle. Symptoms of paresthesias and radial nerve entrapment appear along the distribution of the radial nerve on the posterior forearm and hand.

Olecranon Bursitis

Swelling of the olecranon bursae can cause pain and limited range of motion of the elbow in extension or extreme flexion. Several bursae are associated with the posterior elbow. The subcutaneous olecranon bursa may become inflamed in response to minor trauma or repetitive pressure such as that caused by leaning on a desk or table surface.[11] When the subcutaneous bursa is inflamed, pain is produced or exacerbated as the elbow is moved into flexion. Superficial layers of the skin over the olecranon process compress the already swollen and tender bursa, producing more pain.

Additional bursae are found deep to and within the triceps muscle tendon near its insertion on the olecranon process. When one or more of these bursae are inflamed and swollen, movement of the elbow into extension, especially movement against resistance, causes compression and pain in the bursae.

TESTING AND ADJUSTING THE ELBOW, WRIST, AND HAND

When a patient has problems involving the elbow, wrist, or hand, perform Isolation and Stress Tests and adjustments as necessary for the following misalignments:

- Lateral distal end of humerus
- Anterior/posterior proximal ulna–elbow supination/pronation
- Pronator quadratus
- Wrist extensors
- Posterior-superior proximal radius and anterior lunate
- Interior lateral ulna and posterior carpals
- Proximal carpals
- Carpal tunnel–separated distal radius/ulna
- Approximated distal radius/ulna
- Trapeziometacarpal joint
- Anterior proximal first metacarpal
- Medial/superior hamate
- Pisiform
- Interphalangeal joints

Bear in mind that the tests for some of these misalignments and neuroarticular dysfunctions are *Stress Tests*, and some are *Isolation Tests*, that is, patient movements or maneuvers performed by the clinician are intended to move the structure or joint into the direction of misalignment. After performing the test, look for shortening or reactivity of the Pelvic Deficient (PD) leg in Position #1. Use a Pressure Test applied in the direction of adjustment to confirm findings based on any of the Stress or Isolation Tests.

Signs and symptoms of elbow, wrist, and hand involvement may be manifestations of shoulder or cervical articular dysfunction, especially when neurovascular compromise plays a role in the clinical presentation. Be alert to aspects of patient history, parameters of the complaint, and examination findings that suggest shoulder or cervical involvement as causative or concurrent factors in elbow, wrist, and hand dysfunction.

Lateral Distal End of Humerus

For any complaints involving the elbow and chronic, unresolving shoulder complaints, after all scapula and shoulder tests have been tested and cleared, perform the Isolation Test for a lateral distal end of the humerus.

Isolation Test.   To isolate for a lateral distal end of the humerus, instruct the patient to push the involved elbow into the table. The patient should be in the Activator Testing position with the palm facing toward the ceiling (Figure 17-1). Look for reactivity of the PD leg in Position #1.

Adjustment.   To adjust for a lateral distal end of the humerus, instruct the patient to externally rotate the arm so the palm is down on the table in a true anatomical position. This will expose the lateral condyle of the humerus to the doctor for contact (Figure 17-2). Line of Drive (LOD) is medial.

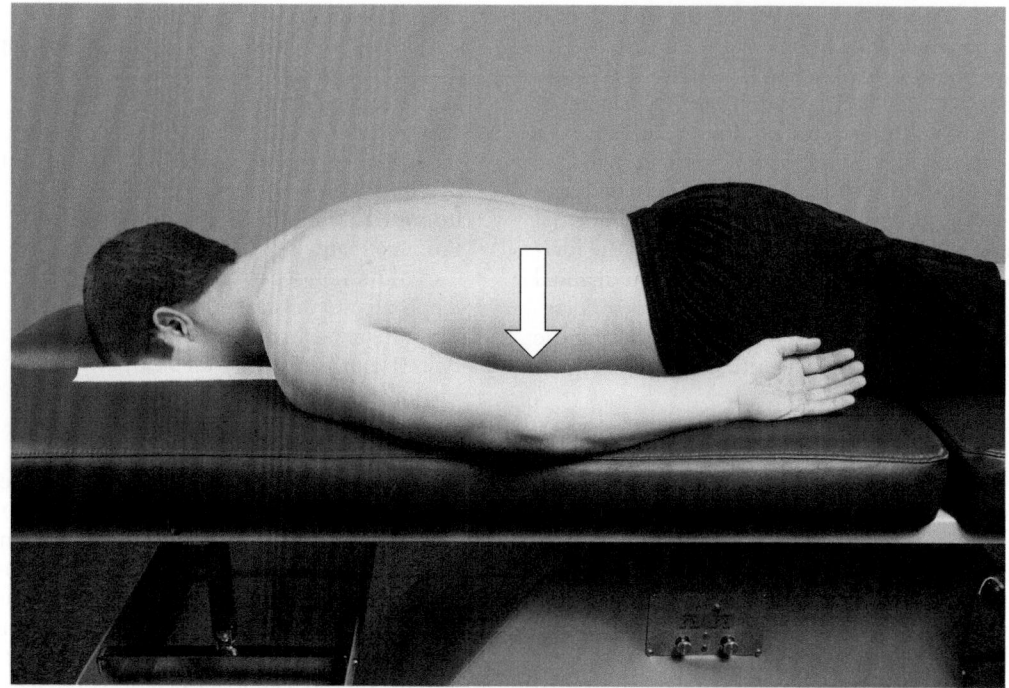

Figure 17-1 Isolation Test for lateral distal humerus. Push elbow into table.

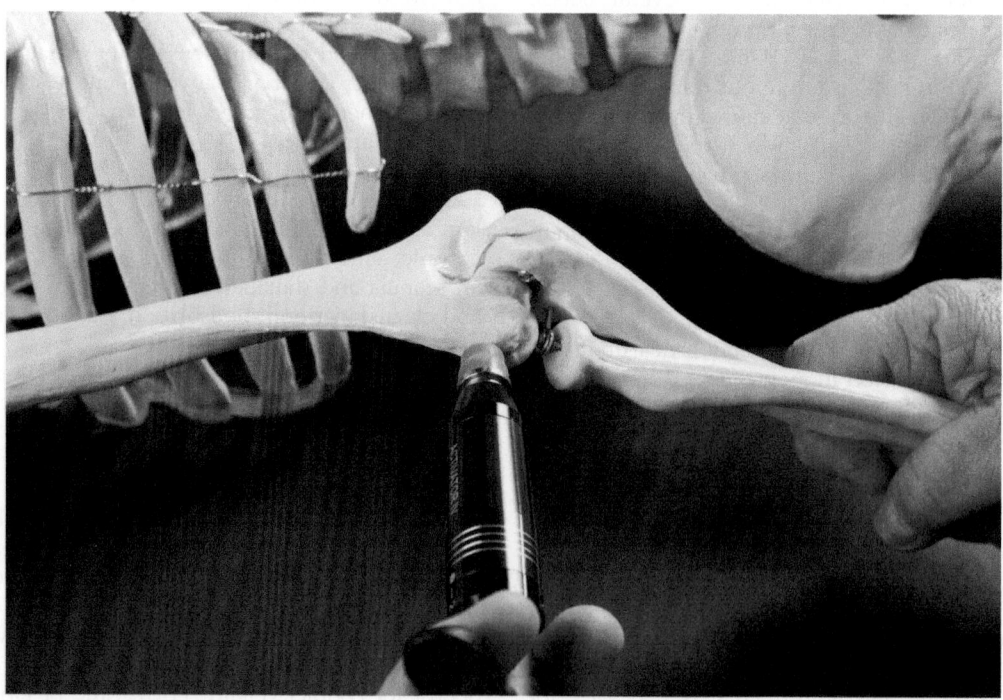

Figure 17-2 Adjustment for lateral distal humerus. Rotate arm so the palm is down. Line of Drive is straight medial.

Anterior/Posterior Proximal Ulna–Elbow Pronation/Supination

This is common in tennis forehand strokes with top spin, golf swing on the hand closest to the top of the club, writing for a prolonged time, carpal tunnel syndrome, and ulnar nerve distribution symptoms.

Isolation Test. Instruct the patient to rest the arm of the involved side off the table slightly to induce at least 30 degrees of flexion in the elbow. Stabilize above the elbow with your hand, and have the patient or the doctor pronate the forearm (Figure 17-3). Check for involvement of a posterior proximal ulna by looking for reactivity of the PD leg in Position #1. Follow the same protocol as was outlined previously, except supinate the forearm (Figure 17-4). Check for involvement of an anterior proximal ulna while looking for reactivity of the PD leg in Position #1.

Adjustment. For pronation, or a posterior proximal ulna, have the patient return to the Activator Testing position with the palm facing away from the table and the elbow in approximately 90 degrees of flexion. Contact the posterior proximal end of the ulna, and adjust with the LOD superior and medial, directed through the shaft of the humerus (Figure 17-5).

For supination, or an anterior proximal ulna, have the patient return to the Activator Testing position with the palm facing away from the table and the elbow in approximately 30 degrees of flexion. Contact the anterior proximal end of the ulna, and adjust with the LOD inferior (distal) and anatomically medial (Figure 17-6).

CLINICAL TIP: The anterior-posterior proximal ulna can be a difficult test to remember, as can the direction of supination and pronation. If you hold a bowl of soup, you are in the supination position. Pouring out the soup is pronation. A clue is to keep your **P**'s together. With **P**ronation of the forearm, the involvement is a **P**osterior, **P**roximal ulna. Test this one first so you can remember it, and then check supination of the forearm for involvement of the anterior proximal ulna.

Pronator Quadratus

With symptoms and complaints of carpal tunnel syndrome, as well as forearm, wrist, and hand problems, consider involvement of the pronator quadratus.

Isolation Test. After clearing the wrist and shoulder tests, instruct the patient to pronate the involved hand to full range of motion (Figure 17-7), and look for reactivity of the PD leg in Position #1 for involvement.

Adjustment. There are two contact points on the radial side of the forearm.

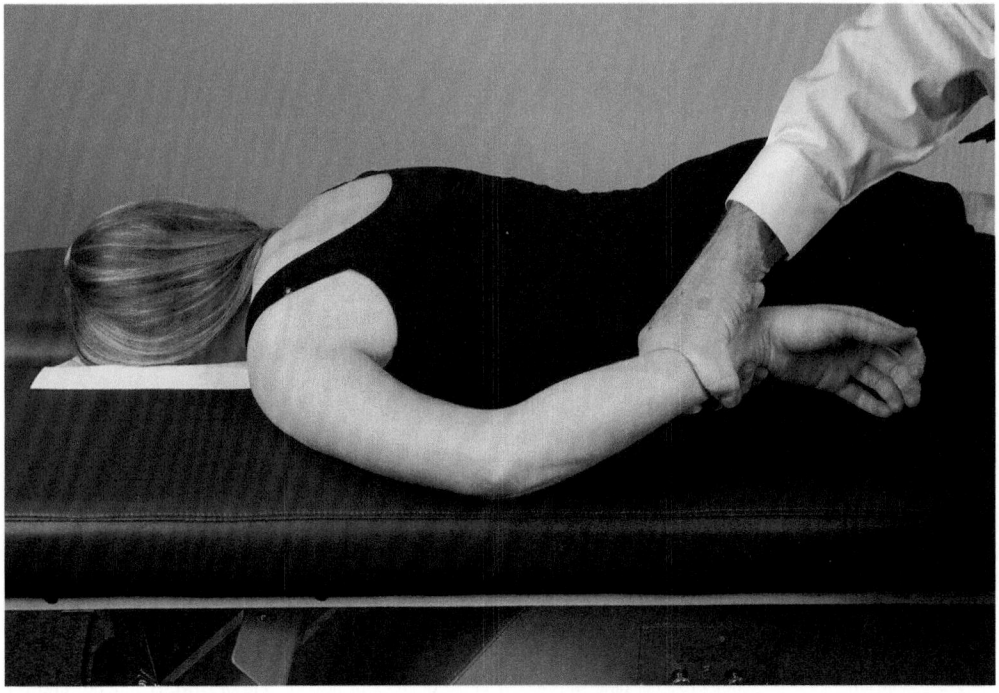

Figure 17-3 Stress Test for posterior proximal ulna. Doctor pronates the forearm.

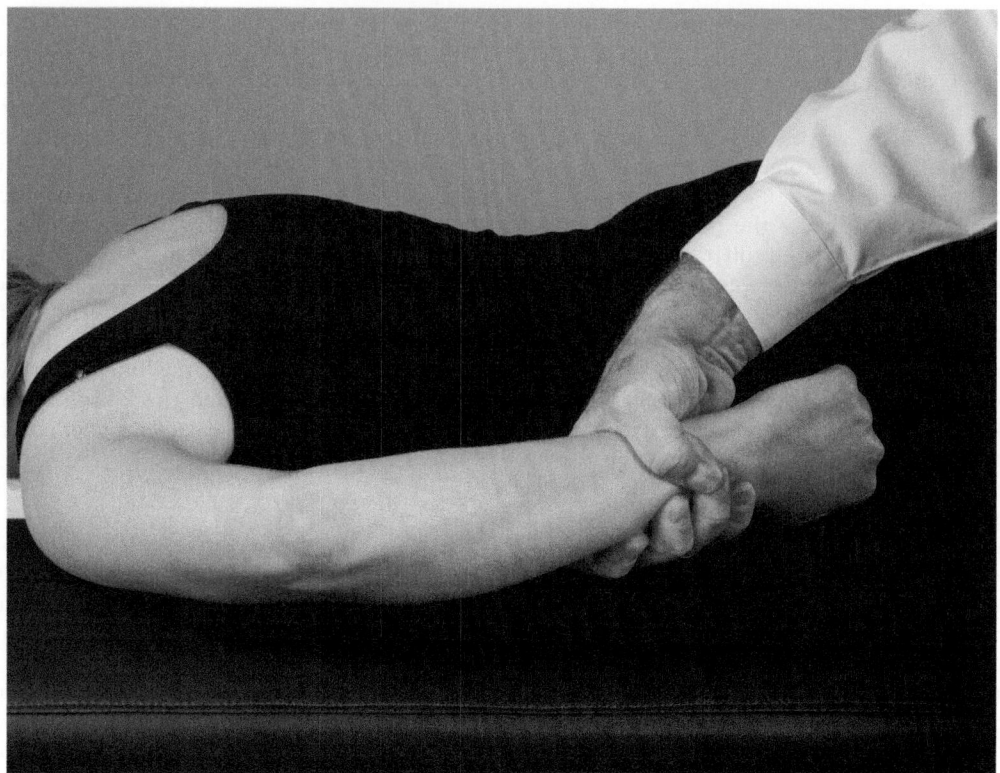

Figure 17-4 Stress Test for anterior proximal ulna. Doctor supinates the forearm.

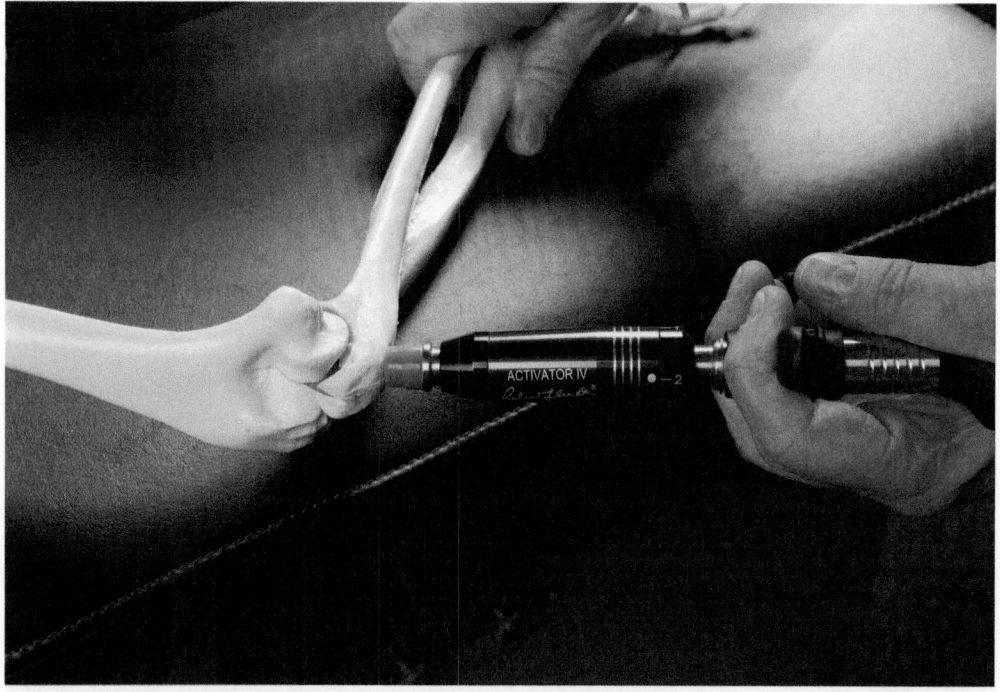

Figure 17-5 Adjustment for posterior proximal ulna with elbow at 90 degrees of flexion. Line of Drive is superior and medial, directed through the shaft of the humerus.

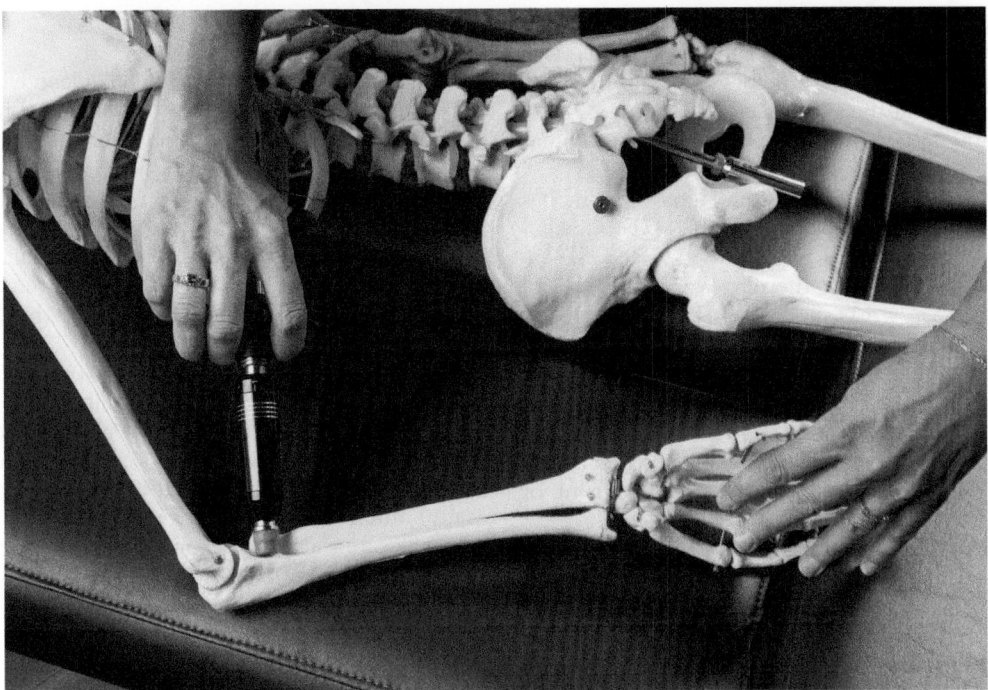

Figure 17-6 Adjustment for anterior proximal ulna with elbow at 30 degrees of flexion. Line of Drive is lateral and slightly inferior.

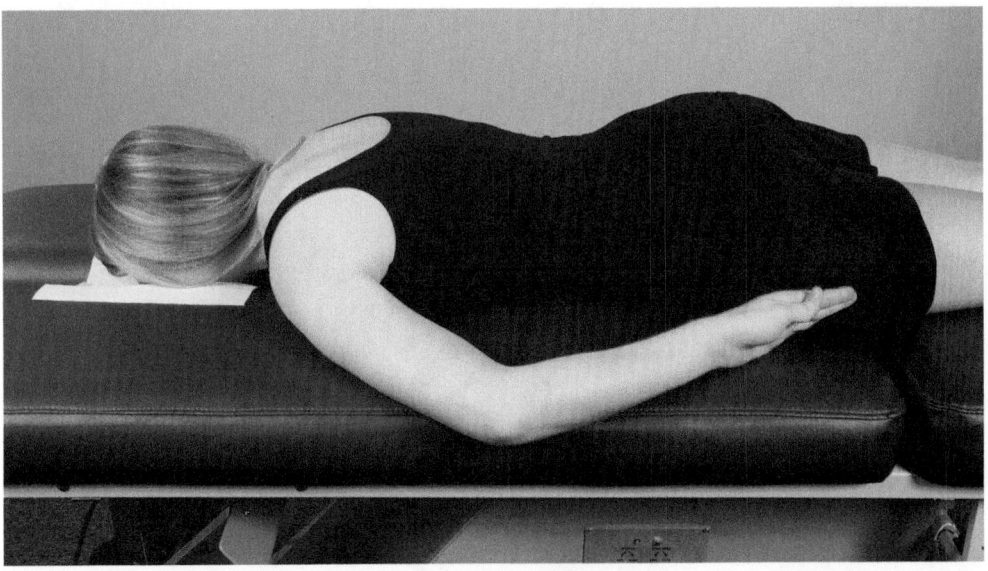

Figure 17-7 Isolation Test for pronator quadratus; patient maximally pronates the forearm.

Step One: Contact 1½ inches proximal from the wrist, and the LOD is lateral (Figure 17-8).

Step Two: Contact 3 inches proximal from the wrist, and the LOD is lateral (Figure 17-9).

Contact points three and four are on the ulnar side of the forearm.

Step Three: Contact the ulna 1½ inches proximal to the wrist, and the LOD is medial (Figure 17-10).

Step Four: Contact the ulna 3 inches proximal to the wrist, and the LOD is medial (Figure 17-11).

Wrist Extensors

For patients who present with complaints of tennis elbow–related symptoms and proximal forearm pain, consider testing for involvement of the wrist extensor muscles.

Isolation Test. After checking and clearing the posterior superior proximal radius, instruct the patient to extend the affected wrist against resistance of the doctor (Figure 17-12). Look for reactivity of the PD leg in Position #1 for involvement.

Adjustment. Place the involved arm on the table next to the head with the palm down on the table. Contact 1½ inches distal to the end of the elbow crease, and the LOD is anatomically anterior (Figure 17-13).

Posterior-Superior Proximal Radius and Anterior Lunate

When a patient experiences lateral epicondylitis or difficulty completing full pronation or supination of the forearm, consider a posterior-superior proximal radius and a corresponding anterior lunate.

Isolation Test. To isolate for a posterior-superior proximal radius, ask the patient to make a fist with the hand on the side of involvement (Figure 17-14). Look for reactivity of the PD leg in Position #1.

Adjustment. Adjust for a posterior-superior proximal radius and anterior lunate in two steps. First, place the patient's forearm alongside the head. Contact the posterior aspect of the proximal head of the radius. The LOD is (anatomically) anterior and inferior (Figure 17-15).

To locate the contact point for adjustment of the posterior-superior radius, ask the patient to pronate and supinate the forearm and hand. The head of the radius will be palpable as a bony prominence that rolls in the annular ligament with supination and pronation. If the patient has active lateral epicondylitis, avoid discomfort to the patient by taking a superior-to-inferior (proximal-to-distal) tissue pull over the radial head with the thumb of the stabilization hand. Use the thumb to stabilize the instrument during the adjustment.

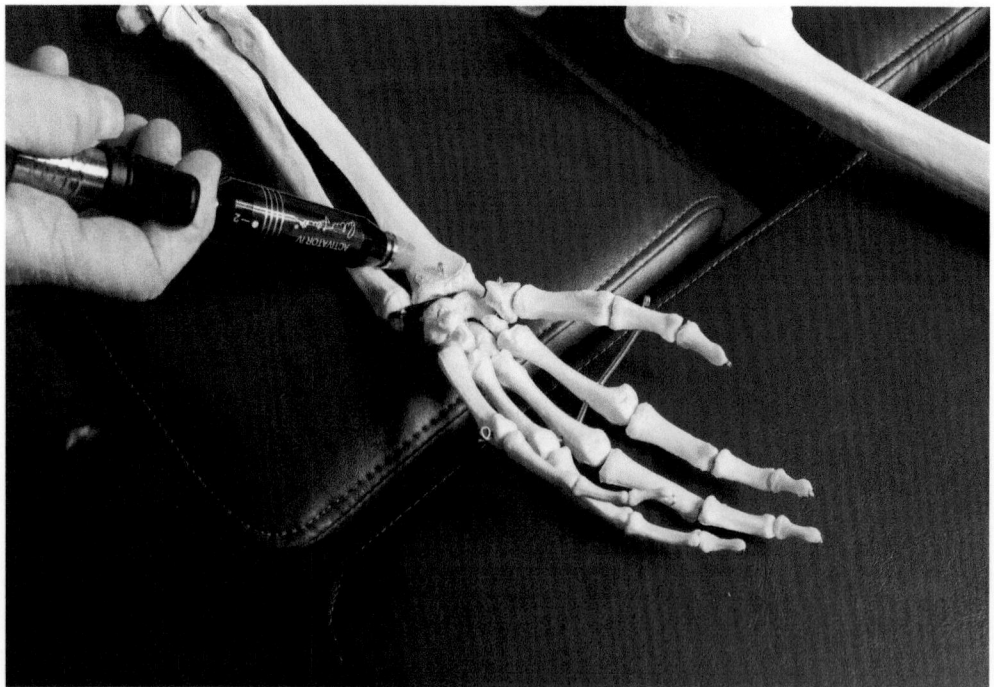

Figure 17-8 Adjustment for pronator quadratus. Step One: Contact 1½ inches proximal from the wrist on the radial side. Line of Drive is lateral.

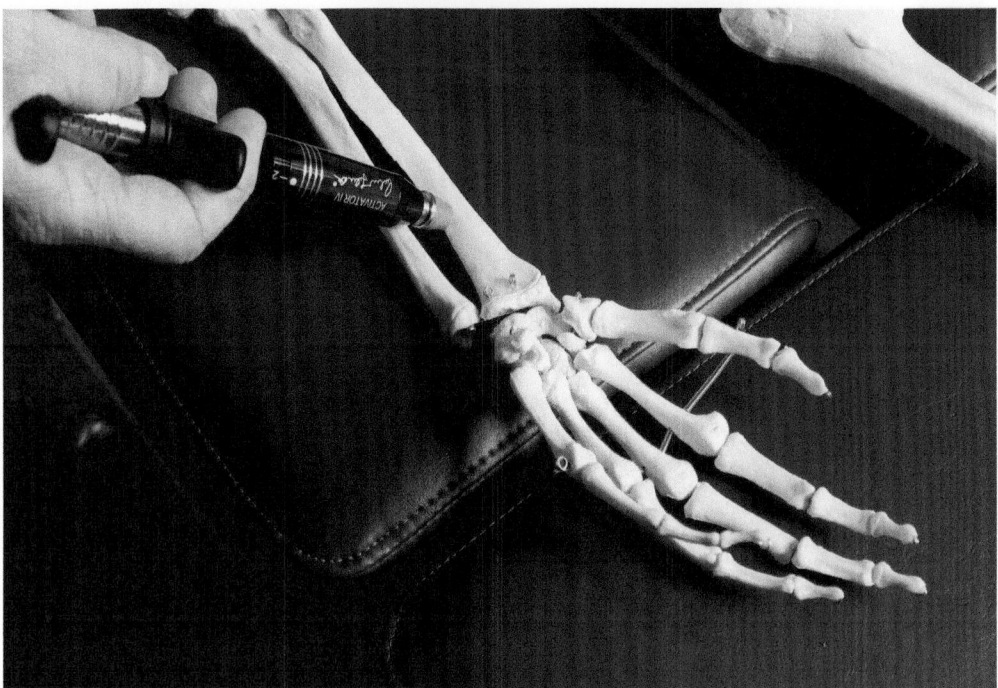

Figure 17-9 Adjustment for pronator quadratus. Step Two: Contact 3 inches proximal from the wrist on the radial side. Line of Drive is lateral.

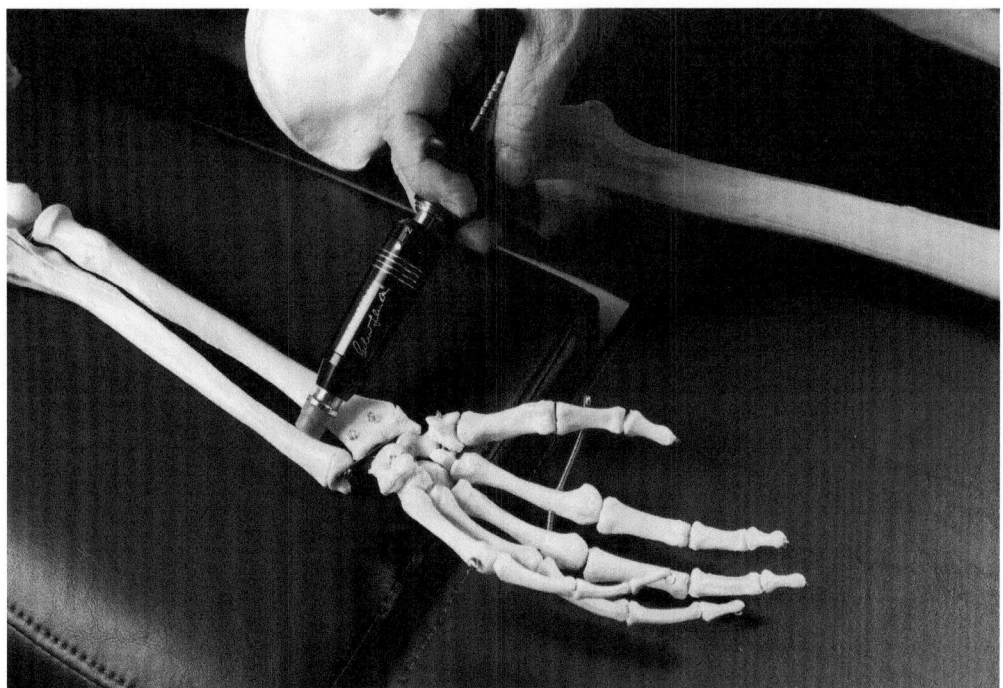

Figure 17-10 Adjustment for pronator quadratus. Step Three: Contact the ulna 1½ inches proximal to the wrist. Line of Drive is medial.

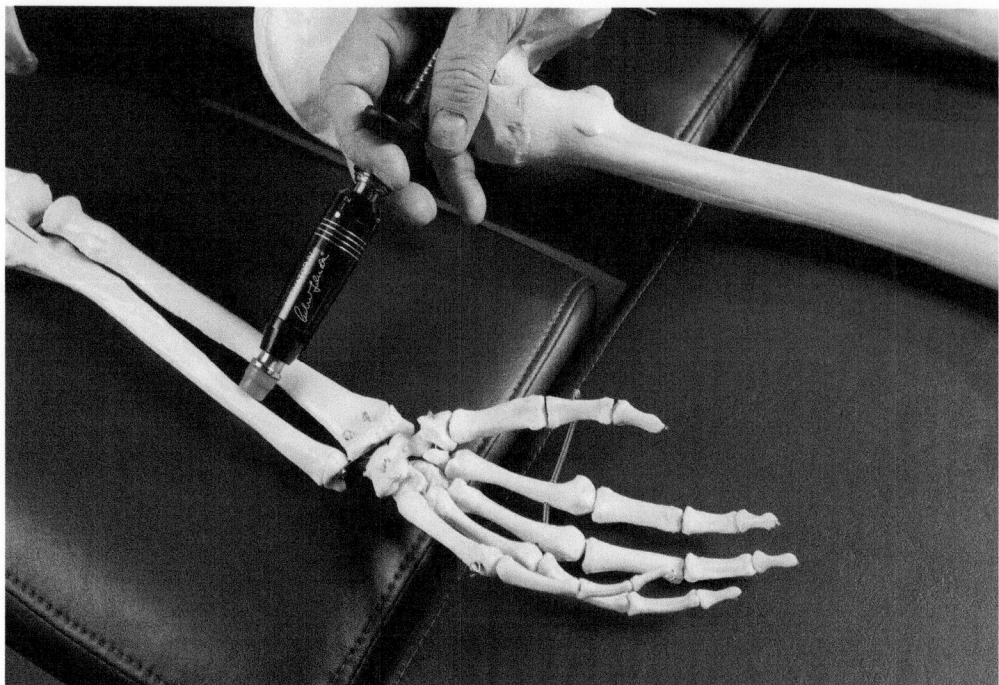

Figure 17-11 Adjustment for pronator quadratus. Step Four: Contact the ulna 3 inches proximal to the wrist. Line of Drive is medial.

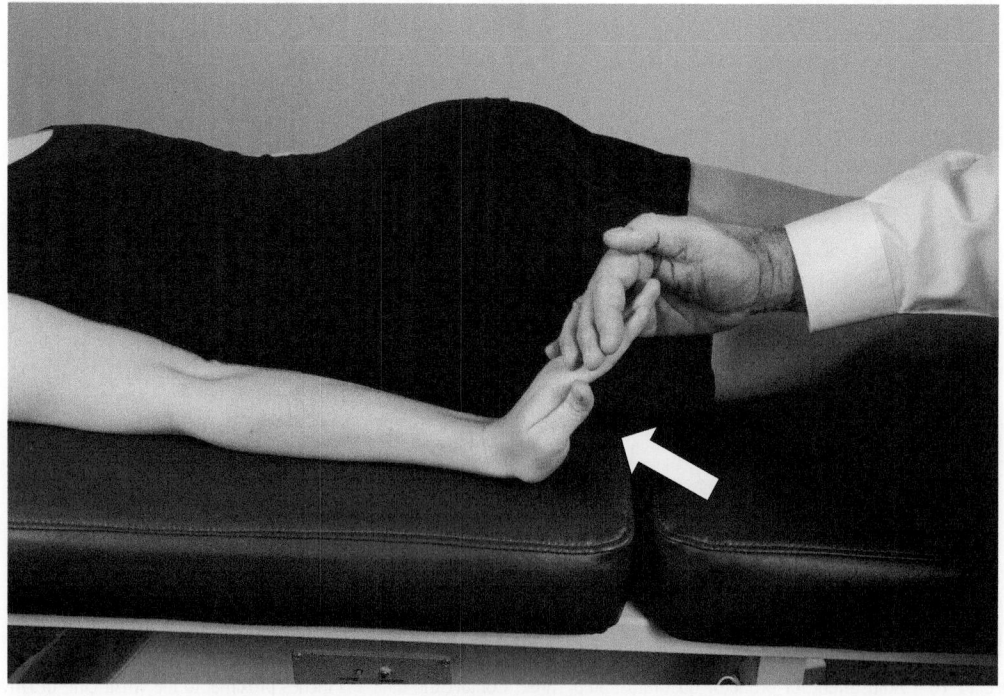

Figure 17-12 Isolation Test for wrist extensors; resist wrist extension.

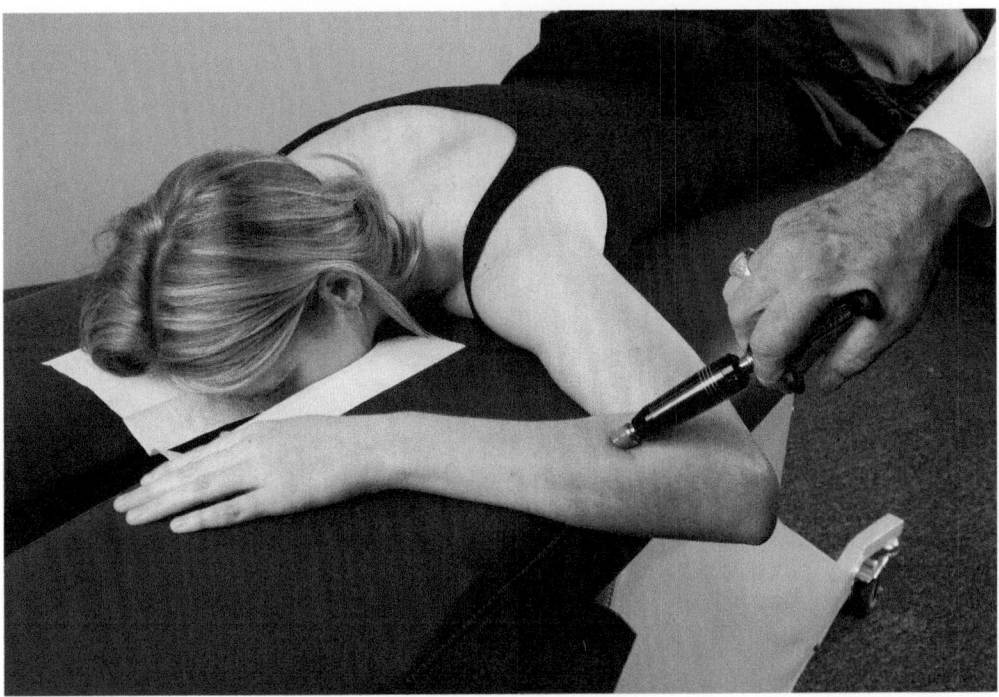

Figure 17-13 Adjustment for wrist extensors. Line of Drive is anatomically anterior.

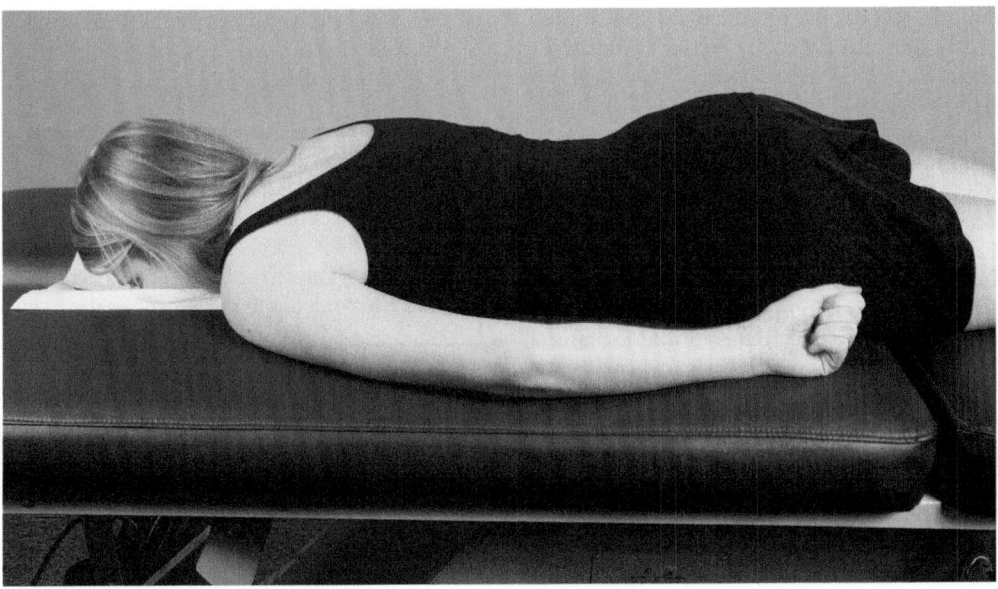

Figure 17-14 Isolation Test for posterior-superior proximal radius and anterior lunate.

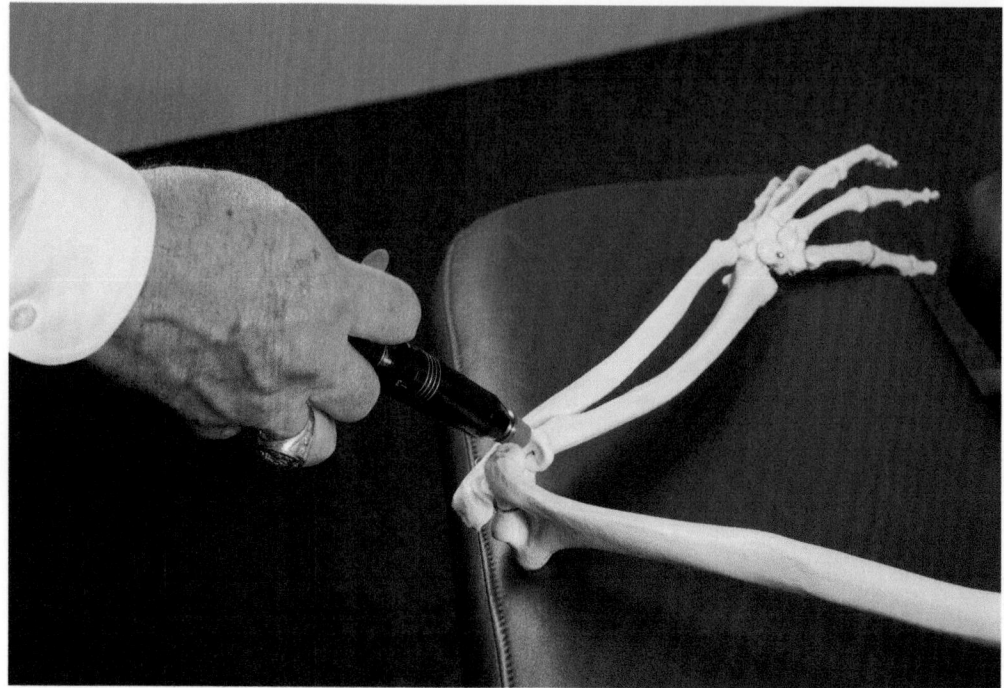

Figure 17-15   Adjustment for posterior-superior proximal radius. Line of Drive is anterior and inferior.

Next, place the arm down at the patient's side with the forearm and wrist pronated so the palm of the hand faces the ceiling. Contact the anterior aspect of the lunate by positioning the instrument on the volar aspect of the wrist just distal to the wrist crease. The LOD is straight posterior (Figure 17-16).

Inferior Lateral Ulna and Posterior Carpals

When a patient exhibits signs and symptoms of medial epicondylitis, or when there is pain on flexion of the wrist, consider an inferior medial ulna and corresponding posterior carpals.

Isolation Test.   To isolate for an inferior lateral ulna, ask the patient to flex the wrist on the involved hand (Figure 17-17). Look for reactivity of the PD leg in Position #1.

Adjustment.   Adjust for an inferior lateral ulna and posterior carpals in two steps. First, position the patient's arm at the side of the body with the wrist pronated so the palm of the hand faces the ceiling. The shoulder should be in slight abduction and the elbow slightly flexed. Contact the anterior aspect of the ulna just distal to the olecranon. The LOD is superior (proximal) and anatomically medial (Figure 17-18).

Next, place the patient's hand palm down on the table. The LOD is straight anterior on each posterior carpal (two to three thrusts, depending on the hand size of the patient). (Figures 17-18, 17-19, and 17-20 are illustrated on right side for photographic reasons.)

> **Clinical Observations**
>
> Most cases of lateral epicondylitis involve strain injury to the common extensor and supinator muscles of the forearm.[13] Pain and reactive hypertonicity or spasm of these muscles may contribute to posterior superior misalignment of the radius.

Proximal Carpals

When a patient reports wrist pain, especially with limited wrist extension and increased pain upon extension, consider involvement of the proximal carpals.

Isolation Test.   Ask the patient to extend the wrist, and look for PD leg reactivity in Position #1 (Figure 17-21).

Adjustment.   Adjustment involves multiple contacts and thrust on the posterior aspect of the proximal carpal row. Make sure that contact and adjustments avoid the lunate. Depending on

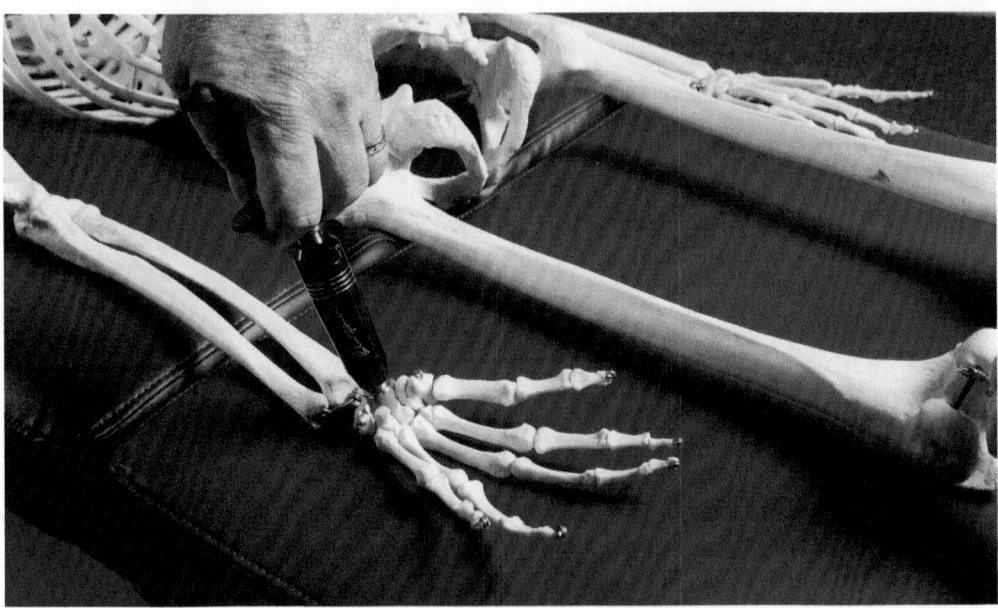

Figure 17-16 Adjustment for anterior lunate. Line of Drive is straight posterior.

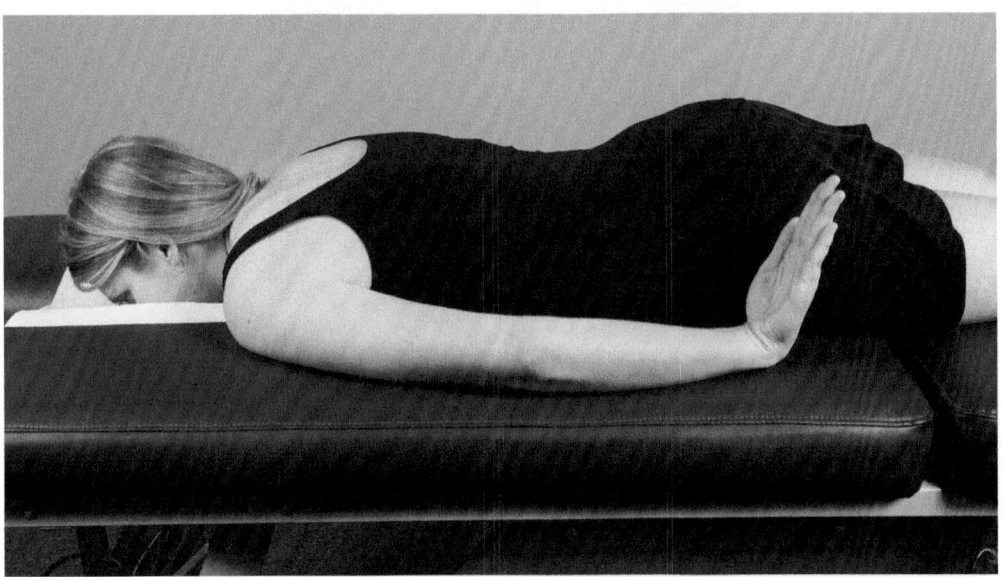

Figure 17-17 Isolation Test for inferior medial ulna and posterior distal carpals.

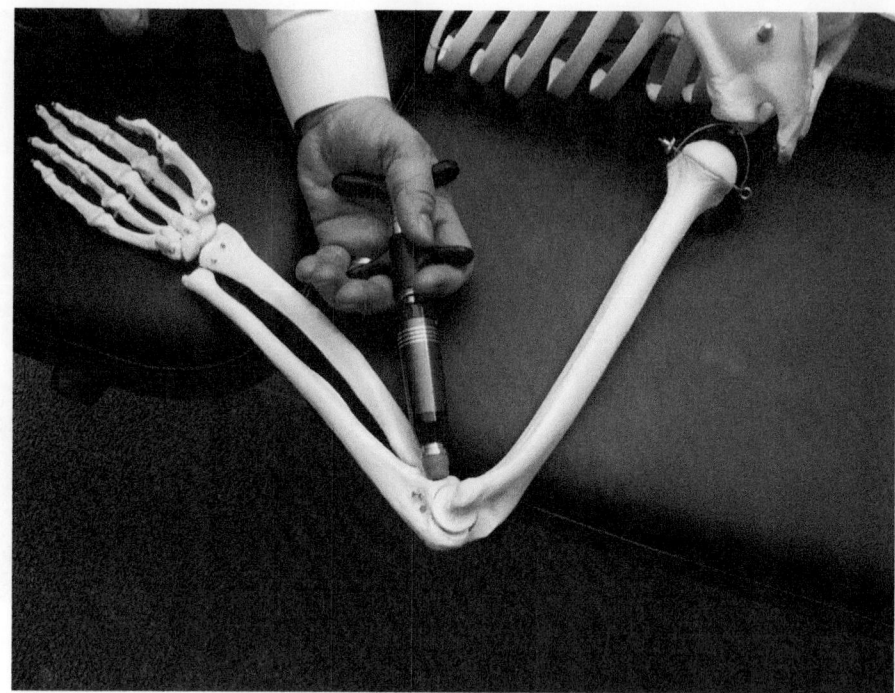

Figure 17-18   Adjustment for inferior medial ulna. Line of Drive is superior and lateral.

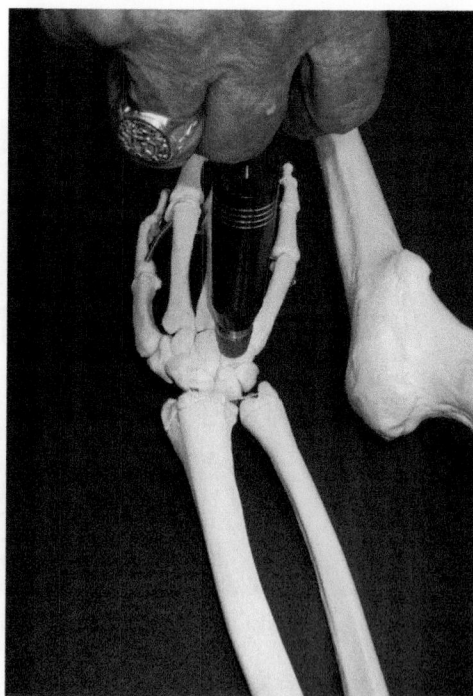

Figure 17-19   Adjustment for posterior carpals, one of two contacts. Line of Drive is anterior.

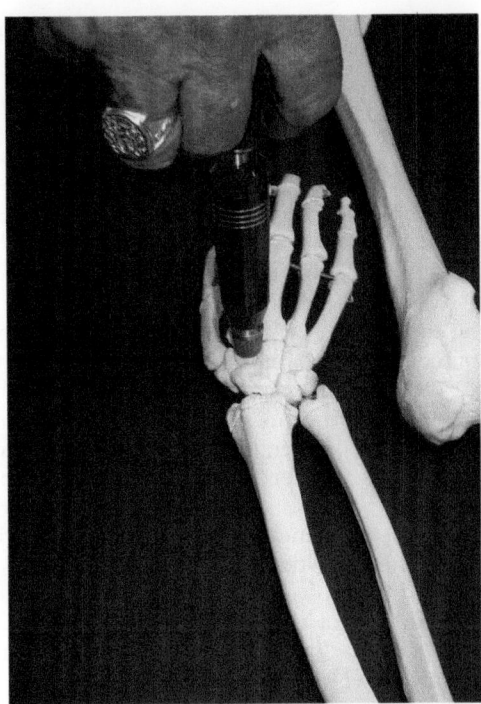

Figure 17-20 Adjustment for posterior carpals, two of two contacts. Line of Drive is anterior.

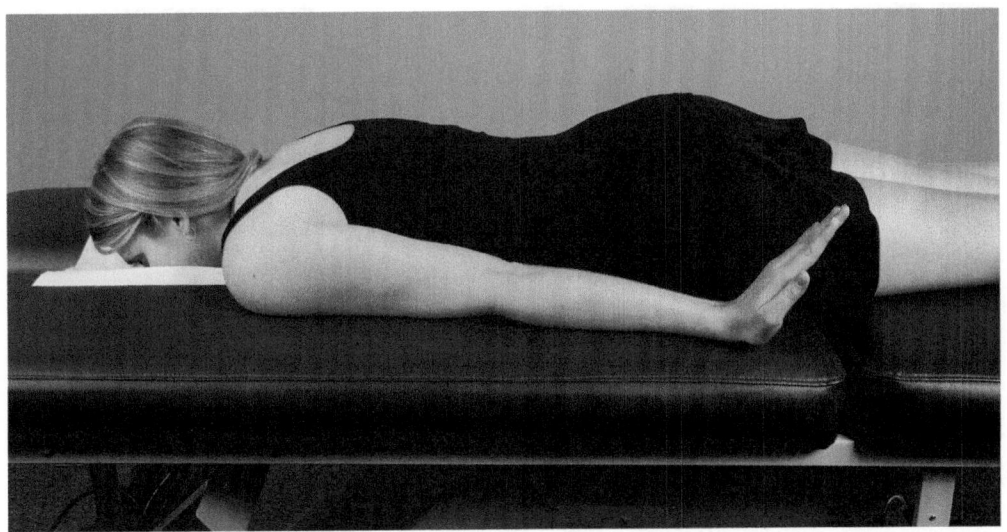

Figure 17-21 Isolation for posterior, proximal carpals.

the size of the wrist, two to three thrusts should be performed on the individual bones of the proximal carpal row. The LOD is anterior and inferior (Figures 17-22 and 17-23).

Carpal Tunnel–Separated Distal Radius and Ulna

When a patient presents with symptoms of carpal tunnel syndrome, such as numbness and tingling into the first three digits with or without weakness, or if the diagnosis of entrapment of the median nerve in the carpal tunnel has been concluded on the basis of outcomes of nerve conduction studies or positive orthopedic tests such as the Tinel tap at the wrist, prayer sign, or Phalen's/reverse Phalen's test, consider adjusting the attachments of the flexor retinaculum.

Isolation Test. To isolate the carpal tunnel area, instruct the patient to press together the tips of the thumb and fifth digit on the involved side (Figure 17-24). Look for reactivity of the PD leg in Position #1.

Adjustment. To adjust for carpal tunnel involvement, use two thrusts. With the patient's palm up, first contact the lateral aspect of the distal radius. The LOD is anatomically lateral to medial (the ulnar direction) (Figure 17-25). The second contact is on the medial aspect

of the distal ulna, and the LOD is anatomically medial to lateral (in the radial direction) (Figure 17-26).[21]

Clinical Observations

Stenosing tenosynovitis of the tendon sheaths of the abductor pollicis longus and extensor pollicis brevis is the key characteristic of DeQuervain's disease. A diagnostic test for the condition is Finkelstein's test, during which the patient forms a fist with the thumb wrapped inside the fingers. The examiner then passively deviates the hand and wrist to the ulnar side. Sharp pain with the maneuver suggests soft tissue swelling and impingement of stenosing synovitis. Because the Activator Method Isolation Test for a trapeziometacarpal joint is clearly modeled on Finkelstein"s test, be alert to patient reports of pain during the maneuver.

Recurrent trapeziometacarpal joint dysfunction may result from repetitive motion injury to the hand. Activities that require forceful gripping of tools or operation of vibrating equipment may cause or exacerbate thumb joint instability and dysfunction. If equipment or operation technique is not changed, more serious vascular occlusion or nerve entrapment may develop.[21]

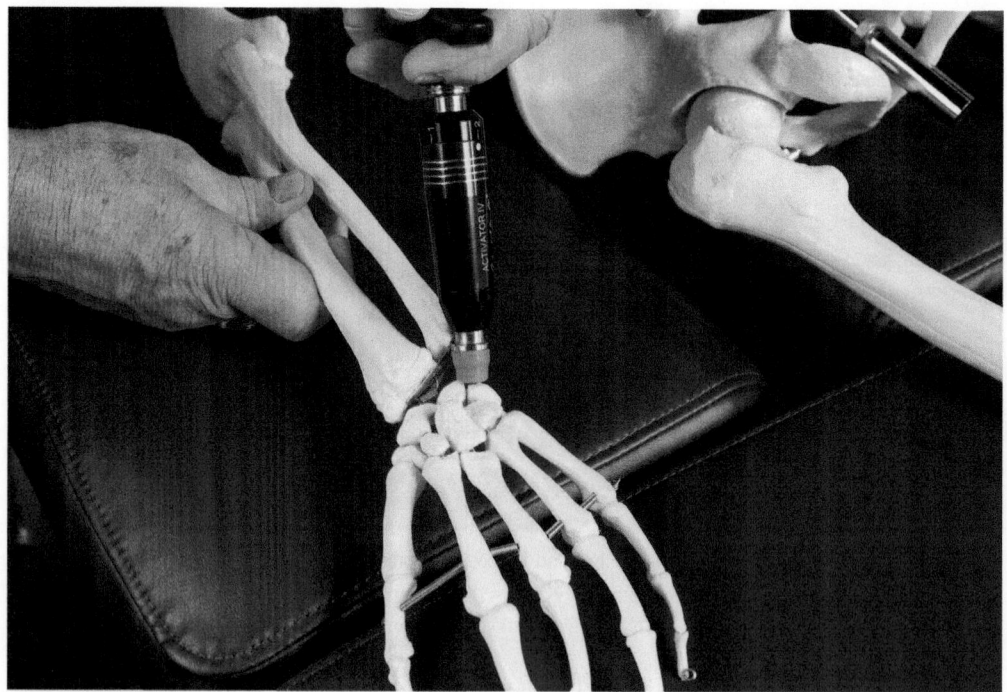

Figure 17-22 Adjustment for posterior, proximal carpals, one of two contacts. Line of Drive is anterior and inferior.

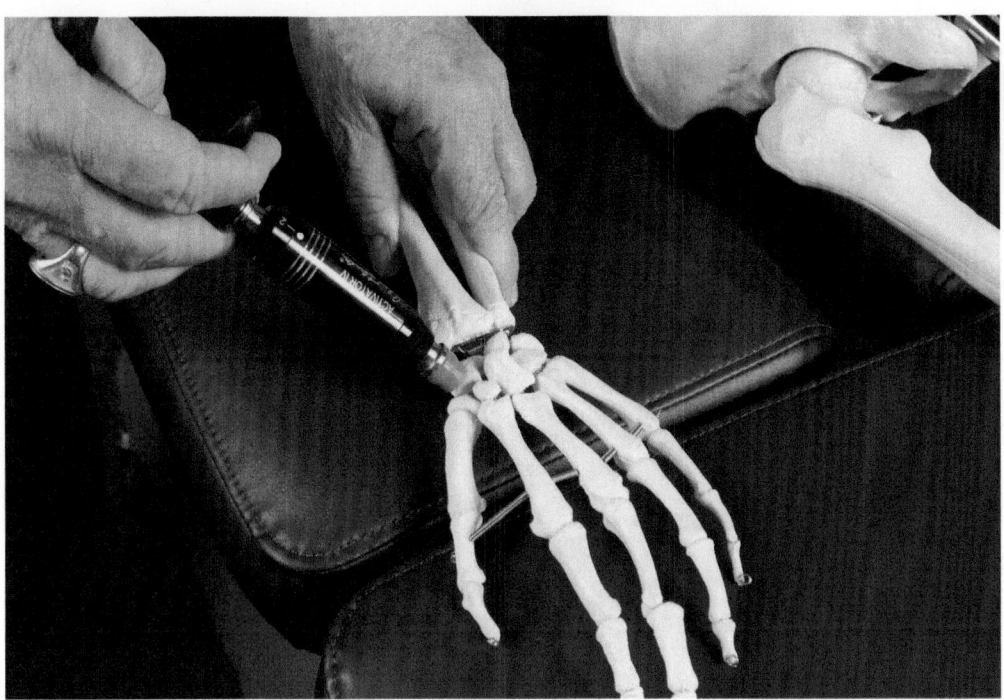

Figure 17-23 Adjustment for posterior, proximal carpals, two of two contacts. Line of Drive is anterior and inferior.

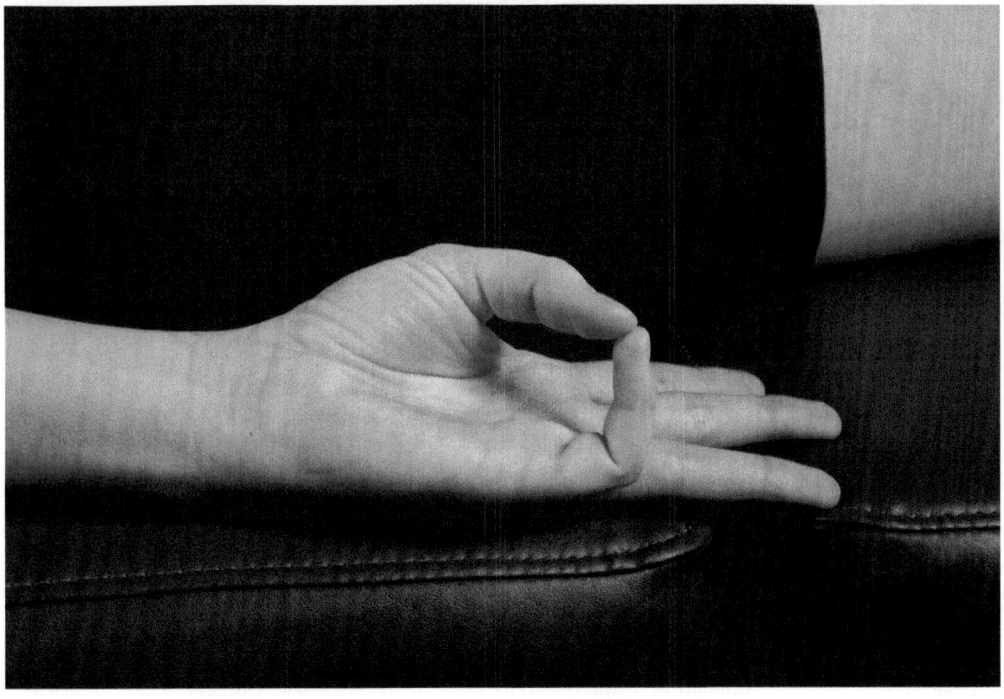

Figure 17-24 Isolation for carpal tunnel (approximated radius and ulna).

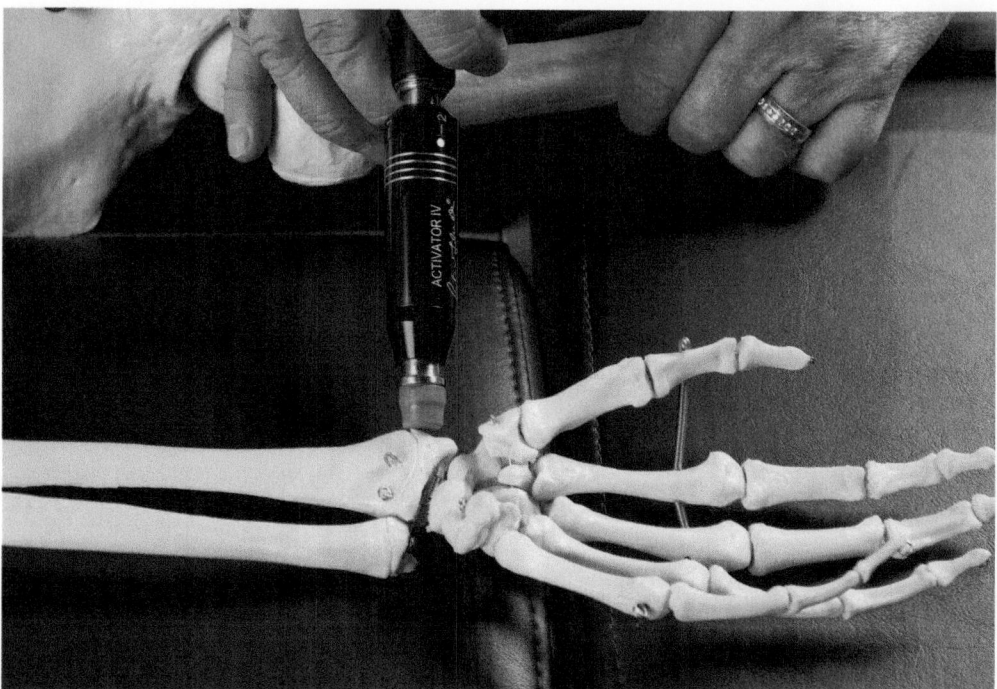

Figure 17-25 Adjustment for carpal tunnel. Step One: Contact the lateral aspect of the distal radius. Line of Drive is anatomically lateral to medial (the ulnar direction).

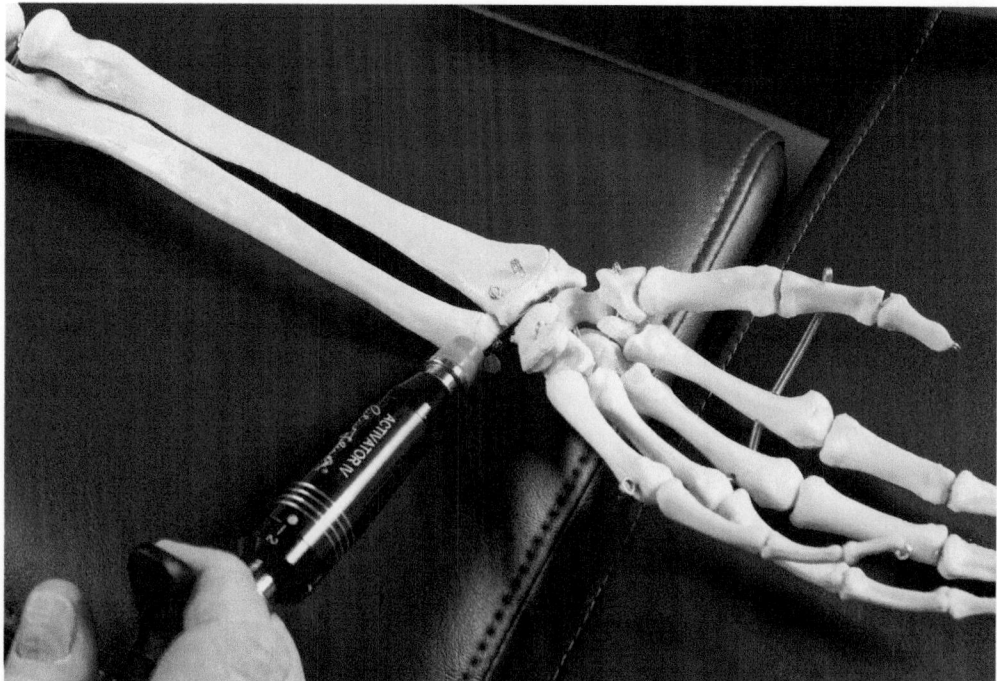

Figure 17-26 Adjustment for carpal tunnel. Step Two: Contact the medial aspect of the distal ulna. Line of Drive medial to lateral (in the radial direction).

Approximated Distal Radius and Ulna

Involvement of an approximated distal radius and ulna includes symptoms and complaints of pain in the wrist, and burning-type pain in the wrist with or without signs and symptoms of carpal tunnel syndrome.

Stress Test. The doctor uses the thumb and first finger to "compress" the distal end of the radius and ulna together (Figure 17-27). Look for reactivity of the PD leg in Position #1 for involvement.

Adjustment. There are two thrusts in opposition to the Stress Test, one each on the palmar side of the medial distal aspects of the radius and ulna (Figures 17-28 and 17-29). The doctor is contacting the inner aspects of the distal radius and ulnar bones from the palmar side and adjusts them out and downward toward the table, "separating the radius and ulna." The LOD is in a lateral-to-posterior LOD at approximately 45 to 60 degrees.

Trapeziometacarpal Joint

When a patient experiences hand pain in the region of the anatomical snuffbox or has suffered stenosing tenosynovitis or DeQuervain's syndrome, consider neuroarticular dysfunction at the trapeziometacarpal joint. This involvement also should be considered when active or passive ulnar deviation of the wrist causes pain at or near the base of the first metacarpal. This joint is the most commonly affected of the wrist and hand in the patient with osteoarthritis.

Isolation Test. To isolate the trapeziometacarpal joint, instruct the patient to lay the thumb of the involved hand across the palm of the hand. Then ask the patient to form a fist with the hand by wrapping the fingers around the thumb. This is the orthopedic test for DeQuervain's syndrome, known as Finkelstein's test (Figure 17-30). Look for reactivity of the PD leg in Position #1.

Adjustment. To adjust the trapeziometacarpal joint, place the tip of the instrument on the base of the first metacarpal, on the dorsal surface in the floor of the anatomical snuffbox. The LOD is inferior (distal) along the longitudinal axis of the first metacarpal (Figures 17-31 and 17-32).

The dysfunctional trapeziometacarpal joint may be painful on touch or deep palpation. To minimize discomfort for the patient, take a distal tissue pull over the snuffbox with the thumb of the free hand. Use the thumb to stabilize the tip of the instrument during the adjustment.

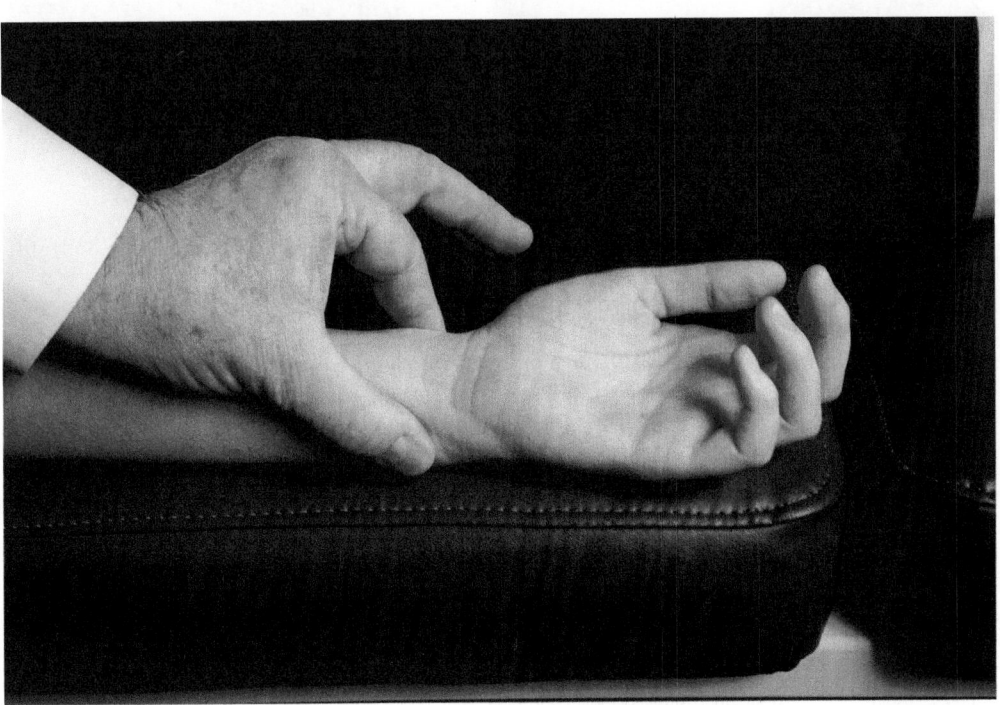

Figure 17-27 Stress Test for distal approximated radius and ulna.

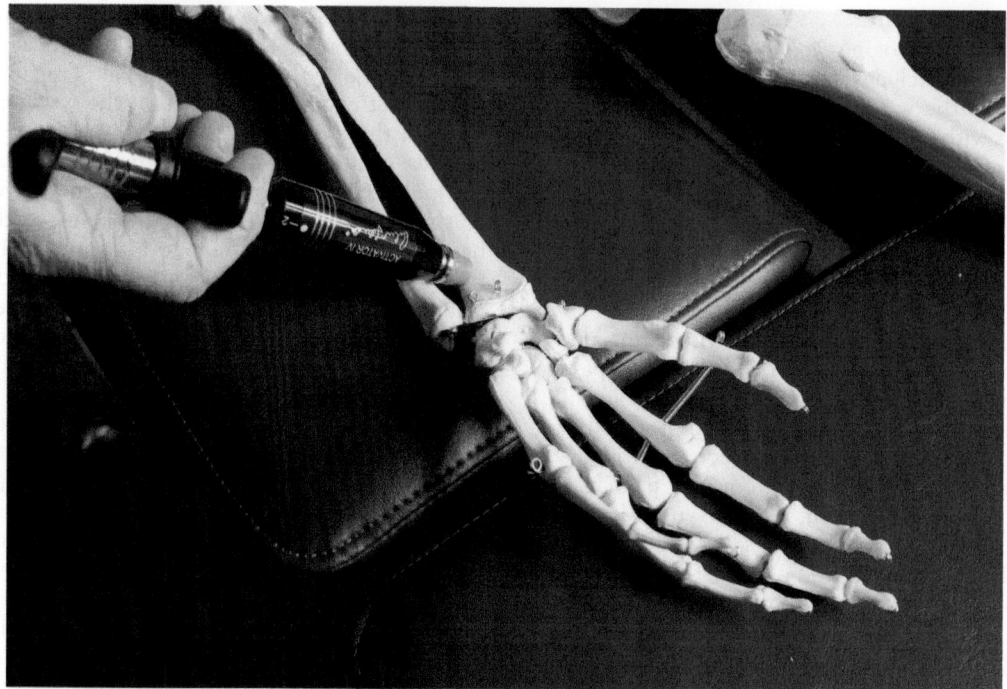

Figure 17-28 Adjustment for distal approximated radius and ulna. Step One: Contact the distal radius on the palmar side. Line of Drive (LOD) is in a lateral-to-posterior LOD, 45 to 60 degrees.

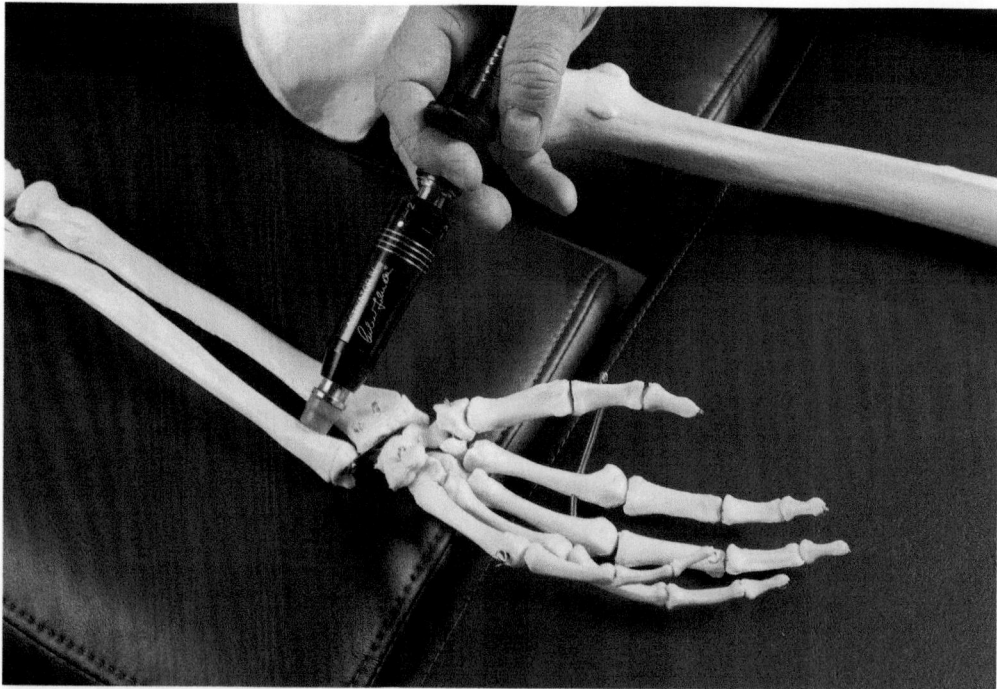

Figure 17-29 Adjustment for distal approximated radius and ulna. Step Two: Contact the distal ulna on the palmar side. Line of Drive (LOD) is in a medial-to-posterior LOD, 45 to 60 degrees.

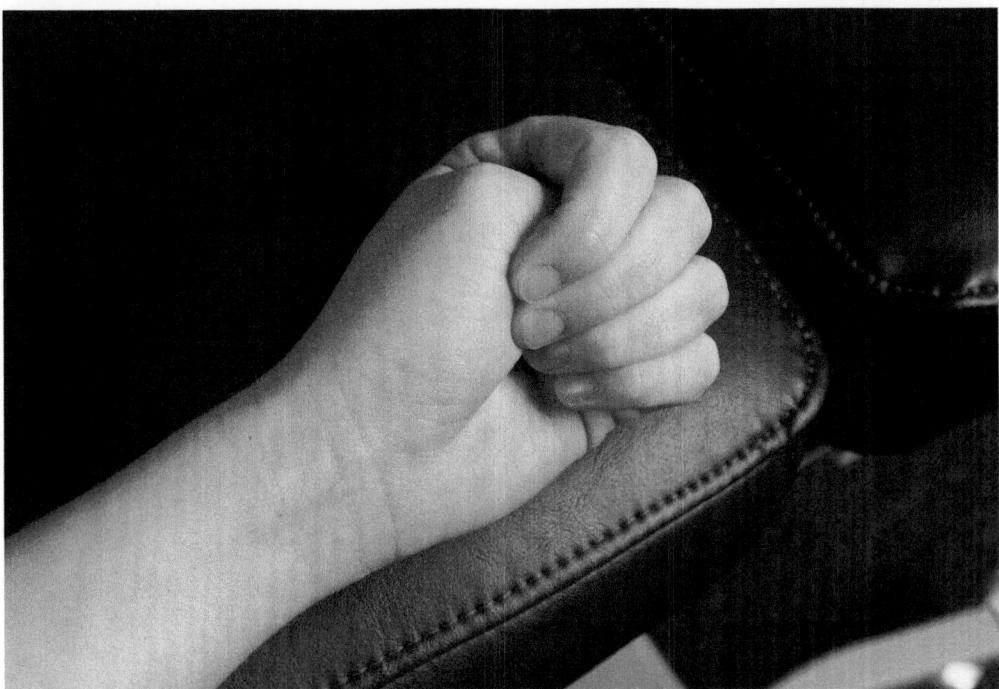

Figure 17-30 Isolation Test for trapeziometacarpal joint; lay the thumb across the palm of the hand and form a fist over the thumb.

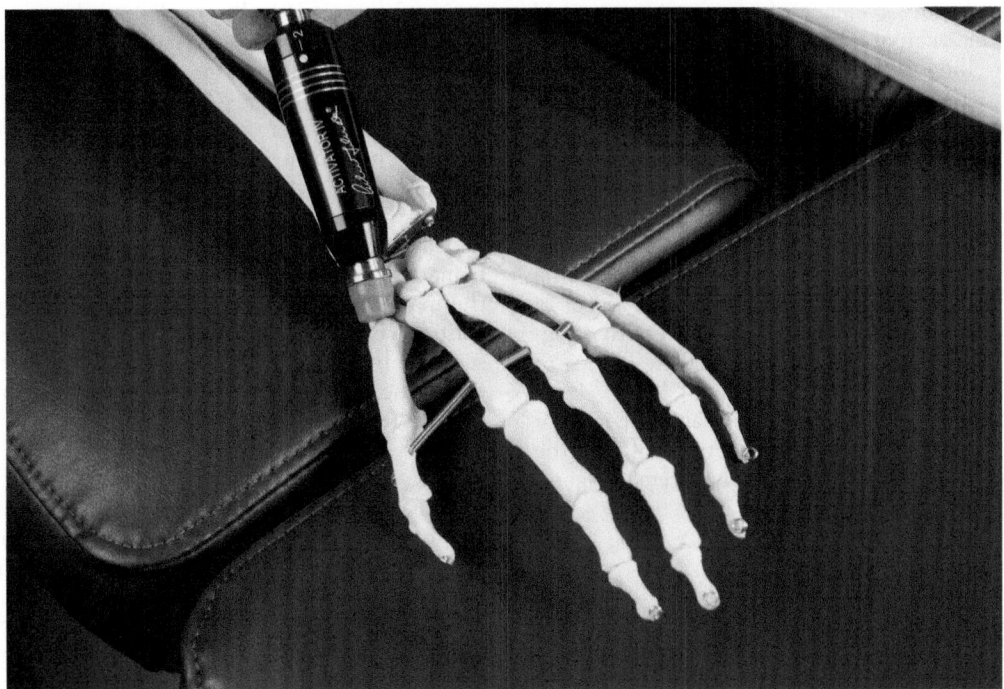

Figure 17-31 Adjustment for trapeziometacarpal joint. Line of Drive is inferior (distal) along the longitudinal axis of the first metacarpal.

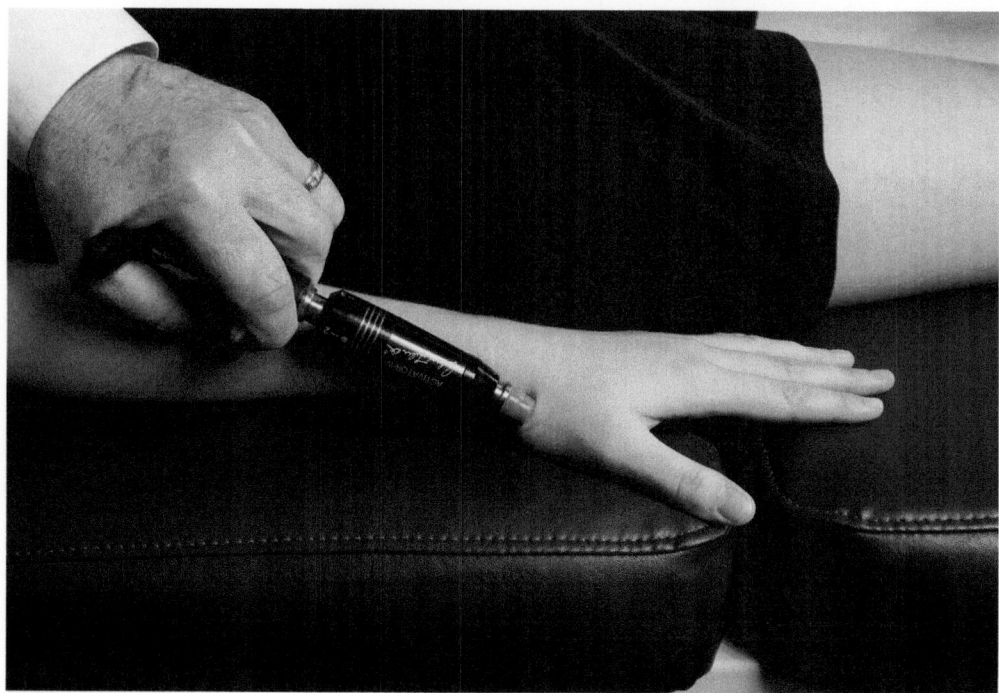

Figure 17-32 Adjustment for trapeziometacarpal joint. Contact the anatomical snuffbox. Line of Drive is inferior (distal) along the longitudinal axis of the first metacarpal.

Anterior Proximal First Metacarpal

Consider involvement of an anterior proximal first metacarpal when the patient reports pain or swelling to the proximal aspect of the thumb. The patient also can be involved in activities that stress the joint in extension, or hyperextension. Examples would include athletes who catch a ball and massage therapists who fail to lock their thumb in the neutral position when addressing trigger points.

Stress Test. The doctor gently distracts the distal thumb while pushing the dorsal aspect of the proximal first metacarpal anteriorly (Figure 17-33). Look for reactivity of the PD leg in Position #1 for involvement.

Adjustment. Contact the anterior-inferior aspect of the proximal first metacarpal, and the LOD is posterior and slightly lateral (Figures 17-34 and 17-35).

Medial Superior Hamate

When a patient reports hand and wrist pain, consider assessment of a medial superior hamate. The ulnar nerve may be compressed in the canal of Guyon, located between the hook of the hamate and the pisiform.

Stress Test. To Stress Test the hamate, push it in the anatomically medial and superior direction (Figure 17-36). To palpate the hamate, slide lateral and inferior (distal) from the pisiform. Look for reactivity of the PD leg in Position #1. If there was no reactivity, Stress Test the hamate in the opposite direction, and push it in the anatomically lateral and superior direction (Figure 17-37).

Adjustment. To adjust a medial superior hamate, contact the hamate with the tip of the instrument. The LOD is lateral and inferior (distal) (Figure 17-38). To adjust for a lateral superior hamate, contact the hamate with the tip of the instrument. The LOD is medial and inferior (distal) (Figure 17-39).

Pisiform

Patient complaints of hand, wrist, or finger pain, loss of grip strength, carpal tunnel syndrome, and tenderness on the pisiform are indications for testing.

Stress Test. The doctor pinches together the thenar and hypothenar, approximating the first and fifth metacarpals (Figure 17-40). Look for reactivity of the PD leg in Position #1 for involvement.

Text continued on p. 509

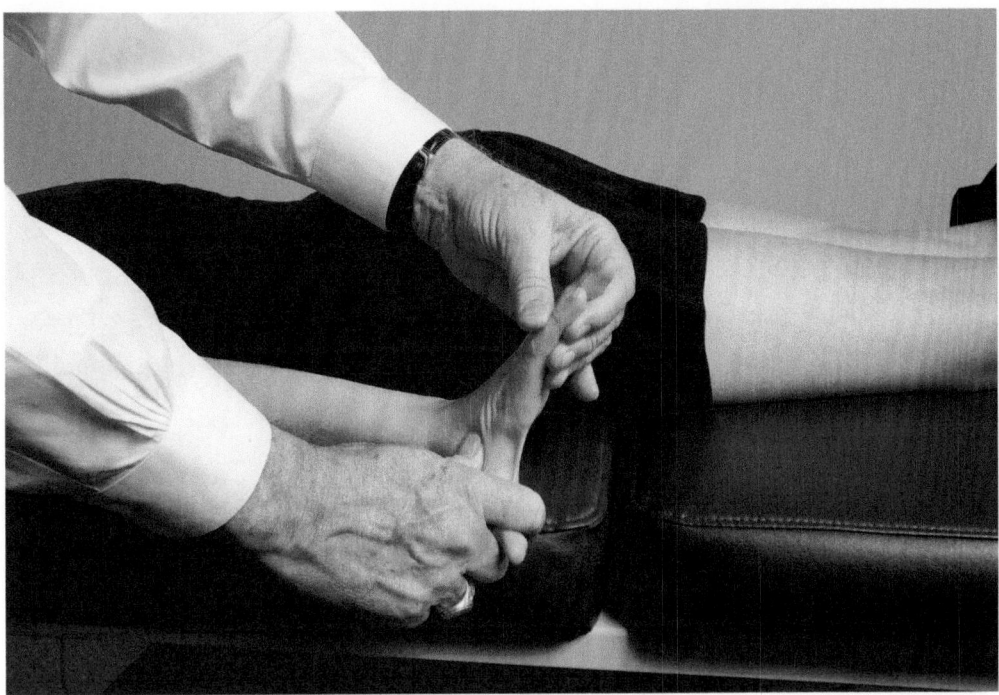

Figure 17-33 Stress Test for anterior proximal first metacarpal; doctor gently distracts the distal thumb while pushing the dorsal aspect of the proximal first metacarpal anteriorly.

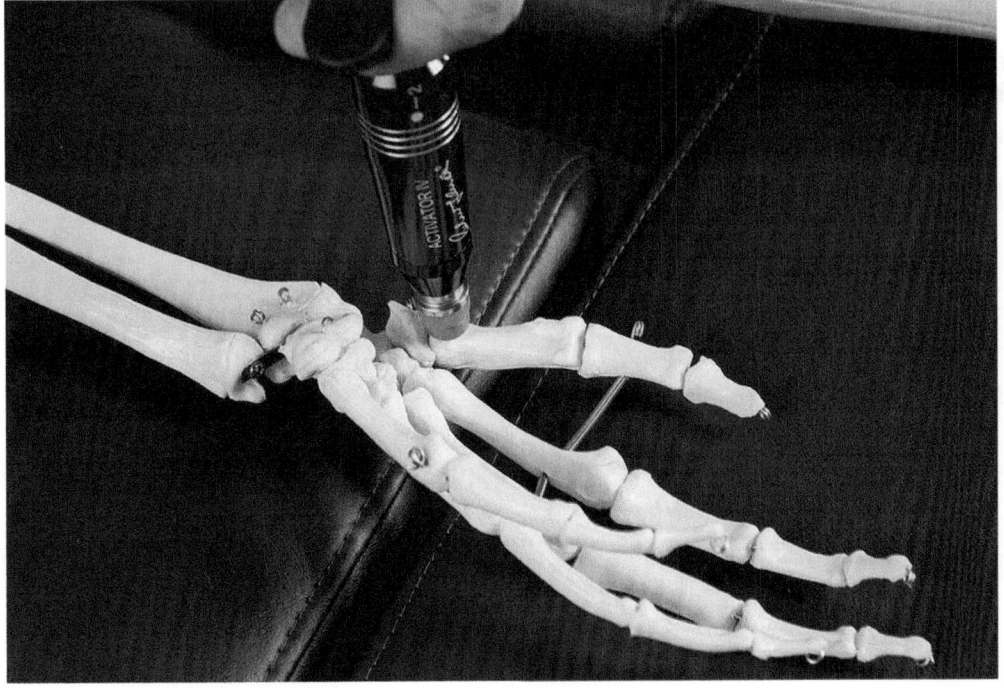

Figure 17-34 Adjustment for anterior proximal first metacarpal. Line of Drive is posterior and slightly lateral.

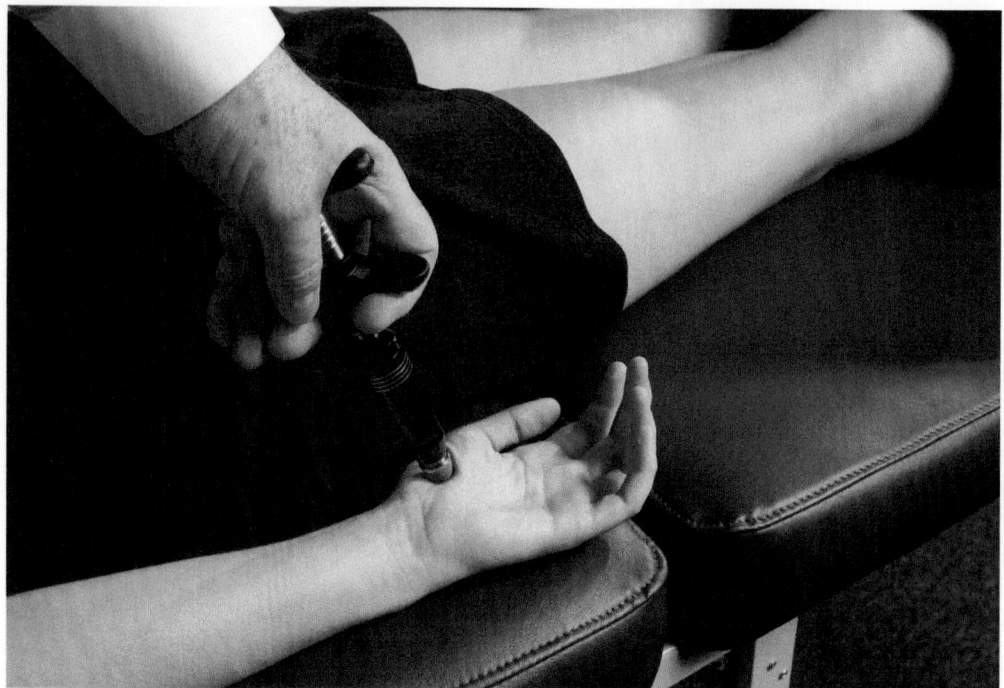

Figure 17-35   Adjustment for anterior proximal first metacarpal. Line of Drive is posterior and slightly lateral.

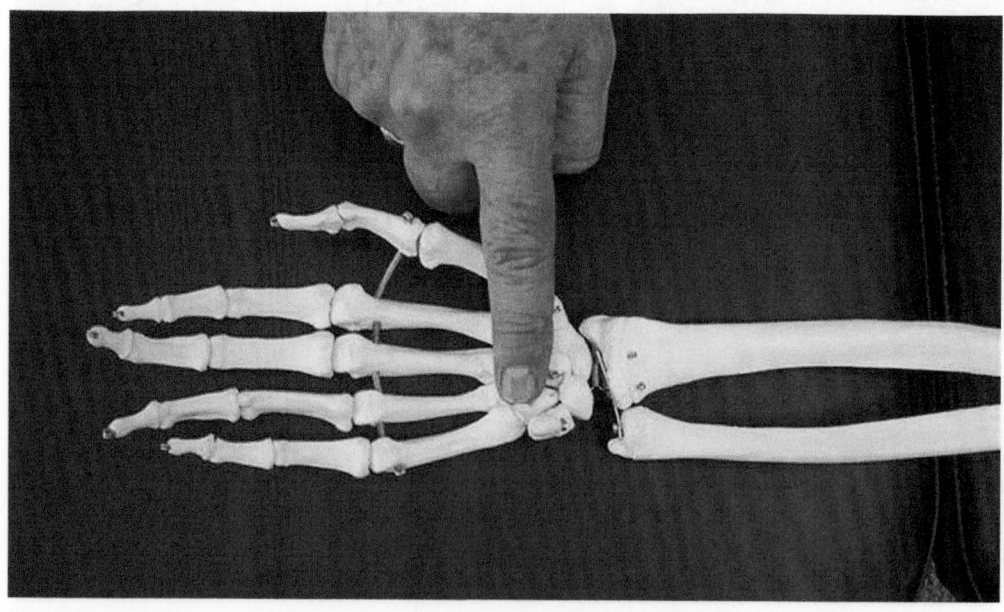

Figure 17-36   Stress Test for medial superior hamate.

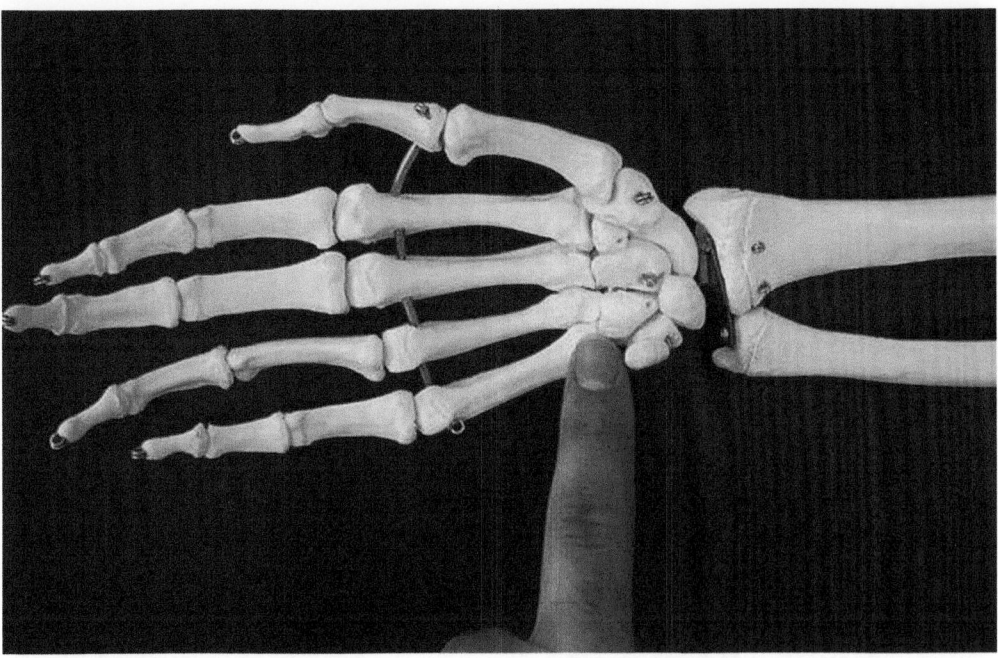

Figure 17-37   Stress Test for lateral superior hamate.

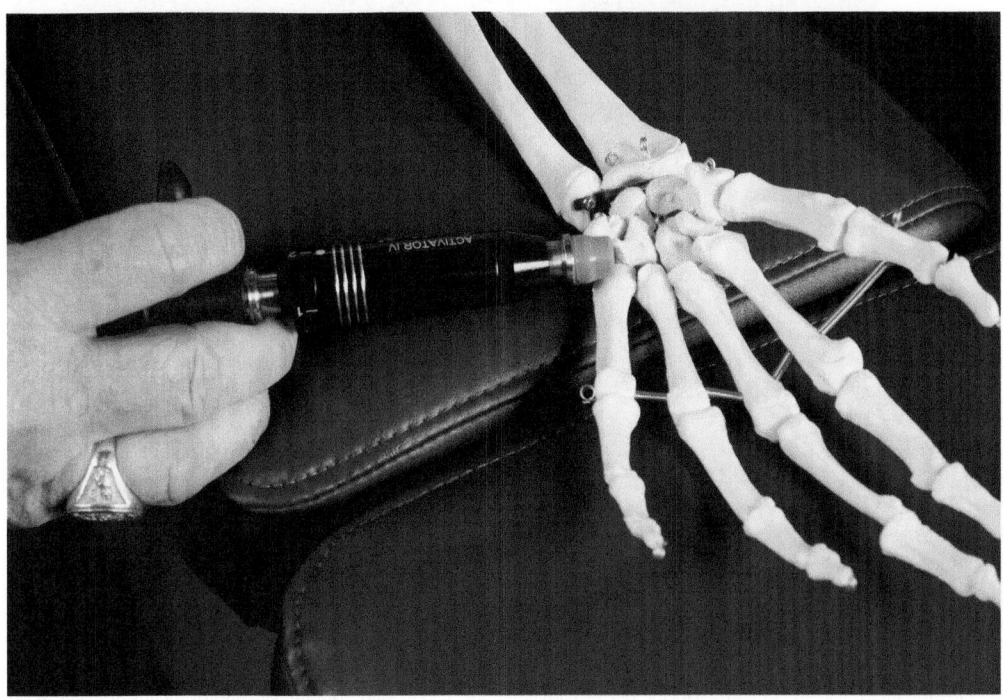

Figure 17-38   Adjustment for medial superior hamate. Line of Drive is lateral and inferior (distal).

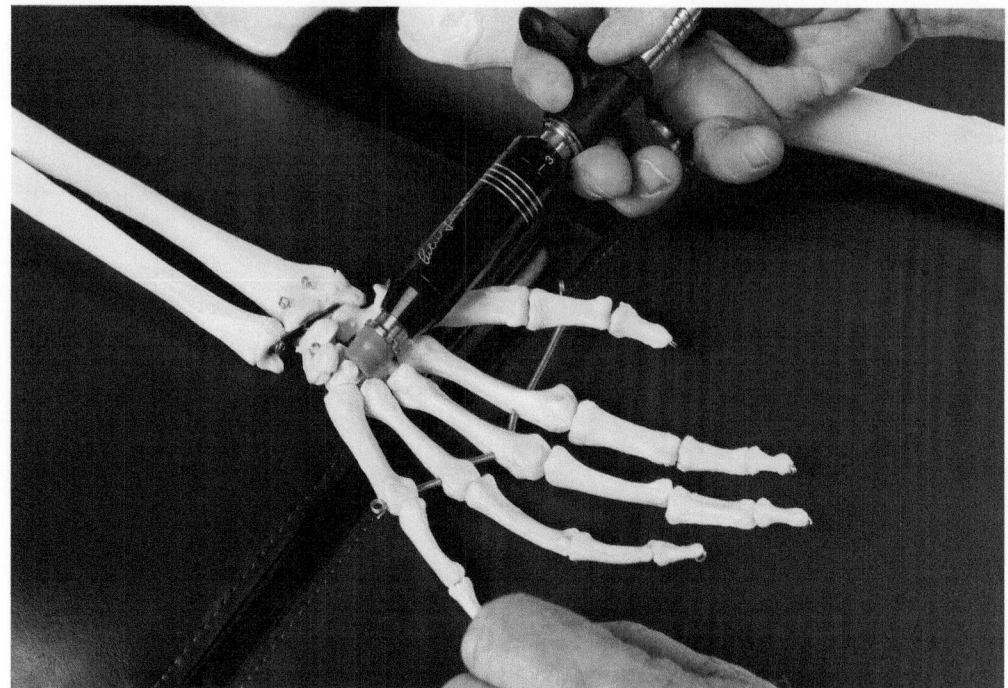

Figure 17-39 Adjustment for lateral superior hamate. Line of Drive is medial and inferior (distal).

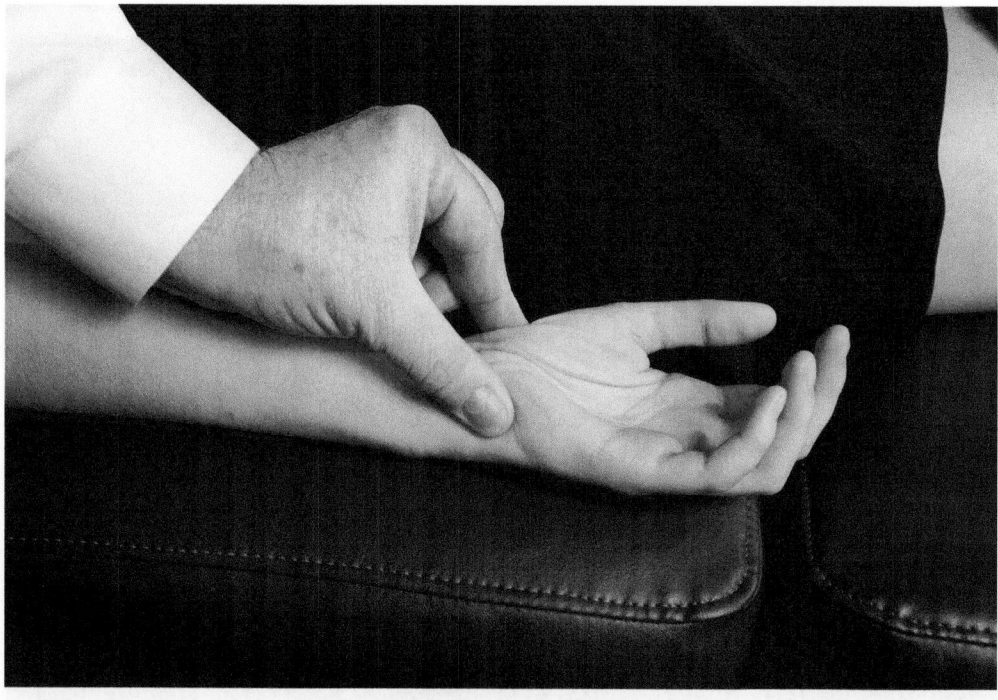

Figure 17-40 Stress Test for pisiform. Doctor pinches together the thenar and hypothenar, approximating the first and fifth metacarpals.

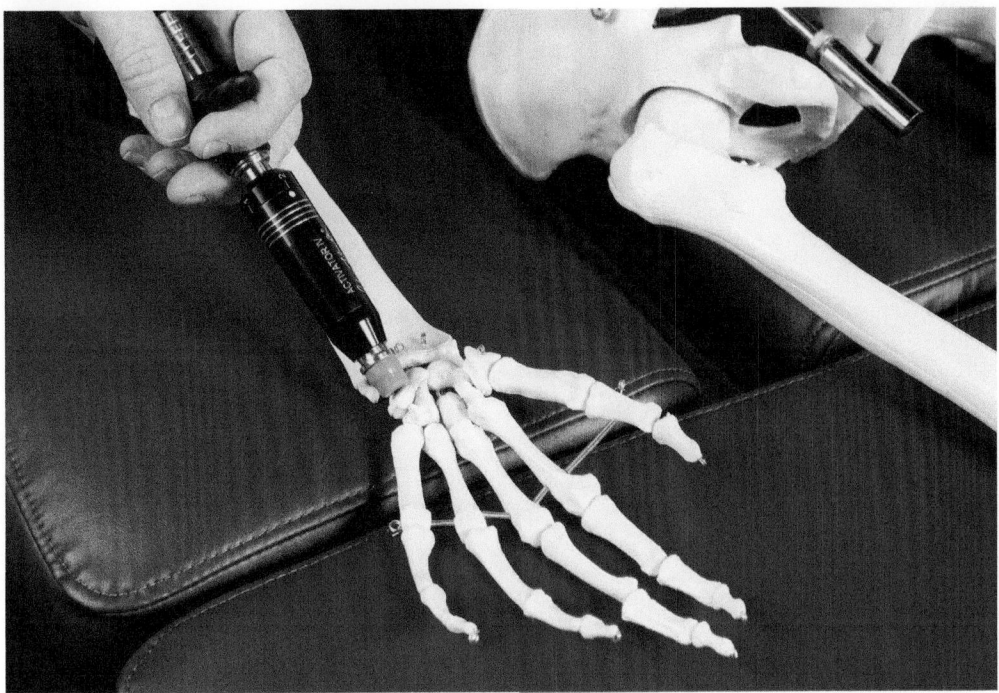

Figure 17-41 Adjustment for pisiform. Line of Drive is toward the shaft of the fourth (ring) finger.

Adjustment. Contact the superior portion of the pisiform, and the LOD is toward the shaft of the fourth (ring) finger (Figure 17-41).

Interphalangeal Joints

In patients who display the typical signs and symptoms of osteoarthritis in the hands and fingers, it is common to see the proximal and distal interphalangeal joints (PIPs and DIPs) of the second digits affected. Typically, the PIP is radially deviated and the DIP is ulnar deviated.

Stress Test. To stress the interphalangeal joints of the affected finger, push the PIP and the DIP toward midline simultaneously (Figure 17-42). Look for reactivity of the PD leg in Position #1.

Adjustment. To adjust for the interphalangeal joints, make one thrust on two contacts. Contact the radial aspect of the PIP with the tip of the instrument while stabilizing the middle phalanx with your free hand. The LOD is in the ulnar (medial) direction (Figures 17-43 and 17-44). Next, contact the ulnar aspect of the DIP with the tip of the instrument while stabilizing the middle phalanx with your free hand. The LOD is in the radial (lateral) direction (Figures 17-45 and 17-46).

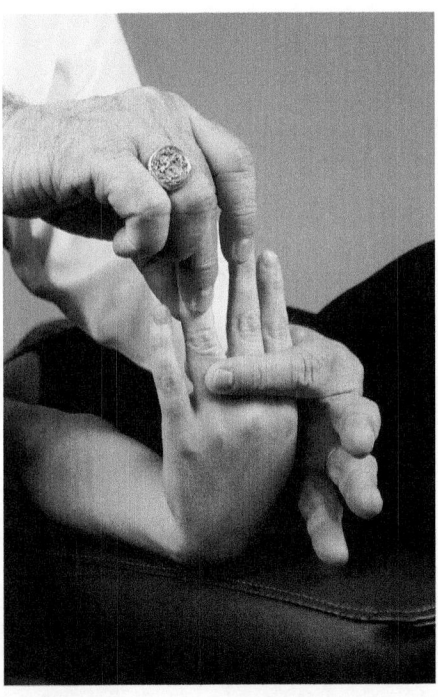

Figure 17-42 Stress Test for interphalangeal joints. Push the proximal interphalangeal joint and the distal interphalangeal joint toward midline simultaneously.

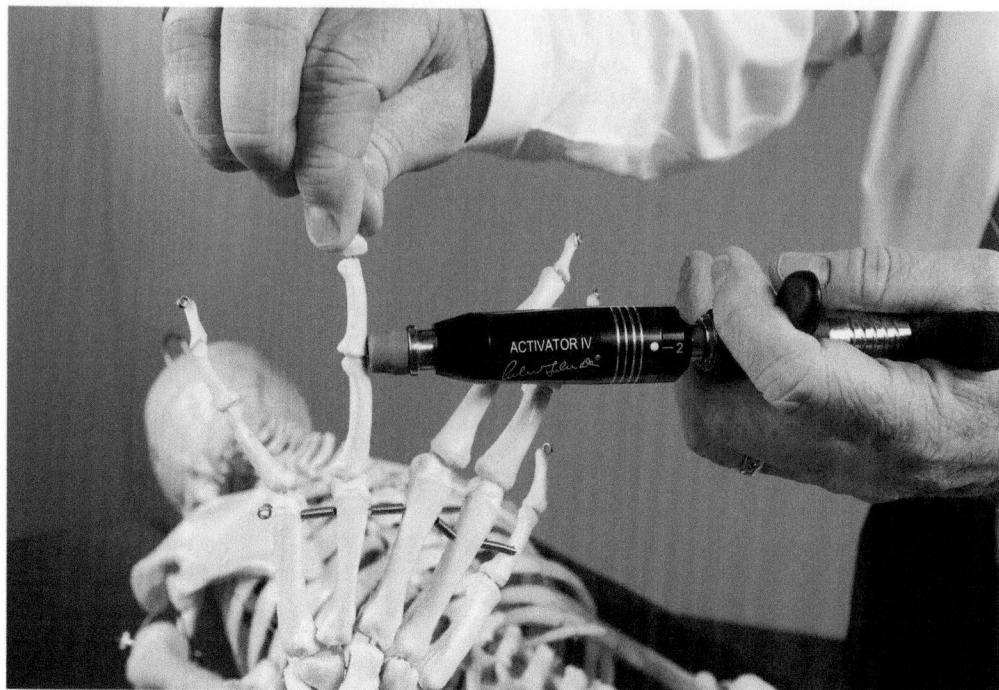

Figure 17-43 Adjustment for interphalangeal joints. Step One: Contact the radial aspect of the proximal interphalangeal joint while stabilizing the middle phalanx. Line of Drive is in the ulnar (medial) direction.

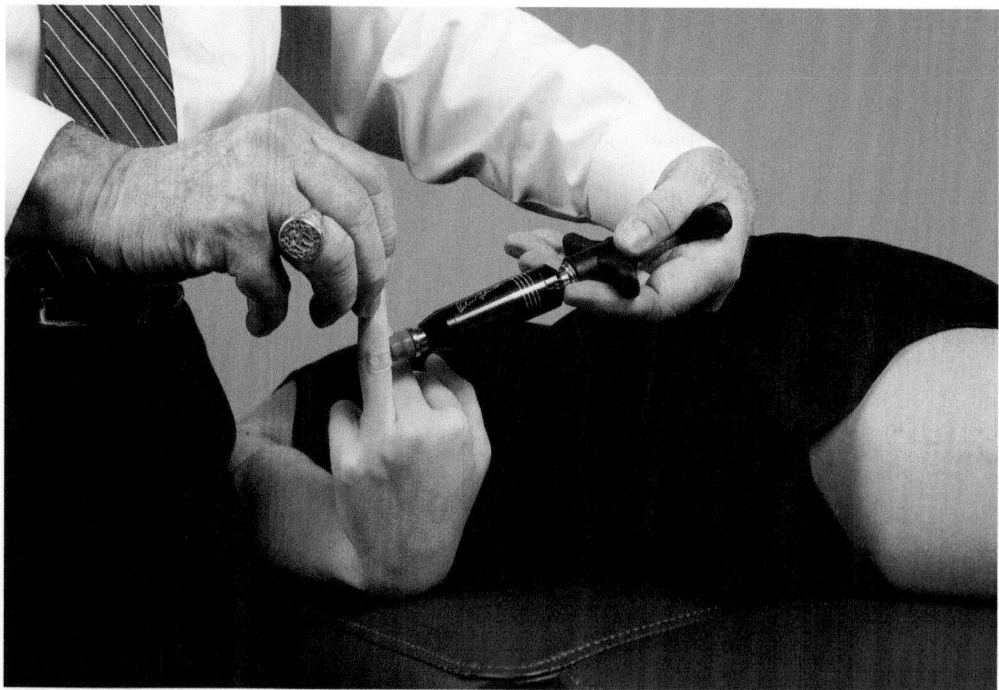

Figure 17-44 Adjustment for interphalangeal joints. Step One: Contact the radial aspect of the proximal interphalangeal joint while stabilizing the middle phalanx. Line of Drive is in the ulnar (medial) direction.

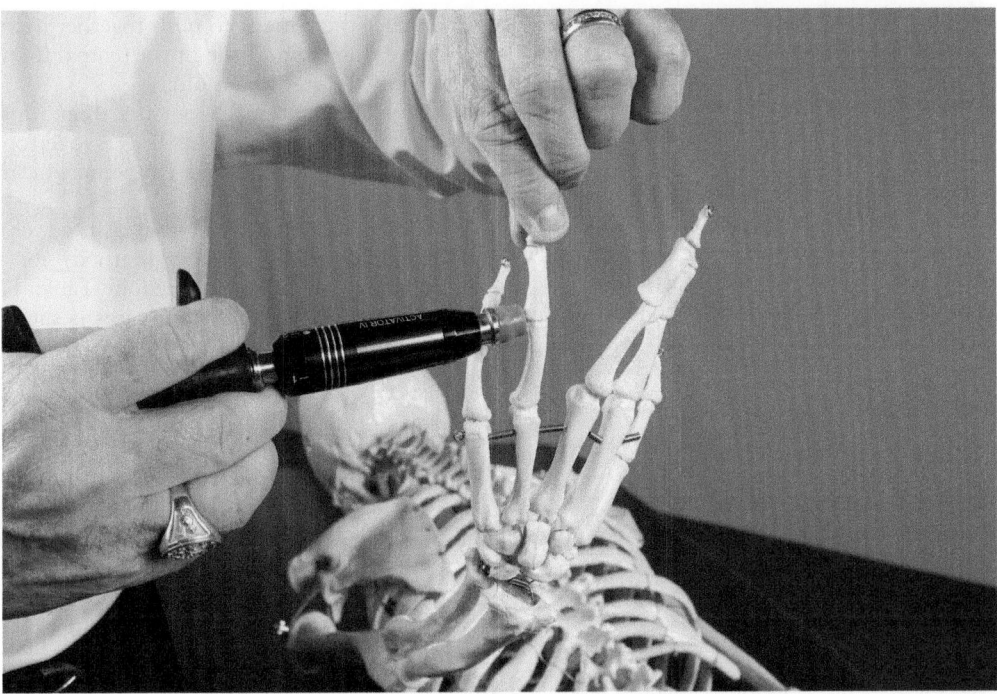

Figure 17-45   Adjustment for interphalangeal joints. Step Two: Contact the ulnar aspect of the distal interphalangeal joint while stabilizing the middle phalanx. Line of Drive is in the radial (lateral) direction.

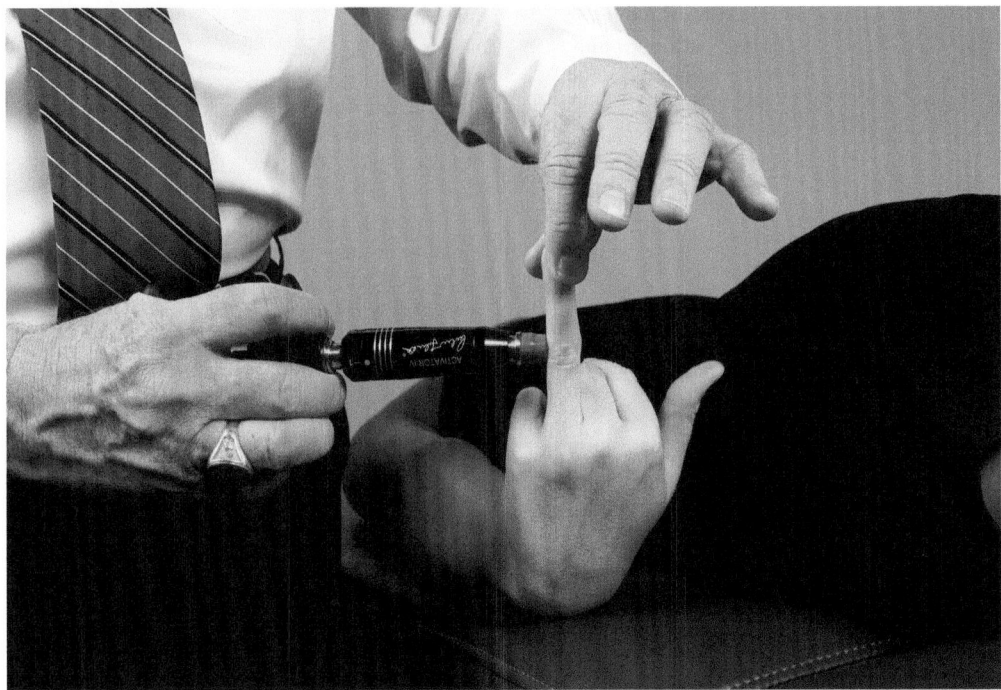

Figure 17-46   Adjustment for interphalangeal joints. Step Two: Contact the ulnar aspect of the distal interphalangeal joint while stabilizing the middle phalanx. Line of Drive is in the radial (lateral) direction.

Sequential Wrist and Hand Involvement

This sequence of testing involves the most common hand and wrist involvements and can be easily remembered by the doctor and patient. Consider this sequence with all wrist and hand complaints:

1. Instruct the patient to make a fist (posterior-superior proximal radius and anterior lunate).
2. Instruct the patient to flex the wrist (inferior lateral ulna and posterior carpals).
3. Instruct the patient to extend the wrist in the opposite direction (proximal carpals).

4. Instruct the patient to push together the tips of the thumb and little finger (carpal tunnel–separated distal radius/ulna).
5. Instruct the patient to put the thumb inside the hand and close the fingers overtop of the thumb, making a fist (trapeziometacarpal joint).

Mechanical force, manually assisted chiropractic adjusting (Activator Method) for the elbow and wrist is summarized in Table 17-1. Sequential testing for forearm cases is summarized in Box 17-3.

Table 17-1   Summary Table of Tests and Adjustments for the Elbow, Wrist, and Hands

Articular Dysfunction	Test	Adjustment Segmental Contact Point	Adjustment Line of Drive
Lateral Distal Humerus	Instruct patient to push involved elbow into the table	Roll arm so hand is palm down (supinate); lateral distal humerus	Medial
Posterior Proximal Ulna (Pronation)	Elbow in 30 degrees of flexion; doctor or patient pronates forearm	Elbow at 90 degrees of flexion, posterior proximal ulna	Superior and medial through shaft of humerus
Anterior Proximal Ulna (Supination)	Elbow in 30 degrees of flexion; doctor or patient supinates the forearm	Elbow at 30 degrees of flexion, anterior proximal ulna	Inferior (distal) and anatomically medial
Pronator Quadratus	Instruct patient to fully pronate hand to end range	*Anterior Radius*	
		Step One: 1½ inches proximal to wrist crease	Lateral
		Step Two: 3 inches proximal to wrist crease	Lateral
		Anterior Ulna	
		Step Three: 1½ inches proximal to wrist crease	Medial
		Step Four: 3 inches proximal to wrist crease	Medial
Wrist Extensors	Instruct patient to extend wrist against resistance of doctor	Place patient with hand palm down by head, 1½ inches distal to the end of the elbow crease in extensor muscle belly	Anterior
Posterior-Superior Proximal Radius and Anterior Lunate	Instruct patient to make a fist on involved hand	*Step One:* Posterior-superior proximal radius	Anterior and inferior
		Step Two: Anterior aspect of lunate	Posterior
Inferior Lateral Ulna and Posterior Carpals	Instruct patient to flex wrist on involved hand	*Step One:* Anterior aspect of proximal ulna	Lateral and slightly superior
		Step Two: Posterior carpals	Anterior

Table 17-1	**Summary Table of Tests and Adjustments for the Elbow, Wrist, and Hands—cont'd**		
		ADJUSTMENT	
Articular Dysfunction	**Test**	**Segmental Contact Point**	**Line of Drive**
Proximal Carpals	Instruct the patient to extend the wrist	Contact the posterior aspect of each proximal carpal, excluding the lunate	Anterior and inferior
Carpal Tunnel– Separated Distal Radius/Ulna	Instruct the patient to squeeze the tips of the first and fifth digits on the involved side	*Patient's Palm Is Up* *Step One*: Lateral aspect of distal radius *Step Two*: Medial aspect of distal ulna	Lateral to medial (ulnar direction) Medial to lateral (radial direction)
Approximate Distal Radius/Ulna	Stress by squeezing radius and ulna together	*Step One*: Palmar, distal, medial aspect of radius *Step Two*: Palmar, distal, medial aspect of ulna	Lateral Medial
Trapeziometacarpal Joint	Instruct patient to lay thumb of involved hand across palm of hand, form a fist, and squeeze	Base of first metacarpal in anatomical snuffbox	Distal along longitudinal axis of first metacarpal
Anterior Proximal First Metacarpal	Stress base of thumb anterior with distal thumb distraction	Anterior proximal first metacarpal	Posterior and slightly lateral
Medial Superior Hamate	Stress hamate in the medial and superior directions	Hamate	Lateral and inferior
Pisiform	Stress pads of palm together	Superior aspect of pisiform	Toward shaft of fourth finger
Interphalangeal Joints	Stress the PIP and the DIP by pushing the joints toward the midline	*Step One*: radial side of PIP *Step Two*: ulnar side of DIP	Medial Lateral

DIP, Distal interphalangeal joint; *PIP*, proximal interphalangeal joint.

Box 17-3	**Sequential Testing of the Elbow, Wrist, and Hand**

1. Posterior-Superior Proximal Radius and Anterior Lunate (Make a Fist)
2. Inferior Lateral Ulna and Posterior Carpals (Flex the Wrist)
3. Proximal Carpals (Extend the Wrist)
4. Carpal Tunnel (Thumb and Little Fingertips Together)
5. Trapeziometacarpal Joint (Thumb Inside with Closed Fist Overtop)
6. Lateral Distal Humerus (Patient Pushes Elbow into Table)
7. Posterior (Pronation) Proximal Ulna (Doctor Flexes Elbow and Pronates Forearm)
8. Anterior (Supination) Proximal Ulna (Doctor Flexes Elbow and Supinates Forearm)
9. Wrist Extensors (Patient Resists Wrist Extension)
10. Pronator Quadratus (Maximal Pronation Attempt)

RELATED RESEARCH

Related published research for the elbow, wrist, and hand is presented in Box 17-4.

Box 17-4

Reference: Bradley S, Polkinghorn DC. A novel method for assessing elbow pain resulting from epicondylitis. J Chiropr Med. 2002;1:117-21.

ABSTRACT
OBJECTIVE
To describe a novel orthopedic test (Polk's test) that can assist the clinician in differentiating between medial and lateral epicondylitis, two of the most common causes of elbow pain. This test has not been described previously in the literature.

CLINICAL FEATURES
The testing procedure described in this paper is easy to learn and simple to perform and may provide the clinician with a quick and effective method of differentiating between lateral and medial epicondylitis. The test also helps to elucidate normal activities of daily living that the patient may unknowingly be performing on a repetitive basis that are hindering recovery. The results of this simple test allow the clinician to make immediate lifestyle recommendations to the patient that should improve and hasten response to subsequent treatment. It may be used in conjunction with other orthopedic testing procedures because it correlates well with other clinical tests for assessing epicondylitis.

CONCLUSION
The use of Polk's test may help the clinician to differentiate diagnostically between lateral and medial epicondylitis and supply information relative to the selection of proper instructions for the patient to follow as part of the treatment program. Further research, performed in an academic setting, should prove helpful in more thorough evaluation of the merits of this test. In the meantime, clinical experience over the years suggests that the practicing physician should find a great deal of clinical usefulness in performing this simple, yet effective, diagnostic procedure.

POLK'S TEST

There are two phases to the test, both starting with the patient seated and the elbow flexed. The patient is instructed to lift an object of approximately 5 lb (2.5 kg suggestive) in two different ways.

Phase one is with the patient grasping the object with the palm facing the floor (pronation of the forearm). The patient is instructed to lift the object up (Figure 17-47). Pain produced at the elbow upon lifting the object is suggestive of lateral epicondylitis. The pain is due to the strain imposed at the attachment site of the extensor/supinator muscle group. The patient, by trying to hold the book up against gravity, involves resistance to attempted dorsiflexion of the wrist, which is mediated by the extensor/supinators, and is the most common finding of the two phases.

Phase two is performed the same, with the patient seated and the elbow flexed, but now he or she is grasping the object with the palm up (supination of the forearm). When attempting to lift the object (Figure 17-48) in this position, imposed forces are at the attachment site of the flexor/pronators muscle group. Pain upon lifting and holding up the object is suggestive of medial epicondylitis.

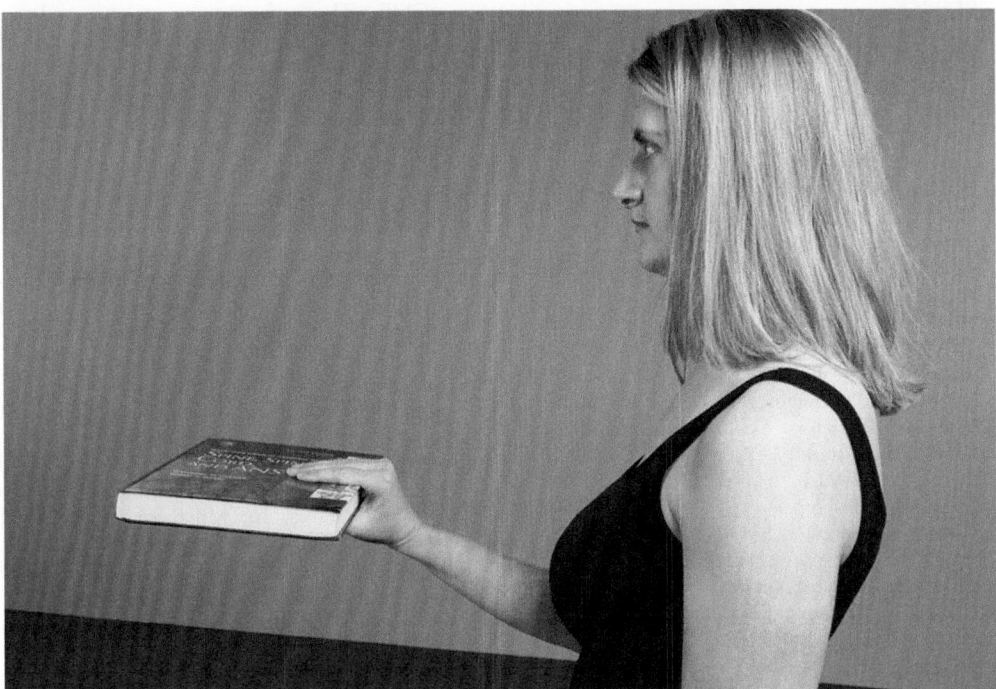

Figure 17-47   Polk's test for lateral epicondylitis. Patient should be seated with the elbow flexed, palm down (forearm pronated) as he or she attempts to lift the book.

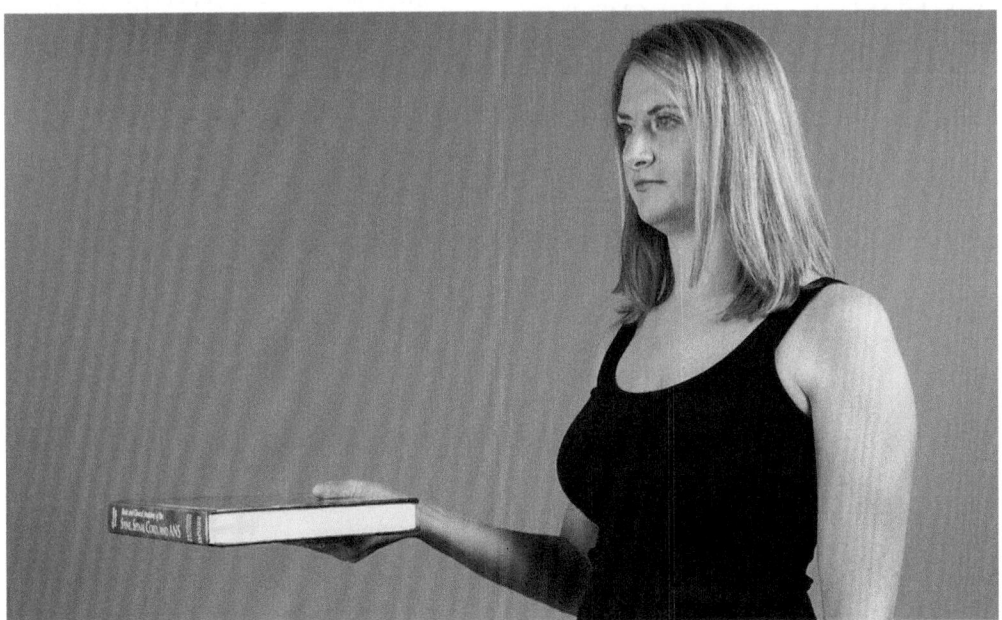

Figure 17-48   Polk's test for medial epicondylitis. Patient should be seated with the elbow flexed, palm up (forearm supination) as he or she attempts to lift the book.

REFERENCES

1. Pascarelli E, Quilter D. Repetitive strain injury: a computer user's guide. New York: Wiley; 1994.
2. Ireland DCR. Australian experience with cumulative trauma disorders. In: Millender LH, Louis DS, Simmons BP, editors. Occupational disorders of the upper extremity. New York: Churchill Livingstone; 1992.
3. Terrono AL, Millender LH. Evaluation and management of occupational wrist disorders. In: Millender LH, Louis DS, Simmons BP, editors. Occupational disorders of the upper extremity. New York: Churchill Livingstone; 1992.
4. Simmons BP, Wyman ET Jr. Occupational injuries of the elbow. In: Millender LH, Louis DS, Simmons BP, editors. Occupational disorders of the upper extremity. New York: Churchill Livingstone; 1992.
5. Cherniack M. Upper extremity disorders. In: Rosenstock L, Cullen MR, editors. Textbook of clinical occupational and environmental medicine. Philadelphia: Saunders; 1994.
6. Cipriano JJ. Photographic manual of regional orthopaedic tests. Baltimore: Williams & Wilkins; 1985.
7. Evans RC. Illustrated essentials in orthopedic physical assessment. St. Louis: Mosby; 1994.
8. Hoppenfeld S. Physical examination of the spine and extremities. Norwalk (CT): Appleton-Century-Crofts; 1976.
9. Clemente CD. Gray's anatomy. 30th American ed. Philadelphia: Lea & Febiger; 1985.
10. Leach RE, Miller JK. Lateral and medial epicondylitis of the elbow. Clin Sports Med. 1987;6(2): 259-72.
11. Chase J, Carnine K. Injuries to the upper limb. In: McLatchie GR, Lennox CME, Percy EC, Davies J: The soft tissues: trauma and sports injuries. London: Butterworth-Heinemann; 1993.
12. Percy EC. Risks and athletic injuries in North American sports. In: McLatchie GR, Lennox CME. The soft tissues: trauma and sports injuries. London: Butterworth-Heinemann; 1993.
13. Adebajo AO, Hazelman BL. Incidence, nature and economic effects of soft tissue injury. In: McLatchie GR, Lennox CME, editors. The soft tissues: trauma and sports injuries. London: Butterworth-Heinemann; 1993.
14. Pecina M, Bojanic I. Overuse injuries of the musculoskeletal system. Boca Raton (FL): CRC Press; 1993.
15. Coonrad RW, Hooper RW. Tennis elbow: its course, natural history, conservative, and surgical management. J Bone Joint Surg Am 1973;55 (6):1177-82.
16. Gruchow HW, Pelletier BS. An epidemiologic study of tennis elbow. Am J Sports Med. 1979;7(4):234-8.
17. Armstrong TJ. Cumulative trauma disorders of the upper limb and identification of work-related factors. In: Millender LH, Louis DS, Simmons BP, editors. Occupational disorders of the upper extremity. New York: Churchill Livingstone; 1992.
18. Wilson FD, Andrews JR, Blackburn TA, McCluskey G. Valgus extension overload in the pitching elbow. Am J Sports Med. 1983;11(2):83-8.
19. Andrews JR, Whiteside JA, Wilk KE. Rehabilitation of throwing and racquet sport injuries. In: Buschbacher RM, Braddom RL, editors. Sports medicine and rehabilitation: a sport-specific approach. Philadelphia: Hanley & Belfus; and St. Louis: Mosby; 1994.
20. Magee DJ. Forearm, wrist, and hand. In: Orthopedic physical assessment. Philadelphia: Saunders; 1987. p. 107-41.
21. Punnett L, Rosenman KD. Hand-arm vibration syndrome. In: Weeks JL, Levy BS, Wagner GR, editors. Preventing occupational disease and injury. Washington (DC): American Public Health Association; 1991.

Charlotte J. Watts

ACTIVATOR QUICK NOTES KEY

Bold & Large Font	Basic Scan Protocol (Track I)
Plain Font	Advanced Protocol (Track II)
Italics Font	*Track III Protocol*
LOD	Line of Drive
A	Anterior
P	Posterior
S	Superior
I	Inferior
M	Medial
L	Lateral
X/X/X Example: A/I/M	Combined LOD Anterior/Inferior/Medial
S/L Rule	Short/Long Rule
LPJ	Lamina Pedicle Junction
SP	Spinous Process
TVP	Transverse Process
AC	Acromioclavicular Joint
EAM	External Auditory Meatus
PD	Pelvic Deficiency
OPD	Opposite of Pelvic Deficiency
*	*Remember the contralateral rib adjustment
Split	1. if "A" adjust this
Cells	2. if "B" adjust this
Bold Lines	Contain Information & Instructions

BASIC PROTOCOL

REVISED 11-5-07

*Please Note: **ONLY ONE THRUST** at each segmental contact point!

Possibility #1: PD lengthens in Position #2, begin protocol with: Pressure Test in this order: **PD Medial Knee, OPD Medial Knee, PD Lateral Knee, OPD Lateral Knee** (see below)
Possibility #2: PD gets shorter in Position #2 begin protocol with: the **L4 Isolation Test.**
Possibility #3: Legs are even in Position #1 and even in Position #2, begin protocol with: **Pubic Bone Isolation Test.**

PRESSURE TEST: A light pressure applied in the direction of Correction. (Look for Improvement in Position #1)
STRESS TEST: A light pressure applied in the direction of Subluxation. (Look for Reactivity in Position # 1)

Subluxation	*Test*	*Adjustment*
PD Medial knee joint & Talus	Pressure Test PD medial collateral ligament lateral and inferior & if there is improvement in the leg lengths in Position #1, adjust…	1. Contact medial border of PD talus inferior to medial malleolus – LOD is **P/S/L** 2. Contact PD medial knee joint space – LOD is **L/I**
OPD Medial knee joint & Talus	Pressure Test OPD medial collateral ligament lateral and inferior & if there is improvement in the leg lengths Position #1, adjust…	1. Contact medial border of OPD talus inferior to medial malleolus – LOD is **P/S/L** 2. Contact OPD medial knee joint space – LOD is **L/I**
PD Lateral knee joint & Cuboid	Pressure Test PD lateral collateral ligament medial and inferior & if there is improvement in the leg lengths Position #1, adjust…	1. Contact inferior lateral aspect of PD cuboid – LOD is **P/S/M** 2. Contact PD lateral knee joint – LOD is **M/I**
OPD Lateral knee joint & Cuboid	Pressure Test OPD lateral collateral ligament medial and inferior & if there is improvement in the leg lengths Position #1, adjust…	1. Contact inferior lateral aspect of OPD cuboid – LOD is **P/S/M** 2. Contact OPD lateral knee joint – LOD is **M/I**

After Knees and Feet:
- If legs are uneven in Position #1 go to **OPD Ilium and Pressure Test** for an AS Ilium Subluxation.
- If legs are even in Position #1 but uneven in Position #2 go to **OPD Ilium and Pressure Test** for an AS Ilium Subluxation.
- If legs are even in Position #1 and even in Position #2 go to **Pubic Bone Isolation Test**.
  +*The Goal is to have the legs EVEN in Position #1 **AND** Position #2.*

AS Ilium	Pressure Test crest of OPD ilium I/M & if there is improvement in the leg lengths in Position #1, adjust…	1. Contact base of sacrum on OPD side
		  – LOD is **A/I**
		2. Contact OPD crest of ilium
		  – LOD is **I/M**
		3. Contact OPD ischial tuberosity (posterior aspect)
		  – LOD is **A/I**

PI Ilium	Pressure Test with a firm <u>thumb</u> contact, under PD sacrotuberous ligament P/S/L & if there is improvement in the leg lengths in Position #1, adjust…	1. Contact PD spine of ischium
		  – LOD is **P/L/S**
		2. Contact PD sacrotuberous ligament
		  – LOD is **P/L/S**
		3. Contact PD iliac fossa
		  – LOD is **A/S**

ISOLATION TEST: Specific *active* movements performed <u>by the patient</u> that assist in the location and evaluation of subluxated motion segments of the spine and extremities. Utilize the Short/Long Rule.

SHORT/LONG RULE: **PD LENGTHENS in Position #2 adjust the PD side.**
PD gets SHORTER in Position #2 adjust the OPD side.
>*Check Position #2 even if there is no change in Position #1. Position #2 is <u>more sensitive</u> than Position #1 alone.*
+*The Goal is to have the legs EVEN in Position #1 **AND** Position #2.*

Sup. or **Inf.** **pube**	Instruct patient to squeeze knees together. If PD leg lengthens in Position #2. --- If PD leg shortens in Position #2.	Contact PD pubic bone, superior aspect – LOD is **Inferior** Contact OPD pubic bone, inferior aspect – LOD is **Superior**
L5	Instruct patient to place PD forearm on low back (OPD arm remains at the side of the body), Compare Position #1 to Position #2	Contact L5 inferior articular process on side indicated by S/L Rule – LOD is **A/S**
L4	Instruct patient to place OPD forearm on low back (PD arm remains at the side of the body), Compare Position #1 to Position #2	Contact L4 inferior articular process on side indicated by S/L Rule – LOD is **A/S**
L2	Instruct patient to place both forearms on low back, *palms up*, Compare Position #1 to Position #2	Contact L2 inferior articular process on side indicated by S/L Rule – LOD is **A/S**
T12	Instruct patient to place the PD forearm on the table superior and lateral to the head (OPD arm remains at the side of the body), Compare Position #1 to Position #2	Contact the T12 transverse process on side indicated by S/L Rule – LOD is **A/S/M**
T12 –Rib If clinically Indicated	Repeat T-12 Isolation Test and instruct patient to inhale and hold, Compare Position #1 to Position #2	Contact body of T12 rib ½ inch lateral to transverse process on side of rib involvement indicated by S/L Rule – LOD is **L/I** along the shaft of the **rib**
T8*	Instruct patient to place both forearms on the table superior and lateral to the head, Compare Position #1 to Position #2	1. Contact the T8 transverse process on side indicated by S/L Rule – LOD is **A/S/M** 2. Proceed to T8 contralateral **rib*** – LOD is **L/I** along the shaft of the **rib**
T6*	Instruct the patient to turn face toward PD side and rest head on table (both arms remain at the sides of the body), Compare Position #1 to Position #2	1. Contact the T6 transverse process on side indicated by S/L Rule– LOD is **A/S/M** 2. Proceed to T6 contralateral **rib*** – LOD is **L/I** along the shaft of the **rib**
T4*	Instruct the patient to <u>keep face turned to PD side</u>, lift **PD** shoulder off the table, then relax. (both arms remain at the sides of the body), Compare Position #1 to Position #2	1. Contact the T4 transverse process on side indicated by S/L Rule – LOD is **A/S/M** 2. Proceed to T4 contralateral **rib*** – LOD is **L/I** along the shaft of the **rib**

T1	Instruct patient to keep face turned to PD side, and shrug both shoulders toward ears, then relax (both arms remain at the sides of the body), Compare Position #1 to Position #2	Contact the T1 transverse process on side indicated by S/L Rule – LOD is **A/S/M. Separately** Test T1 rib
T1 Rib Re-Test For Bilateral	Instruct the patient to keep the face turned to PD side, shrug up & roll both shoulders back and down in circular motion, Compare Position #1 to Position #2	In facedown, neutral position, contact body of the rib (½ inch lateral to the transverse process) on side indicated by the S/L Rule – LOD is **Inferior**

SCAPULA RULE: The inferior angle of the scapula *"points"* to the longest leg in POSITION # 2 !

Medial Or Lateral Scapula	1. Instruct the patient to keep face turned to PD side and squeeze **PD elbow** against the side of the body, use **Scapula Rule (above)**… 2. Instruct the patient to keep face turned to PD side and squeeze **OPD elbow** against the side of the body, use **Scapula Rule (above)**…	**Medial Scapula Adjustment:** *"MURL"* 1. Ala of scapula (distal 1/3 of ala) – LOD is **Lateral**. 2. Humerus (proximal 1/3, lateral aspect) – LOD is **Superior** 3. Radius (proximal) – LOD is **Anterior/Inferior** (toward thumb) 4. Lunate (anterior aspect) – LOD is **Posterior**
	Mnemonic: **M**-Medial <u>Scapula</u> -**Lat** **L**-Lateral <u>Scapula</u>-**Med** **U**-Up on humerus -**Sup** **D**-Down on humerus -**Inf** **R**-Radius -**A/I** **U**-Ulna -**S/M** **L**-Lunate -**Post** **C**-Carpals (<u>not</u> lunate) -**Ant**	**Lateral Scapula Adjustment:** *"LDUC"* 1. Ala of scapula (distal 1/3 of ala) – LOD is **Medial** 2. Humerus (proximal 1/3, lateral aspect) – LOD is **Inferior** 3. Ulna (ant. prox. shaft) – LOD is **Superior/Medial** (toward olecranon) 4. Carpals (post. distal row; avoid Lunate) – LOD is **Anterior**

REMEMBER: Test and adjust scapula **before** moving to the cervical spine!

C7	Instruct the patient to turn face down (neutral position), from the PD side, *active motion by the patient*, Compare Position #1 to Position #2	Contact C7 lamina-pedicle junction on side indicated by S/L Rule – LOD is **A/S/M**
C5	Instruct the patient to lift head and look at the wall in front (*extend neck*), then relax, Compare Position #1 to Position #2	Contact C5 lamina-pedicle junction on side indicated by S/L Rule – LOD is **A/S/M**
C1 (Translation)	Instruct the patient to tuck chin toward chest (*flex neck*) and then relax, Compare Position #1 to Position #2	*Lowest Setting* – Contact **C1** TVP lateral-most aspect
or	If PD leg lengthens in position #2, Subluxation is **C1** on **PD side**.	**PD side** – LOD is straight **Medial**
C2	If PD leg shortens in position #2, Subluxation is **C2** on **OPD side**.	Contact **C2** lamina-pedicle junction on **OPD side** – LOD is **A/S/M**
Post Occ. Re-Test For Bilateral	Instruct the patient to push face gently into table, then relax, Compare Position #1 to Position #2	*Lowest Setting* -Contact posterior aspect of occiput at inferior nuchal line on the side indicated by S/L Rule, **protect the arch of atlas** – LOD is **straight Anterior** – Re-test to check for Bilateral subluxation

ADVANCED PROTOCOL

REVISED 11-5-07

*Please Note: **ONLY ONE THRUST** at each segmental contact point!

Possibility #1: PD lengthens in Position #2, begin protocol with: Pressure Test in this order: **PD Medial Knee, OPD Medial Knee, PD Lateral Knee, OPD Lateral Knee** (see below)		
Possibility #2: PD gets shorter in Position #2 begin protocol with: the **L4 Isolation Test.**		
Possibility #3: Legs are even in Position #1 and even in Position #2, begin protocol with: **Pubic Bone Isolation Test.**		

PRESSURE TEST: A light pressure applied in the direction of Correction. *(Look for Improvement in Position #1)*
STRESS TEST: A light pressure applied in the direction of Subluxation. *(Look for Reactivity in Position # 1)*

Listing	Test	Adjustment
PD Medial Knee joint & Talus	Pressure Test PD medial collateral ligament lateral and inferior & if there is improvement in the leg lengths in Position #1, adjust…	1. Contact medial border of PD talus inferior to medial malleolus – LOD is **P/S/L** 2. Contact PD medial knee joint space – LOD is **L/I**
OPD Medial Knee joint & Talus	Pressure Test OPD medial collateral ligament lateral and inferior & if there is improvement in the leg lengths Position #1, adjust…	1. Contact medial border of OPD talus inferior to medial malleolus – LOD is **P/S/L** 2. Contact OPD medial knee joint space – LOD is **L/I**
PD Lateral Knee joint & Cuboid	Pressure Test PD lateral collateral ligament medial and inferior & if there is improvement in the leg lengths Position #1, adjust…	1. Contact inferior lateral aspect of PD cuboid – LOD is **P/S/M** 2. Contact PD lateral knee joint – LOD is **M/I**
OPD Lateral Knee joint & Cuboid	Pressure Test OPD lateral collateral ligament medial and inferior & if there is improvement in the leg lengths Position #1, adjust…	1. Contact inferior lateral aspect of OPD cuboid – LOD is **P/S/M** 2. Contact OPD lateral knee joint – LOD is **M/I**

After Knees and Feet:
- If legs are uneven in Position #1 go to **OPD Ilium and Pressure Test** for an AS Ilium Subluxation.
- If legs are even in Position #1 but uneven in Position #2 go to **OPD Ilium and Pressure Test** for an AS Ilium Subluxation.
- If legs are even in Position #1 and even in Position #2 go to **Pubic Bone Isolation Test**.

*+The Goal is to have the legs EVEN in Position #1 **AND** Position #2.*

AS Ilium	Pressure Test crest of OPD ilium I/M & if there is improvement in the leg lengths in Position #1, adjust…	1. Contact base of sacrum on OPD side – LOD is **A/I** 2. Contact OPD crest of ilium – LOD is **I/M** 3. Contact OPD ischial tuberosity (posterior aspect) – LOD is **A/I**
PI Ilium	Pressure Test with a firm <u>thumb</u> contact, under PD sacrotuberous ligament P/S/L & if there is improvement in the leg lengths in Position #1, adjust…	1. Contact PD spine of ischium – LOD is **P/L/S** 2. Contact PD sacrotuberous ligament – LOD is **P/L/S** 3. Contact PD iliac fossa – LOD is **A/S**

ISOLATION TEST: Specific *active* movements performed <u>by the patient</u> that assist in the location and evaluation of subluxated motion segments of the spine and extremities. Utilize the Short/Long Rule.

SHORT/LONG RULE: **PD LENGTHENS in Position #2, relative to Position #1, adjust the PD side.**
PD gets SHORTER in Position #2, relative to Position #1, adjust the OPD side.
>Check Position #2 even if there is no change in Position #1. Position #2 is <u>more sensitive</u> than Position #1 alone.
*+The Goal is to have the legs EVEN in Position #1 **AND** Position #2.*

Sup. *or* **Inf. pube**	Instruct patient to squeeze knees together.	
	If PD leg lengthens in Position #2.	Contact PD pubic bone, superior aspect – LOD is **Inferior**
	If PD leg shortens in Position #2.	Contact OPD pubic bone, inferior aspect – LOD is **Superior**

Anterior Pubic Bone	Instruct patient to push PD pube/hip into the table, Look for Reactivity in Position #1	Contact anterior aspect of PD pubic bone – LOD is **Posterior**
	Instruct patient to push OPD pube/hip into the table, Look for Reactivity in Position #1	Contact anterior aspect of OPD pubic bone – LOD is **Posterior**
Lateral Pubic Bone	*Instruct patient to squeeze knees together.* *Use Position #4 to test for laterality,* *Compare Position #1 to Position #2*	*Contact ¾ inch lateral to the pubic symphysis on the side indicated by the S/L rule* *– LOD is **Medial***

ADVANCED PELVIS: *Either do Advanced Pelvis after testing/adjusting the AS, PI, and Pubes or complete the protocol through to the occiput and then come back to the pelvis. If you are returning to the pelvis, re-isolate it by having the patient squeeze their knees together again. The pubes should be clear because you already addressed the superior/inferior pube subluxations. After checking for even legs in Position #1 and #2 proceed on, to Position #3, test for Sup. or Inf. Sacrum.*

Superior or Inferior Sacrum Position #3 (AKA: Ant or Post Sacral Base)	Doctor, Flex both legs past 90° (past Position #2)	
	If PD leg lengthens in Position #3, indicates SUPERIOR sacrum (ANTERIOR sacral base)	Contact superior aspect of S3 – LOD is **A/I**
	If PD leg shortens in Position #3, indicates INFERIOR sacrum (POSTERIOR sacral base)	Contact inferior aspect of S1 – LOD is **A/S**
Lateral Sacrum Position #4	Doctor, Flex PD knee past **90°** ("cock" PD leg), compare Position #1 to Position #2… *Or see: Alternative Lateral Sacrum*	Contact inferior-lateral aspect of S3 on the side indicated by the S/L rule – LOD is **Medial/Superior**
Alternative Lateral Sacrum	*Doctor stabilizes Sacral Base, Instruct patient to lift each thigh off table keeping knee extended. Sacrum is lateral to side of most restriction in hip extension*	*Contact inferior-lateral aspect of S3 on the side of most restriction in hip extension.* *– LOD is **Medial/Superior***
Clockwise or Counter-Clockwise Sacral Rotation	*Doctor places palm on sacrum, fingers pointing superior, with firm contact rotate in **clockwise** direction (Stress Test)* *Look for Reactivity in Position #1*	*1. Contact lateral to 1st sacral tubercle on the right side* *– LOD is **A/S/M*** *2. Contact lateral to 3rd sacral tubercle on the left side* *– LOD is **A/I/M***
	*Doctor places palm on sacrum, fingers pointing superior, with firm contact rotate in **counter-clockwise** direction (Stress Test)* *Look for Reactivity in Position #1*	*1. Contact lateral to 1st sacral tubercle on the left side* *– LOD is **A/S/M*** *2. Contact lateral to 3rd sacral tubercle on the right side* *– LOD is **A/I/M***
Sacral Segments	*Doctor, Stress Test Anterior, on the PD side of the sacrum in a stroking motion (S to I)* *Look for Reactivity in Position #1*	*Pressure Test individual segments on the OPD side anteriorly* *Look for the segment that improvements in Position #1* *adjust that segment(s) – LOD is **Anterior***
	Doctor, Stress Test Anterior, on the OPD side of the sacrum in a stroking motion (S to I) *Look for Reactivity in Position #1*	*Pressure Test individual segments on the PD side anteriorly* *Look for the segment that improvements in Position #1* *adjust that segment(s) – LOD is **Anterior***
Piriformis	*Doctor, Flex knee to 90°, bring the lower leg across the midline, externally rotating the hip, ask the patient to push lower leg (medial) against your hand, then relax* *Look for Reactivity in Position #1* *(See Hip for Femur tests to be evaluated prior)*	*1. Contact ½ inch lateral to the sacral border* *– LOD is **A/I/L** into Piriformis Muscle* *2. Contact ½ inch medial to the greater trochanter* *– LOD is **A/I/L** into Piriformis Muscle* *3. Contact insertion of Piriformis at the greater trochanter* *– LOD is **A/I/L***
Quadratus Lumborum	*Instruct the patient to reach toward the knee on the affected side, thus laterally flexing the lumbar spine* *Look for Reactivity in Position #1* *Retest for bilateral involvement*	*1. Contact the superior attachment of the muscle at 12th rib* *– LOD is **Superior and slightly medial*** *2. Second contact is on the inferior attachment at the iliac crest* *– LOD is **Inferior and slightly lateral***
Lateral Coccyx	Instruct patient to squeeze buttocks muscles tight, then relax, Compare Position #1 to Position #2	Contact Sacro-coccyx <u>ligament</u>, lateral to the base of coccyx on side indicated by S/L Rule – LOD is **S/L/P**
Anterior or Posterior Base of Coccyx *(Sup. or Inf.)*	*Doctor, Stress Test Base of Coccyx push lightly with stroking motion Anterior-Superior* *Look for Reactivity in Position #1*	*Contact Base of Coccyx with thumb, Activator on Thumb* *– LOD is **Inferior/Anterior***
	Doctor, Stress Test Base of Coccyx push lightly with stroking motion Anterior-Inferior *Look for Reactivity in Position #1*	*Contact Base of Coccyx with thumb, Activator on Thumb* *– LOD is **Superior/Anterior***

When testing for **IN Ilium or A/I Sacrum** and **EX Ilium or P/S Sacrum** (see test below) You must Recall: _Which ilium subluxation/s you corrected in the Basic Scan?_ Then you will be able to correlate the previous subluxation of the ilium or sacrum to the additional testing to fine tune the Pelvis.		
If PD **L**engthens in Position #2, indicates I**L**ium. (see test below)	PI ilium tends to subluxate IN (PIIN)	
	AS ilium tends to subluxate EX (ASEX)	
If PD **S**hortens in Position #2, indicates **S**acrum (see test below)	PI ilium tends to have an A/I Sacrum (Contact Sacrotuberous Ligament)	
	AS ilium tends to have a P/S Sacrum (Contact Sacral Base)	

IN Ilium or A/I Sacrum	Doctor, lift and extend patient's **PD** thigh off the table (support tibia also)	
	if PD **L**engthens in Position #2, indicates IN I**L**ium	Contact medial border of PSIS on the PD side – LOD is **Lateral**
	if PD **S**hortens in Position #2, indicates A/I **S**acrum	Contact under sacrotuberous ligament on PD side – LOD is **P/S/L**
EX Ilium or P/S Sacrum	Doctor, lift and extend patient's **OPD** thigh off the table (support tibia also)	
	if PD **L**engthens in Position #2, indicates EX I**L**ium	Contact lateral border of PSIS on the OPD side – LOD is **Medial**
	if PD **S**hortens in Position #2, indicates P/S **S**acrum	Contact base of sacrum on OPD side – LOD is **A/I**
Bilat. Lat. Iliums .	Doctor, Stress Test laterally on both PSIS simultaneously, Look for Reactivity in Position #1	Contact lateral aspect of each PSIS – LOD is **Medial** on both PSIS
Bilat. Lat. Ischial Tuberosities	Doctor, Stress Test laterally on both ischial tuberosities simultaneously, Look for Reactivity in Position #1	Contact lateral aspect of each ischial tuberosity – LOD is **Medial** on both ischial tuberosities
Bilat. Med. Ischial Tuberosities	_Doctor, Stress Test medially on both ischial tuberosities simultaneously, Look for Reactivity in Position #1_	_Contact medial aspect of each ischial tuberosity – LOD is **Lateral** on both ischial tuberosities_

Utilize Position #3, #4 and #5 when segments are adjusted for involvement and/or are related to the patient's chief complaint. If a segment is adjusted in Basic Protocol then, "fine-tune" the segment by also testing that vertebral level in Position #3 (adjust what you find) and Position #4 (adjust what you find). If it is a chief complaint area or the legs are not balancing then test in Position #5 (adjust what you find). If the legs are still not balancing, then test the vertebral level **superior** to it. Otherwise, **test only the Basic vertebral levels**.
Position #3, #4 and #5 are done when the patient is in the Isolation Test for that particular vertebral level.
Adjust as you find the subluxation/facilitation in the spine. Do not save them up and then adjust them all at one time.

Position #3: Superiority (Flexion) or Inferiority (Extension): Flex both legs past 90° (past Position #2)	
If PD leg lengthens in Position #3, indicates SUPERIOR spinous	Contact superior aspect of the spinous process – LOD is **Inferior**
If PD leg shortens in Position #3, indicates INFERIOR spinous	Contact Inferior aspect of the spinous process – LOD is **Superior**

Position #4: Laterality: Flex PD knee past 90° ("cock" PD leg), Compare Position #1 to Position #2, use S/L Rule.	Go to the side indicated by S/L Rule: Contact PD lamina-pedicle junction on side indicated by S/L Rule, Thumb on OPD side of spinous, to prevent rotation
If PD leg lengthens in Position #2, indicates PD LATERALITY	– LOD is **Medial**
If PD leg shortens in Position #2, indicates OPD LATERALITY	Contact OPD lamina-pedicle junction on side indicated by S/L rule, Thumb on PD side of spinous, to prevent rotation –LOD is **Medial**

Position #5: Facet Syndrome: While the patient is in the Isolation Test, the Doctor will Dorsiflex both feet simultaneously. Compare Position #1 to Position #2, use S/L Rule	Go to the side indicated by S/L Rule: 1. Contact inferior articular process / TVP / LPJ of the level tested – LOD is **A/S, A/S/M, A/S/M** 2. Contact superior articular process / TVP / LPJ of segment inferior to the level tested – LOD is **A/I, A/I/M, A/I/M**

L5	Instruct patient to place PD forearm on low back (OPD arm remains at the side of the body), Compare Position #1 to Position #2	Contact L5 inferior articular process on side indicated by S/L Rule – LOD is **A/S**
L4	Instruct patient to place OPD forearm on low back (PD arm remains at the side of the body), Compare Position #1 to Position #2	Contact L4 inferior articular process on side indicated by S/L Rule – LOD is **A/S**
L3	Instruct patient to lift PD hip off the table, then relax (Both arms remains at the sides of the body), Compare Position #1 to Position #2	Contact L3 inferior articular process on side indicated by S/L Rule – LOD is **A/S**
L2	Instruct patient to place both forearms on low back, *palms up* Compare Position #1 to Position #2	Contact L2 inferior articular process on side indicated by S/L Rule – LOD is **A/S**
L1	Instruct patient to place the PD forearm on the table superior and lateral to the head and OPD forearm remains on the low back, Compare Position #1 to Position #2	Contact L1 inferior articular process on side indicated by S/L Rule – LOD is **A/S**

Additional Rib Testing *(see end of Quick Notes)*

T12	Instruct patient to place the PD forearm on the table superior and lateral to the head (OPD arm remains at the side of the body), Compare Position #1 to Position #2	Contact the T12 transverse process on side indicated by S/L Rule – LOD is **A/S/M**
T12 –Rib If clinically Indicated	Repeat T-12 Isolation Test and instruct patient to inhale and hold, Compare Position #1 to Position #2	Contact body of T12 rib ½ inch lateral to transverse process on side of rib involvement indicated by S/L Rule – LOD is **L/I** along the shaft of the **rib**

REMEMBER the ORDER is: T12, T10, T11, T9!

T10*	Instruct the patient to lower PD forearm from T12 test back alongside of body, *active motion by the patient* (OPD arm remains at the side of the body) Compare Position #1 to Position #2	1. Contact the T10 transverse process on side indicated by S/L Rule – LOD is **A/S/M** 2. Proceed to T10 contralateral **rib*** – LOD is **L/I** along the shaft of the **rib**
T11	Instruct patient to place the OPD forearm on the table superior and lateral to the head (PD arm remains at the side of the body), Compare Position #1 to Position #2	Contact the T11 transverse process on side indicated by S/L Rule – LOD is **A/S/M**
T11 – Rib If clinically Indicated	Repeat T-11 Isolation Test and instruct patient to inhale and hold, Compare Position #1 to Position #2	Contact body of T11 rib ½ inch lateral to transverse process on side indicated by S/L Rule – LOD is **L/I** along the shaft of the **rib**
T9*	Instruct the patient to lower OPD forearm from T11 test back alongside of body, *active motion by the patient* (PD arm remains at the side of the body) Compare Position #1 to Position #2	1. Contact the T9 transverse process on side indicated by S/L Rule – LOD is **A/S/M** 2. Proceed to T9 contralateral **rib*** – LOD is **L/I** along the shaft of the **rib**
T8*	Instruct patient to place both forearms on the table superior and lateral to the head, Compare Position #1 to Position #2	1. Contact the T8 transverse process on side indicated by S/L Rule – LOD is **A/S/M** 2. Proceed to T8 contralateral **rib*** – LOD is **L/I** along the shaft of the **rib**
T7*	(both arms back alongside of body), Instruct the patient to raise both shoulders off the table (posteriorly), then relax Compare Position #1 to Position #2	1. Contact the T7 transverse process on side indicated by S/L Rule – LOD is **A/S/M** 2. Proceed to T7 contralateral **rib*** – LOD is **L/I** along the shaft of the **rib**
T6*	Instruct the patient to turn face toward PD side and rest head on table (both arms remain at the sides of the body), Compare Position #1 to Position #2	1. Contact the T6 transverse process on side indicated by S/L Rule – LOD is **A/S/M** 2. Proceed to T6 contralateral **rib*** – LOD is **L/I** along the shaft of the **rib**
T5*	Instruct the patient to <u>keep face turned to PD side</u>, and place the **OPD** forearm on the table superior and lateral to the head (PD arm remains at the side of the body), Compare Position #1 to Position #2	1. Contact the T5 transverse process on side indicated by S/L Rule – LOD is **A/S/M** 2. Proceed to T5 contralateral **rib*** – LOD is **L/I** along the shaft of the **rib**
T4*	Instruct the patient to <u>keep face turned to PD side</u>, lift **PD** shoulder off the table, then relax. (both arms remain at the sides of the body), Compare Position #1 to Position #2	1. Contact the T4 transverse process on side indicated by S/L Rule – LOD is **A/S/M** 2. Proceed to T4 contralateral **rib*** – LOD is **L/I** along the shaft of the **rib**

T3*	Instruct the patient to <u>keep face turned to PD side</u>, and place the **PD** forearm on the table superior and lateral to the head (OPD arm remains at the side of the body), Compare Position #1 to Position #2	1. Contact the T3 transverse process on side indicated by S/L Rule – LOD is **A/S/M** 2. Proceed to T3 contralateral **rib*** – LOD is **L/I** along the shaft of the **rib**
T2*	Instruct the patient to <u>keep face turned to PD side</u>, and bring the **PD** arm back down by the side of the body, *active motion by the patient* (OPD arm remains at the side of the body), Compare Position #1 to Position #2	1. Contact the T2 transverse process on side indicated by S/L Rule – LOD is **A/S/M** 2. Proceed to T2 contralateral **rib*** – LOD is **L/I** along the shaft of the **rib**
T1	Instruct patient to <u>keep face turned to PD side</u>, and shrug both shoulders toward ears, then relax (both arms remain at the sides of the body), Compare Position #1 to Position #2	Contact the T1 transverse process on side indicated by S/L Rule – LOD is **A/S/M**. **Separately** Test T1 rib
T1 Rib Re-Test For Bilateral	Instruct the patient to <u>keep the face turned to PD side</u>, shrug up & roll both shoulders back and down in circular motion, Compare Position #1 to Position #2	In facedown, neutral position, contact body of the rib (½ inch lateral to the transverse process) on side indicated by S/L Rule – LOD is **Inferior**

SCAPULA RULE: The inferior angle of the scapula *"points"* to the longest leg **in POSITION # 2 !**

Medial Or Lateral Scapula	1. Instruct the patient to <u>keep face turned to PD side</u> and squeeze **PD elbow** against the side of the body, use **Scapula Rule (above)**… 2. Instruct the patient to <u>keep face turned to PD side</u> and squeeze **OPD elbow** against the side of the body, use **Scapula Rule (above)**…	**Medial Scapula Adjustment:** *"MURL"* 1. Ala of scapula (distal 1/3 of ala) – LOD is **Lateral**. 2. Humerus (proximal 1/3, lateral aspect) – LOD is **Superior** 3. Radius (proximal) – LOD is **Anterior/Inferior** (toward thumb) 4. Lunate (anterior aspect) – LOD is **Posterior**
	Mnemonic: **M**-Medial <u>Scapula</u> -**Lat** **L**-Lateral <u>Scapula</u>-**Med** **U**-Up on humerus -**Sup** **D**-Down on humerus -**Inf** **R**-Radius -**A/I** **U**-Ulna -**S/M** **L**-Lunate -**Post** **C**-Carpals (<u>not</u> lunate) -**Ant**	**Lateral Scapula Adjustment:** *"LDUC"* 1. Ala of scapula (distal 1/3 of ala) – LOD is **Medial** 2. Humerus (proximal 1/3, lateral aspect) – LOD is **Inferior** 3. Ulna (ant. prox.shaft) – LOD is **Superior/Medial** (toward olecranon) 4. Carpals (post. distal row; avoid Lunate) – LOD is **Anterior**

REMEMBER: *Test and adjust scapula **before** moving to the cervical spine!*

C7	Instruct the patient to turn face down (neutral position), from the PD side, *active motion by the patient*, Compare Position #1 to Position #2	Contact C7 lamina-pedicle junction on side indicated by S/L Rule – LOD is **A/S/M**
C6	Instruct the patient to leave the face down and shrug both shoulders toward the ears, relax, Compare Position #1 to Position #2	Contact C6 lamina-pedicle junction on side indicated by S/L Rule – LOD is **A/S/M**
C6 Enhancement	*Instruct the patient to return the face to PD side, shrug both shoulders and hold while returning the head to neutral, Compare Position #1 to Position #2*	*Contact C6 lamina-pedicle junction on side indicated by S/L Rule* – LOD is **A/S/M**
C5	Instruct the patient to lift head and look at the wall in front (*extend neck*), then relax, Compare Position #1 to Position #2	Contact C5 lamina-pedicle junction on side indicated by S/L Rule – LOD is **A/S/M**
C5 Enhancement	*Instruct the patient to slide their chin up the table and push it into the table, Compare Position #1 to Position #2*	*Contact C5 lamina-pedicle junction on side indicated by S/L Rule – LOD is **A/S/M***
Hidden Posterior C5	*Instruct the patient to shrug shoulders toward ears and hold the shrug, then lift head and look at the wall in front (extend neck), then relax, Look in Position #1 for Reactivity*	*Contact posterior-inferior aspect of C5 Spinous Process – LOD is **A/S***
C4	Instruct the patient to turn the face to the **PD** side and look up to the corner of the ceiling, (*rotate and extend*) then relax, Compare Position #1 to Position #2	Contact C4 lamina-pedicle junction on side indicated by S/L Rule – LOD is **A/S/M**

C3	Instruct the patient to turn the face to the **PD** side and look down to the PD shoulder, *(rotate and flex)* then relax, Compare Position #1 to Position #2	Contact C3 lamina-pedicle junction on side indicated by S/L Rule – LOD is **A/S/M**
C3 OPD Alternative Test	*Instruct the patient to turn the face to the OPD side and look down to the OPD shoulder, (rotate and flex) then relax*	*Contact C3 lamina-pedicle junction on side indicated by S/L Rule* *– LOD is **A/S/M***
C2 - C5 Combo & Position 3	*Testing C2* *1. Instruct the patient to tuck chin toward chest (flexion), Check legs in Position #3*	*If PD lengthens in Position #3 = Superior C2* *Contact superior aspect of C2 spinous process – LOD is **Inferior***
		If PD shortens in Position #3 = Inferior C2 *Contact inferior aspect of C2 spinous process – LOD is **Superior***
	Testing C5 *2. Instruct the patient to tuck chin toward chest (flexion) again, Check legs in Position #3*	*If PD lengthens in Position #3 = Superior C5* *Contact superior aspect of C5 spinous process – LOD is **Inferior***
		If PD shortens in Position #3 = Inferior C5 *Contact inferior aspect of C5 spinous process – LOD is **Superior***
C2	***Before Testing C1 with chin tuck...***	*1. Contact C2 lamina-pedicle junction on side indicated by S/L Rule (Pressure Test to confirm)* *– LOD is **A/S/M***
	1. Instruct the patient to turn face toward OPD Compare Position #1 to Position #2	
	2. If no reaction in test above, instruct patient to return back to neutral, Look for Reactivity in Position #1	*2. Contact C2 lamina-pedicle junction on **PD** side (Pressure Test to confirm) – LOD is **A/S/M***
C1 (Translation) or **C2**	Instruct the patient to tuck chin toward chest *(flex neck)* and then relax, Compare Position #1 to Position #2	
	If PD leg lengthens in Position #2, Subluxation is **C1** on **PD** side.	*LOWEST SETTING*– Contact **C1** TVP lateral-most aspect **PD side** – LOD is straight **Medial**
	If PD leg shortens in Position #2, Subluxation is **C2** on **OPD side.**	Contact **C2** lamina-pedicle junction on **OPD side** – LOD is **A/S/M**
Post Occ. Re-Test For Bilateral	Instruct the patient to push face gently into table, then relax, Compare Position #1 to Position #2	*LOWEST SETTING* -Contact posterior aspect of occiput at inferior nuchal line on side indicated by S/L Rule, **protect the arch of atlas** – LOD is **straight Anterior** – Re-test to check for Bilateral subluxation
Lateral Occiput (C0)	Use Position #4 to test Lateral Occiput, Compare Position #1 to Position #2 *(or see below)*	Contact the lateral aspect of occiput indicated by S/L Rule – LOD is **Medial**
	Instruct the patient to turn their face to the PD side and push head into the table, Look in Position #1 for Reactivity	*Contact PD side lateral aspect of occiput – LOD is **Medial***
	Instruct the patient to turn their face to the OPD side and push head into the table, Look in Position #1 for Reactivity	*Contact OPD side lateral aspect of occiput – LOD is **Medial***
C2 Enhancement	*If C2 showed no reactivity after completing the Cervical Protocol through the occiput...*	*1. Contact C2 lamina-pedicle junction on **PD** side (Pressure Test to confirm) – LOD is **A/S/M***
	1. Instruct patient to slightly tuck chin toward chest and hold while turning face toward PD	
	2. If no reaction, instruct patient to slightly tuck chin toward chest and hold while turning face toward OPD	*2. Contact C2 lamina-pedicle junction on **OPD** side (Pressure Test to confirm) – LOD is **A/S/M***
Cervical Disc with Radiculopathy	*Instruct the patient to laterally flex their head to the involved side Look for Reactivity in Position #1*	*Prior to adjustment, Patient is positioned so they are slightly laterally flexed away from involved side/side tested* *1. Contact lamina-pedicle junction on side tested of involved segment – LOD is **S/M*** *2. Contact lamina-pedicle junction on side tested of the segment below involved segment – LOD is **I/M***

TMJ: adjustments are made with the patient's teeth slightly apart; _LOWEST SETTING;_ Adjust through the thumb/finger; palpate very lightly; do **NOT** contact the condyle, joint capsule, discal attachments or teeth!		
Anterior-Extension TMJ	Instruct patient to open mouth wide, then relax, Compare Position #1 to Position #2	_LOWEST SETTING_ – Patient Prone: face turned to side indicated by **S/L Rule**. Contact ant/inf aspect of neck of coronoid process; through thumb – LOD is straight **P/S** (toward EAM) [note: no Med. or Lat. in the LOD!]
Superior TMJ	Instruct patient to clench or bite down, then relax, Compare Position #1 to Position #2	_LOWEST SETTING_ – Patient Prone: face turned to side indicated by **S/L Rule**. Contact body of ramus (inferior to condyle); through thumb – LOD is straight **Inferior** (down the ramus)
PD Lateral TMJ	Instruct patient to slide the lower jaw to PD side If the legs are reactive in Position #1, Pressure Test to confirm; adjust...	_LOWEST SETTING_ – Patient Prone: face turned to PD side. Contact ramus (halfway between condyle and angle of ramus); through thumb – LOD is straight **Medial**
OPD Lateral TMJ	Instruct patient to slide the lower jaw to OPD side. If the legs are reactive in Position #1, Pressure Test to confirm; adjust...	_LOWEST SETTING_ – Patient Prone: face turned to OPD side. Contact ramus (halfway between condyle and angle of ramus); through thumb – LOD is straight **Medial**
Posterior TMJ	Instruct patient to place the tip of tongue on the **BACK** of the roof of their mouth, then relax, Compare Position #1 to Position #2	_LOWEST SETTING_ – Patient Prone: face remains neutral, Contact is the posterior aspect of the ramus at the angle of the mandible on the side indicated by **S/L Rule**; through index finger – LOD is straight **Anterior**
Anterior TMJ	Instruct patient to jut or protrude their lower jaw forward (into table slot), ("like a bull dog"), then relax, Compare Position #1 to Position #2	_LOWEST SETTING_ – Patient **Supine:** face is in the neutral position. Contact on the mental tubercle, on the side indicated by **S/L Rule**; through thumb – LOD is **Posterior and Superior** toward ipsilateral EAM
Hip: The Doctor is **STRESS TESTING** each joint into neuro-biomechanical dysfunction. If there is **REACTIVITY** in Position #1, confirm by PRESSURE TESTING the joint out of neuro-biomechanical dysfunction, legs will be even again.		
Internal Femur Rotation (or A/I Hip)	Doctor, Flex knee to 90°, bring the lower leg away from midline, internally rotating the hip, (like Hibb's Test) Look for Reactivity in Position #1	Contact anterior aspect of greater trochanter – LOD is **Posterior and Superior** (taking into account the angle of the neck of the femur)
External Femur Rotation (or P/S Hip)	Doctor, Flex knee to 90°, bring the lower leg across the midline, externally rotating the hip, (opposite of Hibb's Test), Look for Reactivity in Position #1	Contact posterior aspect of greater trochanter – LOD is **Anterior and Inferior** (taking into account the angle of the neck of the femur)
Superior Femur	Doctor, Stress Test greater trochanter superior, Look for Reactivity in Position #1	Contact superior aspect of greater trochanter – LOD is **Inferior**
Inferior Femur	Doctor, Stress Test greater trochanter inferior, Look for Reactivity in Position #1	Contact inferior aspect of greater trochanter – LOD is **Superior**
Lateral Proximal Femur	Doctor, Grasp tissue over greater trochanter and pull straight laterally, Look for Reactivity in Position #1	Contact lateral trochanter – LOD is **Medial and Superior** (taking into account the angle of the neck of the femur)
Piriformis	_(May have tested previously, during evaluation of Pelvis/Sacrum.)_ _Doctor, Flex knee to 90°, bring the lower leg across the midline, externally rotating the hip, ask the patient to push lower leg (medial) against your hand, then relax_ _Look for Reactivity in Position #1_ _(Perform after External Femur Rotation)_	_Look for reactivity in Position #1, then adjust:_ 1. _Contact ½ inch lateral to the sacral border – LOD is A/I/L_ 2. _Contact ½ inch medial to the greater trochanter – LOD is A/I/L_ 3. _Contact attachment of the piriformis at the greater trochanter – LOD is A/I/L_
Psoas Muscle Imbalance	Doctor, lift both of the patient's feet a few inches off the table and instruct patient to press both knees into surface of table, relax	Patient **Supine:** Contact belly of psoas muscle on side indicated by S/L Rule – LOD is **P/I/L**
Medial (Int. Rot.) of distal femur	_Doctor, stabilize the proximal tibia and Stress Test the distal femur into internal rotation, Look for Reactivity in Position #1_	_Contact posterior aspect of the medial femoral condyle – LOD is **Anterior**_

Knee: The Doctor is **STRESS TESTING** each joint into neuro-biomechanical dysfunction. If there is **REACTIVITY** in Position #1, confirm by PRESSURE TESTING the joint out of neuro-biomechanical dysfunction, legs will be even again.		
Anterior Proximal Tibia	Doctor, Place your open palm on the gastrocs and Stress Test proximal tibia anterior, Look for Reactivity in Position #1	Flex knee to 90° and contact ½ inch below anterior tibial tuberosity (adj. through Doc finger for pt. comfort) – LOD is **Posterior** (anatomically)
Posterior Proximal Tibia	Doctor, Lift proximal tibia posterior, Look for Reactivity in Position #1 **AVOID** the popliteal fossa during adjustment!	1. Contact posterior aspect of medial tibial condyle – LOD is **Anterior** 2. Contact posterior aspect of lateral tibial condyle – LOD is **Anterior**
Ext. Rot. of Proximal Tibia	Doctor, Grasp gastrocs and Rotate proximal tibia external (reference point is the anterior tibial tuberosity or toes), Look for Reactivity in Position #1	Contact lateral to anterior tibial tuberosity – LOD is lateral to **Medial** (Internal)
Int. Rot. of Proximal Tibia	Doctor, Grasp gastrocs and Rotate proximal tibia internal (reference point is the anterior tibial tuberosity or toes), Look for Reactivity in Position #1	Contact medial to anterior tibial tuberosity – LOD is medial to **Lateral** (External)
Genu Valgus (Lat. Shear)	Doctor, simultaneously push medial tibial condyle laterally and push lateral femoral condyle medially, Look for Reactivity in Position #1	1. Contact lateral tibial condyle (avoid fibula) – LOD is **Medial** 2. Contact medial femoral condyle – LOD is **Lateral**
Genu Varus (Med. Shear)	Doctor, simultaneously push lateral tibial condyle medially and push medial femoral condyle laterally, Look for Reactivity in Position #1	1. Contact medial tibial condyle – LOD is **Lateral** 2. Contact lateral femoral condyle – LOD is **Medial**
Medial Knee joint	Doctor, flex the knee to 90°, compress and externally rotate (reference the toes) the tibia, Look for Reactivity in Position #1	Contact medial collateral ligament in joint space – LOD is **Lateral**
Lateral Knee joint	Doctor, flex the knee to 90°, compress and internally rotate (reference the toes) the tibia, Look for Reactivity in Position #1	Contact lateral collateral ligament in joint space – LOD is **Medial**
Hamstrings	Doctor, flex patient's knee ~30°, Doctor's hand on posterior aspect of distal tibia, instruct the patient to flex knee against resistance, Look for Reactivity in Position #1	1. Contact myotendon junction of the medial hamstrings – LOD is **Anterior** 2. Contact myotendon junction of the lateral hamstring – LOD is **Anterior**
Quadriceps Femoris	Doctor, flex patient's knee ~30°, Doctor's hand on anterior aspect of distal tibia, instruct the patient to straighten knee against resistance, Look for Reactivity in Position #1	Contact Vastus medialis myotendon junction – LOD is **Posterior**
Gastroc-nemius	Doctor, flex patient's knee ~75°, Doctor's hand on plantar surface of foot, instruct the patient to plantar flex against resistance, Look for Reactivity in Position #1	1. Contact medial head of the gastrocnemius ½ inch inferior to the medial tibial condyle – LOD is **Anterior and slightly superior** 2. Contact lateral head of the gastrocnemius ½ inch inferior to the lateral tibial condyle – LOD is **Anterior and slightly superior**
Compressed/ Impinged Femoral-Tibial Joint	**Medial Impingement:** Doctor, grasp the involved posterior-lateral distal tibia with one hand, place the other hand on the posterior-medial distal femur. Doctor, move tibia toward midline, a lateral to medial Stress Test, Look for Reactivity in Position #1	1. Contact medial condyle of the femur – LOD is **Superior and slightly lateral** 2. Contact medial aspect of the proximal tibia – LOD is **Inferior and slightly lateral**
	Lateral Impingement: Doctor, grasp the involved posterior-medial distal tibia with one hand, place the other hand on the posterior-lateral distal femur. Doctor, move the tibia away from mid-line, a medial to lateral Stress Test, Look for Reactivity in Position #1	1. Contact lateral condyle of the femur – LOD is **Superior and slightly medial** 2. Contact lateral aspect of the proximal tibia – LOD is **Inferior and slightly medial**

Inferior Patella	Doctor, Lightly Stress Test patella inferior, Look for Reactivity in Position #1	Flex knee to 45°, Contact inferior border of patella – LOD is **Superior**
Superior Patella	*Doctor, Lightly Stress Test patella superior, Look for Reactivity in Position #1*	*Supine, Contact superior border of patella – LOD is Inferior*
Lateral Patella	Doctor, Lightly Stress Test patella lateral, Look for Reactivity in Position #1	Contact lateral border of patella – LOD is **Medial**
P/S Proximal Fibula	Doctor, Stress Test proximal head of fibula posterior and superior, Look for Reactivity in Position #1	Contact posterior aspect of fibula head – LOD is **A/I** (45° to long axis of fibula)
Lateral Fibula	Doctor, Stress Test with a tissue pull laterally at the proximal 1/3 of the fibula, Look for Reactivity in Position #1	Contact proximal 1/3 of the fibula on the lateral aspect – LOD is **Medial**

Ankle and Foot: STRESS TESTS are still done with the **shoes on** so as to read the leg **REACTIVITY** in Position #1. **Remove the shoe to Adjust!** The Doctor is **STRESS TESTING** each joint into neuro-biomechanical dysfunction. If there is **REACTIVITY** in Position #1, confirm by PRESSURE TESTING the joint out of neuro-biomechanical dysfunction, legs will be even again.

Posterior Distal Fibula	Doctor, Stress Test lateral malleolus posterior, Look for Reactivity in Position #1	Contact posterior aspect of lateral malleolus – LOD is **Anterior**
Anterior Distal Tibia	*Doctor, Stress Test the distal tibia by pulling it anterior, Look for Reactivity in Position #1*	*Contact the anterior distal tibia – LOD is Posterior*
Superior Calcaneus	Doctor, Plantar flex the foot which will Stress Test calcaneus superior, Look for Reactivity in Position #1	Contact posterior aspect of calcaneus (contact at insertion of Achilles Tendon) – LOD is **Inferior**
Inferior Calcaneus	*Doctor, grasp posterior aspect of calcaneus and dorsiflex foot, Look for Reactivity in Position #1*	*Contact inferior aspect of calcaneus – LOD is Superior*
Medial Calcaneus	Doctor, Tap lateral border in a lateral to medial direction, Look for Reactivity in Position #1	Contact medial aspect of calcaneus – LOD is **Lateral**
Lateral Calcaneus	*Doctor, Tap medial border in a medial to lateral direction, Look for Reactivity in Position #1*	*Contact lateral aspect of calcaneus – LOD is Medial*
Posterior Calcaneus	*Doctor, pull calcaneus posterior, Look for Reactivity in Position #1*	*Contact distal to insertion of Achilles tendon – LOD Anterior*
A/L Talus	Doctor, Plantar flex and invert the foot, Look for Reactivity in Position #1	Contact neck of talus in sinus tarsi – LOD is **P/M**
Inf. 1st Metatarsal & Inf. 1st Cuneiform	Doctor, Plantar flex and evert the foot, Look for Reactivity in Position #1	1. Contact inferior or plantar aspect of 1st **metatarsal base** (in the arch) – LOD is **Superior**. 2. Contact inferior border of 1st cuneiform – LOD is **S/L**
A/S Tarsal Navicular	Doctor, Tissue pull A/S over the tarsal navicular (it is located on the Medial aspect of the foot), Look for Reactivity in Position #1	Contact superior aspect of navicular – LOD is **P/I**
Medial Navicular	*Doctor, Stress Test lateral to medial across navicular, Look for Reactivity in Position #1*	*Contact medial tuberosity of the navicular – LOD is S/L*
Inferior or Dropped Metatarsal Heads	Doctor, Push metatarsal heads inferior while Curling the toes dorsally, Look for Reactivity in Position #1.	Contact inferior aspect of metatarsal heads (on as many that palpate inferior) – LOD is **Superior**
Distal 1st Metatarsal and Superior Proximal 1st Phalange	*Doctor, plantar flex at first metatarsal phalangeal joint, Look for Reactivity in Position#1*	*Contact superior aspect of the first metatarsal-phalange joint, While applying distal traction on proximal phalanx – LOD is Inferior*
Hallux Valgus	*Doctor, push distal first phalange lateral, While stabilizing first metatarsal head, Look for Reactivity in Position #1*	*Contact medial aspect first metatarsal-phalangeal joint, While applying distal traction on proximal phalanx – LOD is Lateral*

Shoulder: In the shoulder scan the <u>patient</u> is **<u>STRESS TESTING</u>** each joint into neuro-biomechanical dysfunction. If there is **<u>REACTIVITY</u>** in Position #1, confirm by PRESSURE TESTING the joint out of neuro-biomechanical dysfunction, legs will be even again.

A/I Humerus	Instruct the patient to (extend) lift arm and palm toward the ceiling (end of active ROM) Look for Reactivity in Position #1	Contact anterior aspect of proximal humerus at the intertubercular groove – LOD is **P/S**
Lateral Distal Humerus	*Instruct the patient to push the involved elbow into the table, Look for Reactivity in Position #1*	*Roll the patient's arm so the palm is down on the table, Contact the lateral distal humerus – LOD is **Medial***
External Humerus	Instruct the patient to lock elbow & turn palm over to touch the table (Ext. Rot. of Humerus), Look for Reactivity in Position #1	Contact lateral aspect of greater tubercle – LOD is **A/M**
Internal Humerus	Instruct the patient to lock elbow & now turn the palm in the other direction and turn it further, palm faces away from body (Internal Rotation of Humerus), Look for Reactivity in Position #1	Contact posterior aspect, head of humerus – LOD is **A/M**
Posterior Humerus	Instruct the patient to hang arm over side of table (if not enough fulcrum, STRESS posterior), Look for Reactivity in Position #1	Contact posterior aspect of proximal humerus @ insertion of infraspinatus tendon –LOD is **Anterior**
T2 Rib Involvement	Instruct the patient to stick arm straight out like an airplane with palm up, Look for Reactivity in Position #1	Contact body of T2 rib ½ inch lateral to TVP (on the side you tested) – LOD is **L/I** along the shaft of the rib
T2/T3 Facet Syndrome	Instruct the patient to make a swimming motion (big forward circle), Look for Reactivity in Position #1	1. Contact T2 TVP – LOD is **A/S** 2. Contact T3 TVP – LOD is **A/I**
Superior Scapula	Instruct the patient to place palm of hand on back of neck, Look for Reactivity in Position #1	Contact the S/M aspect of the spine of the scapula – LOD is **Inferior**
Superior Proximal Clavicle	Instruct the patient to place palm of hand on back of neck and push elbow into table, Look for Reactivity in Position #1	Patient **supine** and face turned to ipsilateral side: Contact proximal clavicle – LOD is **I/L**
T3/T4 Facet Syndrome	*Instruct the patient to place hand on back of neck and lift the elbow off the table, Look for Reactivity in Position #1*	*1. Contact T3 TVP – LOD is A/S 2. Contact T4 TVP – LOD is A/I*
Inferior Scapula	*Instruct the patient to return hand/arm to side after testing for Superior Scapula, Look for Reactivity in Position #1*	*Contact inferior medial spine of scapula – LOD is **Superior***
A/C Joint Separation Subluxation	Instruct the patient to place hand on "hip" (crest of ilium) of involved side and push hand medially into body, "Sassy", Look for Reactivity in Position #1	Patient **Supine:** 1. Contact superior aspect of distal clavicle – LOD is **Lateral** (support acromion) 2. Contact lateral aspect of acromion process – LOD is **Medial** (support clavicle)
A/C joint Impingement Subluxation	*Doctor, pinch the distal clavicle and acromion together, Look for Reactivity in Position #1*	*1. Contact posterior distal clavicle – LOD is A/M 2. Contact anterior and superior acromion process – LOD is P/L/I*
I/M Coracoid	Doctor, Stress coracoid process inferior and medial, Look for Reactivity in Position #1	Patient **Supine:** Contact coracoid process – LOD is **S/L** (45° angle)

Additional Clavicle Tests: The Doctor is <u>STRESS TESTING</u> each joint into neuro-biomechanical dysfunction. If there is **REACTIVITY** in Position #1, confirm by PRESSURE TESTING the joint out of neuro-biomechanical dysfunction, legs will be even again.

Superior Distal Clavicle	Instruct the patient to shrug shoulder of involved side toward the ear, then relax, Look for Reactivity in Position #1	Contact superior aspect of distal clavicle just medial to acromioclavicular joint – LOD is **Inferior**
Anterior Distal Clavicle	Doctor, Stress Test distal clavicle anterior, Look for Reactivity in Position #1	Patient **Supine**: Contact anterior aspect of distal clavicle just medial to acromioclavicular joint – LOD is **Posterior**
Posterior Distal Clavicle	Doctor, Stress Test distal clavicle posterior, Look for Reactivity in Position #1	Contact posterior aspect at acromioclavicular joint – LOD is **Anterior**
Lateral Clavicle	Doctor, Stress Test clavicle lateral, Look for Reactivity in Position #1	Contact distal clavicle just medial to acromioclavicular joint – LOD is **Medial**
Inferior Proximal Clavicle	Doctor, Stress Test inferior on proximal clavicle, Look for Reactivity in Position #1	Patient **Supine:** Contact inferior aspect of proximal clavicle – LOD is **S/M**

Shoulder Muscles: Do these Stress Tests after adjusting for neuro-biomechanical dysfunctions of the shoulder on several visits and the patient has reached sub-acute status.

Supra-spinatus	*Instruct the patient to reach (from below) behind their back and up toward the opposite scapula, Look for Reactivity in Position #1*	*1. Contact medial aspect of supraspinatus muscle belly – LOD is* **Inferior** *2. Contact lateral aspect of the supraspinatus muscle belly – LOD is* **Inferior** *3. Contact proximal lateral humerus on musculotendon junction of supraspinatus – LOD is* **Inferior, and slightly medial**
Infra-spinatus	*Instruct the patient to hang forearm over the edge of the table and push the forearm superior (headward) against resistance of the doctor, Look for Reactivity in Position #1*	*1. Contact Lateral aspect of the infraspinatus fossa of the scapula– LOD is* **M/S** *2. Contact Medial aspect of the infraspinatus fossa of the scapula– LOD is* **M/S**
Sub-scapularis	*Instruct the patient to hang forearm over the edge of the table and push the forearm inferior (footward) against resistance of the doctor, Look for Reactivity in Position #1*	*Contact Lateral aspect of the subscapularis under the scapula – LOD is* **Medial and slightly Superior**
Medial (Global) Scapula	*Patient places forearm over low back. Doctor places hand against the lateral distal humerus and patient pushes out against resistance (isometric shoulder abduction), Look for Reactivity in Position #1*	*1. Contact Superior aspect of medial border of scapula – LOD is* **Lateral** *2. Contact Mid-aspect of medial border of scapula – LOD is* **Lateral** *3. Contact Inferior aspect of medial border of scapula – LOD is* **Lateral**

Forearm and Wrist: can be **<u>STRESS TESTED</u>** separate from the Scapula Tests. The Doctor or Patient is **<u>STRESS TESTING</u>** each joint into neuro-biomechanical dysfunction. If there is **REACTIVITY** in Position #1, confirm by PRESSURE TESTING the joint out of neuro-biomechanical dysfunction, legs will be even again.

P/S Radius & Ant. Lunate	Instruct patient to make fist on involved hand, Look for Reactivity in Position #1	1. Contact Head of Radius (Proximal) – LOD is **Anterior/Inferior** (toward thumb) 2. Contact Anterior Lunate – LOD is **Posterior**
I/M Ulna & Posterior Carpals	Instruct patient to flex wrist on involved hand, Look for Reactivity in Position #1	1. Contact anterior proximal Ulna – LOD is (anatomically) **Superior/Medial** (toward olecranon) 2. Contact post. distal row; avoid Lunate – LOD is **Anterior**
Posterior Proximal Ulna (Pronation)	*Elbow in 30° of flexion, Doctor, Stress Test forearm into pronation, Look for Reactivity in Position #1*	*Contact posterior proximal ulna (olecranon), elbow flexed 90° – LOD is* **S/M** *toward (through) shaft of humerus (Keep "P"s together.)*
Anterior Proximal Ulna (Supination)	*Elbow in 30° of flexion, Doctor, Stress Test forearm into supination, Look for Reactivity in Position #1*	*Contact anterior proximal ulna, elbow flexed 30° – LOD is* **I/M**

Pronator Quadratus	*Instruct patient to fully pronate hand to end of range of motion,*
	Look for Reactivity in Position #1
		1. Contact anterior radius 1½ inches proximal to wrist crease
		   – LOD is **Lateral**
		2. Contact anterior radius 3 inches proximal to wrist crease
		   – LOD is **Lateral**
		3. Contact anterior Ulna 1 ½ inches proximal to wrist crease
		   – LOD is **Medial**
		4. Contact anterior Ulna 3 inches proximal to wrist crease
		   – LOD is **Medial**

Carpal Tunnel
Separated
Distal
Radius
& Ulna
	Instruct the patient to squeeze together the tips
	of the thumb and little finger
	(first and fifth digits) on the involved side,
	Look for Reactivity in Position #1
		Patient's arm along side body, palm is up:
		1. Contact lateral aspect of distal radius
		   – LOD is **Medial** (ulnar direction)
		2. Contact medial aspect of distal ulna
		   – LOD is **Lateral** (radial direction)
		(adjustments approximate the radius and ulna)

Approximated Distal Radius & Lunate	*Doctor, Stress Test by squeezing distal radius and ulna together,*
	Look for Reactivity in Position #1
		1. Contact distal, anteriomedial aspect of radius
		   – LOD is **Lateral**
		2. Contact distal, anteriolateral aspect of ulna
		   – LOD is **Medial**
		(adjustments "separate" the radius and ulna)

Wrist Extensors	*Instruct patient to extend wrist against resistance of Doctor,* *Look for Reactivity in Position #1*	*Patient's hand by head, palm down:* *Contact in belly of wrist extensor muscles 1½ inches distal to antecubital fossa* *– LOD is* **Anterior**
Proximal Carpals	*Instruct the patient to extend their wrist,* *Look for Reactivity in Position #1*	*Contact the posterior aspect of each proximal carpal excluding the lunate* *– LOD is* **Anterior and Inferior**

Hand: The Doctor is **STRESS TESTING** each joint into neuro-biomechanical dysfunction. If there is **REACTIVITY** in Position #1, confirm by PRESSURE TESTING the joint out of neuro-biomechanical dysfunction, legs will be even again.

Trapezio- Metacarpal (Thumb) Joint	Instruct patient to lay thumb of involved hand across palm of hand, form a fist and squeeze, Look for Reactivity in Position #1	Contact base of metacarpal in "anatomical snuff box" – LOD is **Distal** along longitudinal axis of first metacarpal
Anterior Proximal First Metacarpal	*Doctor, Stress Test base of thumb anterior with distal distraction of thumb,* *Look for Reactivity in Position #1*	*Contact anterior proximal first metacarpal base* *– LOD is* **Posterior and slightly lateral**
Medial - Superior Hamate	*Doctor, Stress Test hamate in the medial and superior directions,* *Look for Reactivity in Position #1*	*Contact hamate* *– LOD is* **L/I**
Pisiform	*Doctor, Stress Test by approximating thenar and hypothenar together* (palm pads together) *Look for Reactivity in Position #1*	*Contact superior aspect of pisiform* *– LOD is* **L/I** *(toward shaft of fourth finger)*

Additional Rib Testing: These tests maybe done while evaluating the Thoracic Spine or at the end of the adjustment.

Anterior First Rib	*Instruct the patient to push involved shoulder into the table, then relax,* *Look for Reactivity in Position #1*	*Patient* **supine**: *Contact just below the clavicle, 2 inches lateral to the manubrium on the first rib* *LOD is* **P/S**
T3 Rib Involvement	*Instruct the patient to abduct both arms to 90°, palms facing up and hold* ("airplane"), *Compare Position #1 to Position #2*	*Contact T3 rib ½ inch lateral to transverse process on side indicated by S/L Rule* *– LOD is* **L/I** *along the shaft of the rib*
T4 Rib Involvement	*Instruct the patient to abduct both arms to 90°, palms facing up and hold* ("airplane"), *then return arms to their sides on the table* ("airplane landing"), *Compare Position #1 to Position #2*	*Contact T4 rib ½ inch lateral to transverse process on side indicated by S/L Rule* *– LOD is* **L/I** *along the shaft of the rib*

Costo-Vertebral Rib (Post. aspect)	Isolate the involved vertebral segment, adjust accordingly. Instruct the patient to **Inhale** deeply and hold briefly, Compare Position #1 to Position #2	Contact rib (at the level tested) ½ inch lateral to transverse process on side indicated by S/L Rule – LOD is **L/I** along the shaft of the rib
Superior or Inferior Rib Costo-Vertebral (Post. aspect)	Isolate the involved vertebral segment, adjust accordingly. Instruct the patient to **Inhale** deeply and hold briefly, use Position #2 for side indicated by the S/L rule, use Position #3 Superiority or Inferiority of the rib	Contact superior aspect of rib (at the level tested) ½ inch lateral to the transverse process on side indicated by S/L Rule – LOD is **I/A**
	If PD leg lengthens in Position #3, indicates *SUPERIOR* rib	
	If PD leg shortens in Position #3, indicates *INFERIOR* rib	Contact inferior aspect of rib (at the level tested) ½ inch lateral to the transverse process on side indicated by S/L Rule – LOD is **S/A**
Lateral Rib Costo-Vertebral (Post. aspect)	Isolate the involved vertebral segment, adjust accordingly. Instruct the patient to **Inhale** deeply and hold briefly, use Position #4 to test for Laterality of rib on the posterior aspect of the body, Compare Position #1 to Position #2	Contact rib (at the level tested) on lateral aspect of the angle of the rib on side indicated by S/L Rule – LOD is **M/S**
Costo-Sternal Rib (Ant. aspect)	Isolate the involved vertebral segment, adjust accordingly. Instruct the patient to Inhale and then **Exhales** to a deep level of excursion, Compare Position #1 to Position #2	Patient **Supine:** Contact rib ½ inch lateral to the sternum (at the level tested) on side indicated by S/L Rule – LOD is **L/I** along the shaft of the rib
Superior or Inferior Rib Costo-Sternal (Ant. aspect)	Isolate the involved vertebral segment, adjust accordingly. Instruct the patient to Inhale and then **Exhales** to a deep level of excursion, use Position #2 for side indicated by the S/L rule, use Position #3 Superiority or Inferiority of the rib	Patient **Supine:** Contact superior aspect of rib ½ inch lateral to the sternum (at the level tested) on side indicated by S/L Rule – LOD is **I/P**
	If PD leg lengthens in Position #3, indicates *SUPERIOR* rib	
	If PD leg shortens in Position #3, indicates *INFERIOR* rib	Contact inferior aspect of rib ½ inch lateral to the sternum (at the level tested) on side indicated by S/L Rule – LOD is **S/P**
Lateral Rib Costo-Sternal Rib (Ant. aspect)	Isolate the involved vertebral segment, adjust accordingly. Instruct the patient to Inhale and then **Exhales** to a deep level of excursion, use Position #4 to test for Laterality of rib on the anterior aspect of the body, Compare Position #1 to Position #2	Patient **Supine:** Contact rib (at the level tested) ½ inch lateral to the sternum on side indicated by S/L Rule – LOD is **M/S** along the shaft of the rib

Anterior Thorax: The Doctor or Patient is <u>**STRESS TESTING**</u> each of the following into neuro-biomechanical dysfunction. If there is **REACTIVITY** in Position #1, confirm by PRESSURE TESTING, legs will be even again.

Scalenus Anticus	Instruct patient to make fists with both hands, shrug both shoulders, then relax, Compare Position #1 to Position #2	Patient *supine:* Contact scalenus anticus muscle/tendon on side indicated by the S/L Rule, doctor's digit on insertion – LOD is **Inferior**
Superior Manubrium of Sternum	Instruct patient to inhale deeply and hold, Lift head up (extension), then relax, Look for Reactivity in Position #1	Patient *supine:* turn face to one side Contact sternal notch – LOD is **Inferior**

Hiatal Hernia Symptoms	Doctor, gently push superior in the epigastic region near the xiphoid process,
	 Look for Reactivity in Position #1
		Patient *supine:* On Left Abdomen, inferior to rib cage:
		 1. 1 inch inferior to xiphoid process
		    – LOD is **I/L**
		 2. 1 inch inferior and 2 inches lateral to the first contact point
		    – LOD is **I/L**
		 3. 1 inch inferior and 2 inches lateral to the second contact point – LOD is **I/L**

Xiphoid	Patient **supine**, use supine leg analysis, Stress Test, usually inferior, Look for Reactivity in Position #1	Patient *supine:* Contact xiphoid adjust through the doctor's thumb – LOD is Opposite direction of Stress Test

Activator Method (AM) A technique, primarily used by chiropractors, that incorporates a system of analysis with assessment procedures for neuroarticular function and dysfunction and specific treatment with an Activator Instrument. The AM provides a systematic clinical approach to neuroarticular dysfunction through the use of protocols for identifying and treating a wide variety of common complaints of neuromusculoskeletal origin.

Activator Position of Analysis The patient is lying in a prone position with the knees in a slightly flexed position; the ankles and feet are in a neutral relaxed state and extend past the bottom of the table far enough to allow the ankles and feet to move freely. The arms are laying alongside the body in a relaxed position, with the dorsal aspects of the hands against the table and the palms facing up. (This is not considered anatomical position because the palms of the hands are facing backward.)

Allodynia A painful or nociceptive response provoked by normally innocuous stimuli, usually a light mechanical stimulus (tactile allodynia).

Anatomical Position The position assumed when a person is standing erect with arms at the sides and palms forward. Anatomical position is the point of reference used throughout the Activator Method when the direction of subluxations, neuroarticular dysfunctions, and Lines of Drive are described. Of primary importance, the palms of the hands are facing forward. SYN: orthograde position.

Anatomical "True" Short Leg A difference in the size and/or length of the structures between the ground and the femoral head. SYN: leg length discrepancy, Leg Length Inequality, or short leg.

Central Pattern Generator (CPG) The network of neurons that produce patterned motor behavior in the absence of phasic inputs. In higher vertebrates, networks within the spinal cord that generate basic motor behavior patterns underlying walking, hopping, swimming, and scratching, even when isolated from the brain and sensory inputs.

Cold Nociceptors One of the four types of nociceptors that respond to noxious cold stimuli ($<5°$ C).

Crossed Extensor Reflex A coordinated reflex involving an extension of the contralateral leg when a painful stimulus is applied to the skin. This reflex causes the contralateral leg to bear the body's weight while the ipsilateral flexor reflex occurs. Crossed extensor and flexor reflexes are mediated by polysynaptic pathways, while the integrative centers are found in the local spinal cord. These spinally mediated withdrawal reflexes can be reduced or blocked by the descending systems from the higher levels of the brain.

Engram Within the central nervous system, it serves as the physiological basis of memory.

Feed Forward Mechanism Anticipatory motor impulses in the central nervous system predict the effect a movement will have on the body and plan a sequence of muscle activities designed to overcome the potential forces that will be imparted. The prediction involves a coordinated effort of local and global systems to stabilize the spine, allowing for extremity movement, and incorporating the impending speed and resistant forces that will occur during limb movement. Within the central nervous system, it provides the physiological basis of memory.

Feedback Mediated In motor learning, the use of sensory information from contracting muscles to influence subsequent muscular contractions, resulting within the system as a stimulus that may be positive or negative. Positive feedback is the result of the process that intensifies the stimulus. In negative feedback, the process reverses or shuts off the stimulus.

Fictive Locomotion A term used for neural activity when rhythmical patterns of movement occur in the absence of any movements.

Flexor Reflex A coordinated reflex, for example, when the skin of one foot of an individual is stimulated by a mechanical or thermal noxious stimulus, the lower extremity undergoes a coordinated withdrawal. The flexor muscles contract and the extensor muscles relax, facilitating the flexion of the joints so as to escape from injury. Occurs with a crossed extensor reflex.

Hair Follicle Receptors The principal mechanoreceptors of the hairy skin that covers most of the body. There are three separate classes of receptors that innervate different types of hair follicles: hair-guard, hair-tylotrich, and hair-down receptors.

Heat Nociceptors One of the four types of nociceptors that respond selectively to heat or cold. In humans, they respond when the temperature of the receptive field exceeds 45° C—the heat pain threshold.

Hyperalgesia One of the major responses of the nervous system to repetitive noxious stimulation; it creates an extremely increased response to a stimulus that is normally painful and has peripheral and central nervous system origins. Changes in nociceptor sensitivity underlie primary hyperalgesia; the hyperexcitability of spinal dorsal horn neurons underlies centrally mediated hyperalgesia.

Isolation Test Specific *active* movements performed by the patient that assist in the location and evaluation of neuroarticular dysfunctional motion segments of the spine and extremities; movements are performed when leg lengths are balanced. Active motions are thought to facilitate neurological pathways and to increase tension in the musculature or other soft tissues of specific regions of the spine and appendicular skeleton.

Leg Length Analysis (LLA) The Activator Method of assessment for neuroarticular dysfunction and function, based on the assumption that faulty biomechanical behavior of articulations is reflected by differences between and changes in leg lengths. The assessment protocol consists of a series of prone leg length observations and provocative tests designed to evaluate the function of

joints from the feet progressively upward throughout the axial skeleton.

Leg Length Reactivity A tool of analysis that compares the lengths of the legs in non–weight bearing as a patient is lying prone; the appearance of a short leg. The process of evaluating a reactive, dynamic change in comparative leg lengths in the prone or supine position. A phenomenon used as a common clinical test by chiropractors as a sign of "neuromuscular dysfunction" or "nervous system control errors." Because of suprapelvic muscular hyperactivity, or because the nervous system ceases to activate the small spinal stabilization muscles, principally the transverse abdominis and the multifidus, activation of the outer layer muscles may result. In the Activator Method, changes are observed in the relative lengths of legs, at the feet, throughout different stages of ankle and knee flexion, and at times, hip extension. Comparisons of leg length are performed after imposed forces and movements are provided through the use of an Isolation Test, Stress Test, and/or Pressure Test. SYN: unloaded leg length alignment asymmetry, functional short leg.

Line of Drive (LOD) Referenced in anatomical position terms, the direction the Activator Instrument is pointed when an adjustment is performed. The first listing is the primary direction (i.e., posterior and medial). If the LOD is listed with a hyphen (i.e., as posterior-lateral), the direction of the instrument is vectored equally between them.

Long Reflex A reflex involving several segments of the spinal cord. More complex than simple stretch reflexes and involves information processing at higher levels of the central nervous system, including transcortical mechanisms. Long reflexes have a longer latency than do simple stretch reflexes, are more flexible, and can be modified voluntarily; they also have a greater role in error correction, especially when equilibrium is maintained. SYN: intersegmental reflex, long loop reflex.

Mechanical Nociceptors One of the four types of nociceptors that are activated only by strong mechanical stimulation, most effectively with the use of sharp objects.

Mechanochemistry The study of the effect that mechanical forces have on those biochemical processes not directly responsible for regenerative signaling of the nervous system. It involves the balance of tensile loading between outwardly directed forces from extracellular connections and intracellular osmotic pressure and inwardly directed forces from a cell's cytoskeleton; it addresses the ability of these mechanical changes to directly activate biochemical processes.

Meissner's Corpuscle One of the two principal types of mechanoreceptors in the superficial glabrous (hairless) skin. It is a rapidly adapting receptor, which responds at the onset and often also at the termination but not through the duration of the stimulus. It has specialized accessory structures that are thought to be mechanical filters that confer dynamic or static response specificity.

Memory Engram Within the central nervous system, the physiological basis of storage and retrieval of memory. It is the interpretation of sensory input that allows an individual to correlate the nature, intensity, and associated sensations of the immediate stimulus with previous sensory experiences. The major storage site for memory engram appears to be in temporal lobes, which receive thalamocortical projections from the medial thalamic nuclei. Establishment of the memory engram for painful experiences has been noted to be a function of the intensity of the stimulus, the length of time the stimulus lasts, and the frequency with which it is repeated.

Merkel's Receptor One of the two principal types of mechanoreceptors in the superficial glabrous (hairless) skin. It is a slowly adapting mechanoreceptor that responds continuously to a persistent stimulus. It includes specialized accessory structures that are thought to be mechanical filters and that confer dynamic or static response specificity.

Nociceptors Receptors that respond selectively to stimuli that can damage tissue. They respond directly to some noxious stimuli and indirectly to others by means of one or more chemical intermediaries released from cells in the traumatized tissue. Four types of nociceptors are distinguished on the basis of properties of the stimuli. Nociceptive information is carried from the spinal cord to the higher centers in the brain through five major ascending pathways that originate in different laminae of the dorsal horn.

Non-nociceptors Receptors responding to non-noxious stimuli, such as touch, warmth, cold, and limb proprioception. These receptors can be divided into cutaneous and subcutaneous mechanoreceptors, muscle and skeletal mechanoreceptors, and thermal and cool receptors.

Opposite Pelvic Deficiency The long leg determined through Position #1 during initial Leg Length Analysis. Considered the nonreactive leg or non–Pelvic Deficient leg.

Pacinian Corpuscle Encapsulated sensory nerve ending that is a rapidly adapting receptor located in subcutaneous tissue beneath hairy and glabrous skin. It is sensitive to deep or heavy pressure.

Pelvic Deficiency The short leg determined through Position #1 during the initial Leg Length Analysis (LLA) has been designated the *Pelvic Deficient*, or *PD*, leg. This designation is used throughout the LLA for discussion and directions for leg testing in the Activator Method. The short leg also is sometimes referred to as the *reactive* leg because of its tendency to appear shorter or longer during different testing procedures. The PD leg tends to remain the reactive leg throughout the procedure for any given patient visit.

Polymodal Nociceptors One of the four types of nociceptors that respond to several different types of noxious stimuli, such as high-intensity mechanical, hot, cold, and chemical stimuli.

Position #1 The starting position for all Activator Method Leg Length Analyses. In Position #1, the patient's legs rest on an Activator Table, allowing the knees to be in a slightly flexed position and the ankles and feet to be in a neutral relaxed state. Application of the "six-point landing" is used, along with other subtle movements, to identify the Pelvic Deficient leg or leg length reactivity.

Position #2 Leg length test performed with the legs flexed to no more than 90 degrees at the knees. Position #2 is thought to provide more precise information about the location and direction of the neuroarticular dysfunction, specifically to identify the *side of involvement* in the axial skeleton.

Position #3 (Superior and Inferior Spinous Testing) After an Isolation Test, the legs are raised by flexing the knees in the same way that Position #2 is attained; however, continue to raise the legs *until the knees are flexed past 90 degrees* or to the resistance of the patient. If the Pelvic Deficient (PD) leg lengthens in Position #3, the spinous process of the segment tested has misaligned superiorly, or the vertebra is in a flexion malposition. If the PD leg shortens in Position #3, the spinous process of the segment tested has misaligned inferiorly, or the vertebra is in an extension malposition. This test can be used throughout the axial skeleton from the sacrum cephalad through the occiput.

Position #4 (Segmental Laterality) After an Isolation Test, flex the knee on the Pelvic Deficient (PD) side past 90 degrees while the leg Opposite Pelvic Deficiency remains on the table. Return the leg to Position #1 and look for shortening of the PD leg. If the PD leg shortens in Position #1, raise the legs to Position #2. Use the Short/Long Rule to interpret the test. If the PD leg lengthens in Position #2, the test suggests segmental laterality of the vertebra on the side of Pelvic Deficiency. If the PD leg shortens in Position #2, the test suggests segmental laterality of the vertebra on the side Opposite Pelvic Deficiency. Lateral listhesis (a lateral malposition) of a vertebral segment may occur at any level of the spine, possibly involving the sacrum, pubic bone, and occiput. It is considered a "global" lateral malposition of the structure that is being isolated.

Position #5 (Neuroarticular Facet Involvement) After an Isolation Test, and after utilization of Positions #3 and #4 along with any indicated adjustment, the doctor places the palms of their hands on the plantar aspect of the metatarsal-phalangeal junction of both feet and applies headward pressure in a quick manner, producing dorsiflexion of both ankles to the resistance of the patient. Look for Pelvic Deficient leg reactivity or shortening, and then raise the legs to Position #2 to determine the side of neuroarticular dysfunction of the facet by following the Short/Long Rule.

Possibility One During the initial Leg Length Analysis, as the legs are raised into Position #2, inspection of leg lengths reveals that the Pelvic Deficient leg *appears* to have lengthened. This change in leg length is a *relative* change, not an absolute change.

Possibility Two During the initial Leg Length Analysis, as the legs are raised into Position #2, inspection of leg lengths reveals that the Pelvic Deficient leg *appears* to have stayed short or becomes shorter. This change in leg length is a *relative* change, not an absolute change.

Possibility Three During the initial Leg Length Analysis, inspection of leg length does not reveal a short or reactive leg in Position #1, and no lengthening or shortening of one of the legs in Position #2 is noted; the legs are of equal length in Position #1, and in Position #2, they are balanced.

Pressure Test Involves the application of a gentle force to a vertebral segment or extremity joint into the direction of the adjustment; the force is applied in a direction that is directly opposite to the direction of neuroarticular dysfunction. This test confirms the need for adjustment and the direction of the adjustment.

Proprioception Awareness of posture, movement, and changes in equilibrium, and knowledge of position, weight, and resistance of objects in relation to the body. Four main types of peripheral receptors signal limb proprioception: (1) mechanoreceptors located in joint capsules, (2) muscle spindle receptors, that is, mechanoreceptors in muscle that are specialized to signal the length, speed, and stretch of the muscle, (3) stretch-sensitive receptors that help to control excess stretch or force, and (4) Golgi tendon organ involvement in muscle contraction.

Ruffini's Corpuscle Encapsulated sensory nerve ending that is a slowly adapting receptor located in subcutaneous tissue beneath hairy and glabrous skin. It is thought to be a pressure receptor.

Sensitization Phenomenon whereby the repeated application of noxious stimuli causes nearby nociceptors that were previously unresponsive to the stimuli to become responsive.

Short Reflex Reflex involving one or a few segments of the spinal cord; monosynaptic stretch reflexes that involve the stretch of a muscle spindle, generating an afferent impulse from the receptor region of the spindles to excite the alpha motoneurons in the same muscle, resulting in contraction. Short-latency reflexes have been identified in the paraspinal muscles when subjects catch an unexpected mass in their hand.

Short/Long Rule A general guideline used to identify the side of involvement in neuroarticular dysfunction. After an Isolation Test for a spinal segment, leg length reactivity is observed in Position #1, and the legs are raised to Position #2. If the Pelvic Deficient (PD) leg relatively lengthens going to Position #2, this test indicates involvement on the PD side. If the PD leg relatively shortens going to Position #2, this test indicates involvement on the side Opposite Pelvic Deficiency.

Simple Reflex Reflex in which only two or possibly three neurons are interposed between receptor and effector organs; simple responses are inflexible and represent a basic mechanism by which the motor system corrects an error or resists an imposed stretch; this also includes neurological integration.

Stress Test The application of a gentle force on a vertebral motion segment, joint, or other tissue into the direction of neuroarticular dysfunction. The applied force may consist of direct manual pressure or traction on the anatomical structure being tested. A Stress Test also can be performed by passive movement of a structure, such as an extremity, toward its limit of motion in the direction of neuroarticular dysfunction. Stress Tests are used most often to identify and evaluate neuroarticular dysfunction in the upper and lower extremities. When performed, reactivity of the Pelvic

Deficient leg in Position #1 is thought to indicate the presence of neuroarticular dysfunction. A Stress Test is the opposite of a Pressure Test.

Subluxation A partial or incomplete dislocation. Referred to in chiropractic as a "facilitated segment" that responds to various stimuli in a more intense and prolonged manner than is normal owing to the summation of subthreshold stimuli at an involved spinal segment. This brings the segmentally innervated paraspinal muscles closer to threshold.

Subluxation Complex Refers to the relationship of all component structures of the joint (biomechanical), along with its nervous system control, which can cause nerve interference and has the capacity to affect homeostatic mechanisms (see Subluxation). SYN: neuroarticular dysfunction.

Viscerohormonal Response Response to pain that consists of cardiovascular, gastrointestinal, and hormonal changes, manifested by changes such as increased respiratory and heart rates, blood pressure, and gastrointestinal movement.

INDEX

Page numbers followed by *f* indicate figures; *t*, tables; *b*, boxes.

Printed and bound by CPI Group (UK) Ltd, Croydon, CR0 4YY

11/05/2025

01866563-0001